hydroxyzine	meperidine	morphine	nalbuphine	pentobarbital	phenobarbital	promethazine	scopolamine	secobarbital	sodium bicarbonate	thiopental
P	P	P	Y	P		P	P		N	
Y				N	N	Y	Y	N		N
P	P	P		N	N	P	P	N	N	N
P				N					N	
N	N	N	N	N	N	N	N	N	N	N
Y	Y	Y	Y	N		Y	Y	N	N	N
									N	N
■	P	P	Y	N	N	P	P		N	
P	■	N		N	N	P	P		N	N
P	N	■		?	N	?	P		N	N
Y			■	N		Y	Y			
N	N	?	N	■		N	P		?	P
N	N	N			■	N				Y
P	P	?	Y	N	N	■	P			N
P	P	P	Y	P		P	■	N	N	Y
							N	■		
N	N	N		?			N		■	N
	N	N		P	Y	N	Y		N	■

? = conflicting reports on compatibility; mixing not recommended
(A blank space indicates no available data on compatibility.)

Nursing83
DRUG
HANDBOOK™

Nursing83
DRUG
HANDBOOK™

NURSING83 BOOKS™
INTERMED COMMUNICATIONS, INC.
SPRINGHOUSE, PENNSYLVANIA

**NURSING83
DRUG HANDBOOK**™

Intermed Communications Book Division

CHAIRMAN
Eugene W. Jackson

PRESIDENT
Daniel L. Cheney

VICE-PRESIDENT
Timothy B. King

RESEARCH DIRECTOR
Elizabeth O'Brien

PRODUCTION AND PURCHASING DIRECTOR
Bacil Guiley

The clinical procedures described and recommended in this publication are
based on research and consultation with medical and nursing authorities. To
the best of our knowledge, these procedures reflect currently accepted clinical
practice; nevertheless, they can't be considered absolute and universal recommendations. For individual application, treatment recommendations must be
considered in light of the patient's clinical condition and, before administration
of new or infrequently used drugs, in light of latest package-insert information.
The authors and the publisher disclaim responsibility for any adverse effects resulting directly or indirectly from the suggested procedures, from any unde-
tected errors, or from the reader's misunderstanding of the text.

NDH-010183

NURSING83 DRUG HANDBOOK
ISSN 0273-320X
ISBN 0-916730-54-9

Staff for this volume

EDITORIAL DIRECTOR: Helen Klusek Hamilton

CLINICAL DIRECTOR: Minnie Bowen Rose, RN, BSN, MEd

DRUG INFORMATION EDITOR: Larry Neil Gever, RPh, PharmD

CLINICAL EDITOR: Anne Moraca-Sawicki, RN, MSN

COPY CHIEF: Jill Lasker

COPY EDITORS: Andrea F. Barrett, Jo Lennon, Ruth A. Older, Barbara F. Ritter

PRODUCTION ASSISTANT: Sally Johnson

DESIGNER: Kathaleen Motak Singel

ASSISTANT DESIGNER: Christopher Laird

ART PRODUCTION MANAGER: Robert Perry

ART ASSISTANT: Sandra Simms

TYPOGRAPHY MANAGER: David C. Kosten

TYPOGRAPHERS: Ethel Halle, Diane Paluba

TYPOGRAPHY ASSISTANTS: Janice Auch Haber, Nancy Wirs

PRODUCTION MANAGER: Wilbur D. Davidson

EDITORIAL ASSISTANT: Maree E. DeRosa

Special thanks to Edward Quigley for his assistance, and to the following, no longer on the staff, who assisted in preparation of this volume: Linda Roucken; Karen Dyer Vance, RN, BSN; and Pat Weiser.

NURSING83 BOOKS™

NURSING SKILLBOOK® SERIES
Reading EKGs Correctly
Dealing with Death and Dying
Managing Diabetics Properly
Assessing Vital Functions Accurately
Helping Cancer Patients Effectively
Giving Cardiovascular Drugs Safely
Giving Emergency Care Competently
Monitoring Fluid and Electrolytes Precisely
Documenting Patient Care Responsibly
Combatting Cardiovascular Diseases Skillfully
Coping with Neurologic Problems Proficiently
Using Crisis Intervention Wisely
Nursing Critically Ill Patients Confidently

NURSING PHOTOBOOK™ SERIES
Providing Respiratory Care
Managing I.V. Therapy
Dealing with Emergencies
Giving Medications
Assessing Your Patients
Using Monitors
Providing Early Mobility
Giving Cardiac Care
Performing GI Procedures
Implementing Urologic Procedures
Controlling Infection
Ensuring Intensive Care
Coping with Neurologic Disorders
Caring for Surgical Patients
Working with Orthopedic Patients
Nursing Pediatric Patients
Helping Geriatric Patients
Attending Ob/Gyn Patients
Aiding Ambulatory Patients
Carrying Out Special Procedures

NURSE'S REFERENCE LIBRARY® SERIES
Diseases
Diagnostics
Drugs
Assessment
Procedures

***Nursing83* DRUG HANDBOOK™**

CLINICAL CONSULTANTS

Beverly A. Baldwin, RN, MA, Assistant Professor, School of Nursing, University of Maryland, Baltimore.

Heather Boyd-Monk, RN, BSN, Educational Coordinator, Wills Eye Hospital, Philadelphia.

Nancy Burns, RN, PhD, Assistant Professor, University of Texas School of Nursing, Arlington.

Carla J. Burton, RN, BS, Dermatology Nurse Clinician, Beth Israel Hospital, Boston.

Priscilla A. Butts, RN, MSN, Lecturer, University of Pennsylvania, Philadelphia.

Judy Donlen, RNC, MSN, Instructor, Perinatal Graduate Program, University of Pennsylvania School of Nursing, Philadelphia.

Jeanne Dupont, RN, Head Nurse, Emergency Department, Massachusetts Eye and Ear Infirmary, Boston.

DeAnn M. Englert, RN, MSN, Assistant Professor, Louisiana State University Medical Center School of Nursing, New Orleans.

Margarethe Hawken, RN, MA, CNRN, Clinical Nurse Specialist in Neurology and Epilepsy, Seattle Veterans' Administration Medical Center.

Kathleen M. Hawkins, RN, Clinical Nurse Specialist in Dermatology, University of Colorado, Health Sciences Center, Denver.

Carolyn Holt, RN, BSEd, Coordinator, Nursing Staff Development, Columbus-Cuneo-Cabrini Medical Center, Chicago.

Gail D'Onofrio Long, RN, MS, Clinical Nurse Specialist in Medical Intensive Care and Coronary Care, University Hospital, Boston.

Elizabeth A. Phillips, RN, BA, BSN, Administrative Supervisor, Delaware Valley Medical Center, Bristol, Pa.

Despina Seremelis, RN, BSN, Staff, Temple University Hospital, Philadelphia.

Barbara Solomon, RN, MS, Clinical Nurse Expert, Division of Arthritis and Metabolism, National Institute of Health, Bethesda, Md.

Robin Tourigan, RN, MSN, Nurse Clinician, Thomas Jefferson University Hospital, Philadelphia.

Paula Brammer Vetter, RN, BSN, Clinical Instructor in Coronary Intensive Care, Cleveland Clinic Hospital.

Carmen Brochu Wohrle, RN, BS, MS, Assistant Director of Nursing, Deaconess Hospital, Spokane, Wash.

PHARMACY REVIEWERS

ADVISORY BOARD

Contents

Section V

Autonomic Nervous System

Section VI

Respiratory System

Section VII

Gastrointestinal System

Section VIII

Hormones, Hormone Antagonists, and Synthetic Substitutes

Section IX

Fluid and Electrolyte Balance

Section X

Blood

Section XI

Antineoplastics

Section XII

Eye, Ear, Nose, and Throat

FOREWORD

This is the fifth annual edition of the *Nursing83 Drug Handbook*—a best-seller that has become an indispensable tool for the working nurse. And, as I look at this new edition, I know why: With more than 1,000 drugs routinely used in treating patients, nurses simply can't rely on memory alone for the vital information they need to answer the many pharmacologic questions that come up daily in patient care.

During the past year, there have been an unusually large number of important new drugs introduced. And you'll be sure to come in contact with most of these during the course of your practice. With the *Nursing83 Drug Handbook*, you can be confident that you have the drug information you need about these new drugs. This new edition adds a new feature that I'm sure you'll find useful—the identification of oral drugs that may contain alcohol and of those which contain the allergenic coloring agent, tartrazine dye.

In addition to these, you'll find the features that have made this book one of the leading drug references for nurses: its emphasis on each drug's clinical usefulness; its easy-to-use format with indications and dosage, side effects, interactions, and nursing considerations arranged for easy reference; and its single index listing both trade and generic names...and more.

With the *Nursing83 Drug Handbook*, you can quickly validate virtually any form of drug therapy. It's an indispensable source of accurate, up-to-date information you can use with confidence every day.

LUTHER CHRISTMAN, PhD, RN
*Vice-President, Nursing Affairs, and
Dean, College of Nursing, Rush University
Rush-Presbyterian-St. Luke's Medical Center
Chicago*

How to use Nursing83 Drug Handbook

Nursing83 Drug Handbook is meant to fill a very special need. It represents a joint effort by pharmacists and nurses to provide the nursing profession with drug information that focuses directly on what nurses need to know. With this in mind, it emphasizes clinical aspects and does not attempt to replace detailed pharmacology texts. For the same reason, the information is arranged in a format designed to make it readily accessible.

Introductory information
Following this chapter, Chapter 2 explains, in a general way, how drugs work. It also tells about side effects and adverse reactions, and gives general guidelines about drug use in pregnancy and the presence of drugs in breast milk. Chapters 3 and 4 discuss the unique problems of administering drugs to children and the elderly. They offer guidelines you can use to avoid potential pitfalls and minimize problems in these areas. In the remaining chapters, all drugs are classified according to their common, therapeutic uses.

Drug information
Each chapter begins with an alphabetically arranged list of the generic names of drugs described in that chapter. Next, the chapter summarizes each drug's or drug group's mechanism of action. This is followed by a list of selected combination products in which these drugs are found. Specific information on each drug is arranged under five headings: *Name; Indications and*

Dosage; Side Effects; Interactions; and *Nursing Considerations.*

Each drug's generic name is immediately followed by an alphabetic list of bits brand names. Brands available in both the United States and Canada are designated with a diamond (♦); those available *only* in Canada with a double diamond (♦♦). A brand name with no symbol after it is available only in the United States. If a drug is a controlled substance, that too is clearly indicated (example: Controlled Substance Schedule II). Products listed, although generally available, may not be approved by the Food and Drug Administration. The mention of a brand name in no way implies endorsement of that product or guarantees its legality.

The section titled *Indications and Dosage* lists general dosage information for adults and children, as applicable. Children's doses are usually indicated in terms of mg/kg daily. Dosage instructions reflect current clinical trends in therapeutics and can't be considered an absolute and universal recommendation. For individual application, dosage instructions must be considered in context with the patient's clinical condition.

The section titled *Side Effects* lists each drug's commonly observed side effects (and selected rare ones if life-threatening). The most common and life-threatening side effects are italicized for easy reference. An exception to this rule is a side effect that, although it is normally considered quite hazardous, has been reported to be mild and reversible with the drug in question. For example, thrombocytopenia is considered a life-threatening side effect of mithramycin (a chemotherapeutic drug). Conversely, the thrombocytopenia seen with methyldopa (Aldomet) is generally mild and reversible. Hence, thrombocytopenia listed as a side effect of mithramycin is italicized, whereas the same side effect under methyldopa is not. Side effects are grouped according to the body system in which they appear.

The next section, *Interactions*, lists each drug's confirmed, *clinically significant* interactions with other drugs, including additive effects, potentiated effects, and antagonistic effects. Also included are specific suggestions for dealing with dangerous drug interaction (for example, reducing doses or monitoring certain laboratory tests). Drug interactions are listed under the drug that is adversely affected. For example, magnesium trisilicate, an ingredient in antacids, interacts with tetracycline to cause decreased absorption of tetracycline. Therefore, this interaction is listed under tetracycline. To check on the possible effects of using two or more drugs simultaneously, refer to the interaction entry for *each* of the drugs in question.

The final section, *Nursing Considerations*, lists other useful information, starting with contraindications and precautions, followed by monitoring techniques and suggestions for prevention and treatment of side effects. Also included in this column are suggestions for promoting patient comfort, for patient teaching, and for preparing, administering, and storing each drug.

Special information: alcohol and tartrazine content

Many liquid drug preparations for oral use contain alcohol. Although the slight sedative effect that alcohol produces is not harmful in most patients—and can sometimes be beneficial—in some circumstances, alcohol ingestion can be undesirable and even dangerous. Consequently, alcohol-containing oral drugs should be given very cautiously, if at all, to patients who:
- are concomitantly taking potent CNS depressants, such as barbiturates;
- are taking drugs that may produce a disulfiram-type reaction (such as chlorpropamide, metronidazole, and moxalactam);
- are known alcoholics or are taking disulfiram (Antabuse) as part of a treatment program for their alcoholism. Patients taking disulfiram, upon ingestion of alcohol or alcohol-containing drugs, will exhibit severe symptoms that may include blurred vision, confusion, dyspnea, flushing, sweating, and tachycardia.

To help prevent inadvertent and potentially harmful exposure to alcohol, a single asterisk (*) follows the generic name of a drug if its liquid form contains alcohol. In many of the preparations so marked, the alcohol content is small. Nevertheless, in patients who are especially susceptible to develop adverse effects upon exposure to alcohol, these drugs should be avoided.

Tartrazine dye, also known as FD&C Yellow No. 5, is a common coloring agent used in some foods and drugs. Although this substance is usually harmless, it can provoke a severe allergic reaction in susceptible persons. For this reason, most drug manufacturers have begun to eliminate tartrazine from their products, but many drugs still contain this potentially allergenic substance.

The incidence of tartrazine sensitivity is estimated at approximately 1 in 10,000 in the general population, but somewhat higher in persons with asthma and/or sensitivity to aspirin. Why this is so is unknown. The most common symptoms of tartrazine sensitivity are urticaria, rhinorrhea, asthma (or exacerbation of existing asthma) and angioedema. Acutely sensitive persons may develop allergic vascular purpura, tachycardia, dyspnea, and chest pain. These allergic symptoms generally subside spontaneously upon discontinuation of the tartrazine containing drug, but occasionally require treatment with antihistamines or epinephrine.

Avoiding exposure to tartrazine is not simply a matter of avoiding yellow-colored drugs because this substance may be present in many other color blends, such as turquoise, green, and maroon. You can be sure to prevent exposure to tartrazine only by carefully checking the specific content of any drug preparation. To this end, this volume signals tartrazine content. The name of every brand drug that may contain tartrazine will be followed by a double asterisk (**). If you suspect tartrazine sensitivity in a patient receiving such a drug, inform the doctor and contact the pharmaceutical manufacturer to determine which dosage forms contain tartrazine.

Drug actions, reactions, and interactions explained

Administration of any drug provokes a series of physiochemical events within the body. The first event, when a drug combines with cell drug receptors, is known as the drug action. What follows as a result of this action of the drug is known as the drug effect. Depending upon the number of different cellular drug receptors affected by a given drug, a drug effect can be local or systemic, or both. For example, the antipeptic ulcer drug Tagamet (cimetidine) acts solely by blocking histamine receptor cells in the parietal cells of the stomach. This is known as a local drug effect because the drug action is sharply limited to one area and does not spread to other parts of the body. On the other hand, diphenhydramine (Benadryl) produces a systemic effect in that it blocks histamine receptors in widespread areas of the body. In other words, local drug effects are specific to a limited number of organ systems, whereas systemic drug effects are generalized and affect different and diverse organ systems.

Three factors modify drug action
1. Absorption
Before a drug can act within the body, it must be absorbed into the bloodstream—usually after oral administration, the most frequently used route. Before a drug contained in a tablet or capsule can be absorbed, the dosage form must disintegrate, that is, break into smaller particles. Then, these smaller particles can dissolve in gastric juices. Only after so dissolving can a drug be absorbed into the bloodstream.

Once absorbed and circulating in the bloodstream, it is said to be bioavailable or ready to produce a drug effect. Of course, whether such absorption is complete or partial depends on several factors: the drug's physiochemical effects, dosage form, route of administration, its interactions with other substances in the gastrointestinal tract, and various patient characteristics. These same factors also determine the speed of absorption. Thus, oral solutions and elixirs, which bypass the need for disintegration and dissolution, are usually absorbed more rapidly. Drugs administered intramuscularly must first be absorbed through the muscle into the bloodstream. Rectal suppositories must dissolve to be absorbed through the rectal mucosa. Of course, drugs administered intravenously are placed directly into the circulation and are completely and immediately bioavailable.

2. Distribution
After absorption, a drug moves from the bloodstream into various fluids and tissues within the body; this is distribution. Individual patient variations can greatly alter the amount of drug that is distributed throughout the body. For example, in an edematous patient, a given dose must be distributed to a larger volume than in a nonedematous patient; the amount of drug must sometimes be increased to account for this. Remember, the dosage should be decreased when the edema is corrected. Conversely, in an extremely dehydrated patient, the drug will be distributed to a much smaller volume, so the dose must then be decreased. The total area to

which a drug is distributed is known as volume of distribution. Patients who are particularly obese may present another problem when considering drug distribution. Some drugs—such as digoxin, gentamicin, and tobramycin—are not well distributed to fatty tissue. Therefore, dosing based on actual body weight may lead to overdose and serious toxicity. In some cases, dosing must be based on lean body weight, which may be estimated from actuarial tables that give average weight range for height.

3. Metabolism and excretion (drug elimination)

Most drugs are metabolized in the liver and excreted by the kidneys. Hepatic diseases may affect one or more of the metabolic functions of the liver. Therefore, in patients with hepatic disease, the metabolism of a drug may be increased, decreased, or unchanged. Clearly, all patients with hepatic disease must be monitored closely for drug effect and toxicity. Some drugs (digoxin, gentamicin) are eliminated almost unchanged by the kidneys. For safe use of such drugs, renal function must be adequate or the drug will accumulate, producing toxic effects. Some drugs can alter the effect and excretion of other drugs. For example, they can stimulate hepatic metabolizing enzymes to speed up the rate of metabolism and change the drug effect. Or, they can block or promote renal excretion of other drugs, causing them to accumulate and enhance their effects, or causing them to be too rapidly excreted and so diminish their effects. Some slight elimination takes place by way of perspiration, saliva, breast milk, and so on. (Certain volatile anesthetics, however—halothane, for instance—are eliminated primarily by exhalation.)

The rate at which a drug is metabolized varies with the individual. In some patients, drugs are metabolized so quickly that their blood and tissue levels prove therapeutically inadequate. In others, the rate of metabolism is so slow that ordinary doses can produce toxic results.

Other modifying factors

An important factor that influences a drug's action and effect is its *binding to plasma proteins,* especially albumin, and other tissue components. Because only free, unbound drug can act in the body, such binding greatly influences effectiveness and duration of effect.

The *patient's age* is another important factor. Elderly patients usually have decreased hepatic function, less muscle mass, and diminished renal function. Consequently, lower doses and sometimes longer dosage intervals are needed to avoid toxicity in the elderly. With similar consequences, neonates have underdeveloped metabolic enzyme systems and inadequate renal function. They need highly individualized dosage and careful monitoring.

Underlying disease can also markedly affect drug action and effect. For example, acidosis may cause insulin resistance. Genetic diseases such as glucose-6-phosphate dehydrogenase (G-6-PD) deficiency and hepatic porphyria may turn drugs into toxins with serious consequences. Patients with G-6-PD deficiency may develop hemolytic anemia when given sulfonamides or a number of other drugs. A genetically susceptible patient can develop an acute porphyria attack if given a barbiturate. Also, patients who have highly active hepatic enzyme systems (for example, rapid acetylators), when treated with isoniazid, can develop hepatitis from the rapid intrahepatic buildup of a toxic metabolite.

Things to consider about administration

1. Dosage forms do matter. Some tablets and capsules are too large to be readily swallowed by very ill patients. You may then request an oral solution or elixir of the same drug, but bear in mind that because a liquid is more easily and completely absorbed, it produces higher blood levels than a tablet. When a potentially toxic drug is given, the increased amount absorbed could cause toxicity. One example of this is digoxin tablets versus digoxin elixir. Sometimes a change in dosage form requires a change in dose.

2. *Routes of administration are not therapeutically interchangeable*. For example, phenytoin (Dilantin) is readily absorbed orally but is slowly and erratically absorbed intramuscularly. On the other hand, carbenicillin must be given parenterally because oral administration yields inadequate blood levels to treat systemic infections. However, it can be given orally to treat urinary tract infections because it concentrates in the urine.

3. *The timing of drug administration can be important*. Sometimes giving an oral drug during or shortly after mealtime decreases the amount of drug absorbed. This is not clinically significant with most drugs and may in fact be desirable with irritating drugs such as aspirin or phenylbutazone. But penicillins and tetracyclines should not be scheduled for administration at mealtimes because certain foods can inactivate them. If in doubt about the effect of food on a certain drug, check with a pharmacist.

4. *Consider the patient's age, height, and weight*. The doctor will need this information when calculating the dose for many drugs. It should be accurately recorded on the patient's chart. This chart should also include current laboratory data, especially kidney and liver function studies, so the doctor can consider them and adapt dosage as needed.

5. *Watch for metabolic changes*. Monitor for any physiologic change that might alter drug effect. Examples: depressed respiratory function and the development of acidosis or alkalosis.

6. *Know the patient's history*. Whenever possible, obtain a comprehensive family history from the patient or his family. Ask about past reactions to drugs, possible genetic traits that might alter drug response, and the current use of other drugs. Multiple drug therapy can dramatically change the effects of many drugs. These are known as drug interactions.

Drug interactions

When one drug administered in combination with or shortly after another drug alters the effect of one or both drugs, this is known as a drug interaction. Usually, the effect of one drug is increased or decreased. For instance, one drug may inhibit or stimulate the metabolism or excretion of the other; or it may release another from plasma protein-binding sites, freeing it for further action.

Combination therapy is based upon drug interaction. One drug, for example, may be given in order to potentiate another. Probenecid, which blocks the excretion of penicillin, is sometimes given with penicillin to maintain adequate blood levels of penicillin for a longer period. Often two drugs with similar action are given together precisely because of the additive effect that results. Aspirin and codeine, for instance, both analgesics, are often given in combination because together they provide greater relief from pain than either alone.

Drug interactions are sometimes used to prevent or antagonize certain side effects. Hydrochlorothiazide and spironolactone, both diuretics, are often administered in combination, because the former is potassium-depleting, while the latter is potassium-sparing.

But not all drug interactions are beneficial. Multiple drugs can interact to produce effects that are often undesirable and sometimes hazardous. Harmful drug interactions decrease efficacy or increase toxicity. A hypertensive patient well controlled with guanethidine may see his blood pressure rise to its former high level if he takes the antidepressant amitriptyline (Elavil) at the same time. Such a drug effect is known as antagonism. Drug combinations that produce these effects when used together should be avoided if possible. Another kind of inhibiting effect occurs when a tetracycline drug is administered with calcium- or magnesium-containing drugs or foods (i.e., antacids or milk). These combine with tetracycline in the gastrointestinal tract and cause inadequate absorption of tetracycline.

Side effects

Any drug effect other than what is therapeutically intended can be called a side effect. It may be expected and benign, or unexpected and potentially harmful. For example, during hay fever season, a patient may have to contend with the drowsiness caused by chlorpheniramine to get relief from hay fever symptoms. In such a case, the dose may be adjusted up or down to balance therapeutic effect with side effect.

A side effect may be tolerated for a necessary therapeutic effect, or it may be hazardous and unacceptable and require discontinuation of the drug. Some side effects subside with continued use. As an example, the drowsiness associated with methyldopa (Aldomet) and the orthostatic hypotension associated with prazosin (Minipress) usually subside after several days, as the patient develops a tolerance to these effects. But many side effects are dose-related and lessen or disappear only if dosage is reduced. Although most side effects are not therapeutically desirable, an occasional one can be put to clinical use. An outstanding example of this is the drowsiness associated with diphenhydramine (Benadryl), which makes it clinically useful as a mild hypnotic.

Hypersensitivity, a term sometimes used interchangeably with drug allergy, is the result of an antigen-antibody immune reaction that occurs in the body when a drug is given to a susceptible patient. One of the most dangerous of all drug hypersensitivities is penicillin allergy. In its severest form, penicillin anaphylaxis can rapidly become fatal.

Rarely, idiosyncratic reactions occur. These are highly unpredictable, individual, and unusual. Probably the best known idiosyncratic drug reaction is the aplastic anemia caused by the antibiotic chloramphenicol (Chloromycetin). This reaction appears in only 1 out of 40,000 patients, but when it does, it is often fatal. A more common idiosyncratic reaction is extreme sensitivity to very low doses of a drug, or insensitivity to higher-than-normal doses.

To deal with side effects correctly, you need to be alert to even minor changes in the patient's clinical status. Such minor changes may be an early warning of pending toxicity. Listen to the patient's complaints about his reactions to a drug, and consider each complaint objectively. You may be able to reduce undesirable side effects in several ways. Obviously, dosage reduction often helps. But often so does a simple rescheduling of the same dose. For example, pseudoephedrine (Sudafed) may produce stimulation that will be no problem if it's given early in the day; similarly, the drowsiness that occurs with antihistamines or tranquilizers can be totally harmless if the dose is given at bedtime. Most important, your patient needs to be told what side effects to expect so he won't become worried or even stop taking the drug on his own. Of course, the patient should report any unusual or unexpected side effects to the doctor.

Recognizing drug allergies or serious idiosyncratic reactions can sometimes be lifesaving. Ask each patient about drugs he is taking or has taken in the past and what, if any, unusual effects he experienced from taking them. If a patient claims to be allergic to a drug, ask him to tell you exactly what happens when he takes it. He may be calling a harmless side effect such as upset stomach, an allergic reaction, or he may have a true tendency to anaphylaxis. In either case, you and the doctor need to know this. Of course, you must record and report any clinical changes throughout the patient's hospital stay. If you suspect a hazardous side effect, withhold the drug until you can check with the pharmacist and the doctor.

Toxic reactions

Chronic drug toxicities are generally due to cumulative effect and the resulting buildup of the drug in the body. These effects may be extensions of the desired therapeutic effect. For example, guanethidine-induced norepinephrine depletion produces a desired antihypertensive effect, but in larger doses, this same biochemical action often produces orthostatic hypotension.

Drug toxicities usually occur when drug blood levels rise due to impaired metabolism or excretion. For example, blood levels of theophylline rise when hepatic dysfunction impairs metabolism of the drug. Similarly, digoxin toxicity can follow impaired renal function because digoxin is eliminated from the body almost exclusively by the kidneys (via glomerular filtration). Of course, toxic blood levels also follow excessive dosage. Aspirin tinnitus (ringing in ears) is usually a sign that the safe dose has been exceeded.

Most drug toxicity is predictable and dose-related; fortunately, most drug toxicity is also readily reversible upon dosage adjustment. So it's essential to monitor patients carefully for physiological changes that might alter drug effect. Watch especially for impaired hepatic and renal function. Warn the patient about signs of pending toxicity, and tell him what to do if a toxic reaction occurs. Also, be sure to emphasize the importance of taking a drug exactly as prescribed. Warn the patient about serious problems that could arise if he changes the dose or the schedule for taking it.

Drugs and pregnancy

Ever since the thalidomide tragedy of the late 1950s—when thousands of malformed infants were born after their mothers used this mild sedative-hypnotic during pregnancy—use of drugs during pregnancy has been a source of serious medical concern and controversy. To identify drugs that may cause such teratogenic effects, preclinical drug studies always include tests on pregnant laboratory animals. These tests do point out gross teratogenicity but do not clearly establish safety. Because different species react to drugs in different ways, animal studies do not rule out possible teratogenic effects in humans. For example, the preliminary studies on thalidomide gave no warning of teratogenic effects, and it was subsequently released for general use in Europe.

To prevent such tragedies, just about every drug now carries a special warning on the official package insert. Such warnings state that safety in human pregnancy has not been established and use of the drug in pregnancy requires the expected therapeutic benefit be weighed against possible hazard to mother and child. With the exception of vitamins and minerals, no drug is approved caveat-free for use in pregnancy. Even Bendectin (a combination of the antihistamine doxylamine and the vitamin pyridoxine), for which nausea and vomiting of pregnancy is an official indication, carries a warning for cautious use during pregnancy.

What about the placental barrier? Once thought to protect the fetus from drug effects, the placenta isn't actually much of a barrier at all. Except for drugs with exceptionally large molecular structure, almost every drug administered to a pregnant woman crosses the placenta and enters the fetal circulation. An example of such large molecular size is heparin, the injectable anticoagulant. Theoretically, then, heparin could be used in a pregnant woman without fear of harming the fetus—but even heparin carries a warning for cautious use in pregnancy. Conversely, just because a drug crosses the placenta doesn't necessarily mean it's harmful to the fetus.

Actually, only one factor—stage of fetal development—seems clearly related to exaggerated risk during pregnancy. During two stages of pregnancy—the first and the third trimesters—the fetus is especially vulnerable to damage from maternal use of drugs. During these times, *all* drugs should be given with extreme caution. The most sensitive period for drug-induced fetal malformation is the first trimester, when fetal organs are differentiating (organogenesis). During this time, *all* drugs should be withheld unless doing so would jeopardize the mother's health. Theoretically, during this sensitive time, even aspirin could harm the fetus. So, strongly advise your patient to avoid *all* self-prescribed drugs during early pregnancy.

The other time of special fetal sensitivity to drugs is the last trimester. The reason? At birth, when separated from his mother, the newborn must rely on his own metabolism to eliminate any remaining drug. Because his detoxifying systems are not fully developed, any residual drug may take a long time to be metabolized—and thus may induce prolonged toxic reactions. Consequently, drugs should be used only when absolutely necessary during the last 3 months of pregnancy.

Of course, in many circumstances, pregnant women must continue to take certain drugs. For example, an epileptic woman who is well controlled with an anticonvulsant should continue to take it even during pregnancy. Or a pregnant woman with a bacterial infection must receive antibiotics. In such cases, the potential risk to the fetus is overbalanced by the mother's need.

Following these general guidelines can prevent indiscriminate and potentially harmful use of drugs in pregnancy:

● Before a drug is prescribed for a woman of childbearing age, she should be asked the date of her last menstrual period and whether there is a possibility she is pregnant.

● Especially during the first and the third trimesters, a pregnant patient should avoid *all* drugs except those *essential* to maintain the pregnancy or maternal health.

● Topical drugs are not exempt from the warning against indiscriminate use during pregnancy. Many topically applied drugs can be absorbed in large enough amounts to be harmful to the fetus.

● When a pregnant patient needs *any* drug, the doctor should prescribe the *safest* possible drug in the *lowest* possible dose to minimize any harmful effect to the fetus.

● Every pregnant patient should check with her doctor before taking *any* drug.

Drugs and lactation

Most drugs a nursing mother takes do appear in breast milk. Drug levels in breast milk tend to be high when blood levels are high—generally, shortly after taking each dose. Therefore, the mother should be advised to breast-feed *before* taking medication, not *after*.

Nevertheless, with very few exceptions, a mother who wishes to breast-feed may continue to do so with her doctor's permission. The exceptions: Breast-feeding should be temporarily interrupted and replaced with bottle-feeding when the mother must take...

● tetracyclines
● chloramphenicol
● sulfonamides (during first 2 weeks postpartum)
● oral anticoagulants

- iodine-containing drugs
- antineoplastics.

To protect her infant, a nursing mother should avoid taking drugs indis- criminately. If she needs to take a drug to maintain her own health, she should first check with her doctor to be sure of taking the safest drug at the safest dose.

Drug therapy in children

A child's absorption, distribution, metabolism, and excretion undergo profound changes that affect drug dosage. To ensure optimal drug effect and minimal toxicity, consider these factors when administering drugs to a child.

Absorption

Drug absorption in children depends on the form of the drug; its physical properties; other drugs or substances, such as food, taken simultaneously; physiologic changes; and concurrent disease.

• The pH of neonatal gastric fluid is neutral or slightly acidic and becomes more acidic as the infant matures. This affects drug absorption. For example, nafcillin and penicillin G, erratically absorbed or malabsorbed in an adult due to degradation by gastric acid, are better absorbed in an infant due to low gastric acidity.

• Various infant formulas or milk products may increase gastric pH and impede absorption of acidic drugs. So, if possible, give a child oral medications when his stomach is empty.

• Gastric emptying time and transit time through the small intestine—longer in children than in adults—can affect absorption. Also, intestinal hypermotility (as in diarrhea) can diminish the drug's absorption.

• A child's comparatively thin epidermis allows increased absorption of topical drugs.

Distribution

As with absorption, changes in body weight and physiology during childhood can significantly influence a drug's distribution and effects. In a premature infant, body fluid makes up about 85% of total body weight; in a full-term infant, 55% to 70%; and in an adult, 50% to 55%. Extracellular fluid (mostly blood) comprises 40% of a neonate's body weight, compared with 20% in an adult. Intracellular fluid remains fairly constant throughout life and has little effect on drug dosage.

Since most drugs travel through extracellular fluid to reach their receptors, however, extracellular fluid volume influences a water-soluble drug's concentration and effect. Children have a larger proportion of fluid to solid body weight, so their distribution area is proportionately greater.

Because the proportion of fat to lean body mass increases with age, the distribution of fat-soluble drugs is more limited in children than adults. As a result, a drug's lipid- or water-solubility affects the dosage for a child.

Binding to plasma proteins
As the result of a decrease in either albumin concentration or intermolecular attraction between drug and plasma protein, many drugs are less bound to plasma proteins in infants than in adults.

Furthermore, preparations that bind plasma proteins may displace endogenous compounds, such as bilirubin or free fatty acids. Conversely, an endogenous compound may displace a weakly bound drug. For example, displacement of bound bilirubin can cause a rise in unbound bilirubin, which can lead to increased risk of kernicterus at normal bilirubin levels.

Since only unbound, or free, drug has a pharmacologic effect, any alteration in ratio of protein-bound to unbound active drug can greatly influence effect.

Several diseases, such as malnutrition and nephrotic syndrome, can also decrease plasma protein and increase the concentration of unbound drug, intensifying the drug's effect or producing toxicity.

Metabolism
A newborn infant's ability to metabolize a drug depends on the integrity of his hepatic enzyme system, his intrauterine exposure to the drug, and the nature of the drug itself.

Certain metabolic mechanisms are underdeveloped in neonates. Glucuronidation, the mechanism that neutralizes drugs, for example, is insufficiently developed to permit full pediatric doses until the infant is 1 month old. Because of this, the use of chloramphenicol in a newborn infant may cause gray baby syndrome, illustrating the newborn's inability to metabolize the drug. Use of chloramphenicol in neonates, therefore, requires decreased dosage (25 mg/kg daily) and monitoring of blood levels.

Conversely, intrauterine exposure to drugs may induce precocious development of hepatic enzyme mechanisms, increasing the infant's capacity to metabolize potentially harmful substances.

Older children can metabolize some drugs (theophylline, for example) more rapidly than adults. This ability may be due to their increased hepatic metabolic activity. Larger doses than those recommended for adults may be required.

Also, preparations given concurrently to a child may alter hepatic metabolism and induce release of hepatic enzymes. Phenobarbital, for example, can induce hepatic enzyme production and accelerate metabolism of drugs given concurrently.

Excretion
Renal excretion of a drug is the net effect of glomerular filtration, active tubular secretion, and passive tubular reabsorption. Because so many drugs are excreted in the urine, the degree of renal development or presence of renal disease can profoundly affect a child's dosage requirements. If a child is unable to excrete a drug renally, drug accumulation and possible toxicity may result unless dosage is reduced.

Physiologically, an infant's kidneys differ from an adult's in that they have:
• high resistance to blood flow and subsequent decreased renal fraction of cardiac output.
• incomplete glomerular and tubular development and short, incomplete loops of Henle. (A child's glomerular filtration reaches adult values by age 2½ to 5 months; his tubular secretion may reach adult values by age 7 to 12 months.)
• low glomerular filtration rate. (Penicillins are eliminated by this route.)
• decreased ability to concentrate urine or reabsorb various filtered compounds.
• reduced ability by the proximal tubules to secrete organic acids.

Calculating and monitoring pediatric dosages
When calculating pediatric dosages, don't use formulas that modify adult dosages: a child is not a scaled-down version of an adult. Pediatric dosages should be calculated on the basis of either body weight (mg/kg) or body-surface area (mg/m^2).
• Reevaluate dosages at regular intervals to ensure necessary adjustments as the child develops.
• Although useful for adults and older children, don't use dosages based on body-surface area in premature or full-

term infants. Use the body-weight method instead.

• Don't exceed the maximum adult dose when calculating amounts per kilogram of body weight (except with certain drugs, such as theophylline, if indicated).

• Obtain an accurate maternal drug history—prescription and nonprescription drugs, vitamins, and herbs or other health foods taken during pregnancy. In utero exposure may harm the neonate and hinder subsequent drug therapy.

• Drugs passed through breast milk can also have adverse effects on the nursing infant. Before a drug is prescribed for a breast-feeding mother, the potential effects on the infant should be investigated. For example, sulfa drugs given to a breast-feeding mother for a urinary tract infection appear in breast milk and may cause kernicterus at lower-than-normal levels of unconjugated bilirubin. Also, high concentrations of isoniazid appear in breast milk. Since this drug is metabolized by the liver, an infant's immature hepatic enzyme mechanisms cannot metabolize the drug, and the infant may suffer central nervous system (CNS) toxicity.

Oral medications

• *When giving oral medication to an infant,* administer it in liquid form if possible. For accuracy, measure and give the preparation by syringe; never use a vial or cup.

• Lift the patient's head to prevent aspiration of the medication, and press down on his chin to prevent choking.

• You may also place the drug in a nipple and allow the infant to suck the contents.

• *If the patient is a toddler,* explain how you're going to give him the medication. If possible, have the parents enlist the child's cooperation.

• Don't mix medication with food or call it "candy" even if it has a pleasant taste.

• Let the child drink liquid medication

from a calibrated medication cup rather than from a spoon: it's easier and more accurate. If the preparation is available only in tablet form, crush it and mix it with a compatible syrup. (Check with the pharmacist to make sure tablet can be crushed without losing its effectiveness.)

• *If the patient's an older child* who can swallow a tablet or capsule by himself, have him place the medication on the back of his tongue and swallow it with water or fruit juice. Remember, milk or milk products may interfere with drug absorption.

Intravenous infusions

When administering I.V. infusions to children, note the following special considerations.

Protecting the insertion site

In infants, use a peripheral vein or a scalp vein in the temporal region for I.V. infusions. The scalp vein is safest since the needle is not likely to be dislodged; however, the head must be shaved around the site. Disfigurement may also result from the needle and infiltrated fluids. For these reasons, the scalp veins are not used as frequently today as they were in the past.

The extremities are the most accessible insertion sites; however, since patients tend to move about, take these precautions:

• Protect the insertion site to prevent catheter or needle dislodgment.

• Use a padded arm board to minimize dislodgment.

• Place the clamp out of the child's reach; if extension tubing is used to allow the child greater mobility, securely tape the connection.

• Restrain the child only when necessary.

• To allay anxiety, give a simple explanation to the child who must be restrained while asleep.

Maintaining flow rate and fluid balance

While administering a continuous I.V. infusion to a child, monitor flow rate and check the patient's condition and insertion site at least hourly—more frequently when giving medication intermittently.

Adjust the flow rate only while the patient is composed; crying and other emotional upset can constrict blood vessels. Flow rate may be retarded if a pump isn't used. Flow should be adequate because some drugs (calcium, for example) can be very irritating at low flow rates.

Making dilutions

Some drugs are hyperosmolar; in infants, these drugs must be diluted to prevent radical changes in fluid that might induce CNS hemorrhage. Sodium bicarbonate, for example, must be diluted to half strength to lower osmolality and lessen the risk of CNS bleeding.

In general, however, use the minimum amount of compatible fluid over the shortest recommended period of time. Remember also to check the total daily fluid intake and the amount allotted to medication.

Intramuscular injections

If indicated, intramuscular injections are preferred when the drug cannot be given by other parenteral routes and rapid absorption is necessary.

• In children under 2 years, the vastus lateralis muscle is the preferred injection site; in older children, either the ventrogluteal area or the gluteus medius muscle can be used.

• To determine correct needle size, consider the patient's age, muscle mass, and nutritional status, and the drug's viscosity; record and rotate injection sites.

• Explain to the patient that the injection will hurt, but that the medication will help him. Restrain him during the injection and comfort him afterward.

Dermatomucosal medications

• Use ear drops warmed to room temperature; cold drops can cause considerable pain and possible vertigo.

• To administer drops, turn the patient on his side with the affected ear up. If he is younger than 3 years, pull the pinna down and back; if he is older than 3 years, pull the pinna up and back.

• Avoid using inhalants in very small children: obtaining their cooperation is difficult.

• Before attempting to administer medication through a metered-dose nebulizer to an older child, explain the inhaler to him. First have him hold the nebulizer upside down and close his lips around the mouthpiece. Then have him exhale; pinch his nostrils shut; and when he starts to inhale, release one dose of medication into his mouth. Have the patient continue inhaling until his lungs feel full.

• Most inhaled agents are not useful if taken orally; therefore, if you doubt the patient's ability to use the inhalant correctly, don't use it.

Parenteral nutrition

Intravenous nutrition is given to patients who can't or won't take adequate food orally and to patients with hypermetabolic conditions who need I.V. supplementation. The latter group includes premature infants and children who have burns or other major trauma, intractable diarrhea, malabsorption syndromes, gastrointestinal abnormalities, emotional disorders such as anorexia nervosa, and congenital abnormalities.

Before fat emulsions are administered to infants and children, however, potential benefits must be weighed against possible risks.

Fats—supplied as 10% or 20% emulsions—are administered both peripherally and centrally. Their use is limited by the child's ability to metabolize them. An infant or child with a diseased liver cannot efficiently metabolize fats, for example.

Some fats, however, must be supplied both to prevent essential fatty acid deficiency and to permit normal growth and development. A minimum of calories (2% to 4%) must be supplied as linoleic acid—an essential fatty acid found in lipids. In the infant, fats are essential for normal neurologic development.

Nevertheless, fat solutions may decrease oxygen perfusion and may adversely affect patients with pulmonary disease. This risk can be minimized by supplying only the minimum fat needed for essential fatty acid requirements and not the usual intake of 40% to 50% of the patient's total calories.

Fatty acids can also displace bilirubin bound to serum albumin, causing a rise in free, unconjugated bilirubin and an increased risk of kernicterus. However, fat solutions may interfere with some bilirubin assays and cause falsely elevated levels. To avoid this complication, a blood sample should be drawn 4 hours after infusion of the lipid emulsion; or if the emulsion is introduced over 24 hours, the blood sample should be centrifuged before the assay is performed.

Drug therapy in the elderly

If you're providing drug therapy for elderly patients, you'll want to understand physiologic and pharmacokinetic changes that may alter drug dosage; common adverse reactions; and compliance problems in the elderly.

Physiologic changes affecting drug action

As a person ages, gradual changes occur in his anatomy and physiology. Some of these age-related changes may alter the therapeutic and toxic effects of medications.

Body composition
Proportions of fat, lean tissue, and water in the body change with age. Total body mass and lean body mass tend to decrease; the proportion of body fat tends to increase.

Varying from person to person, these changes in body composition affect the relationship between a drug's concentration and solubility in the body.

For example, a *water-soluble drug*, such as gentamicin, is *not* distributed to fat. Since there's relatively less lean tissue in an elderly person, more drug remains in the blood, and toxic levels can result. Likewise, pentobarbital, which is distributed *only* to fat, may produce lower blood levels in the elderly patient.

Gastrointestinal function
In the elderly, decreases in gastric acid secretion and gastrointestinal motility slow emptying of stomach contents and movement of intestinal contents through the entire tract. Furthermore, although inconclusive, research shows the elderly may have more difficulty absorbing medications. This is a particularly significant problem with drugs having a narrow therapeutic range, such as digoxin, in which any change in absorption can be crucial.

Hepatic function
The liver's ability to metabolize certain drugs decreases with age. This is probably due to diminished blood flow to the liver, which results from the age-related decrease in cardiac output. When an elderly patient takes certain sleep medications, such as secobarbital, his liver's reduced ability to metabolize the drug may produce a hangover effect due to central nervous system depression. Elimination of these medications is highly dependent on the liver.

Decreased hepatic function may cause:
• more intense drug effects due to higher blood levels
• longer-lasting drug effects due to prolonged blood concentrations
• greater incidence of drug toxicity.

Renal function
Although an elderly person's renal function is usually sufficient to eliminate excess body fluid and waste, his ability to eliminate some medications may be reduced by 50% or more.

Many medications commonly used by the elderly, such as digoxin, are excreted primarily through the kidneys. If the kidneys' ability to excrete the drug is decreased, high blood concentrations may result. Digoxin toxicity, therefore, is relatively common.

Drug dosages can be modified to compensate for age-related decreases in renal function. Aided by laboratory tests, such as BUN and serum creatinine, clinical pharmacists and doctors can adjust medication dosages so the patient receives the expected therapeutic benefits without the risk of toxicity. Observe your patient for signs of toxicity. A patient taking digoxin, for example, may experience anorexia, nausea, and vomiting.

Adverse drug reactions
As compared with younger people, the elderly reportedly experience twice as many adverse drug reactions, relating to greater drug consumption, poor compliance, and physiologic changes.

Signs and symptoms of adverse drug reactions—confusion, weakness, and lethargy—are often mistakenly attributed to senility or disease. If the adverse reaction isn't identified, the patient may continue to receive the drug. Furthermore, he may receive unnecessary additional medication to treat complications caused by the original medication.

Although any medication can cause adverse reactions, most of the serious reactions in the elderly are caused by relatively few medications. Be particularly alert for toxicities resulting from diuretics, digoxin, corticosteroids, sleep medications, and nonprescription drugs.

Diuretic toxicity
Because total body water decreases with age, normal doses of potassium-wasting diuretics, such as hydrochlorothiazide and furosemide, may result in fluid loss and even dehydration in an elderly patient.

These diuretics may deplete serum potassium, causing weakness in the patient; and they may raise blood uric acid and glucose levels, complicating preexisting gout and diabetes mellitus.

Digoxin toxicity
As the body's renal function and rate of excretion decline, digoxin concentrations in the blood may build to toxic levels, causing nausea, vomiting, diarrhea, and—most serious—cardiac arrhythmias. Try to prevent severe toxicity by observing your patient for early signs such as appetite loss, confusion, or depression.

Corticosteroid toxicity
Elderly patients on corticosteroids may experience short-term effects including fluid retention and psychological manifestations ranging from mild euphoria to acute psychotic reactions. Long-term toxic effects, such as osteoporosis, can be especially severe in elderly patients who have been taking prednisone or related steroidal compounds for months or even years. To prevent serious toxicity, carefully monitor patients on long-term regimens. Observe them for subtle changes in appearance, mood, and mobility, as well as for signs of impaired healing and fluid and electrolyte disturbances.

Sleep medication toxicity
In some cases, sedatives or sleeping aids, such as flurazepam, cause excessive sedation or residual drowsiness.

Nonprescription drug toxicity
When aspirin and aspirin-containing analgesics are used in moderation, toxicity is minimal, but prolonged ingestion may cause gastrointestinal irritation and gradual blood loss resulting in severe anemia. Although anemia from chronic aspirin consumption can affect all age groups, the elderly may be less able to compensate because of their already reduced iron stores.

Laxatives may cause diarrhea in elderly patients who are extremely sensitive to drugs such as bisacodyl. Chronic oral use of mineral oil as a lubricating laxative may result in lipid pneumonia due to aspiration of small residual oil droplets in the patient's mouth.

Patient noncompliance

Approximately one third of the elderly fail to comply with their prescribed drug therapy. They may fail to take prescribed doses or to follow the correct schedule; they may take medications prescribed for previous disorders, discontinue medications prematurely, or use p.r.n. medications indiscriminately.

Review your patient's medication regimen with him. Be sure he understands the medication amount, and the time and frequency of doses. Also, explain how he should take each medication, that is, with food or water, or by itself.

Give your patient whatever help you can to avoid drug therapy problems, and refer him to his doctor or pharmacist if he needs further information.

Amebicides and trichomonacides

carbarsone
chloroquine hydrochloride
chloroquine phosphate
diiodohydroxyquin
emetine hydrochloride
metronidazole
metronidazole hydrochloride
paromomycin sulfate

MECHANISM OF ACTION

• Carbarsone is an organic arsenic derivative with amebicidal activity in the intestinal lumen, possibly due to inhibition of sulfhydryl enzymes.
• Chloroquine is mainly an antimalarial. Its mechanism of action as an amebicide is unknown, but it is useful in the treatment of extraintestinal amebiasis.
• Diiodohydroxyquin is an iodine derivative with amebicidal activity in the intestinal lumen. Its precise mechanism of action is unknown.
• Emetine kills *Entamoeba histolytica* by a mechanism related to the inhibition of protein synthesis.
• Metronidazole is a direct-acting trichomonacide and amebicide that works at both intestinal and extraintestinal sites.
• Paromomycin is an aminoglycoside antibiotic that acts as an amebicide in intestinal sites, effective in the presence or absence of bacteria. Its specific mechanism of action is unknown.

COMBINATION PRODUCTS
None.

carbarsone

INDICATIONS & DOSAGE
Intestinal amebiasis—
Adults: 250 mg P.O. b.i.d. or t.i.d. for 10 days. Rectal (as retention enema): 2 g dissolved in 200 ml warm 2% sodium bicarbonate solution, every other night for 5 doses. Discontinue oral therapy when enema is given.
Children: average total dose is 75 mg/kg P.O. daily in 3 divided doses over 10-day period. Recommended total varies according to age—2 to 4 years, 2 g total; 5 to 8 years, 3 g total; 9 to 12 years, 4 g total; and over 12 years, 5 g total.

SIDE EFFECTS
Blood: *agranulocytosis.*
CNS: neuritis, convulsions, *hemorrhagic encephalitis.*
EENT: sore throat, retinal edema, visual disturbances.
GI: epigastric pain and burning, irritation, *nausea, vomiting,* diarrhea, anorexia, constipation, increased motility, abdominal cramps.
GU: polyuria, albuminuria, kidney damage.
Hepatic: hepatomegaly, jaundice, hepatitis.
Skin: eruptions, *exfoliative dermatitis,* pruritus.
Other: edema of wrists, ankles, and knees; weight loss; splenomegaly.

INTERACTIONS
None significant.

NURSING CONSIDERATIONS

• Contraindicated as initial treatment in patients with hepatic or renal disease; in patients with contracted visual or color fields; and in patients with known hypersensitivity or intolerance to any arsenical treatment.

• Don't exceed recommended dose; toxicity may result. If second treatment is needed, allow at least 10 days between courses.

• Divide carbarsone capsule to obtain required dose. Give in ½ glass orange juice or milk, in small amount of 1% sodium bicarbonate solution, or in jelly or other food.

• Discontinue upon first sign of intolerance or toxicity. Fatal exfoliative dermatitis has been reported.

• Tell patient to report any unusual symptoms, even post-treatment.

• Liver function tests should precede therapy. Careful inspection of skin, vision testing, and palpation of liver and spleen should be repeated regularly.

• Monitor intake/output. Notify doctor of number, frequency, and character of stools.

• If ordered, give a cleansing enema before giving carbarsone enema.

• Deliver stool specimen to lab promptly; movements of parasites are seen only when stool is warm. Amebic cysts in stool indicate need for additional therapy. Stool specimen should be studied 1 week after stopping therapy and monthly for 1 year. To help prevent reinfestation, instruct patient in proper hygiene.

---

chloroquine hydrochloride
Aralen HCl

chloroquine phosphate
Aralen Phosphate♦, Chlorocon, Roquine

INDICATIONS & DOSAGE

Extraintestinal amebiasis—
Adults: 160 to 200 mg chloroquine (hydrochloride) base I.M. daily for no more than 10 to 12 days. As soon as possible, substitute 1 g (600 mg base) chloroquine phosphate P.O. daily for 2 days; then 500 mg (300 mg base) daily for at least 2 to 3 weeks. Treatment is usually combined with an effective intestinal amebicide.

Children: 10 mg/kg of chloroquine (hydrochloride) base for 2 to 3 weeks. Maximum 300 mg daily.

Rheumatoid arthritis—
250 mg chloroquine phosphate daily with evening meal.

SIDE EFFECTS

Blood: *agranulocytosis.*
CNS: mild and transient headache, neuromyopathy, psychic stimulation, fatigue, irritability, nightmares, convulsions, dizziness.
EENT: *visual disturbances* (blurred vision; difficulty in focusing; reversible corneal changes; generally irreversible, sometimes progressive or delayed retinal changes, e.g., narrowing of arterioles; macular lesions; pallor of optic disk; optic atrophy; patchy retinal pigmentation, often leading to blindness), ototoxicity, nerve deafness, vertigo, tinnitus.
GI: anorexia, abdominal cramps, diarrhea, nausea, vomiting.
Skin: pruritus, lichen planus-like eruptions, skin and mucosal pigmentary changes, pleomorphic skin eruptions.

INTERACTIONS
None significant.

NURSING CONSIDERATIONS

• Contraindicated in patients with retinal or visual field changes, porphyria. Use with extreme caution in presence of severe GI, neurologic, or blood disorders. Drug concentrates in liver; use cautiously in patients with hepatic disease or alcoholism. Use with caution in patients with G-6-PD deficiency or psoriasis; drug may exacerbate these conditions.

Italicized side effects are common or life-threatening.
*Liquid form contains alcohol.   **May contain tartrazine.

• Complete blood cell counts and liver function studies should be made periodically during prolonged therapy; if severe disorder appears that is not attributable to disease under treatment, drug may need to be discontinued.

• Overdosage can quickly produce toxic symptoms: headache, visual disturbances, drowsiness, cardiovascular collapse, and convulsions, followed by respiratory and cardiac arrest. Children are extremely susceptible to toxicity; avoid long-term treatment.

• Baseline and periodic ophthalmologic examinations needed. Report blurred vision, increased sensitivity to light, or muscle weakness. Check periodically for muscle weakness after long-term use. Audiometric examinations recommended before, during, and after therapy, especially if long term.

• To prevent exacerbated drug-induced dermatoses, warn patient to avoid excessive exposure to sun.

• Each ml parenteral solution containing 50 mg dihydrochloride salt = 40 mg chloroquine base; each 500 mg tablet phosphate = 300 mg chloroquine base.

diiodohydroxyquin
Gynovules◆◆, Inserfem, Yodoxin

INDICATIONS & DOSAGE
Intestinal amebiasis—
Adults: 630 to 650 mg P.O. t.i.d. for 20 days. Total daily dose should not exceed 2 g.
Children: usual dose: 30 to 40 mg/kg of body weight daily in 2 to 3 divided doses for 20 days.
Additional courses of diiodohydroxyquin therapy should not be repeated before a resting interval of 2 to 3 weeks.

SIDE EFFECTS
Blood: *agranulocytosis.*
CNS: neurotoxicity, dysesthesia, weakness, vertigo, malaise, headache, agita-

tion, retrograde amnesia, ataxia, peripheral neuropathy.
EENT: optic neuritis, optic atrophy, loss of vision.
GI: anorexia, nausea, vomiting, abdominal cramps, diarrhea, increased motility, constipation, epigastric burning and pain, gastritis, anal irritation and itching.
Skin: pruritus, hives, papular and pustular eruptions, urticaria, discoloration of hair and nails.
Other: thyroid enlargement, fever, chills, generalized furunculosis, hair loss.

INTERACTIONS
None significant.

NURSING CONSIDERATIONS
• Contraindicated in patients with known hypersensitivity to 8-hydroxyquinoline derivatives or iodine-containing preparations. Diiodohydroxyquin causes hepatic damage in such patients. Also contraindicated in patients with hepatic or renal disease, or preexisting optic neuropathy.

• Patient should have periodic ophthalmologic examinations during treatment.

• Give after meals. Crush tablets and mix with applesauce or chocolate syrup.

• Record intake/output and color and amount of stool. Send warm specimens to lab frequently.

• Watch for diarrhea during the first 2 or 3 days of treatment. Notify doctor if it continues past 3 days.

• Advise patient not to discontinue the medication prematurely. Tell him to notify doctor if skin rash occurs.

emetine hydrochloride

INDICATIONS & DOSAGE
Acute fulminating amebic dysentery—
Adults: 1 mg/kg daily up to 60 mg daily (1 or 2 doses) deep S.C. or I.M. 3

---

to 5 days to control symptoms. Give another antiamebic drug simultaneously.
Children: 1 mg/kg daily in 2 doses I.M. for up to 5 days. Maximum 60 mg daily.
Amebic hepatitis and abscess—
Adults: 60 mg daily (1 or 2 doses) deep S.C. or I.M. for 10 days.
Children: 1 mg/kg daily in 2 doses I.M. for up to 5 days. Maximum 60 mg daily.

SIDE EFFECTS
CNS: dizziness, headache, mild sensory disturbances, central or peripheral nerve function changes, neuromuscular symptoms (weakness, aching, stiffness, tenderness, pain, tremors).
CV: *acute toxicity*—can occur at any dose (hypotension, tachycardia, precordial pain, dyspnea, *EKG abnormalities,* gallop rhythm, cardiac dilatation, severe acute degenerative myocarditis, pericarditis, congestive failure).
GI: *nausea, vomiting, diarrhea,* abdominal cramps, loss of sense of taste.
Metabolic: decreased serum potassium levels.
Skin: eczematous, urticarial purpuric lesions.
Local: skeletal muscle stiffness, aching, tenderness, muscle weakness at injection site, cellulitis.
Other: edema.

INTERACTIONS
None significant.

NURSING CONSIDERATIONS
• Contraindicated in patients with cardiac or renal disease, except those with amebic abscess or hepatitis not controlled by chloroquine; patients who have received a course of emetine less than 6 to 8 weeks previously; children, except for severe dysentery unresponsive to other amebicides; and in those with polyneuropathy or muscle disease. Use with caution in elderly or debilitated patients, patients with hypotension, or those about to undergo surgery.

• Record pulse rate and blood pressure 2 to 3 times daily. Discontinue use if drug produces tachycardia, precipitous fall in blood pressure, neuromuscular symptoms, marked gastrointestinal effects, or considerable weakness. Weakness and muscle symptoms usually precede more serious symptoms and serve as a guide for avoiding toxicity.
• Don't exceed recommended dose or extend therapy beyond 10 days. Patient confined to bed during treatment and for several days thereafter.
• Drug may alter EKG tracings for 6 weeks. EKG should be taken before therapy, after fifth dose, upon completion, and 1 week after therapy. Patterns can resemble those of myocardial infarction. First and most consistent change is T wave inversion.
• Deep S.C. administration is preferred; I.M. acceptable, but I.V. route is dangerous and contraindicated. Injections cause necrosis and edema. Rotate sites and apply warm soaks.
• Record intake/output; odor and consistency of stools; and presence of mucus, blood, or other foreign matter. Send warm specimens to lab frequently. Repeat fecal examinations at 3-month intervals to assure elimination of amebae. Patients with acute amebic dysentery often become asymptomatic carriers. Check family members and suspected contacts.
• Suspect emetine-induced reaction if stools increase in number following initial relief of diarrhea.
• To help prevent reinfection, instruct patient in proper hygiene.
• Drug is very irritating. Avoid contact with eyes and mucous membranes.
• Restoration of body fluids and nutrients is an important adjunct to therapy.

Italicized side effects are common or life-threatening.
*Liquid form contains alcohol.   **May contain tartrazine.

metronidazole
Flagyl♦, Metryl, Neo-Tric♦♦,
Novonidazol♦♦, Satric, Trikacide♦♦

metronidazole hydrochloride
Flagyl I.V., Flagyl I.V. R.T.U.,
Metro I.V.

INDICATIONS & DOSAGE
Amebic hepatic abscess—
Adults: 500 to 750 mg P.O. t.i.d. for 5
to 10 days.
Children: 35 to 50 mg/kg daily (in
3 doses) for 10 days.
Intestinal amebiasis—
Adults: 750 mg P.O. t.i.d. for 5 to
10 days.
Children: 35 to 50 mg/kg daily (in
3 doses) for 10 days.
Follow this therapy with oral
diiodohydroxyquin.
Trichomoniasis—
Adults (both male and female):
250 mg P.O. t.i.d. for 7 days or 2 g
P.O. in single dose; 4 to 6 weeks should
elapse between courses of therapy.
Refractory trichomoniasis—
Women: 250 mg P.O. b.i.d. for
10 days.
*Treatment of bacterial infections caused
by anaerobic microorganisms—*
Adults: Loading dose is 15 mg/kg I.V.
infused over 1 hour (approximately 1 g
for a 70-kg adult). Maintenance dose is
7.5 mg/kg I.V. or P.O. q 6 hours (approximately 500 mg for a 70-kg adult).
The first maintenance dose should be
administered 6 hours following the
loading dose.
Giardiasis—
Adults: 250 mg P.O. t.i.d. for 5 days.
Children: 5 mg/kg P.O. t.i.d. for 5
days.

SIDE EFFECTS
Blood: leukopenia, neutropenia.
CNS: vertigo, headache, ataxia, incoordination, confusion, irritability,
depression, restlessness, weakness, fatigue, drowsiness, insomnia, sensory
neuropathy, paresthesias of extremities,
psychic stimulation, neuromyopathy.
CV: EKG change (flattened T wave).
GI: abdominal cramping, stomatitis,
nausea, vomiting, anorexia, diarrhea,
constipation, proctitis, dry mouth.
GU: darkened urine, polyuria, dysuria,
pyuria, incontinence, cystitis, decreased libido, dyspareunia, dryness of
vagina and vulva, sense of pelvic pressure.
Skin: pruritus, flushing.
Local: *thrombophlebitis after I.V. infusion.*
Other: overgrowth of nonsusceptible
organisms, especially *Candida* (glossitis, furry tongue), metallic taste, fever.

INTERACTIONS
Alcohol: disulfiram-like reaction (nausea, vomiting, headache, cramps,
flushing). Don't use together.
Disulfiram: acute psychoses and confu-
sional states. Don't use together.

NURSING CONSIDERATIONS
Warning: This drug has been shown to
be carcinogenic in mice and possibly
rats. Unnecessary use should be
avoided.
• Use cautiously in patients with a history of blood dyscrasia or CNS disorder, and in patients with retinal or visual field changes. Use with caution in
patients with hepatic disease or alcoholism; in conjunction with known hepatotoxic drugs.
• Tell patients to avoid alcohol or
alcohol-containing medications for
48 hours after therapy is completed.
• Give with meals to minimize GI distress.
• Tell patients metallic taste and dark
or red-brown urine are possible.
• Record number and character of
stools when used in the treatment of
amebiasis. Metronidazole should be
used only after *Trichomonas vaginalis*
has been confirmed by wet smear or
culture or *Entamoeba histolytica* has

been identified. Asymptomatic sexual partners of patients being treated for *T. vaginalis* infection should be treated simultaneously to avoid reinfection. Instruct patient in proper hygiene.
• The I.V. form should be administered by slow infusion only. Don't give I.V. push.
• Follow package instructions carefully when mixing the I.V. solution.

paromomycin sulfate
Humatin

INDICATIONS & DOSAGE
Intestinal amebiasis, acute and chronic—
Adults and children: 25 to 35 mg/kg daily P.O. in 3 doses for 5 to 10 days after meals.
Tapeworms (fish, beef, pork, dog)—
Adults: 1 g P.O. q 15 minutes for 4 doses.
Children: 11 mg/kg P.O. q 15 minutes for 4 doses.

SIDE EFFECTS
Blood: eosinophilia.
CNS: headache, vertigo.
EENT: ototoxicity.
GI: anorexia, *nausea, vomiting, epigastric pain and burning, abdominal cramps,* diarrhea, constipation, increased motility, steatorrhea, pruritus ani, malabsorption syndrome.

GU: hematuria, nephrotoxicity.
Skin: rash, exanthema, pruritus.
Other: overgrowth of nonsusceptible organisms.

INTERACTIONS
None significant.

NURSING CONSIDERATIONS
• Contraindicated in patients with impaired renal function or intestinal obstruction. Use with caution in patients with ulcerative lesions of the bowel to avoid inadvertent absorption and resulting renal toxicity. Poorly absorbed orally, but will accumulate with renal impairment or ulcerative lesions.
• Ask about history of sensitivity to drug before giving first dose.
• Administer after meals.
• Emphasize personal hygiene, particularly handwashing before eating and after defecation.
• Criterion of cure is absence of amebae in stools examined weekly for 6 weeks after treatment and thereafter at monthly intervals for 2 years. Examine feces of family members or suspected contacts.
• Avoid high doses or prolonged therapy.
• Watch for signs of superinfection (continued fever and other signs of new infections, especially monilial infections).

Italicized side effects are common or life-threatening.
∗Liquid form contains alcohol.   ∗∗May contain tartrazine.

Anthelmintics

diethylcarbamazine citrate
gentian violet
mebendazole
oxamniquine
niclosamide
piperazine adipate
piperazine citrate
piperazine phosphate
piperazine tartrate
pyrantel pamoate
pyrvinium pamoate
quinacrine hydrochloride
thiabendazole

MECHANISM OF ACTION

• Diethylcarbamazine appears to sensitize the worms to phagocytosis by the reticuloendothelial system.

• Mebendazole appears to selectively and irreversibly inhibit uptake of glucose and other nutrients in susceptible helminths.

• Niclosamide inhibits the metabolic process of oxidative phosphorylation in tapeworms.

• Oxamniquine reduces the egg load of *Schistosoma mansoni,* but its exact mechanism of action is unknown.

• Piperazine and pyrantel block neuromuscular action, paralyzing the worm and causing its expulsion by normal peristalsis.

• Pyrvinium, a cyanine dye, appears to destroy parasites by preventing them from using exogenous carbohydrates.

• Quinacrine inhibits deoxyribonucleic acid metabolism.

• Mechanism of action of gentian violet and thiabendazole is unknown.

COMBINATION PRODUCTS
None.

---

diethylcarbamazine citrate
Hetrazan

INDICATIONS & DOSAGE
Ascariasis (roundworm)—
Adults: 13 mg/kg P.O. daily for 7 days.
Children: 6 to 10 mg/kg P.O. t.i.d. for 7 to 10 days.
Loiasis, dipetalonemiasis, onchocerciasis, Bancroftian or Malayan filariasis—
Adults and children:
2 mg/kg P.O. t.i.d. for 3 to 4 weeks.
Repeat if necessary.
Tropical (pulmonary) eosinophilia—
Adults and children:
13 mg/kg P.O. daily for 4 to 7 days.

SIDE EFFECTS
Blood: leukocytosis, eosinophilia.
CNS: *headache, malaise, weakness,* lassitude, syncope.
CV: tachycardia, tachypnea, hypotension.
GI: anorexia, nausea, vomiting.
Skin: pruritus, dermatitis, bullous eruptions.
Other: arthralgia, myalgia, joint pain, swelling and edema of face, severe pedal edema, fever, lymphadenitis, sweating, cough.

INTERACTIONS
None significant.

NURSING CONSIDERATIONS
• Use with caution in patients with

---

hypertension; severe hepatic, renal, or cardiac disease; and in children under 1 year of age. Treat patients with recent history of malaria with an antimalarial agent first to prevent relapse in asymptomatic malarial infections.

• Administer carefully to avoid or control allergic or other untoward reactions. Minimize allergic reactions by giving with corticosteroids, antihistamines, or aspirin.
• Inform patient that side effects will usually be minor and transient.
• Instruct patient in good hygiene.
• Give immediately after meals. Drug has sweet but unpleasant taste.

gentian violet

INDICATIONS & DOSAGE
Pinworms—
Adults: 60 mg P.O. t.i.d. 7 to 10 days.
Children: 2 mg/kg P.O. daily in 2 to 3 doses for 8 to 10 days, not to exceed 90 mg/day. Discontinue treatment after 7 to 10 days. Resume if needed.

SIDE EFFECTS
CNS: headache, dizziness, lassitude.
GI: nausea, diarrhea, vomiting (purple), abdominal cramps.

INTERACTIONS
None significant.

NURSING CONSIDERATIONS
• Use with caution in patients with cardiac, hepatic, renal, or GI disease.
• Tablets must be taken whole with water. Give with meals.
• Patient should abstain from alcohol during treatment.
• If nausea and vomiting occur, stop treatment for 1 to 2 days; resume at reduced dosage and notify doctor. Warn that skin, clothing, vomitus, and feces will be stained purple.
• Instruct patient in good hygiene.

mebendazole
Vermox♦

INDICATIONS & DOSAGE
Pinworms—
Adults and children over 2 years: 100 mg P.O. as a single dose. If infection persists 3 weeks later, repeat treatment.
Roundworm, whipworm, hookworm—
Adults and children over 2 years: 100 mg P.O. b.i.d. for 3 days. If infection persists 3 weeks later, repeat treatment.

SIDE EFFECTS
GI: occasional, transient abdominal pain and diarrhea in massive infection and expulsion of worms.

INTERACTIONS
None significant.

NURSING CONSIDERATIONS
• Tablets may be chewed, swallowed whole, or crushed and mixed with food.
• No dietary restrictions, laxatives, or enemas necessary.
• To avoid reinfection, wash perianal area daily. Change undergarments and bedclothes daily. Wash hands and clean fingernails after bowel movements and before meals. Treat all family members.

niclosamide
Niclocide

INDICATIONS & DOSAGE
Tapeworms (fish and beef)—
Adults: 4 tablets (2 g) chewed thoroughly as a single dose.
Children (more than 34 kg): 3 tablets (1.5 g) chewed thoroughly as a single dose.
Children (11 to 34 kg): 2 tablets (1.0 g) chewed thoroughly as a single dose.
Dwarf Tapeworm—

Italicized side effects are common or life-threatening.
∗Liquid form contains alcohol.   ∗∗May contain tartrazine.

Adults: 4 tablets chewed thoroughly as a single daily dose for 7 days.
Children (more than 34 kg): 3 tablets chewed thoroughly on the first day, then 2 tablets for the next 6 days.
Children (11 to 34 kg): 2 tablets chewed thoroughly on the first day, then one tablet daily for the next 6 days.

SIDE EFFECTS
CNS: drowsiness, dizziness, headache
EENT: oral irritation, bad taste in mouth
GI: *nausea, vomiting, anorexia,* diarrhea
Skin: rash, pruritis ani

INTERACTIONS
None reported.

NURSING CONSIDERATIONS
• Instruct patient to chew tablets thoroughly and wash down with water; for smaller children, the tablets can be crushed and mixed with water or applesauce.
• Tablets should be taken as a single dose after breakfast.
• A mild laxative should be administered to cleanse the bowel prior to initiation of niclosamide therapy. This is only desirable in patients who are constipated.
• When treating dwarf tapeworms, urge patient to drink fruit juices. This helps to eliminate the accumulated intestinal mucus under which they lodge.

oxamniquine
Vansil

INDICATIONS & DOSAGE
Treatment of schistosomiasis caused by Schistosoma mansoni—
Adults and children: 12 to 15 mg/kg given as a single oral dose.

SIDE EFFECTS
CNS: convulsions, *dizziness, drowsiness, headache.*

GI: nausea, vomiting, abdominal pain, anorexia.
Skin: urticaria.

INTERACTIONS
None significant

NURSING CONSIDERATIONS
• There are no known contraindications.
• Use cautiously in patients with a history of convulsive conditions. Epileptiform convulsions have rarely been observed within the first few hours after ingestion. Patients with history of convulsions should be kept under medical supervision.
• Instruct patient to avoid driving and other hazardous activities if he's dizzy or drowsy.
• Gastrointestinal tolerance is improved if you give the drug after meals.
• Although *S. mansoni* infection is rare in the United States and Canada, travelers or immigrants from such areas as Puerto Rico, Latin America, and Africa may have contracted the infection from contaminated water.

piperazine adipate
Entacyl♦♦

piperazine citrate
Antepar♦, Bryrel, Pin-Tega Tabs, Pipril, Ta-Verm, Vermazine

piperazine phosphate
Antepar Phosphate

piperazine tartrate
Razine Tartrate

INDICATIONS & DOSAGE
Pinworms—
Adults and children: 65 mg/kg P.O. daily 7 to 8 days. Maximum daily dose is 2.5 g.
Roundworm—
Adults: 3.5 g P.O. in single doses for 2 consecutive days.

Children: 75 mg/kg P.O. daily in single dose for 2 consecutive days. Maximum daily dose: 3.5 g.

SIDE EFFECTS
CNS: ataxia, tremors, choreiform movements, muscular weakness, myoclonus, hyporeflexia, paresthesias, convulsions, sense of detachment, EEG abnormalities, memory defect, headache, vertigo.
EENT: nystagmus, blurred vision, paralytic strabismus, cataracts with visual impairment, lacrimation, difficulty in focusing, rhinorrhea.
GI: *nausea, vomiting,* diarrhea, abdominal cramps.
Skin: urticaria, photodermatitis, *erythema multiforme,* purpura, eczematous skin reactions.
Other: arthralgia, fever, bronchospasm.

INTERACTIONS
None significant.

NURSING CONSIDERATIONS
• Contraindicated in patients with hepatic and/or renal impairment, or convulsive disorders. Use with caution in patients with severe malnutrition or anemia.
• Discontinue if CNS or significant GI reactions occur.
• Because of potential neurotoxicity, avoid prolonged or repeated treatment, especially in children.
• No dietary restrictions, laxatives, or enemas necessary.
• May be taken with food.
• To avoid reinfection, wash perianal area daily. Change undergarments and bedclothes daily. Wash hands and clean fingernails before meals and after bowel movements. Treat all family members.
• Protect drug from air, light, and moisture.

pyrantel pamoate
Antiminth, Combantrin••

INDICATIONS & DOSAGE
Roundworm and pinworm—
Adults and children over 2 years: single dose of 11 mg/kg P.O. Maximum dose 1 g. For pinworm, dose should be repeated in 2 weeks.

SIDE EFFECTS
CNS: headache, dizziness, drowsiness, insomnia.
GI: anorexia, nausea, vomiting, gastralgia, cramps, diarrhea, tenesmus.
Hepatic: transient elevation of SGOT.
Skin: rashes.
Other: fever, weakness.

INTERACTIONS
None significant.

NURSING CONSIDERATIONS
• Use cautiously in severe malnutrition or anemia, or in hepatic dysfunction. Treat for anemia, dehydration, or malnutrition before giving drug.
• No dietary restrictions, laxatives, or enemas necessary.
• May be taken with food. Shake well before pouring.
• To avoid reinfection, wash perianal area daily. Change undergarments and bedclothes daily. Wash hands and clean fingernails before meals and after bowel movements. Treat all family members.
• Protect drug from light. Store below 30° C. (86° F.).

pyrvinium pamoate
Pamovin••, Povan, Pyr-Pam••, Vanquin••

INDICATIONS & DOSAGE
Pinworm—
Adults and children: 5 mg/kg P.O. single dose (maximum 350 mg). Repeat in 2 weeks if needed.

Italicized side effects are common or life-threatening.
*Liquid form contains alcohol.　　**May contain tartrazine.

SIDE EFFECTS
GI: nausea, vomiting, cramping, diarrhea (vomiting more common with suspension than with tablets).
Skin: photosensitivity, *erythema multiforme*.

INTERACTIONS
None significant.

NURSING CONSIDERATIONS
• Safe use in children who weigh less than 36 kg not established.
• Swallow tablets whole to avoid staining teeth. May be taken with food.
• Warn that drug stains fabrics, skin, vomitus, and stools bright red.
• No dietary restrictions, laxatives, or enemas necessary.
• To avoid reinfection, wash perianal area daily. Change undergarments and bedclothes daily. Wash hands and clean fingernails before meals and after bowel movements. Treat all family members.
• Protect drug from light.

quinacrine hydrochloride
Atabrine

INDICATIONS & DOSAGE
Treatment of giardiasis—
Adults: 100 mg P.O. for 5 to 7 days.
Children: 7 mg/kg/day P.O. given in 3 divided doses after meals for 5 days. Maximum 300 mg/day. If necessary, the dosage may be repeated in 2 weeks.

SIDE EFFECTS
CNS: *headache, dizziness,* nervousness, vertigo, mood shifts, nightmares.
GI: *diarrhea, anorexia, nausea, abdominal cramps,* vomiting.
Skin: pleomorphic skin eruptions.

INTERACTIONS
None significant.

NURSING CONSIDERATIONS
• Contraindicated if primaquine is being given concurrently since primaquine toxicity could be increased.
• Use with extreme caution in patients with porphyria or psoriasis; may exacerbate these conditions.
• Use with caution in patients with hepatic disease, alcoholism, severe renal or cardiac disease, psychosis, G-6-PD deficiency, and in those over 60 years or under 1 year.
• Give after meals with large glass of water, tea, or fruit juice to reduce GI irritation. Bitter taste may be disguised by jam or honey.
• Nausea and vomiting after large doses may be lessened by taking sodium bicarbonate with each dose.
• Collect all of stool after treatment. Don't put toilet paper in bedpan. Look for the scolex (attachment organ), which will be stained yellow from drug.
• Warn patients about temporary yellow color of skin and urine; it is not jaundice.
• Patient should be on a bland, nonfat, semisolid diet for 24 hours, and should fast after the evening meal before treatment.
• Quinacrine is not as effective as metronidazole in the treatment of giardiasis.
• Keep out of reach of children; drug is highly toxic.
• Induce emesis for overdose.

thiabendazole
Mintezol♦

INDICATIONS & DOSAGE
Systemic infection with pinworm, roundworm, threadworm, whipworm, cutaneous larva migrans, and trichinosis—
Adults or children: 25 mg/kg P.O. in 2 doses daily. Maximum dose is 3 g daily.
Cutaneous infestations with larva migrans (creeping eruption)—
Adults and children: 25 mg/kg P.O. b.i.d. for 2 to 5 days. Maximum 3 g

daily. If lesions persist after 2 days, repeat course.

Pinworm—2 doses daily for 1 day; repeat in 7 days.

Roundworm, threadworm, whipworm—2 doses daily for 2 successive days.

Trichinosis—2 doses daily for 2 to 4 successive days.

SIDE EFFECTS
CNS: impaired mental alertness, impaired physical coordination, *drowsiness, giddiness,* headache, dizziness.
GI: anorexia, *nausea, vomiting,* diarrhea, epigastric distress.
Skin: rash, pruritus, *erythema multiforme.*
Other: lymphadenopathy, fever, flushing, chills.

INTERACTIONS
None significant.

NURSING CONSIDERATIONS
• Use with caution in patients with hepatic or renal dysfunction, severe malnutrition, anemia, and in patients who are vomiting. Supportive therapy indicated for anemic, dehydrated, or malnourished patients. In children under 15 kg, weigh benefits of therapy against risks.
• Warn that medication may cause drowsiness and dizziness.
• Give after meals. Shake suspension before measuring; chew tablets before swallowing.
• Laxatives, enemas, and diet restrictions not needed.
• To avoid reinfection, wash perianal area daily. Change undergarments and bedclothes daily. Wash hands and clean fingernails before meals and after bowel movements. Treat all family members.

Italicized side effects are common or life-threatening.
*Liquid form contains alcohol.   **May contain tartrazine.

Antifungals

amphotericin B
flucytosine
griseofulvin microsize
griseofulvin ultramicrosize
ketoconazole
miconazole
nystatin

MECHANISM OF ACTION

• Amphotericin B and nystatin probably act by binding to sterols in the fungal cell membrane, altering cell permeability and allowing leakage of intracellular components. They may also inhibit glycolysis and protein synthesis.

• Flucytosine appears to penetrate fungal cells, where it is converted to fluorouracil, a known metabolic antagonist. Flucytosine is incorporated into fungal ribonucleic acid (RNA) and causes defective protein synthesis.

• Griseofulvin arrests fungal cell activity by disrupting its mitotic spindle structure.

• Miconazole and ketoconazole inhibit purine transport, and deoxyribonucleic acid, RNA, and protein synthesis; and they increase cell-wall permeability, making the fungus more susceptible to osmotic pressure.

COMBINATION PRODUCTS

ACHROSTATIN-V: nystatin 250,000 units and tetracycline HCl 250 mg.
DECLOSTATIN TABS: nystatin 500,000 units and demeclocycline HCl 300 mg.
DECLOSTATIN CAPS: nystatin 250,000 units and demeclocycline HCl 150 mg.
MYSTECLIN-F CAPS: tetracycline HCl 250 mg and amphotericin B 50 mg buffered with potassium metaphosphate.
MYSTECLIN-F CAPS: tetracycline HCl 125 mg and amphotericin B 25 mg buffered with potassium metaphosphate.
MYSTECLIN-F SYRUP: tetracycline HCl 125 mg and amphotericin B 25 mg per 5 ml buffered with potassium metaphosphate.
TERRASTATIN CAPS: nystatin 250,000 units and oxytetracycline 250 mg.
TETRASTATIN CAPS: nystatin 250,000 units and tetracycline HCl 250 mg.

---

amphotericin B
Fungizone♦

INDICATIONS & DOSAGE

Systemic fungal infections (histoplasmosis, coccidioidomycosis, blastomycosis, cryptococcosis, disseminated moniliasis, aspergillosis, phycomycosis), meningitis—
Adults and children: initially, 1 mg in 250 ml of 5% dextrose in water infused over 2 to 4 hours; or 0.25 mg/kg daily by slow infusion over 6 hours. Increase gradually as patient tolerance develops to maximum 1 mg/kg daily. Therapy must not exceed 1.5 mg/kg. If drug is discontinued for 1 week or more, administration must resume with initial dose and again increase gradually.
Topical (3% cream, lotion, ointment): apply liberally and rub well into affected area b.i.d. to q.i.d.
Intrathecal: 25 mcg/0.1 ml diluted with 10 to 20 ml of cerebrospinal fluid and administered by barbotage 2 or 3 times

---

weekly. Initial dose should not exceed 100 mcg.
Coccidioidal arthritis—
Adults: 5 to 15 mg into joint spaces.

SIDE EFFECTS
Blood: normochromic, normocytic anemia.
CNS: headache, peripheral neuropathy; with intrathecal administration— peripheral nerve pain, paresthesias.
GI: *anorexia, weight loss, nausea,* vomiting, dyspepsia, diarrhea, epigastric cramps.
GU: abnormal renal function with *hypokalemia, azotemia, hyposthenuria,* renal tubular acidosis, nephrocalcinosis; with large doses—permanent renal impairment, anuria, oliguria.
Local: burning, stinging, irritation, tissue damage with extravasation, *thrombophlebitis,* pain at site of injection.
Other: arthralgia, myalgia, muscle weakness secondary to hypokalemia, *fever, chills,* malaise, generalized pain.

INTERACTIONS
None significant.

NURSING CONSIDERATIONS
• Use cautiously in patients with impaired renal function.
• Use parenterally only in hospitalized patients, under close supervision, when diagnosis of potentially fatal fungal infection has been confirmed.
• Monitor vital signs; fever may appear 1 to 2 hours after start of I.V. infusion and should subside within 4 hours of discontinuation.
• Monitor intake/output; report change in urine appearance or volume. Renal damage usually reversible if drug is stopped with first sign of dysfunction.
• Obtain liver and renal function studies weekly. If BUN exceeds 40 mg/ 100 ml, or if serum creatinine exceeds 3 mg/100 ml, doctor may reduce or stop drug until renal function improves. Monitor CBC weekly. Stop drug if

Bromsulphalein, alkaline phosphatase, or bilirubin levels become elevated.
• Monitor potassium levels closely. Report any signs of hypokalemia. Check calcium and magnesium levels periodically.
• In the dry state, store at 2° to 8° C. (35.6° to 46.4° F.). Protect from light. Expires 2 years after date of manufacture. Reconstitute with 10 ml sterile water only. Mixing with solutions containing sodium chloride, other electrolytes, or bacteriostatic agents such as benzyl alcohol causes precipitation. Do not use if solution contains precipitate or foreign matter. Use aseptic technique.
• Appears to be compatible with limited amounts of heparin sodium, hydrocortisone sodium succinate, and methylprednisolone sodium succinate.
• Reconstituted solution is stable for 1 week under refrigeration or 24 hours at room temperature. It has 24 hour stability in room light.
• Recommended infusion solution is 10 mg/100 ml of 5% dextrose in water.
• An initial test dose may be prescribed: 1 mg is added to 50 to 150 ml 5% dextrose in water and infused over 20 to 30 minutes.
• Severity of some side effects can be reduced by premedication with aspirin, antihistamines, antiemetics, or small doses of corticosteroids; addition of phosphate buffer and heparin to the solution; and alternate-day dose schedule. For severe reactions, drug may have to be stopped for varying periods.
• For I.V. infusion, an in-line membrane with mean pore diameter larger than 1 micron can be used. Infuse very slowly; rapid infusion may result in cardiovascular collapse. Warn patient of discomfort at infusion site and other potential side effects. Advise patient that several months of therapy may be needed to assure adequate response.
• Antibiotics should be given separately; don't mix or piggyback with amphotericin B.

Italicized side effects are common or life-threatening.
*Liquid form contains alcohol.   **May contain tartrazine.

- Topical preparations may stain clothing.

flucytosine
Ancobon, Ancotil♦♦

INDICATIONS & DOSAGE
For severe fungal infections caused by susceptible strains of Candida *(including septicemia, endocarditis, urinary tract and pulmonary infections) and* Cryptococcus *(meningitis, pulmonary infection, and possible urinary tract infections)*—

Adults and children weighing more than 50 kg: 50 to 150 mg/kg daily q 6 hours P.O.
Children weighing less than 50 kg: 1.5 to 4.5 g/m²/day in 4 divided doses P.O.
Severe infections such as meningitis may require doses up to 250 mg/kg.

SIDE EFFECTS
Blood: anemia, leukopenia, bone marrow depression, thrombocytopenia.
CNS: dizziness, drowsiness, confusion, headache.
GI: *nausea, vomiting, diarrhea,* abdominal bloating.
Hepatic: elevated SGOT, SGPT.
Metabolic: elevated serum alkaline phosphatase, BUN, serum creatinine.
Skin: occasional rash.

INTERACTIONS
None significant.

NURSING CONSIDERATIONS
- Use with extreme caution in patients with impaired hepatic or renal function, or bone marrow depression.
- Hematologic tests and renal and liver function studies should precede therapy and should be repeated at frequent intervals thereafter. Before treatment, susceptibility tests should establish that organism is flucytosine-sensitive. Tests should be repeated weekly to monitor drug resistance.
- Flucytosine is well absorbed from the GI tract. Nausea, vomiting, stomach upset are reduced if capsules given over a 15-minute period.
- Monitor intake and output; report any marked change.
- If possible, blood level assays of drug should be performed regularly to maintain flucytosine at therapeutic level (25 to 120 mcg/ml). Higher blood levels may be toxic.
- Drug is often combined with amphotericin B; use may be synergistic.
- Store in light-resistant containers.
- Inform patient that adequate response may take weeks or months.

griseofulvin microsize
Fulvicin-U/F♦, Grifulvin V, Grisactin, Grisovin-FP♦♦, Grisowen

griseofulvin ultramicrosize
Fulvicin P/G, Grisactin-Ultra, Gris-PEG

INDICATIONS & DOSAGE
Ringworm infections of skin, hair, nails (tinea corporis, tinea pedis, tinea cruris, tinea barbae, tinea capitis, and tinea unguium) when caused by Trichophyton, Microsporum, *or* Epidermophyton—
Adults: 500 mg (microsize) P.O. daily in single or divided doses. Severe infections may require up to 1 g daily.
Children: 10 mg/kg daily (microsize).
Adults: 125 to 165 mg tablet (ultramicrosize) P.O. b.i.d. or 250 to 330 mg daily. Resistant fungal infections of tinea pedis and tinea unguium may require divided daily dose of 500 to 660 mg.
Children: 5 mg/kg daily P.O. (ultramicrosize).

SIDE EFFECTS
Blood: leukopenia, *granulocytopenia (requires discontinuation of drug).*
CNS: headaches (in early stages of treatment), fatigue with large doses,

occasional mental confusion, impaired performance of routine activities, psychotic symptoms.
GI: nausea, vomiting, excessive thirst, flatulence, diarrhea.
Metabolic: porphyria.
Skin: rash, urticaria, photosensitive reactions (may aggravate lupus erythematosus).
Other: estrogen-like effects in children, oral thrush.

INTERACTIONS
Barbiturates: decreased griseofulvin absorption. Divide into 3 doses of griseofulvin per day.

NURSING CONSIDERATIONS
• Contraindicated in patients with porphyria or hepatocellular failure. Since griseofulvin is a penicillin derivative, cross-sensitivity is possible. Use cautiously in penicillin-sensitive patients. Use only when topical treatment fails to arrest mycotic disease.
• CBC should be repeated regularly.
• Advise patient that prolonged treatment may be needed to control infection and prevent relapse, even if symptoms abate in first few days of therapy. Tell patient to keep skin clean and dry and to maintain good hygiene. Caution him to avoid intense sunlight.
• Most effectively absorbed and causes least GI distress when given after high-fat meal.
• Effective treatment of tinea pedis may require concomitant use of topical agent.
• Diagnosis of infecting organism should be verified in lab. Continue drug until clinical and laboratory examinations confirm complete eradication.
• Because griseofulvin ultramicrosize is dispersed in polyethylene glycol (PEG), it is absorbed more rapidly and completely than microsize preparations and is effective at one half to two thirds the usual griseofulvin dose.

ketoconazole
Nizoral

INDICATIONS & DOSAGE
Treatment of systemic candidiasis, chronic mucocandidiasis, oral thrush, candiduria, coccidioidomycosis, histoplasmosis, chromomycosis, and paracoccidioidomycosis—
Adults and children over 40 kg: Initially, 200 mg P.O. daily single dose. Dosage may be increased to 400 mg once daily in patients who don't respond to lower dosage.
Children (less than 20 kg): 50 mg (¼ tablet) daily single dose.
Children (20 to 40 kg): 100 mg (½ tablet) daily single dose.

SIDE EFFECTS
CNS: headache, nervousness, dizziness.
GI: *nausea, vomiting,* abdominal pain, diarrhea, constipation.
Hepatic: elevated liver enzymes, *fatal hepatotoxicity.*
Skin: itching.

INTERACTIONS
Antacids, anticholinergics, cimetidine: decreased absorption of ketoconazole. Wait at least 2 hours after ketoconazole dose before administering these drugs.

NURSING CONSIDERATIONS
• Contraindicated in patients with fungal meningitis since ketoconazole penetrates poorly into the cerebrospinal fluid.
• Ketoconazole is not effective in patients with achlorhydria. The drug requires acidity for dissolution and absorption. Instruct patient to dissolve each tablet in 4 ml aqueous solution of 0.2 N hydrochloric acid; and, to avoid contact with teeth, to sip the mixture through a straw (glass or plastic). Tell patient to follow with a glass of water.
• Make sure patient understands that treatment should be continued until all

clinical and laboratory tests indicate that active fungal infection has subsided. If drug is discontinued too soon, infection will reoccur. Minimum treatment for candidiasis is 7 to 14 days. Minimum treatment for other systemic fungal infections is 6 months.

• Reassure patient that, although nausea is common early in therapy, it will subside.

• Monitor for elevated liver enzymes and nausea that does not subside. May be sign of hepatoxicity.

• Ketoconazole represents a major advance since it is the most effective oral antifungal drug available and it produces the least side effects.

miconazole
Monistat I.V.

INDICATIONS & DOSAGE
Treatment of systemic fungal infections (coccidioidomycosis, candidiasis, cryptococcosis, paracoccidioidomycosis), chronic mucocutaneous candidiasis—
Adults: 200 to 3,600 mg per day. Doses may vary with diagnosis and with infective agent. May divide daily dose over 3 infusions, 200 to 1,200 mg per infusion. Repeated courses may be needed due to relapse or reinfection.
Children: 20 to 40 mg/kg per day. Do not exceed 15 mg/kg per infusion.

SIDE EFFECTS
Blood: transient decreases in hematocrit, thrombocytopenia.
CNS: dizziness, drowsiness.
GI: *nausea, vomiting,* diarrhea.
Metabolic: *transient decrease in serum sodium.*
Skin: *pruritic rash.*
Local: *phlebitis at injection site.*

INTERACTIONS
None significant.

NURSING CONSIDERATIONS
• Rapid injection of undiluted miconazole may produce arrhythmia.

• Acute cardiorespiratory arrest has occurred with the first dose. A doctor should be present when the first dose is administered.

• Premedication with antiemetic may lessen nausea and vomiting.

• Avoid administration at mealtime in order to lessen GI side effects.

• Lesser incidence and severity of side effects with this drug may offer a significant advantage over other antifungals.

• Pruritic rash may persist for weeks after drug is discontinued.

• In treatment of fungal meningitis and urinary bladder infections, must be supplemented with intrathecal administration and bladder irrigation, respectively.

• I.V. infusion should be given over 30 to 60 minutes.

• Inform patient that adequate response may take weeks or months.

• Monitor levels of hemoglobin, hematocrit, electrolytes, and lipids regularly. Transient elevations in serum cholesterol and triglycerides may be due to castor oil vehicle.

nystatin
Mycostatin♦, Nadostine♦♦, Nilstat♦, O-V Statin

INDICATIONS & DOSAGE
Gastrointestinal infections—
Adults: 500,000 to 1,000,000 units as oral tablets, t.i.d.
Treatment of oral, vaginal, and intestinal infections caused by Candida albicans (Monilia) *and other* Candida *species—*
Adults: 400,000 to 600,000 units oral suspension q.i.d. for oral candidiasis.
Children and infants over 3 months: 250,000 to 500,000 units oral suspension q.i.d.
Newborn and premature infants:

100,000 units oral suspension q.i.d.
Vaginal infections—
Adults: 100,000 units, as vaginal tablets, inserted high into vagina, daily or b.i.d. for 14 days.

SIDE EFFECTS
GI: transient nausea, vomiting, diarrhea (usually with large oral dosage).

INTERACTIONS
None significant.

NURSING CONSIDERATIONS
- Nystatin is virtually nontoxic and nonsensitizing when used orally, vaginally, topically; but advise patient to report redness, swelling, or irritation.
- Vaginal tablets can be used by pregnant women up to 6 weeks before term to prevent thrush in newborn. Continue therapy during menstruation. Instruct patient to wash applicator thoroughly after each use.
- Explain that use of antibiotics, oral contraceptives, and corticosteroids; diabetes; reinfection by sexual partner; and tight-fitting panty hose are predisposing factors of vaginal infection.
- For treatment of oral candidiasis (thrush): Be sure the mouth is clean of food debris before administering drug, then tell patient to hold suspension in mouth for several minutes before swallowing. When treating infants, swab medication on oral mucosa. Instruct patient in good oral hygiene techniques. Tell patient overuse of mouthwash or poorly fitting dentures, especially in older patients, may alter flora and promote infection.
- Advise patient to continue medication for 1 to 2 weeks after symptomatic improvement to ensure against reinfection. Consult doctor for exact length of therapy.
- Immunosuppressed patients sometimes take vaginal tablets (100,000 units) by mouth as this provides prolonged contact with oral mucosa.
- Instruct patient in careful hygiene for affected areas.
- Store in tightly closed, light-resistant containers in cool place.
- Not effective against systemic infections.

Italicized side effects are common or life-threatening.
*Liquid form contains alcohol.   **May contain tartrazine.

Antimalarials

chloroquine hydrochloride
chloroquine phosphate
hydroxychloroquine sulfate
primaquine phosphate
pyrimethamine
quinine sulfate

MECHANISM OF ACTION
- The 4-aminoquinoline compounds bind to, and alter the properties of, both microbial and mammalian deoxyribonucleic acid.
- Primaquine phosphate is a gametocidal drug that destroys exoerythrocytic forms and prevents delayed primary attack. Its precise mechanism of action is unknown.
- Pyrimethamine inhibits the enzyme dihydrofolate reductase, thereby impeding reduction of folic acid.
- Quinine's exact mechanism of action is unknown, but the drug is often referred to as a generalized protoplasmic poison.

COMBINATION PRODUCTS
ARALEN PHOSPHATE WITH PRIMA-QUINE PHOSPHATE: chloroquine phosphate 500 mg (300 mg base) and primaquine phosphate 79 mg (45 mg base).
FANSIDAR: sulfadoxine 500 mg and pyrimethamine 25 mg.

chloroquine hydrochloride
Aralen HCl, Roquine

chloroquine phosphate
Aralen Phosphate♦, Chlorocon

INDICATIONS & DOSAGE
Suppressive prophylaxis and treatment of acute attacks of malaria due to Plasmodium vivax, Plasmodium malariae, Plasmodium ovale, *and susceptible strains of* Plasmodium falciparum—
Adults: initially, 600 mg (base) P.O., then 300 mg P.O. at 6, 24, and 48 hours. Or 160 to 200 mg (base) I.M. initially; repeat in 6 hours if needed. Switch to oral therapy as soon as possible.
Children: initially, 10 mg (base)/kg P.O., then 5 mg (base)/kg dose P.O. at 6, 24, and 48 hours (do not exceed adult dose). Or 5 mg (base)/kg I.M. initially; repeat in 6 hours if needed. Switch to oral therapy as soon as possible.
Malaria suppressive treatment—
Adults and children: 5 mg (base)/kg P.O. (not to exceed 300 mg) weekly on same day of the week (begin 2 weeks before entering endemic area and continue for 8 weeks after leaving). If treatment begins after exposure, double the initial dose (600 mg for adults, 10 mg/kg for children) in 2 divided doses, P.O. 6 hours apart.

SIDE EFFECTS
Blood: *agranulocytosis,* hemolytic anemia.
CNS: mild and transient headache,

neuromyopathy, psychic stimulation, fatigue, irritability, nightmares, convulsions, dizziness.

EENT: *visual disturbances* (blurred vision; difficulty in focusing; reversible corneal changes; generally irreversible, sometimes progressive or delayed, retinal changes, e.g., narrowing of arterioles; macular lesions; pallor of optic disk; optic atrophy; patchy retinal pigmentation, often leading to blindness), ototoxicity (nerve deafness, vertigo, tinnitus).

GI: anorexia, abdominal cramps, diarrhea, nausea, vomiting.

Skin: pruritus, lichen planus-like eruptions, skin and mucosal pigmentary changes, pleomorphic skin eruptions.

INTERACTIONS
None significant.

NURSING CONSIDERATIONS
• Contraindicated in patients with retinal or visual field changes, porphyria. Use with extreme caution in presence of severe GI, neurologic, or blood disorders. Drug concentrates in liver; use cautiously in patients with hepatic disease or alcoholism. Use with caution in patients with G-6-PD deficiency or psoriasis; drug may exacerbate these conditions.

• Complete blood cell counts and liver function studies should be made periodically during prolonged therapy; if severe blood disorder appears that is not attributable to disease under treatment, drug may need to be discontinued.

• Overdosage can quickly lead to toxic symptoms: headache, drowsiness, visual disturbances, cardiovascular collapse and convulsions, followed by respiratory and cardiac arrest. Children are extremely susceptible to toxicity; avoid long-term treatment.

• Baseline and periodic ophthalmologic examinations needed. Report blurred vision, increased sensitivity to light, or muscle weakness. Check periodically for ocular muscle weakness after long-term use. Audiometric examinations recommended before, during, and after therapy, especially if long term.

• Give drug immediately before or after meals on same day each week.

• To avoid exacerbated drug-induced dermatoses, warn patient to avoid excessive exposure to sun.

• Each ml parenteral solution containing 50 mg dihydrochloride salt = 40 mg chloroquine base; each 500 mg tablet phosphate = 300 mg chloroquine base.

hydroxychloroquine sulfate
Plaquenil Sulfate♦

INDICATIONS & DOSAGE
Suppressive prophylaxis of attacks of malaria due to Plasmodium vivax, Plasmodium malariae, Plasmodium ovale, *and susceptible strains of* Plasmodium falciparum—

Adults and children: for suppression: 5 mg (base)/kg body weight P.O. (not to exceed 310 mg) weekly on same day of the week (begin 2 weeks prior to entering and continue for 8 weeks after leaving endemic area). If not started prior to exposure, double initial dose (620 mg for adults, 10 mg/kg for children) in 2 divided doses P.O. 6 hours apart.

Treatment of acute malarial attacks—
Adults and children over 15 years: initially, 800 mg (sulfate) P.O., then 400 mg after 6 to 8 hours, then 400 mg daily for 2 days (total 2 g sulfate salt).

Children 11 to 15 years: 600 mg (sulfate) P.O. stat, then 200 mg 8 hours later, then 200 mg 24 hours later (total 1 g sulfate salt).

Children 6 to 10 years: 400 mg (sulfate) P.O. stat, then 2 doses of 200 mg at 8-hour intervals (total 800 mg sulfate salt).

Children 2 to 5 years: 400 mg (sul-

Italicized side effects are common or life-threatening.
*Liquid form contains alcohol.   **May contain tartrazine.

fate) P.O. stat, then 200 mg 8 hours later (total 600 mg sulfate salt).

Children under 1 year: 100 mg (sulfate) P.O. stat; then 3 doses of 100 mg 6 to 9 hours apart (total 400 mg sulfate salt).

Lupus erythematosus (chronic discoid and systemic)—

Adults: 400 mg P.O. daily or b.i.d., continued for several weeks or months, depending on response. Prolonged maintenance—200 to 400 mg P.O. daily.

Rheumatoid arthritis—

Adults: initially, 400 to 600 mg P.O. daily. When good response occurs (usually in 4 to 12 weeks), cut dosage in half.

SIDE EFFECTS

Blood: *agranulocytosis, leukopenia,* thrombocytopenia, *aplastic anemia.*

CNS: irritability, nightmares, ataxia, convulsions, psychic stimulation, toxic psychosis, vertigo, tinnitus, nystagmus, lassitude, fatigue, dizziness, hypoactive deep-tendon reflexes, skeletal muscle weakness.

EENT: visual disturbances (blurred vision; difficulty in focusing; reversible corneal changes; generally irreversible, sometimes progressive or delayed, retinal changes, e.g., narrowing of arterioles; macular lesions; pallor of optic disk; optic atrophy; visual field defects; patchy retinal pigmentation, often leading to blindness), ototoxicity (irreversible nerve deafness, tinnitus, labyrinthitis).

GI: anorexia, abdominal cramps, diarrhea, nausea, vomiting.

Skin: pruritus, lichen planus-like eruptions, skin and mucosal pigmentary changes, pleomorphic skin eruptions.

Other: weight loss, bleaching of hair.

INTERACTIONS
None significant.

NURSING CONSIDERATIONS
• Contraindicated in patients with retinal or visual field changes, or porphyria. Use with extreme caution in presence of severe GI, neurologic, or blood disorders. Drug concentrates in the liver; use cautiously in patients with hepatic disease or alcoholism. Use with caution in patients with G-6-PD deficiency or psoriasis; drug may exacerbate these conditions.

• Complete blood cell counts and liver function studies should be made periodically during prolonged therapy; if severe blood disorder appears that is not attributable to disease under treatment, consider discontinuing.

• Overdosage can quickly lead to toxic symptoms: headache, drowsiness, visual disturbances, cardiovascular collapse and convulsions, followed by respiratory and cardiac arrest. Children are extremely susceptible to toxicity; avoid long-term treatment.

• Baseline and periodic ophthalmologic examinations needed. Report blurred vision, increased sensitivity to light, or muscle weakness. Check periodically for ocular muscle weakness after long-term use. Audiometric examinations recommended before, during, and after therapy, especially if long term.

• Give drug immediately before or after meals on same day of each week.

• 100 mg sulfate salt = 77.5 mg hydroxychloroquine base.

primaquine phosphate

INDICATIONS & DOSAGE
Radical cure of relapsing vivax malaria, eliminating symptoms and infection completely; prevention of relapse—
Adults: 15 mg (base) P.O. daily for 14 days. (26.3 mg tablet = 15 mg of base).

SIDE EFFECTS
Blood: leukopenia, hemolytic anemia in G-6-PD deficiency, methemoglobinemia in NADH methemoglobin reduc-

tase deficiency, leukocytosis, mild anemia, *granulocytopenia, agranulocytosis.*
EENT: disturbances of visual accommodation.
GI: nausea, vomiting, epigastric distress, abdominal cramps.
Skin: urticaria.

INTERACTIONS
None significant.

NURSING CONSIDERATIONS
• Contraindicated in patients with lupus erythematosus and rheumatoid arthritis; in patients taking bone marrow suppressants and potentially hemolytic drugs.
• Use with a fast-acting blood schizonticide, such as amodiaquine or chloroquine. Use full dose to reduce possibility of drug-resistant strains.
• Caucasians taking more than 30 mg daily, dark-skinned patients taking more than 15 mg (base) daily, and patients with severe anemia or suspected sensitivity should have frequent blood studies and urine examinations. Sudden fall in hemoglobin concentration, erythrocyte or leukocyte count, or marked darkening of the urine suggests impending hemolytic reactions.
• Observe closely for tolerance in patients with previous idiosyncrasy (manifested by hemolytic anemia, methemoglobinemia, or leukopenia); family or personal history of favism; erythrocytic G-6-PD deficiency or NADH methemoglobin reductase deficiency.
• Administer drug with meals or with antacids.

pyrimethamine
Daraprim♦, Fansidar (with sulfadoxine)

INDICATIONS & DOSAGE
Malaria prophylaxis and transmission control (pyrimethamine)—

Adults and children over 10 years: 25 mg P.O. weekly.
Children 4 to 10 years: 12.5 mg P.O. weekly.
Children under 4 years: 6.25 mg P.O. weekly.
Continue in all age groups at least 10 weeks after leaving endemic areas.
Acute attacks of malaria (Fansidar)—
Adults: 2 to 3 tablets as a single dose, either alone or in sequence with quinine or primaquine.
Children 9 to 14 years: 2 tablets.
Children 4 to 8 years: 1 tablet.
Children under 4 years: ½ tablet.
Malaria prophylaxis (Fansidar)—
Adults: 1 tablet weekly, or 2 tablets every 2 weeks.
Children 9 to 14 years: ¾ tablet weekly, or 1½ tablets every 2 weeks.
Children 4 to 8 years: ½ tablet weekly, or 1 tablet every 2 weeks.
Children under 4 years: ¼ tablet weekly, or ½ tablet every 2 weeks.
Acute attacks of malaria (pyrimethamine)—
not recommended alone in nonimmune persons; use with faster-acting antimalarials, such as chloroquine, for 2 days to initiate transmission control and suppressive cure.
Adults and children over 15 years: 25 mg P.O. daily for 2 days.
Children under 15 years: 12.5 mg P.O. daily for 2 days.
Toxoplasmosis (pyrimethamine)—
Adults: initially, 100 mg P.O., then 25 mg P.O. daily for 4 to 5 weeks; during same time give 1 g sulfadiazine P.O. q 6 hours.
Children: initially, 1 mg/kg P.O., then 0.25 mg/kg daily for 4 to 5 weeks, along with 100 mg sulfadiazine/kg P.O. daily, divided q 6 hours.

SIDE EFFECTS
Blood: *agranulocytosis, aplastic anemia,* megaloblastic anemia, bone marrow suppression, leukopenia, thrombocytopenia, pancytopenia.

Italicized side effects are common or life-threatening.
*Liquid form contains alcohol.   **May contain tartrazine.

CNS: stimulation and convulsions (acute toxicity).
GI: anorexia, vomiting, diarrhea, atrophic glossitis.
Skin: rashes, *erythema multiforme (Stevens-Johnson syndrome)*.

INTERACTIONS
Folic acid and para-aminobenzoic acid: decreased antitoxoplasmic effects. May require dosage adjustment.

NURSING CONSIDERATIONS
• Sulfadoxine, an ingredient in Fansidar, is a sulfonamide; therefore, this combination is contraindicated in porphyria. Use cautiously in patients with impaired hepatic or renal function, severe allergy or bronchial asthma, or G-6-PD deficiency.
• Contraindicated in chloroquine-resistant malaria. Use cautiously in patients with convulsive disorders; smaller doses may be needed. Also use cautiously following treatment with chloroquine.
• Dosages required to treat toxoplasmosis approach toxic levels. Twice-weekly blood counts, including platelets, are required. If signs of folic or folinic acid deficiency develop, dosage should be reduced or discontinued while patient receives parenteral folinic acid (leucovorin) until blood counts become normal.
• Do not exceed recommended dosage.
• Give with meals to minimize GI distress.
• The first dose of Fansidar, when taken prophylactically, should be taken 1 to 2 days before traveling to an endemic area.

---

quinine sulfate
Coco-Quinine**, Quinamm

INDICATIONS & DOSAGE
Malaria due to Plasmodium falciparum *(chloroquine-resistant)—*

Adults: 650 mg P.O. q 8 hours for 10 days, with 25 mg pyrimethamine q 12 hours for 3 days, and with 500 mg sulfadiazine q.i.d. for 5 days.

SIDE EFFECTS
Blood: hemolytic anemia, thrombocytopenia, agranulocytosis, hypoprothrombinemia.
CNS: severe headache, apprehension, excitement, confusion, delirium, syncope, hypothermia, convulsions (with toxic doses).
CV: hypotension, *cardiovascular collapse* with overdosage or rapid I.V. administration.
EENT: altered color perception, photophobia, blurred vision, night blindness, amblyopia, scotoma, diplopia, mydriasis, optic atrophy, tinnitus, impaired hearing.
GI: epigastric distress, diarrhea, nausea, vomiting.
GU: renal tubular damage, anuria.
Skin: rashes, pruritus.
Local: thrombosis at infusion site.
Other: asthma, flushing.

INTERACTIONS
Sodium bicarbonate: elevates quinine levels by decreasing quinine excretion. Use together cautiously.

NURSING CONSIDERATIONS
• Contraindicated in patients with G-6-PD deficiency. Use with caution in patients with cardiovascular conditions.
• Discontinue if any signs of idiosyncrasy or toxicity occur.
• Has been used as a treatment for nocturnal leg cramps.
• Quinine is no longer used for acute attacks of malaria due to *Plasmodium vivax* or for suppression of malaria due to organism resistance.
• Administer after meals to minimize GI distress.
• May interefere with laboratory determinations of urine catecholamines and steroids.

Antituberculars and antileprotics

capreomycin sulfate
cycloserine
dapsone
ethambutol hydrochloride
ethionamide
isoniazid (INH)
para-aminosalicylic acid
sodium aminosalicylate
pyrazinamide
rifampin
streptomycin sulfate
sulfoxone sodium

MECHANISM OF ACTION

• Cycloserine inhibits cell-wall biosynthesis by inhibiting the utilization of amino acids (bacteriostatic).

• Dapsone (bactericidal) and sulfoxone (bacteriostatic) are thought to inhibit folic acid biosynthesis.

• Ethambutol interferes with the synthesis of RNA, thus inhibiting protein metabolism (bacteriostatic).

• Isoniazid inhibits cell-wall biosynthesis by interfering with lipid and DNA synthesis (bactericidal).

• Para-aminosalicylic acid inhibits the enzymes responsible for folic acid biosynthesis (bacteriostatic).

• Rifampin inhibits DNA-dependent RNA polymerase, thus impairing ribonucleic acid synthesis (bactericidal).

• Streptomycin inhibits protein synthesis by binding to 30S ribosomal subunits (bactericidal).

• The mechanism of action of capreomycin (bactericidal), ethionamide (bacteriostatic), and pyrazinamide (bactericidal) is not known.

COMBINATION PRODUCTS

RIFAMATE: isoniazid 150 mg and rifampin 300 mg.
TEEBACONIN AND VITAMIN B_6: isoniazid 100 mg and pyridoxine HCl 10 mg.

---

capreomycin sulfate
Capastat Sulfate

INDICATIONS & DOSAGE

Adjunctive treatment in pulmonary tuberculosis—

Adults: 15 mg/kg/day up to 1 g I.M. daily injected deeply into large muscle mass for 60 to 120 days; then 1 g 2 to 3 times weekly for a period of 18 to 24 months. Maximum dose should not exceed 20 mg/kg daily. Must be given in conjunction with another antitubercular drug.

SIDE EFFECTS

Blood: eosinophilia, leukocytosis, leukopenia.
CNS: headache.
EENT: *ototoxicity* (tinnitus, vertigo, hearing loss).
GU: *nephrotoxicity* (elevated BUN and nonprotein nitrogen, proteinuria, casts, red blood cells, leukocytes; tubular necrosis, decreased creatinine clearance).
Local: pain, induration, excessive bleeding and sterile abscesses at injection site.
Metabolic: hypokalemia.

INTERACTIONS

None significant.

NURSING CONSIDERATIONS
- Contraindicated in patients receiving other ototoxic or nephrotoxic drugs. Use cautiously in patients with impaired renal function, history of allergies, or hearing impairment.
- Considered a "second-line" drug in the treatment of tuberculosis.
- Drug is never given I.V.; may cause neuromuscular blockade.
- Evaluate patient's hearing before and during therapy. Notify doctor if patient complains of tinnitus, vertigo, hearing impairment.
- Monitor renal function (output, specific gravity, urinalysis, BUN, serum creatinine) before and during therapy; notify doctor of decreasing renal function. Dose must be reduced in renal impairment.
- Monitor serum potassium levels and hepatic function periodically.
- Reconstituted solutions can be stored for 48 hours at room temperature or 14 days if refrigerated. Straw- or dark-colored solution does not indicate a loss in potency.

cycloserine
Seromycin

INDICATIONS & DOSAGE
Adjunctive treatment in pulmonary or extrapulmonary tuberculosis—
Adults: initially, 250 mg P.O. every 12 hours for 2 weeks; then, if blood levels are below 25 to 30 mcg/ml and there are no clinical signs of toxicity, dose is increased to 250 mg P.O. q 8 hours for 2 weeks. If optimum blood levels are still not achieved, and there are no signs of clinical toxicity, then dose is increased to 250 mg P.O. q 6 hours. Maximum dose 1 g/day. If CNS toxicity occurs, drug is discontinued for 1 week, then resumed at 250 mg daily for 2 weeks. If no serious toxic effects occur, dose is increased by 250 mg increments every 10 days until blood level of 25 to 30 mcg/ml is obtained.

SIDE EFFECTS
CNS: drowsiness, headache, tremor, dysarthria, vertigo, confusion, loss of memory, *possible suicidal tendencies and other psychotic symptoms, nervousness, hallucinations, depression,* hyperirritability, paresthesias, paresis, hyperreflexia.
Other: hypersensitivity (allergic dermatitis).

INTERACTIONS
Isoniazid: monitor for CNS toxicity (dizziness or drowsiness).

NURSING CONSIDERATIONS
- Contraindicated in patients with seizure disorders, depression or severe anxiety, severe renal insufficiency, or chronic alcoholism. Use cautiously in patients with impaired renal function; reduced dosage required.
- Considered a "second-line" drug in the treatment of tuberculosis.
- Obtain specimen for culture and sensitivity tests before therapy begins and periodically thereafter to detect possible resistance.
- Serious neurologic effects can be precipitated by ingestion of alcohol; warn patient not to drink.
- Toxic reactions may occur with blood levels above 30 mcg/ml.
- Pyridoxine, anticonvulsants, tranquilizers, or sedatives may help to relieve side effects.
- Observe for personality changes.
- Monitor hematologic tests and renal and liver function studies.
- Instruct patient to take drug exactly as prescribed; warn against discontinuing use without doctor's consent.

dapsone
Avlosulfon♦

INDICATIONS & DOSAGE
All forms of leprosy—
Adults: 100 mg P.O. daily for indefi-

Unmarked trade names available in the United States only.
♦ Also available in Canada.   ♦♦ Available in Canada only.

nite period, plus rifampin 600 mg daily
for 3 months.

SIDE EFFECTS
Blood: anemia, especially hemolytic;
methemoglobinemia; possible leuko-
penia.
CNS: psychosis, headache, dizziness,
lethargy, severe malaise, paresthesias.
EENT: tinnitus, allergic rhinitis.
GI: anorexia, abdominal pain, nausea,
vomiting.
Hepatic: hepatitis.
Skin: allergic dermatitis (generalized
or fixed maculopapular rash).

INTERACTIONS
Probenecid: elevates levels of dapsone.
Use together with extreme caution.

NURSING CONSIDERATIONS
• Use cautiously in chronic renal, hepatic, or cardiovascular disease; refractory types of anemia.
• Therapy should be interrupted if
generalized, diffuse dermatitis occurs.
• Dapsone dosage should be reduced
or temporarily discontinued if hemoglobin falls below 9 g/dl; if leukocyte
count falls below 5,000/mm³; if erythrocyte count falls below 2.5 million/
mm³ or remains low.
• Patient should receive hematinics
during dapsone therapy.
• Antihistamines may help to combat
dapsone-induced allergic dermatitis.
• Erythema nodosum type of lepra reaction may occur during therapy as a
result of *Mycobacterium leprae* bacilli
(malaise, fever, painful inflammatory
induration in the skin and mucosa, iritis, neuritis). In severe cases, therapy
should be stopped and glucocorticoids
given cautiously.
• Obtain CBC before treatment and
monitor frequently throughout therapy
(weekly for the first month, monthly
for 6 months, and semiannually thereafter).

ethambutol hydrochloride
Etibi♦♦, Myambutol♦

INDICATIONS & DOSAGE
*Adjunctive treatment in pulmonary tu-
berculosis—*
Adults and children over 13 years:
initial treatment for patients who have
not received previous antitubercular
therapy 15 mg/kg P.O. daily single
dose.
Re-treatment: 25 mg/kg P.O. daily single dose for 60 days with at least one
other antitubercular drug; then decrease to 15 mg/kg P.O. daily single
dose.

SIDE EFFECTS
CNS: headache, dizziness, mental confusion, possible hallucinations, peripheral neuritis (numbness and tingling of
extremities).
EENT: optic neuritis (vision loss and
loss of color discrimination, especially
red and green).
GI: anorexia, nausea, vomiting, abdominal pain.
Metabolic: *elevated uric acid.*
Other: anaphylactoid reactions, fever,
malaise, bloody sputum.

INTERACTIONS
None significant.

NURSING CONSIDERATIONS
• Contraindicated in patients with optic neuritis and in children under
13 years. Use cautiously in patients
with impaired renal function, cataracts,
recurrent eye inflammations, gout, and
diabetic retinopathy.
• Dose must be reduced in renal impairment.
• Perform visual acuity and color discrimination tests before and during
therapy.
• Always monitor serum uric acid; observe patient for symptoms of gout.
• Instruct patient to take this drug exactly as prescribed; warn against dis-

continuing use without doctor's consent.

---

ethionamide
Trecator SC

INDICATIONS & DOSAGE
Adjunctive treatment in pulmonary or extrapulmonary tuberculosis (when primary therapy with streptomycin, isoniazid, and para-aminosalicylic acid cannot be used or has failed)—
Adults: 500 mg to 1 g P.O. daily in divided doses. Concomitant administration of other effective antitubercular drugs and pyridoxine recommended.
Children: 12 to 15 mg/kg P.O. daily in 3 to 4 doses. Maximum dose 750 mg.

SIDE EFFECTS
Blood: thrombocytopenia.
CNS: *peripheral neuritis,* psychic disturbances (especially mental depression).
CV: postural hypotension.
GI: *anorexia,* metallic taste in mouth, nausea, vomiting, sialorrhea, *epigastric distress,* diarrhea, stomatitis, weight loss.
Hepatic: jaundice, hepatitis, elevated SGOT and SGPT.
Skin: rash, *exfoliative dermatitis.*

INTERACTIONS
None significant.

NURSING CONSIDERATIONS
• Contraindicated in patients with severe hepatic damage. Use cautiously in patients with diabetes mellitus.
• Culture and sensitivity tests should be performed before starting therapy. Stop drug if skin rash occurs; may progress to exfoliative dermatitis.
• Monitor hepatic function.
• Give with meals or antacids to minimize GI effects. Patient may require antiemetic.
• Pyridoxine may be ordered to prevent neuropathy.

• Instruct patient to take this drug exactly as prescribed; warn against discontinuing drug without doctor's consent.
• Warn patient to avoid excess alcohol ingestion because it may make him more vulnerable to liver damage.

---

isoniazid (INH)
Hyzyd, Isotamine♦♦, Laniazid, Nydrazid**, Rimifon♦♦, Rolazid, Teebaconin

INDICATIONS & DOSAGE
Primary treatment against actively growing tubercle bacilli—
Adults: 5 mg/kg P.O. or I.M. daily single dose, up to 300 mg/day, continued for 9 months to 2 years.
Infants and children: 10 to 20 mg/kg P.O. or I.M. daily single dose, up to 300 to 500 mg/day, continued for 18 months to 2 years. Concomitant administration of at least one other effective antitubercular drug is recommended.
Preventive therapy against tubercle bacilli of those closely exposed or those with positive skin test whose chest X-rays and bacteriologic studies are consistent with nonprogressive tuberculous disease—
Adults: 300 mg P.O. daily single dose, continued for 1 year.
Infants and children: 10 mg/kg P.O. daily single dose, up to 300 mg/day, continued for 1 year.

SIDE EFFECTS
Blood: *agranulocytosis,* hemolytic anemia, *aplastic anemia,* eosinophilia, leukopenia, neutropenia, thrombocytopenia, methemoglobinemia, pyridoxine-responsive hypochromic anemia.
CNS: *peripheral neuropathy* (especially in the malnourished, alcoholics, diabetics, and slow acetylators), usually preceded by paresthesias of hands and feet, psychosis.
GI: nausea, vomiting, epigastric dis-

tress, constipation, dryness of the mouth.
Hepatic: *hepatitis, occasionally severe and sometimes fatal, especially in the elderly.*
Metabolic: hyperglycemia, metabolic acidosis.
Local: irritation at injection site.
Other: rheumatic syndrome and systemic lupus erythematosus–like syndrome; hypersensitivity (fever, rash, lymphadenopathy, vasculitis).

INTERACTIONS
Aluminum-containing antacids and laxatives: may decrease the rate and amount of isoniazid absorbed. Give isoniazid at least 1 hour before antacid or laxative.
Disulfiram: neurologic symptoms, including changes in behavior and coordination, may develop with concomitant isoniazid use. Avoid concomitant use.

NURSING CONSIDERATIONS
• Contraindicated in patients with acute hepatic disease, or isoniazid-associated hepatic damage. Use cautiously in patients with chronic non–isoniazid-associated hepatic disease, seizure disorder (especially those taking phenytoin), severe renal impairment, chronic alcoholism; in elderly patients; in slow acetylator phenotypes (approximately 50% of Blacks and Caucasians).
• Monitor hepatic function if clinical signs of hepatic dysfunction occur during therapy. Tell patient to notify doctor immediately if symptoms of hepatic impairment occur (loss of appetite, fatigue, malaise, jaundice, dark urine).
• Alcohol may be associated with increased incidence of isoniazid-related hepatitis. Discourage use.
• Pyridoxine should be given to prevent peripheral neuropathy, especially in malnourished patients.
• Instruct patient to take this drug exactly as prescribed; warn against discontinuing drug without doctor's consent.
• Store drug at room temperature.
• Advise patient to take with food if GI irritation occurs.
• Reportedly effective when used investigationally to treat arthritis.

para-aminosalicylic acid
PAS, Nemasol Sodium♦♦

sodium aminosalicylate
Parasal Sodium, Pasdium

INDICATIONS & DOSAGE
Treatment of tuberculosis (para-aminosalicylic acid)—
Adults: 10 to 12 g P.O. daily, divided in 2 or 3 doses.
Children: 200 to 300 mg/kg P.O. daily, divided in 3 or 4 doses.
Treatment of tuberculosis (sodium aminosalicylate)—
Adults: 14 to 16 g P.O. daily, divided in 3 or 4 doses.
Children: 240 to 360 mg/kg P.O. daily, divided in 3 or 4 doses.

SIDE EFFECTS
Blood: *leukopenia, agranulocytosis,* eosinophilia, thrombocytopenia, hemolytic anemia.
CNS: encephalopathy.
CV: vasculitis.
GI: *nausea, vomiting,* diarrhea, abdominal pain.
GU: albuminuria, hematuria, crystalluria.
Hepatic: *jaundice, hepatitis.*
Metabolic: acidosis; hypokalemia.
Skin: rash.
Other: infectious mononucleosis–like syndrome, fever, lymphadenopathy.

INTERACTIONS
Ascorbic acid, ammonium chloride: acidify urine, increasing possibility of para-aminosalicylic acid crystalluria. Avoid if possible.
Probenecid: may increase levels of

Italicized side effects are common or life-threatening.
✱Liquid form contains alcohol.   ✱✱May contain tartrazine.

para-aminosalicylic acid. Use together cautiously.
Rifampin: para-aminosalicylic acid may interfere with absorption of rifampin. Give these drugs 8 to 12 hours apart.
Diphenhydramine: inhibits para-aminosalicylic acid absorption. Monitor for decreased para-aminosalicylic acid effect.

NURSING CONSIDERATIONS
• Use cautiously in patients with impaired renal function, decreased hepatic function, and gastric ulcers.
• Sodium aminosalicylate should not be given to patients on sodium-restricted diets. A 15-g dose provides 1.6 g sodium.
• Give with meals or antacid to reduce gastrointestinal distress. Tell patient to swallow enteric-coated tablets whole and not with antacids.
• Monitor renal, hematopoietic, hepatic functions, and serum electrolytes.
• Tell patient to notify doctor at once if symptoms of hepatic impairment (loss of appetite, fatigue, malaise, jaundice, dark urine), fever, sore throat, or skin rash occurs.
• Instruct patient to take any of these drugs exactly as prescribed; warn against discontinuing drug without doctor's consent.
• Protect from water, heat, and sun; don't use if drug turns brown or purple.
• Concomitant administration of at least one other effective antitubercular drug is recommended.

pyrazinamide
Tebrazid♦♦

INDICATIONS & DOSAGE
Treatment of tuberculosis (when primary and secondary antitubercular drugs cannot be used or have failed)—
Adults: 20 to 35 mg/kg P.O. daily, divided in 3 to 4 doses. Maximum dose 3 g daily.

SIDE EFFECTS
Blood: sideroblastic anemia, possible bleeding tendency due to thrombocytopenia.
GI: anorexia, nausea, vomiting.
GU: dysuria.
Hepatic: hepatitis.
Metabolic: interference with control in diabetes mellitus, *hyperuricemia*.
Other: malaise, fever, arthralgia.

INTERACTIONS
None significant.

NURSING CONSIDERATIONS
• Contraindicated in patients with severe hepatic disease. Use cautiously in patients with diabetes mellitus or gout.
• Nearly 100% excreted in urine; reduced dose needed in patients with renal impairment.
• Perform liver function studies and examination for jaundice, liver tenderness, or enlargement before and frequently during therapy.
• Watch closely for signs of gout and of hepatic impairment (loss of appetite, fatigue, malaise, jaundice, dark urine, liver tenderness). Call doctor at once.
• Monitor hematopoietic studies and serum uric acid levels.
• When used with surgical management of tuberculosis, start pyrazinamide 1 to 2 weeks before surgery and continue for 4 to 6 weeks postoperatively.

rifampin
Rifadin♦, Rimactane♦

INDICATIONS & DOSAGE
Primary treatment in pulmonary tuberculosis—
Adults: 600 mg P.O. daily single dose 1 hour before or 2 hours after meals.
Children over 5 years: 10 to 20 mg/kg P.O. daily single dose 1 hour before or 2 hours after meals. Maximum dose 600 mg daily. Concomitant administra-

tion of other effective antitubercular drugs is recommended.
Meningococcal carriers—
Adults: 600 mg P.O. twice daily for 2 days.
Children over 5 years: 10 mg/kg twice daily P.O., not to exceed 600 mg/dose.

SIDE EFFECTS
Blood: thrombocytopenia, transient leukopenia, hemolytic anemia.
CNS: headache, fatigue, *drowsiness,* ataxia, dizziness, mental confusion, generalized numbness.
GI: epigastric distress, anorexia, nausea, vomiting, abdominal pain, diarrhea, flatulence, sore mouth and tongue.
Metabolic: hyperuricemia.
Hepatic: *serious hepatotoxicity as well as transient abnormalities in liver function tests.*
Skin: pruritus, urticaria, rash.
Other: flu-like syndrome.

INTERACTIONS
Para-aminosalicylic acid: may interfere with absorption of rifampin. Give these drugs 8 to 12 hours apart.
Probenecid: may increase rifampin levels. Use cautiously.

NURSING CONSIDERATIONS
• Contraindicated in patients with clinically active hepatitis.
• Use cautiously in patients with hepatic disease or in those receiving other hepatotoxic drugs.
• Monitor hepatic function, hematopoietic studies, and serum uric acid levels.
• Warn patient about drowsiness and the possibility of red-orange discoloration of urine, feces, saliva, sweat, sputum, and tears. Soft contact lenses may be permanently stained.
• Tell patient to take this drug exactly as prescribed and to report side effects. Warn against discontinuing use without doctor's consent.

• Give 1 hour before or 2 hours after meals for optimal absorption; however, if GI irritation occurs, patient may take rifampin with meals.
• Increases enzyme activity of liver; may require increased doses of warfarin, corticosteroids, oral contraceptives, and oral hypoglycemics. See each drug entry for specific drug interactions.

----

streptomycin sulfate

INDICATIONS & DOSAGE
Primary treatment in tuberculosis—
Adults: with normal renal function, 1 g I.M. daily for 2 to 3 months, then 1 g 2 or 3 times a week. Inject deeply into upper outer quadrant of buttocks.
Children: with normal renal function, 20 mg/kg daily in divided doses injected deeply into large muscle mass. Give concurrently with other antitubercular agents, but *not* with capreomycin, and continue until sputum specimen becomes negative.

SIDE EFFECTS
CNS: *transient paresthesias,* especially circumoral; lassitude; muscle weakness.
EENT: *ototoxicity* (damage to vestibular and auditory portions of 8th cranial nerve, severe headache, *nausea, vomiting, vertigo,* ataxia, *tinnitus, roaring and sense of fullness in the ears,* hearing loss), optic nerve dysfunction (blurred vision, amblyopia).
GU: *nephrotoxicity* (transient proteinuria, increase in BUN and serum creatinine levels); nephrotoxicity less common than with other aminoglycosides.
Local: pain, irritation at injection site.
Other: respiratory depression, muscle weakness, systemic lupus erythematosus syndrome, *hypersensitivity* (rash, fever, urticaria, pruritus, angioneurotic edema).

Italicized side effects are common or life-threatening.
*Liquid form contains alcohol.   **May contain tartrazine.

INTERACTIONS

Other aminoglycosides, methoxyflurane: may increase streptomycin's ototoxic and nephrotoxic effects. Use cautiously.
Ethacrynic acid, furosemide: may increase streptomycin's ototoxic effects. Monitor carefully.
Dimenhydrinate: may mask symptoms of ototoxicity. Use together cautiously.

NURSING CONSIDERATIONS

• Contraindicated in patients with labyrinthine disease; hypersensitivity to any of the aminoglycosides; or those receiving other ototoxic or nephrotoxic drugs, neuromuscular blocking agents, and general anesthetics. Use cautiously in elderly patients and in those with impaired renal function.
• Monitor renal function studies.
• Test patient's hearing before, during, and 6 months after therapy. Notify doctor if patient complains of tinnitus, roaring noises, fullness in ears.
• Observe for respiratory depression.
• To minimize renal damage, patient should be well hydrated; encourage increased fluid intake during therapy.
• Watch for signs of superinfection (continued fever and other signs of new infections, especially of the upper respiratory tract).
• Very sensitizing topically. Protect hands when preparing drug.
• In primary treatment of tuberculosis, streptomycin is discontinued when sputum becomes negative.

---

sulfoxone sodium
Diasone Sodium♦

INDICATIONS & DOSAGE

Lepromatous and tuberculoid leprosy—
Adults: weeks 1 and 2: 330 mg P.O. 2 times a week; weeks 3 and 4: 330 mg 4 times a week; week 5 and following weeks: 330 mg daily for 6 days, skip a day and continue.

Children 4 years and older: give ½ the adult dose.

SIDE EFFECTS

Blood: possible leukopenia, *anemia, especially hemolytic;* methemoglobinemia.
CNS: psychosis, headache, dizziness, lethargy, severe malaise, paresthesias.
EENT: tinnitus, allergic rhinitis.
GI: anorexia, *abdominal pain,* nausea, vomiting.
Skin: allergic dermatitis (generalized or fixed maculopapular rash).
Other: hepatitis, drug fever, lepra reaction.

INTERACTIONS

None significant.

NURSING CONSIDERATIONS

• Use cautiously in chronic renal, hepatic, or cardiovascular disease, or refractory anemias.
• Therapy should be interrupted if generalized, diffuse dermatitis occurs.
• Sulfoxone sodium should be reduced or temporarily discontinued if hemoglobin falls below 9 g/dl; if leukocyte count falls below 5,000/mm³; if erythrocyte count falls below 2.5 million/mm³ or remains low.
• Patient should receive hematinics during sulfoxone sodium therapy.
• Antihistamines may help combat sulfoxone induced allergic dermatitis.
• A lepra reaction may occur during sulfoxone therapy as a result of circulating antigens caused by disintegrating *Mycobacterium leprae* bacilli (malaise, fever, painful areas of inflammatory induration in the skin and mucosa, iritis, neuritis). In severe cases, therapy should be interrupted and glucocorticoids given cautiously.
• With severe or frequent drug fever, interrupt therapy or reduce dosage.
• To minimize stomach upset, give drug with meals.
• Protect drug from light.

Unmarked trade names available in the United States only.
♦ Also available in Canada.   ♦♦ Available in Canada only.

10

Aminoglycosides

amikacin sulfate
gentamicin sulfate
kanamycin sulfate
neomycin sulfate
streptomycin sulfate
tobramycin sulfate

MECHANISM OF ACTION
Aminoglycosides act directly on the ribosomes of susceptible organisms. By binding directly to the 30S ribosomal subunit, they inhibit protein synthesis. Generally, they are bactericidal in high concentrations and bacteriostatic in low concentrations.

COMBINATION PRODUCTS
NEOSPORIN G.U. IRRIGANT: 40 mg neomycin sulfate and 200,000 units polymixin B sulfate/ml.

amikacin sulfate
Amikin♦

INDICATIONS & DOSAGE
Serious infections caused by sensitive Pseudomonas aeruginosa, Escherichia coli, Proteus, Klebsiella, Serratia, Enterobacter, Acinetobacter, Providencia, Citrobacter, Staphylococcus—
Adults and children with normal renal function: 15 mg/kg/day divided q 8 to 12 hours I.M. or I.V. infusion (in 100 to 200 ml 5% dextrose in water run in over 30 to 60 minutes). May be given by direct I.V. push if necessary.
Neonates with normal renal function: initially, 10 mg/kg I.M. or I.V. infusion (in 5% dextrose in water run in over 1 to 2 hours), then 7.5 mg/kg q 12 hours I.M. or I.V. infusion.
Meningitis—
Adults: systemic therapy as above; may also use up to 4 mg intrathecally or intraventricularly daily.
Children: systemic therapy as above; may also use 1 to 2 mg intrathecally daily.
Serious urinary tract infections—
Adults: 250 mg I.M. b.i.d.
Adults with impaired renal function: initially, 7.5 mg/kg. Subsequent doses and frequency determined by blood amikacin levels and renal function studies.

SIDE EFFECTS
CNS: headache, lethargy.
EENT: *ototoxicity (tinnitus, vertigo, hearing loss).*
GI: nausea, vomiting.
GU: *nephrotoxicity (cells or casts in urine, oliguria, proteinuria, decreased creatinine clearance, increased BUN and serum creatinine levels).*
Skin: rash, urticaria.

INTERACTIONS
I.V. ethacrynic acid, I.V. furosemide: increase ototoxicity. Use cautiously.
Dimenhydrinate: may mask symptoms of ototoxicity. Use with caution.
Carbenicillin and mezlocillin: amikacin antagonism. Don't mix together in I.V. Schedule 1 hour apart.
Other aminoglycosides, methoxyflurane: increase ototoxicity and nephrotoxicity. Use together cautiously.

Italicized side effects are common or life-threatening.
*Liquid form contains alcohol.   **May contain tartrazine.

NURSING CONSIDERATIONS

- Use cautiously in patients with impaired renal function, in neonates and infants, and elderly patients.
- Obtain specimen for culture and sensitivity before first dose. Therapy may begin pending test results.
- Weigh patient and obtain baseline renal function studies before therapy begins.
- Monitor renal function (output, specific gravity, urinalysis, BUN, creatinine levels, and creatinine clearance). Notify doctor of signs of decreasing renal function.
- Patient should be well hydrated while taking drug to minimize chemical irritation of the renal tubules.
- Evaluate patient's hearing before and during therapy. Notify doctor if patient complains of tinnitus, vertigo, hearing loss.
- Watch for superinfection (continued fever and other signs of new infections, especially of upper respiratory tract).
- Usual duration of therapy is 7 to 10 days. If no response after 3 to 5 days, therapy should be stopped and new specimens obtained for culture and sensitivity.
- Peak blood levels that are above 35 mcg/ml and trough levels that are above 10 mcg/ml are associated with higher incidence of toxicity.
- After I.V. infusion, flush line with normal saline solution.
- Amikacin is usually reserved for gentamicin-resistant organisms.
- Draw blood for peak amikacin level 1 hour after I.M. injection and 1 hour after I.V. infusion begins; for trough levels, draw blood just before next dose.
- Don't collect blood in a heparinized tube.

gentamicin sulfate
Apagen, Bristagen, Cidomycin♦♦, Garamycin♦, U-Gencin

INDICATIONS & DOSAGE

Serious infections caused by sensitive Pseudomonas aeruginosa, Escherichia coli, Proteus, Klebsiella, Serratia, Enterobacter, Citrobacter, Staphylococcus—

Adults with normal renal function: 3 mg/kg daily in divided doses q 8 hours I.M. or I.V. infusion (in 50 to 200 ml of normal saline solution or 5% dextrose in water infused over 30 minutes to 2 hours). May be given by direct I.V. push if necessary. For life-threatening infections, patient may receive up to 5 mg/kg daily in 3 to 4 divided doses.

Children with normal renal function: 2 to 2.5 mg/kg I.M. or I.V. infusion q 8 hours.

Infants and neonates over 1 week with normal renal function: 2.5 mg/kg q 8 hours I.M. or I.V. infusion.

Neonates under 1 week: 2.5 mg/kg I.V. q 12 hours. For I.V. infusion, dilute in normal saline solution or 5% dextrose in water and infuse over 30 minutes to 2 hours.

Meningitis—
Adults: systemic therapy as above; may also use 4 to 8 mg intrathecally daily.
Children: systemic therapy as above; may also use 1 to 2 mg intrathecally daily.

Endocarditis prophylaxis for dental and other respiratory tract procedures—
Adults: 1.5 mg/kg I.M. 30 to 60 minutes before procedure. Given with penicillin G.
Children: 2.5 mg/kg I.M. 30 to 60 minutes before procedure. Given with penicillin G.

Endocarditis prophylaxis for GI or GU procedure or surgery—
Adults: 1.5 mg/kg I.M. or I.V. 30 to 60 minutes before procedure or surgery and q 8 hours after, for 2 doses. Given

with aqueous penicillin G or ampicillin.

Children: 2.5 mg/kg I.M. or I.V. 30 to 60 minutes before procedure or surgery and q 8 hours after, for 2 doses. Given with aqueous penicillin G or ampicillin.

Patients with impaired renal function: initial dose is same as for those with normal renal function. Subsequent doses and frequency determined by renal function studies.

Posthemodialysis to maintain therapeutic blood levels—

Adults: 1 to 1.7 mg/kg I.M. or I.V. infusion after each dialysis.

Children: 2 mg/kg I.M. or I.V. infusion after each dialysis.

SIDE EFFECTS
CNS: headache, lethargy.
EENT: *ototoxicity (tinnitus, vertigo, hearing loss).*
GI: nausea, vomiting.
GU: *nephrotoxicity (cells or casts in the urine, oliguria, proteinuria, decreased creatinine clearance, increased BUN, nonprotein nitrogen, and serum creatinine levels).*
Skin: rash, urticaria.

INTERACTIONS
I.V. ethacrynic acid, I.V. furosemide: increase ototoxicity. Use cautiously.
Dimenhydrinate: may mask symptoms of ototoxicity. Use with caution.
Carbenicillin and mezlocillin: gentamicin antagonism. Don't mix together in I.V. Schedule 1 hour apart.
Cephalosporins: increase nephrotoxicity. Use together cautiously.
Other aminoglycosides, methoxyflurane: increase ototoxicity and nephrotoxicity. Use together cautiously.

NURSING CONSIDERATIONS
• Use cautiously in patients with impaired renal function, and in neonates, infants, and elderly patients.
• Obtain specimen for culture and sen-

sitivity before first dose. Therapy may begin pending test results.
• Weigh patient and obtain baseline renal function studies before therapy begins.
• Monitor renal function (output, specific gravity, urinalysis, BUN, creatinine levels, and creatinine clearance). Notify doctor of signs of decreasing renal function.
• Patient should be well hydrated while taking drug to minimize chemical irritation of the renal tubules.
• After completing I.V. infusion, flush the line with normal saline solution.
• Evaluate patient's hearing before and during therapy. Notify doctor if patient complains of tinnitus, vertigo, hearing loss.
• Watch for superinfection (continued fever and other signs of new infections, especially of upper respiratory tract).
• Usual duration of therapy is 7 to 10 days. If no response in 3 to 5 days, therapy should be stopped and new specimens obtained for culture and sensitivity.
• Peak blood levels above 12 mcg/ml and trough levels (those drawn just before next dose) above 2 mcg/ml are associated with higher incidence of toxicity.
• Draw blood for peak gentamicin level 1 hour after I.M. injection and 1 hour after I.V. infusion begins; for trough levels, draw blood just before next dose.
• Don't collect blood in a heparinized tube.
• Hemodialysis (8 hours) removes up to 50% of drug from blood.
• Endocarditis prophylaxis is recommended for all patients with rheumatic or congenital heart disease or prosthetic heart valve.
• Intrathecal form (without preservatives) should be used when intrathecal administration is indicated.

Italicized side effects are common or life-threatening.
*Liquid form contains alcohol.   **May contain tartrazine.

kanamycin sulfate
Kantrex♦, Klebcil

INDICATIONS & DOSAGE

Serious infections caused by sensitive Escherichia coli, Proteus, Enterobacter aerogenes, Klebsiella pneumoniae, Serratia marcescens, Acinetobacter—
Adults and children with normal renal function: 15 mg/kg daily divided q 8 to 12 hours deep I.M. into upper outer quadrant of buttocks or I.V. infusion (diluted 500 mg/200 ml of normal saline solution or 5% dextrose in water infused at 60 to 80 drops/minute). Maximum daily dose 1.5 g.
Neonates: 15 mg/kg daily I.M. or I.V. divided q 12 hours.
Adjunctive treatment in hepatic coma—
Adults: 8 to 12 g daily P.O. in divided doses.
Preoperative bowel sterilization—
Adults: 1 g P.O. q 1 hour for 4 doses, then q 4 hours for 4 doses; or 1 g P.O. q 1 hour for 4 doses, then q 6 hours for 36 to 72 hours.
Intraperitoneal irrigation—
500 mg in 20 ml sterile distilled water instilled via catheter into wound after patient fully recovered from anesthesia and neuromuscular blocking agent effects.
*Wound irrigation—*up to 2.5 mg/ml in normal saline irrigation solution.

SIDE EFFECTS

CNS: headache, lethargy.
EENT: *ototoxicity (tinnitus, vertigo, hearing loss).*
GI: nausea, vomiting.
GU: *nephrotoxicity (cells or casts in the urine, oliguria, proteinuria, decreased creatinine clearance, increased BUN and serum creatinine levels).*
Skin: rash, urticaria.

INTERACTIONS

Ethacrynic acid, furosemide: increase ototoxicity. Use cautiously.

Dimenhydrinate: may mask symptoms of ototoxicity. Use with caution.
Other aminoglycosides, methoxyflurane: increase ototoxicity and nephrotoxicity. Don't use together.

NURSING CONSIDERATIONS

• Oral use contraindicated in patients with intestinal obstruction; in treatment of systemic infection. Use cautiously in patients with impaired renal function and in the elderly.
• Obtain specimen for culture and sensitivity before first dose. Therapy may begin pending test results.
• Weigh patient and obtain baseline renal function studies before therapy begins.
• Monitor renal function (output, specific gravity, urinalysis, BUN, creatinine levels, and creatinine clearance). Notify doctor of signs of decreasing renal function.
• Patient should be well hydrated while taking drug to minimize chemical irritation of the renal tubules.
• Evaluate patient's hearing before and during therapy. Notify doctor if patient complains of tinnitus, vertigo, hearing loss.
• Watch for superinfection (continued fever and other signs of new infection, especially of upper respiratory tract).
• If no response in 3 to 5 days, therapy should be stopped and new specimens obtained for culture and sensitivity.
• Peak blood levels over 30 mcg/ml are associated with increased incidence of toxicity.

neomycin sulfate
Mycifradin Sulfate♦, Neobiotic

INDICATIONS & DOSAGE

Infectious diarrhea caused by enteropathogenic Escherichia coli—
Adults: 50 mg/kg daily P.O. in 4 divided doses for 2 to 3 days.
Children: 50 to 100 mg/kg daily P.O. divided q 4 to 6 hours for 2 to 3 days.

Suppression of intestinal bacteria preoperatively—
Adults: 1 g P.O. q 1 hour for 4 doses, then 1 g q 4 hours for the balance of the 24 hours.
Children: 40 to 100 mg/kg daily P.O. divided q 4 to 6 hours. First dose should be preceded by saline cathartic.
Adjunctive treatment in hepatic coma—
Adults: 1 to 3 g P.O. q.i.d. for 5 to 6 days; or 200 ml of 1% or 100 ml of 2% solution as enema retained for 20 to 60 minutes q 6 hours.

SIDE EFFECTS
CNS: headache, lethargy.
EENT: *ototoxicity (tinnitus, vertigo, hearing loss).*
GI: nausea, vomiting.
GU: *nephrotoxicity (cells or casts in the urine, oliguria, proteinuria, decreased creatinine clearance, increased BUN and serum creatinine levels).*
Skin: rash, urticaria.

INTERACTIONS
Ethacrynic acid, furosemide: increase ototoxicity. Use cautiously.
Dimenhydrinate: may mask symptoms of ototoxicity. Use with caution.
Other aminoglycosides, methoxyflurane: increase ototoxicity and nephrotoxicity. Use together cautiously.

NURSING CONSIDERATIONS
• Contraindicated in patients with intestinal obstruction. Use cautiously in patients with impaired renal function, ulcerative bowel lesions, and in elderly patients.
• Oral therapy not recommended for systemic infection; parenteral dosage form available for I.M. use but not recommended because of extreme ototoxicity and nephrotoxicity.
• Weigh patient and obtain baseline renal function studies before therapy begins.
• Monitor renal function (output, specific gravity, urinalysis, BUN, creatinine levels, and creatinine clearance).

Notify doctor of signs of decreasing renal function.
• Patient should be well hydrated while taking drug to minimize chemical irritation of the renal tubules.
• Watch for respiratory depression in patients with renal disease, hypocalcemia, or neuromuscular diseases, such as myasthenia gravis.
• Evaluate hearing of patient with hepatic or renal disease before and during prolonged therapy. Notify doctor if patient complains of tinnitus, vertigo, hearing loss. Onset of deafness may occur several weeks after drug is stopped.
• Watch for superinfection (continued fever and other signs of new infections, especially of upper respiratory tract).
• Sometimes used in the treatment of high blood cholesterol.
• Nonabsorbable at recommended dosage. However, more than 4 g of neomycin per day may be systemically absorbed and lead to nephrotoxicity.
• Available in combination with polymyxin B as a urinary bladder irrigant.

streptomycin sulfate

INDICATIONS & DOSAGE
Streptococcal endocarditis—
Adults: 10 mg/kg I.M. (maximum 0.5 g) q 12 hours for 2 weeks with penicillin.
Treatment of tuberculosis—
Adults: initially, 0.75 to 1 g I.M. daily for 60 to 90 days, then 1 g 2 to 3 times weekly.
Patients with impaired renal function: initial dose is same as for those with normal renal function. Subsequent doses and frequency determined by renal function study results.
Enterococcal endocarditis—
Adults: 1 g I.M. q 12 hours for 2 weeks, then 500 mg I.M. q 12 hours for 4 weeks with penicillin.
Tularemia—
Adults: 1 to 2 g I.M. daily in divided doses injected deep into upper outer

---

Italicized side effects are common or life-threatening.
*Liquid form contains alcohol.   **May contain tartrazine.

quadrant of buttocks. Continue until patient is afebrile for 5 to 7 days.

SIDE EFFECTS
EENT: *ototoxicity (tinnitus, vertigo, hearing loss).*
GU: some nephrotoxicity (not nearly as frequent as with other aminoglycosides).
Local: pain, irritation, and sterile abscesses at injection site.
Skin: *exfoliative dermatitis.*
Other: *hypersensitivity* (rash, fever, urticaria, and angioneurotic edema).

INTERACTIONS
Dimenhydrinate: may mask symptoms of streptomycin-induced ototoxicity. Use together cautiously.
Ethacrynic acid, furosemide: increase ototoxicity. Use cautiously.
Other aminoglycosides, methoxyflurane: may increase streptomycin's ototoxic and nephrotoxic effects. Use cautiously.

NURSING CONSIDERATIONS
• Contraindicated in labyrinthine disease. Use cautiously in patients with impaired renal function and in the elderly.
• Obtain specimen for culture and sensitivity before first dose except when treating tuberculosis. Therapy may begin pending test results.
• Patient should be well hydrated while taking drug to minimize chemical irritation of the renal tubules.
• Evaluate patient's hearing before, during, and 6 months after therapy. Notify doctor if patient complains of tinnitus, roaring noises, or fullness in ears.
• Watch for superinfection (continued fever and other signs of new infections, especially of upper respiratory tract) and respiratory depression.
• Peak blood concentrations over 25 mcg/ml are associated with increased incidence of toxicity.
• Endocarditis prophylaxis is recommended for all patients with rheumatic or congenital heart disease or with prosthetic heart valve. Patients should receive prophylactic antibiotics during GI or GU procedures or surgery, or during upper respiratory tract procedures.

---

tobramycin sulfate
Nebcin♦

INDICATIONS & DOSAGE
Serious infections caused by sensitive strains of Escherichia coli, Proteus, Klebsiella, Enterobacter, Serratia, Staphylococcus aureus, Pseudomonas, Citrobacter, Providencia—
Adults and children with normal renal function: 3 mg/kg I.M. or I.V. daily divided q 8 hours. Up to 5 mg/kg I.M. or I.V. daily divided q 6 to 8 hours for life-threatening infections.
Neonates under 1 week: up to 4 mg/kg I.M. or I.V. daily divided q 12 hours. For I.V. use, dilute in 50 to 100 ml normal saline solution or 5% dextrose in water for adults and less volume for children. Infuse over 20 to 60 minutes.
Patients with impaired renal function: initial dose is same as for those with normal renal function. Subsequent doses and frequency determined by renal function study results.

SIDE EFFECTS
CNS: headache, lethargy.
EENT: *ototoxicity (tinnitus, vertigo, hearing loss).*
GI: nausea, vomiting.
GU: *nephrotoxicity (cells or casts in the urine, oliguria, proteinuria, decreased creatinine clearance, increased BUN and serum creatinine levels).*
Skin: rash, urticaria.

INTERACTIONS
I.V. ethacrynic acid, I.V. furosemide: increase ototoxicity. Use cautiously.
Dimenhydrinate: may mask symptoms of ototoxicity. Use with caution.
Carbenicillin and mezlocillin: tobramy-

cin antagonism. Don't mix together in I.V. Schedule 1 hour apart.
Cephalosporins: increase nephrotoxicity. Use together cautiously.
Other aminoglycosides, methoxyflurane: increase ototoxicity and nephrotoxicity. Use together cautiously.

NURSING CONSIDERATIONS

• Use cautiously in patients with impaired renal function and in the elderly.
• Obtain specimen for culture and sensitivity before first dose. Therapy may begin pending test results.
• Weigh patient and obtain baseline renal function studies before starting therapy.
• Usual duration of therapy is 7 to 10 days.
• Monitor renal function (output, specific gravity, urinalysis, BUN, creatinine, and creatinine clearance). Notify doctor of signs of decreasing renal function.

• Patient should be well hydrated while taking drug to minimize chemical irritation of the renal tubules.
• Evaluate patient's hearing before and during therapy. Notify doctor if patient complains of tinnitus, vertigo, hearing loss.
• Watch for superinfection (continued fever and other signs of new infections, especially of upper respiratory tract).
• Peak blood levels over 12 mcg/ml are associated with increased incidence of toxicity.
• Draw blood for peak tobramycin level 1 hour after I.M. injection and 1 hour after I.V. infusion begins; draw blood for trough level just before next dose.
• Don't collect blood in a heparinized tube.
• After I.V. infusion, flush line with normal saline solution.
• Recent studies indicate tobramycin is less nephrotoxic than gentamicin.

11

Penicillins

amoxicillin trihydrate
ampicillin
ampicillin sodium
azlocillin sodium
bacampicillin
carbenicillin disodium
carbenicillin indanyl sodium
cloxacillin sodium
cyclacillin
dicloxacillin sodium
hetacillin
hetacillin potassium
methicillin sodium
mezlocillin sodium
nafcillin sodium
oxacillin sodium
penicillin G benzathine
penicillin G potassium
penicillin G procaine
penicillin G sodium
penicillin V
penicillin V potassium
piperacillin sodium
ticarcillin disodium

MECHANISM OF ACTION
Penicillins are thought to be bactericidal against microorganisms by inhibiting cell-wall synthesis during active multiplication. They are more effective against young, rapidly dividing organisms than against mature resting cells that are not in the process of cell-wall formation.

Bacteria resist penicillin by producing penicillinases—enzymes that convert penicillin to inactive penicilloic acid. The penicillinase-resistant penicillins (cloxacillin, dicloxacillin, methicillin, nafcillin, and oxacillin) resist these enzymes.

COMBINATION PRODUCTS
None.

amoxicillin trihydrate
Amoxil♦, Larotid, Polymox♦, Robamox, Sumox, Trimox, Utimox

INDICATIONS & DOSAGE
Systemic infections, acute and chronic urinary tract infections caused by susceptible strains of gram-positive and gram-negative organisms—
Adults: 750 mg to 1.5 g P.O. daily, divided into doses given q 8 hours.
Children: 20 to 40 mg/kg P.O. daily, divided into doses given q 8 hours.
Uncomplicated gonorrhea—
Adults: 3 g P.O. with 1 g probenecid given as a single dose.
Uncomplicated urinary tract infections due to susceptible organisms—
Adults: 3 g P.O. given as a single dose.

SIDE EFFECTS
Blood: anemia, thrombocytopenia, thrombocytopenic purpura, eosinophilia, leukopenia.
GI: *nausea,* vomiting, *diarrhea.*
Other: *hypersensitivity (erythematous maculopapular rash, urticaria, anaphylaxis),* overgrowth of nonsusceptible organisms.

INTERACTIONS
Probenecid: increases blood levels of penicillin. Probenecid is often used for this purpose.
Chloramphenicol, erythromycin, tetracyclines: antibiotic antagonism. Give

Unmarked trade names available in the United States only.
♦ Also available in Canada. ♦♦ Available in Canada only.

penicillins at least 1 hour before bacteriostatic antibiotics.

NURSING CONSIDERATIONS
• Use cautiously in patients with other drug allergies, especially to cephalosporins (possible cross-allergenicity); and in patients with mononucleosis— high incidence of maculopapular rash in those receiving amoxicillin.
• Obtain cultures for sensitivity tests before first dose. Unnecessary to wait for results before beginning therapy.
• Before giving amoxicillin, ask patient if he's had any allergic reactions to penicillin. However, a negative history of penicillin allergy is no guarantee against a future allergic reaction.
• Tell patient to take medication exactly as prescribed, even after he feels better. Entire quantity prescribed should be taken.
• Give with food to prevent GI distress.
• Large doses may cause increased yeast growths. Report symptoms to doctor.
• With prolonged therapy, bacterial and fungal superinfection may occur, especially in the elderly, debilitated, or those with low resistance to infection due to immunosuppressives or irradiation. Close observation essential.
• Check expiration date. Warn patient never to use leftover penicillin for a new illness or to share penicillin with family and friends.
• Tell patient to call the doctor if rash, fever, or chills develop. A rash is the most common allergic reaction. The rash is most common if the patient is also taking allopurinol.
• Amoxicillin and ampicillin have similar clinical applications.

ampicillin
Amcill, Ampilean♦♦, Omnipen, Pfizerpen A, Roampicillin

ampicillin sodium
Omnipen-N, Pen A/N, Polycillin-N, Totacillin-N

INDICATIONS & DOSAGE
Systemic infections, acute and chronic urinary tract infections caused by susceptible strains of gram-positive and gram-negative organisms—
Adults: 1 to 4 g P.O. daily, divided into doses given q 6 hours; 2 to 12 g I.M. or I.V. daily, divided into doses given q 4 to 6 hours.
Children: 50 to 100 mg/kg P.O. daily, divided into doses given q 6 hours; or 100 to 200 mg/kg I.M. or I.V. daily, divided into doses given q 6 hours.
Meningitis—
Adults: 8 to 14 g I.V. daily for 3 days, then I.M. divided q 3 to 4 hours.
Children: up to 300 mg/kg I.V. daily for 3 days, then I.M. divided q 4 hours.
Uncomplicated gonorrhea—
Adults: 3.5 g P.O. with 1 g probenecid given as a single dose.

SIDE EFFECTS
Blood: anemia, thrombocytopenia, thrombocytopenic purpura, eosinophilia, leukopenia.
GI: *nausea,* vomiting, *diarrhea,* glossitis, stomatitis.
Local: pain at injection site, vein irritation, thrombophlebitis.
Other: *hypersensitivity (erythematous maculopapular rash, urticaria, anaphylaxis),* overgrowth of nonsusceptible organisms.

INTERACTIONS
Probenecid: increases blood levels of penicillin. Probenecid is often used for this purpose.
Chloramphenicol, erythromycin, tetracyclines: antibiotic antagonism. Give

---

penicillins at least 1 hour before bacteriostatic antibiotics.

NURSING CONSIDERATIONS
● Use cautiously in patients with other drug allergies, especially to cephalosporins (possible cross-allergenicity); and in patients with mononucleosis—high incidence of maculopapular rash in those receiving ampicillin.
● Obtain cultures for sensitivity tests before first dose. Unnecessary to wait for results before beginning therapy.
● Before giving ampicillin, ask patient if he's had any allergic reactions to penicillin. However, a negative history of penicillin allergy is no guarantee against a future allergic reaction.
● Tell patient to take medication exactly as prescribed, even after he feels better. Entire quantity prescribed should be taken.
● Tell the patient to call the doctor if rash, fever, or chills develop. A rash is the most common allergic reaction. Rash is most common if the patient is also taking allopurinol.
● When given orally, drug may cause GI disturbances. Food may interfere with absorption, so give 1 to 2 hours before meals or 2 to 3 hours after.
● Don't give I.M. or I.V. unless infection is severe or patient can't take oral dose.
● Dosage should be altered in patients with impaired hepatic and renal functions.
● When giving I.V., mix with 5% dextrose in water or a saline solution. Don't mix with other drugs or solutions: they might be incompatible.
● Give I.V. intermittently to prevent vein irritation. Change site every 48 hours.
● Large doses may cause increased yeast growths. Report symptoms to doctor.
● With prolonged therapy, bacterial or fungal superinfection may occur, especially in the elderly, debilitated, or those with low resistance to infection

due to immunosuppressives or irradiation. Close observation is essential.
● Check expiration date. Warn patient never to use leftover penicillin for a new illness or to share penicillin with family and friends.
● Initial dilution in vial is stable for 1 hour. Follow manufacturer's direction for stability data when ampicillin is further diluted for I.V. infusion.

azlocillin sodium
Azlin

INDICATIONS & DOSAGE
Serious infections caused by susceptible strains of Pseudomonas aeruginosa—
Adults: 200 to 350 mg/kg daily I.V. given in 4 to 6 divided doses. Usual dose is 3 g q 4 (18 g daily). Maximum daily dosage is 24 g. May be administered by I.V. intermittent infusion or by direct slow I.V. injection.
Children (with acute exacerbation of cystic fibrosis): 75 mg/kg q 4 hours (450 mg/kg daily). Maximum daily dosage is 24 g.
Azlocillin should not be used in neonates.

SIDE EFFECTS
Blood: *bleeding with high doses,* neutropenia, eosinophilia, leukopenia, *thrombocytopenia.*
CNS: neuromuscular irritability, headache, dizziness.
GI: nausea, diarrhea.
Local: pain at injection site, vein irritation, phlebitis.
Metabolic: *hypokalemia.*
Other: *hypersensitivity (edema, fever, chills, rash, pruritus, urticaria, anaphylaxis),* overgrowth of nonsusceptible organisms.

INTERACTIONS
Gentamicin, tobramycin: chemically incompatible. Don't mix together in I.V. solution. Give 1 hour apart.
Chloramphenicol, erythromycin, tetra-

cyclines: antibiotic antagonism. Give penicillins at least 1 hour before bacteriostatic antibiotics.

NURSING CONSIDERATIONS
• Use cautiously in patients hypersensitive to drugs, especially to cephalosporins (possible cross-allergenicity), and in those with bleeding tendencies, uremia, or hypokalemia.
• Obtain cultures for sensitivity tests before starting therapy. Unnecessary to wait for results before starting therapy.
• Before giving azlocillin, ask patient if he's had allergic reactions to penicillin. A negative history of penicillin allergy, however, is no guarantee against future allergic reactions.
• Dosage should be altered in patients with impaired hepatic and renal functions.
• Check CBC frequently. Drug may cause thrombocytopenia.
• Monitor serum potassium level.
• Patient with high serum level of this drug may have convulsions. Take seizure precautions.
• When giving I.V., mix with 5% dextrose in water or other suitable I.V. fluids.
• Give I.V. intermittently to prevent vein irritation. Change site every 48 hours.
• Large doses may cause increased yeast growths. Report symptoms to doctor.
• Almost always used with another antibiotic, such as gentamicin.
• With prolonged therapy, superinfections may occur, especially in the elderly or debilitated, or in those patients with low resistance to infection due to immunosuppressors or irradiation. Monitor patient closely.
• Check drug expiration date.
• Azlocillin is less likely to cause hypokalemia than similar antibiotics, such as carbenicillin and ticarcillin.
• Drug may be better suited to patients on salt-free diets than carbenicillin and ticarcillin (contains 2.17 mEq Na$^+$/g of azlocillin).

bacampicillin
Spectrobid

INDICATIONS & DOSAGE
Upper and lower respiratory tract infections due to streptococci, pneumococci, staphylococci, and Hemophilus influenzae; *urinary tract infections due to* Escherichia coli, Proteus mirabilis, *and* Streptococcus faecalis; *skin infections due to streptococci and susceptible staphylococci—*
Adults and children weighing more than 25 kg: 400 to 800 mg P.O. q 12 hours.
Gonorrhea—
Usual dosage is 1.6 g plus 1 g probenecid given as a single dose.
Not recommended for children under 25 kg.

SIDE EFFECTS
Blood: anemia, thrombocytopenia, thrombocytopenic purpura, eosinophilia, leukopenia.
GI: *nausea,* vomiting, *diarrhea,* glossitis, stomatitis.
Other: *hypersensitivity (erythematous maculopapular rash, urticaria, anaphylaxis),* overgrowth of nonsusceptible organisms.

INTERACTIONS
Probenecid: increased blood levels of bacampicillin or other penicillins. Probenecid is often used for this purpose.
Chloramphenicol, erythromycin, tetracyclines: antibiotic antagonism. Administer penicillins at least 1 hour before bacteriostatic antibiotics.

NURSING CONSIDERATIONS
• Use cautiously in patients with other drug allergies, especialy to cephalosporins (possible cross-allergenicity).
• Obtain cultures for sensitivity tests

before first dose. Unnecessary to wait for results before beginning therapy.
• Before giving bacampicillin, ask patient if he's had any previous allergic reactions to penicillin. However, a negative history of penicillin allergy is no guarantee against a future allergic reaction.
• Bacampicillin is especially formulated to produce high blood levels of antibiotic when administered twice daily.
• Diarrhea may occur less frequently with bacampicillin than with ampicillin.
• Tell patient to take medication even after he feels better. Entire quantity prescribed should be taken.
• Tell patient to call the doctor if rash, fever, or chills develop. A rash is the most common allergic reaction.
• With prolonged therapy, bacterial or fungal superinfection may occur, especially in the elderly or the debilitated, and in those with low resistance to infection due to immunosuppressors or irradiation. Close observation is essential.
• Check expiration date. Warn patient never to use leftover penicillin products for a new illness or to share penicillin with family and friends.
• Unlike ampicillin, bacampicillin may be taken with meals without fear of diminished drug absorption. Give with food to prevent GI distress.

carbenicillin disodium
Geopen, Pyopen♦

INDICATIONS & DOSAGE

Systemic infections caused by susceptible strains of gram-positive and especially gram-negative organisms (Proteus, Pseudomonas aeruginosa)—
Adults: 30 to 40 g daily I.V. infusion, divided into doses given q 4 to 6 hours.
Children: 300 to 500 mg/kg daily I.V. infusion, divided into doses given q 4 to 6 hours.

Urinary tract infections—
Adults: 200 mg/kg daily I.M. or I.V. infusion, divided into doses given q 4 to 6 hours.
Children: 50 to 200 mg/kg daily I.M. or I.V. infusion, divided into doses given q 4 to 6 hours.

SIDE EFFECTS

Blood: *bleeding with high doses,* neutropenia, eosinophilia, leukopenia, *thrombocytopenia.*
CNS: neuromuscular irritability.
GI: nausea.
Local: pain at injection site, vein irritation, phlebitis.
Metabolic: *hypokalemia.*
Other: hypersensitivity *(edema, fever, chills, rash, pruritus, urticaria, anaphylaxis),* overgrowth of nonsusceptible organisms.

INTERACTIONS

Probenecid: increases blood levels of penicillin. Probenecid is often used for this purpose.
Gentamicin, tobramycin: chemically incompatible. Don't mix together in I.V. Give 1 hour apart.
Chloramphenicol, erythromycin, tetracyclines: antibiotic antagonism. Give penicillins at least 1 hour before bacteriostatic antibiotics.

NURSING CONSIDERATIONS

• Use cautiously in patients with other drug allergies, especially to cephalosporins (possible cross-allergenicity); and in those with bleeding tendencies, uremia, hypokalemia. Use cautiously in patients on sodium-restricted diets; contains 4.7 mEq sodium/g.
• Obtain cultures for sensitivity tests before first dose. Unnecessary to wait for test results before beginning therapy.
• Before giving carbenicillin, ask patient if he's had any allergic reactions to penicillin. However, a negative history of penicillin allergy is no guarantee against a future allergic reaction.

- Dosage should be altered in patients with impaired hepatic and renal function. Patients with impaired renal function are susceptible to nephrotoxicity. Monitor intake and output.
- Check CBC frequently. Drug may cause thrombocytopenia.
- Monitor serum potassium. Patients may develop hypokalemia due to large amount of sodium in the preparation.
- If patient has high blood level of this drug, he may have convulsions. Be prepared by keeping side rails up on bed.
- When giving I.V., mix with 5% dextrose in water or other suitable I.V. fluids.
- Give I.V intermittently to prevent vein irritation. Change site every 48 hours.
- Almost always used with another antibiotic, such as gentamicin.
- Large doses may cause increased yeast growths. Report symptoms to doctor.
- With prolonged therapy, other superinfections may occur, especially in the elderly, debilitated, or those with low resistance to infection due to immunosuppressives or irradiation. Close observation is essential.
- Check expiration date; do not use any penicillin that is outdated.

carbenicillin indanyl sodium
Geocillin, Geopen Oral♦♦

INDICATIONS & DOSAGE
Urinary tract infection and prostatitis caused by susceptible strains of gram-negative organisms—
Adults: 382 to 764 mg P.O. q.i.d. Not recommended for children.

SIDE EFFECTS
Blood: leukopenia, neutropenia, eosinophilia, anemia, thrombocytopenia.
GI: *nausea,* vomiting, *diarrhea, flatulence, abdominal cramps, unpleasant taste.*

Other: *hypersensitivity (rash, chills, fever, urticaria, pruritus, anaphylaxis),* overgrowth of nonsusceptible organisms.

INTERACTIONS
None significant.

NURSING CONSIDERATIONS
- Use cautiously in patients with other drug allergies, especially to cephalosporins (possible cross-allergenicity).
- Obtain cultures for sensitivity tests before first dose. Unnecessary to wait for test results before starting therapy.
- Before giving carbenicillin, ask patient if he's had any allergic reactions to penicillin. However, a negative history of penicillin allergy is no guarantee against a future allergic reaction.
- Tell patient to take medication exactly as prescribed, even after he feels better. Entire quantity prescribed should be taken.
- Tell patient to call the doctor if he develops rash, fever, or chills. A rash is the most common allergic reaction.
- When given orally, drug may cause GI disturbances. Food may interfere with absorption, so give 1 to 2 hours before meals or 2 to 3 hours after.
- Large doses may cause increased yeast growths. Report symptoms to doctor.
- With prolonged therapy, other superinfections may occur, especially in the elderly, debilitated, or those with low resistance to infection due to immunosuppressives or irradiation. Close observation is essential.
- Check expiration date. Warn patient never to use leftover penicillin for a new illness or to share penicillin with family and friends.
- Use only in patients whose creatinine clearance is 10 ml/minute or more.
- Excellent treatment for *Pseudomonas* urinary tract infections in ambulatory patients.
- May be useful in treatment of cystitis, but not pyelonephritis.

Italicized side effects are common or life-threatening.
*Liquid form contains alcohol. **May contain tartrazine.

• Not effective for any systemic infection because blood levels are nil.

cloxacillin sodium
Bactopen♦♦, Cloxapen♦,
Novocloxin♦♦, Orbenin♦♦,
Tegopen♦

INDICATIONS & DOSAGE
Systemic infections caused by penicillinase-producing staphylococci—
Adults: 2 to 4 g P.O. daily, divided into doses given q 6 hours.
Children: 50 to 100 mg/kg P.O. daily, divided into doses given q 6 hours.

SIDE EFFECTS
Blood: eosinophilia.
GI: *nausea,* vomiting, *epigastric distress, diarrhea.*
Other: *hypersensitivity (rash, urticaria, chills, fever, sneezing, wheezing, anaphylaxis),* overgrowth of nonsusceptible organisms.

INTERACTIONS
Probenecid: increases blood levels of penicillin. Probenecid is often used for this purpose.
Chloramphenicol, erythromycin, tetracyclines: antibiotic antagonism. Give penicillins at least 1 hour before bacteriostatic antibiotics.

NURSING CONSIDERATIONS
• Use with caution in patients with other drug allergies, especially to cephalosporins (possible cross-allergenicity).
• Obtain cultures for sensitivity tests before first dose. Unnecessary to wait for test results before starting therapy.
• Before giving cloxacillin, ask patient if he's had any allergic reactions to penicillin. However, a negative history of penicillin allergy is no guarantee against a future allergic reaction.
• Tell patient to take medication exactly as prescribed, even if he feels bet-

ter. Entire quantity prescribed should be taken.
• Tell patient to call the doctor if rash, fever, or chills develop. A rash is the most common allergic reaction.
• When given orally, drug may cause GI disturbances. Food may interfere with absorption, so give 1 to 2 hours before meals or 2 to 3 hours after.
• Large doses may cause increased yeast growths. Report symptoms to doctor.
• With prolonged therapy, other superinfections may occur, especially in the elderly, debilitated, or those with low resistance to infection due to immunosuppressives or irradiation. Close observation is essential.
• Check expiration date. Warn patient never to use leftover penicillin for a new illness or to share penicillin with family and friends.

cyclacillin
Cyclapen-W

INDICATIONS & DOSAGE
Systemic and urinary tract infections caused by susceptible strains of gram-positive and gram-negative organisms—
Adults: 250 to 500 mg P.O. q.i.d. in equally spaced doses.
Children: 50 to 100 mg/kg daily in equally divided doses.

SIDE EFFECTS
Blood: anemia, thrombocytopenia, thrombocytopenic purpura, leukopenia, neutropenia, eosinophilia.
GI: *nausea,* vomiting, *diarrhea.*
Other: *hypersensitivity (edema, fever, chills, rash, pruritus, urticaria, anaphylaxis),* overgrowth of nonsusceptible organisms.

INTERACTIONS
Probenecid: increases blood levels of penicillin. Probenecid is often used for this purpose.
Chloramphenicol, erythromycin, tetra-

Unmarked trade names available in the United States only.
♦ Also available in Canada.   ♦♦ Available in Canada only.

cyclines: antibiotic antagonism. Give penicillins at least 1 hour before bacteriostatic antibiotics.

NURSING CONSIDERATIONS
• Contraindicated in patients allergic to other penicillins.
• Obtain cultures for sensitivity tests before first dose. Unnecessary to wait for test results before starting therapy.
• Before giving cyclacillin, ask patient if he's had any allergic reactions to penicillin. However, a negative history of penicillin allergy is no guarantee against a future allergic reaction.
• Tell patient he must take all medication exactly as prescribed, for as long as ordered, even after he feels better.
• Patients with renal insufficiency should receive less drug in accordance with their creatinine clearance level.
• Large doses of penicillin may cause increased yeast growths. Watch for signs and symptoms, and report to doctor.
• With prolonged therapy, bacterial and fungal superinfection may occur, especially in the elderly, debilitated, or those with low resistance to infection due to immunosuppressives or irradiation. Close observation is essential.
• Check expiration date before giving this drug. Warn patient never to use leftover penicillin for a new illness or to share his penicillin with family and friends.
• Tell patient to call the doctor if he develops rash, fever, chills. A rash is the most common allergic reaction.

---

diclocacillin sodium
Dycill, Dynapen♦, Pathocil

INDICATIONS & DOSAGE
Systemic infections caused by penicillinase-producing staphylococci—
Adults: 1 to 2 g daily P.O. or I.M., divided into doses given q 6 hours.
Children: 25 to 50 mg/kg P.O. or I.M.

daily, divided into doses given q 6 hours.

SIDE EFFECTS
Blood: eosinophilia.
GI: *nausea,* vomiting, *epigastric distress,* flatulence, *diarrhea.*
Other: *hypersensitivity (pruritus, urticaria, rash, anaphylaxis),* overgrowth of nonsusceptible organisms.

INTERACTIONS
Chloramphenicol, erythromycin, tetracyclines: antibiotic antagonism. Give penicillins at least 1 hour before bacteriostatic antibiotics.
Probenecid: increases blood levels of penicillin. Probenecid is often used for this purpose.

NURSING CONSIDERATIONS
• Use cautiously in patients allergic to cephalosporins (possible cross-allergenicity).
• Obtain cultures for sensitivity tests before first dose. Unnecessary to wait for test results before starting therapy.
• Before giving diclocacillin, ask patient if he's had any allergic reactions to penicillin. However, a negative history of penicillin allergy is no guarantee against a future allergic reaction.
• Tell patient to take medication exactly as prescribed, even if he feels better. Entire quantity prescribed should be taken.
• Tell patient to call the doctor if rash, fever, or chills develop. A rash is the most common allergic reaction.
• When given orally, drug may cause GI disturbances. Food may interfere with absorption, so give 1 to 2 hours before meals or 2 to 3 hours after.
• Don't give I.M. unless infection is severe or patient can't take oral dose.
• Large doses may cause increased yeast growths. Report symptoms to doctor.
• With prolonged therapy, other superinfections may occur, especially in the elderly, debilitated, or those with low

---

Italicized side effects are common or life-threatening.
∗Liquid form contains alcohol.   ∗∗May contain tartrazine.

resistance to infection due to immuno-suppressives or irradiation. Close observation is essential.

• Periodic assessments of renal, hepatic, and hematopoietic function should be made when therapy is prolonged.

• Check expiration date. Warn patient never to use leftover penicillin for a new illness or to share penicillin with family and friends.

hetacillin
Versapen

hetacillin potassium
Versapen K

INDICATIONS & DOSAGE
Systemic infections caused by susceptible strains of gram-positive and gram-negative organisms—
Adults: 225 to 450 mg P.O. q.i.d.
Children: 22.5 to 45 mg/kg P.O. daily, divided into doses given q 6 hours.

SIDE EFFECTS
Blood: thrombocytopenia, thrombocytopenic purpura, eosinophilia, leukopenia.
GI: vomiting, *nausea, epigastric distress, diarrhea,* glossitis, stomatitis.
Local: pain at injection site, vein irritation, phlebitis.
Other: *hypersensitivity (chills, fever, anaphylaxis, maculopapular rash, urticaria),* overgrowth of nonsusceptible organisms.

INTERACTIONS
Chloramphenicol, erythromycin, tetracyclines: antibiotic antagonism. Give penicillins at least 1 hour before bacteriostatic antibiotics.
Probenecid: increased blood levels of penicillin. Probenecid is often used for this purpose.

NURSING CONSIDERATIONS
• Contraindicated in patients with

mononucleosis. Use cautiously in patients with other drug allergies, especially to cephalosporins (possible cross-allergenicity), or with gastrointestinal disturbances.

• Obtain cultures for sensitivity tests before first dose. Unnecessary to wait for test results before beginning therapy.

• Before giving hetacillin, ask patient if he's had any allergic reactions to penicillin. However, a negative history of penicillin allergy is no guarantee against a future allergic reaction.

• Tell patient to take medication exactly as prescribed, even if he feels better. Entire quantity prescribed should be taken.

• Tell patient to call the doctor if rash, fever, or chills develop. A rash is the most common allergic reaction.

• When given orally, drug may cause GI disturbances. Food may interfere with absorption, so give 1 to 2 hours before meals or 2 to 3 hours after.

• Large doses may cause increased yeast growths. Report symptoms to doctor.

• With prolonged therapy, other superinfections may occur, especially in the elderly, debilitated, or those with low resistance to infection due to immuno-suppressives or irradiation. Close observation is essential.

• Check expiration date. Warn patient never to use leftover penicillin for a new illness or to share penicillin with family and friends.

• Very similar to ampicillin.

methicillin sodium
Celbenin, Staphcillin♦

INDICATIONS & DOSAGE
Systemic infections caused by penicillinase-producing staphylococci—
Adults: 4 to 12 g I.M. or I.V. daily, divided into doses given q 4 to 6 hours.
Children: 100 to 200 mg/kg I.M. or

I.V. daily, divided into doses given q
4 to 6 hours.

SIDE EFFECTS
Blood: *eosinophilia,* hemolytic anemia,
transient neutropenia.
CNS: neuropathy, convulsions with
high doses.
GI: glossitis, stomatitis.
GU: interstitial nephritis.
Local: *vein irritation, thrombophlebitis.*
Other: *hypersensitivity (chills, fever,
edema, rash, urticaria, anaphylaxis),*
overgrowth of nonsusceptible organisms.

INTERACTIONS
*Chloramphenicol, erythromycin, tetra-
cyclines:* antibiotic antagonism. Give
penicillins at least 1 hour before bacteriostatic antibiotics.
Probenecid: increases blood levels of
penicillin. Probenecid is often used for
this purpose.

NURSING CONSIDERATIONS
• Use cautiously in patients with other
drug allergies, especially to cephalosporins (possible cross-allergenicity),
and in infants.
• Obtain cultures for sensitivity tests
before first dose. Unnecessary to wait
for test results before starting therapy.
• Before giving methicillin, ask patient
if he's had any allergic reactions to penicillin. However, a negative history of
penicillin allergy is no guarantee
against a future allergic reaction.
• If ordered 4 times a day, be sure to
give every 6 hours—even during the
night.
• Urinalysis should be done frequently
to monitor renal function.
• If patient has high blood level of this
drug, he may have convulsions. Be prepared by keeping side rails up on bed.
• Dosage should be altered in patients
with impaired hepatic and renal functions.
• When giving I.V., mix with a normal

saline solution. Don't mix with others
because methicillin may be inactivated.
Initial dilution must be made with sterile water for injection.
• Give I.V. intermittently to prevent
vein irritation. Change site every
48 hours.
• Large doses may cause increased
yeast growths. Report symptoms to
doctor.
• With prolonged therapy, other superinfections may occur, especially in the
elderly, debilitated, or those with low
resistance to infection due to immunosuppressives or irradiation. Close observation is essential.
• Periodic assessment of hepatic, is
renal, and hematopoietic function required during prolonged therapy.
• Check expiration date.

---

mezlocillin sodium
Mezlin

INDICATIONS & DOSAGE
*Systemic infections caused by suscepti-
ble strains of gram-positive and especially gram-negative organisms* (Proteus, Pseudomonas aeruginosa)—
Adults: 200 to 300 mg/kg daily I.V. or
I.M. given in 4 to 6 divided doses.
Usual dose is 3 g q 4 hours or 4 g q 6
hours. For very serious infections, up
to 24 g daily may be administered.
Children to age 12: 50 mg/kg q 4
hours by I.V. infusion or direct I.V. injection.

SIDE EFFECTS
Blood: *bleeding with high doses,* neu-
tropenia, eosinophilia, leukopenia,
thrombocytopenia.
CNS: neuromuscular irritability.
GI: nausea, diarrhea.
Local: pain at injection site, vein irrita-
tion, phlebitis.
Metabolic: *hypokalemia.*
Other: *hypersensitivity (edema, fever,
chills, rash, pruritus, urticaria, ana-*

Italicized side effects are common or life-threatening.
*Liquid form contains alcohol.   **May contain tartrazine.

phylaxis), overgrowth of nonsusceptible organisms.

INTERACTIONS
Gentamicin, tobramycin: chemically incompatible. Don't mix together in I.V. solution. Give 1 hour apart.
Chloramphenicol erythromycin, tetracyclines: antibiotic antagonism. Give penicillins at least 1 hour before bacteriostatic antibiotics.

NURSING CONSIDERATIONS
• Use cautiously in patients hypersensitive to drugs, especially to cephalosporins (possible cross-hypersensitivity), and those with bleeding tendencies, uremia, hypokalemia.
• Obtain cultures for sensitivity tests before starting therapy. Unnecessary to wait for culture and sensitivity results before starting therapy.
• Before giving mezlocillin, ask patient if he's had allergic reactions to penicillin. A negative history of penicillin allergy, however, is no guarantee against future allergic reaction.
• Dosage should be altered in patients with impaired hepatic and renal function.
• Check CBC frequently. Drug may cause thrombocytopenia.
• Monitor serum potassium level.
• Patient with high serum level of this drug may have convulsions. Take seizure precautions.
• When giving I.V., mix with 5% dextrose in water or other suitable I.V. fluids.
• Give I.V. intermittently to prevent vein irritation. Change site every 48 hours.
• Large doses may cause increased yeast growths. Report symptoms to doctor.
• Almost always used with another antibiotic, such as gentamicin.
• With prolonged therapy, superinfections may occur, especially in the elderly or debilitated, or those with low resistance to infection due to immuno-

suppressors or irradiation. Monitor patient closely.
• Check drug expiration date.
• Compared with similar antibiotics such as carbenicillin and ticarcillin, mezlocillin is less likely to cause hypokalemia.
• Drug may be better suited to patients on salt-free diets than carbenicillin and ticarcillin (contains 1.85 mEq Na/g of mezlocillin).

nafcillin sodium
Nafcil, Unipen♦

INDICATIONS & DOSAGE
Systemic infections caused by penicillinase-producing staphylococci—
Adults: 2 to 4 g P.O. daily, divided into doses given q 6 hours; 2 to 12 g I.M. or I.V. daily, divided into doses given q 4 to 6 hours.
Children: 50 to 100 mg/kg P.O. daily, divided into doses given q 4 to 6 hours; or 100 to 200 mg/kg I.M. or I.V. daily, divided into doses given q 4 to 6 hours.

SIDE EFFECTS
Blood: transient leukopenia, neutropenia, granulocytopenia, thrombocytopenia with high doses.
GI: *nausea,* vomiting, diarrhea.
Local: *vein irritation, thrombophlebitis.*
Other: *hypersensitivity (chills, fever, rash, pruritus, urticaria, anaphylaxis).*

INTERACTIONS
Chloramphenicol, erythromycin, tetracyclines: antibiotic antagonism. Give penicillins at least 1 hour before bacteriostatic antibiotics.
Probenecid: increases blood levels of penicillin. Probenecid is often used for this purpose.

NURSING CONSIDERATIONS
• Use cautiously in patients with other drug allergies, especially to cephalosporins (possible cross-allergenicity),

and in those with gastrointestinal distress.

• Obtain cultures for sensitivity tests before first dose. Unnecessary to wait for test results before starting therapy.

• Before giving nafcillin, ask patient if he's had any allergic reactions to penicillin. However, a negative history of penicillin allergy is no guarantee against a future allergic reaction.

• Tell patient to take medication exactly as prescribed, even if he feels better. Entire quantity prescribed should be taken.

• Tell patient to call the doctor if rash, fever, or chills develop. A rash is the most common allergic reaction.

• When given orally, drug may cause GI disturbances. Food may interfere with absorption, so give 1 to 2 hours before meals or 2 to 3 hours after.

• Don't give I.M. or I.V. unless infection is severe or patient can't take oral dose.

• When giving I.V., mix with 5% dextrose in water or a saline solution.

• Give I.V. intermittently to prevent vein irritation. Change site every 48 hours.

• Large doses may cause increased yeast growths. Report symptoms to doctor.

• With prolonged therapy, other superinfections may occur, especially in the elderly, debilitated, or those with low resistance to infection due to immunosuppressives or irradiation. Close observation is essential.

• Check expiration date. Warn patient never to use leftover penicillin for a new illness or to share penicillin with family and friends.

oxacillin sodium
Bactocill, Prostaphilin♦

INDICATIONS & DOSAGE
Systemic infections caused by penicillinase-producing staphylococci—
Adults: 2 to 4 g P.O. daily, divided into doses given q 6 hours; 2 to 12 g I.M. or I.V. daily, divided into doses given q 4 to 6 hours.
Children: 50 to 100 mg/kg P.O. daily, divided into doses given q 6 hours; 100 to 200 mg/kg I.M. or I.V. daily, divided into doses given q 4 to 6 hours.

SIDE EFFECTS
Blood: granulocytopenia, thrombocytopenia, eosinophilia, hemolytic anemia, transient neutropenia.
CNS: neuropathy.
GI: oral lesions.
GU: interstitial nephritis.
Hepatic: hepatitis.
Local: *thrombophlebitis.*
Other: *hypersensitivity (fever, chills, rash, urticaria, anaphylaxis),* overgrowth of nonsusceptible organisms.

INTERACTIONS
Probenecid: increases blood levels of penicillin. Probenecid is often used for this purpose.
Chloramphenicol, erythromycin, tetracyclines: antibiotic antagonism. Give penicillins at least 1 hour before bacteriostatic antibiotics.

NURSING CONSIDERATIONS
• Use cautiously in patients with other drug allergies, especially to cephalosporins (possible cross-allergenicity), in premature newborns, and in infants.

• Obtain cultures for sensitivity tests before first dose. Unnecessary to wait for test results before starting therapy.

• Before giving oxacillin, ask patient if he's had any allergic reactions to penicillin. However, a negative history of penicillin allergy is no guarantee against a future allergic reaction.

• Tell the patient to take medication exactly as prescribed, even if he feels better. The entire quantity prescribed should be taken.

• Tell patient to call the doctor if rash, fever, or chills develop. A rash is the most common allergic reaction.

• When given orally, drug may cause

GI disturbances. Food may interfere with absorption, so give 1 to 2 hours before meals or 2 to 3 hours after.
• Don't give I.M. or I.V. unless infection is severe or patient can't take oral dose.
• Periodic liver function studies are indicated; watch for elevated SGOT and SGPT.
• When giving I.V., mix with 5% dextrose in water or a saline solution.
• Give I.V. intermittently to prevent vein irritation. Change site every 48 hours.
• Large doses may cause increased yeast growths. Report symptoms to doctor.
• With prolonged therapy, other superinfections may occur, especially in the elderly, debilitated, or those with low resistance to infection due to immunosuppressives or irradiation. Close observation is essential.
• Check expiration date. Warn patient never to use leftover penicillin for a new illness or to share penicillin with family and friends.

penicillin G benzathine
Bicillin L-A♦, Megacillin Suspension♦♦, Permapen

INDICATIONS & DOSAGE
Congenital syphilis—
Children under age 2: 50,000 units/kg I.M. as a single dose.
Group A streptococcal upper respiratory infections—
Adults: 1.2 million units I.M. in a single injection.
Children over 27 kg: 900,000 units I.M. in a single injection.
Children under 27 kg: 300,000 to 600,000 units I.M. in a single injection.
Prophylaxis of poststreptococcal rheumatic fever—
Adults and children: 1.2 million units I.M. once a month or 600,000 units twice a month.

Syphilis of less than 1 year's duration—
Adults: 2.4 million units I.M. in a single dose.
Syphilis of more than 1 year's duration—
Adults: 2.4 million units I.M. weekly for 3 successive weeks.

SIDE EFFECTS
Blood: eosinophilia, hemolytic anemia, thrombocytopenia, leukopenia.
CNS: neuropathy, convulsions with high doses.
Local: pain and sterile abscess at injection site.
Other: *hypersensitivity (maculopapular and exfoliative dermatitis, chills, fever, edema, anaphylaxis).*

INTERACTIONS
Chloramphenicol, erythromycin, tetracyclines: antibiotic antagonism. Give penicillins at least 1 hour before bacteriostatic antibiotics.
Probenecid: increases blood levels of penicillin. Probenecid is often used for this purpose.

NURSING CONSIDERATIONS
• Use cautiously in patients with other drug allergies, especially to cephalosporins (possible cross-allergenicity).
• Obtain cultures for sensitivity tests before first dose. Unnecessary to wait for test results before beginning therapy.
• Before giving penicillin, ask patient if he's had any allergic reactions to this drug. However, a negative history of penicillin allergy is no guarantee against a future allergic reaction.
• Tell patient to call the doctor if rash, fever, or chills develop. Fever and eosinophilia are the most common allergic reactions.
• Shake medication well before injection.
• Never give I.V. Inadvertent I.V. administration has caused cardiac arrest and death.

• Very slow absorption time makes allergic reactions difficult to treat.
• Inject deeply into upper outer quadrant of buttocks in adults; in midlateral thigh in infants and small children.
• Check expiration date.

penicillin G potassium
Arcocillin, Biotic-T, Burcillin-G, Cryspen, Deltapen, Falapen♦♦, Hyasorb, Hylenta♦♦, Ka-Pen♦♦, Lanacillin, Megacillin♦♦, Novopen-G♦, Parcillin, Pensorb, Pentids**, P-50♦♦, Pfizerpen

INDICATIONS & DOSAGE
Moderate to severe systemic infections—
Adults: 1.6 to 3.2 million units P.O. daily, divided into doses given q 6 hours (1 mg = 1,600 units); 1.2 to 24 million units I.M. or I.V. daily, divided into doses given q 4 hours.
Children: 25,000 to 100,000 units/kg P.O. daily, divided into doses given q 6 hours; or 25,000 to 300,000 units/kg I.M. or I.V. daily, divided into doses given q 4 hours.

SIDE EFFECTS
Blood: hemolytic anemia, leukopenia, thrombocytopenia.
CNS: neuropathy, convulsions with high doses.
Metabolic: possible severe potassium poisoning with high doses (hyperreflexia, convulsions, coma).
Local: *thrombophlebitis, pain at injection site.*
Other: *hypersensitivity (rash, urticaria, maculopapular eruptions, exfoliative dermatitis, chills, fever, edema, anaphylaxis),* overgrowth of nonsusceptible organisms.

INTERACTIONS
Chloramphenicol, erythromycin, tetracyclines: antibiotic antagonism. Give penicillins at least 1 hour before bacteriostatic antibiotics.
Probenecid: increases blood levels of penicillin. Probenecid is often used for this purpose.

NURSING CONSIDERATIONS
• Use cautiously in patients with other drug allergies, especially to cephalosporins (possible cross-allergenicity).
• Obtain cultures for sensitivity tests before first dose. Unnecessary to wait for results before beginning therapy.
• Before giving penicillin, ask patient if he's had any allergic reactions to this drug. However, a negative history of penicillin allergy is no guarantee against a future allergic reaction.
• Tell patient to take medication exactly as prescribed, even if he feels better.
• Tell patient to call the doctor if rash, fever, or chills develop. A rash is the most common allergic reaction.
• When given orally, drug may cause GI disturbances. Food may interfere with absorption, so give 1 to 2 hours before meals or 2 to 3 hours after.
• Don't give I.M. or I.V. unless infection is severe or patient can't take oral dose. Extremely painful when given I.M. Inject deep into large muscle.
• If patient has high blood level of this drug, he may have convulsions. Be prepared by keeping side rails up on bed.
• When giving I.V., mix with 5% dextrose in water or a saline solution.
• Give I.V. intermittently to prevent vein irritation. Change site every 48 hours.
• Large doses may cause increased yeast growths. Report symptoms to doctor.
• With prolonged therapy, other superinfections may occur, especially in the elderly, debilitated, or those with low resistance to infection due to immunosuppressives or irradiation. Close observation is essential.
• Check expiration date. Warn patient never to use leftover penicillin for a new illness or to share penicillin with family and friends.

Italicized side effects are common or life-threatening.
*Liquid form contains alcohol.   **May contain tartrazine.

penicillin G procaine
Ayercillin♦♦, Crysticillin A.S.,
Duracillin A.S., Pfizerpen A.S.,
Wycillin♦

INDICATIONS & DOSAGE
Moderate to severe systemic infections—
Adults: 600,000 to 1.2 million units
I.M. daily given as a single dose.
Children: 300,000 units I.M. daily
given as a single dose.
Uncomplicated gonorrhea—
Adults and children over 12 years:
give 1 g probenecid; then 30 minutes
later give 4.8 million units of penicillin
G procaine I.M., divided into two in-
jection sites.
Pneumococcal pneumonia—
Adults and children over 12 years:
300,000 to 600,000 units I.M. daily q
6 to 12 hours.

SIDE EFFECTS
Blood: thrombocytopenia, hemolytic
anemia, leukopenia.
CNS: arthralgia, convulsions.
Other: *hypersensitivity (rash, urticaria, chills, fever, edema, prostration,
anaphylaxis),* overgrowth of nonsusceptible organisms.

INTERACTIONS
*Chloramphenicol, erythromycin, tetra-
cyclines:* antibiotic antagonism. Give
penicillins at least 1 hour before bacteriostatic antibiotics.
Probenecid: increases blood levels of
penicillin. Probenecid is often used for
this purpose.

NURSING CONSIDERATIONS
• Contraindicated in patients with
hypersensitivity to procaine. Use cautiously in patients with other drug allergies, especially to cephalosporins (possible cross-allergenicity).
• Obtain cultures for sensitivity tests
before first dose. Unnecessary to wait
for test results before beginning
therapy.

• Before giving penicillin, ask patient
if he's had any allergic reactions to this
drug. However, a negative history of
penicillin allergy is no guarantee
against a future allergic reaction.
• Tell patient to call doctor if rash, fever, or chills develop. A rash is the
most common allergic reaction.
• Give deep I.M. in upper outer quadrant of buttocks in adults; in midlateral
thigh in small children. Do not give
subcutaneously.
• Never give I.V. Inadvertent I.V.
administration has caused death, due
to CNS toxicity from procaine.
• Large doses may cause increased
yeast growths. Report symptoms to
doctor.
• Due to slow absorption rate, allergic
reactions are hard to treat.
• With prolonged therapy, other superinfections may occur, especially in the
elderly, debilitated, or those with low
resistance to infection due to immunosuppressives or irradiation. Close observation is essential.
• Periodic evaluations of renal and
hematopoietic function are recommended.
• Check expiration date.

penicillin G sodium
Crystapen♦♦

INDICATIONS & DOSAGE
Moderate to severe systemic infections—
Adults: 1.2 to 24 million units daily
I.M. or I.V., divided into doses given q
4 hours.
Children: 25,000 to 300,000 units/kg
daily I.M. or I.V., divided into doses
given q 4 hours.

SIDE EFFECTS
Blood: hemolytic anemia, leukopenia,
thrombocytopenia.
CNS: arthralgia, neuropathy, convulsions.
CV: *congestive heart failure with high
doses.*

Unmarked trade names available in the United States only.
♦ Also available in Canada.   ♦♦ Available in Canada only.

Local: *vein irritation, pain at injection site, thrombophlebitis.*
Other: *hypersensitivity (chills, fever, edema, maculopapular rash, exfoliative dermatitis, urticaria, anaphylaxis),* overgrowth of nonsusceptible organisms.

INTERACTIONS
Chloramphenicol, erythromycin, tetracyclines: antibiotic antagonism. Give penicillins at least 1 hour before bacteriostatic antibiotics.
Probenecid: increases blood levels of penicillin. Probenecid is often used for this purpose.

NURSING CONSIDERATIONS
• Contraindicated in patients on sodium restriction. Use cautiously in patients with other drug allergies, especially to cephalosporins (possible cross-allergenicity).
• Obtain cultures for sensitivity tests before first dose. Unnecessary to wait for test results before beginning therapy.
• Before giving penicillin, ask patient if he's had any allergic reactions to this drug. However, a negative history of penicillin allergy is no guarantee against a future allergic reaction.
• If patient has high blood level of this drug, he may have convulsions. Be prepared by keeping side rails up on bed.
• When giving I.V., mix with 5% dextrose in water or a saline solution.
• Give I.V. intermittently to prevent vein irritation. Change site every 48 hours.
• Large doses may cause increased yeast growths. Report symptoms to doctor.
• With prolonged therapy, other superinfections may occur, especially in the elderly, debilitated, or those with low resistance to infection due to immunosuppressives or irradiation. Close observation is essential.
• Monitor vital signs frequently.
• Monitor serum sodium.

• Check expiration date.

---

penicillin V
Biotic Powder, Ledercillin VK♦, Pfizerpen VK♦, Robicillin-VK, SK-Penicillin VK, Uticillin VK, V-Pen

penicillin V potassium
Betapen VK, Biotic-V-Powder, Bopen V-K, Cocillin V-K, Lanacillin VK, Ledercillin VK♦, LV, Nadopen-V♦♦, Novopen-V♦♦, Penapar VK, Penbec-V♦♦, Pen-Vee-K♦, Pfizerpen VK, PVF K♦♦, Uticillin VK, V-Cillin K♦, Veetids**

INDICATIONS & DOSAGE
Mild to moderate systemic infections—
Adults: 250 to 500 mg (400,000 to 800,000 units) P.O. q 6 hours.
Children: 15 to 50 mg/kg (25,000 to 90,000 units/kg) P.O. daily, divided into doses given q 6 to 8 hours.
Endocarditis prophylaxis for dental surgery—
Adults: 0.5 g P.O. q 6 hours for 8 doses after procedure. Parenteral penicillin or P.O. penicillin V is given 30 to 60 minutes before procedure.
Children under 30 kg: ½ of the adult dose.

SIDE EFFECTS
Blood: eosinophilia, hemolytic anemia, leukopenia, thrombocytopenia.
CNS: neuropathy.
GI: *epigastric distress,* vomiting, diarrhea, *nausea.*
Other: *hypersensitivity (rash, urticaria, chills, fever, edema, anaphylaxis),* overgrowth of nonsusceptible organisms.

INTERACTIONS
Chloramphenicol, erythromycin, tetracyclines: antibiotic antagonism. Give penicillins at least 1 hour before bacteriostatic antibiotics.
Neomycin: decreases absorption of penicillin. Give penicillin by injection.

Italicized side effects are common or life-threatening.
*Liquid form contains alcohol.   **May contain tartrazine.

Probenecid: increases blood levels of penicillin. Probenecid is often used for this purpose.

NURSING CONSIDERATIONS

• Use cautiously in patients with other drug allergies, especially to cephalosporins (possible cross-allergenicity) and GI disturbances.

• Obtain cultures for sensitivity tests before first dose. Unnecessary to wait for test results before beginning therapy.

• Before giving penicillin, ask patient if he's had any allergic reactions to this drug. However, a negative history of penicillin allergy is no guarantee against a future allergic reaction.

• Tell patient to take medication exactly as prescribed, even if he feels better. Entire quantity prescribed should be taken.

• Tell patient to call the doctor if rash, fever, or chills develop. A rash is the most common allergic reaction.

• May cause GI disturbances. Food may interfere with absorption, so give 1 to 2 hours before meals or 2 to 3 hours after.

• Large doses may cause increased yeast growths. Report symptoms to doctor.

• Patients being treated for streptococcal infections should take the drug until the full 10-day course is completed.

• With prolonged therapy, other superinfections may occur, especially in the elderly, debilitated, or those with low resistance to infection due to immunosuppressives or irradiation. Close observation is essential.

• Periodic renal and hematopoietic function studies are recommended in patients receiving prolonged therapy.

• Check expiration date. Warn patient never to use leftover penicillin for a new illness or to share penicillin with family and friends.

piperacillin sodium
Pipracil

INDICATIONS & DOSAGE
*Systemic infections caused by susceptible strains of gram-positive and especially gram-negative organisms (*Proteus, Pseudomonas aeruginosa*)—*
Adults and children over 12 years:
100 to 300 mg/kg daily divided q 4 to 6 hours I.V. or I.M. Doses for children under 12 years not established.

SIDE EFFECTS
Blood: *bleeding with high doses,* neutropenia, eosinophilia, leukopenia, *thrombocytopenia.*
CNS: neuromuscular irritability, headache, dizziness.
GI: nausea, diarrhea.
Local: pain at injection site, vein irritation, phlebitis.
Metabolic: *hypokalemia.*
Other: *hypersensitivity (edema, fever, chills, rash, pruritus, urticaria, anaphylaxis),* overgrowth of nonsusceptible organisms.

INTERACTIONS
Gentamicin, tobramycin: chemically incompatible. Don't mix together in I.V. solution. Give 1 hour apart.
Chloramphenicol, erythromycin, tetracyclines: antibiotic antagonism. Give penicillins at least 1 hour before bacteriostatic antibiotics.

NURSING CONSIDERATIONS
• Use cautiously in patients hypersensitive to drugs, especially to cephalosporins (possible cross-hypersensitivity), and those with bleeding tendencies, uremia, hypokalemia.

• Obtain cultures for sensitivity tests before starting therapy. Unnecessary to wait for culture and sensitivity results before starting therapy.

• Before giving piperacillin, ask patient if he's had allergic reactions to penicillin. A negative history of peni-

---
Unmarked trade names available in the United States only.
♦ Also available in Canada.   ♦ ♦ Available in Canada only.

cillin allergy, however, is no guarantee against future allergic reaction.
• Dosage should be altered in patients with impaired hepatic and renal function.
• Check CBC frequently. Drug may cause thrombocytopenia.
• Monitor serum potassium level.
• Patient with high serum level of this drug may have convulsions. Take seizure precautions.
• When giving I.V., mix with 5% dextrose in water or other suitable I.V. fluids.
• Give I.V. intermittently to prevent vein irritation. Change site every 48 hours.
• Large doses may cause increased yeast growths. Report symptoms to doctor.
• Almost always used with another antibiotic, such as gentamicin.
• With prolonged therapy, superinfections may occur, especially in the elderly or debilitated, or those with low resistance to infection due to immunosuppressors or irradiation. Monitor patient closely.
• Check drug expiration date.
• Compared with similar antibiotics, such as carbenicillin and ticarcillin, piperacillin is less likely to cause hypokalemia.
• Drug may be better suited to patients on salt-free diets than carbenicillin and ticarcillin (contains 1.98 mEq Na/g of piperacillin).
• Piperacillin has shown greater activity against *Pseudomonas aeruginosa* than carbenicillin, ticarcillin, or mezlocillin.

---

ticarcillin disodium
Ticar

INDICATIONS & DOSAGE
Severe systemic infections caused by susceptible strains of gram-positive and especially gram-negative organisms (Pseudomonas, Proteus)—

Adults: 18 g I.V. or I.M. daily, divided into doses given q 4 to 6 hours.
Children: 200 to 300 mg/kg I.V. or I.M. daily, divided into doses given q 4 to 6 hours.

SIDE EFFECTS
Blood: leukopenia, neutropenia, eosinophilia, *thrombocytopenia,* hemolytic anemia.
CNS: convulsions, neuromuscular excitability.
GI: nausea, diarrhea.
Metabolic: *hypokalemia.*
Local: pain at injection site, vein irritation, phlebitis.
Other: *hypersensitivity (rash, pruritus, urticaria, chills, fever, edema, anaphylaxis),* overgrowth of nonsusceptible organisms.

INTERACTIONS
Chloramphenicol, erythromycin, tetracyclines: antibiotic antagonism. Give penicillins at least 1 hour before bacteriostatic antibiotics.
Probenecid: increases blood levels of penicillin. Probenecid is often used for this purpose.
Gentamicin, tobramycin: chemically incompatible. Don't mix together in I.V. Give 1 hour apart.

NURSING CONSIDERATIONS
• Use cautiously in patients with other drug allergies, especially to cephalosporins (possible cross-allergenicity); and in patients with impaired renal function, hemorrhagic conditions, hypokalemia, or sodium restrictions (contains 5.2 mEq sodium/g).
• Obtain cultures for sensitivity tests before first dose. Unnecessary to wait for test results before beginning therapy.
• Before giving ticarcillin, ask patient if he's had any allergic reactions to penicillin. However, a negative history of penicillin allergy is no guarantee against a future allergic reaction.
• Dosage should be decreased in pa-

Italicized side effects are common or life-threatening.
*Liquid form contains alcohol.   **May contain tartrazine.

tients with impaired hepatic and renal functions.

• Check CBC frequently. Drug may cause thrombocytopenia.

• If patient has high blood level of this drug, he may develop convulsions. Be prepared by keeping side rails up on bed.

• When giving I.V., mix with 5% dextrose in water or other suitable I.V. fluids.

• Give I.V. intermittently to prevent vein irritation. Change site every 48 hours.

• Administer deep I.M. into large muscle.

• Large doses may cause increased yeast growths. Report symptoms to doctor.

• Almost always used with another antibiotic, such as gentamicin.

• With prolonged therapy, other super-infections may occur, especially in the elderly, debilitated, or those with low resistance to infection due to immuno-suppressives or irradiation. Close observation is essential.

• Monitor serum potassium.

• Check expiration date.

12

Cephalosporins

cefaclor
cefadroxil monohydrate
cefamandole naftate
cefazolin sodium
cefotaxime
cefoxitin sodium
cephalexin monohydrate
cephaloglycin dihydrate
cephalothin sodium
cephapirin sodium
cephradine
moxalactam disodium

MECHANISM OF ACTION
Cephalosporins are either bactericidal or bacteriostatic, depending on organism susceptibility and reproduction rate, drug dose, and blood and tissue concentrations. They inhibit cell-wall synthesis, thereby making the wall less osmotically stable. They are more effective against young, rapidly dividing organisms than against mature, resting cells that are not in the process of cell-wall formation.

COMBINATION PRODUCTS
None.

cefaclor
Ceclor

INDICATIONS & DOSAGE
Treatment of infections of respiratory or urinary tracts, skin, and soft tissue; and otitis media due to Hemophilus influenzae, Streptococcus pneumoniae, Streptococcus pyogenes, Escherichia coli, Proteus mirabilis, Klebsiella *species, and staphylococci—*

Adults: 250 to 500 mg P.O. q 8 hours. Total daily dose should not exceed 4 g.
Children: 20 mg/kg daily P.O. in divided doses q 8 hours. In more serious infections, 40 mg/kg daily are recommended, not to exceed 1 g per day.

SIDE EFFECTS
Blood: transient leukopenia, lymphocytosis, anemia, eosinophilia.
CNS: dizziness, headache, somnolence.
GI: *nausea,* vomiting, diarrhea, anorexia.
GU: red and white cells in urine, vaginal moniliasis, vaginitis.
Skin: *maculopapular rash,* dermatitis.
Other: hypersensitivity, fever.

INTERACTIONS
Probenecid: may inhibit excretion and increase blood levels of cefaclor. Use together cautiously.

NURSING CONSIDERATIONS
• Contraindicated in hypersensitivity to other cephalosporins. Use cautiously in patients with impaired renal status and in those with history of sensitivity to penicillin. Ask patient if he's had any reaction to previous cephalosporin or penicillin therapy before administering first dose.
• Prolonged use may result in overgrowth of nonsusceptible organisms. Careful observation of patient for superinfection is essential.
• Obtain cultures for sensitivity tests before first dose, but therapy may begin pending test results.
• Major clinical use appears to be in

treating otitis media caused by *H. influenzae* when resistant to ampicillin or amoxicillin.
• Tell patient to take medication exactly as prescribed, even after he feels better.
• Call doctor if skin rash develops.
• Store reconstituted suspension in refrigerator. Stable for 14 days if refrigerated. Shake well before using.
• Drug may be taken with meals.
• Cefaclor is a relatively expensive antibiotic and should be used only when the organism is resistant to other agents.
• If ordered, total daily dose of cefaclor may be administered twice daily rather than 3 times daily with similar therapeutic results.

cefadroxil monohydrate
Duricef, Ultracef

INDICATIONS & DOSAGE
Treatment of urinary tract infections caused by Escherichia coli, Proteus mirabilis, *and* Klebsiella *species; infections of skin and soft tissue; and streptococcal pharyngitis—*
Adults: 500 mg to 2 g P.O. per day, depending on the infection being treated. Usually given in once-daily or b.i.d. dosage.
Children: 30 mg/kg daily in 2 divided doses.

SIDE EFFECTS
Blood: transient neutropenia, eosinophilia, leukopenia, anemia.
CNS: dizziness, headache, malaise, paresthesias.
GI: *nausea*, anorexia, vomiting, *diarrhea*, glossitis, *dyspepsia*, abdominal cramps, anal pruritus, tenesmus, oral candidiasis (thrush).
GU: genital pruritus, moniliasis.
Skin: *maculopapular and erythematous rashes.*
Other: dyspnea.

INTERACTIONS
Probenecid: may inhibit excretion and increase blood levels of cefadroxil. Use together cautiously.

NURSING CONSIDERATIONS
• Contraindicated in hypersensitivity to other cephalosporins. Use cautiously in patients with impaired renal status and in those with history of sensitivity to penicillin. Ask patient if he's had any reaction to previous cephalosporin or penicillin therapy before administering first dose.
• Prolonged use may result in overgrowth of nonsusceptible organisms. Careful observation of patient for superinfection is essential.
• Obtain cultures for sensitivity tests before first dose, but therapy may begin pending test results.
• If creatinine clearance is below 50 ml/minute, dosage interval should be lengthened so drug doesn't accumulate.
• Tell patient to take medication exactly as prescribed, even after he feels better.
• Call doctor if skin rash develops.
• Absorption not delayed by presence of food.
• Longer half-life permits twice-daily dosing.

cefamandole naftate
Mandol

INDICATIONS & DOSAGE
Treatment of serious infections of respiratory and genitourinary tracts, skin and soft-tissue infections, bone and joint infections, septicemia, and peritonitis due to Escherichia coli *and other coliform bacteria,* Staphylococcus aureus *(penicillinase- and nonpenicillinase-producing),* Staphyloccus epidermidis, *group A beta-hemolytic streptococci,* Klebsiella, Hemophilus influenzae, Proteus mirabilis, *and* Enterobacter *species—*

Adults: 500 mg to 1 g q 4 to 8 hours. In life-threatening infections, up to 2 g q 4 hours may be needed.

Infants and children: 50 to 100 mg/kg daily in equally divided doses q 4 to 8 hours. May be increased to total daily dose of 150 mg/kg (not to exceed maximum adult dose) for severe infections. Total daily dosage is same for I.M. or I.V. administration and depends on susceptibility of organism and severity of infection. In patients with impaired renal function, doses or frequency of administration must be modified according to degree of renal impairment, severity of infection, susceptibility of organism, and blood levels of drug. Should be injected deep I.M. into a large muscle mass, such as gluteus or lateral aspect of thigh.

SIDE EFFECTS

Blood: transient neutropenia, eosinophilia, hemolytic anemia, hypoprothrombinemia.
CNS: headache, malaise, paresthesias, dizziness.
GI: nausea, anorexia, vomiting, *diarrhea,* glossitis, dyspepsia, abdominal cramps, tenesmus, anal pruritus, oral candidiasis (thrush).
GU: nephrotoxicity, genital pruritus and moniliasis.
Skin: *maculopapular and erythematous rashes, urticaria.*
Local: *at injection site—pain, induration, sterile abscesses,* temperature elevation, tissue sloughing; *phlebitis and thrombophlebitis with I.V. injection.*
Other: *hypersensitivity,* dyspnea.

INTERACTIONS

Ethyl alcohol: may cause a disulfiram-like reaction. Warn patients not to drink alcohol for several days after discontinuing cefamandole.
Probenecid: may inhibit excretion and increase blood levels of cefamandole. Use together cautiously.

NURSING CONSIDERATIONS

• Contraindicated in hypersensitivity to other cephalosporins. Use cautiously in patients with impaired renal status and in those with history of sensitivity to penicillin. Ask patient if he's had any reaction to previous cephalosporin or penicillin therapy before administering first dose.
• Prolonged use may result in overgrowth of nonsusceptible organisms. Careful observation of patient for superinfection is essential.
• Obtain cultures for sensitivity tests before first dose, but therapy may begin pending test results.
• Cephalosporin of choice for treatment of *Enterobacter* sepsis.
• Not as effective as cefoxitin in treating anaerobic infections.
• For most cephalosporin-sensitive organisms, cefamandole offers little advantage over previously available agents.
• For I.V. use, reconstitute 1 g with 10 ml of sterile water for injection, 5% dextrose or 0.9% sodium chloride for injection. May be combined with the following intravenous fluids: 0.9% sodium chloride injection, 5% dextrose injection, 10% dextrose injection, 5% dextrose and 0.9% sodium chloride injection, 5% dextrose and 0.45% sodium chloride injection, 5% dextrose and 0.2% sodium chloride injection, or sodium lactate injection.
• I.M. cefamandole is not as painful as cefoxitin. Does not require addition of lidocaine.
• After reconstitution, remains stable for 24 hours at room temperature or 96 hours under refrigeration.

cefazolin sodium
Ancef♦, Kefzol♦

INDICATIONS & DOSAGE

Treatment of serious infections of respiratory and genitourinary tracts, skin and soft-tissue infections, bone and

---

Italicized side effects are common or life-threatening.
∗Liquid form contains alcohol.   ∗∗May contain tartrazine.

joint infections, septicemia, and endo-carditis due to Escherichia coli, *Entero-bacteriaceae, gonococci,* Hemophilus influenzae, Klebsiella, Proteus mirabi-lis, Staphylococcus aureus, Streptococ-cus pneumoniae, *and group A beta-he-molytic streptococci; and perioperative prophylaxis—*
Adults: 250 mg I.M. or I.V. q 8 hours to 1 g q 6 hours.
Children over 1 month: 8 to 16 mg/kg I.M. or I.V. q 8 hours, or 6 to 12 mg/kg q 6 hours.
Total daily dosage is same for I.M. or I.V. administration and depends on sus-ceptibility of organism and severity of infection. In patients with impaired renal function, doses or frequency of administration must be modified ac-cording to degree of renal impairment, severity of infection, susceptibility of organism, and serum levels of drug. Should be injected deep I.M. into a large muscle mass, such as gluteus or lateral aspect of thigh.

SIDE EFFECTS
Blood: transient neutropenia, leuko-penia, eosinophilia, anemia.
CNS: dizziness, headache, malaise, paresthesias.
GI: nausea, anorexia, vomiting, *diar-rhea,* glossitis, dyspepsia, abdominal cramps, anal pruritus, tenesmus, oral candidiasis (thrush).
GU: nephrotoxicity, genital pruritus and moniliasis, vaginitis.
Skin: *maculopapular and erythema-tous rashes, urticaria.*
Local: *at injection site—pain, indura-tion, sterile abscesses,* tissue sloughing; *phlebitis and thrombophlebitis with I.V. injection.*
Other: *hypersensitivity,* dyspnea.

INTERACTIONS
Probenecid: may increase blood levels of cephalosporins. Use together cau-tiously.

NURSING CONSIDERATIONS
• Use cautiously in patients with im-paired renal status and in those with history of sensitivity to penicillin. Ask patient if he's ever had any reaction to cephalosporin or penicillin therapy be-fore administering first dose.
• Avoid doses greater than 4 g daily in patients with severe renal impairment.
• Prolonged use may result in over-growth of nonsusceptible organisms. Watch carefully for superinfection.
• Obtain cultures for sensitivity tests before first dose, but therapy may begin pending test results.
• Because of long duration of effect, most infections can be treated with a single dose q 8 hours.
• For I.M. administration, reconstitute with sterile water, bacteriostatic water, or 0.9% sodium chloride solution as follows: 2 ml to 250-mg vial; 2 ml to 500-mg vial; 2.5 ml to 1-g vial. Shake well until dissolved. Resultant concen-tration: 125 mg/ml, 225 mg/ml, 330 mg/ml, respectively.
• Not as painful as other cephalospo-rins when given I.M.
• Alternate injection sites if I.V. ther-apy lasts longer than 3 days. Use of small I.V. needles in the larger avail-able veins may be preferable.
• For I.V. administration, reconstituted cefazolin sodium is diluted in 50 to 100 ml of 0.9% sodium chloride injec-tion, 5% or 10% dextrose injection, 5% dextrose in lactated Ringer's, 5% dex-trose and 0.9% sodium chloride, 5% dextrose and 0.45% or 0.2% sodium chloride, lactated Ringer's injection, Normosol-M in 5% dextrose in water, Ionosol B with 5% dextrose, or Plasma-Lyte with 5% dextrose.
• Reconstituted cefazolin sodium is stable for 24 hours at room tempera-ture, for 96 hours under refrigeration.
• About 40% to 75% of patients re-ceiving cephalosporins show a false-positive direct Coombs' test; only a few of these indicate hemolytic anemia.
• Urine glucose tests with Benedict's

Qualitative Reagent, Clinitest, or Fehling's solution may cause false-positive reaction during cephalosporin therapy. Clinistix, Diastix, and Tes-Tape are not affected.

cefotaxime
Claforan

INDICATIONS & DOSAGE
Treatment of serious infections of the lower respiratory and urinary tracts, gynecological infections, bacteremia, septicemia, and skin infections. Among susceptible microorganisms are streptococci, including Streptococcus pneumoniae *and* pyogenes; Staphylococcus aureus *(penicillinase- and nonpenicillinase-producing);* Staphylococcus epidermidis; Escherichia coli; Klebsiella *species;* Hemophilus influenzae; Enterobacter *species;* Proteus *species; and* Peptostreptococcus *species—*
Adults: usual dose is 1 g I.V. or I.M. q 6 to 8 hours. Up to 12 g daily can be administered in life-threatening infections.

Total daily dosage is same for I.M. or I.V. administration and depends on susceptibility of organism and severity of infection. In patients with impaired renal function, doses or frequency of administration must be modified according to degree of renal impairment, severity of infection, susceptibility of organism, and blood levels of drug. Should be injected deep I.M. into a large muscle mass, such as gluteus or lateral aspect of thigh.

SIDE EFFECTS
Blood: transient neutropenia, eosinophilia, hemolytic anemia.
CNS: headache, malaise, paresthesias, dizziness.
GI: nausea, anorexia, vomiting, diarrhea, glossitis, dyspepsia, abdominal cramps, tenesmus, anal pruritus, oral candidiasis (thrush).

GU: nephrotoxicity, genital pruritus and moniliasis.
Skin: *maculopapular and erythematous rashes, urticaria.*
Local: *at injection site–pain, induration, sterile abscesses, temperature elevation, tissue slough; phlebitis and thrombophlebitis with I.V. injection.*
Other: hypersensitivity, dyspnea.

INTERACTIONS
Probenecid: may inhibit excretion and increase blood levels of cefotaxime. Use together cautiously.

NURSING CONSIDERATIONS
• Contraindicated in hypersensitivity to other cephalosporins. Use cautiously in patients with impaired renal function and in those with history of sensitivity to penicillin. Ask patient if he's had any reaction to previous cephalosporin or penicillin therapy before administering first dose.
• Prolonged use may result in overgrowth of nonsusceptible organisms. Careful observation of patient for superinfection is essential.
• Obtain cultures for sensitivity tests before therapy, but therapy may begin pending results of cultures and sensitivity tests.
• Cefotaxime is the first of the so-called "third-generation" cephalosporins. It's said to have increased antibacterial activity against gram-negative microorganisms.
• Some doctors may prescribe cefotaxime in clinical situations in which they formerly prescribed aminoglycosides. However, this drug is not effective against infections caused by *Pseudomonas* organisms.
• For I.V. use, reconstitute with at least 10 ml sterile water for injection. Reconstituted solutions may be further diluted with sterile water for injection; 0.9% sodium chloride; 5% or 10% dextrose and 0.9% sodium chloride; 5% dextrose and 0.45% sodium chloride injection; 5% dextrose and 0.2% so-

---

Italicized side effects are common or life-threatening.
*Liquid form contains alcohol.   **May contain tartrazine.

dium chloride injection and lactated Ringer's solution.

cefoxitin sodium
Mefoxin

INDICATIONS & DOSAGE

Treatment of serious infection of respiratory and genitourinary tracts, skin and soft-tissue infections, bone and joint infections, bloodstream and intra-abdominal infections due to Escherichia coli *and other coliform bacteria,* Staphylococcus aureus *(penicillinase- and nonpenicillinase-producing),* Staphylococcus epidermidis, *strepto-cocci,* Klebsiella, Hemophilus influenzae, *and* Bacteroides *species, including* B. fragilis—

Adults: 1 to 2 g q 6 to 8 hours for un-complicated forms of infection. Up to 12 g daily in life-threatening infections.
Children: 80 to 160 mg/kg daily.
Total daily dosage is same for I.M. or I.V. administration and depends on susceptibility of organism and severity of infection. In patients with impaired renal function, doses or frequency of administration must be modified according to degree of renal impairment, severity of infection, susceptibility of organism, and blood levels of drug. Should be injected deep I.M. into a large muscle mass, such as gluteus or lateral aspect of thigh.

SIDE EFFECTS

Blood: transient neutropenia, eosinophilia, hemolytic anemia.
CNS: headache, malaise, paresthesias, dizziness.
GI: nausea, anorexia, vomiting, *diarrhea*, glossitis, dyspepsia, abdominal cramps, tenesmus, anal pruritus, oral candidiasis (thrush).
GU: nephrotoxicity, genital pruritus and moniliasis.
Skin: *maculopapular and erythematous rashes, urticaria.*
Local: *at injection site—pain, indura-tion, sterile abscesses, tissue sloughing; phlebitis and thrombophlebitis with I.V. injection.*
Other: *hypersensitivity,* dyspnea, elevated temperature.

INTERACTIONS

Probenecid: may inhibit excretion and increase blood levels of cefoxitin. Use together cautiously.

NURSING CONSIDERATIONS

• Contraindicated in hypersensitivity to other cephalosporins. Use cautiously in patients with impaired renal status and in those with history of sensitivity to penicillin. Ask patient if he's had any reaction to previous cephalosporin or penicillin therapy before administering first dose.
• Prolonged use may result in over-growth of nonsusceptible organisms. Observe patient for superinfection.
• Obtain cultures for sensitivity tests before first dose, but therapy may begin pending test results.
• A very useful cephalosporin when anaerobic or mixed aerobic-anaerobic infection is suspected, especially *B. fragilis.*
• For most cephalosporin-sensitive organisms, cefoxitin offers little advantage over previously available agents.
• For I.V. use, reconstitute 1 g with at least 10 ml of sterile water for injection, and 2 g with 10 to 20 ml. Solutions of 5% dextrose and 0.9% sodium chloride for injection can also be used. These primary solutions can be further diluted with the following solutions: Ringer's injection, lactated Ringer's injection, 5% dextrose in lactated Ringer's injection, 5% or 10% invert sugar in water, 10% invert sugar in saline solution, 5% sodium bicarbonate injection, Aminosol 5% solution, Normosol-M in 5% dextrose in water, Ionosol B with 5% dextrose, Polyonic M 56 in 5% dextrose.
• I.M. injection can be reconstituted

with 0.5% or 1% lidocaine HCl (without epinephrine) to minimize pain.
• May cause false-positive result for urine glucose with Clinitest tablets.
• May be useful in the treatment of resistant gonorrhea.
• After reconstitution, remains stable for 24 hours at room temperature or 1 week under refrigeration.

cephalexin monohydrate
Ceporex♦♦, Keflex♦

INDICATIONS & DOSAGE
Treatment of infections of respiratory or genitourinary tract, skin and soft-tissue infections, bone and joint infections, and otitis media due to Escherichia coli *and other coliform bacteria, group A beta-hemolytic streptococci,* Hemophilus influenzae, Klebsiella, Proteus mirabilis, Streptococcus pneumoniae, *and staphylococci—*
Adults: 250 mg to 1 g P.O. q 6 hours.
Children: 6 to 12 mg/kg P.O. q 6 hours. Maximum 25 mg/kg q 6 hours.

SIDE EFFECTS
Blood: transient neutropenia, eosinophilia, anemia.
CNS: dizziness, headache, malaise, paresthesias.
GI: *nausea, anorexia,* vomiting, *diarrhea,* glossitis, dyspepsia, abdominal cramps, anal pruritus, tenesmus, oral candidiasis (thrush).
GU: genital pruritus and moniliasis, vaginitis.
Skin: *maculopapular and erythematous rashes, urticaria.*
Other: *hypersensitivity,* dyspnea.

INTERACTIONS
Probenecid: may increase blood levels of cephalosporins. Use together cautiously.

NURSING CONSIDERATIONS
• Use cautiously in patients with impaired renal status and in those with history of sensitivity to penicillin. Ask patient if he's had any reaction to previous cephalosporin or penicillin therapy before administering first dose.
• Prolonged use may result in overgrowth of nonsusceptible organisms. Watch closely for superinfection.
• Obtain cultures for sensitivity tests before first dose, but therapy may begin pending test results.
• Tell patient to take medication exactly as prescribed, even after he feels better. Group A beta-hemolytic streptococcal infections should be treated for a minimum of 10 days.
• Call doctor if skin rash develops.
• Preparation of oral suspension: add required amount of water to powder in two portions. Shake well after each addition. After mixing, store in refrigerator. Stable for 14 days without significant loss of potency. Keep tightly closed and shake well before using.
• About 40% to 75% of patients receiving cephalosporins show a false-positive direct Coombs' test, but only a few of these indicate hemolytic anemia.
• Urine glucose tests with Benedict's Qualitative Reagent, Clinitest, or Fehling's solution may give false-positive results during cephalosporin therapy. Clinistix, Diastix, and Tes-Tape are not affected.

cephaloglycin dihydrate
Kafocin

INDICATIONS & DOSAGE
Treatment of acute and chronic urinary-tract infections, including cystitis, pyelitis, pyelonephritis, and asymptomatic bacteriuria when due to susceptible strains of Escherichia coli, Klebsiella, Enterobacter, Proteus, *staphylococci, and enterococci—*
Adults: 250 to 500 mg P.O. q 6 hours.

Italicized side effects are common or life-threatening.
*Liquid form contains alcohol.   **May contain tartrazine.

SIDE EFFECTS

Blood: transient neutropenia, eosinophilia, anemia.

CNS: dizziness, headache, malaise, paresthesias.

GI: *nausea, anorexia, vomiting, diarrhea,* glossitis, dyspepsia, abdominal cramps, anal pruritus, tenesmus, oral candidiasis (thrush).

GU: genital pruritus and moniliasis, vaginitis.

Skin: *maculopapular and erythematous rashes, urticaria.*

Other: *hypersensitivity,* dyspnea.

INTERACTIONS

Probenecid: may increase blood levels of cephalosporins. Use together cautiously.

NURSING CONSIDERATIONS

• Use cautiously in patients with impaired renal function and in those with history of sensitivity to penicillin. Ask patient if he's had any reaction to previous cephalosporin or penicillin therapy before administering first dose.

• Cephaloglycin blood levels are low; used only for urinary tract infections.

• Prolonged use may result in overgrowth of nonsusceptible organisms. Watch for superinfection.

• Obtain cultures for sensitivity tests before first dose, but therapy may begin pending test results.

• Tell patient to take medication exactly as prescribed, even after he feels better.

• About 40% to 75% of patients receiving cephalosporins show a false-positive direct Coombs' test, but only a few of these indicate hemolytic anemia.

• Urine glucose tests with Benedict's Qualitative Reagent, Clinitest, or Fehling's solution may give false-positive results during cephalosporin therapy. Clinistix, Diastix, and Tes-Tape are not affected.

cephalothin sodium
Keflin Neutral♦

INDICATIONS & DOSAGE

Treatment of serious infections of respiratory, genitourinary, or gastrointestinal tract; skin and soft-tissue infections (including peritonitis); bone and joint infections; septicemia; endocarditis; and meningitis due to Escherichia coli *and other coliform bacteria,* Enterobacteriaceae, enterococci, gonococci, group A beta-hemolytic streptococci, Hemophilus influenzae, Klebsiella, Proteus mirabilis, Salmonella, Staphylococcus aureus, Shigella, Streptococcus pneumoniae, *staphylococci, and* Streptococcus viridans—

Adults: 500 mg to 1 g I.M. or I.V. (or intraperitoneally) q 4 to 6 hours; in life-threatening infections, up to 2 g q 4 hours.

Children: 14 to 27 mg/kg I.V. q 4 hours, or 20 to 40 mg/kg q 6 hours; dose should be proportionately less in accordance with age, weight, and severity of infection.

Dosage schedule is determined by degree of renal impairment, severity of infection, and susceptibility of causative organism. Should be injected deep I.M. into a large muscle mass, such as gluteus or lateral aspect of thigh. I.V. route is preferable in severe or life-threatening infections.

SIDE EFFECTS

Blood: transient neutropenia, eosinophilia, hemolytic anemia.

CNS: headache, malaise, paresthesias, dizziness.

GI: nausea, anorexia, vomiting, *diarrhea,* glossitis, dyspepsia, abdominal cramps, tenesmus, anal pruritus, oral candidiasis (thrush).

GU: nephrotoxicity, genital pruritus and moniliasis.

Skin: maculopapular and erythematous rashes, urticaria.

Local: *at injection site—pain, indura-*

tion, sterile abscesses, tissue sloughing; phlebitis and thrombophlebitis with I.V. injection.
Other: *hypersensitivity,* dyspnea, temperature elevation.

INTERACTIONS
Probenecid: may increase blood levels of cephalosporins. Use together cautiously.

NURSING CONSIDERATIONS
• Use cautiously in patients with impaired renal function and in those with history of sensitivity to penicillin. Ask patient if he's had any reaction to previous cephalosporin or penicillin therapy before administering first dose.
• Obtain cultures for sensitivity tests before first dose, but therapy may begin pending test results.
• Prolonged use may result in overgrowth of nonsusceptible organisms. Watch for superinfection.
• Drug causes severe pain when administered I.M.; avoid this route if possible.
• When giving this drug I.V., check frequently for vein irritation and phlebitis. Alternate injection sites if I.V. therapy lasts longer than 3 days. Use of small I.V. needle in the larger available veins may be preferable. Addition of a small concentration of heparin (100 units) may reduce incidence of phlebitis.
• For I.M. administration, reconstitute each gram of cephalothin sodium with 4 ml of sterile water for injection, providing 500 mg in each 2.2 ml. If vial contents do not dissolve completely, add an additional 0.2 to 0.4 ml diluent, and warm contents slightly.
• For I.V. administration, dilute contents of 4-g vial with at least 20 ml of sterile water for injection, 5% dextrose injection, or 0.9% sodium chloride injection and add to one of following I.V. solutions: acetated Ringer's injection, 5% dextrose injection, 5% dextrose in lactated Ringer's injection, Ionosol B in

5% dextrose in water, lactated Ringer's injection, Normosol-N in 5% dextrose in water, Plasma-Lyte injection, Plasma-Lyte-N injection in 5% dextrose, Ringer's injection, or 0.9% sodium chloride injection. Choose solution and fluid volume according to patient's fluid and electrolyte status.
• About 40% to 75% of patients receiving cephalosporins show a false-positive direct Coombs' test; only a few of these indicate hemolytic anemia.
• Urine glucose tests with Benedict's Qualitative Reagent, Clinitest, or Fehling's solution may give false-positive results during cephalosporin therapy. Clinistix, Diastix, and Tes-Tape are not affected.

---

cephapirin sodium
Cefadyl♦

INDICATIONS & DOSAGE
Serious infections of respiratory, genitourinary, or gastrointestinal tract; skin and soft-tissue infections; bone and joint infections (including osteomyelitis); septicemia; endocarditis due to Streptococcus pneumoniae, Escherichia coli, *group A beta-hemolytic streptococci,* Hemophilus influenzae, Klebsiella, Proteus mirabilis, Staphylococcus aureus, *and* Streptococcus viridans—
Adults: 500 mg to 1 g I.V. or I.M. q 4 to 6 hours up to 12 g daily.
Children over 3 months: 10 to 20 mg/kg I.V. or I.M. q 6 hours; dose depends on age, weight, and severity of infection.
Should be injected deep I.M. into a large muscle mass, such as gluteus or lateral aspect of thigh. Depending upon causative organism and severity of infection, patients with reduced renal function may be treated adequately with a lower dose (7.5 to 15 mg/kg q 12 hours). Patients with severely reduced renal function and who are to be dialyzed should receive same dose just

---

Italicized side effects are common or life-threatening.
∗Liquid form contains alcohol.   ∗∗May contain tartrazine.

before dialysis and q 12 hours thereafter.

SIDE EFFECTS
Blood: transient neutropenia, eosinophilia, anemia.
CNS: dizziness, headache, malaise, paresthesias.
GI: nausea, anorexia, vomiting, *diarrhea,* glossitis, dyspepsia, abdominal cramps, tenesmus, anal pruritus, oral candidiasis (thrush).
GU: nephrotoxicity, genital pruritus and moniliasis, vaginitis.
Skin: *maculopapular and erythematous rashes, urticaria.*
Local: *at injection site—pain, induration, sterile abscesses, tissue sloughing; phlebitis and thrombophlebitis with I.V. injection.*
Other: *hypersensitivity,* dyspnea.

INTERACTIONS
Probenecid: may increase blood levels of cephalosporins. Use together cautiously.

NURSING CONSIDERATIONS
• Use cautiously in patients with impaired renal function and in those with a history of sensitivity to penicillin. Ask patient if he's had any reaction to previous cephalosporin or penicillin therapy before administering first dose.
• Prolonged use may result in overgrowth of nonsusceptible organisms. Watch for superinfection.
• Obtain cultures for sensitivity tests before first dose, but therapy may begin pending test results.
• For I.M. administration, reconstitute 1-g vial with 2 ml sterile water for injection or bacteriostatic water for injection so that 1.2 ml contains 500 mg of cephapirin. I.M. injection is painful; prepare patient for this.
• When giving this drug I.V., check frequently for vein irritation and phlebitis. Alternate injection sites if I.V. therapy lasts longer than 3 days. Use of small I.V. needles in the larger available veins may be preferable.
• Prepare I.V. infusion using dextrose injection, sodium chloride injection, or bacteriostatic water for injection as diluent: 20 ml yields 1 g per 10 ml; 50 ml yields 1 g per 25 ml; 100 ml yields 1 g per 50 ml.
• I.V. infusion with Y-tubing: during infusion of cephapirin solution, it is desirable to stop other solution. Check volume of cephapirin solution carefully so that calculated dose is infused. When Y-tubing is used, dilute 4-g vial with 40 ml of diluent.
• Compatible with following infusion solutions: sodium chloride injection, 5% dextrose in water, sodium lactate injection, 5% dextrose in normal saline solution, 10% invert sugar in normal saline solution, 10% invert sugar in water, 5% dextrose and 0.2% sodium chloride injection, lactated Ringer's with 5% dextrose, 5% dextrose and 0.45% sodium chloride injection, Ringer's injection, lactated Ringer's injection, 10% dextrose injection, sterile water for injection, 20% dextrose injection, 5% sodium chloride in water, and 5% dextrose in Ringer's injection.
• Reconstituted cephapirin is stable and compatible for 10 days under refrigeration and for 24 hours at room temperature.
• About 40% to 75% of patients receiving cephalosporins show a false-positive direct Coombs' test, but only a few indicate hemolytic anemia.
• Urine glucose tests with Benedict's Qualitative Reagent, Clinitest, or Fehling's solution may give false-positive results during cephalosporin therapy. Clinistix, Diastix, and Tes-Tape are not affected.

cephradine
Anspor, Velosef♦**

INDICATIONS & DOSAGE
Serious infection of respiratory, geni-

tourinary, or gastrointestinal tract; skin and soft-tissue infections; bone and joint infections; septicemia; endocarditis; and otitis media due to Escherichia coli *and other coliform bacteria, group A beta-hemolytic streptococci,* Hemophilus influenzae, Klebsiella, Proteus mirabilis, Staphylococcus aureus, Streptococcus pneumoniae, *staphylococci, and* Streptococcus viridans—
Adults: 500 mg to 1 g I.M. or I.V. 2 to 4 times daily; do not exceed 8 g daily. Or 250 to 500 mg P.O. q 6 hours. Severe or chronic infections may require larger and/or more frequent doses (up to 1 g P.O. q 6 hours).
Children over 1 year: 6 to 12 mg/kg P.O. q 6 hours. 12 to 25 mg/kg I.M. or I.V. q 6 hours.
Otitis media—19 to 25 mg/kg P.O. q 6 hours. Do not exceed 4 g daily.
All patients, regardless of age and weight: larger doses (up to 1 g q.i.d.) may be given for severe or chronic infections. Parenteral therapy may be followed by oral. Injections should be given deep I.M. into a large muscle mass, such as gluteus or lateral aspect of thigh.

SIDE EFFECTS
Blood: transient neutropenia, eosinophilia.
CNS: dizziness, headache, malaise, paresthesias.
GI: *nausea, anorexia,* vomiting, heartburn, glossitis, dyspepsia, abdominal cramping, *diarrhea,* tenesmus, anal pruritus, oral candidiasis (thrush).
GU: genital pruritus and moniliasis, vaginitis.
Skin: *maculopapular and erythematous rashes, urticaria.*
Local: *at injection site—pain, induration, sterile abscesses, tissue sloughing; phlebitis and thrombophlebitis with I.V. injection.*
Other: *hypersensitivity,* dyspnea.

INTERACTIONS
Probenecid: may increase blood levels of cephalosporins. Use together cautiously.

NURSING CONSIDERATIONS
• Use cautiously in patients with impaired renal function and in those with a history of sensitivity to penicillin. Ask patient if he's had any reaction to previous cephalosporin or penicillin therapy before administering first dose.
• Obtain cultures for sensitivity tests before first dose, but therapy may begin pending test results.
• Prolonged use may result in overgrowth of nonsusceptible organisms. Watch for superinfection.
• When giving this drug I.V., check frequently for vein irritation and phlebitis. Alternate injection sites if I.V. therapy lasts longer than 3 days. Use of small I.V. needle in the larger available veins may be preferable.
• Tell patient to take medication exactly as prescribed, even after he feels better. Group A beta-hemolytic streptococcal infections should be treated for a minimum of 10 days.
• I.M. injection is painful.
• For I.M. administration, reconstitute with sterile water for injection or with bacteriostatic water for injection as follows: 1.2 ml to 250-mg vial; 2 ml to 500-mg vial; 4 ml to 1-g vial. I.M. solutions must be used within 2 hours if kept at room temperature and within 24 hours if refrigerated. Solutions may vary in color from light straw to yellow without affecting potency.
• When preparing cephradine for intravenous administration, when available, use preparation specifically supplied for infusion. Follow specific product directions carefully when reconstituting.
• About 40% to 75% of patients receiving cephalosporins show a false-positive direct Coombs' test, but only a few indicate hemolytic anemia.
• Urine glucose tests with Benedict's Qualitative Reagent, Clinitest, or Fehling's solution may give false-positive

---

Italicized side effects are common or life-threatening.
＊Liquid form contains alcohol.　　＊＊May contain tartrazine.

results during cephalosporin therapy. Clinistix, Diastix, and Tes-Tape are not affected.

moxalactam disodium
Moxam

INDICATIONS & DOSAGE
Treatment of serious infections of lower respiratory and urinary tract, gynecologic infections, bacteremia, septicemia, and skin infections.
Susceptible microorganisms include Streptococcus pneumoniae *and* pyogenes; Staphylococcus aureus *(penicillinase- and nonpenicillinase-producing);* Staphylococcus epidermidis; Escherichia coli; Klebsiella; Hemophilus influenzae; Enterobacter; Proteus; *some* Pseudomonas *species; and* Peptostreptococcus.

Adults: Usual daily dose is 2 to 6 g I.M. or I.V. administered in divided doses q 8 hours for 5 to 10 days, or up to 14 days. Up to 12 g daily may be needed in life-threatening infections or in infections due to less susceptible organisms.
Children: 50 mg/kg I.M. or I.V. q 6 to 8 hours.
Neonates: 50 mg/kg I.M. or I.V. q 8 to 12 hours.
Total daily dosage is same for I.M. or I.V. administration and depends on susceptibility of organism and severity of infection. In patients with impaired renal function, doses or frequency of administration must be modified according to degree of impairment, severity of infection, susceptibility of organism, and blood levels of drug. Should be injected deep I.M. into the gluteus or lateral aspect of thigh.

SIDE EFFECTS
Blood: transient neutropenia, eosinophilia, hemolytic anemia, hypoprothrombinemia
CNS: headache, malaise, paresthesias, dizziness.
GI: nausea, anorexia, vomiting, *diarrhea,* glossitis, dyspepsia, abdominal cramps, tenesmus, pruritus ani, oral candidiasis (thrush).
GU: nephrotoxicity, genital moniliasis.
Skin: *maculopapular and erythematous rashes, urticaria.*
Local: *pain at injection site, induration, sterile abscesses, tissue sloughing; phlebitis and thrombophlebitis with I.V. injection.*
Other: *hypersensitivity,* dyspnea, elevated temperature.

INTERACTIONS
Ethyl alcohol: may cause a disulfiram-like reaction. Warn patients not to drink alcohol for several days after discontinuing moxalactam.
Probenecid: may inhibit excretion and increase blood levels of moxalactam. Use together cautiously.

NURSING CONSIDERATIONS
• Contraindicated in hypersensitivity to other cephalosporins. Use cautiously in patients with impaired renal function and in those with history of sensitivity to penicillin. Before administering first dose, ask patient if he's had any reaction to cephalosporin or penicillin.
• Prolonged use may result in overgrowth of nonsusceptible organisms. Monitor closely for superinfection.
• Obtain cultures for sensitivity tests before therapy. Unnecessary to wait for culture and sensitivity results before starting therapy.
• Moxalactam is one of the third generation cephalosporins. It's said to have increased antibacterial activity against gram-negative organisms. Doctors may prescribe moxalactam in clinical situations in which they formerly prescribed aminoglycosides.
• For direct intermittent I.V. administration, add 10 ml of sterile water for injection, 5% dextrose injection, or 0.9% NaCl injection/g of moxalactam.

13

Tetracyclines

demeclocycline hydrochloride
doxycycline hyclate
methacycline hydrochloride
minocycline hydrochloride
oxytetracycline hydrochloride
tetracycline hydrochloride
tetracycline phosphate complex

MECHANISM OF ACTION

Tetracyclines are thought to exert bacteriostatic effect by binding to the 30S ribosomal subunit of microorganisms, thus inhibiting protein synthesis.

COMBINATION PRODUCTS

MYSTECLIN-F CAPS: tetracycline HCl 250 mg and amphotericin B 50 mg buffered with potassium metaphosphate.
MYSTECLIN-F SYRUP: tetracycline HCl 125 mg and amphotericin B 25 mg per 5 ml, buffered with potassium metaphosphate.
For additional combinations, see Chapter 15, URINARY TRACT ANTISEPTICS.

demeclocycline hydrochloride

Declomycin♦, Ledermycin

INDICATIONS & DOSAGE

Infections caused by susceptible gram-negative and gram-positive organisms, trachoma, rickettsiae—
Adults: 150 mg P.O. q 6 hours or 300 mg P.O. q 12 hours.
Children over 8 years: 6 to 12 mg/kg P.O. daily, divided q 6 to 12 hours.
Gonorrhea—
Adults: 600 mg P.O. initially, then 300 mg P.O. q 12 hours for 4 days (total 3 g).
Syndrome of inappropriate ADH (a hyposmolar state)—
Adults: 600 to 1200 mg P.O. daily in divided doses.

SIDE EFFECTS

Blood: neutropenia, eosinophilia.
CV: pericarditis.
EENT: dysphagia, glossitis.
GI: anorexia, *nausea, vomiting, diarrhea,* enterocolitis, anogenital inflammation.
Metabolic: *increased BUN,* diabetes insipidus syndrome (polyuria, polydipsia, weakness).
Skin: *maculopapular and erythematous rashes, photosensitivity, increased pigmentation, urticaria.*
Other: hypersensitivity.

INTERACTIONS

Antacids (including $NaHCO_3$) and laxatives containing aluminum, calcium, and magnesium; food, milk, or other dairy products: decrease antibiotic absorption. Give antibiotic 1 hour before or 2 hours after any of the above.
Ferrous sulfate and other iron products, zinc: decrease antibiotic absorption. Give demeclocycline 3 hours after or 2 hours before iron administration.
Methoxyflurane: may cause nephrotoxicity with tetracyclines. Monitor carefully.

NURSING CONSIDERATIONS

- Use with extreme caution in impaired renal or hepatic function. Use of these drugs during last half of pregnancy and

Italicized side effects are common or life-threatening.
*Liquid form contains alcohol. **May contain tartrazine.

in children younger than 8 years may cause permanent discoloration of teeth, enamel defects, and retardation of bone growth.

• Obtain cultures before starting therapy.

• Check expiration date. Outdated or deteriorated demeclocycline may cause nephrotoxicity.

• Do not expose these drugs to light or heat; store in tight container.

• Watch for overgrowth of nonsusceptible organisms. Check patient's tongue for signs of monilia infection. Stress good oral hygiene. If superinfection occurs, drug should be discontinued.

• Observe patient for diarrhea, which may result from local irritation or superinfection.

• Warn patient to avoid direct sunlight and ultraviolet light. A sunscreen may help prevent photosensitivity reactions. Photosensitivity persists for some time after discontinuation of drug.

• Effectiveness is reduced when taken with milk or other dairy products, food, antacids, or iron products. Explain this to patient. Tell patient to take each dose with a full glass of water on an empty stomach, at least 1 hour before meals or 2 hours afterward. Give at least 1 hour before bedtime to prevent esophagitis.

• Instruct patient to take medication for as long as prescribed, exactly as prescribed, even after he feels better. Treat streptococcal infections for at least 10 days.

---

doxycycline hyclate
Doxychel, Vibramycin♦, Vibra Tabs

INDICATIONS & DOSAGE
Infections caused by sensitive gram-negative and gram-positive organisms, trachoma, rickettsiae—
Adults: 100 mg P.O. q 12 hours on first day, then 100 mg P.O. daily; or 200 mg I.V. on first day in 1 or 2 infusions, then 100 to 200 mg I.V. daily.

Children over 8 years (under 45 kg): 4.4 mg/kg P.O. or I.V. daily, divided q 12 hours first day, then 2.2 to 4.4 mg/kg daily. Over 45 kg, same as adults. Give I.V. infusion slowly (minimum time 1 hour). Infusion must be completed within 12 hours (within 6 hours in lactated Ringer's solution or 5% dextrose in lactated Ringer's solution).
Gonorrhea in patients allergic to penicillin—
Adults: 200 mg P.O. initially, followed by 100 mg P.O. at bedtime, and 100 mg P.O. b.i.d. for 3 days; or 300 mg P.O. initially and repeat dose in 1 hour.
Primary or secondary syphilis in patients allergic to penicillin—
Adults: 300 mg P.O. daily in divided doses for 10 days.

SIDE EFFECTS
Blood: neutropenia, eosinophilia.
CNS: intracranial hypertension.
CV: pericarditis.
EENT: sore throat, glossitis, dysphagia.
GI: anorexia, *epigastric distress, nausea,* vomiting, *diarrhea,* enterocolitis, anogenital inflammation.
Skin: *maculopapular and erythematous rashes, photosensitivity, increased pigmentation, urticaria.*
Local: thrombophlebitis.
Other: hypersensitivity.

INTERACTIONS
Antacids (including NaHCO$_3$) and laxatives containing aluminum, magnesium, or calcium: decrease antibiotic absorption. Give antibiotic 1 hour before or 2 hours after any of the above.
Ferrous sulfate and other iron products, zinc: decrease antibiotic absorption. Give doxycycline 3 hours after or 2 hours before iron administration.
Phenobarbital, carbamazepine, alcohol: decrease antibiotic effect. Avoid if possible.

NURSING CONSIDERATIONS
• Use of these drugs during last half of

---

pregnancy and in children younger than
8 years may cause permanent discoloration of teeth, enamel defects, and retardation of bone growth.
• Patient may develop thrombophlebitis with I.V. administration.
• Obtain cultures before starting therapy.
• Check expiration date.
• Don't expose drug to light or heat.
Protect from sunlight during infusion.
• Watch for overgrowth of nonsusceptible organisms. Check patient's tongue
for signs of monilia infection. Stress
good oral hygiene. If superinfection occurs, drug should be discontinued.
• Observe patient for diarrhea, which
may result from local irritation or superinfection.
• May be taken with milk or food if GI
side effects develop.
• Do not give with antacids.
• Tell patient to take medication exactly as prescribed, even after he feels
better. Treat streptococcal infections
for at least 10 days.
• Reconstitute powder for injection
with sterile water for injection. Use
10 ml in 100-mg vial and 20 ml in 200-
mg vial. Dilute solution to 100 to 1,000
ml before giving. Do not infuse solutions more concentrated than 1 mg/ml.
• Reconstituted solution is stable for 72
hours refrigerated.
• Doxycycline may be used in patients
with renal impairment; does not accumulate or cause a significant rise in
BUN.
• May cause false-positive reading of
Clinitest; false-negative reading of
Clinistix or Tes-Tape.
• Should not be taken within 1 hour of
bedtime because of increased incidence
of dysphagia.

methacycline hydrochloride
Rondomycin

INDICATIONS & DOSAGE
Infections caused by sensitive gram-
negative and gram-positive organisms,
trachoma, rickettsiae—
Adults: 150 mg P.O. q 6 hours or
300 mg q 12 hours.
Children over 8 years: 6 to 12 mg/kg
P.O. daily, divided q 6 hours to q
12 hours.
Gonorrhea in patients sensitive to
penicillin—
Adults: 900 mg P.O. initially, then
300 mg P.O. q.i.d. for total of 5.4 g.
Syphilis in patients sensitive to
penicillin—
Adults: total dose of 18 to 24 g in
equally divided doses over 10 to
15 days.

SIDE EFFECTS
Blood: neutropenia, eosinophilia.
CV: pericarditis.
EENT: dysphagia, glossitis.
GI: anorexia, *epigastric distress, nau-*
sea, vomiting, *diarrhea,* enterocolitis,
anogenital inflammation.
Metabolic: increased BUN.
Skin: *maculopapular and erythema-*
tous rashes, photosensitivity, urticaria.
Other: hypersensitivity.

INTERACTIONS
Antacids (including NaHCO₃) and lax-
atives containing aluminum, magne-
sium, or calcium; food, milk, or other
dairy products: decrease antibiotic absorption. Give antibiotic 1 hour before
or 2 hours after any of the above.
Ferrous sulfate and other iron products,
zinc: decrease antibiotic absorption.
Give tetracyclines 3 hours after or 2
hours before iron administration.

NURSING CONSIDERATIONS
• Use with extreme caution in patients
with impaired renal or hepatic function.
Use during last half of pregnancy and in
children younger than 8 years may
cause permanent discoloration of teeth,
enamel defects, and retardation of bone
growth.
• Obtain cultures before starting therapy.

- Check expiration date. Outdated or deteriorated methacycline may cause nephrotoxicity.
- Do not expose these drugs to light or heat.
- Watch for overgrowth of nonsusceptible organisms. Check patient's tongue for signs of monilia infection. Stress good oral hygiene. If superinfection occurs, drug should be discontinued.
- Observe patient for diarrhea, which may result from local irritation or superinfection.
- Warn patient to avoid direct sunlight and ultraviolet light. A sunscreen may help prevent photosensitivity reactions. Photosensitivity persists for considerable time after discontinuation of drug.
- Effectiveness is reduced when taken with milk or other dairy products, food, antacids, or iron products. Explain this to patient. Tell patient to take each dose with a full glass of water on an empty stomach, at least 1 hour before meals or 2 hours afterward. Give at least 1 hour before bedtime to prevent esophagitis.
- Instruct patient to take medication exactly as prescribed, even after he feels better. Treat streptococcal infections for at least 10 days.

---

minocycline hydrochloride
Minocin♦*, Ultramycin♦♦, Vectrin*

INDICATIONS & DOSAGE
Infections caused by sensitive gram-negative and gram-positive organisms, trachoma, amebiasis—
Adults: initially, 200 mg P.O., I.V.; then 100 mg q 12 hours or 50 mg P.O. q 6 hours.
Children over 8 years: initially, 4 mg/kg P.O., I.V.; then 4 mg/kg P.O. daily, divided q 12 hours. Give I.V. in 500 to 1,000 ml solution without calcium, over 6 hours.
Gonorrhea in patients sensitive to penicillin—

Adults: initially, 200 mg, then 100 mg q 12 hours for 4 days.
Syphilis in patients sensitive to penicillin—
Adults: initially, 200 mg, then 100 mg q 12 hours for 10 to 15 days.
Meningococcal carrier state—
100 mg P.O. q 12 hours for 5 days.

SIDE EFFECTS
Blood: neutropenia, eosinophilia.
CNS: *light-headedness, dizziness from vestibular otxicity.*
CV: pericarditis.
EENT: dysphagia, glossitis.
GI: *anorexia,* epigastric distress, *nausea,* vomiting, *diarrhea,* enterocolitis, inflammatory lesions in anogenital region.
Metabolic: increased BUN.
Skin: *maculopapular and erythematous rashes, photosensitivity, increased pigmentation, urticaria.*
Local: *thrombophlebitis.*
Other: hypersensitivity.

INTERACTIONS
Antacids (including NaHCO$_3$) or laxatives containing aluminum, magnesium, or calcium: decrease antibiotic absorption. Give antibiotic 1 hour before or 2 hours after any of the above.
Ferrous sulfate or other iron products, zinc: decrease antibiotic absorption. Tetracyclines should be given 3 hours after or 2 hours before iron administration.
Methoxyflurane: may cause severe nephrotoxicity with tetracyclines. Monitor carefully.

NURSING CONSIDERATIONS
- Use with extreme caution in patients with impaired renal or hepatic function. Use during last half of pregnancy and in children younger than 8 years may cause permanent discoloration of teeth, enamel defects, and retardation of bone growth.
- Patient may develop thrombophlebi-

---

tis with I.V. administration of this drug. Avoid extravasation.

• Obtain cultures before starting therapy.

• Check expiration date.

• Do not expose these drugs to light or heat. Keep cap tightly closed.

• Watch for overgrowth of nonsusceptible organisms. Check patient's tongue for signs of monilia infection. Stress good oral hygiene. If superinfection occurs, drug should be discontinued.

• Observe patient for diarrhea, which may result from local irritation or superinfection.

• May be taken with food. Tell patient to take medication exactly as prescribed, even after he feels better. Treat streptococcal infections for at least 10 days, syphilis for 10 to 15 days, gonorrhea for at least 4 days, and meningococcal carriers for 5 days.

• Reconstitute 100 mg powder with 5 ml sterile water for injection, with further dilution of 500 to 1,000 ml for I.V. infusion. Stable for 24 hours at room temperature.

• Vestibular toxicity resulting in dizziness may commonly occur with this drug.

---

oxytetracycline hydrochloride
Dalimycin, Oxlopar, Oxy-Kesso-Tetra, Oxytetraclor, Terramycin♦, Uri-tet

INDICATIONS & DOSAGE
Infections caused by sensitive gram-negative and gram-positive organisms, trachoma, rickettsiae—
Adults: 250 mg P.O. q 6 hours; 100 mg I.M. q 8 to 12 hours; 250 mg I.M. q 12 hours; or 250 to 500 mg I.V. q 6 to 12 hours.
Children over 8 years: 25 to 50 mg/kg P.O. daily, divided q 6 hours; 15 to 25 mg/kg I.M. daily, divided q 8 to 12 hours; or 10 to 20 mg/kg I.V. daily, divided q 12 hours.

Brucellosis—
Adults: 500 mg P.O. q.i.d. for 3 weeks with streptomycin 1 g I.M. q 12 hours first week, once daily second week.
Syphilis in patients sensitive to penicillin—
Adults: 30 to 40 g total dose P.O., divided equally over 10 to 15 days.
Gonorrhea in patients sensitive to penicillin—
Adults: initially, 1.5 g P.O. followed by 0.5 g q.i.d. for a total of 9 g.

SIDE EFFECTS
Blood: neutropenia, eosinophilia.
CNS: intracranial hypertension.
CV: pericarditis.
EENT: dysphagia, glossitis.
GI: *anorexia, nausea,* vomiting, *diarrhea,* enterocolitis, anogenital inflammation.
Metabolic: *increased BUN.*
Skin: *maculopapular and erythematous rashes, urticaria, photosensitivity, increased pigmentation.*
Local: *irritation after I.M. injection, thrombophlebitis.*
Other: hypersensitivity.

INTERACTIONS
Antacids (including NaHCO₃) and laxatives containing aluminum, magnesium, or calcium; food, milk, or other dairy products: decrease antibiotic absorption. Give antibiotic 1 hour before or 2 hours after any of the above.
Ferrous sulfate and other iron products, zinc: decrease antibiotic absorption. Give tetracyclines 3 hours after or 2 hours before iron administration.
Methoxyflurane: may cause severe nephrotoxicity with tetracyclines. Monitor carefully.

NURSING CONSIDERATIONS
• Use with extreme caution in patients with impaired renal or hepatic function. Use during last half of pregnancy and in children younger than 8 years may cause permanent discoloration of teeth,

---

enamel defects, and retardation of bone growth.
- Patient may develop thrombophlebitis with I.V. administration. Avoid extravasation.
- Obtain cultures before starting therapy.
- Check expiration date. Outdated or deteriorated oxytetracycline may cause nephrotoxicity.
- Do not expose these drugs to light or heat.
- Inject I.M. dose deeply. Warn that it may be painful. Rotate sites. I.M. preparations contain a local anesthetic; ask patient about hypersensitivity to local anesthetics.
- Watch for overgrowth of nonsusceptible organisms. Check patient's tongue for signs of monilia infection. Stress good oral hygiene. If superinfection occurs, drug should be discontinued.
- Observe patient for diarrhea, which may result from local irritation or superinfection.
- Warn patient to avoid direct sunlight and ultraviolet light. A sunscreen may help prevent photosensitivity reactions. Photosensitivity persists for considerable time after discontinuation of drug.
- Effectiveness is reduced when taken with milk or other dairy products, food, antacids, or iron products. Explain this to patient. Tell patient to take each dose with a full glass of water on an empty stomach, at least 1 hour before meals or 2 hours afterward. Give at least 1 hour before bedtime to prevent esophagitis.
- Tell patient to take medication exactly as prescribed, even after he feels better.
- For I.V. use, reconstitute 250 mg and 500 mg powder for injection with 10 ml sterile water.
- Dilute to at least 100 ml in 5% dextrose in water, normal saline solution, or Ringer's solution. Do not mix with any other drug.
- Store reconstituted solutions in refrigerator. Stable for 48 hours.

- May cause false-positive reading of Clinitest; false-negative reading of Clinistix or Tes-Tape.

tetracycline hydrochloride

Achromycin♦, Amer-Tet, Bicycline, Cefracycline♦♦, Centet-250, Cycline, Cyclopar, Maso-Cycline, Medicycline♦♦, Neo-Tetrine♦♦, Nor-Tet 500, Novotetra♦♦, Panmycin**, Partrex, Piracaps, Retet, Robitet, Sarocycline, Scotrex, SK-Tetracycline*, Sumycin♦, T-250, Tet-Cy, Tetra-C, Tetrachel, Tetraclor, Tetra-Co, Tetracrine♦♦, Tetracyn♦, Tetralan, Tetralean♦♦, Tetram, Tetram S, Tetramax, Trexin, Triacycline♦♦

tetracycline phosphate complex

Tetrex♦

INDICATIONS & DOSAGE

Infections caused by sensitive gram-negative and gram-positive organisms, trachoma, rickettsiae, Mycoplasma, *and* Chlamydia—
Adults: 250 to 500 mg P.O. q 6 hours; 250 mg I.M. daily or 150 mg I.M. q 12 hours; or 250 to 500 mg I.V. q 8 to 12 hours (I.M. and I.V. hydrochloride salt only).
Children over 8 years: 25 to 50 mg/kg P.O. daily, divided q 6 hours; 15 to 25 mg/kg daily (maximum 250 mg) I.M. single dose or divided q 8 to 12 hours; or 10 to 20 mg/kg I.V. daily, divided q 12 hours.
Brucellosis—
Adults: 500 mg P.O. q 6 hours for 3 weeks with streptomycin 1 g I.M. q 12 hours week 1 and daily week 2.
Gonorrhea in patients sensitive to penicillin—
Adults: initially,1.5 g P.O., then 500 mg q 6 hours for total of 9 g.
Syphilis in patients sensitive to penicillin—

Unmarked trade names available in the United States only.
♦ Also available in Canada.   ♦♦ Available in Canada only.

Adults: 30 to 40 g total in equally divided doses over 10 to 15 days.
Acne—
Adults and adolescents: initially, 250 mg P.O. q 6 hours, then 125 to 500 mg P.O. daily or every other day.
Shigellosis—
Adults: 2.5 g P.O. in 1 dose.

SIDE EFFECTS
Blood: neutropenia, eosinophilia.
CNS: dizziness, headache, intracranial hypertension.
CV: pericarditis.
EENT: sore throat, glossitis, dysphagia.
GI: anorexia, *epigastric distress, nausea,* vomiting, *diarrhea,* stomatitis, enterocolitis, inflammatory lesions in anogenital region.
Hepatic: hepatotoxicity with doses given I.V.
Metabolic: *increased BUN.*
Skin: *maculopapular and erythematous rashes, urticaria, photosensitivity, increased pigmentation.*
Local: *irritation after I.M. injection, thrombophlebitis.*

INTERACTIONS
Antacids (including NaHCO$_3$) and laxatives containing aluminum, magnesium, or calcium; food, milk, or other dairy products: decrease antibiotic absorption. Give antibiotic 1 hour before or 2 hours after any of the above.
Ferrous sulfate and other iron products, zinc: decrease antibiotic absorption. Give tetracyclines 3 hours after or 2 hours before iron administration.
Methoxyflurane: may cause severe nephrotoxicity with tetracyclines. Monitor carefully.

NURSING CONSIDERATIONS
• Use with extreme caution in patients with impaired renal or hepatic function. Use during last half of pregnancy and in children younger than 8 years may cause permanent discoloration of teeth,

enamel defects, and retardation of bone growth.
• Obtain cultures before starting therapy.
• Effectiveness reduced when taken with milk or other dairy products, food, antacids, or iron products. Explain this to patient. Tell patient to take each dose with a full glass of water on an empty stomach, at least 1 hour before meals or 2 hours afterward. Give at least 1 hour before bedtime to prevent esophagitis.
• Patient may develop thrombophlebitis with I.V. administration. Avoid extravasation.
• Check expiration date. Outdated or deteriorated tetracycline may cause nephrotoxicity.
• Discard I.M. solutions after 24 hours because they deteriorate. Exception: discard Achromycin solution in 12 hours.
• Do not expose these drugs to light or heat.
• Inject I.M. dose deeply. Warn patient that it may be painful. Rotate sites. I.M. preparations often contain a local anesthetic; ask patient about hypersensitivity to local anesthetics.
• Watch for overgrowth of nonsusceptible organisms. Check patient's tongue for signs of monilia infection. Stress good oral hygiene. If superinfection occurs, drug should be discontinued.
• Observe patient for diarrhea, which may result from local irritation or superinfection.
• Warn patient to avoid direct sunlight and ultraviolet light. A sunscreen may help prevent photosensitivity reactions. Photosensitivity persists for some time after discontinuation of drug.
• Tell patient to take medication exactly as prescribed, even after he feels better. Treat streptoccocal infections for at least 10 days.
• For I.V. use, reconstitute 100 mg and 250 mg powder for injection with 5 ml sterile water; with 10 ml for 500 mg. Dilute in 100 to 1,000 ml volume of

---

Italicized side effects are common or life-threatening.
*Liquid form contains alcohol.   **May contain tartrazine.

5% dextrose in 0.9% saline solution. Refrigerate diluted solution for I.V. use and use within 24 hours. Exception: use Achromycin solution immediately.
• Do not mix tetracycline solution with any other I.V. additive.
• For I.M. use, reconstitute 100 mg powder for injection with 2 ml sterile water for injection. Concentration will be 50 mg/ml. Amount of diluent for 250-mg injection varies according to brand. Check with pharmacy or follow manufacturer's instructions.
• May cause false-positive reading of Clinitest; false-negative reading of Clinistix or Tes-Tape.

14

Sulfonamides

co-trimoxazole
sulfacytine
sulfadiazine
sulfamethizole
sulfamethoxazole
sulfapyridine
sulfasalazine
sulfisoxazole

MECHANISM OF ACTION
Sulfonamides have a broad spectrum of antibacterial action and are bacteriostatic. Chemically similar to para-aminobenzoic acid (PABA), these drugs competitively inhibit dihydropteroate synthetase, a bacterial enzyme responsible for incorporation of PABA into dihydrofolic acid (folic acid). This mechanism blocks folic-acid synthesis. Hence, nucleic acids—essential building blocks of the bacterial cell—cannot be synthesized. Bacteria are susceptible because they must synthesize their own folic acid.

COMBINATION PRODUCTS
AZO GANTANOL: sulfamethoxazole 500 mg and phenazopyridine hydrochloride 100 mg.
AZO GANTRISIN: sulfisoxazole 500 mg and phenazopyridine hydrochloride 50 mg.
AZOTREX: sulfamethizole 250 mg, tetracycline phosphate complex equivalent to 125 mg tetracycline HCl activity, and phenazopyridine hydrochloride 50 mg.
SULADYNE: sulfamethizole 125 mg, sulfadiazine 125 mg, and phenazopyridine hydrochloride 75 mg.
THIOSULFIL-A: sulfamethizole 250 mg and phenazopyridine hydrochloride 50 mg.
TRIPLE SULFA: sulfadiazine 167 mg, sulfamerazine 167 mg, and sulfamethazine 167 mg.
UROBIOTIC-250: sulfamethizole 250 mg, oxytetracycline (as the hydrochloride) 250 mg, and phenazopyridine hydrochloride 50 mg.

---

co-trimoxazole
(sulfamethoxazole-trimethoprim)
Bactrim♦*, Bactrim DS♦, Bactrim I.V. Infusion, Septra♦*, Septra DS♦ Septra I.V. Infusion

INDICATIONS & DOSAGE
Urinary tract infections and shigellosis—
Adults: 160 mg trimethoprim/800 mg sulfa q 12 hours for 10 to 14 days in urinary tract infections and for 5 days in shigellosis.
Children: 8 mg/kg trimethoprim/ 40 mg/kg sulfa per 24 hours, in 2 divided doses q 12 hours (10 days for urinary tract infections; for 5 days in shigellosis).
Otitis media—
Children: 8 mg/kg trimethoprim/ 40 mg/kg sulfa per 24 hours, in 2 divided doses q 12 hours for 10 days.
Pneumocystis carinii pneumonitis—
Adults and children: 20 mg/kg trimethoprim/ 100 mg/kg sulfa per 24 hours, in equally divided doses q 6 hours for 14 days.
Chronic bronchitis—
Adults: 160 mg trimethoprim/800 mg sulfa q 12 hours for 10 to 14 days. Not

Italicized side effects are common or life-threatening.
*Liquid form contains alcohol.   **May contain tartrazine.

recommended for infants less than 2 months old.

SIDE EFFECTS
Blood: *agranulocytosis, aplastic anemia,* megaloblastic anemia, thrombocytopenia, leukopenia, hemolytic anemia.
CNS: headache, mental depression, convulsions, hallucinations.
GI: *nausea, vomiting, diarrhea,* abdominal pain, anorexia, stomatitis.
GU: toxic nephrosis with oliguria and anuria, crystalluria, hematuria.
Hepatic: jaundice.
Skin: *erythema multiforme (Stevens-Johnson syndrome), generalized skin eruption, epidermal necrolysis, exfoliative dermatitis,* photosensitivity, urticaria, pruritus.
Other: *hypersensitivity, serum sickness, drug fever, anaphylaxis.*

INTERACTIONS
Ammonium chloride, ascorbic acid, paraldehyde: doses sufficient to acidify urine may cause precipitation of sulfonamide and crystalluria. Don't use together.

NURSING CONSIDERATIONS
• Contraindicated in patients with porphyria. Use cautiously and in reduced dosages in patients with impaired hepatic or renal function and in those with severe allergy or bronchial asthma, G-6-PD deficiency, blood dyscrasias.
• I.V. infusion must be diluted in 5% dextrose in water prior to administration. Don't mix with other drugs or solutions.
• I.V. infusion must be infused slowly over 60 to 90 minutes. Don't give by rapid infusion or bolus injection. Must be used within 2 hours of mixing; don't refrigerate solution.
• This combination is often used in extremely ill immunosuppressed patients when prescribed for treatment of *Pneumocystis* pneumonia.

• Oral suspension available for patients who cannot swallow large tablets.
• Note that the "DS" product means "double strength."
• Promptly report skin rash, sore throat, fever, or mouth sores—early signs of blood dyscrasias.
• Used effectively for treatment of chronic bacterial prostatitis.
• Used prophylactically for recurrent urinary tract infections in women.
• Most side effects develop within 2 weeks of onset of therapy.

sulfacytine
Renoquid

INDICATIONS & DOSAGE
Urinary tract infections—
Adults: initially, 500 mg P.O., then 250 mg P.O. q.i.d. for 10 days.

SIDE EFFECTS
Blood: *agranulocytosis, aplastic anemia,* megaloblastic anemia, thrombocytopenia, leukopenia, hemolytic anemia.
CNS: headache, mental depression, convulsions, hallucinations.
GI: *nausea, vomiting, diarrhea,* abdominal pain, anorexia, stomatitis.
GU: toxic nephrosis with oliguria and anuria, crystalluria, hematuria.
Hepatic: jaundice.
Skin: *erythema multiforme (Stevens-Johnson syndrome), generalized skin eruption, epidermal necrolysis, exfoliative dermatitis,* photosensitivity, urticaria, pruritus.
Other: *hypersensitivity, serum sickness, drug fever, anaphylaxis.*

INTERACTIONS
Ammonium chloride, ascorbic acid, paraldehyde: doses sufficient to acidify urine may cause precipitation of sulfonamide and crystalluria. Don't use together.
PABA-containing drugs: inhibit antibacterial action. Don't use together.

NURSING CONSIDERATIONS

• Contraindicated in porphyria. Use cautiously and in reduced dosages in patients with impaired hepatic or renal function, bronchial asthma, history of multiple allergies, G-6-PD deficiency, blood dyscrasias.

• Tell patient to drink a full glass of water with each dose and to drink plenty of water throughout the day to prevent crystalluria. Monitor fluid intake and urinary output. Intake should be sufficient to produce output of 1,500 ml daily (between 3,000 and 4,000 ml daily for adults).

• To aid in prevention of crystalluria, sodium bicarbonate may be administered to alkalinize urine. Monitor urine pH daily.

• Tell patient to take medication for as long as prescribed, even after he feels better. Warn patient to avoid direct sunlight and ultraviolet light to prevent photosensitivity reaction.

• Monitor urine cultures, CBCs, and urinalyses before and during therapy.

• Tell patient to report early signs of blood dyscrasias (sore throat, fever, pallor) immediately and to stop taking drug.

---

sulfadiazine
Microsulfon

INDICATIONS & DOSAGE

Urinary tract infection—
Adults: initially, 2 to 4 g P.O., then 500 mg to 1 g P.O. q 6 hours.
Children: initially, 75 mg/kg or 2 g/m² P.O., then 150 mg/kg or 4 g/m² P.O. in 4 to 6 divided doses daily. Maximum daily dose 6 g.
Rheumatic fever prophylaxis, as an alternative to penicillin—
Children over 30 kg: 1 g P.O. daily.
Children under 30 kg: 500 mg P.O. daily.
Adjunctive treatment in toxoplasmosis—
Adults: 4 g P.O. in divided doses q 6 hours for 3 to 4 weeks, discontinued for 1 week; given with pyrimethamine 25 mg P.O. daily for 3 to 4 weeks.
Children: 100 mg/kg P.O. in divided doses q 6 hours for 3 to 4 weeks; given with pyrimethamine 2 mg/kg daily for 3 days, then 1 mg/kg daily for 3 to 4 weeks.

SIDE EFFECTS

Blood: *agranulocytosis, aplastic anemia,* megaloblastic anemia, thrombocytopenia, leukopenia, hemolytic anemia.
CNS: headache, mental depression, convulsions, hallucinations.
GI: *nausea, vomiting, diarrhea,* abdominal pain, anorexia, stomatitis.
GU: toxic nephrosis with oliguria and anuria, crystalluria, hematuria.
Hepatic: jaundice.
Skin: *erythema multiforme (Stevens-Johnson syndrome), generalized skin eruption, epidermal necrolysis, exfoliative dermatitis,* photosensitivity, urticaria, pruritus.
Local: irritation, extravasation.
Other: *hypersensitivity, serum sickness, drug fever, anaphylaxis.*

INTERACTIONS

Ammonium chloride, ascorbic acid, paraldehyde: doses sufficient to acidify urine may cause precipitation of sulfonamide and crystalluria. Don't use together.
PABA-containing drugs: inhibit antibacterial action. Don't use together.

NURSING CONSIDERATIONS

• Contraindicated in patients with porphyria or in infants younger than 2 months (except in congenital toxoplasmosis). Use cautiously in reduced doses in patients with impaired hepatic or renal function, bronchial asthma, history of multiple allergies, G-6-PD deficiency, blood dyscrasias.

• Tell patient to drink a full glass of water with each dose and to drink plenty of water throughout the day to

---

Italicized side effects are common or life-threatening.
*Liquid form contains alcohol.   **May contain tartrazine.

prevent crystalluria. Monitor fluid intake and urinary output. Intake should be sufficient to produce output of 1,500 ml daily (between 3,000 and 4,000 ml daily for adults). To aid in prevention of crystalluria, sodium bicarbonate may be administered to alkalinize urine. Monitor urine pH daily.
• Tell patient to take medication for as long as prescribed, even if he feels better. Warn patient to avoid direct sunlight and ultraviolet light to prevent photosensitivity reaction.
• Give drug on schedule to maintain constant blood level.
• Watch for signs of blood dyscrasias (purpura, ecchymosis, sore throat, fever, pallor). Report them immediately.
• Monitor urine cultures, CBCs, and urinalyses before and during therapy.
• Folic or folinic acid may be used during rest periods in toxoplasmosis therapy to reverse hematopoietic depression and/or anemia associated with pyrimethamine and sulfadiazine.
• Protect drug from light.

---

sulfamethizole
Bursul, Microsul, Sulfasol, Sulfstat, Sulfurine, Thiosulfil♦, Unisul, Uri-Pak, Urifon, Utrasul

INDICATIONS & DOSAGE
Urinary tract infections only—
Adults: 500 mg to 1 g P.O. t.i.d. to q.i.d.
Children over 2 months: 30 to 45 mg/kg P.O. daily, divided into doses given q 6 hours.

SIDE EFFECTS
Blood: *agranulocytosis, aplastic anemia,* megaloblastic anemia, thrombocytopenia, leukopenia, hemolytic anemia.
CNS: headache, mental depression, convulsions, hallucinations.
GI: *nausea, vomiting, diarrhea,* abdominal pain, anorexia, stomatitis.

GU: toxic nephrosis with oliguria and anuria, crystalluria, hematuria.
Hepatic: jaundice.
Skin: *erythema multiforme (Stevens-Johnson syndrome), generalized skin eruption, epidermal necrolysis, exfoliative dermatitis,* photosensitivity, urticaria, pruritus.
Other: *hypersensitivity, serum sickness, drug fever, anaphylaxis.*

INTERACTIONS
Ammonium chloride, ascorbic acid, paraldehyde: doses sufficient to acidify urine may cause precipitation of sulfonamide and crystalluria. Don't use together.
PABA-containing drugs: inhibit antibacterial action. Don't use together.

NURSING CONSIDERATIONS
• Contraindicated in porphyria. Use cautiously and in reduced dosages in patients with impaired hepatic or renal function, blood dyscrasias, G-6-PD deficiency, asthma, history of multiple allergies.
• Tell patient to drink a full glass of water with each dose and to drink plenty of water throughout the day to prevent crystalluria. Monitor fluid intake and urinary output. Intake should be sufficient to produce output of 1,500 ml daily (between 3,000 and 4,000 ml daily for adults). To aid in prevention of crystalluria, sodium bicarbonate may be administered to alkalinize urine. Monitor urine pH daily.
• Tell patient to take medication for as long as prescribed, even after he feels better. Warn patient to avoid direct sunlight and ultraviolet light to prevent photosensitivity reaction. Instruct patient to report early signs of blood dyscrasias (sore throat, fever, pallor) immediately and to stop taking drug.
• Monitor urine cultures, CBCs, and urinalyses before and during therapy.

---

sulfamethoxazole
Gantanol♦, Urobak

INDICATIONS & DOSAGE
Urinary tract and systemic infections—
Adults: initially, 2 g P.O., then 1 g P.O. b.i.d. up to t.i.d. for severe infections.
Children and infants over 2 months: initially, 50 to 60 mg/kg P.O., then 25 to 30 mg/kg b.i.d. Maximum dose should not exceed 75 mg/kg daily.

SIDE EFFECTS
Blood: *agranulocytosis, aplastic anemia,* megaloblastic anemia, thrombocytopenia, leukopenia, hemolytic anemia.
CNS: headache, mental depression, convulsions, hallucinations.
GI: *nausea, vomiting, diarrhea,* abdominal pain, anorexia, stomatitis.
GU: toxic nephrosis with oliguria and anuria, crystalluria, hematuria.
Hepatic: jaundice.
Skin: *erythema multiforme (Stevens-Johnson syndrome), generalized skin eruption, epidermal necrolysis, exfoliative dermatitis,* photosensitivity, urticaria, pruritus.
Other: *hypersensitivity, serum sickness, drug fever, anaphylaxis.*

INTERACTIONS
Ammonium chloride, ascorbic acid, paraldehyde: doses sufficient to acidify urine may cause precipitation of sulfonamide and crystalluria. Don't use together.
PABA-containing drugs: inhibit antibacterial action. Don't use together.

NURSING CONSIDERATIONS
• Contraindicated in patients with porphyria or in infants younger than 2 months (except in congenital toxoplasmosis). Use cautiously and in reduced dosages in patients with impaired hepatic or renal function and in those with severe allergy or bronchial asthma, G-6-PD deficiency, blood dyscrasias.
• Tell patient to drink a full glass of water with each dose and to drink plenty of water during the day to prevent crystalluria. Monitor fluid intake/urinary output. Intake should be sufficient to produce output of 1,500 ml daily (between 3,000 and 4,000 ml daily for adults). To aid in prevention of crystalluria, sodium bicarbonate may be administered to alkalinize urine. Monitor urine pH daily.
• Tell patient to take medication for as long as prescribed, even after he feels better. Warn patient to avoid direct sunlight and ultraviolet light to prevent photosensitivity reaction.
• Monitor urine cultures, CBCs, and urinalyses before and during therapy.
• Sulfamethoxazole is also used in adjunctive therapy for treatment of toxoplasmosis following therapy with other first-line agents.
• Instruct patient to report early signs of blood dyscrasias (sore throat, fever, pallor) immediately and to stop taking the drug.

sulfapyridine
Dagenan♦♦

INDICATIONS & DOSAGE
Dermatitis herpetiformis—
Adults: 500 mg P.O. q.i.d. until improvement noted, then decrease dose by 500 mg every 3 days until minimum effective maintenance dose achieved.

SIDE EFFECTS
Blood: *agranulocytosis, aplastic anemia,* megaloblastic anemia, thrombocytopenia, leukopenia, hemolytic anemia.
CNS: headache, mental depression, convulsions, hallucinations.
GI: *nausea, vomiting, diarrhea,* abdominal pain, anorexia, stomatitis.
GU: toxic nephrosis with oliguria and anuria, crystalluria, hematuria.

Italicized side effects are common or life-threatening.
*Liquid form contains alcohol.   **May contain tartrazine.

Hepatic: jaundice.
Skin: *erythema multiforme (Stevens-Johnson syndrome), generalized skin eruption, epidermal necrolysis, exfoliative dermatitis,* photosensitivity, urticaria, pruritus.
Other: *hypersensitivity, serum sickness, drug fever, anaphylaxis.*

INTERACTIONS

Ammonium chloride, ascorbic acid, paraldehyde: doses sufficient to acidify urine may cause precipitation of sulfonamide and crystalluria. Don't use together.
PABA-containing drugs: inhibit antibacterial action. Don't use together.

NURSING CONSIDERATIONS

• Contraindicated in porphyria. Use cautiously and in reduced dosages in patients with impaired hepatic or renal function, G-6-PD deficiency, history of multiple allergies, asthma, blood dyscrasias.
• Tell patient to drink a full glass of water with each dose and to drink plenty of water during the day to prevent crystalluria. Monitor fluid intake/urinary output. Intake should be sufficient to produce output of 1,500 ml daily (between 3,000 and 4,000 ml daily for adults).
• Alkalinization of the urine may decrease the danger of crystalluria but may greatly increase renal tubular reabsorption of the drug, sustained blood levels, and risk of toxicity.
• Tell patient to take medication for as long as prescribed, even after he feels better. Warn patient to avoid direct sunlight and ultraviolet light to prevent photosensitivity reaction.
• Monitor urine cultures, CBCs, and urinalyses before and during therapy.
• Sulfapyridine is an intermediate-acting sulfonamide with a high potential for toxicity; its use is restricted to treatment of dermatitis herpetiformis when sulfone therapy is contraindicated.

• Tell patient to report any side effects at once and to stop drug.

sulfasalazine
Azulfidine, Azulfidine En-Tabs, SAS-500

INDICATIONS & DOSAGE
Mild to moderate ulcerative colitis, adjunctive therapy in severe ulcerative colitis—
Adults: initially, 3 to 4 g P.O. daily in evenly divided doses; usual maintenance dose is 1.5 to 2 g P.O. daily in divided doses q 6 hours. May need to start with 1 to 2 g initially, with a gradual increase in dose to minimize side effects.
Children over 2 years: initially, 40 to 60 mg/kg P.O. daily, divided into 3 to 6 doses; then 30 mg/kg daily in 4 doses. May need to start at lower dose if gastrointestinal intolerance occurs.

SIDE EFFECTS
Blood: *agranulocytosis, aplastic anemia,* megaloblastic anemia, thrombocytopenia, leukopenia, hemolytic anemia.
CNS: headache, mental depression, convulsions, hallucinations.
GI: *nausea, vomiting, diarrhea,* abdominal pain, anorexia, stomatitis.
GU: toxic nephrosis with oliguria and anuria, crystalluria, hematuria.
Hepatic: jaundice, hepatoxicity.
Skin: *erythema multiforme (Stevens-Johnson syndrome), generalized skin eruption, epidermal necrolysis, exfoliative dermatitis,* photosensitivity, urticaria, pruritus.
Other: *hypersensitivity, serum sickness, drug fever, anaphylaxis.*

INTERACTIONS
None significant.

NURSING CONSIDERATIONS
• Contraindicated in porphyria. Use cautiously and in reduced dosages in

---

patients with impaired hepatic or renal function and in those with severe allergy or bronchial asthma, G-6-PD deficiency.

• Instruct patient to take medication for as long as prescribed, even after he feels better. Warn patient to avoid direct sunlight and ultraviolet light to prevent photosensitivity reaction.

• Colors alkaline urine orange-yellow.

• Side effects are usually those affecting GI tract. Minimize symptoms by spacing doses evenly and administering after food intake.

• Also available as an oral suspension.

sulfisoxazole
Barazole, Gantrisin♦, G-Sox, J-Sul, Lipo Gantrisin, Novosoxazole♦♦, Rosoxol, SK-Soxazole, Sosol, Soxa, Soxomide, Sulfagan, Sulfizin, Urisoxin, Urizole, Velmatrol

INDICATIONS & DOSAGE
Urinary tract and systemic infections—
Adults: initially, 2 to 4 g P.O., then 1 to 2 g P.O. q.i.d.; extended-release suspension 4 to 5 g P.O. q 12 hours.
Children over 2 months: initially, 75 mg/kg P.O. daily or 2 g/m² P.O. daily in divided doses q 6 hours, then 150 mg/kg or 4 g/m² P.O. daily in divided doses q 6 hours; extended-release suspension 60 to 70 mg/kg P.O. q 12 hours.
Adults and children over 2 months: parenteral dosages (sulfisoxazole diolamine) initially, 50 mg/kg or 1.125 g/m² by slow I.V. injection, then 100 mg/kg daily or 2.25 g/m² daily in divided doses q 6 hours by slow I.V. injection. 40% solution must be diluted to a concentration of 5% for I.V. use.

SIDE EFFECTS
Blood: *agranulocytosis, aplastic anemia,* megaloblastic anemia, thrombocytopenia, leukopenia, hemolytic anemia.

CNS: headache, mental depression, convulsions, hallucinations.
GI: *nausea, vomiting, diarrhea,* abdominal pain, anorexia, stomatitis.
GU: toxic nephrosis with oliguria and anuria, crystalluria, hematuria.
Hepatic: jaundice.
Skin: *erythema multiforme (Stevens-Johnson syndrome), generalized skin eruption, epidermal necrolysis, exfoliative dermatitis,* photosensitivity, urticaria, pruritus.
Other: *hypersensitivity, serum sickness, drug fever, anaphylaxis.*

INTERACTIONS
PABA-containing drugs: inhibit antibacterial action. Don't use together.
Ammonium chloride, ascorbic acid, paraldehyde: doses sufficient to acidify urine may cause crystalluria and precipitation of sulfonamide. Don't use together.

NURSING CONSIDERATIONS
• Contraindicated in patients with porphyria and in infants younger than 2 months (except in congenital toxoplasmosis). Use cautiously in patients with impaired hepatic or renal function, severe allergy or bronchial asthma, G-6-PD deficiency.

• Tell patient to drink a full glass of water with each dose and to drink plenty of water throughout the day to prevent crystalluria. Monitor fluid intake and urinary output. Intake should be sufficient to produce output of 1,500 ml daily (between 3,000 and 4,000 ml daily for adults). To aid in prevention of crystalluria, sodium bicarbonate may be administered to alkalinize urine. Monitor urine pH daily.

• Tell patient to take medication for as long as prescribed, even after he feels better. Warn patient to avoid direct sunlight and ultraviolet light to prevent photosensitivity reaction.

• Monitor urine cultures, CBCs, and urinalyses before and during therapy.

• Parenteral form can be given I.M. or

Italicized side effects are common or life-threatening.
∗Liquid form contains alcohol.   ∗∗May contain tartrazine.

subcutaneously, but these routes are discouraged. Administration of this form with parenteral fluids is not recommended. Diluents other than sterile distilled water may cause precipitation.

• Gantrisin suspension and Lipo Gantrisin suspension cannot be interchanged, since the latter is an extended-release preparation.

• Sulfisoxazole/pyrimethamine combination is used to treat toxoplasmosis.

• Tell patient to report early signs of blood dyscrasias (sore throat, fever, pallor) immediately and to stop taking drug.

• When given preoperatively, the patient should receive a low-residue diet and a minimal number of enemas and cathartics.

• Although often given, initial loading dose is not pharmacologically necessary.

15

Urinary tract antiseptics

cinoxacin
methenamine hippurate
methenamine mandelate
methylene blue
nalidixic acid
nitrofurantoin
nitrofurantoin macrocrystals

MECHANISM OF ACTION

In acid urine, methenamines are hydrolyzed to ammonia and to formaldehyde, which is responsible for antibacterial action against gram-positive and gram-negative organisms. Mandelic and hippuric acids, with which methenamines are combined, are also antibacterial by unknown mechanisms.

Methylene blue is a mildly antiseptic dye. High concentrations convert the ferrous iron of reduced hemoglobin to ferric iron to form methemoglobin. This mechanism is the basis for its use as an antidote in cyanide poisoning. Low concentrations of methylene blue can hasten conversion of methemoglobin to hemoglobin.

Nalidixic acid and cinoxacin are bacteriostatic, inhibiting DNA biosynthesis in microorganisms.

Nitrofurantoin is bacteriostatic in low concentration and possibly bactericidal in high concentration. It is presumed to interfere with bacterial enzyme systems.

COMBINATION PRODUCTS

AZO GANTANOL: sulfamethoxazole 500 mg and phenazopyridine HCl 100 mg.

AZO GANTRISIN: sulfisoxazole 500 mg and phenazopyridine HCl 50 mg.

AZO-MANDELAMINE: methenamine mandelate 500 mg and phenazopyridine HCl 50 mg.

AZOTREX: tetracycline phosphate complex equivalent to 125 mg tetracycline HCl activity, sulfamethizole 250 mg, and phenazopyridine HCl 50 mg.

CYSTEX: methenamine 162 mg, salicylamide 65 mg, sodium salicylate 97 mg, and benzoic acid 32 mg.

CYSTISED (IMPROVED): methenamine 40.8 mg, phenyl salicylate 18.1 mg, atropine sulfate 0.03 mg, hyoscyamine 0.03 mg, benzoic acid 4.5 mg, methylene blue 5.4 mg, and gelsemium 6.1 mg.

HEXALOL: methenamine 40.8 mg, phenyl salicylate 18.1 mg, atropine sulfate 0.03 mg, hyoscyamine 0.03 mg, benzoic acid 4.5 mg, and methylene blue 5.4 mg.

METHENAMINE AND SODIUM BIPHOSPHATE: methenamine 325 mg and sodium biphosphate 325 mg.

PROSED: methylene blue 5.4 mg, methenamine 40.8 mg, phenyl salicylate 18.1 mg, atropine sulfate 0.03 mg, hyoscyamine 0.03 mg, and benzoic acid 4.5 mg.

SULADYNE: sulfamethizole 125 mg, sulfadiazine 125 mg, and phenazopyridine HCl 75 mg.

THIOSULFIL-A: sulfamethizole 250 mg and phenazopyridine HCl 50 mg.

URO-PHOSPHATE: methenamine 300 mg and sodium acid phosphate 500 mg. Sugar coated.

UROQUID-ACID: methenamine mandelate 350 mg and sodium acid phosphate 200 mg.

UROQUID-ACID NO. 2: methenamine

Italicized side effects are common or life-threatening.
∗Liquid form contains alcohol.   ∗∗May contain tartrazine.

mandelate 500 mg and sodium acid phosphate 500 mg.

cinoxacin
Cinobac

INDICATIONS & DOSAGE
Treatment of initial and recurrent urinary tract infections caused by susceptible strains of Escherichia coli, Klebiella, Enterobacter, Proteus mirabilis, Proteus vulgaris, *and* Proteus morgani, Serratia, *and* Citrobacter—
Adults and children 12 years or older: 1 g daily, in two to four divided doses for 7 to 14 days.
Not recommended for children under age 12.

SIDE EFFECTS
CNS: *dizziness, headache,* drowsiness, insomnia, convulsions.
EENT: sensitivity to light.
GI: *nausea, vomiting, abdominal pain,* diarrhea.
Skin: rash, urticaria, pruritus, photosensitivity.

INTERACTIONS
Probenecid: may decrease urinary levels of cinoxacin by inhibiting renal tubular secretion. Monitor for increased toxicity and reduced antibacterial effectiveness.

NURSING CONSIDERATIONS
• Contraindicated in patients who are hypersensitive to nalidixic acid. Use cautiously in patients with impaired renal and hepatic function.
• Not effective against *Pseudomonas,* enterococci, or staphylococci.
• Obtain clean-catch urine specimen for culture and sensitivity before starting therapy and repeat p.r.n.
• High urine levels permit twice-daily dosing.
• Report CNS side effects to doctor immediately. They indicate serious tox-

icity and usually mean that administration of drug should be stopped.
• Cinoxacin should be taken with meals to help decrease GI side effects.
• Resistant bacteria may emerge with this drug.
• Warn patient about photophobic effects of drug, and advise him to avoid very bright sunlight.

methenamine hippurate
Hiprex, Hip-Rex♦♦, Urex

methenamine mandelate
Mandacon, Mandelamine♦, Mandelets, Mandelurine♦♦, Methandine♦♦, Prov-U-Sep, Sterine♦♦

INDICATIONS & DOSAGE
Long-term prophylaxis or suppression of chronic urinary tract infections—
Adults and children over 12 years: 1 g P.O. q 12 hours.
Children 6 to 12 years: 500 mg to 1 g P.O. q 12 hours.
Urinary tract infections, infected residual urine in patients with neurogenic bladder—
Adults: 1 g P.O. q.i.d. after meals.
Children 6 to 12 years: 500 mg P.O. q.i.d. after meals.
Children under 6 years: 50 mg/kg divided in 4 doses after meals.

SIDE EFFECTS
GU: with high doses, urinary tract irritation, dysuria, frequency, albuminuria, hematuria.
Hepatic: elevated liver enzymes.
Skin: rashes.

INTERACTIONS
Alkalinizing agents: inhibit methenamine action. Don't use together.
Acetazolamide: antagonizes methenamine effect. Use together cautiously.

NURSING CONSIDERATIONS
• Contraindicated in patients with

renal insufficiency, severe hepatic disease, or severe dehydration.
• Ineffective against *Candida* infection.
• Oral suspension contains vegetable oil. Administer cautiously to elderly or debilitated patients, because aspiration could cause lipid pneumonia.
• Monitor intake and output. Intake should be at least 1,500 to 2,000 ml daily.
• Obtain a clean-catch urine specimen for culture and sensitivity tests before starting therapy, and repeat p.r.n.
• Limit intake of alkaline foods, such as vegetables, milk, peanuts, fruits, and fruit juices, except cranberry, plum, and prune juices. These juices or ascorbic acid may be used to acidify urine.
• Warn patient not to take antacids, including Alka-Seltzer and sodium bicarbonate.
• Maintain urine pH at 5.5 or less. Use Nitrazine paper to check pH.
• *Proteus* and *Pseudomonas* tend to raise urine pH; urinary acidifiers are usually necessary when treating these infections.
• Obtain liver function studies periodically during long-term therapy.
• Administer after meals to minimize GI upset.
• If rash appears, hold dose and contact doctor.

methylene blue
MG-Blue, Urolene Blue, Wright's Stain

INDICATIONS & DOSAGE
Cystitis, urethritis—
Adults: 65 mg P.O. b.i.d. or t.i.d. after meals with glass of water.
Methemoglobinemia and cyanide poisoning—
Adults and children: 1 to 2 mg/kg of 1% sterile solution slow I.V.

SIDE EFFECTS
Blood: anemia (long-term use).

GI: nausea, vomiting, diarrhea.
GU: dysuria, bladder irritation.
Other: fever (large doses).

INTERACTIONS
None significant.

NURSING CONSIDERATIONS
• Contraindicated in patients with renal insufficiency.
• Monitor intake and output carefully. Intake should be at least 2,000 ml daily.
• Monitor hemoglobin; possibility of anemia from accelerated destruction of erythrocytes.
• Turns urine and stool blue-green.
• Seldom used as urinary tract antiseptic.
• I.V. form has been used to treat nitrite intoxication.

nalidixic acid
NegGram♦

INDICATIONS & DOSAGE
Acute and chronic urinary tract infections caused by susceptible gram-negative organisms (Proteus, Klebsiella, Enterobacter, *and* Escherichia coli)—
Adults: 1 g P.O. q.i.d. for 7 to 14 days; 2 g daily for long-term use.
Children over 3 months: 55 mg/kg P.O. daily divided q.i.d. for 7 to 14 days; 33 mg/kg daily for long-term use.

SIDE EFFECTS
Blood: eosinophilia.
CNS: drowsiness, weakness, headache, dizziness, vertigo, convulsions in epileptics.
EENT: sensitivity to light, change in color perception, diplopia, blurred vision.
GI: *abdominal pain, nausea, vomiting,* diarrhea.
Skin: pruritus, photosensitivity, urticaria, rash.

Italicized side effects are common or life-threatening.
*Liquid form contains alcohol.   **May contain tartrazine.

Other: angioedema, fever, chills, increased intracranial pressure and bulging fontanelles in infants and children.

INTERACTIONS
Nitrofurantoin: may antagonize nalidixic acid effect. Use together cautiously.

NURSING CONSIDERATIONS
●Contraindicated in patients with convulsive disorders. Use with caution in impaired hepatic or renal function, or severe cerebral arteriosclerosis. Should be used very cautiously in prepubertal children; erosion of cartilage of immature animals has been reported.
● Not effective against *Pseudomonas*.
● Tell the patient to report visual disturbances; these usually disappear with reduced dose.
● Obtain clean-catch urine specimen for culture and sensitivity tests before starting therapy and repeat p.r.n.
● Obtain CBC, renal and liver function studies during long-term therapy.
● Resistant bacteria may emerge within the first 48 hours of therapy.
● May cause a false-positive Clinitest reaction. Use Clinistix or Tes-Tape to monitor urine glucose. Also gives false elevations in urine vanillylmandelic acid (VMA) and 17-ketosteroids. Repeat tests after therapy completed.
● Avoid undue exposure to sunlight due to photosensitivity. Patient may continue to be photosensitive for as long as 3 months after drug is discontinued.

nitrofurantoin
Furadantin, Furalan, Furatine♦♦, Furantoin, Ivadantin, J-Dantin, Nephronex♦♦, Nifuran♦♦, Nitrex, Novofuran♦♦, Sarodant

nitrofurantoin macrocrystals
Macrodantin♦

INDICATIONS & DOSAGE
Pyelonephritis, pyelitis, and cystitis due to susceptible Escherichia coli, Staphylococcus aureus, *enterococci; certain strains of* Klebsiella, Proteus, *and* Enterobacter—
Adults and children over 12 years: 50 to 100 mg P.O. q.i.d. with meals. Or, 180 mg I.M. or I.V. b.i.d. in patients over 55 kg; 5 to 7 mg/kg daily I.M. or I.V. in patients under 55 kg.
Children 1 month to 12 years: 5 to 7 mg/kg P.O. daily, divided q.i.d.

SIDE EFFECTS
Blood: hemolysis in patients with G-6-PD deficiency (reversed after stopping drug).
CNS: peripheral neuropathy, headache, dizziness, drowsiness, ascending polyneuropathy with high doses or renal impairment.
GI: anorexia, *nausea, vomiting,* abdominal pain, *diarrhea.*
Hepatic: hepatitis.
Skin: maculopapular, erythematous, or eczematous eruption; pruritus; urticaria.
Other: asthmatic attacks in patients with history of asthma; *anaphylaxis;* drug fever; overgrowth of nonsusceptible organisms in the urinary tract; *pulmonary sensitivity reactions (cough, chest pains, fever, chills, dyspnea).*

INTERACTIONS
None significant.

NURSING CONSIDERATIONS

• Contraindicated in patients with moderate to severe renal impairment, anuria, oliguria, creatinine clearance under 40 ml/minute; in patients with G-6-PD deficiency.

• Obtain a clean-catch urine specimen for culture and sensitivity tests before starting therapy and repeat p.r.n.

• Give with food or milk to minimize GI distress.

• I.M. route painful and should not be used for more than 5 days.

• Dilute I.V. nitrofurantoin to 500 ml of suitable I.V. solution before administering. Constitute in sterile water without preservatives.

• Monitor intake/output carefully. May turn urine brown or darker.

• Store in amber container. Keep away from metals other than stainless steel or aluminum to avoid precipitate formation. Warn patients not to use pillboxes made of these materials.

• Continue treatment for 3 days after sterile urine specimens have been obtained.

• Monitor pulmonary status.

• May cause false-positive results with urine sugar test using copper sulfate reduction method (Clinitest) but not with glucose oxidase tests (Tes-Tape, Diastix, Clinistix).

16

Miscellaneous anti-infectives

amantadine hydrochloride
bacitracin
chloramphenicol
chloramphenicol palmitate
chloramphenicol sodium succinate
clindamycin hydrochloride
clindamycin palmitate hydrochloride
clindamycin phosphate
colistimethate sodium
erythromycin base
erythromycin estolate
erythromycin ethylsuccinate
erythromycin gluceptate
erythromycin lactobionate
erythromycin stearate
furazolidone
lincomycin hydrochloride
novobiocin calcium
novobiocin sodium
polymyxin B sulfate
spectinomycin dihydrochloride
trimethoprim
troleandomycin phosphate
vancomycin hydrochloride
vidarabine monohydrate

MECHANISM OF ACTION

- Amantadine is thought to interfere with influenza A virus penetration into susceptible cells.
- Bacitracin, colistimethate, polymyxin B, and vancomycin all hinder bacterial cell-wall synthesis, damaging the bacterial plasma membrane and making the cell more vulnerable to osmotic pressure.
- Chloramphenicol, clindamycin, lincomycin, erythromycin, and troleandomycin inhibit bacterial protein synthesis by binding to the 50S subunit of the ribosome.
- Furazolidone's mechanism of action is unknown.
- Novobiocin interferes with bacterial cell-wall, protein, and nucleic acid synthesis.
- Trimethoprim interferes with the action of dihydrofolate reductase, inhibiting bacterial synthesis of folic acid.
- Vidarabine, as its phosphorylated metabolite, becomes incorporated into viral deoxyribonucleic acid and inhibits viral multiplication.

COMBINATION PRODUCTS

None.

amantadine hydrochloride

Symmetrel♦

INDICATIONS & DOSAGE

Prophylaxis or symptomatic treatment of influenza type A virus, respiratory tract illnesses—

Adults and children over 9 years: 200 mg P.O. daily in a single dose or divided b.i.d.

Children 1 to 9 years: 4.4 to 8.8 mg/kg P.O. daily, divided b.i.d. or t.i.d. Don't exceed 150 mg daily.

Treatment should continue for 24 to 48 hours after symptoms disappear. Prophylaxis should start as soon as possible after initial exposure and continue for at least 10 days after exposure. May continue prophylactic treatment up to 90 days for repeated or suspected exposures if influenza vaccine unavailable. If used with influenza vaccine, con-

Unmarked trade names available in the United States only.
♦ Also available in Canada. ♦♦ Available in Canada only.

tinue dose for 2 to 3 weeks until protection from vaccine develops.

SIDE EFFECTS
CNS: depression, fatigue, confusion, dizziness, psychosis, hallucinations, anxiety, irritability, ataxia, insomnia, weakness, headache.
CV: peripheral edema, orthostatic hypotension, congestive heart failure.
GI: anorexia, nausea, constipation, vomiting, dry mouth.
GU: urinary retention.

INTERACTIONS
None significant.

NURSING CONSIDERATIONS
• Use cautiously in patients with history of epilepsy, congestive heart failure, peripheral edema, hepatic disease, mental illness, eczematoid rash, renal impairment, orthostatic hypotension, cardiovascular disease, and in elderly patients.
• For best absorption, drug should be taken after meals.
• Instruct patient to report side effects to the doctor, especially dizziness, depression, anxiety, nausea, and urinary retention.
• Monitor electrolyte balance and urinary output.
• If orthostatic hypotension occurs, instruct patient not to stand or change positions too quickly.
• If insomnia occurs, dose should be taken several hours before bedtime.
• Prophylactic use recommended for patients who can't receive influenza virus vaccine.

bacitracin

INDICATIONS & DOSAGE
Pneumonia or empyema caused by susceptible staphylococci—
Infants over 2.5 kg: 1,000 units/kg I.M. daily, divided q 8 to 12 hours.

Infants under 2.5 kg: 900 units/kg I.M. daily, divided q 8 to 12 hours. Although the FDA approves the use of bacitracin in infants only, adults with susceptible staphylococcal infections may receive 10,000 to 25,000 units I.M. q 6 hours (maximum 25,000 units/dose, 100,000 units daily).

SIDE EFFECTS
Blood: blood dyscrasias, eosinophilia.
GI: nausea, vomiting, anorexia, diarrhea, rectal itching or burning.
GU: nephrotoxicity *(albuminuria, cylindruria, oliguria, anuria,* increased BUN, tubular and glomerular necrosis).
Skin: urticaria, rash.
Local: *pain at injection site.*
Other: superinfection, fever, *anaphylaxis.*

INTERACTIONS
None significant.

NURSING CONSIDERATIONS
• Contraindicated in patients with impaired renal function. Use cautiously in myasthenia gravis or neuromuscular disease.
• Culture and sensitivity test should be done before starting treatment and p.r.n.
• For I.M. administration only. Give deep I.M.; injection may be painful; dilute in solution containing sodium chloride and 2% procaine hydrochloride (if hospital policy permits). Do not give if patient is sensitive to procaine or PABA derivatives.
• Maintain adequate fluid intake, and monitor urinary output closely. If intake or output decreases, notify the doctor.
• Obtain baseline renal function studies before starting therapy. Monitor renal function (BUN, serum creatinine, creatinine clearance, urinalysis) daily during therapy. Notify doctor of any change.
• Concentration of bacitracin should be

Italicized side effects are common or life-threatening.
*Liquid form contains alcohol.   **May contain tartrazine.

between 5,000 and 10,000 units/ml. Store in refrigerator. Drug is inactivated at room temperature.
• Report side effects to the doctor immediately.
• May be used with neomycin as a bowel prep, or in solution as a wound irrigating agent.
• Urine pH should be kept above 6.0.
• Prolonged therapy may result in overgrowth of nonsusceptible organisms, especially *Candida albicans*.

---

chloramphenicol

chloramphenicol palmitate

chloramphenicol sodium succinate
Chloromycetin♦, Mychel, Novochlorocap♦♦

INDICATIONS & DOSAGE
Hemophilus influenzae *meningitis, acute* Salmonella typhi *infection, severe infections caused by sensitive* Salmonella *species,* Rickettsia, *lymphogranuloma, psittacosis, various sensitive gram-negative organisms causing meningitis, bacteremia, or other serious infections—*
Adults and children: 50 to 100 mg/kg P.O. or I.V. daily, divided q 6 hours. Maximum dose is 100 mg/kg daily.
Premature infants and neonates (2 weeks or younger): 25 mg/kg P.O. or I.V. daily, divided q 6 hours. I.V. route must be used to treat meningitis.

SIDE EFFECTS
Blood: *aplastic anemia,* hypoplastic anemia, *granulocytopenia,* thrombocytopenia.
CNS: headache, mild depression, confusion, delirium, peripheral neuropathy with prolonged therapy.
CV: *cardiovascular collapse in newborns ("gray syndrome").*
EENT: optic neuritis (in patients with

cystic fibrosis), glossitis, decreased visual acuity.
GI: nausea, vomiting, stomatitis, diarrhea, enterocolitis.
Other: infections by nonsusceptible organisms, hypersensitivity reaction (fever, rash, urticaria, *anaphylaxis*), *gray baby syndrome in premature and newborn infants (abdominal distention, gray cyanosis, vasomotor collapse, respiratory distress, death within a few hours of onset of symptoms).*

INTERACTIONS
Penicillins: antagonize antibacterial effect. Give penicillin at least 1 hour before.
Acetaminophen: elevates chloramphenicol levels. Monitor for chloramphenicol toxicity.

NURSING CONSIDERATIONS
• Use cautiously in patients with impaired hepatic or renal function, and with other drugs causing bone marrow depression or blood disorders. *Don't use for infections caused by organisms susceptible to other agents or for trivial infections such as colds; use only when clearly indicated for severe infection.*
• Culture and sensitivity test may be done concurrently with first dose and p.r.n.
• Monitor CBC, platelets, serum iron, and reticulocytes before and every 2 days during therapy. Stop drug immediately if anemia, reticulocytopenia, leukopenia, or thrombocytopenia develops.
• Instruct patient to report side effects to the doctor, especially nausea, vomiting, diarrhea, fever, confusion, sore throat, or mouth sores.
• Tell patient to take medication for as long as prescribed, exactly as directed, even after he feels better.
• Give I.V. slowly over 1 minute. Check injection site daily for phlebitis and irritation.
• Reconstitute 1-g vial of powder for injection with 10 ml sterile water for in-

jection. Concentration will be 100 mg/
ml. Stable for 30 days at room temperature, but refrigeration recommended.
Do not use cloudy solutions.
• Watch for evidence of superinfection
by nonsusceptible organisms.

clindamycin hydrochloride

clindamycin palmitate hydrochloride

clindamycin phosphate
Cleocin, Dalacin C♦♦

INDICATIONS & DOSAGE
*Infections caused by sensitive staphylo-
cocci, streptococci, pneumococci,* Bacteroides, Fusobacterium, Clostridium
perfringens, *and other sensitive aerobic
and anaerobic organisms—*
Adults: 150 to 450 mg P.O. q 6 hours;
or 300 mg I.M. or I.V. q 6, 8, or
12 hours. Up to 2,700 mg I.M. or I.V.
daily, divided q 6, 8, or 12 hours. May
be used for severe infections.
Children over 1 month: 8 to 25 mg/kg
P.O. daily, divided q 6 to 8 hours; or 15
to 40 mg/kg I.M. or I.V. daily, divided
q 6 hours.

SIDE EFFECTS
Blood: transient leukopenia, eosinophilia, thrombocytopenia.
GI: *nausea,* vomiting, abdominal pain,
*diarrhea, pseudomembranous entero-
colitis,* esophagitis, flatulence, anorexia, *bloody or tarry stools.*
Hepatic: elevated SGOT, alkaline
phosphatase, bilirubin.
Skin: maculopapular rash, urticaria.
Local: *pain,* induration, *sterile abscess
with I.M. injection;* thrombophlebitis,
erythema, and pain after I.V. administration.
Other: unpleasant or bitter taste, *anaphylaxis.*

INTERACTIONS
Erythromycin: antagonist that may

block access of clindamycin to its site
of action; don't use together.

NURSING CONSIDERATIONS
• Contraindicated in patients with
known hypersensitivity to the antibiotic
congener lincomycin; also in patients
with history of GI disease, especially
colitis. Use cautiously in newborns and
patients with renal or hepatic disease,
asthma, or significant allergies.
• Monitor renal, hepatic, and hematopoietic functions during prolonged therapy.
• Culture and sensitivity test should be
performed before starting treatment
and p.r.n.
• Don't use in meningitis. Drug does
not penetrate CSF.
• Don't refrigerate reconstituted oral
solution, as it will thicken. Drug is stable for 2 weeks at room temperature.
• Instruct patient to report side effects
to the doctor, especially diarrhea. Warn
patient not to treat such diarrhea himself.
• Don't give diphenoxylate compound
(Lomotil) to treat drug-induced diarrhea. May prolong and worsen diarrhea.
• Give deep I.M. Rotate sites. Warn
that I.M. injection may be painful.
Doses greater than 600 mg per injection are not recommended.
• When giving I.V., check site daily for
phlebitis and irritation. For I.V. infusion, dilute each 300 mg in 50 ml solution, and give no faster than 30 mg/
minute.
• I.M. injection may cause CPK levels
to rise due to muscle irritation.
• Topical form is now available to treat
acne.

colistimethate sodium
Colistin Sulfate, Coly-Mycin M♦,
Coly-Mycin S Oral

INDICATIONS & DOSAGE
Enterocolitis caused by sensitive Esche-

Italicized side effects are common or life-threatening.
*Liquid form contains alcohol.   **May contain tartrazine.

richia coli, *sensitive* Shigella, *gastroenteritis*—
Adults and children: 2.5 to 5 mg/kg I.M. or I.V. daily, divided q 6 to 12 hours. Maximum daily dose not to exceed 5 mg/kg daily in patients with normal renal function.
Infants and children: 5 to 15 mg/kg P.O. daily, divided q 6 to 8 hours.
Severe infections, especially of urinary tract, caused by sensitive Pseudomonas, Enterobacter, E. coli, *and* Klebsiella—

SIDE EFFECTS
CNS: *circumoral and lingual paresthesias;* paresthesias of extremities; neuromuscular blockage with respiratory arrest, especially in patients with impaired renal function; dizziness; slurring of speech.
GI: nausea, vomiting, discomfort.
GU: *nephrotoxicity* (decreased urine output, increased BUN and serum creatinine).
Skin: pruritus, urticaria.
Local: pain at I.M. site.
Other: "drug fever," overgrowth of nonsusceptible organisms.

INTERACTIONS
None significant.

NURSING CONSIDERATIONS
• Contraindicated in patients with known hypersensitivity to the antibiotic congener polymyxin B. Use cautiously in renal impairment.
• Give deep I.M. Rotate sites. Warn that I.M. injection may be painful.
• Use sterile water for injection to reconstitute. When mixing, swirl solution gently to avoid frothing. Always prepare I.V. infusion fresh. Use within 24 hours.
• When giving I.V., check site daily for phlebitis and irritation. For direct I.V. administration, inject ½ daily dose over 3 to 5 minutes at 12-hour intervals.
• For continuous I.V. infusion, directly inject ½ daily dose over 3 to 5 minutes.

Add the remaining ½ to 5% dextrose, 5% dextrose in 0.9% sodium chloride, 5% dextrose in 0.45% sodium chloride, 5% dextrose in 0.225% sodium chloride, 10% invert sugar, lactated Ringer's injection, or 0.9% sodium chloride solution; then infuse 1 to 2 hours later at rate of 5 mg/hour.
• Monitor renal function closely (BUN, creatinine clearance, urinary output). Discontinue if BUN increases and urinary output decreases.
• Report side effects immediately, especially speech impairment or paresthesias. Watch for signs of superinfection.
• Store reconstituted oral suspension at 2° to 15° C. (35.6° to 59° F.), and use within 7 days.

erythromycin base
E-Mycin♦, Ery-Tab, Eryc, Erythromid♦♦, Ethril 500, Ilotycin♦, Novorythro♦♦, Robimycin♦, Staticin

erythromycin estolate
Ilosone♦, Novorythro♦♦

erythromycin ethylsuccinate
E.E.S., Erythrocin♦, Pediamycin, Wyamycin Liquid

erythromycin gluceptate
Ilotycin♦

erythromycin lactobionate
Erythrocin♦

erythromycin stearate
Bristamycin, E-Biotic, Ethril**, Erypar, Erythrocin♦, Novorythro♦♦, Pfizer E, SK-Erythromycin, Wintrocin, Wyamycin

INDICATIONS & DOSAGE
Acute pelvic inflammatory disease caused by Neisseria gonorrhoeae—
Women: 500 mg I.V. (erythromycin gluceptate, lactobionate) q 6 hours for

3 days, then 250 mg (erythromycin base, estolate, stearate) or 400 mg (erythromycin ethylsuccinate) P.O. q 6 hours for 7 days.

Endocarditis prophylaxis for dental procedures—

Adults: 1 g (erythromycin base, estolate, stearate) P.O. before procedure, followed by 250 mg P.O. q 6 hours for 8 doses afterward; or 1,200 mg (erythromycin ethylsuccinate) P.O. before procedure, followed by 400 mg P.O. q 6 hours for 8 doses afterward.

Children: 20 mg/kg (oral erythromycin salts) P.O.1½ to 2 hours before procedure, then 10 mg/kg q 6 hours for 8 doses.

Intestinal amebiasis—

Adults: 250 mg (erythromycin base, estolate, stearate) P.O. q 6 hours for 10 to 14 days.

Children: 30 to 50 mg/kg (erythromycin base, estolate, stearate) P.O. daily, divided q 6 hours for 10 to 14 days.

Mild-to-moderately severe respiratory tract, skin, and soft-tissue infections caused by sensitive group A beta-hemolytic streptococci, Diplococcus pneumoniae, Mycoplasma pneumoniae, Corynebacterium diphtheriae, Bordetella pertussis, Listeria monocytogenes—

Adults: 250 to 500 mg (erythromycin base, estolate, stearate) P.O. q 6 hours; or 400 to 800 mg (erythromycin ethylsuccinate) P.O. q 6 hours; or 15 to 20 mg/kg I.V. daily, as continuous infusion or divided q 6 hours.

Children: 30 mg/kg to 50 mg/kg (oral erythromycin salts) P.O. daily, divided q 6 hours; or 15 to 20 mg/kg I.V. daily, divided q 4 to 6 hours.

Syphilis—

Adults: 500 mg (erythromycin base, estolate, stearate) P.O. q.i.d. for 15 days.

Legionnaire's Disease—

Adults: 500 mg to 1 g I.V or P.O. q 6 hours for 21 days.

SIDE EFFECTS

EENT: hearing loss with high doses I.V.

GI: *abdominal pain and cramping, nausea, vomiting, diarrhea.*

Hepatic: cholestatic jaundice (with erythromycin estolate).

Skin: urticaria, rashes.

Local: *venous irritation, thrombophlebitis following I.V. injection.*

Other: overgrowth of nonsusceptible bacteria or fungi; *anaphylaxis;* fever.

INTERACTIONS

Clindamycin, lincomycin: may be antagonistic. Don't use together.

Penicillins: antagonize antibacterial effect. Give penicillin at least 1 hour before.

NURSING CONSIDERATIONS

• Erythromycin estolate contraindicated in hepatic disease. Use other erythromycin salts cautiously in patients with impaired hepatic function.

• Culture and sensitivity test should be performed before starting treatment and p.r.n.

• For best absorption, instruct patient to take oral form of drug with a full glass of water 1 hour before or 2 hours after meals. If tablets are coated, they may be taken with meals. Tell patient not to drink fruit juice with medication. Chewable erythromycin tablets should not be swallowed whole.

• When administering suspension, be sure to note the concentration.

• May cause overgrowth of nonsusceptible bacteria or fungi. Watch for signs and symptoms of superinfection.

• Tell patient to take medication for as long as prescribed, exactly as directed, even after he feels better. Treat streptococcal infections for 10 days.

• Report side effects, especially nausea, abdominal pain, or fever.

• Erythromycin estolate may cause serious hepatotoxicity in adults (reversible cholestatic jaundice). Monitor hepatic function (increased levels of bili-

---

Italicized side effects are common or life-threatening.
*Liquid form contains alcohol.   **May contain tartrazine.

rubin, SGOT, SGPT, alkaline phosphatase may occur). Other erythromycin salts cause hepatotoxicity to a lesser degree.
• I.V. dose should be administered over 20 to 60 minutes. Reconstitute according to manufacturer's directions and dilute each 250 mg in at least 100 ml 0.9% normal saline solution.
• Erythromycin lactobionate should not be administered with other drugs.
• Topical form now available to treat acne.
• A 333 mg enteric-coated tablet that is supposed to decrease GI irritation is now available. May be taken with meals.

furazolidone
Furoxone

INDICATIONS & DOSAGE
Gastroenteritis, adjunctive therapy in cholera—
Adults: 100 mg P.O. q.i.d.
Children 5 to 12 years: 25 to 50 mg P.O. q.i.d.
Children 1 to 4 years: 17 to 25 mg P.O. q.i.d.
Infants 1 month to 1 year: 8 to 17 mg P.O. q.i.d. Dosage based on 5 mg/kg daily; maximum dose 8.8 mg/kg daily.

SIDE EFFECTS
Blood: hemolytic anemia in infants under 1 month and patients with G-6-PD deficiency; *agranulocytosis.*
CNS: headache, malaise.
GI: nausea, vomiting, abdominal pain, diarrhea.
Other: hypersensitivity reaction (arthralgia, fever, hypotension, rash, urticaria, angioedema), hypoglycemia.

INTERACTIONS
None significant.

NURSING CONSIDERATIONS
• Tell patient to take medication ex-

actly as directed, even after he feels better.
• Report side effects to doctor, especially fever, rash, and abdominal pain.
• Store medication in dark place at 2° to 15° C. (36.5° to 59° F.).
• Drug may turn urine brown. Flushing, nausea, sweating, tachycardia, dyspnea may occur following ethanol ingestion. Tell patient not to drink alcohol or use alcohol-containing medication.
• If patient is taking drug for more than 5 days, instruct him not to eat broad beans, cheese, pickled herring, chicken livers, yeast extracts, or fermented products. Drug is similar to monoamine oxidase inhibitor.
• May cause false-positive urine glucose with Benedict's reagent.
• Frequent blood and urine studies should be performed on patients with G-6-PD deficiency to detect hemolysis.

lincomycin hydrochloride
Lincocin♦

INDICATIONS & DOSAGE
Respiratory tract, skin and soft-tissue, and urinary tract infections; osteomyelitis, septicemia, caused by sensitive group A beta-hemolytic streptococci, pneumococci, and staphylococci—
Adults: 500 mg P.O. q 6 to 8 hours (not to exceed 8 g daily); or 600 mg I.M. daily or q 12 hours; or 600 mg to 1 g I.V. q 8 to 12 hours (not to exceed 8 g daily).
Children over 1 month: 30 to 60 mg/kg P.O. daily, divided q 6 to 8 hours; or 10 mg/kg I.M. daily or divided q 12 hours; or 10 to 20 mg/kg I.V. daily, divided q 6 to 8 hours. For I.V. infusion, dilute to 100 ml; infuse over 1 hour to avoid hypotension.

SIDE EFFECTS
Blood: *neutropenia, leukopenia,* thrombocytopenia, purpura.
CNS: dizziness, headache.

Unmarked trade names available in the United States only.
♦ Also available in Canada.   ♦ ♦ Available in Canada only.

CV: hypotension with rapid I.V. infusion.
EENT: glossitis, tinnitus.
GI: nausea, vomiting, *persistent diarrhea*, abdominal cramps, enterocolitis, stomatitis, pruritus ani.
GU: vaginitis.
Hepatic: cholestatic jaundice.
Skin: rashes, urticaria.
Local: pain at injection site.
Other: hypersensitivity, angioedema.

INTERACTIONS
Antidiarrheal medication (kaolin, pectin, attapulgite): reduce oral absorption of lincomycin by as much as 90%. Antidiarrheals should be avoided or given at least 2 hours before lincomycin.

NURSING CONSIDERATIONS
• Contraindicated in known hypersensitivity to clindamycin. Use cautiously in patients with history of GI disorders (especially colitis); asthma or significant allergies; hepatic or renal disease; and endocrine or metabolic disorders.
• Culture and sensitivity tests should be done before starting treatment and p.r.n.
• For best absorption, instruct patient to take drug with a full glass of water 1 hour before or 2 hours after meals.
• Tell patient to take medication exactly as directed, even after he feels better.
• Tell patient to report side effects to doctor, especially diarrhea. Warn him not to treat diarrhea himself. Watch for signs of superinfection, especially when therapy exceeds 10 days.
• Never treat drug-induced diarrhea with diphenoxylate compound (Lomotil); it may prolong or worsen diarrhea.
• Give deep I.M. Rotate sites. Warn that I.M. injection may be painful.
• When giving I.V., check site daily for phlebitis and irritation. Rotate infusion sites regularly.
• Monitor blood pressure in patients receiving the drug parenterally.
• Monitor hepatic function (increased

levels of alkaline phosphatase, SGOT, SGPT, bilirubin may occur).
• Monitor CBC and platelets. Stop drug immediately if neutropenia, leukopenia, or other blood disorders develop.

novobiocin calcium

novobiocin sodium
Albamycin*

INDICATIONS & DOSAGE
Serious infections from sensitive Staphylococcus aureus *and* Proteus *when other antibiotics are contraindicated—*
Adults: 250 to 500 mg P.O. q 6 hours, or 500 mg to 1 g q 12 hours (not to exceed 2 g daily).
Children: 15 to 45 mg/kg P.O. daily, divided q 6 hours.

SIDE EFFECTS
Blood: pancytopenia, *leukopenia, agranulocytosis,* anemia, thrombocytopenia, eosinophilia.
GI: nausea, vomiting, anorexia, diarrhea, intestinal hemorrhage.
Hepatic: jaundice, hepatitis.
Skin: urticaria, *maculopapular dermatitis.*
Local: pain at injection site.
Other: *erythema multiforme,* fever in hypersensitivity reactions, swollen joints, overgrowth of nonsusceptible organisms.

INTERACTIONS
None significant.

NURSING CONSIDERATIONS
• Use cautiously in patients with hepatic disease or blood disorders. Do not use in infants, as it may cause kernicterus.
• Culture and sensitivity tests should be done before starting treatment and p.r.n.
• For best absorption, instruct patient

Italicized side effects are common or life-threatening.
*Liquid form contains alcohol.   **May contain tartrazine.

to take drug with a full glass of water
1 hour before or 2 hours after meals.
• Tell patient to take medication for as
long as prescribed exactly as directed,
even after he feels better.
• Report side effects, especially skin
rash, fever, jaundice, or GI distress,
which may indicate blood dyscrasia.
Stop drug immediately and notify the
doctor.
• Monitor hepatic function (bilirubin,
SGOT, SGPT, and alkaline phosphatase).
• Monitor CBC, and platelet, reticulocyte counts before and during therapy.

polymyxin B sulfate
Aerosporin♦

INDICATIONS & DOSAGE
*Acute urinary tract infections or septi-
cemia caused by sensitive* Pseudomonas
aeruginosa, *or when other antibiotics
are ineffective or contraindicated; bacteremia caused by sensitive* Enterobacter aerogenes *and* Klebsiella pneumoniae, *or acute urinary tract infections
caused by* Escherichia coli—
Adults and children: 15,000 to
25,000 units/kg daily I.V. infusion, divided q 12 hours; or 25,000 to 30,000
units/kg daily, divided q 4 to 8 hours.
I.M. not advised due to severe pain at
injection site.
Meningitis caused by sensitive P. aeruginosa *or* Hemophilus influenzae *when
other antibiotics ineffective or contraindicated—*
Adults and children over 2 years:
50,000 units intrathecally once daily
for 3 to 4 days, then 50,000 units every
other day for at least 2 weeks after cerebrospinal fluid tests are negative and
cerebrospinal fluid sugar is normal.
Children under 2 years: 20,000 units
intrathecally once daily for 3 to 4 days,
then 25,000 units every other day for at
least 2 weeks after cerebrospinal fluid
tests are negative and cerebrospinal
fluid sugar is normal.

SIDE EFFECTS
CNS: irritability, drowsiness, facial
flushing, weakness, ataxia, respiratory
paralysis, headache and meningeal irritation with intrathecal administration,
peripheral and perioral paresthesias,
convulsions, *coma.*
EENT: blurred vision.
GU: nephrotoxicity (albuminuria, cylindruria, hematuria, proteinuria, decreased urine output, increased BUN).
Skin: urticaria.
Local: *pain at I.M. injection site.*
Other: hypersensitivity reactions with
fever, *anaphylaxis.*

INTERACTIONS
None significant.

NURSING CONSIDERATIONS
• Use cautiously in patients with impaired renal function or myasthenia
gravis.
• Give only to hospitalized patients under constant medical supervision.
• For meningitis, must give intrathecally to achieve adequate cerebrospinal
fluid levels.
• Give deep I.M. Warn that injection
may be painful. If patient isn't allergic
to procaine, use 1% procaine (if hospital policy permits) as diluent to decrease pain. Rotate sites.
• Don't give solution containing local
anesthetics I.V. or intrathecally.
• When giving I.V., check site daily for
phlebitis and irritation. Dilute each
500,000 units in 300 to 500 ml 5% dextrose in water; infuse over 60 to 90
minutes. Rotate I.V. sites regularly.
• Parenteral solutions should be refrigerated and used within 72 hours.
• Monitor renal function (BUN, serum
creatinine, creatinine clearance, urinary output) before and during therapy.
Intake should be sufficient to maintain
output at 1,500 ml/day (between 3,000
and 4,000 ml/day for adults).
• Discontinue therapy if BUN increases and urinary output decreases.
• Notify doctor immediately if patient

develops fever, CNS side effects, rash, or symptoms of nephrotoxicity.
• If patient is scheduled for surgery, notify anesthesiologist of preoperative treatment with this drug since neuromuscular blockade can occur.

spectinomycin dihydrochloride
Trobicin♦

INDICATIONS & DOSAGE
Gonorrhea—
Adults: 2 to 4 g I.M. single dose injected deeply into the upper outer quadrant of the buttock.

SIDE EFFECTS
CNS: insomnia, dizziness.
GI: nausea.
GU: decreased urine output.
Skin: urticaria.
Local: pain at injection site.
Other: fever, chills (may mask or delay symptoms of incubating syphilis).

INTERACTIONS
None significant.

NURSING CONSIDERATIONS
• Not effective in the treatment of syphilis.
• Serologic test for syphilis should be done before treatment dose and 3 months after.
• Use 20G needle to administer drug. The 4-g dose (10 ml) should be divided into two 5-ml injections—one in each buttock.
• Shake vial vigorously after reconstitution and before withdrawing dose. Store at room temperature after reconstitution and use within 24 hours.
• Should be reserved for penicillin-resistant strains of gonorrhea.

trimethoprim
Proloprim, Trimpex

INDICATIONS & DOSAGE
Treatment of uncomplicated urinary tract infections caused by susceptible strains of Escherichia coli, Proteus mirabilis, Klebsiella, *and* Enterobacter *species—*
Adults: 100 mg P.O. every 12 hours for 10 days.
Not recommended for children under 12 years.

SIDE EFFECTS
Blood: thrombocytopenia, leukopenia, megaloblastic anemia, methemoglobinemia.
GI: epigastric distress, nausea, vomiting, glossitis.
Skin: *rash, pruritus, exfoliative dermatitis.*
Other: fever.

INTERACTIONS
None significant.

NURSING CONSIDERATIONS
• Contraindicated in documented megaloblastic anemia due to folate deficiency.
• Clinical signs such as sore throat, fever, pallor, or purpura may be early indications of serious blood disorders. Complete blood counts should be done routinely. Prolonged use of trimethoprim at high doses may cause bone marrow depression.
• Dose should be decreased in patients with severely impaired renal function. Give cautiously to patients with impaired hepatic function.
• To be of benefit, full course of therapy must be completed.

Italicized side effects are common or life-threatening.
∗Liquid form contains alcohol.   ∗∗May contain tartrazine.

troleandomycin phosphate
Tao

INDICATIONS & DOSAGE
*Sensitive pneumococcal pneumonia or
group A beta-hemolytic streptococcal
respiratory tract infection—*
Adults: 250 to 500 mg P.O. q 6 hours.
Children: 6.6 to 11 mg/kg P.O. daily,
q 6 hours.

SIDE EFFECTS
GI: *nausea,* vomiting, diarrhea, dis-
comfort.
Hepatic: cholestatic jaundice.
Skin: urticaria and rashes in hypersen-
sitivity reactions.
Other: *anaphylaxis.*

INTERACTIONS
None significant.

NURSING CONSIDERATIONS
• Use cautiously in patients with hepatic impairment.
• Drug is not recommended for routine
use.
• For best absorption, instruct patient
to take drug with a full glass of water 1
hour before or 2 hours after meals.
• Tell patient to take medication for as
long as prescribed, exactly as directed,
even after he feels better. Treat streptococcal infections at least 10 days.
• Monitor hepatic function (bilirubin,
SGOT, SGPT, and alkaline phosphatase).
• Report side effects, especially abdominal pain, nausea, or jaundice.

vancomycin hydrochloride
Vancocin♦

INDICATIONS & DOSAGE
*Severe staphylococcal infections when
other antibiotics ineffective or contraindicated—*
Adults: 500 mg I.V. q 6 hours, or l g q
12 hours.

Children: 44 mg/kg I.V. daily, divided
q 6 hours.
Neonates: 10 mg/kg I.V. daily, divided
q 6 to 12 hours.
*Antibiotic-associated pseudomembran-
ous and staphylococcal enterocolitis—*
Adults: 500 mg P.O. in 30 ml water q 6
hours for 7 to 10 days.
Children: 44 mg/kg P.O. daily, divided
q 6 hours with 30 ml water.

SIDE EFFECTS
Blood: transient eosinophilia.
EENT: tinnitus, ototoxicity (deafness).
GI: nausea.
GU: nephrotoxicity (hyaline casts in
urine, albuminuria, increased BUN).
Local: *pain or thrombophlebitis with
I.V. administration, necrosis.*
Other: chills, fever, *anaphylaxis,*
overgrowth of nonsusceptible or-
ganisms.

INTERACTIONS
None significant.

NURSING CONSIDERATIONS
• Contraindicated in patients receiving
other neurotoxic, nephrotoxic, or ototoxic drugs. Use cautiously in patients
with impaired hepatic or renal function;
also in those with preexisting hearing
loss; in patients over 60 years; and in
patients with allergies to other antibiotics.
• Tell patient to take medication exactly as directed, even after he feels
better. Treat staphylococcal endocarditis for at least 4 weeks.
• Patients should receive auditory
function tests before and during
therapy.
• Tell patient to report side effects at
once, especially dizziness, fullness or
ringing in ears. Stop drug immediately
if these occur.
• Do not give drug I.M.
• For I.V. infusion, dilute in 200 ml sodium chloride injection or 5% glucose
solution and infuse over 20 to 30 minutes. Check site daily for phlebitis and

irritation. Report pain at infusion site. Avoid extravasation. Severe irritation and necrosis can result.
• Refrigerate I.V. solution after reconstitution and use within 96 hours.
• Monitor renal function (BUN, serum creatinine, urinalysis, creatinine clearance, urinary output) before and during therapy. Watch for signs of superinfection.
• Oral preparation stable for 2 weeks if refrigerated.
• Has been used recently to treat pseudomembranous enterocolitis caused by clindamycin.

---

vidarabine monohydrate
Vira-A

INDICATIONS & DOSAGE
Herpes simplex virus encephalitis—
Adults and children (including neonates): 15 mg/kg daily for 10 days. Slowly infuse the total daily dose by I.V. infusion at a constant rate over 12- to 24-hour period. Avoid rapid or bolus injection.

SIDE EFFECTS
Blood: anemia, neutropenia, thrombocytopenia.
CNS: tremor, dizziness, hallucinations, confusion, psychosis, ataxia.
GI: *anorexia, nausea,* vomiting, diarrhea.
Hepatic: elevated SGOT, bilirubin.
Skin: pruritus, rash.
Local: pain at injection site.
Other: weight loss.

INTERACTIONS
Allopurinol: concurrent therapy increases risk of CNS side effects.

NURSING CONSIDERATIONS
• Will reduce mortality caused by herpes simplex virus encephalitis from 70% to 28%. No evidence that vidarabine is effective in encephalitis due to other viruses.
• Don't give I.M. or subcutaneously because of low solubility and poor absorption.
• Monitor hematologic tests, such as hemoglobin, hematocrit, WBC, and platelets during therapy. Also monitor renal and liver function studies.
• Patient with impaired renal function may need dosage adjustment.
• Once in solution, vidarabine is stable at room temperature for at least 2 weeks.
• Use with an I.V. filter.
• Must be diluted to a concentration of less than 0.5 mg/ml.
• Any intravenous solution is suitable as a diluent.

Italicized side effects are common or life-threatening.
*Liquid form contains alcohol.   **May contain tartrazine.

17

Cardiotonic glycosides

deslanoside
digitalis leaf
digitoxin
digoxin
gitalin
lanatoside C
ouabain

MECHANISM OF ACTION
• Cardiotonic glycosides act directly on the myocardium to increase the force of contraction (produce a positive inotropic effect) by two mechanisms:
   They promote movement of calcium from extracellular to intracellular cytoplasm. The force of contraction is directly related to the concentration of calcium in the myocardial cytoplasm.
   They also inhibit adenosinetriphosphatase (ATPase), the enzyme that regulates potassium and sodium electrolyte concentrations in myocardial cells. Inhibition of ATPase increases intracellular sodium concentration, which in turn increases the force of contraction.
• The glycosides decrease conduction velocity through the atrioventricular (AV) node to slow heart rate.
• They prolong the effective refractory period of the AV node by both direct and sympatholytic effects on the sinoatrial (SA) node.

COMBINATION PRODUCTS
None.

deslanoside
Cedilanid-D

INDICATIONS & DOSAGE
Congestive heart failure, paroxysmal atrial tachycardia, atrial fibrillation and flutter—
Adults: loading dose 1.2 to 1.6 mg I.M. or I.V. in 2 divided doses over 24 hours; for maintenance, use another glycoside. Not recommended for children.

SIDE EFFECTS
The following are signs of toxicity that may occur with all cardiotonic glycosides:
CNS: *fatigue, generalized muscle weakness, agitation, hallucinations,* headache, malaise, dizziness, vertigo, stupor, paresthesias.
CV: *increased severity of congestive heart failure, arrhythmias (most commonly conduction disturbances with or without AV block, premature ventricular contractions, and supraventricular arrhythmias),* hypotension.
Toxic effects on heart may be life-threatening and require immediate attention.
EENT: *yellow-green halos around visual images, blurred vision,* light flashes, photophobia, diplopia.
GI: *anorexia, nausea,* vomiting, diarrhea.

INTERACTIONS
Amphotericin B, carbenicillin, ticarcillin, corticosteroids, and diuretics, including chlorthalidone, ethacrynic acid, furosemide, metolazone, and

---

thiazides: hypokalemia, predisposing patient to digitalis toxicity. Monitor serum potassium.
Parenteral calcium, thiazides: hypercalcemia and hypomagnesemia, predisposing patient to digitalis toxicity. Monitor serum calcium and serum magnesium.

NURSING CONSIDERATIONS
• Contraindicated in presence of any digitalis-induced toxicity; ventricular fibrillation; ventricular tachycardia unless caused by congestive heart failure. Administering calcium salts to digitalized patient is contraindicated. Calcium affects cardiac contractility and excitability in much the same way that glycosides do and may lead to serious arrhythmias in digitalized patient. Use with extreme caution in the elderly, and in patients with acute myocardial infarction, incomplete AV block, chronic constrictive pericarditis, idiopathic hypertrophic subaortic stenosis, renal insufficiency, severe pulmonary disease, or hypothyroidism.
• Hypothyroid patients are very sensitive to glycosides; hyperthyroid patients may need larger doses.
• Obtain baseline data (heart rate and rhythm, blood pressure, electrolytes) before giving first dose.
• Question patient about recent use of cardiotonic glycosides (within the previous 2 to 3 weeks) before administering a loading dose. Always divide loading dose over first 24 hours unless clinical situation indicates otherwise.
• Use only for rapid digitalization, not maintenance.
• Dose is adjusted to patient's clinical condition and is monitored by serum levels of cardiotonic glycoside, calcium, potassium, magnesium, and by EKG.
• Take apical-radial pulse for a full minute. Record and report to doctor any significant changes (sudden increase or decrease in rate, pulse deficit, irregular beats, and particularly regu-

larization of a previously irregular rhythm). Check blood pressure and obtain 12-lead EKG with these changes.
• Observe eating pattern. Ask patient about nausea, vomiting, anorexia, visual disturbances, and other symptoms of toxicity.
• I.M. injection is painful; give I.V. if possible.
• Monitor serum potassium carefully. Take corrective action *before* hypokalemia occurs.

digitalis leaf

INDICATIONS & DOSAGE
Congestive heart failure, paroxysmal atrial tachycardia, atrial fibrillation and flutter—
Adults: loading dose 1.2 to 1.8 g P.O. in divided doses over 24 hours; usual maintenance 100 mg P.O. daily. Not recommended for children.

SIDE EFFECTS
The following are signs of toxicity that may occur with all cardiotonic glycosides:
CNS: *fatigue, generalized muscle weakness, agitation, hallucinations,* headache, malaise, dizziness, vertigo, stupor, paresthesias.
CV: *increased severity of congestive heart failure, arrhythmias (most commonly conduction disturbances with or without AV block, premature ventricular contractions, and supraventricular arrhythmias),* hypotension.
Toxic effects on heart may be life-threatening and require immediate attention.
EENT: *yellow-green halos around visual images, blurred vision,* light flashes, photophobia, diplopia.
GI: *anorexia, nausea,* vomiting, diarrhea.

INTERACTIONS
Para-aminosalicylic acid, antacids, cholestyramine, kaolin-pectin, neomycin, colestipol: decreased absorption of

---

Italicized side effects are common or life-threatening.
*Liquid form contains alcohol.   **May contain tartrazine.

digitoxin, the main active component of the digitalis leaf. Schedule doses as far as possible from administration of digitalis leaf.

Amphotericin B, carbenicillin, ticarcillin, corticosteroids, and diuretics, including chlorthalidone, ethacrynic acid, furosemide, metolazone, and thiazides: hypokalemia, predisposing patient to digitalis toxicity. Monitor serum potassium.

Parenteral calcium, thiazides: hypercalcemia and hypomagnesemia, predisposing patient to digitalis toxicity. Monitor serum calcium and serum magnesium.

Phenylbutazone, phenobarbital, phenytoin, rifampin: faster metabolism and shorter duration of action of digitoxin. Observe for underdigitalization.

NURSING CONSIDERATIONS

• Contraindicated in presence of any digitalis-induced toxicity; ventricular fibrillation; ventricular tachycardia unless caused by congestive heart failure. Administering calcium salts to digitalized patient is contraindicated. Calcium affects cardiac contractility and excitability in much the same way that glycosides do and may lead to serious arrhythmias in digitalized patient. Use with extreme caution in patients with acute myocardial infarction, incomplete AV block, chronic constrictive pericarditis, idiopathic hypertrophic subaortic stenosis, renal insufficiency, severe pulmonary disease, hypothyroidism, and in the elderly.

• Hypothyroid patients are very sensitive to glycosides; hyperthyroid patients may need larger doses.

• Obtain baseline data (heart rate and rhythm, blood pressure, electrolytes) before giving first dose.

• Question patient about recent use of cardiotonic glycosides (within the previous 2 to 3 weeks) before administering a loading dose. Always divide loading dose over first 24 hours unless clinical situation indicates otherwise.

• Dose is adjusted to patient's clinical condition and is monitored by serum levels of cardiotonic glycoside, calcium, potassium, magnesium, and by EKG.

• Take apical-radial pulse for a full minute. Record and report to doctor any significant changes (sudden increase or decrease in rate, pulse deficit, irregular beats, and particularly regularization of a previously irregular rhythm). Check blood pressure and obtain 12-lead EKG with these changes.

• Observe eating pattern. Ask patient about nausea, vomiting, anorexia, visual disturbances, and other symptoms of toxicity.

• Monitor serum potassium carefully. Take corrective action *before* hypokalemia occurs.

• Digitalis leaf is a long-acting drug; watch for cumulative effects.

• Instruct patient and responsible family member about drug action, dosage regimen, how to take pulse, reportable signs, and follow-up plans.

• Therapeutic blood levels of digitoxin (the active agent in the leaf) range from 25 to 35 ng/ml.

digitoxin
Crystodigin, De-Tone, Purodigin**♦

INDICATIONS & DOSAGE
Congestive heart failure, paroxysmal atrial tachycardia, atrial fibrillation and flutter—
Adults: loading dose 1.2 to 1.6 mg I.V. or P.O. in divided doses over 24 hours; maintenance 0.1 mg daily.
Children 2 to 12 years: loading dose 0.03 mg/kg or 0.75 mg/m² I.M., I.V., or P.O. in divided doses over 24 hours; maintenance $^1/_{10}$ loading dose or 0.003 mg/kg or 0.075 mg/m² daily. Monitor closely for toxicity.
Children 1 to 2 years: loading dose 0.04 mg/kg over 24 hours in divided doses; maintenance 0.004 mg/kg daily. Monitor closely for toxicity.

Unmarked trade names available in the United States only.
♦ Also available in Canada.   ♦ ♦ Available in Canada only.

Children 2 weeks to 1 year: loading dose 0.045 mg/kg I.M., I.V., or P.O. in divided doses over 24 hours; maintenance 0.0045 mg/kg daily. Monitor closely for toxicity.

Premature infants, neonates, severely ill older infants: loading dose 0.022 mg/kg I.M., I.V., or P.O. in divided doses over 24 hours; maintenance 0.0022 mg/kg daily. Monitor closely for toxicity.

SIDE EFFECTS
The following are signs of toxicity that may occur with all cardiotonic glycosides:

CNS: *fatigue, generalized muscle weakness, agitation, hallucinations,* headache, malaise, dizziness, vertigo, stupor, paresthesias.

CV: *increased severity of congestive heart failure, arrhythmias (most commonly conduction disturbances with or without AV block, premature ventricular contractions, and supraventricular arrhythmias),* hypotension.
Toxic effects on heart may be life-threatening and require immediate attention.

EENT: *yellow-green halos around visual images, blurred vision,* light flashes, photophobia, diplopia.

GI: *anorexia, nausea,* vomiting, diarrhea.

INTERACTIONS
Para-aminosalicylic acid, antacids, cholestyramine, colestipol, kaolin-pectin, neomycin: decreased absorption of oral digitoxin. Schedule doses as far as possible from oral digitoxin administration.
Amphotericin B, carbenicillin, ticarcillin, corticosteroids, and diuretics, including chlorthalidone, ethacrynic acid, furosemide, metolazone, and thiazides: hypokalemia, predisposing patient to digitalis toxicity. Monitor serum potassium.
Parenteral calcium, thiazides: hypercalcemia and hypomagnesemia, predisposing patient to digitalis toxicity. Monitor serum calcium and serum magnesium.
Phenylbutazone, phenobarbital, phenytoin, rifampin: faster metabolism and shorter duration of digitoxin. Observe for underdigitalization.
Cimetidine: decreased digitoxin metabolism. Monitor for digitoxin toxicity.

NURSING CONSIDERATIONS
• Contraindicated in presence of any digitalis-induced toxicity; ventricular fibrillation; ventricular tachycardia unless caused by congestive heart failure. Administering calcium salts to digitalized patient is contraindicated. Calcium affects cardiac contractility and excitability in much the same way that glycosides do and may lead to serious arrhythmias in digitalized patient. Use with extreme caution in patients with acute myocardial infarction, incomplete AV block, chronic constrictive pericarditis, idiopathic hypertrophic subaortic stenosis, severe pulmonary disease, hypothyroidism, and in the elderly.
• Hypothyroid patients are very sensitive to glycosides; hyperthyroid patients may need larger doses.
• Obtain baseline data (heart rate and rhythm, blood pressure, electrolytes) before giving first dose.
• Question patient about recent use of cardiotonic glycosides (within the previous 2 to 3 weeks) before administering a loading dose. Always divide loading dose over first 24 hours unless clinical situation indicates otherwise.
• Dose is adjusted to patient's clinical condition and is monitored by serum levels of cardiotonic glycoside, calcium, potassium, magnesium, and by EKG.
• Take apical-radial pulse for a full minute. Record and report to doctor any significant changes (sudden increase or decrease in rate, pulse deficit, irregular beats, and particularly

---

Italicized side effects are common or life-threatening.
∗Liquid form contains alcohol.   ∗∗May contain tartrazine.

regularization of a previously irregular rhythm). Check blood pressure and obtain 12-lead EKG with these changes.
• Observe eating pattern. Ask patient about nausea, vomiting, anorexia, visual disturbances, and other symptoms of toxicity.
• Watch closely for signs of toxicity, especially in children and the elderly.
• Monitor serum potassium carefully. Take corrective action *before* hypokalemia occurs.
• I.M. injection is painful; give I.V. if parenteral route is necessary.
• Digitoxin is a long-acting drug; watch for cumulative effects.
• Protect solution from light.
• Instruct patient and responsible family member about drug action, dosage regimen, how to take pulse, reportable signs, and follow-up plans.
• Don't substitute one brand for another.
• Therapeutic blood levels of digitoxin range from 25 to 35 ng/ml.

digoxin
Lanoxin*♦, Masoxin

INDICATIONS & DOSAGE
Congestive heart failure, atrial fibrillation and flutter, paroxysmal atrial tachycardia—
Adults: loading dose 0.5 to 1 mg I.V. or P.O. in divided doses over 24 hours; maintenance 0.125 to 0.5 mg I.V. or P.O. daily (average 0.25 mg). Larger doses are often needed for treatment of arrhythmias, depending on patient response.
Children over 2 years: loading dose 0.04 to 0.06 mg/kg P.O. divided q 8 hours over 24 hours; I.V. loading dose 0.025 to 0.04 mg/kg; maintenance 0.02 mg/kg P.O. daily divided q 12 hours.
Children 1 month to 2 years: loading dose 0.06 to 0.075 mg/kg P.O. divided into three doses over 24 hours;

I.V. loading dose 0.035 to 0.05 mg/kg; maintenance 0.02 to 0.025 mg/kg P.O. daily divided q 12 hours.
Neonates under 1 month: loading dose 0.05 mg/kg P.O. divided q 8 hours over 24 hours; I.V. loading dose 0.015 to 0.04 mg/kg; maintenance 0.0167 mg/kg P.O. daily divided q 12 hours.
Premature infants: loading dose 0.04 mg/kg I.V. divided into 3 doses over 24 hours; maintenance 0.0133 mg/kg I.V. daily divided q 12 hours.

SIDE EFFECTS
The following are signs of toxicity that may occur with all cardiotonic glycosides:
CNS: *fatigue, generalized muscle weakness, agitation, hallucinations, headache, malaise, dizziness, vertigo, stupor, paresthesias.*
CV: *increased severity of congestive heart failure, arrhythmias (most commonly conduction disturbances with or without AV block, premature ventricular contractions, and supraventricular arrhythmias), hypotension.*
Toxic effects on heart may be life-threatening and require immediate attention.
EENT: *yellow-green halos around visual images, blurred vision, light flashes, photophobia, diplopia.*
GI: *anorexia, nausea, vomiting, diarrhea.*

INTERACTIONS
Para-aminosalicylic acid, antacids, cholestyramine, colestipol, kaolin-pectin, neomycin: decreased absorption of oral digoxin. Schedule doses as far as possible from oral digoxin administration.
Quinidine, nifedipine, and verapamil: increased digoxin blood levels. Monitor for toxicty.
Amphotericin B, carbenicillin, ticarcillin, corticosteroids, and diuretics, including chlorthalidone, ethacrynic

acid, furosemide, metolazone, and thiazides: hypokalemia, predisposing patient to digitalis toxicity. Monitor serum potassium.

Parenteral calcium, thiazides: hypercalcemia and hypomagnesemia, predisposing patient to digitalis toxicity. Monitor serum calcium and serum magnesium.

Amiloride: inhibits and increases digoxin excretion. Monitor for altered digoxin effect.

NURSING CONSIDERATIONS

• Contraindicated in presence of any digitalis-induced toxicity; ventricular fibrillation; ventricular tachycardia unless caused by congestive heart failure. Administering calcium salts to digitalized patient is contraindicated. Calcium affects cardiac contractility and excitability in much the same way that glycosides do and may lead to serious arrhythmias in digitalized patient. Use with extreme caution in the elderly, and in patients with acute myocardial infarction, incomplete AV block, chronic constrictive pericarditis, idiopathic hypertrophic subaortic stenosis, renal insufficiency, severe pulmonary disease, or hypothyroidism. Dose must be reduced in renal impairment.

• Hypothyroid patients are very sensitive to glycosides; hyperthyroid patients may need larger doses.

• Obtain baseline data (heart rate and rhythm, blood pressure, electrolytes) before giving first dose.

• Question patient about recent use of cardiotonic glycosides (within the previous 2 to 3 weeks) before administering a loading dose. Always divide loading dose over first 24 hours unless clinical situation indicates otherwise.

• Dose is adjusted to patient's clinical condition and is monitored by serum levels of cardiotonic glycoside, calcium, potassium, magnesium, and by EKG.

• Take apical-radial pulse for a full minute. Record and report to doctor any significant changes (sudden increase or decrease in rate, pulse deficit, irregular beats, and particularly regularization of a previously irregular rhythm). Check blood pressure and obtain 12-lead EKG with these changes.

• Observe eating pattern. Ask patient about nausea, vomiting, anorexia, visual disturbances, and other symptoms of toxicity.

• Monitor serum potassium carefully. Take corrective action *before* hypokalemia occurs.

• Withhold for 1 to 2 days before elective electrocardioversion. Adjust dose after cardioversion.

• Instruct patient and responsible family member about drug action, dosage regimen, how to take pulse, reportable signs, and follow-up plans.

• Don't substitute one brand for another.

• Therapeutic blood levels of digoxin range from 0.5 to 2.5 ng/ml.

---

gitalin
Gitaligin**

INDICATIONS & DOSAGE

Congestive heart failure, atrial fibrillation and flutter, paroxysmal atrial tachycardia—
Adults: loading dose 2.5 mg P.O. initially, then 0.75 mg q 6 hours until therapeutic effect is attained (not to exceed 6 mg total in 24 hours); maintenance 0.25 to 1.25 mg daily. Not recommended for children.

SIDE EFFECTS

The following are signs of toxicity that may occur with all cardiotonic glycosides:
CNS: *fatigue, generalized muscle weakness, agitation, hallucinations,* headache, malaise, dizziness, vertigo, stupor, paresthesias.
CV: *increased severity of congestive*

Italicized side effects are common or life-threatening.
*Liquid form contains alcohol.   **May contain tartrazine.

heart failure, arrhythmias (most commonly conduction disturbances with or without AV block, premature ventricular contractions, and supraventricular arrhythmias), hypotension.
Toxic effects on heart may be life-threatening and require immediate attention.
EENT: *yellow-green halos around visual images, blurred vision,* light flashes, photophobia, diplopia.
GI: *anorexia, nausea,* vomiting, diarrhea.

INTERACTIONS
Para-aminosalicylic acid, antacids, cholestyramine, colestipol, kaolin-pectin, neomycin: decreased absorption of oral gitalin. Schedule doses as far as possible from oral gitalin administration.
Amphotericin B, carbenicillin, ticarcillin, corticosteroids, and diuretics, including chlorthalidone, ethacrynic acid, furosemide, metolazone, and thiazides: hypokalemia, predisposing patient to digitalis toxicity. Monitor serum potassium.
Parenteral calcium, thiazides: hypercalcemia and hypomagnesemia, predisposing patient to digitalis toxicity. Monitor serum calcium and serum magnesium.

NURSING CONSIDERATIONS
• Contraindicated in presence of any digitalis-induced toxicity; ventricular fibrillation; ventricular tachycardia unless caused by congestive heart failure. Administering calcium salts to digitalized patient is contraindicated. Calcium affects cardiac contractility and excitability in much the same way that glycosides do and may lead to serious arrhythmias in digitalized patient. Use with extreme caution in the elderly, and in patients with acute myocardial infarction, incomplete AV block, chronic constrictive pericarditis, idiopathic hypertrophic subaortic stenosis, renal insufficiency, severe

pulmonary disease, or hypothyroidism.
• Hypothyroid patients are very sensitive to glycosides; hyperthyroid patients may need larger doses.
• Obtain baseline data (heart rate and rhythm, blood pressure, electrolytes) before giving first dose.
• Question patient about recent use of cardiotonic glycosides (within the previous 2 to 3 weeks) before administering a loading dose. Always divide loading dose over first 24 hours unless clinical situation indicates otherwise.
• Dose is adjusted to patient's clinical condition and is monitored by serum levels of cardiotonic glycoside, calcium, potassium, magnesium, and by EKG.
• Take apical-radial pulse for a full minute. Record and report to doctor any significant changes (sudden increase or decrease in rate, pulse deficit, irregular beats, and particularly regularization of a previously irregular rhythm). Check blood pressure and obtain 12-lead EKG with these changes.
• Observe eating pattern. Ask patient about nausea, vomiting, anorexia, visual disturbances, and other symptoms of toxicity.
• Monitor serum potassium carefully. Take corrective action *before* hypokalemia occurs.
• Gitalin is a long-acting drug; watch for cumulative effects.
• Withhold for 1 to 2 days before elective electrocardioversion. Adjust dose after cardioversion.
• Instruct patient and responsible family member about drug action, dosage regimen, how to take pulse, reportable signs, and follow-up plans.

lanatoside C

INDICATIONS & DOSAGE
Congestive heart failure, atrial fibril-

lation and flutter, paroxysmal atrial tachycardia—
Adults: average total dose for digitalization is 10 mg P.O. given as follows: loading dose. First day, 3.5 mg; second day, 2.5 mg; third day, 2 mg; thereafter 1.5 mg per day until digitalization obtained; maintenance 0.5 to 1.5 mg daily.
Not recommended for children.

SIDE EFFECTS
The following are signs of toxicity that may occur with all cardiotonic glycosides:
CNS: *fatigue, generalized muscle weakness, agitation, hallucinations,* headache, malaise, dizziness, vertigo, stupor, paresthesias.
CV: *increased severity of congestive heart failure, arrhythmias (most commonly conduction disturbances with or without AV block, premature ventricular contractions, and supraventricular arrhythmias),* hypotension.
Toxic effects on heart may be life-threatening and require immediate attention.
EENT: *yellow-green halos around visual images, blurred vision,* light flashes, photophobia, diplopia.
GI: *anorexia, nausea,* vomiting, diarrhea.

INTERACTIONS
Para-aminosalicylic acid, antacids, cholestyramine, kaolin-pectin, neomycin, colestipol: decreased absorption of digoxin formed in stomach from lanatoside C. Schedule doses as far as possible from lanatoside C administration.
Amphotericin B, carbenicillin, ticarcillin, corticosteroids, and diuretics, including chlorthalidone, ethacrynic acid, furosemide, metolazone, and thiazides: hypokalemia, predisposing patient to digitalis toxicity. Monitor serum potassium.
Parenteral calcium, thiazides: hypercalcemia and hypomagnesemia, predisposing patient to digitalis toxicity. Monitor serum calcium and serum magnesium.

NURSING CONSIDERATIONS
• Contraindicated in presence of any digitalis-induced toxicity; ventricular fibrillation; ventricular tachycardia unless caused by congestive heart failure. Administering calcium salts to digitalized patient is contraindicated. Calcium affects cardiac contractility and excitability in much the same way that glycosides do and may lead to serious arrhythmias in digitalized patient. Use with extreme caution in patients with acute myocardial infarction, incomplete AV block, chronic constrictive pericarditis, idiopathic hypertrophic subaortic stenosis, renal insufficiency, severe pulmonary disease, hypothyroidism; and in the elderly. Dose should be reduced in renal impairment.
• Hypothyroid patients are very sensitive to glycosides; hyperthyroid patients may need larger doses.
• Obtain baseline data (heart rate and rhythm, blood pressure, electrolytes) before giving first dose.
• Question patient about recent use of cardiotonic glycosides (within the previous 2 to 3 weeks) before administering a loading dose. Always divide loading dose over first 24 hours unless clinical situation indicates otherwise.
• Dose is adjusted to patient's clinical condition and is monitored by serum levels of cardiotonic glycoside, calcium, potassium, magnesium, and by EKG.
• Take apical-radial pulse for a full minute. Record and report to doctor any significant changes (sudden increase or decrease in rate, pulse deficit, irregular beats, and particularly regularization of a previously irregular rhythm). Check blood pressure and obtain 12-lead EKG with these changes.
• Observe eating pattern. Ask patient

Italicized side effects are common or life-threatening.
*Liquid form contains alcohol.   **May contain tartrazine.

about nausea, vomiting, anorexia, visual disturbances, and other symptoms of toxicity.
• Monitor serum potassium carefully. Take corrective action *before* hypokalemia occurs.
• Withhold for 1 to 2 days before elective electrocardioversion. Adjust dose after cardioversion.
• Instruct patient and responsible family member about drug action, dosage regimen, how to take pulse, reportable signs, and follow-up plans.

ouabain

INDICATIONS & DOSAGE
Congestive heart failure, atrial fibrillation and flutter, paroxysmal atrial tachycardia—
Adults: loading dose 0.25 to 0.5 mg by slow I.V. injection. Additional 0.1 mg doses may be given every hour until a therapeutic effect is achieved or a total of 1 mg is given. For maintenance, use another glycoside. Not recommended for children.

SIDE EFFECTS
The following are signs of toxicity that may occur with all cardiotonic glycosides:
CNS: *fatigue, generalized muscle weakness, agitation, hallucinations,* headache, malaise, dizziness, vertigo, stupor, paresthesias.
CV: *increased severity of congestive heart failure, arrhythmias (most commonly conduction disturbances with or without AV block, premature ventricular contractions, and supraventricular arrhythmias),* hypotension.
Toxic effects on heart may be life-threatening and require immediate attention.
EENT: *yellow-green halos around visual images, blurred vision,* light flashes, photophobia, diplopia.
GI: *anorexia, nausea,* vomiting, diarrhea.

INTERACTIONS
Amphotericin B, carbenicillin, ticarcillin, corticosteroids, and diuretics, including chlorthalidone, ethacrynic acid, furosemide, metolazone, and thiazides: hypokalemia, predisposing patient to toxicity. Monitor serum potassium.
Parenteral calcium, thiazides: hypercalcemia and hypomagnesemia, predisposing patient to toxicity. Monitor serum calcium and serum magnesium.

NURSING CONSIDERATIONS
• Contraindicated in presence of any digitalis-induced toxicity; ventricular fibrillation; ventricular tachycardia unless caused by congestive heart failure. Administering calcium salts to digitalized patient is contraindicated. Calcium affects cardiac contractility and excitability in much the same way that glycosides do and may lead to serious arrhythmias in digitalized patient. Use with extreme caution in patients with acute myocardial infarction, incomplete AV block, chronic constrictive pericarditis, idiopathic hypertrophic subaortic stenosis, renal insufficiency, severe pulmonary disease, hypothyroidism; and in the elderly. Dose should be reduced in renal impairment.
• Hypothyroid patients are very sensitive to glycosides; hyperthyroid patients may need larger doses.
• Obtain baseline data (heart rate and rhythm, blood pressure, electrolytes) before giving first dose.
• Question patient about recent use of cardiotonic glycosides (within the previous 2 to 3 weeks) before administering a loading dose. Always divide loading dose over first 24 hours unless clinical situation indicates otherwise.
• Use only for rapid digitalization, not maintenance.
• Dose is adjusted to patient's clinical condition and is monitored by serum levels of cardiotonic glycoside, cal-

cium, potassium, magnesium, and by EKG.

• Take apical-radial pulse for a full minute. Record and report to doctor any significant changes (sudden increase or decrease in rate, pulse deficit, irregular beats, and, particularly, regularization of a previously irregular rhythm). Check blood pressure and obtain 12-lead EKG with these changes.

• Observe eating pattern. Ask patient about nausea, vomiting, anorexia, visual disturbances, and other symptoms of toxicity.

• I.M. route is painful; absorption is unpredictable. Not recommended.

• Monitor serum potassium carefully. Take corrective action *before* hypokalemia occurs.

18

Antiarrhythmics

atropine sulfate
bretylium tosylate
disopyramide
disopyramide phosphate
lidocaine hydrochloride
nifedipine
phenytoin
phenytoin sodium
procainamide hydrochloride
propranolol hydrochloride
quinidine bisulfate
quinidine gluconate
quinidine polygalacturonate
quinidine sulfate
verapamil

MECHANISM OF ACTION

• Group I drugs (disopyramide, procainamide, and quinidine) decrease sodium transport through cardiac tissues, slowing conduction through the AV node. These drugs also prolong the effective refractory period and decrease automaticity.
• Group II drugs (lidocaine and phenytoin) increase conduction block against reentry impulses but have little effect on conduction velocity. They stabilize reentry ventricular arrhythmias associated with MI; phenytoin may also combat arrhythmias due to digitalis toxicity.
• Group III drugs (beta blockers) decrease conduction of impulses through the AV node and increase the effective refractory period. In addition to their beta blockade, group III drugs also have reentry blocking effects similar to those of group II. Propranolol, the only beta blocker approved for use as an antiarrhythmic, is effective for supra-

ventricular arrhythmias and, to a lesser extent, for ventricular arrhythmias.
• The group IV drug bretylium was originally thought to act as an anti-adrenergic agent whose action is mediated through the sympathetic division of the autonomic nervous system. Bretylium initially exerts short-lived adrenergic stimulatory effects (caused by release of norepinephrine) on the cardiovascular system. When norepinephrine is depleted, the adrenergic blocking actions predominate. Recent pharmacologic studies indicate that bretylium's action may be due to its large quaternary ammonium structure.
• The group V agents verapamil and nifedipine selectively inhibit the myocardial cell-membrane transport of calcium by blocking the inward current (slow channel) of calcium into cardiac muscle. Impulse transmission through the AV node is delayed, and the spontaneous rhythmicity of the sinoatrial (SA) node is depressed.
• Among the unclassified drugs in this category, atropine blocks the vagal effects on the SA node, relieving severe nodal or sinus bradycardia, or AV block. Increased conduction through the AV node speeds heart rate.

COMBINATION PRODUCTS
None.

atropine sulfate

INDICATIONS & DOSAGE
Bradycardia, bradyarrhythmia (junctional or escape rhythm)—

Adults: usually 0.5 to 1 mg I.V. push; repeat q 5 minutes, to maximum 2 mg. Lower doses (less than 0.5 mg) can cause bradycardia.
Children: 0.01 mg/kg dose up to maximum 0.4 mg; or 0.3 mg/m^2 dose; may repeat q 4 to 6 hours.

SIDE EFFECTS
Blood: leukocytosis.
CNS: *with doses greater than 5 mg—headache, restlessness,* ataxia, disorientation, hallucinations, delirium, coma, *insomnia, dizziness.*
CV: *1 to 2 mg—tachycardia, palpitations; greater than 2 mg—extreme tachycardia, angina.*
EENT: *1 mg—slight mydriasis,* photophobia; *2 mg—blurred vision, mydriasis.*
GI: *dry mouth (common even at low doses),* thirst, *constipation,* nausea, vomiting.
GU: *urinary retention.*
Skin: 2 mg—flushed, dry skin; 5 mg or more—hot, dry, reddened skin.

INTERACTIONS
Methotrimeprazine: may produce extrapyramidal symptoms. Monitor patient carefully.

NURSING CONSIDERATIONS
• Side effects vary considerably with dose. Most common are dry mouth (which can be treated with pilocarpine syrup) and thirst. Recommend sucking sour hard candy.
• Watch for tachycardia in cardiac patients; report to doctor.
• Antidote for atropine overdose is physostigmine salicylate.
• Other anticholinergic drugs may increase vagal blockage.
• Monitor closely for urinary retention in elderly males with benign prostatic hypertrophy (BPH). These are high-risk patients for this effect.

bretylium tosylate
Bretylol

INDICATIONS & DOSAGE
Ventricular fibrillation—
Adults: 5 mg/kg by rapid I.V. injection. If necessary, increase dose to 10 mg/kg and repeat q 15 to 30 minutes until 30 mg/kg have been given.
Other ventricular arrhythmias—
Adults: initially, 500 mg diluted to 50 ml with 5% dextrose in water or normal saline solution and infused I.V. over more than 8 minutes at 5 to 10 mg/kg. Dose may be repeated in 1 to 2 hours. Thereafter, dose q 6 to 8 hours.
I.V. maintenance—
Adults: infused in diluted solution of 500 ml 5% dextrose in water or normal saline solution at 1 to 2 mg/minute.
I.M. injection—
Adults: 5 to 10 mg/kg undiluted. Repeat in 1 to 2 hours if needed. Thereafter, repeat q 6 to 8 hours.
Not recommended for children.

SIDE EFFECTS
CNS: *vertigo, dizziness, lightheadedness, syncope* (usually secondary to hypotension).
CV: *severe hypotension (especially orthostatic), bradycardia,* anginal pain.
GI: severe nausea, vomiting (with rapid infusion).

INTERACTIONS
All antihypertensives: may potentiate hypotension. Monitor blood pressure.

NURSING CONSIDERATIONS
• Contraindicated in digitalis-induced arrhythmias. Use cautiously in patients with fixed cardiac output, aortic stenosis, and pulmonary hypertension to avoid severe and sudden drop in blood pressure.
• Monitor blood pressure, heart rate and rhythm frequently. Notify doctor immediately of any significant change.

Italicized side effects are common or life-threatening.
*Liquid form contains alcohol.   **May contain tartrazine.

If supine systolic blood pressure falls below 75 mmHg, notify doctor, who may order norepinephrine or dopamine, or volume expansion to raise blood pressure.
• Keep patient in the supine position until tolerance to hypotension develops.
• Follow dosage directions carefully to avoid nausea and vomiting.
• Give I.V. injections for ventricular fibrillation as rapidly as possible. Do not dilute.
• Rotate I.M. injection sites to prevent tissue damage, and don't exceed 5-ml volume in any one site.
• To be used with other cardioresuscitative measures such as CPR, countershock, epinephrine, sodium bicarbonate, and lidocaine.
• Avoid subtherapeutic doses (less than 5 mg/kg), since such doses may cause hypotension.
• Ventricular tachycardia and other ventricular arrhythmias respond less rapidly to treatment than ventricular fibrillation does.
• Dosage should be decreased in renal impairment.
• Monitor carefully if pressor amines (sympathomimetics) are given to correct hypotension, as bretylium potentiates pressor amines.
• Ineffective treatment for atrial arrhythmias.
• Has been used investigationally to treat hypertension.
• Observe for increased anginal pain in susceptible patients.
• Observe patient for side effects and notify doctor if any occur.

disopyramide
Rythmodan♦

disopyramide phosphate
Norpace♦

INDICATIONS & DOSAGE
Premature ventricular contractions (unifocal, multifocal, or coupled); ventric-ular tachycardia not severe enough to require electrocardioversion—
Adults: Usual maintenance dose 150 to 200 mg P.O. q 6 hours; for patients who weigh less than 50 kg or those with renal, hepatic, or cardiac impairment—100 mg P.O. q 6 hours. Recommended doses in advanced renal insufficency: Creatinine clearance 15 to 40 ml/minute: 100 mg q 10 hours; creatinine clearance 5 to 15 ml/minute: 100 mg q 20 hours; creatinine clearance 1 to 5 ml/minute: 100 mg q 30 hours.
Children 12 to 18 years: 6 to 15 mg/kg daily.
Children 4 to 12 years: 10 to 15 mg/kg daily.
Children 1 to 4 years: 10 to 20 mg/kg daily.
Children less than 1 year: 10 to 30 mg/kg daily.
All children's doses should be divided into equal amounts and given every 6 hours.

SIDE EFFECTS
CNS: dizziness, agitation, depression, fatigue, muscle weakness, syncope.
CV: *hypotension, congestive heart failure, heart block.*
EENT: *blurred vision, dry eyes, dry nose.*
GI: nausea, vomiting, anorexia, bloating, abdominal pain, *constipation, dry mouth.*
GU: *urinary retention and hesitancy.*
Hepatic: cholestatic jaundice.
Metabolic: hypoglycemia.
Skin: rash in 1% to 3% of patients.

INTERACTIONS
phenytoin: increases disopyramides metabolism. Monitor for decreased antiarrhytmic effect.

NURSING CONSIDERATIONS
• Contraindicated in cardiogenic shock or second- or third-degree heart block with no pacemaker. Use very cautiously, and avoid, if possible, in congestive heart failure. Use cautiously in

underlying conduction abnormalities, urinary tract diseases (especially prostatic hypertrophy), hepatic or renal impairment, myasthenia gravis, narrow-angle glaucoma. Adjust dosage in renal insufficiency.

• Discontinue if heart block develops, if QRS complex widens by more than 25%, or if Q-T interval lengthens by more than 25% above baseline.

• Correct any underlying electrolyte abnormalities before use.

• Watch for recurrence of arrhythmias; check for side effects; notify doctor.

• Check apical pulse before administering drug. Notify doctor if pulse rate is slower than 60 beats per minute (bpm) or faster than 120 bpm.

• Teach patient the importance of taking drug on time, exactly as prescribed. To do this, he may have to use an alarm clock for night doses.

• Relieve discomfort of dry mouth by chewing gum or hard candy.

• Manage constipation with proper diet or bulk laxatives.

• Use of disopyramide with other antiarrhythmics may cause further myocardial depression.

• Pharmacist may prepare disopyramide suspension. 100 mg capsules are used to prepare suspension with cherry syrup. May be best for young children.

lidocaine hydrochloride
Lido Pen Auto-Injector, Xylocaine♦

INDICATIONS & DOSAGE
Ventricular arrhythmias from myocardial infarction, cardiac manipulation, or cardiotonic glycosides; ventricular tachycardia—
Adults: 50 to 100 mg (1 to 1.5 mg/kg) I.V. bolus at 25 to 50 mg/minute. Give half this amount to elderly or lightweight patients, and to those with congestive heart failure or hepatic disease. Repeat bolus q 3 to 5 minutes until arrhythmias subside or side effects develop. Don't exceed 300 mg total bolus

during a 1-hour period. Simultaneously, begin constant infusion: 1 to 4 mg/minute. Use lower dose in elderly patients, those with congestive heart failure or hepatic disease, or patients who weigh less than 50 kg. If single bolus has been given, repeat smaller bolus 15 to 20 minutes after start of infusion to maintain therapeutic serum level. After 24 hours of continuous infusion, decrease rate by half.
I.M. administration: 200 to 300 mg in deltoid muscle only.

SIDE EFFECTS
CNS: *confusion, tremors,* lethargy, *stupor, restlessness,* slurred speech, euphoria, depression, *light-headedness,* muscle twitching, *convulsions.*
CV: *hypotension,* bradycardia, further arrhythmias.
EENT: *tinnitus, blurred or double vision.*
Other: *anaphylaxis,* soreness at injection site, sensations of cold, diaphoresis.

INTERACTIONS
Barbiturates: may decrease patient's response to lidocaine. Adjust dose.
Cimetidine: decreased metabolism of lidocaine. Monitor for toxicity.
Phenytoin: additive cardiac depressant effects. Monitor carefully.
Procainamide: may increase neurologic side effects. Monitor carefully.

NURSING CONSIDERATIONS
• Contraindicated in complete or second-degree heart block. Use of lidocaine with epinephrine (for local anesthesia) to treat arrhythmias contraindicated. Use with caution in elderly patients, those with congestive heart failure, renal or hepatic disease, or patients who weigh less than 50 kg. Such patients will need a reduced dose.
• In many severely ill patients, convulsions may be the first clinically apparent sign of toxicity.
• If toxic signs (dizziness) occur, stop

Italicized side effects are common or life-threatening.
*Liquid form contains alcohol.   **May contain tartrazine.

drug at once and notify doctor. Continued infusion could lead to convulsions and coma. Give oxygen via nasal cannula, if not contraindicated. Keep oxygen and CPR equipment handy.
• Patients receiving infusions must be *attended at all times*, and be on a cardiac monitor. Use an infusion pump or a microdrip system and timer for monitoring infusion precisely. Never exceed an infusion rate of 4 mg/minute, if possible. A faster rate greatly increases risk of toxicity.
• Monitor patient's response, especially blood pressure, serum electrolytes, BUN, and creatinine. Notify doctor promptly if abnormalities develop.
• A bolus dose not followed by infusion will have a short-lived effect.
• A patient who has received lidocaine I.M. will show a sevenfold increase in serum CPK level. Such CPK originates in the skeletal muscle, not the heart. Test isoenzymes if using I.M. route.
• Used investigationally to treat refractory status epilepticus.

nifedipine
Procardia

INDICATIONS & DOSAGE
Management of vasospastic (also called Prinzmetals or variant angina) and classic chronic stable angina pectoris—
Adults: Starting dose is 10 mg P.O. t.i.d.
Usual effective dose range is 10 to 20 mg t.i.d. Some patients may require up to 30 mg q.i.d. Maximum daily dose is 180 mg.

SIDE EFFECTS
CNS: *dizziness, light-headedness, flushing, headache,* weakness, syncope.
CV: peripheral edema, hypotension, palpitations.
EENT: nasal congestion.
GI: *nausea, heartburn,* diarrhea.
Other: muscle cramps, dyspnea.

INTERACTIONS
Propranolol (and other beta blockers): may cause heart failure. Use together cautiously.

NURSING CONSIDERATIONS
• Use cautiously in patients with congestive heart failure or hypotension.
• Monitor blood pressure regularly, especially of patients who are also taking beta blockers or antihypertensives.
• Patient may briefly develop anginal exacerbation when beginning drug therapy or at times of dosage increase. Reassure him that this symptom is temporary.
• Although rebound effect hasn't been observed when drug is stopped, dosage should still be reduced slowly under doctor's supervision.
• If patient is kept on nitrate therapy while drug dosage is being titrated, urge him to continue his compliance. Sublingual nitroglycerin, especially, may be taken as needed when anginal symptoms are acute.
• Nifedipine was the first commercially available oral calcium blocker.

phenytoin
Dilantin Infatab♦, Dilantin Pediatric

phenytoin sodium
Dantoin♦♦, Dihycon, Dilantin♦, Di-Phen, Diphenylan Sodium, Toin Unicelles

INDICATIONS & DOSAGE
Ventricular arrhythmias unresponsive to lidocaine or procainamide; supraventricular and ventricular arrhythmias induced by cardiotonic glycosides—
Adults: loading dose 1 g P.O. divided over first 24 hours, followed by 500 mg daily for 2 days, then maintenance dose 300 mg P.O. daily; 250 mg I.V. over 5 minutes until arrhythmias subside, side effects develop, or 1 g has been given. Infusion rate should never exceed 50 mg/minute (slow I.V. push).

Alternate method: 100 mg I.V. q
15 minutes until side effects develop,
arrhythmias are controlled, or 1 g has
been given. May also administer entire
loading dose of 1 g I.V. slowly at
25 mg/minute. Can be diluted in normal saline solution. I.M. dose not recommended because of pain and erratic
absorption.
Children: 3 to 8 mg/kg P.O. or slow
I.V. daily or 250 mg/m^2 daily given as
single dose or divided in 2 doses.

SIDE EFFECTS
Blood: thrombocytopenia, leukopenia,
*agranulocytosis, pancytopenia, lymph-
adenopathy,* megaloblastic anemia.
CNS: *ataxia,* slurred speech, insomnia, headache, muscle twitching,
lethargy.
CV: *severe hypotension, vascular collapse (with rapid I.V. infusions greater
than 50 mg/minute),* vasodilation, asystole, ventricular fibrillation, AV block.
EENT: *nystagmus, diplopia,* blurred
vision.
GI: *gingival hyperplasia, nausea, vomiting,* constipation.
Metabolic: hyperglycemia.
Skin: rash (*morbilliform* most common), dermatitis (bullous, *exfoliative,
purpuric*), lupus erythematosus, Stevens-Johnson syndrome.

INTERACTIONS
*Alcohol, barbiturates, folic acid, loxap-
ine succinate:* monitor for decreased
phenytoin activity.
*Oral anticoagulants, antihistamines,
chloramphenicol, diazepam, diazoxide,
disulfiram, isoniazid, phenylbutazone,
phenyramidol, salicylates, sulfamethizole, valproate:* monitor for increased
phenytoin activity.

NURSING CONSIDERATIONS
• Contraindicated in heart block, sinus
bradycardia, Stokes-Adams attacks.
Use cautiously in congestive heart failure, hepatic or renal dysfunction, elderly or debilitated patients, hypotension, myocardial insufficiency, respiratory depression. Cardiac patients on
thyroid replacement therapy should be
given I.V. phenytoin cautiously to prevent supraventricular tachycardia.
• Administer drug slow I.V. push, not
to exceed 50 mg/minute in adults.
• Monitor blood pressure and EKG.
Notify doctor if side effects occur.
• Don't mix with 5% dextrose I.V.
fluids, as crystallization will occur.
Flush I.V. line with saline solution before and after administration.
• Watch patients on phenytoin and
other antiarrhythmics (disopyramide,
quinidine, procainamide, propranolol)
closely for signs of additive cardiac
depression.
• Phenytoin can be diluted in normal
saline solution and infused without precipitation. Such infusions should not
take longer than 1 hour.
• Shake oral suspensions well to make
dosage uniform. After giving suspension by nasogastric tube, flush tube
with water to facilitate passage to stomach.
• Give drug with food or large glass of
water to minimize gastric irritation.
• Avoid I.M. route of administration.
• Teach patient importance of taking
drug on time, exactly as prescribed.
• Dose should be decreased in hepatic
dysfunction.
• Blood levels greater than 20 mcg/ml
may be toxic. The difference between
therapeutic and toxic levels of phenytoin in the blood is very slight. If toxic
symptoms occur, draw blood to determine drug level.
• Stress need for good oral hygiene to
minimize gingival hyperplasia.
• Patients with uremia may require
dose adjustment for stabilization.
• Patients concurrently on phenytoin
and barbiturates, prednisone, or isoniazid should have phenytoin blood levels
checked frequently. Observe for phenytoin toxicity and for failure to respond adequately to phenytoin.

Italicized side effects are common or life-threatening.
∗Liquid form contains alcohol.   ∗∗May contain tartrazine.

- Patients concurrently on digitoxin and phenytoin may need larger doses.
- Warn patient not to drink alcohol as he may lose control of previously stable antiarrhythmic effects.

procainamide hydrochloride
Procan, Procan SR, Pronestyl♦**, Pronestyl-SR, Sub-Quin

INDICATIONS & DOSAGE
Premature ventricular contractions, ventricular tachycardia, atrial arrhythmias unresponsive to quinidine, paroxysmal atrial tachycardia—
Adults: 100 mg q 5 minutes slow I.V. push, no faster than 25 to 50 mg/minute until arrhythmias disappear, side effects develop, or 1 g has been given. When arrhythmias disappear, give continuous infusion of 2 to 6 mg/minute. Usual effective dose 500 to 600 mg. If arrhythmias recur, repeat bolus as above and increase infusion rate; 0.5 to 1 g I.M. q 4 to 8 hours until oral therapy begins.
Loading dose for atrial fibrillation or paroxysmal atrial tachycardia—
Adults: 1 to 1.25 g P.O. If arrhythmias persist after 1 hour, give additional 750 mg. If no change occurs, give 500 mg to 1 g q 2 hours until arrhythmias disappear or side effects occur. Maintenance 0.5 to 1 g q 4 to 6 hours.
Loading dose for ventricular tachycardia—
Adults: 1 g P.O. Maintenance 50 mg/kg daily given at 3-hour intervals; average 250 to 500 mg q 3 hours.
Note: Sustained-release tablet may be used for maintenance dosing when treating ventricular tachycardia, atrial fibrillation, and paroxysmal atrial tachycardia. Dose is 500 mg to 1 g q 6 hours.

SIDE EFFECTS
Blood: thrombocytopenia, *agranulocy-*
tosis, hemolytic anemia, *increased ANA titer.*
CNS: hallucinations, confusion, convulsions, depression.
CV: *severe hypotension, bradycardia,* AV block, ventricular fibrillation (after parenteral use).
GI: *nausea, vomiting, anorexia, diarrhea, bitter taste.*
Skin: *maculopapular rash.*
Other: *fever, lupus erythematosus syndrome (especially after prolonged administration),* myalgia.

INTERACTIONS
None significant.

NURSING CONSIDERATIONS
- Contraindicated in patients with hypersensitivity to procaine and related drugs; with complete, second-, or third-degree heart block unassisted by electrical pacemaker; or with myasthenia gravis. Use with caution in congestive heart failure or other conduction disturbances, such as bundle branch block or cardiotonic glycoside intoxication, or with hepatic or renal insufficiency.
- Patients receiving infusions must be *attended at all times.* Use an infusion pump or a microdrip system and timer to monitor the infusion precisely.
- Monitor blood pressure and EKG continuously during I.V. administration. Watch for prolonged Q-T and Q-R intervals, heart block, or increased arrhythmias. If these occur, withhold drug, obtain rhythm strip, and notify doctor immediately.
- Keep patient in supine position for I.V. administration.
- Watch closely for side effects and notify doctor if they occur. Instruct patient to report fever, rash, muscle pain, diarrhea, or pleuritic chest pain.
- Decrease dose in hepatic and renal dysfunction, and give over 6 hours. Half-life of procainamide is increased as much as threefold in these states.
- Patient with congestive heart failure

has a lower volume of distribution and can be treated with lower doses.

• Positive antinuclear antibody titer common in about 60% of patients who don't have symptoms of lupus erythematosus syndrome. This response seems related to prolonged use, not dosage.

• After long-standing atrial fibrillation, restoration of normal rhythm may result in thromboembolism, due to dislodgment of thrombi from atrial wall. Anticoagulation usually advised before restoration of normal sinus rhythm.

• Stress importance of taking drug exactly as prescribed. Patient may have to set an alarm clock for night doses.

propranolol hydrochloride
Inderal♦

INDICATIONS & DOSAGE

Supraventricular, ventricular, and atrial arrhythmias; tachyarrhythmias due to excessive catecholamine action during anesthesia, hyperthyroidism, and pheochromocytoma; angina—
Adults: 1 to 3 mg I.V. diluted in 50 ml 5% dextrose in water or normal saline solution infused slowly, not to exceed 1 mg/minute. After 3 mg have been infused, another dose may be given in 2 minutes; subsequent doses no sooner than q 4 hours. Usual maintenance 10 to 80 mg P.O. t.i.d. or q.i.d.

SIDE EFFECTS

CNS: *fatigue, lethargy,* vivid dreams, hallucinations.
CV: *bradycardia, hypotension, congestive heart failure,* peripheral vascular disease.
GI: nausea, vomiting, diarrhea.
Metabolic: hypoglycemia without tachycardia.
Skin: rash.
Other: *increased airway resistance,* fever.

INTERACTIONS

Insulin, hypoglycemic drugs (oral): can alter requirements for these drugs in previously stabilized diabetics. Monitor for hypoglycemia.
Cardiotonic glycosides: cause excessive bradycardia and increased depressant effect on myocardium. Use together cautiously.
Aminophylline: antagonizes beta-blocking effects of propranolol. Use together cautiously.
Isoproterenol, glucagon: antagonizes propranolol effect. May be used therapeutically and in emergencies.
Cimetidine: inhibits propranolol's metabolism. Monitor for greater beta-blocking effect.
Epinephrine: Severe vasocontriction. Monitor blood pressure and observe patient carefully.

NURSING CONSIDERATIONS

• Contraindicated in asthma or allergic rhinitis; during ethyl ether anesthesia; in sinus bradycardia and in heart block greater than first degree; in cardiogenic shock; in right ventricular failure secondary to pulmonary hypertension. Use with caution in patients with congestive heart failure, diabetes mellitus, or respiratory disease.

• Always withdraw drug slowly. Abrupt withdrawal might precipitate myocardial infarction or aggravate angina, thyrotoxicosis, pheochromocytoma. Abrupt withdrawal in thyrotoxicosis may exacerbate hyperthyroidism or precipitate thyroid storm. In thyrotoxicosis, propranolol may mask clinical signs of hyperthyroidism.

• *Don't discontinue before surgery for pheochromocytoma.* Before any surgical procedure, notify anesthesiologist that patient is receiving propranolol.

• Double-check dose and route. I.V. doses much smaller than P.O.

• Check apical pulse rate and blood pressure before giving drug. If you detect extremes in pulse rate, withhold drug and notify doctor at once. Severe bradycardia may be treated with atropine 0.25 to 1 mg I.V.

Italicized side effects are common or life-threatening.
*Liquid form contains alcohol.   **May contain tartrazine.

• After long-standing atrial fibrillation, restoration of normal sinus rhythm may result in thromboembolism due to dislodgment of thrombi from atrial wall. Anticoagulation often advised before restoration of normal atrial rhythm.

• Monitor blood pressure, EKG, heart rate and rhythm frequently, especially during I.V. administration. When propranolol is used with other antihypertensives, monitor blood pressure while patient is sitting and standing.

• Monitor patient daily for weight gain and development of peripheral edema.

• Auscultate patient's lungs for rales and his heart for gallop rhythm or for third or fourth heart sounds. If these develop, notify doctor at once.

---

quinidine bisulfate
(66% quinidine base)
Biquin Durules♦♦

quinidine gluconate
(62% quinidine base)
Duraquin, Quinaglute Dura-Tabs♦, Quinate♦♦

quinidine polygalacturonate
(60.5% quinidine base)
Cardioquin♦

quinidine sulfate
(83% quinidine base)
CinQuin, Quine, Quinidex Extentabs♦, Quinora, SK-Quinidine Sulfate

---

INDICATIONS & DOSAGE
Atrial flutter or fibrillation—
Adults: 200 mg quinidine sulfate or equivalent base P.O. q 2 to 3 hours for 5 to 8 doses with subsequent daily increases until sinus rhythm is restored or toxic effects develop. Administer quinidine only after digitalization to avoid increasing AV conduction. Maximum 3 to 4 g daily.

Paroxysmal supraventricular tachycardia—
Adults: 400 to 600 mg I.M. gluconate q 2 to 3 hours until toxic side effects develop or arrhythmia subsides.
Premature atrial and ventricular contractions; paroxysmal atrioventricular junctional rhythm; paroxysmal atrial tachycardia; paroxysmal ventricular tachycardia; maintenance after cardioversion of atrial fibrillation or flutter—
Adults: test dose 50 to 200 mg P.O., then monitor vital signs before beginning therapy. Quinidine sulfate or equivalent base 200 to 400 mg P.O. q 4 to 6 hours; or initially, quinidine gluconate 600 mg I.M., then up to 400 mg q 2 hours, p.r.n.; or quinidine gluconate 800 mg I.V. diluted in 40 ml 5% dextrose in water, infused at 1 mg/minute.
Children: test dose 2 mg/kg; 3 to 6 mg/kg q 2 to 3 hours for 5 doses P.O. daily.

SIDE EFFECTS
Blood: *hemolytic anemia, thrombocytopenia, agranulocytosis.*
CNS: *vertigo, headache, lightheadedness,* confusion, restlessness, cold sweat, pallor, fainting.
CV: *premature ventricular contractions; severe hypotension; SA and AV block; ventricular fibrillation, tachycardia; aggravated congestive heart failure; EKG changes (particularly widening of QRS complex, notched P waves, widened Q-T interval, ST segment depression).*
EENT: *tinnitus,* excessive salivation, blurred vision.
GI: *diarrhea, nausea, vomiting,* anorexia, abdominal pains.
Skin: rash, petechial hemorrhage of buccal mucosa, pruritus.
Other: angioedema, acute asthmatic attack, respiratory arrest, *fever, cinchonism.*

INTERACTIONS
Acetazolamide, antacids, sodium bicarbonate: may increase quinidine blood

---

levels due to alkaline urine. Monitor for increased effect.

Barbiturates, phenytoin, rifampin: may antagonize quinidine activity. Monitor for decreased quinidine effect.

Verapamil: don't use together in patients with cardiomyopathy. May result in hypotension.

NURSING CONSIDERATIONS
• Contraindicated in cardiotonic glycoside toxicity when AV conduction is grossly impaired; complete AV block with AV nodal or idioventricular pacemaker. Use with caution in myasthenia gravis. Anticholinergic drug doses may have to be increased.
• May increase toxicity of digitalis derivatives. Use with caution in patients previously digitalized. Monitor digoxin levels.
• Dosage varies—some patients may require drug q 4 hours, others q 6 hours. Titrate dose by both clinical response and blood levels.
• When changing route of administration, alter dosage to compensate for variations in quinidine base content.
• Dose should be decreased in congestive heart failure and hepatic disease.
• Check apical pulse rate and blood pressure before starting therapy. If you detect extremes in pulse rate, withhold drug and notify doctor at once.
• Lidocaine may be effective in treating quinidine-induced arrhythmias, since it increases AV conduction.
• GI side effects, especially diarrhea, are signs of toxicity. Notify doctor. Check quinidine blood levels, which are toxic when greater than 8 mcg/ml. GI symptoms may be decreased by giving with meals. Monitor drug response carefully.
• Instruct patient to notify doctor if skin rash, fever, unusual bleeding, bruising, ringing in ears, or visual disturbance occurs.
• After long-standing atrial fibrillation, restoration of normal sinus rhythm may result in thromboembolism due to

dislodgment of thrombi from atrial wall. Anticoagulation often advised before restoration of normal atrial rhythm.
• Never use discolored (brownish) quinidine solution.

verapamil
Calan, Isoptin

INDICATIONS & DOSAGE
Treatment of atrial arrhythmias—
Adults: 0.075 to 0.15 mg/kg (5 to 10 mg) I.V. push over 60 seconds with EKG and blood pressure monitoring. Repeat dose in 30 minutes if no response. Follow bolus injection with maintenance infusion of 0.005 mg/kg/minute.
Children 1 to 15 years: 0.1 to 0.3 mg/kg and I.V. bolus over 2 minutes.
Children less than 1 year: 0.1 to 0.2 mg/kg as I.V. bolus over 2 minutes. Dose can be repeated in 30 minutes if no response.
Management of vasospastic (also called Prinzmetal's or variant) angina and classic chronic, stable angina pectoris—
Adults: starting dose is 80 mg P.O. t.i.d. or q.i.d. Dosage may be increased at weekly intervals. Some patients may require up to 480 mg daily.

SIDE EFFECTS
CNS: dizziness, headache, fatigue.
CV: *transient hypotension, heart failure,* bradycardia, AV block, ventricular asystole, peripheral edema.
GI: *constipation,* nausea (primarily from oral form).
Hepatic: elevated liver enzymes.

INTERACTIONS
Propranolol (and other beta blockers) disopyramide: may cause heart failure. Use together cautiously.
Quinidine: don't use together in patients with cardiomyopathy. May result in hypotension.

Italicized side effects are common or life-threatening.
∗Liquid form contains alcohol.   ∗∗May contain tartrazine.

NURSING CONSIDERATIONS

• Contraindicated in patients with advanced heart failure, AV block, severe left ventricular dysfunction, cardiogenic shock, sinus node disease, and severe hypotension.

• Use cautiously in patients with myocardial infarction followed by coronary occlusion, sick sinus syndrome, impaired AV conduction, and heart failure with atrial tachyarrhythmia.

• Liver function tests should be done periodically.

• Patients with severely compromised cardiac function or those receiving beta blockers should receive lower doses of verapamil. Monitor these patients very closely.

• In older patients, I.V. doses should be administered over at least 3 minutes to minimize the risk of adverse effects.

• Notify doctor if such signs of congestive heart failure as swelling of hands and feet or shortness of breath occur.

• If patient is kept on nitrate therapy while drug dosage of oral verapamil is being titrated, urge him to continue his compliance. Sublingual nitroglycerin, especially, may be taken as needed when anginal symptoms are acute.

• Oral verapamil is also used investigationally as a treatment for hypertension.

• A new and very effective drug for treatment of supraventricular arrhythmias. Not very effective for ventricular arrhythmias.

19

Antihypertensives

alseroxylon
atenolol
captopril
clonidine hydrochloride
cryptenamine acetate
cryptenamine tannate
deserpidine
diazoxide
guanethidine sulfate
hydralazine hydrochloride
mecamylamine hydrochloride
methyldopa
metoprolol tartrate
metyrosine
minoxidil
nadolol
nitroprusside sodium
pargyline hydrochloride
phenoxybenzamine
    hydrochloride
phentolamine hydrochloride
phentolamine methanesulfonate
prazosin hydrochloride
propranolol hydrochloride
rauwolfia serpentina
rescinnamine
reserpine
timolol maleate
trimethaphan camsylate

MECHANISM OF ACTION

Antihypertensives are classified as sympatholytics or vasodilators. *Among the sympatholytics:*

• Cryptenamine (veratrum alkaloid) stimulates pressor receptors in the heart and carotid sinus.

• Alseroxylon, desperidine, guanethidine, rauwolfia, rescinnamine, and reserpine act peripherally, inhibiting norepinephrine release and depleting norepinephrine stores in adrenergic nerve endings.

• Captopril, metyrosine, and pargyline are enzyme inhibitors. Captopril, by inhibiting angiotensin-converting enzyme, prevents pulmonary conversion of angiotensin I to angiotensin II. Metyrosine inhibits tyrosine hydroxylase, and pargyline inhibits monoamine oxidase.

• Clonidine inhibits the central vasomotor centers, thereby decreasing sympthetic outflow.

• Mecamylamine, a ganglionic blocker, competes with acetylcholine for cholinergic receptors.

• Methyldopa, an alpha-adrenergic stimulator, alters sympathetic outflow.

• Atenolol, metoprolol, nadolol, propranolol, and timolol block response to beta stimulation and depress renin secretion.

• Phentolamine and phenoxybenzamine are alpha blockers and competitively block alpha-adrenergic receptors.

• Trimethaphan, a ganglionic blocker, stabilizes postsynaptic membranes.

Among the vasodilators:

• Diazoxide and hydralazine directly relax arteriolar smooth muscle.

• Minoxidil, nitroprusside, and prazosin relax both arteriolar and venous smooth muscle.

COMBINATION PRODUCTS

ALDOCLOR-150: chlorothiazide 150 mg and methyldopa 250 mg.
ALDOCLOR-250: chlorothiazide 250 mg and methyldopa 250 mg.
ALDORIL-15♦: hydrochlorothiazide 15 mg and methyldopa 250 mg.

Italicized side effects are common or life-threatening.
*Liquid form contains alcohol.   **May contain tartrazine.

ANTIHYPERTENSIVES **143**

ALDORIL-25♦: hydrochlorothiazide 25 mg and methyldopa 250 mg.

ALDORIL D30: hydrochlorothiazide 30 mg and methyldopa 500 mg.

ALDORIL D50: hydrochlorothiazide 50 mg and methyldopa 500 mg.

APRESAZIDE 25/25: hydrochlorothiazide 25 mg and hydralazine HCl 25 mg.

APRESAZIDE 50/50: hydrochlorothiazide 50 mg and hydralazine HCl 50 mg.

APRESAZIDE 100/50: hydrochlorothiazide 50 mg and hydralazine HCl 100 mg.

APRESOLINE-ESIDRIX: hydrochlorothiazide 15 mg and hydralazine HCl 25 mg.

COMBIPRES 0.1♦: chlorthalidone 15 mg and clonidine HCl 0.1 mg.

COMBIPRES 0.2: chlorthalidone 15 mg and clonidine HCl 0.2 mg.

DEMI-REGROTON: chlorthalidone 25 mg and reserpine 0.125 mg.

DIUPRES-250: chlorothiazide 250 mg and reserpine 0.125 mg.

DIUPRES-500: chlorothiazide 500 mg and reserpine 0.125 mg.

DIUTENSEN: methyclothiazide 2.5 mg and cryptenamine 2 mg (as tannate).

DIUTENSEN-R: methyclothiazide 2.5 mg and reserpine 0.1 mg.

ENDURONYL: methyclothiazide 5 mg and deserpidine 0.25 mg.

ENDURONYL-FORTE: methyclothiazide 5 mg and deserpidine 0.5 mg.

ESIMIL: hydrochlorothiazide 25 mg and guanethidine monosulfate 10 mg.

EUTRON FILMTABS: methyclothiazide 5 mg and pargyline HCl 25 mg.

EXNA-R TABLETS: benzthiazide 50 mg and reserpine 0.125 mg.

HYDROMOX-R: quinethazone 50 mg and reserpine 0.125 mg.

HYDROPRES-25♦: hydrochlorothiazide 25 mg and reserpine 0.125 mg.

HYDROPRES-50♦: hydrochlorothiazide 50 mg and reserpine 0.125 mg.

HYDROSERP: hydrochlorothiazide 50 mg and reserpine 0.125 mg.

HYDROTENSIN-25 TABLETS: hydrochlorothiazide 25 mg and reserpine 0.125 mg.

HYDROTENSIN-50: hydrochlorothiazide 50 mg and reserpine 0.125 mg.

HYSTON TABLETS: hydrochlorothiazide 15 mg and hydralazine 25 mg.

INDERIDE 40/25: propranolol HCl 40 mg and hydrochlorothiazide 25 mg.

INDERIDE 80/25: propranolol HCl 80 mg and hydrochlorothiazide 25 mg.

METATENSIN TABLETS: trichlormethiazide 2 or 4 mg and reserpine 0.1 mg.

NAQUIVAL: trichlormethiazide 4 mg and reserpine 0.1 mg.

NATURETIN W/K 2.5 mg♦: bendroflumethiazide 2.5 mg and potassium chloride 500 mg.

NATURETIN W/K 5 mg♦: bendroflumethiazide 5 mg and potassium chloride 500 mg.

ORETICYL FORTE: hydrochlorothiazide 25 mg and deserpidine 0.25 mg.

ORETICYL 25: hydrochlorothiazide 25 mg and deserpidine 0.125 mg.

ORETICYL 50: hydrochlorothiazide 50 mg and deserpidine 0.125 mg.

RAUTRAX**: flumethiazide 400 mg, potassium chloride 400 mg, and powdered rauwolfia serpentina 50 mg.

RAUTRAX-N**: bendroflumethiazide 4 mg, powdered rauwolfia serpentina 50 mg, and potassium chloride 400 mg.

RAUZIDE**: bendroflumethiazide 4 mg and powdered rauwolfia serpentina 50 mg.

REGROTON: chlorthalidone 50 mg and reserpine 0.25 mg.

RENESE-R: polythiazide 2 mg and reserpine 0.25 mg.

SALUTENSIN♦: hydroflumethiazide 50 mg and reserpine 0.125 mg.

SALUTENSIN DEMI: hydroflumethiazide 25 mg and reserpine 0.125 mg.

SER-AP-ES♦: hydrochlorothiazide 15 mg, reserpine 0.1 mg, and hydralazine HCl 25 mg.

SERPASIL-APRESOLINE #1: reserpine 0.1 mg and hydralazine HCl 25 mg.

SERPASIL-APRESOLINE #2♦: reserpine 0.2 mg and hydralazine HCl 50 mg.

Unmarked trade names available in the United States only.
♦ Also available in Canada.   ♦♦ Available in Canada only.

SERPASIL-ESIDRIX #1✦: hydrochloro-thiazide 25 mg and reserpine 0.1 mg (called Serpasil-Esidrix 25 in Canada).
SERPASIL-ESIDRIX #2✦: hydrochloro-thiazide 50 mg and reserpine 0.1 mg (called Serpasil-Esidrix 50 in Canada).
THIASERP-250: chlorothiazide 250 mg and reserpine 0.125 mg.
TIMOLIDE 10/25: timolol maleate 10 mg and hydrochlorothiazide 25 mg.
UNIPRES: hydrochlorothiazide 15 mg, reserpine 0.1 mg, and hydralazine HCl 25 mg.

alseroxylon
Raudolfin, Rauwiloid

INDICATIONS & DOSAGE
Mild, labile hypertension—
Adults: initially, 4 mg P.O. daily as a single dose or divided in 2 doses for 1 to 3 weeks. Maintenance dose: 2 mg or less daily. No dosing recommendations for children.

SIDE EFFECTS
CNS: mental confusion, *depression, drowsiness, nervousness, anxiety,* insomnia, *nightmares,* sedation.
CV: *orthostatic hypotension, bradycardia.*
EENT: *mouth dryness, nasal stuffiness,* glaucoma.
GI: *hypersecretion of gastric acid, nausea, vomiting,* gastrointestinal bleeding.
Skin: *pruritus, rash.*
Other: *impotence, weight gain.*

INTERACTIONS
MAO inhibitors: may cause excitability and hypertension. Avoid if possible.

NURSING CONSIDERATIONS
• Use cautiously in patients with severe cardiac or cerebrovascular disease, peptic ulcer, ulcerative colitis, renal disease, gallstones, or mental depressive disorders, or in those undergoing surgery.

• Use cautiously in patients taking other antihypertensive drugs.
• Monitor patient's blood pressure and pulse rate frequently.
• Teach patient about his disease and therapy. Explain why it's important to take this drug exactly as prescribed, even when he's feeling well. Tell outpatient not to discontinue this drug suddenly, but to call the doctor if such unpleasant side effects as mental depression, nightmares, or insomnia develop. Watch patient closely for signs of mental depression.
• Effect of drug may last for 10 days after discontinuation.
• Warn patient that this drug can cause drowsiness.
• Warn female patient to notify doctor if she becomes pregnant.
• Inform patient that orthostatic hypotension can be minimized by rising slowly and avoiding sudden position changes. Mouth dryness can be relieved with sugarless chewing gum, sour hard candy, or ice chips.
• Tell patient to contact doctor if relief is needed for nasal stuffiness.
• Give this drug with meals.
• Patient should weigh himself daily and notify doctor of any weight gain.
• One mg of alseroxylon is approximately equal to 0.1 mg of reserpine.

atenolol
Tenormin

INDICATIONS & DOSAGE
Treatment of hypertension—
Adults: initially, 50 mg P.O. daily single dose. Dosage may be increased to 100 mg once daily after 7 to 14 days. Dosages greater than 100 mg are unlikely to produce further benefit.

SIDE EFFECTS
CNS: fatigue, lethargy.
CV: *bradycardia, hypotension, congestive heart failure,* peripheral vascular disease.

Italicized side effects are common or life-threatening.
✦Liquid form contains alcohol.   ✦✦May contain tartrazine.

GI: nausea, vomiting, diarrhea.
Metabolic: hypoglycemia without tachycardia.
Skin: rash.
Other: fever.

INTERACTIONS

Insulin, hypoglycemic drugs (oral): can alter dosage requirements in previously stablilized diabetics. Observe patient carefully.
Cardiac glycosides: excessive bradycardia and increased depressant effect on myocardium. Use together cautiously.

NURSING CONSIDERATIONS

• Contraindicated in sinus bradycardia and greater than first degree conduction block, and cardiogenic shock.
• Use cautiously in patients with cardiac failure.
• Similar to metoprolol, atenolol is a cardioselective beta blocker. Although atenolol can be used in patients with bronchospastic diseases such as asthma and emphysema, the drug should still be used cautiously in such patients–especially when 100 mg are given.
• Dosage should be reduced if patient has renal insufficiency.
• Once-a-day dosage encourages patient compliance. Counsel your patient to take the drug at a regular time every day. Drug can be dispensed in a 28-day calendar pack.
• Always check patient's apical pulse before giving this drug; if slower than 60 beats per minute (bpm), hold drug and call doctor.
• Monitor blood pressure frequently. If patient develops severe hypotension, administer a vasopressor.
• Don't discontinue abruptly; can exacerbate angina and MI.
• Teach patient about his disease and therapy. Explain the importance of taking this drug, even when he's feeling well. Tell patient not to discontinue drug suddenly, but to call doctor if unpleasant side effects dvelop.

• This drug masks common signs of shock and hypoglycemia.
• Atenolol, as well as other beta blockers, is being prescribed to decrease mortality following myocardial infarction.

captopril
Capoten

INDICATIONS & DOSAGE

Treatment of severe hypertension—
Adults: 25 mg t.i.d. initially. If blood pressure isn't satisfactorily controlled in 1 to 2 weeks, dose may be increased to 50 mg t.i.d. If not satisfactorily controlled after another 1 to 2 weeks, a diuretic should be added to regimen. If further blood pressure reduction is necessary, dose may be raised to as high as 150 mg t.i.d. while continuing the diuretic. Maximum dose is 450 mg daily.

SIDE EFFECTS

Blood: *leukopenia, agranulocytosis, pancytopenia.*
CNS: dizziness, fainting.
CV: *tachycardia,* hypotension, angina pectoris, congestive heart failure.
EENT: *loss of taste (dysgeusia).*
GU: *proteinuria, nephrotic syndrome, membranous glomerulopathy, renal failure,* urinary frequency.
GI: anorexia.
Skin: *urticarial rash, maculopapular rash,* pruritus.
Other: fever, angioedema of face and extremities, transient increases in liver enzymes.

INTERACTIONS

None significant

NURSING CONSIDERATIONS

• Use cautiously in patients with impaired renal function or serious autoimmune disease (particularly systemic lupus erythematosus), or those who have been exposed to other drugs

---

known to affect white cell counts or immune response.

• Proteinuria and nephrotic syndrome may occur in patients who are on captopril therapy. Those who develop persistent proteinuria or proteinuria that exceeds 1 g daily should have their captopril therapy reevaluated.

• Monitor patient's blood pressure and pulse rate frequently.

• Perform WBC and differential counts before starting treatment, every 2 weeks for the first 3 months of therapy, and periodically thereafter.

• Advise patients to report any sign of infection (sore throat, fever).

• Because captopril may cause serious side effects, it should be reserved for those patients who have developed undesirable side effects from or failed to respond to other antihypertensive drugs. Commonly used in patients who fail to respond to "triple-drug therapy" (a diuretic, a beta blocker, and a vasodilator).

• Although captopril can be used alone, its beneficial effects are increased when a thiazide diuretic is added.

• May cause dizziness or fainting; advise patients to avoid sudden postural changes.

• Question patient about impaired taste sensation.

• Should be taken 1 hour before meals since food in the GI tract may reduce absorption.

clonidine hydrochloride ♦

INDICATIONS & DOSAGE
Essential, renal, and malignant hypertension—
Adults: initially, 0.1 mg P.O. b.i.d. Then increase by 0.1 to 0.2 mg daily on a weekly basis. Usual dose range: 0.2 to 0.8 mg daily in divided doses. Infrequently, doses as high as 2.4 mg daily. No dosing recommendations for children.

To supress abstinence symptoms during narcotics withdrawl—
Adults: 0.1 mg P.O. t.i.d.

SIDE EFFECTS
CNS: *drowsiness,* dizziness, fatigue, sedation, nervousness, headache.
CV: orthostatic hypotension, bradycardia.
EENT: *mouth dryness.*
GI: *constipation.*
GU: urinary retention.
Other: impotence.

INTERACTIONS
Tricyclic antidepressants and MAO inhibitors: may decrease antihypertensive effect. Use together cautiously.
Propranolol and other beta blockers: paradoxical hypertensive response. Monitor carefully.

NURSING CONSIDERATIONS
• Use cautiously in patients with severe coronary insufficiency, myocardial infarction, cerebral vascular disease, chronic renal failure, or history of depression, or in those taking other antihypertensives.

• Monitor blood pressure and pulse rate frequently. Dosage is usually adjusted to patient's blood pressure and tolerance.

• May be given to rapidly lower blood pressure in some hypertensive emergency situations.

• Reduce dose gradually over 2 to 4 days. If discontinued abruptly, this drug may cause severe hypertension.

• Teach patient about his disease and therapy. Explain why it's important to take this drug exactly as prescribed, even when he's feeling well. Tell outpatient not to discontinue this drug suddenly, but to call the doctor if unpleasant side effects develop. Warn that this drug can cause drowsiness, but that tolerance to this side effect will develop.

• Inform patient that orthostatic hypotension can be minimized by rising slowly and avoiding sudden position

changes. Mouth dryness can be relieved with sugarless chewing gum, sour hard candy, or ice chips.
• Last dose should be taken immediately before retiring.
• Has been used investigationally for migraine headache prophylaxis and treatment of dysmenorrhea.

cryptenamine acetate
Unitensen Aqueous

cryptenamine tannate
Unitensen, Unitensyl♦♦

INDICATIONS & DOSAGE
Mild to moderate hypertension, toxemia—
Adults: initially, 2 mg P.O. b.i.d., increased at weekly intervals, depending on response. Total daily dose not to exceed 12 mg daily. I.V. (for hypertensive crises and convulsive toxemia)—0.5 ml (130 CSR units) diluted to 20 ml with 5% dextrose in water. Administer at infusion rate of 1 ml/minute. When giving this drug I.V., record blood pressure approximately every minute.

SIDE EFFECTS
CNS: mental confusion.
CV: *orthostatic hypotension,* cardiac arrhythmias, *bradycardia.*
EENT: blurred vision, excessive salivation, unpleasant taste.
GI: *nausea, vomiting,* epigastric burning, hiccups.
Other: respiratory depression, bronchial constriction.

INTERACTIONS
Anesthetic agents: may cause additive hypotensive effect. Observe patient carefully.
Tricyclic antidepressants: may diminish hypotensive response. Avoid if possible.

NURSING CONSIDERATIONS
• Contraindicated in patients with pheochromocytoma. Use cautiously in patients with angina, cerebrovascular disease, bronchial asthma, or renal insufficiency, or in those taking other antihypertensives.
• Monitor blood pressure and pulse rate closely. If severe hypotension develops, stop infusion and notify doctor, as he may use phenylephrine or ephedrine to counteract effect. Hypotension should dissipate in 60 to 90 minutes. If patient develops bradycardia, he may require atropine. Notify doctor promptly.
• The range between therapeutic and toxic doses of this drug is narrow. Call doctor immediately if side effects develop.
• Teach patient about his disease and therapy. Explain why it's important to take this drug exactly as prescribed, even when he's feeling well. Tell outpatient not to discontinue this drug suddenly, but to call the doctor if unpleasant side effects develop.
• Inform patient that orthostatic hypotension can be minimized by rising slowly and avoiding sudden position changes. Unpleasant taste can be relieved with sugarless chewing gum, sour hard candy, or ice chips.

deserpidine
Harmonyl**

INDICATIONS & DOSAGE
Mild essential hypertension—
Adults: 0.25 mg P.O. t.i.d. to q.i.d. for up to 2 weeks, then maintenance dose of 0.25 mg once daily may be adequate. No dosing recommendations for children.

SIDE EFFECTS
CNS: mental confusion, *depression, drowsiness, nervousness,* anxiety, nightmares, sedation.
CV: bradycardia.
EENT: *mouth dryness, nasal stuffiness,* glaucoma.

GI: *hypersecretion of gastric acid, nausea, vomiting,* gastrointestinal bleeding.
Skin: pruritus, rash.
Other: *impotence, weight gain.*

INTERACTIONS
MAO inhibitors: may cause excitability and hypertension. Avoid if possible.

NURSING CONSIDERATIONS
• Contraindicated in patients with mental depression. Use cautiously in patients with severe cardiac or cerebrovascular disease, peptic ulcer, ulcerative colitis, gallstones, or mental depressive disorders; in patients undergoing surgery; and in patients taking other antihypertensives or anticonvulsants.
• Monitor patient's blood pressure and pulse rate frequently.
• Teach patient about his disease and therapy. Explain why it's important to take this drug exactly as prescribed, even when he's feeling well. Tell outpatient not to discontinue this drug suddenly, but to call the doctor if unpleasant side effects, such as mental depression, insomnia, or loss of appetite, develop. Warn that drug can cause drowsiness.
• Watch patient closely for signs of mental depression. Warn him to notify doctor promptly if he starts having nightmares.
• Tell patient to avoid alcohol and to follow prescribed diet.
• Mouth dryness can be relieved with chewing gum, sour hard candy, or ice chips. Tell patient to contact doctor if relief is needed for nasal stuffiness.
• Give this drug with meals to increase absorption.
• Patient should weigh himself daily and notify doctor of any weight gain.

diazoxide
Hyperstat♦ (I.V. only)

INDICATIONS & DOSAGE
Hypertensive crisis—

Adults: 300 mg I.V. bolus push, administered in 30 seconds or less into peripheral vein. Repeat at intervals of 4 to 24 hours, p.r.n. Mini-boluses of 1 to 3 mg/kg repeated at intervals of 5 to 15 minutes or infusions of 15 mg/minute are equally effective. Switch to therapy with oral antihypertensives as soon as possible.
Children: 5 mg/kg I.V. rapid bolus push.

SIDE EFFECTS
CNS: *headaches,* dizziness, light-headedness, euphoria.
CV: *sodium and water retention, orthostatic hypotension,* sweating, flusing, warmth, angina, myocardial ischemia, arrhythmias, EKG changes.
GI: *nausea, vomiting,* abdominal discomfort.
Metabolic: *hyperglycemia,* hyperuricemia.
Local: inflammation and pain from extravasation.

INTERACTIONS
Hydralazine: may cause severe hypotension. Use together cautiously.
Thiazide diuretics: may increase the effects of diazoxide. Use together cautiously.

NURSING CONSIDERATIONS
• Use cautiously in patients with impaired cerebral or cardiac function, diabetes, or uremia, or in those taking other antihypertensives.
• Monitor blood pressure frequently. Notify doctor immediately if severe hypotension develops. Keep norepinephrine available.
• Monitor patient's intake and output carefully. If fluid or sodium retention develops, doctor may want to order diuretics.
• Take care to avoid extravasation.
• This drug may alter requirements for insulin, diet, or oral hypoglycemic drugs in previously controlled diabetics. Monitor blood glucose daily.

Italicized side effects are common or life-threatening.
✱Liquid form contains alcohol.   ✱✱May contain tartrazine.

• Weigh patient daily. Notify doctor of any weight increase.

• Watch diabetics closely for signs of severe hyperglycemia or hyperosmolar nonketotic coma. Insulin may be needed.

• Check patient's uric acid levels frequently. Report abnormalities to doctor.

• Inform patient that orthostatic hypotension can be minimized by rising slowly and avoiding sudden position changes. Instruct patient to remain supine for 30 minutes after injection.

• Infusion of diazoxide has been shown to be as effective as a bolus in some patients.

guanethidine sulfate
Ismelin♦

INDICATIONS & DOSAGE
For moderate to severe hypertension; usually used in combination with other antihypertensives—
Adults: initially, 10 mg P.O. daily. Increase by 10 mg at weekly to monthly intervals, p.r.n. Usual dose is 25 to 50 mg daily. Some patients may require up to 300 mg.
Children: initially, 200 mcg/kg P.O. daily. Increase gradually every 1 to 3 weeks to maximum of 8 times initial dose.

SIDE EFFECTS
CNS: *dizziness, weakness, syncope.*
CV: *orthostatic hypotension, bradycardia,* congestive heart failure, arrhythmias.
EENT: *nasal stuffiness,* mouth dryness.
GI: *diarrhea.*
Other: *edema, weight gain, inhibition of ejaculation.*

INTERACTIONS
Levodopa, alcohol: may increase hypotensive effect of guanethidine. Use together cautiously.

MAO inhibitors, ephedrine, levarterenol, methylphenidate, tricyclic antidepressants, amphetamines, phenothiazines: may inhibit the antihypertensive effect of guanethidine. Adjust dose accordingly.

NURSING CONSIDERATIONS
• Contraindicated in patients with pheochromocytoma. Use cautiously in patients with severe cardiac disease, recent MI, cerebrovascular disease, peptic ulcer, impaired renal function, or bronchial asthma, or in those taking other antihypertensives.

• Discontinue drug 2 to 3 weeks before elective surgery to reduce the possibility of vascular collapse and cardiac arrest during anesthesia.

• Teach patient about his disease and therapy. Explain why it's important to take this drug exactly as prescribed, even when he's feeling well. Tell patient not to discontinue this drug suddenly, but to call the doctor if unpleasant side effects develop.

• Tell outpatient to avoid strenuous exercise, and warn that hot showers may cause hypotensive reaction.

• Inform patient that orthostatic hypotension can be minimized by rising slowly and avoiding sudden position changes. Mouth dryness can be relieved with sugarless chewing gum, sour hard candy, or ice chips.

• Give this drug with meals to increase absorption.

• If patient develops diarrhea, doctor may prescribe atropine or paregoric.

hydralazine hydrochloride
Apresoline♦, Dralzine**, Hydralyn, Rolazine

INDICATIONS & DOSAGE
Essential hypertension (oral, alone or in combination with other antihypertensives); to reduce afterload in severe congestive heart failure (with nitrates); and

severe essential hypertension (parenteral to lower blood pressure quickly)—
Adults: initially, 10 mg P.O. q.i.d.; gradually increased to 50 mg q.i.d. Maximum recommended dosage is 200 mg daily, but some patients may require 300 to 400 mg daily.
I.V.—20 to 40 mg given slowly and repeated as necessary, generally q 4 to 6 hours. Switch to oral antihypertensives as soon as possible.
I.M.—20 to 40 mg repeated as necessary, generally q 4 to 6 hours. Switch to oral antihypertensives as soon as possible.
Children: initially, 0.75 mg/kg P.O. daily in 4 divided doses (25 mg/m² daily). May increase gradually to 10 times this dose, if necessary.
I.V.—give slowly 1.7 to 3.5 mg/kg daily or 50 to 100 mg/m² daily in 4 to 6 divided doses.
I.M.—1.7 to 3.5 mg/kg daily or 50 to 100 mg/m² daily in 4 to 6 divided doses.

SIDE EFFECTS
CNS: peripheral neuritis, *headache*, dizziness.
CV: orthostatic hypotension, *tachycardia*, arrhythmias, *angina, palpitations, sodium retention*.
GI: *nausea, vomiting, diarrhea, anorexia*.
Skin: rash.
Other: *lupus erythematosus-like syndrome, weight gain*.

INTERACTIONS
Diazoxide: may cause severe hypotension. Use together cautiously.

NURSING CONSIDERATIONS
• Use cautiously in patients with cardiac disease or in those taking other antihypertensives.
• Monitor patient's blood pressure and pulse rate frequently.
• Watch patient closely for signs of lupus erythematosus-like syndrome (sore throat, fever, muscle and joint aches,

skin rash). Call doctor immediately if any of these develop.
• Teach patient about his disease and therapy. Explain why it's important to take this drug exactly as prescribed, even when he's feeling well. Tell outpatient not to discontinue this drug suddenly, but to call the doctor if unpleasant side effects develop.
• Inform patient that orthostatic hypotension can be minimized by rising slowly and avoiding sudden position changes.
• Give this drug with meals to increase absorption.
• Compliance may be improved by administering this drug b.i.d. Check with doctor.
• Complete blood count, LE cell preparation, and antinuclear antibody titer determinations should be done before therapy and periodically during long-term therapy.

---

mecamylamine hydrochloride
Inversine

INDICATIONS & DOSAGE
For moderate to severe essential hypertension and uncomplicated malignant hypertension—
Adults: initially, 2.5 mg P.O. b.i.d. Increase by 2.5 mg daily every 2 days. Average daily dose 25 mg given in 3 divided doses. No dosing recommendations for children.

SIDE EFFECTS
CNS: *paresthesias,* sedation, *fatigue, tremor, choreiform movements,* convulsions, psychic changes, dizziness, *weakness, headaches.*
CV: *orthostatic hypotension.*
EENT: *mouth dryness,* glossitis, dilated pupils, *blurred vision.*
GI: *anorexia,* nausea, vomiting, *constipation, adynamic ileus, diarrhea.*
GU: urinary retention.
Other: decreased libido, impotence.

Italicized side effects are common or life-threatening.
*Liquid form contains alcohol.   **May contain tartrazine.

INTERACTIONS

Sodium bicarbonate and acetazol-amide: may increase effect of mecamy-lamine. Use together cautiously. Watch for increased hypotensive effects and toxicity.

NURSING CONSIDERATIONS

• Contraindicated in patients with recent MI, or uremia, chronic pyelonephritis. Use cautiously in patients with lower urinary tract pathology, renal insufficiency, glaucoma, pyloric stenosis, coronary insufficiency, or cerebrovascular insufficiency, or in those taking other antihypertensives.

• Effects of this drug are increased by high environmental temperature, fever, stress, or severe illness.

• Don't withdraw this drug suddenly; rebound hypertension may occur. Tell outpatient to call the doctor if unpleasant side effects develop.

• Monitor patient's blood pressure frequently while he's standing.

• Give with meals for better absorption. Don't restrict sodium intake.

• If patient develops constipation from this drug, the doctor may want him to take milk of magnesia. Instruct patient to avoid bulk laxatives.

• Teach the patient about his disease and therapy. Explain why it's important to take this drug exactly as prescribed, even when he's feeling well.

• Inform patient that orthostatic hypotension can be minimized by rising slowly and avoiding sudden position changes. Mouth dryness can be relieved with sugarless chewing gum, sour hard candy, or ice chips.

---

methyldopa

Aldomet♦, Dopamet♦♦,
Medimet-250♦♦, Novomedopa♦♦

INDICATIONS & DOSAGE

For sustained mild to severe hypertension; should not be used for acute treatment of hypertensive emergencies—

Adults: initially, 250 mg P.O. b.i.d. to t.i.d. in first 48 hours. Then increase as needed every 2 days. May give entire daily dose in the evening or at bedtime. Dosages may need adjustment if other antihypertensive drugs are added to or deleted from therapy.
Maintenance dosages—500 mg to 2 g daily in 2 to 4 divided doses. Maximum recommended daily dose is 3 g.
I.V.—500 mg to 1 g q 6 hours, diluted in 5% dextrose in water, and administered over 30 to 60 minutes. Switch to oral antihypertensives as soon as possible.
Children: initially, 10 mg/kg daily P.O. in 2 to 3 divided doses; or 20 to 40 mg/kg daily I.V. in 4 divided doses. Increase dose daily until desired response occurs. Maximum daily dose 65 mg/kg.

SIDE EFFECTS

Blood: *hemolytic anemia,* reversible granulocytopenia, thrombocytopenia.
CNS: *sedation,* headache, asthenia, weakness, dizziness, *decreased mental acuity,* involuntary choreoathetotic movements, psychic disturbances, depression, nightmares.
CV: bradycardia, *orthostatic hypotension,* aggravated angina, myocarditis, *edema and weight gain.*
EENT: *dry mouth, nasal stuffiness.*
GI: diarrhea, pancreatitis.
Hepatic: *hepatic necrosis.*
Other: gynecomastia, lactation, skin rash, drug-induced fever, impotence.

INTERACTIONS

Norepinephrine, phenothiazines, tricyclic antidepressants, amphetamines: possible hypertensive effects. Monitor carefully.

NURSING CONSIDERATIONS

• Use cautiously in patients receiving other antihypertensives or MAO inhibitors. Monitor blood pressure and pulse rate frequently.

• Observe patient for side effects, par-

---

ticularly unexplained fever. Report side effects to doctor.
• If patient requires blood transfusion, make sure he gets direct and indirect Coombs' tests to avoid cross-matching problems.
• Monitor blood studies (complete blood count) before and during therapy.
• If patient has been on this drug for several months, positive reaction to direct Coombs' test indicates hemolytic anemia.
• Weigh patient daily. Notify doctor of any weight increase. Salt and water retention may occur but can be relieved with diuretics.
• Tell patient that urine may turn dark in toilet bowls treated with bleach.
• Teach patient about his disease and therapy. Explain why it's important to take this drug exactly as prescribed, even when he's feeling well. Tell outpatient not to stop this drug suddenly, but to call the doctor if unpleasant side effects develop. Once-daily dosage administered at bedtime will minimize drowsiness during daytime. Check with doctor.
• Inform patient that orthostatic hypotension can be minimized by rising slowly and avoiding sudden position changes. Mouth dryness can be relieved with sugarless chewing gum, sour hard candy, or ice chips.

metoprolol tartrate
Betaloc◆◆, Lopresor◆◆, Lopressor

INDICATIONS & DOSAGE
For hypertension; may be used alone or in combination with other antihypertensives—
Adults: 50 mg b.i.d. P.O. initially. Up to 200 to 400 mg daily in 2 to 3 divided doses. No dosage recommendations for children.

SIDE EFFECTS
CNS: fatigue, lethargy.
CV: *bradycardia, hypotension, conges-*

tive heart failure, peripheral vascular disease.
GI: nausea, vomiting, diarrhea.
Metabolic: hypoglycemia without tachycardia.
Skin: rash.
Other: fever.

INTERACTIONS
Insulin, hypoglycemic drugs (oral): can alter dosage requirements in previously stabilized diabetics. Observe patient carefully.
Cardiotonic glycosides: excessive bradycardia and increased depressant effect on myocardium. Use together cautiously.

NURSING CONSIDERATIONS
• Use cautiously in patients with heart block, congestive heart failure, diabetes, or respiratory disease, or in those taking other antihypertensives. Always check patient's apical pulse rate before giving this drug. If it's slower than 60 beats per minute (bpm), hold drug and call doctor immediately.
• Although most patients with asthma and bronchitis can take his drug without fear of worsening their condition, higher dosages should be used cautiously in those patients.
• Monitor blood pressure frequently. If patient develops severe hypotension, administer a vasopressor as ordered.
• Teach patient about his disease and therapy. Explain why it's important to take this drug, even when he's feeling well. Tell outpatient not to discontinue this drug suddenly; abrupt discontinuation can exacerbate angina and MI. Instruct patient to call doctor if unpleasant side effects develop.
• Food may increase absorption of metoprolol. Give consistently with meals.
• Metaprolol, as well as other beta blockers, is being prescribed to decrease mortality following myocardial infarction.

Italicized side effects are common or life-threatening.
*Liquid form contains alcohol.   **May contain tartrazine.

metyrosine
Demser

INDICATIONS & DOSAGE
Preoperative preparation of patients with pheochromocytoma; management of such patients when surgery is contra-indicated; to control or prevent hypertension before or during pheochromocytomectomy—

Adults and children over 12 years: 2150 mg P.O. q.i.d. May be increased by 250 to 500 mg q day to a maximum of 4 g daily in divided doses. When used for preoperative preparation, optimally effective dosage should be given for at least 5 to 7 days.

SIDE EFFECTS
CNS: *sedation,* extrapyramidal symptoms, such as speech difficulty and tremors, disorientation.
GI: *diarrhea,* nausea, vomiting, abdominal pain.
GU: *crystalluria,* hematuria.
Other: impotence, hypersensitivity.

INTERACTIONS
Phenothiazines and haloperidol: increased inhibition of catecholamine synthesis may result in extrapyramidal symptoms. Use cautiously.

NURSING CONSIDERATIONS
• During surgery, monitor blood pressure and EKG continuously. If a serious arrhythmia occurs during anesthesia and surgery, treatment with a beta-blocking drug or lidocaine may be necessary.
• Warn patient that sedation almost always occurs in those treated with metyrosine. Sedation usually subsides after several days' treatment.
• Instruct patient to increase daily fluid intake to prevent crystalluria. Daily urine volume should be 2,000 ml or more.
• Tell patient to notify doctor if any of the listed side effects occur.

• Insomnia may occur when metyrosine is stopped.
• If patient's hypertension is not adequately controlled by metyrosine, an alpha-adrenergic blocking agent, such as phenoxybenzamine, should be added to the regimen.
• Available as 250-mg capsules.

---

minoxidil
Loniten

INDICATIONS & DOSAGE
Treatment of severe hypertension—
Adults: 5 mg P.O. initially as a single dose. Effective dosage range is usually 10 to 40 mg daily. Maximum dose 100 mg daily.
Children (under 12 years): 0.2 mg/kg as a single daily dose. Effective dosage range usually 0.25 to 1.0 mg/kg daily. Maximum dose is 50 mg.

SIDE EFFECTS
CV: *edema, tachycardia, pericardial effusion and tamponade, congestive heart failure,* EKG changes.
Skin: rash, *Stevens-Johnson syndrome.*
Other: *hypertrichosis* (elongation, thickening, and enhanced pigmentation of fine body hair), breast tenderness.

INTERACTIONS
Guanethidine: severe orthostatic hypotension. Advise patient to stand up slowly.

NURSING CONSIDERATIONS
• Contraindicated in patients with pheochromocytoma.
• A potent vasodilator: Use only when other antihypertensives have failed.
• About 8 out of 10 patients will experience hypertrichosis within 3 to 6 weeks of beginning treatment. Unwanted hair can be controlled with a depilatory or shaving. Assure patient that extra hair will disappear within 1 to 6 months of stopping minoxidil.

Advise patient, however, not to discontinue drug without doctor's consent.

• Drug is usually prescribed with a beta-blocking drug to control tachycardia and a diuretic to counteract fluid retention. Make sure patient complies with total treatment regimen.

• A patient package insert (PPI) has been prepared by the manufacturer of minoxidil, describing in layman's terms the drug and its side effects. Be sure your patient receives this insert and reads it thoroughly. Provide an oral explanation also.

• Available as a 2.5-mg and 10-mg tablet.

nadolol
Corgard♦

INDICATIONS & DOSAGE
Treatment of hypertension—
Adults: 40 mg P.O. once daily, initially. Dosage may be increased in 40- to 80-mg increments until optimum response occurs. Usual maintenance dosage range: 80 to 320 mg once daily. Doses of 640 mg may be necessary in rare cases.
Long-term management of angina pectoris—
Adults: 40 mg P.O. once daily, initially. Dosage may be increased in 40- to 80-mg increments until optimum response occurs. Usual maintenance dosage range: 80 to 240 mg once daily.

SIDE EFFECTS
CNS: fatigue, lethargy.
CV: *bradycardia, hypotension, congestive heart failure,* peripheral vascular disease.
GI: nausea, vomiting, diarrhea.
Metabolic: hypoglycemia without tachycardia.
Skin: rash.
Other: *increased airway resistance,* fever.

INTERACTIONS
Insulin, hypoglycemic drugs (oral): can alter dosage requirements in previously stabilized diabetics. Observe patient carefully.
Cardiotonic glycosides: excessive bradycardia and increased depressant effect on myocardium. Use together cautiously.
Epinephrine: Severe vasoconstriction. Monitor blood pressure and observe patient carefully.

NURSING CONSIDERATIONS
• Contraindicated in patients with bronchial asthma, sinus bradycardia and greater than first degree conduction block, and cardiogenic shock.

• Use cautiously in patients with heart failure, chronic bronchitis, and emphysema.

• Always check patient's apical pulse before giving this drug. If slower than 60 beats per minute (bpm), hold drug and call doctor.

• Monitor blood pressure frequently. If patient develops severe hypotension, administer a vasopressor as ordered.

• Don't discontinue abruptly: can exacerbate angina and MI.

• Teach patient about his disease and therapy. Explain why it's important to take this drug, even when he's feeling well. Tell outpatient not to discontinue drug suddenly, but to call doctor if unpleasant side effects develop.

• This drug masks common signs of shock and hypoglycemia.

• May be given without regard to meals.

nitroprusside sodium
Nipride♦, Nitropress

INDICATIONS & DOSAGE
To lower blood pressure quickly in hypertensive emergencies; to control hypotension during anesthesia; to reduce preload and afterload in cardiac

---

pump failure or cardiogenic shock; may be used with or without dopamine—
Adults: 50-mg vial diluted with 2 to 3 ml of 5% dextrose in water I.V. and then added to 250, 500, or 1,000 ml 5% dextrose in water. Infuse at 0.5 to 10 mcg/kg/minute.

Average dose: 3 mcg/kg/minute. Maximum infusion rate: 10 mcg/kg/minute. Patients taking other antihypertensive drugs along with nitroprusside are very sensitive to this drug. Adjust dosage accordingly.

SIDE EFFECTS
The following effects generally indicate overdosage:
CNS: *headache, dizziness,* ataxia, loss of consciousness, coma, weak pulse, absent reflexes, widely dilated pupils, *restlessness, muscle twitching, diaphoresis.*
CV: distant heart sounds, palpitations, dyspnea, shallow breathing.
GI: *vomiting, nausea, abdominal pain.*
Metabolic: acidosis.
Skin: pink color.

INTERACTIONS
None significant.

NURSING CONSIDERATIONS
• Use cautiously in patients with hypothyroidism or hepatic or renal disease, or in those receiving other antihypertensives.
• Due to light sensitivity, wrap I.V. solution in foil. It's not necessary to wrap the tubing in foil. Fresh solution should have faint brownish tint. Discard after 4 hours.
• Obtain baseline vital signs before giving this drug, and find out what parameters the doctor wants to achieve.
• Check blood pressure every 5 minutes at start of infusion and every 15 minutes thereafter. If severe hypotension occurs, turn off I.V. nitroprusside—effects of drug quickly reversed. Notify doctor. If possible, an arterial

pressure line should be started. Regulate drug flow to specified level.
• Don't use bacteriostatic water for injection or sterile saline solution for reconstitution.
• Infuse with automatic infusion pump.
• This drug is best run piggyback through a peripheral line with no other medication. Don't adjust rate of main I.V. line while drug is running. Even small bolus of nitroprusside can cause severe hypotension.
• This drug can cause cyanide toxicity, so check serum thiocyanate levels every 72 hours. Watch for signs of thiocyanate toxicity: profound hypotension, metabolic acidosis, dyspnea, headache, loss of consciousness, ataxia, vomiting. If these occur, discontinue drug immediately and notify doctor.

---

pargyline hydrochloride
Eutonyl

INDICATIONS & DOSAGE
For moderate to severe hypertension, usually given in combination with other drugs—
Adults: initially, 25 to 50 mg P.O. once daily, if not receiving any other antihypertensive drugs. Then increase dosage by 10 mg daily at weekly intervals. Maximum daily dosage 200 mg. Usual daily dose for patients over 65 years or those who've had sympathectomy: 10 to 25 mg. When used in combination with other drugs, total daily dose of pargyline should not exceed 25 mg. No dosage recommendations for children.

SIDE EFFECTS
CNS: *tremors,* convulsions, choreiform movements, psychic changes, *nightmares, hyperexcitability, sweating,* dizziness, fainting, drowsiness.
CV: palpitations, *orthostatic hypotension,* fluid retention.
EENT: *mouth dryness,* optic damage.

GI: *nausea, vomiting, increased appetite, constipation.*
Other: impotence.

INTERACTIONS
Amphetamines, ephedrine, levodopa, metaraminol, methotrimeprazine, methylphenidate, phenylephrine, phenylpropanolamine, pseudoephedrine: enhanced pressor effects. Use together cautiously.
Alcohol, barbiturates, and other sedatives; tranquilizers; narcotics; dextromethorphan; tricyclic antidepressants: unpredictable interactions. Should be used with caution and in reduced dosage.

NURSING CONSIDERATIONS
• Contraindicated in patients with advanced renal failure, pheochromocytoma, hyperthyroidism, or Parkinson's disease; in patients who are hyperactive and hyperexcitable. Use cautiously in patients who are receiving other antihypertensives, or who have hepatic disease.
• Discontinue this drug at least 2 weeks before elective surgery.
• Hypotensive effects of this drug are increased by high temperatures, fever, stress, or severe illness. If patient develops severe hypotension, counteract with ephedrine or phenylephrine.
• Monitor blood pressure and pulse rate frequently. Take blood pressure while patient is standing.
• Patient should have periodic ophthalmic evaluations during therapy.
• If patient is scheduled for surgery and has been taking this drug, be sure narcotic dosages are reduced.
• This drug may require up to several weeks to reach optimal effect.
• Warn patient not to take any other medications, including over-the-counter cold remedies, without first asking doctor.
• This drug is an MAO inhibitor. Tell patient not to eat foods with high tyramine content: for example, aged

cheese, chianti wine, sour cream, canned figs, raisins, chicken livers, yeast extract, pickled herring.
• Teach patient about his disease and therapy. Explain why it's important to take this drug exactly as prescribed, even when he's feeling well. Tell outpatient not to discontinue this drug suddenly, but to call the doctor if unpleasant side effects develop.
• Inform patient that orthostatic hypotension can be minimized by rising slowly and avoiding sudden position changes. Mouth dryness can be relieved with sugarless chewing gum, sour hard candy, or ice chips.

phenoxybenzamine hydrochloride
Dibenzyline

INDICATIONS & DOSAGE
To control hypertension and sweating secondary to pheochromocytoma; may be used in combination with propranolol to control excessive tachycardia—
Adults: initially, 10 mg P.O. daily. Increase by 10 mg daily every 4 days. Maintenance dose: 20 to 60 mg daily.
Children: initially, 0.2 mg/kg or 6 mg/m^2 P.O. daily in a single dose. Maintenance dose: 12 to 36 mg/m^2 daily as a single dose or in divided doses.

SIDE EFFECTS
CNS: lethargy, drowsiness.
CV: *orthostatic hypotension, tachycardia,* shock.
EENT: *nasal stuffiness, dry mouth, miosis.*
GI: vomiting, abdominal distress.
Other: *impotence.*

INTERACTIONS
None significant.

NURSING CONSIDERATIONS
• Use cautiously in patients with cerebrovascular or coronary insufficiency,

---

advanced renal disease, respiratory disease.
• Watch patient closely for side effects, and call doctor promptly if they occur. If severe hypotension develops, patient may require levarterenol to counteract effect.
• Nasal congestion, miosis, and impotence usually decrease with continued therapy.
• Patient with tachycardia may require concurrent propranolol therapy.
• Monitor patient's heart rate and blood pressure frequently.
• This drug may take several weeks to achieve optimal effect.
• Monitor respiratory status carefully. This drug may aggravate symptoms of pneumonia and asthma.
• Teach patient about his disease and therapy. Explain why it's important to take this drug exactly as prescribed, even when he's feeling well. Tell outpatient not to discontinue this drug suddenly, but to call the doctor if unpleasant side effects develop.
• Inform patient that orthostatic hypotension can be minimized by rising slowly and avoiding sudden position changes. Mouth dryness can be relieved with sugarless chewing gum, sour hard candy, or ice chips.
• Used investigationally to treat chronic urinary retention.
• Small initial doses are increased gradually until desired effect is obtained. Patient should be observed at each dose for at least 4 days.

phentolamine hydrochloride
Regitine

phentolamine methanesulfonate
Regitine, Rogitine♦♦

INDICATIONS & DOSAGE
To aid in diagnosis of pheochromocytoma; to control or prevent hypertension

before or during pheochromocytomectomy—
Adults: P.O. therapeutic dose: 50 mg q.i.d.
I.V. diagnostic dose: 5 mg, with close monitoring of blood pressure.
Before surgical removal of tumor, give 2 to 5 mg I.M. or I.V. During surgery, patient may need small I.V. doses (1 mg) or small I.M. doses (3 mg).
Children: P.O. therapeutic dose: 5 mg/ kg daily or 150 mg/m² daily in 4 to 6 divided doses.
I.V. diagnostic dose: 0.1 mg/kg or 3 mg/m² as single dose, with close monitoring of blood pressure.
Before surgical removal of tumor give 1 mg I.V. or 3 mg I.M.
During surgery, patient may need small I.V. doses (1 mg).

SIDE EFFECTS
CNS: *dizziness, weakness, flushing.*
CV: *hypotension,* shock, *arrhythmias,* palpitations, *tachycardia,* angina pectoris.
GI: *diarrhea,* abdominal pain, *nausea, vomiting,* hyperperistalsis.
Other: *nasal stuffiness,* hypoglycemia.

INTERACTIONS
None significant.

NURSING CONSIDERATIONS
• Contraindicated in patients with angina, coronary artery disease, and history of MI. Use cautiously in patients with gastritis or peptic ulcer and in those receiving other antihypertensives.
• When this drug is given for diagnostic test, check patient's blood pressure first. Make frequent blood pressure checks during administration.
• Diagnosis positive for pheochromocytoma if severe hypotension results from I.V. test dose.
• Administer levarterenol to counteract severe hypotensive effect of this drug. Don't administer epinephrine to raise blood pressure, as this may cause further drop.

• Don't give sedatives or narcotics 24 hours before diagnostic test.

prazosin hydrochloride
Minipress♦

INDICATIONS & DOSAGE
For mild to moderate hypertension; used alone or in combination with a diuretic or other antihypertensive drugs; also used to decrease afterload in severe chronic congestive heart failure—
Adults: P.O. test dose: 1 mg given before bedtime to prevent "first-dose syncope." Initial dose: 1 mg t.i.d. Increase dosage slowly. Maximum daily dose 20 mg. Maintenance dose: 3 to 20 mg daily in 3 divided doses. A few patients have required dosages larger than this (up to 40 mg daily). If other antihypertensive drugs or diuretics are added to this drug, decrease prazosin dosage to 1 to 2 mg t.i.d. and retitrate.

SIDE EFFECTS
CNS: *dizziness,* headache, drowsiness, weakness, *"first-dose syncope,"* depression.
CV: orthostatic hypotension, *palpitations.*
EENT: blurred vision, dry mouth.
GI: vomiting, diarrhea, abdominal cramps, constipation, *nausea.*
GU: priapism.

INTERACTIONS
Propranolol and other beta blockers: syncope with loss of consciousness may occur more frequently. Advise patient to sit or lie down if he feels dizzy.

NURSING CONSIDERATIONS
• Use cautiously in patients receiving other antihypertensive drugs.
• Monitor patient's blood pressure and pulse rate frequently.
• If initial dose is greater than 1 mg, patient may develop severe syncope with loss of consciousness (first-dose syncope). Increase dosage slowly. Instruct patient to sit or lie down if he experiences dizziness.
• Teach patient about his disease and therapy. Explain why it's important to take this drug exactly as prescribed, even when he's feeling well. Tell outpatient not to discontinue this drug suddenly, but to call the doctor if unpleasant side effects develop.
• Inform patient that orthostatic hypotension can be minimized by rising slowly and avoiding sudden position changes. Mouth dryness can be relieved with sugarless chewing gum, sour hard candy, or ice chips.
• Compliance *may* be improved by giving this drug once a day. Check with doctor.

propranolol hydrochloride
Inderal♦

INDICATIONS & DOSAGE
Hypertension (usually used with thiazide diuretics)—
Adults: initial treatment of hypertension: 80 mg P.O. daily in 2 to 4 divided doses. Increase at 3- to 7-day intervals to maximum daily dose of 640 mg. Usual maintenance dose for hypertension: 160 to 480 mg daily. No dosing recommendations for children.

SIDE EFFECTS
CNS: *fatigue, lethargy,* vivid dreams, hallucinations.
CV: *bradycardia, hypotension, congestive heart failure,* peripheral vascular disease.
GI: nausea, vomiting, diarrhea.
Metabolic: hypoglycemia without tachycardia.
Skin: rash.
Other: *increased airway resistance,* fever.

INTERACTIONS
Insulin, hypoglycemic drugs (oral): can alter requirements for these drugs in

previously stabilized diabetics. Monitor
for hypoglycemia.
Cardiotonic glycosides: excessive
bradycardia and increased depressant
effect on myocardium. Use together
cautiously.
Aminophylline: antagonized beta-
blocking effects of propranolol. Use together cautiously.
Isoproterenol, glucagon: antagonized
propranolol effect. May be used therapeutically and in emergencies.
Cimetidine: inhibits propranolol's metabolism. Monitor for greater beta-
blocking effect.
Epinephrine: severe vasoconstriction.
Monitor blood pressure and observe patient carefully.

NURSING CONSIDERATIONS
• Contraindicated in diabetes mellitus,
asthma, allergic rhinitis; during ethyl
ether anesthesia; in sinus bradycardia
and heart block greater than first degree; in cardiogenic shock; in right ventricular failure secondary to pulmonary
hypertension. Use with caution in patients with congestive heart failure or
respiratory disease, and in patients taking other antihypertensive drugs.
• Always check patient's apical pulse
rate before giving this drug. If you detect extremes in pulse rates, hold medication and call the doctor immediately.
• Monitor blood pressure frequently. If
patient develops severe hypotension,
notify doctor. He may prescribe a vasopressor.
• Teach patient about his disease and
therapy. Explain why it's important to
take this drug exactly as prescribed,
even when he's feeling well. Tell outpatient not to discontinue this drug suddenly; abrupt discontinuation can exacerbate angina and MI. Tell patient to
call doctor if unpleasant side effects develop.
• This drug masks common signs of
shock and hypoglycemia.
• Food may increase the absorption of

propranolol. Give consistently with
meals.
• Inderal tablets are now manufactured
as a six-sided tablet with a raised "I"
imprint.
• Compliance may be improved by administering this drug on a twice-daily
basis. Check with doctor.
• Propranolol, as well as other beta
blockers, is being prescribed to decrease mortality following myocardial
infarction.
• Has also been used to treat aggression and rage, stage fright, recurrent GI
bleeding, and menopausal symptoms.

rauwolfia serpentina
HBP, Hiwolfia, Hyper-Rauw,
Hywolfia, Rau, Raudixin♦**, Rauja,
Raumason, Rauneed, Raupoid,
Rauserpin, Rausertina, Rauval,
Rauwoldin, Rawfola, Ru-Hy-T,
Serfia, Serfolia, T-Rau, Wolfina

INDICATIONS & DOSAGE
Mild to moderate hypertension—
Adults: initially and for 1 to 3 weeks
thereafter, 200 to 400 mg P.O. daily as
a single dose or in 2 divided doses.
Maintenance dose: 50 to 300 mg daily.
No dosing recommendations for chil-
dren.

SIDE EFFECTS
CNS: mental confusion, *depression,
drowsiness, nervousness,* anxiety,
nightmares, sedation, headache.
CV: *orthostatic hypotension, bradycar-
dia, syncope.*
EENT: *mouth dryness, nasal stuffi-
ness,* glaucoma.
GI: *hypersecretion of gastric acid, nau-
sea, vomiting,* gastrointestinal bleeding.
Skin: pruritus, rash.
Other: *impotence, weight gain.*

INTERACTIONS
MAO inhibitors: may cause excitability
and hypertension. Use together cautiously.

NURSING CONSIDERATIONS
• Contraindicated in patients with depression. Use cautiously in patients with severe cardiac or cerebrovascular disease, impaired renal function, peptic ulcer, ulcerative colitis, gallstones; in those undergoing surgery; and in those taking other antihypertensives or tricyclic antidepressants.
• Monitor patient's blood pressure and pulse rate frequently.
• Teach patient about his disease and therapy. Explain why it's important to take this drug exactly as prescribed, even when he's feeling well. Tell outpatient not to discontinue this drug suddenly, but to call the doctor if unpleasant side effects develop. Warn that this drug can cause drowsiness.
• Watch patient closely for signs of mental depression. Warn him to notify doctor promptly if he starts having nightmares.
• Inform patient that orthostatic hypotension can be minimized by rising slowly and avoiding sudden position changes. Mouth dryness can be relieved with sugarless chewing gum, sour hard candy, or ice chips. Tell patient to contact doctor if relief is needed for nasal stuffiness.
• Give this drug with meals.
• Patient should weigh himself daily and notify doctor of any weight gain.
• Effects of this drug may last for 10 days after it's discontinued.

---

rescinnamine
Anaprel, Moderil

INDICATIONS & DOSAGE
For mild to moderate hypertension; may be used alone or in combination with other antihypertensives—
Adults: initially, 0.5 mg b.i.d. Maintenance dose: 0.25 to 0.5 mg daily. No dosing recommendations for children.

SIDE EFFECTS
CNS: mental confusion, *depression, drowsiness, nervousness, anxiety, nightmares,* sedation, parkinsonism.
CV: *orthostatic hypotension, bradycardia, syncope.*
EENT: *mouth dryness, nasal stuffiness,* glaucoma.
GI: *hypersecretion of gastric acid, nausea, vomiting,* gastrointestinal bleeding.
Skin: pruritus, rash.
Other: *impotence, weight gain.*

INTERACTIONS
MAO inhibitors: may cause excitability and hypertension. Use together cautiously.

NURSING CONSIDERATIONS
• Contraindicated in patients with depression. Use cautiously in patients with severe cardiac or cerebrovascular disease, peptic ulcer, ulcerative colitis, gallstones, or in those undergoing surgery. Also use cautiously in patients taking other antihypertensives.
• Monitor patient's blood pressure and pulse rate frequently.
• Teach patient about his disease and therapy. Explain why it's important to take this drug exactly as prescribed, even when he's feeling well. Tell outpatient not to discontinue this drug suddenly, but to call the doctor if unpleasant side effects develop. Warn that this drug can cause drowsiness.
• Watch patient closely for signs of mental depression. Warn him to notify doctor promptly if he starts having nightmares.
• Inform patient that orthostatic hypotension can be minimized by rising slowly and avoiding sudden position changes. Mouth dryness can be relieved with sugarless chewing gum, sour hard candy, or ice chips. Tell patient to contact doctor if relief is needed for nasal stuffiness.
• Give this drug with meals.
• Patient should weigh himself daily and notify doctor of any weight gain.

Italicized side effects are common or life-threatening.
∗Liquid form contains alcohol.   ∗∗May contain tartrazine.

- Effects of this drug may last for 10 days after it's discontinued.

reserpine

Arcum R-S, Bonapene, Broserpine, De Serpa, Elserpine, Hyperine, Maso-Serpine, Rau-Sed, Rauserpin, Releserp-5, Reserjen, Reserfia♦♦, Reserpanca♦♦, Reserpaneed, Reserpoid* **, Rolserp, Sandril, Serp, Serpalan, Serpena, Serpanray, Serpasil♦*, Serpate, Sertabs, Sertina, Tensin, T-Serp, Zepine

INDICATIONS & DOSAGE

Mild to moderate essential hypertension (oral); hypertensive emergencies (parenteral)—
Adults: initially, 0.5 mg P.O. daily for 1 to 2 weeks. Maintenance dose: 0.1 to 0.5 mg daily.
I.M—initially, 0.5 to 1 mg, followed by doses of 2 to 4 mg at 2-hour intervals. Maximum recommended dose 4 mg.
Children: 0.07 mg/kg or 2 mg/m^2 with hydralazine I.M. every 12 to 24 hours.

SIDE EFFECTS

CNS: mental confusion, *depression, drowsiness, nervousness, anxiety, nightmares,* sedation.
CV: *orthostatic hypotension, bradycardia, syncope.*
EENT: *mouth dryness, nasal stuffiness,* glaucoma.
GI: *hyperacidity, nausea, vomiting,* gastrointestinal bleeding.
Skin: pruritus, rash.
Other: *impotence, weight gain.*

INTERACTIONS

MAO inhibitors: may cause excitability and hypertension. Use together cautiously.

NURSING CONSIDERATIONS

- Contraindicated in patients with depression. Use cautiously in patients with severe cardiac or cerebrovascular disease, peptic ulcer, ulcerative colitis, gallstones, mental depressive disorders; in those undergoing surgery; and in those taking other antihypertensive drugs.
- Monitor patient's blood pressure and pulse rate frequently.
- Teach patient about his disease and therapy. Explain why it's important to take this drug exactly as prescribed, even when he's feeling well. Tell outpatient not to discontinue this drug suddenly, but to call doctor if unpleasant side effects develop. Warn that this drug can cause drowsiness.
- Warn female patient to notify doctor if she becomes pregnant.
- Watch patient closely for signs of mental depression. Warn him to notify doctor promptly if he starts having nightmares.
- Inform patient that orthostatic hypotension can be minimized by rising slowly and avoiding sudden position changes. Mouth dryness can be relieved with sugarless chewing gum, sour hard candy, or ice chips. Tell patient to contact doctor if relief is needed for nasal stuffiness.
- Give this drug with meals.
- Patient should weigh himself daily and notify doctor of any weight gain.
- Effects of this drug may last for 10 days after it's discontinued.
- Parenteral form erratically absorbed; commonly replaced by other antihypertensives for hypertensive emergencies.

timolol maleate

Blocadren

INDICATIONS & DOSAGE

Hypertension—
Adults: Initial dosage is 10 mg P.O. b.i.d.
Usual daily maintenance dosage is 20 to 40 mg. Maximum daily dosage is 60 mg. Drug is used either alone or in combination with diuretics.
Myocardial infarction—

Adults: Recommended dosage for long-term prophylaxis in survivors of acute myocardial infarction (MI) is 10 mg P.O. b.i.d.

SIDE EFFECTS
CNS: fatigue, lethargy, vivid dreams.
CV: *bradycardia, hypotension, congestive heart failure (CHF)*, peripheral vascular disease.
GI: nausea, vomiting, diarrhea.
Metabolic: hypoglycemia without tachycardia.
Skin: rash.
Other: *increased airway resistance*, fever.

INTERACTIONS
Insulin, hypoglycemic drugs (oral): can alter requirements for these drugs in previously stabilized diabetics. Monitor for hypoglycemia.
Cardiac glycosides: excessive bradycardia and increased depressant effect on myocardium. Use together cautiously.

NURSING CONSIDERATIONS
• Contraindicated in diabetes mellitus, asthma, allergic rhinitis; during ethyl ether anesthesia; in sinus bradycardia and heart block greater than first degree; in cardiogenic shock; in right ventricular failure secondary to pulmonary hypertension. Use with caution in CHF and respiratory disease, and in patients taking other antihypertensives.
• Always check patient's apical pulse rate before giving this drug. If you detect extremes in pulse rates, withhold medication and call the doctor immediately.
• Monitor blood pressure frequently. If patient develops severe hypotension, notify doctor. He may prescribe a vasopressor.
• Instruct patient about the disease and therapy. Explain the importance of taking drug exactly as prescribed, even when he's feeling well. Tell patient not to discontinue drug suddenly: abrupt discontinuation can exacerbate angina

and MI. Tell patient to call doctor if unpleasant side effects develop.
• This drug masks common signs of shock and hypoglycemia.
• If patient is taking the drug for hypertension, warn him not to increase the dosage without first consulting his doctor. At least 7 days should intervene between increases in dosage.
• Timolol is the first beta blocker approved for use in post-MI patients. Like other beta blockers, it prolongs survival of MI patients.

---

trimethaphan camsylate
Arfonad♦

INDICATIONS & DOSAGE
To lower blood pressure quickly in hypertensive emergencies; for controlled hypotension during surgery—
Adults: 500 mg (10 ml) diluted in 500 ml dextrose 5% in water to yield concentration of 1 mg/ml I.V. Start I.V. drip at 1 to 2 mg/minute and titrate to achieve desired hypotensive response. Range: 0.3 mg to 6 mg/minute.

SIDE EFFECTS
CNS: dilated pupils, *extreme weakness*.
CV: *severe orthostatic hypotension, tachycardia*.
GI: anorexia, *nausea, vomiting, dry mouth*.
GU: *urinary retention*.
Other: respiratory depression.

INTERACTIONS
None significant.

NURSING CONSIDERATIONS
• Contraindicated in patients with anemia, respiratory insufficiency. Use cautiously in patients with arteriosclerosis; cardiac, hepatic, or renal disease; degenerative CNS disorders; Addison's disease; diabetes. Also use cautiously in patients receiving glucocorticoids; or in those receiving other antihypertensives.

Italicized side effects are common or life-threatening.
*Liquid form contains alcohol.   **May contain tartrazine.

- Monitor patient's blood pressure and vital signs frequently.
- May require elevation of the head of the bed for maximal effect.
- If extreme hypotension occurs, discontinue drug and call doctor. Use phenylephrine or mephentermine to counteract hypotension.
- Watch closely for respiratory distress, especially if large doses are used.

- Use infusion pump to administer this drug slowly.
- Discontinue drug before wound closure in surgery to allow blood pressure to return to normal.
- Position patient to avoid cerebral anoxia.
- Patient should receive oxygen therapy during use of this agent.

20

Vasodilators

amyl nitrite
cyclandelate
dipyridamole
erythrityl tetranitrate
ethaverine hydrochloride
isosorbide dinitrate
isoxsuprine hydrochloride
mannitol hexanitrate
nicotinyl alcohol
nitroglycerin
nylidrin hydrochloride
papaverine hydrochloride
pentaerythritol tetranitrate
tolazoline hydrochloride

MECHANISM OF ACTION

• Some peripheral vasodilators directly relax smooth muscle. This effect may be due to the inhibition of phosphodiesterase, resulting in increased concentrations of cylic adenosine monophosphate, which causes the vasodilation.
• Other peripheral vasodilators have a different mechanism of action. Tolazoline blocks alpha receptors; isoxsuprine and nylidrin stimulate beta receptors. Although isoxsuprine originally was thought only to stimulate beta receptors, newer evidence indicates that it may also be a direct-acting peripheral vasodilator.
• Coronary vasodilation occurs in normal but not in diseased arteries. Thus, the assumption that coronary vasodilators relieve angina by dilating coronary arteries is only partly correct. Coronary vasodilators cause a pooling of venous blood, which decreases the heart's workload by lowering ventricular diastolic pressure and by reducing the stretching of myocardial fibers.

• Dipyridamole, originally classified as a coronary vasodilator, has no value in treating acute attacks of angina. In fact, evidence is lacking that its long-term use is beneficial in preventing chronic angina. It does, however, inhibit platelet adhesion in patients with prosthetic heart valves.
• Nitrates are effective in chronic congestive heart failure refractory to standard therapy. The dilating effect of nitrates on venous circulation ultimately produces more efficient contraction.

COMBINATION PRODUCTS

CARTRAX 10: pentaerythritol tetranitrate 10 mg and hydroxyzine HCl 10 mg.
CARTRAX 20: pentaerythritol tetranitrate 20 mg and hydroxyzine HCl 10 mg.
COROVAS TYMCAPS: pentaerythritol tetranitrate 30 mg and secobarbital 50 mg.
DEAPRIL-ST: dihydroergocornine mesylate 0.167 mg, dihydroergocristine mesylate 0.167 mg, and dihydroergocryptine mesylate 0.167 mg.
EQUANITRATE 10: pentaerythritol tetranitrate 10 mg and meprobamate 200 mg.
EQUANITRATE 20: pentaerythritol tetranitrate 20 mg and meprobamate 200 mg.
HYDERGINE: dihydroergocornine mesylate 0.167 mg, dihydroergocristine mesylate 0.167 mg, and dihydroergocryptine mesylate 0.167 mg.
ISORDIL WITH PHENOBARBITAL: isosorbide dinitrate 10 mg and phenobarbital 15 mg.

Italicized side effects are common or life-threatening.
*Liquid form contains alcohol.   **May contain tartrazine.

MILTRATE-10: pentaerythritol tetranitrate 10 mg and meprobamate 200 mg.
MILTRATE-20: pentaerythritol tetranitrate 20 mg and meprobamate 200 mg.
PAPAVATRAL L.A. CAPSULES: pentaerythritol tetranitrate 50 mg and ethaverine HCl 30 mg.
PERITRATE WITH PHENOBARBITAL: pentaerythritol tetranitrate 10 mg and phenobarbital 15 mg.
PERITRATE WITH PHENOBARBITAL: pentaerythritol tetranitrate 20 mg and phenobarbital 15 mg.

amyl nitrite

INDICATIONS & DOSAGE
Antidote for cyanide poisoning—
0.2 or 0.3 ml by inhalation for 30 to 60 seconds q 5 minutes until conscious.
Relief of angina pectoris, bronchospasm, biliary spasm—
Adults and children: 0.2 to 0.3 ml by inhalation (one glass ampul inhaler), p.r.n.

SIDE EFFECTS
Blood: methemoglobinemia.
CNS: *headache, sometimes with throbbing;* dizziness; weakness.
CV: *orthostatic hypotension, tachycardia,* flushing, palpitations, fainting.
GI: nausea, vomiting.
Skin: cutaneous vasodilation.
Other: hypersensitivity reactions.

INTERACTIONS
None significant.

NURSING CONSIDERATIONS
• Contraindicated in hypersensitivity to nitrites. Use with caution in cerebral hemorrhage, hypotension, head injury, and glaucoma.
• Watch for orthostatic hypotension. Have patient sit down and avoid rapid position changes while inhaling drug.
• Extinguish all cigarettes before use, or ampul may ignite.
• Wrap ampul in cloth and crush. Hold

near patient's nose and mouth so vapor is inhaled.
• Effective within 30 seconds but has a short duration of action (4 to 8 minutes).
• Keeping the head low, deep breathing, and movement of extremities may help relieve dizziness, syncope, or weakness from postural hypotension.
• Drug is often abused. Claimed to have aphrodisiac benefits. Sometimes called "Amy."

cyclandelate
Cyclanfor, Cyclospasmol♦

INDICATIONS & DOSAGE
Adjunct in intermittent claudication, arteriosclerosis obliterans, vasospasm and muscular ischemia associated with thrombophlebitis, nocturnal leg cramps, Raynaud's phenomenon, selected cases of ischemic cerebral vascular disease—
Adults: initially, 200 mg P.O. q.i.d. (before meals and h.s.); maximum 400 mg P.O. q.i.d. When clinical response is noted, decrease dosage gradually until maintenance dosage is reached. Maintenance dose 400 to 800 mg daily in divided doses.

SIDE EFFECTS
CNS: *headache, tingling of the extremities, dizziness.*
CV: *mild flushing,* tachycardia.
GI: pyrosis, eructation, nausea, heartburn.
Other: *sweating.*

INTERACTIONS
None significant.

NURSING CONSIDERATIONS
• Use with extreme caution in severe obliterative coronary artery or cerebrovascular disease, since circulation to these diseased areas may be compromised by vasodilatory effects of the drug elsewhere (coronary steal syn-

drome). Use with caution in patients with glaucoma, hypotension.

• Give with food or antacids to lessen GI distress.

• Use in conjunction with, not as a substitute for, appropriate medical or surgical therapy for peripheral or cerebrovascular disease.

• Short-term therapy of little benefit. Instruct patient to expect long-term treatment and to continue to take medication.

• Side effects usually disappear after several weeks of therapy.

dipyridamole
Persantine♦**

INDICATIONS & DOSAGE
Long-term therapy for chronic angina pectoris, prevention of recurrent transient ischemic attack—
Adults: 50 mg P.O. t.i.d. at least 1 hour before meals, to maximum of 400 mg daily.
Inhibition of platelet adhesion in patients with prosthetic heart valves, in combination with warfarin—
Adults: 100 to 400 mg P.O. daily.
Transient ischemic attack—
Adults: 100 mg P.O. daily as a single dose.

SIDE EFFECTS
CNS: *headache, dizziness,* weakness.
CV: flushing, fainting, *hypotension.*
GI: *nausea,* vomiting, diarrhea.
Skin: rash.

INTERACTIONS
None significant.

NURSING CONSIDERATIONS
• Use with caution in hypotension, anticoagulant therapy.
• Observe for side effects, especially with large doses. Monitor blood pressure.
• Administer 1 hour before meals.
• Watch for signs of bleeding, pro-

longed bleeding time (large doses, long-term).

• Clinical response to antianginal therapy may not be evident before second or third month. Tell patient to continue drug despite lack of observable response.

erythrityl tetranitrate
Anginar, Cardilate♦

INDICATIONS & DOSAGE
Prophylaxis and long-term management of frequent or recurrent anginal pain, reduced exercise tolerance associated with angina pectoris—
Adults: 5 mg sublingually or buccally t.i.d. or 10 mg P.O., a.c. chewed t.i.d., increasing in 2 to 3 days if needed.

SIDE EFFECTS
CNS: *headache, sometimes with throbbing; dizziness;* weakness.
CV: *orthostatic hypotension, tachycardia, flushing, palpitations,* fainting.
GI: nausea, vomiting.
Local: sublingual burning.
Skin: cutaneous vasodilation.
Other: hypersensitivity reactions.

INTERACTIONS
None significant.

NURSING CONSIDERATIONS
• Contraindicated in hypersensitivity to nitrites, head trauma, cerebral hemorrhage, severe anemia. Use with caution in hypotension.
• Monitor blood pressure, and intensity and duration of response to drug.
• May cause headaches, especially at first. Treat headache with aspirin or acetaminophen. Dosage may need to be reduced temporarily, but tolerance usually develops.
• Tell patient to take medication regularly, even long-term, if ordered, and to keep it easily accessible at all times. Physiologically necessary but not habit-forming.

Italicized side effects are common or life-threatening.
*Liquid form contains alcohol.   **May contain tartrazine.

• Additional dose may be taken before anticipated stress or at bedtime if angina is nocturnal.

• Advise patient to avoid alcoholic beverages; they may produce unpleasant disulfiram-like side effects.

• May cause orthostatic hypotension. Patient should get out of bed, go up and down stairs, and change position slowly; he should lie down at first sign of dizziness.

• Teach patient to take sublingual tablet at first sign of attack. He should wet the tablet with saliva, place it under the tongue until completely absorbed, and sit down and rest. Burning sensation indicates potency. Dose may be repeated every 10 to 15 minutes for a maximum of three doses. If no relief, patient should call doctor or go to hospital emergency room. If patient complains of tingling sensation with drug placed sublingually, he may try holding tablet in buccal pouch.

• Teach patient to take oral tablet on empty stomach, either ½ hour before or 1 to 2 hours after meals; to swallow oral tablets whole; and chew chewable tablets thoroughly before swallowing.

• Drug should not be discontinued abruptly—coronary vasospasm may occur.

• Store medication in cool place, in tightly closed container, away from light. To assure freshness, replace supply every 3 months. Remove cotton from container, since it absorbs drug.

---

ethaverine hydrochloride
Cebral, Circubid, Etalent, Ethaquin, Ethatab, Ethavex, Isovex, Myoquin, Pavaspan, Rolidiol, Spasodil

INDICATIONS & DOSAGE
Long-term treatment of peripheral and cerebrovascular insufficiency associated with arterial spasm; spastic conditions of gastrointestinal and genitourinary tracts—
Adults: 100 to 200 mg P.O. t.i.d. or

150 mg of sustained-release preparation P.O. q 12 hours.

SIDE EFFECTS
CNS: *headache,* drowsiness.
CV: *hypotension, flushing,* sweating, vertigo, cardiac depression, arrhythmias.
GI: *nausea; anorexia; abdominal distress; dryness of throat;* constipation; diarrhea.
Hepatic: jaundice, altered liver function tests.
Skin: rash.
Other: respiratory depression, malaise, lassitude.

INTERACTIONS
None significant.

NURSING CONSIDERATIONS
• Contraindicated in complete AV dissociation and in severe hepatic disease. Use with caution in women who are pregnant or of childbearing age, and in patients with glaucoma or pulmonary embolus; may precipitate arrhythmias.

• Hold dose and call doctor if signs of hepatic hypersensitivity develop (gastrointestinal symptoms, altered liver function tests, jaundice, eosinophilia).

• Monitor and record vital signs during therapy.

• FDA has announced this drug may not be effective for disease states indicated.

---

isosorbide dinitrate
Angidil, Coronex♦♦, Dilatrate-SR, Iso-Bid, Iso-D, Isosorb, Isordil♦, Onset, Sorate, Sorbitrate

INDICATIONS & DOSAGE
Treatment of acute anginal attacks (sublingual and chewable only); prophylaxis in situations likely to cause attacks; treatment of chronic ischemic heart disease (by preload reduction); adjunct with other vasodilators, such as hydralazine and prazosin, in treatment

---

of severe chronic congestive heart failure—

Adults:

Sublingual form—2.5 to 10 mg under the tongue for prompt relief of anginal pain, repeated q 2 to 3 hours during acute phase, or q 4 to 6 hours for prophylaxis.

Chewable form—5 to 10 mg, p.r.n., for acute attack or q 2 to 3 hours for prophylaxis but only after initial test dose of 5 mg to determine risk of severe hypotension.

Oral form—5 to 30 mg P.O. q.i.d. for prophylaxis only (use smallest effective dose); sustained-release forms 40 mg P.O. q 6 to 12 hours.

SIDE EFFECTS
CNS: *headache, sometimes with throbbing; dizziness;* weakness.
CV: *orthostatic hypotension, tachycardia, palpitations, ankle edema,* fainting.
GI: nausea, vomiting.
Local: sublingual burning.
Skin: cutaneous vasodilation, *flushing.*
Other: hypersensitivity reactions.

INTERACTIONS
None significant.

NURSING CONSIDERATIONS
• Contraindicated in hypersensitivity to nitrites, head trauma, cerebral hemorrhage, severe anemia. Use with caution in hypotension.
• Monitor blood pressure, and intensity and duration of response to drug.
• May cause headaches, especially at first. Treat headache with aspirin or acetaminophen. Dosage may need to be reduced temporarily, but tolerance usually develops.
• Tell patient to take medication regularly, even long-term, if ordered, and to keep it easily accessible at all times. Physiologically necessary but not habit-forming.
• Additional dose may be taken before

anticipated stress or at bedtime if angina is nocturnal.
• Advise patient to avoid alcoholic beverages; they may produce unpleasant disulfiram-like side effects.
• May cause orthostatic hypotension. Patient should get out of bed, go up and down stairs, and change position slowly; he should lie down at first sign of dizziness.
• Teach patient to take sublingual tablet at first sign of attack. He should wet the tablet with saliva, place it under the tongue until completely absorbed, and sit down and rest. Burning sensation indicates potency. Dose may be repeated every 10 to 15 minutes for a maximum of three doses. If no relief, patient should call doctor or go to hospital emergency room. If patient complains of tingling sensation with drug placed sublingually, he may try holding tablet in buccal pouch.
• Warn patient not to confuse sublingual with oral form.
• Teach patient to take oral tablet on empty stomach, either ½ hour before or 1 to 2 hours after meals; to swallow oral tablets whole; and to chew chewable tablets thoroughly before swallowing.
• Drug should not be discontinued abruptly—coronary vasospasm may occur.
• Store in cool place, in tightly closed container, away from light.
• Has been used investigationally in treatment of congestive heart failure.

---

isoxsuprine hydrochloride
Rolisox, Vasodilan♦, Vasoprine

INDICATIONS & DOSAGE
Adjunct for relief of symptoms associated with cerebrovascular insufficiency, peripheral vascular diseases (such as arteriosclerosis obliterans, thromboangiitis obliterans, Raynaud's disease)—
Adults: 10 to 20 mg P.O. t.i.d. or q.i.d.; initially, 5 to 10 mg I.M. b.i.d.

Italicized side effects are common or life-threatening.
*Liquid form contains alcohol.   **May contain tartrazine.

or t.i.d. in severe or acute conditions, to maximum of 10 mg. Intramuscular doses greater than 10 mg may be associated with hypotension and tachycardia and are not recommended.

SIDE EFFECTS
CNS: *dizziness,* nervousness, weakness, trembling, *light-headedness.*
CV: *hypotension, tachycardia, transient palpitations.*
GI: vomiting, abdominal distress, intestinal distention.
Skin: severe rash.

INTERACTIONS
None significant.

NURSING CONSIDERATIONS
• Contraindicated in immediate postpartum period, arterial bleeding; I.M. contraindicated in hypotension or tachycardia.
• Safe use in pregnancy and lactation not established, although drug has been used to inhibit contractions in premature labor.
• Do not give intravenously.
• Observe for hypotension and tachycardia with parenteral use. Monitor blood pressure and pulse rate.
• Discontinue if rash develops.

mannitol hexanitrate
Mannex, Vascunitol

INDICATIONS & DOSAGE
Chronic prophylaxis against attacks of angina pectoris—
Adults: 15 to 60 mg P.O. q 4 to 6 hours.

SIDE EFFECTS
CNS: *headache, sometimes with throbbing; dizziness;* weakness, increased intracranial pressure.
CV: *orthostatic hypotension, tachycardia, flushing, palpitations,* fainting.
EENT: rise in intraocular tension.
GI: nausea, vomiting.

Local: sublingual burning.
Skin: cutaneous vasodilation.
Other: hypersensitivity.

INTERACTIONS
None significant.

NURSING CONSIDERATIONS
• Contraindicated in head trauma, cerebral hemorrhage, severe anemia. Use with caution in hypotension.
• Monitor blood pressure, and intensity and duration of response to drug.
• Medication may cause headaches, especially at first. Treat headache with aspirin or acetaminophen. Dosage may need to be reduced temporarily, but tolerance usually develops.
• Tell patient to take medication regularly, even long-term, if ordered. Physiologically necessary but not habit-forming.
• Additional doses may be taken before anticipated stress or at bedtime if angina is nocturnal.
• Alcoholic beverages should be avoided, since they may produce unpleasant disulfiram-like side effects.
• Medication may cause orthostatic hypotension. Patient should get out of bed, go up and down stairs, or change position slowly; he should lie down at first sign of dizziness.
• Store medication in cool dark place in tightly covered container.
• Effective within 15 to 30 minutes; duration 4 to 6 hours.

nicotinyl alcohol
Roniacol♦

INDICATIONS & DOSAGE
Treatment of conditions of deficient circulation, such as peripheral vascular disease, vascular spasm, varicose ulcers, decubital ulcers, Ménière's syndrome, vertigo—
Adults: 50 to 100 mg regular tablets P.O. b.i.d. or t.i.d. (may increase to 150 to 200 mg P.O. t.i.d. or q.i.d.);

150 to 300 mg sustained-release tablets P.O. b.i.d.; 5 to 10 ml of elixir P.O. t.i.d.

SIDE EFFECTS
CNS: paresthesias.
CV: *transient flushing.*
GI: *gastric irritation.*
Skin: minor rashes.
Other: allergic reactions.

INTERACTIONS
Clonidine: may inhibit vasodilation. Observe for lack of response.

NURSING CONSIDERATIONS
• Contraindicated in active peptic ulcer or gastritis.
• Tolerance to side effects develops with continued therapy.

---

nitroglycerin
Ang-O-Span, Cardabid, Corobid, Glyceryl Trinitrate, Gly-Trate, Nitro-Bid, Nitro-Bid I.V., Nitrocap, Nitrocels, Nitro-Dial, Nitrodisc, Nitro-Dur, Nitroglyn, Nitrol♦, Nitro-Lyn, Nitrong♦, Nitrospan, Nitrostabilin♦♦, Nitrostat♦, Nitrostat I.V., Nyglycon, Transderm-Nitro, Trates, Tridil, Susadrin

---

INDICATIONS & DOSAGE
Prophylaxis against chronic anginal attacks—
Adults: 1 sustained-release capsule q 8 to 12 hours; or 2% ointment: Start with ½ inch ointment, increasing with ½-inch increments until headache occurs, then decreasing to previous dose. Range of dosage with ointment 2 to 5 inches. Usual dose 1 to 2 inches; transmucosal tablet (Susadrin) may be administered under the upper lip or buccally (between cheek and gum) at a dose of 1 mg t.i.d. Alternatively, transdermal disc or pad (Nitrodisc, Nitro-Dur, or Transderm-Nitro) may be applied to hairless site once daily.
Relief of acute angina pectoris, prophylaxis to prevent or minimize anginal attacks when taken immediately prior to stressful events—
Adults: 1 sublingual tablet (gr $^1/_{400}$, $^1/_{200}$, $^1/_{150}$, $^1/_{100}$) dissolved under the tongue or in the buccal pouch immediately upon indication of anginal attack. May repeat q 5 minutes for 15 minutes.
To control hypertension associated with surgery; to treat congestive heart failure associated with myocardial infarction; to relieve angina pectoris in acute situations; to produce controlled hypotension during surgery (by I.V. infusion)—
Adults: Initial infusion rate is 5 mcg/ minute. May be increased by 5 mcg/ minute q 3 to 5 minutes until a response is noted. If a 20 mcg/minute rate doesn't produce a response, dosage may be increased by as much as 20 mcg/minute q 3 to 5 minutes.

SIDE EFFECTS
CNS: *headache, sometimes with throbbing; dizziness;* weakness.
CV: *orthostatic hypotension, tachycardia, flushing, palpitations,* fainting.
GI: nausea, vomiting.
Skin: cutaneous vasodilation.
Local: sublingual burning.
Other: hypersensitivity reactions.

INTERACTIONS
None significant.

NURSING CONSIDERATIONS
• Contraindicated in hypersensitivity to nitrites, head trauma, cerebral hemorrhage, severe anemia. Use with caution in hypotension.
• Monitor blood pressure, and intensity and duration of response to drug.
• May cause headaches, especially at first. Treat headache with aspirin or acetaminophen. Dosage may need to be reduced temporarily, but tolerance usually develops.
• Tell patient to take medication regularly, even long-term, if ordered, and to keep it easily accessible at all times.

Italicized side effects are common or life-threatening.
∗Liquid form contains alcohol.   ∗∗May contain tartrazine.

Physiologically necessary but not habit-forming.

• Additional dose may be taken before anticipated stress or at bedtime if angina is nocturnal.

• Advise patient to avoid alcoholic beverages; they may produce unpleasant disulfiram-like side effects.

• May cause orthostatic hypotension. Patient should get out of bed, go up and down stairs, and change position slowly; he should lie down at first sign of dizziness.

• Teach patient to take sublingual tablet at first sign of attack. He should wet the tablet with saliva; place it under the tongue until completely absorbed and sit down and rest. Burning sensation indicates potency. Dose may be repeated every 10 to 15 minutes for a maximum of three doses. If no relief, patient should call doctor or go to hospital emergency room. If patient complains of tingling sensation with drug placed sublingually, he may try holding tablet in buccal pouch.

• Teach patient to take oral tablet on empty stomach, either ½ hour before or 1 to 2 hours after meals; to swallow oral tablets whole; and to chew chewable tablets thoroughly before swallowing.

• Store in cool dark place, in tightly closed container. To assure freshness, replace supply every 3 months. Remove cotton from container, since it absorbs drug.

• To apply ointment, spread in uniform thin layer on any nonhairy area. Do not rub in. Cover with plastic film to aid absorption and to protect clothing.

• Transdermal dosage forms can be applied to any hairless part of the skin except distal parts of the arms or legs, because absorption will not be maximal at these sites.

• The various brands of transdermal nitroglycerin products have different total content and surface area specifications. Don't interchange brands on same patient without first consulting doctor or pharmacist.

• Doctor may prescribe nitroglycerin by its chemical name, glyceryl trinitrate (GTN).

• When administering as an intravenous infusion, be sure to use the special nonabsorbing tubing supplied by the manufacturer, because up to 80% of the drug can be adsorbed by regular plastic tubing. Also, be sure to prepare in a glass bottle or container.

nylidrin hydrochloride
Arlidin♦, Pervadil♦♦, Rolidrin

INDICATIONS & DOSAGE
To increase blood supply in vasospastic disorders (arteriosclerosis obliterans, thromboangiitis obliterans, diabetic vascular disease, night leg cramps, Raynaud's phenomenon and disease, ischemic ulcer, frostbite, acrocyanosis, acroparesthesia, sequelae of thrombophlebitis); and in circulatory disturbances of the middle ear (primary cochlear ischemia, cochlear striae, vascular ischemia, macular or ampullar ischemia); other disturbances due to labyrinth artery spasm or obstruction—
Adults: 3 to 12 mg P.O. t.i.d. or q.i.d.

SIDE EFFECTS
CNS: trembling, *nervousness*, weakness, *dizziness (not associated with labyrinth artery insufficiency).*
CV: *palpitations, hypotension,* flushing.
GI: *nausea, vomiting.*

INTERACTIONS
None significant.

NURSING CONSIDERATIONS
• Contraindicated in acute myocardial infarction, paroxysmal tachycardia, angina pectoris, thyrotoxicosis. Use with caution in uncompensated heart disease or peptic ulcer.

papaverine hydrochloride
BP-Papaverine, Cerebid, Cerespan, Cirbed, Delapav, Kavrin, Lapav*, Meta-Kaps, Myobid, Papacon, Papalease, PapKaps-150, P-A-V, Pavabid, Pavacap, Pavacen, Pavaclor, Pavacron, Pavadel, Pavadur, Pavadyl, Pavakey S.A., Pava-lyn, Pava-Par, Pava-Rx, Pavasule, Pavatime, Pava-Wol, Paverolan, Pavex, PT-300, Ro-Papav, S.M.R.-Kaps, Vasal, Vasocap, Vasospan, Vazosan

INDICATIONS & DOSAGE
Relief of cerebral and peripheral ischemia associated with arterial spasm and myocardial ischemia; treatment of smooth-muscle spasm (coronary occlusion, angina pectoris, sequelae of peripheral and pulmonary embolism, certain cerebral angiospastic states); and visceral spasms (biliary, ureteral, or gastrointestinal colic)—
Adults: 60 to 300 mg P.O. 1 to 5 times daily, or 150 to 300 mg sustained-release preparations q 8 to 12 hours; 30 to 120 mg I.M. or I.V. q 3 hours, as indicated.

SIDE EFFECTS
CNS: *headache.*
CV: *increased heart rate, increased blood pressure* (with parenteral use), depressed AV and intraventricular conduction, arrhythmias.
GI: constipation, *nausea.*
Other: *sweating, flushing,* malaise, increased depth of respiration.

INTERACTIONS
None significant.

NURSING CONSIDERATIONS
• Contraindicated for I.V. use in complete AV block. Use with caution in glaucoma.
• Monitor blood pressure, heart rate and rhythm, especially in cardiac disease. Hold dose and notify doctor immediately if changes occur.
• Not often used parenterally, except when immediate effect is desired.
• Give I.V. slowly (over 1 to 2 minutes) to avoid side effects.
• Most effective when given early in the course of a disorder.
• Tell patient to take medication regularly; long-term therapy is required.
• Do not add lactated Ringer's injection to the injectable form; will precipitate.
• FDA has announced this drug may not be effective for disease states indicated.

pentaerythritol tetranitrate
Angijen Green, Arcotrate Nos. 1 & 2, Baritrate, Blaintrate, Desatrate 30, Desatrate 50, Dilar, Duotrate, Kaytrate, Maso-Trol, Nitrin, Penta-Cap-No. 1, Penta-E., Penta-E. S.A., Pentaforte-T, Penta-Tal No. 1 & 2, Pentestan-80, Pentetra, Pentraspan, Pentrate T.D., Pentritol, Pent-T-80, Pentylan, Peritrate♦, PETN, Petro-20 mg, P-T♦♦, P-T-T, Quintrate, Rate, Vasolate, Vasolate-80

INDICATIONS & DOSAGE
Prophylaxis against angina pectoris—
Adults: 10 to 20 mg P.O. q.i.d.; may be titrated upward to 40 mg P.O. q.i.d. ½ hour before or 1 hour after meals and h.s.; 80 mg sustained-release preparations P.O. b.i.d.

SIDE EFFECTS
CNS: *headache, sometimes with throbbing; dizziness;* weakness.
CV: *orthostatic hypotension, tachycardia, flushing, palpitations,* fainting.
GI: nausea, vomiting.
Skin: cutaneous vasodilation.
Other: hypersensitivity reactions.

INTERACTIONS
None significant.

Italicized side effects are common or life-threatening.
*Liquid form contains alcohol.   **May contain tartrazine.

NURSING CONSIDERATIONS
• Contraindicated in head trauma, cerebral hemorrhage, severe anemia. Use with caution in hypotension and glaucoma.
• Monitor blood pressure, and intensity and duration of response to drug.
• Medication may cause headaches, especially at first. Treat with aspirin or acetaminophen. Dosage may need to be reduced temporarily, but tolerance usually develops.
• Medication should be taken regularly, even long-term, if ordered. Physiologically necessary but not habit-forming.
• Additional doses may be taken before anticipated stress or at bedtime for nocturnal angina.
• Not to be used for relief of acute anginal attacks.
• Medication may cause orthostatic hypotension. Patient should get out of bed, go up and down stairs, or change position slowly; he should lie down at first sign of dizziness.
• Drug should not be discontinued abruptly—coronary vasospasm may occur.
• Store medication in cool place in tightly covered, light-resistant container.

---

tolazoline hydrochloride
Tazol, Toloxan, Tolzol

INDICATIONS & DOSAGE
Spastic peripheral vascular disorders associated with acrocyanosis, acroparesthesia, arteriosclerosis obliterans, Buerger's disease, causalgia, diabetic arteriosclerosis, gangrene, endarteritis, sequelae of frostbite, post-thrombotic conditions, Raynaud's disease, scleroderma—
Adults:
*Oral—*25 mg 4 to 6 times daily, gradually increasing to maximum of 50 mg 6 times daily.
*Parenteral—*10 to 50 mg S.C., I.V., or I.M. q.i.d. Start with low dose, increasing gradually until optimal response (as determined by appearance of flushing) is reached.
*Intra-arterial—*50 to 75 mg/injection, depending on response; 1 or 2 injections may be required initially, then dose of 2 or 3 injections weekly to maintain circulation, possibly coupled with oral tolazoline between injections.

SIDE EFFECTS
CV: *arrhythmias, anginal pain, hypertension, flushing,* transient postural vertigo, palpitations.
GI: *nausea, vomiting, diarrhea, epigastric discomfort, exacerbation of peptic ulcer.*
Local: burning at injection site.
Other: weakness, paradoxical response in seriously damaged limbs, increased pilomotor activity, tingling, chilliness, apprehension.

INTERACTIONS
Ethyl alcohol: possible disulfiram reaction from accumulation of acetaldehyde. Use together cautiously.

NURSING CONSIDERATIONS
• Contraindicated in coronary artery disease, active peptic ulcer, or following cerebrovascular accident. Use with caution in patients with history of peptic ulcer disease, gastritis, or known or suspected mitral stenosis.
• Keep patient warm during parenteral administration to increase response.
• Appearance of flushing usually indicates maximum tolerable dose.
• Monitor vital signs. Watch especially for blood pressure changes, arrhythmias.
• Instruct patient to avoid alcohol: chills and flushing may occur.
• Due to risks, technique, and precautions, intra-arterial injection should be done only by experienced personnel, in selected cases, and only after maximum benefit has been achieved with oral and parenteral therapy.

• Warn patient against exposure to cold, which can aggravate tissue damage.
• Often used to distinguish between functional (vasospastic) and organic (obstructive) forms of peripheral vascular disease.

21

Antilipemics

cholestyramine
clofibrate
colestipol hydrochloride
dextrothyroxine sodium
gemfibrozil
niacin
probucol
sitosterols

MECHANISM OF ACTION
• Both cholestyramine and colestipol combine with bile acid to form an insoluble compound that is excreted.
• Clofibrate—used when triglycerides are high and cholesterol levels are only moderately elevated—seems to inhibit biosynthesis of cholesterol at an early stage, but the exact mechanism is unknown.
• Dextrothyroxine accelerates hepatic catabolism of cholesterol and increases bile secretion to lower cholesterol levels. The drug's serious cardiovascular side effects restrict its use to young patients with no history of coronary artery disease.
• Gemfibrozil inhibits peripheral lipolysis and also reduces triglyceride synthesis in the liver.
• Niacin, by an unknown mechanism, decreases synthesis of low-density lipoproteins and inhibits lipolysis in adipose tissue.
• Probucol inhibits cholesterol transport from the intestine and may also decrease cholesterol synthesis. The drug appears to be more effective in patients with mild cholesterol elevations than in those with severe hypercholesterolemia.
• Sitosterols, structurally similar to

cholesterol, competes with it to reduce absorption.

COMBINATION PRODUCTS
None.

cholestyramine
Questran♦**

INDICATIONS & DOSAGE
Primary hyperlipidemia, pruritus, and diarrhea due to excess bile acid—
Adults: 4 g before meals and h.s., not to exceed 32 g daily. Each scoop or packet of Questran contains 4 g cholestyramine.
Children: 240 mg/kg daily P.O. in 3 divided doses with beverage or food. Safe dosage not established for children under 6 years.

SIDE EFFECTS
GI: *constipation,* fecal impaction, hemorrhoids, *abdominal discomfort,* flatulence, *nausea,* vomiting, steatorrhea.
Skin: *rashes,* irritation of skin, tongue, and perianal area.
Other: *vitamin A, D, and K deficiency from decreased absorption;* hyperchloremic acidosis with long-term use or very high dosage.

INTERACTIONS
None significant.

NURSING CONSIDERATIONS
• To mix, sprinkle powder on surface of preferred beverage or wet food. Let stand a few minutes, then stir to obtain uniform suspension.

Unmarked trade names available in the United States only.
♦ Also available in Canada.   ♦ ♦ Available in Canada only.

- Mixing with carbonated beverages may result in excess foaming. To avoid, use large glass, mix slowly.
- Administer all other medications at least 1 hour before or 4 to 6 hours after cholestyramine to avoid blocking their absorption.
- Observe bowel habits; treat constipation as needed. Encourage a diet high in roughage and fluids. If severe constipation develops, decrease dosage, add a stool softener, or discontinue drug.
- Monitor cardiotonic glycoside levels in patients receiving both medications concurrently. Should cholestyramine therapy be discontinued, cardiotonic glycoside toxicity may result unless dosage is adjusted.
- Watch for signs of vitamin A, D, and K deficiency.
- May cause decreased absorption of many drugs due to binding. Check drug interaction list of individual drugs.

clofibrate
Atromid-S♦

INDICATIONS & DOSAGE
Hyperlipidemia and xanthoma tuberosum—
Adults: 2 g P.O. daily in 4 divided doses. Some patients may respond to lower doses as assessed by serum lipid monitoring.
Should not be used in children.

SIDE EFFECTS
Blood: leukopenia.
CNS: fatigue, weakness.
GI: *nausea, diarrhea, vomiting,* stomatitis, *dyspepsia,* flatulence.
GU: decreased libido.
Hepatic: gallstones, *transient and reversible elevations of liver function tests.*
Skin: rashes, urticaria, pruritus, dry skin and hair.
Other: *myalgias and arthralgias,* resembling a flu-like syndrome; *weight gain; polyphagia;* fever.

INTERACTIONS
Oral contraceptives: may antagonize clofibrate's lipid-lowering effect. Monitor blood lipid level.

NURSING CONSIDERATIONS
- Contraindicated in patients with severe renal or hepatic disease.
- Warn patient to report flu-like symptoms to doctor immediately.
- Monitor renal and hepatic function, blood counts, serum electrolyte and blood sugar levels. If liver function tests show steady rise, clofibrate should be discontinued.
- Should not be used indiscriminately. May pose increased risk of gallstones, heart disease, and cancer.
- If significant lipid lowering is not achieved within 3 months, drug should be discontinued.

colestipol hydrochloride
Colestid

INDICATIONS & DOSAGE
Primary hypercholesterolemia and xanthomas—
Adults: 15 to 30 g P.O. daily in 2 to 4 divided doses.

SIDE EFFECTS
GI: *constipation (common, may require decreasing the dosage),* fecal impaction, hemorrhoids, abdominal discomfort, flatulence, nausea, vomiting, steatorrhea.
Skin: rashes, irritation of skin, tongue, and perianal area.
Other: vitamin A, D, and K deficiency from decreased absorption; hyperchloremic acidosis with long-term use or very high dosage.

INTERACTIONS
Oral hypoglycemics: may antagonize response to colestipol. Monitor blood lipid level.

Italicized side effects are common or life-threatening.
*Liquid form contains alcohol.   **May contain tartrazine.

NURSING CONSIDERATIONS
• Administer all other medications at least 1 hour before or 4 to 6 hours after colestipol to avoid blocking their absorption.
• Monitor cardiotonic glycoside levels in patients receiving both medications concurrently. Should colestipol therapy be discontinued, cardiotonic glycoside toxicity may result unless dosage is adjusted.
• Watch for signs of vitamin A, D, and K deficiency.
• Lowering dosage or adding stool softener may relieve constipation.
• May cause decreased absorption of many drugs due to binding. Check drug interaction list of individual drugs.

dextrothyroxine sodium
Choloxin•**

INDICATIONS & DOSAGE
Hyperlipidemia in euthyroid patients, especially when cholesterol and triglyceride levels are elevated—
Adults: initial dose 1 to 2 mg daily, increased by 1 to 2 mg daily at monthly intervals to a total of 4 to 8 mg daily.
Children: initial dose 0.05 mg/kg daily, increased by 0.05 mg/kg daily at monthly intervals to a total of 4 mg daily.

SIDE EFFECTS
CV: palpitations, angina pectoris, arrhythmias, ischemic myocardial changes on EKG, myocardial infarction.
EENT: visual disturbances, ptosis.
GI: nausea, vomiting, diarrhea, constipation, decreased appetite.
Metabolic: *insomnia, weight loss, sweating,* flushing, hyperthermia, hair loss, menstrual irregularities.

INTERACTIONS
None significant.

NURSING CONSIDERATIONS
• Contraindicated in patients with hepatic or renal disease, or iodism. Patients with history of cardiac disease, including arrhythmias, hypertension, or angina pectoris, should receive very small doses.
• May increase need for insulin, diet therapy, or oral hypoglycemics in patients with diabetes.
• If the use of anticoagulants is being considered, discontinue drug 2 weeks before surgery to avoid possible potentiation of anticoagulant effect.
• Observe patient for signs of hyperthyroidism, such as nervousness, insomnia, weight loss. If these occur, dosage should be decreased or drug discontinued.

gemfibrozil
Lopid

INDICATIONS & DOSAGE
Treatment of type IV hyperlipidemia (hypertriglyceridemia) and severe hypercholesterolemia unresponsive to diet and other drugs—
Adults: 1,200 mg P.O. administered in two divided doses. Usual dosage range 900 to 1,500 mg daily.

SIDE EFFECTS
Blood: anemia, leukopenia.
CNS: blurred vision, headache, dizziness.
GI: *abdominal and epigastric pain, diarrhea, nausea,* vomiting, flatulence.
Hepatic: elevated enzymes.
Skin: rash, dermatitis, pruritus.
Other: painful extremities.

INTERACTIONS
None significant.

NURSING CONSIDERATIONS
• Contraindicated in hepatic or severe renal dysfunction, including primary biliary cirrhosis, and in preexisting gallbladder disease.

• CBC and liver function tests should be done periodically during the first 12 months of therapy.
• Gemfibrozil is very closely related to clofibrate both chemically and pharmacologically.
• Instruct patient to take drugs ½ hour before breakfast and dinner.
• Should not be used indiscriminately. May pose risk of gallstones, heart disease, and cancer.
• Patient should adhere strictly to prescribed diet, avoiding saturated fats, cholesterol, sugars.
• Because of possible dizziness and blurred vision, patient should avoid driving or operating machinery until CNS response to drug is determined.

niacin
Diacin**, Niac, Niacalex, Niacels, NICL, Nicobid, Nico-400, Nicolar**, NiCord XL, Nico-Span, Nicotinex, Ni-Span, Tega-Span

INDICATIONS & DOSAGE
Adjunctive treatment of hyperlipidemias, especially associated with hypercholesterolemia—
Adults: 1.5 to 3 g daily in 3 divided doses with or after meals, increased at intervals to 6 g daily.

SIDE EFFECTS
CV: *flushing* (which usually subsides in a few weeks).
GI: *nausea,* dyspepsia, vomiting, diarrhea, anorexia, flatulence, epigastric pain.
Hepatic: liver function test abnormalities.
Metabolic: *glucose intolerance resulting in hyperglycemia in previously well-controlled diabetics, hyperuricemia.*
Skin: *pruritus,* sensation of burning or stinging.

INTERACTIONS
None significant.

NURSING CONSIDERATIONS
• Use cautiously in patients with gout, diabetes, gallbladder or hepatic disease, peptic ulcer.
• Advise patient that pruritus and flushing noted in first few weeks of therapy usually lessen with continued use.
• Begin therapy with small doses; then increase gradually.
• Give with meals to minimize GI irritation. Cold water eases swallowing.
• Blood glucose and liver function tests should be performed routinely during early therapy.

probucol
Lorelco♦

INDICATIONS & DOSAGE
Primary hypercholesterolemia—
Adults: 2 tablets (500 mg total) P.O. b.i.d. with morning and evening meals. Not recommended in children.

SIDE EFFECTS
GI: *diarrhea, flatulence, abdominal pain, nausea, vomiting.*
Other: *hyperhidrosis,* fetid sweat, angioneurotic edema.

INTERACTIONS
None significant.

NURSING CONSIDERATIONS
• Drug's effect is enhanced when taken with food.
• Contraindicated in patients with arrhythmias. Drug should be stopped in any patient whose EKG shows prolonged Q-T interval.

sitosterols
Cytellin*

INDICATIONS & DOSAGE
Adjunctive therapy for hypercholesterolemia or hyperbetalipoproteinemia—
Adults: 15 ml (3 g) P.O. before meals

Italicized side effects are common or life-threatening.
*Liquid form contains alcohol.   **May contain tartrazine.

to a total of 45 ml (9 g) daily. May increase to 30 ml before large or high-fat meals; give fraction of usual dose before snacks.

SIDE EFFECTS
GI: anorexia; *diarrhea;* abdominal cramps; *bulky, light-colored stools;* nausea.

INTERACTIONS
None significant.

NURSING CONSIDERATIONS
• Serum cholesterol levels should be frequently monitored during first few months. If no decrease in cholesterol level occurs within 4 months, the doctor will discontinue the drug.
• Administer other medications 1 hour before or 4 hours after sitosterols.
• Give sitosterols immediately before meals or snacks.
• Mix with milk, tea, coffee, or fruit juice for palatability.
• Maximum therapeutic effect occurs during second and third months of therapy.
• Advise the patient to adhere to a low-cholesterol and low-fat diet throughout treatment.

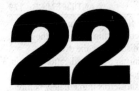

Nonnarcotic analgesics and antipyretics

Salicylates
aspirin
choline magnesium trisalicylate
choline salicylate
magnesium salicylate
salicylamide
salsalate
sodium salicylate
sodium thiosalicylate

Urinary tract analgesics
ethoxazene hydrochloride
phenazopyridine hydrochloride

Miscellaneous
acetaminophen
diflunisal
ethoheptazine citrate
methotrimeprazine
phenacetin
zomepirac sodium

MECHANISM OF ACTION
● Salicylates produce analgesia by an ill-defined effect on the hypothalamus (central action) and by blocking generation of pain impulses (peripheral action). The peripheral action may involve inhibition of prostaglandin synthesis.

Salicylates probably exert their anti-inflammatory effect by inhibiting prostaglandin synthesis; they may also inhibit the synthesis or action of other mediators of the inflammatory response.

They relieve fever by acting on the hypothalamic heat-regulating center to produce peripheral vasodilation. This increases peripheral blood supply and promotes sweating, which leads to loss of heat and cooling by evaporation.

Aspirin also appears to impede clotting by blocking prostaglandin synthetase action, which prevents formation of platelet-aggregating substance thromboxane A_2.
● The exact mechanism of action of the urinary tract analgesics is unknown.
● Among the miscellaneous drugs, acetaminophen and phenacetin produce analgesia by blocking generation of pain impulses. This action is probably due to inhibition of prostaglandin synthesis; it may also be due to inhibition of the synthesis or action of other substances that sensitize pain receptors to mechanical or chemical stimulation.

Both drugs relieve fever by central action in the hypothalamic heat-regulating center.

Ethoheptazine's mechanism of action is unknown.

Methotrimeprazine is thought to suppress sensory impulses by acting on sites in the thalamus, hypothalamus, and reticular activating and limbic systems.

Zomepirac's and diflunisal's mechanisms of action are unknown, but are probably related to inhibition of prostaglandin synthesis.

COMBINATION PRODUCTS
ANACIN: aspirin 400 mg and caffeine 32 mg.
A.P.C.: aspirin 227 mg, phenacetin 162 mg, and caffeine 32 mg.
A.S.A. COMPOUND: aspirin 227 mg, phenacetin 160 mg, and caffeine 32.5 mg.

Italicized side effects are common or life-threatening.
∗Liquid form contains alcohol.   ∗∗May contain tartrazine.

BUTAZOLIDIN ALKA: phenylbutazone 100 mg, dried aluminum hydroxide gel 100 mg, and magnesium trisilicate 150 mg.

DARVOCET-N 50: acetaminophen 325 mg and propoxyphene napsylate 50 mg.

DARVON COMPOUND-65: aspirin 227 mg, phenacetin 162 mg, caffeine 32.4 mg, and propoxyphene HCl 65 mg.

DOLENE AP-65: acetaminophen 650 mg and propoxyphene HCl 65 mg.

DOLENE COMPOUND-65: aspirin 227 mg, phenacetin 162 mg, propoxyphene HCl 65 mg, and caffeine 32.4 mg.

EQUAGESIC: aspirin 250 mg, ethoheptazine citrate 75 mg, and meprobamate 150 mg.

EXCEDRIN TABLETS: aspirin 250 mg, acetaminophen 250 mg, caffeine 65 mg.

FEMCAPS: acetaminophen 324 mg, caffeine 32 mg, ephedrine sulfate 8 mg, and atropine sulfate 0.0325 mg.

FIORINAL: butalbital 50 mg, aspirin 200 mg, phenacetin 130 mg, caffeine 40 mg.

GEMNISYN: aspirin 325 mg, acetaminophen 325 mg

SYNALGOS: promethazine HCl 6.25 mg, aspirin 194.4 mg, phenacetin 162 mg, caffeine 30 mg.

TALWIN COMPOUND CAPLETS: aspirin 325 mg and pentazocine (as HCl) 12.5 mg.

TRILISATE: choline salicylate 293 mg and magnesium salicylate 362 mg.

VANQUISH: aspirin 227 mg, acetaminophen 194 mg, caffeine 33 mg, aluminum hydroxide 25 mg, and magnesium hydroxide 50 mg.

ZACTIRIN: aspirin 325 mg and ethoheptazine citrate 75 mg.

acetaminophen
Acephen, Atasol♦♦, Campain♦♦, Datril, Dolanex, Liquiprin, Paralgin♦♦, Phendex, Robigesic♦♦, Rounox♦♦, Tapar*, Tempra♦*, Tylenol♦* **, Valadol*

INDICATIONS & DOSAGE
Mild pain or fever—
Adults and children over 10 years: 325 to 650 mg P.O. or rectally q 4 hours, p.r.n. Maximum 2.6 g daily.
Children under 1 year: 15 to 60 mg/dose.
Children 1 to 2 years: 60 mg/dose.
Children 2 to 3 years: 120 mg/dose.
Children 3 to 4 years: 180 mg/dose.
Children 4 to 5 years: 240 mg/dose.
Children 5 to 10 years: 325 mg/dose.
May give P.O. or rectally q 4 to 6 hours. Maximum 1.2 g daily.

SIDE EFFECTS
Hepatic: severe hepatotoxicity with large doses.
Skin: rash, urticaria.

INTERACTIONS
Diflunisal: increased acetaminophen blood levels. Don't use together.

NURSING CONSIDERATIONS
• Has no significant anti-inflammatory effect.
• Warn patient that high doses or unsupervised chronic use can cause hepatic damage. Excessive ingestion of alcoholic beverages may hasten hepatotoxicity.
• Has little or no effect on prothrombin time.

aspirin

Acetal♦♦, Acetyl-Sal♦♦, Ancasal♦♦, A.S.A., Aspergum, Aspirjen Jr., Aspirin♦♦, Bayer Timed-Release, Buffinol, Easprin, Ecotrin♦, Empirin, Entrophen♦♦, Measurin, Nova-Phase♦♦, Novasen♦♦, Rhonal♦♦, Sal-Adult♦♦, Sal-Infant♦♦, Supasa♦♦, Triaphen-10♦♦

INDICATIONS & DOSAGE

Adults:
Arthritis—2.6 to 5.2 g P.O. daily in divided doses.
Mild pain or fever—325 to 650 mg P.O. or rectally q 4 hours, p.r.n.
Thromboembolic disorders—325 to 650 mg P.O. daily or b.i.d.
Transient ischemic attacks— 650 mg P.O. b.i.d. or 325 mg q.i.d.

Children:
Arthritis—90 to 130 mg/kg P.O. daily divided q 4 to 6 hours.
Fever—40 to 80 mg/kg P.O. or rectally daily divided q 6 hours, p.r.n.
Mild pain—65 to 100 mg/kg P.O. or rectally daily divided q 4 to 6 hours, p.r.n.

SIDE EFFECTS

Blood: *prolonged bleeding time.*
EENT: *tinnitus and hearing loss (first signs of toxicity).*
GI: *nausea, vomiting, GI distress, occult bleeding.*
Hepatic: abnormal liver function studies, hepatitis.
Skin: *rash,* bruising.
Other: *hypersensitivity manifested by anaphylaxis and/or asthma.*

INTERACTIONS

Ammonium chloride (and other urine acidifiers): increases blood levels of aspirin products. Monitor for aspirin toxicity.
Antacids in high doses (and other urine alkalinizers): decrease levels of aspirin products. Monitor for decreased aspirin effect.

Carbonic anhydrase inhibitors, cimetidine: may elevate salicylate levels. Monitor for toxicity.
Corticosteroids: enhance salicylate elimination. Monitor for decreased salicylate effect.
Oral anticoagulants and heparin: increase risk of bleeding. Avoid using together if possible.

NURSING CONSIDERATIONS

• Contraindicated in GI ulcer, GI bleeding, aspirin hypersensitivity. Use cautiously in patients with hypoprothrombinemia, vitamin K deficiency, bleeding disorders, Hodgkin's disease (may cause profound hypothermia); and in asthmatics with nasal polyps (may cause severe bronchospasm).
• Because of epidemiologic association with Reye's syndrome, the Centers for Disease Control recommend that children with chicken pox or influenza-like illness should not be given salicylates.
• Febrile, dehydrated children can develop toxicity rapidly.
• Give with food, milk, antacid, or large glass of water to reduce GI side effects.
• Warn patients to check with doctor or pharmacist before taking over-the-counter combinations containing aspirin.
• Therapeutic blood salicylate level in arthritis is 20 to 30 mg/100 ml.
• Alcohol may increase gastrointestinal blood loss.
• May cause increase in serum levels of SGOT, SGPT, alkaline phosphatase, and bilirubin. May produce false-negative test results for urine glucose by glucose oxidase methods (Clinistix, Tes-Tape) and false-positive results using Clinitest.
• Keep out of reach of children— aspirin is one of the leading causes of poisoning in children.
• Advise patients receiving large doses of aspirin for an extended period of time to watch for petechiae, bleeding gums, signs of GI bleeding, and to

---

Italicized side effects are common or life-threatening.
∗Liquid form contains alcohol.   ∗∗May contain tartrazine.

maintain adequate fluid intake. Obtain hemoglobin and prothrombin tests periodically.
• Enteric-coated products are slowly absorbed, and are not suitable for acute effects. They do cause less GI bleeding, and may be more suited for long-term therapy.

choline magnesium trisalicylate
Trilisate

INDICATIONS & DOSAGE
Arthritis, mild—
Adults: 1 to 2 teaspoonfuls or tablets, each tablet or teaspoon equal to 500 mg salicylate, b.i.d. Total daily dose can also be given at one time.
Rheumatoid arthritis and osteoarthritis—
Adults: 2 to 3 teaspoonfuls or tablets b.i.d. Each tablet or teaspoonful equal in salicylate content to 650 mg aspirin. Total daily dose can also be given at one time.

SIDE EFFECTS
Blood: *prolonged bleeding time.*
EENT: *tinnitus and hearing loss (first signs of toxicity).*
GI: *nausea, vomiting, GI distress, occult bleeding.*
Hepatic: abnormal liver function studies, hepatitis.
Skin: *rash,* bruising.
Other: *hypersensitivity manifested by anaphylaxis, and/or asthma.*

INTERACTIONS
Ammonium chloride (and other urine acidifiers): increases blood levels of salicylates. Monitor for salicylate toxicity.
Antacids in high doses (and other urine alkalinizers): decrease levels of salicylates. Monitor for decreased salicylate effect.
Carbonic anhydrase inhibitors, cimeti-

dine: may elevate salicylate levels. Monitor for toxicity.
Corticosteroids: enhance salicylate elimination. Monitor for decreased salicylate effect.
Oral anticoagulants and heparin: increase risk of bleeding. Avoid using together if possible.

NURSING CONSIDERATIONS
• Contraindicated in GI ulcer, GI bleeding, aspirin hypersensitivity. Use cautiously in patients with hypoprothrombinemia, vitamin K deficiency, bleeding disorders, Hodgkin's disease (may cause profound hypothermia); and in asthmatics with nasal polyps (may cause severe bronchospasm).
• Because of epidemiologic association with Reye's syndrome, the Centers for Disease Control recommend that children with chicken pox or influenza-like illness should not be given salicylates.
• May cause less GI distress than aspirin. If antacid is needed, give it 2 hours after meals and give choline magnesium trisalicylate before meals.
• May mix drug with water, fruit juice, or carbonated drinks.
• Febrile, dehydrated children can develop toxicity rapidly.
• Warn patient to check with doctor before taking over-the-counter combinations containing aspirin.
• Therapeutic blood salicylate level in arthritis is 20 to 30 mg/100 ml.
• Alcohol may increase gastrointestinal blood loss.
• May cause an increase in serum levels of SGOT, SGPT, alkaline phosphatase, and bilirubin. May produce false-negative test results for urine glucose by glucose oxidase methods (Clinistix, Tes-Tape) and false-positive results using Clinitest.
• Obtain hemoglobin and prothrombin tests periodically in patients receiving large doses over an extended period of time.

choline salicylate
Arthropan♦

INDICATIONS & DOSAGE
Arthritis—
Adults: 5 to 10 ml P.O. q.i.d.
Minor pain or fever—
Adults: 870 mg (5 ml) P.O. q 3 to
4 hours, p.r.n.
Children 3 to 6 years: 105 to 210 mg
P.O. q 4 hours, p.r.n. Each 870 mg
(5 ml) equals 650 mg aspirin.

SIDE EFFECTS
Blood: *prolonged bleeding time.*
EENT: *tinnitus and hearing loss (first signs of toxicity).*
GI: *nausea, vomiting, GI distress, occult bleeding.*
Hepatic: abnormal liver function studies, hepatitis.
Skin: *rash,* bruising.
Other: *hypersensitivity manifested by anaphylaxis and/or asthma.*

INTERACTIONS
Ammonium chloride (and other urine acidifiers): increases blood levels of salicylates. Monitor for salicylate toxicity.
Antacids in high doses (and other urine alkalinizers): decrease levels of salicylates. Monitor for decreased salicylate effect.
Carbonic anhydrase inhibitors, cimetidine: may elevate salicylate levels. Monitor for toxicity.
Corticosteroids: enhance salicylate elimination. Monitor for decreased salicylate effect.
Oral anticoagulants: increase risk of bleeding. Avoid using together if possible.

NURSING CONSIDERATIONS
• Contraindicated in GI ulcer, GI bleeding, aspirin hypersensitivity. Use cautiously in patients with hypoprothrombinemia, vitamin K deficiency, bleeding disorders, Hodgkin's disease

(may cause profound hypothermia); and in asthmatics with nasal polyps (may cause severe bronchospasm).
• Because of epidemiologic association with Reye's syndrome, the Centers for Disease Control recommend that children with chicken pox or influenza-like illness should not be given salicylates.
• May cause less GI distress than aspirin. If antacid is needed, give it 2 hours after meals and give choline salicylate before meals.
• May mix drug with water, fruit juice, or carbonated drinks.
• Febrile, dehydrated children can develop toxicity rapidly.
• Warn patient to check with doctor before taking over-the-counter combinations containing aspirin.
• Therapeutic blood salicylate level in arthritis is 20 to 30 mg/100 ml.
• Alcohol may increase gastrointestinal blood loss.
• May cause an increase in serum levels of SGOT, SGPT, alkaline phosphatase, and bilirubin. May produce false-negative test results for urine glucose by glucose oxidase methods (Clinistix, Tes-Tape) and false-positive results using Clinitest.
• Obtain hemoglobin and prothrombin tests periodically in patients receiving large doses over an extended period of time.

diflunisal
Dolobid

INDICATIONS & DOSAGE
Mild to moderate pain and osteoarthritis—
Adults: 500 to 1000 mg daily in two divided doses, usually q 12 hours. Maximum dosage 1500 mg daily.

SIDE EFFECTS
Blood: prolonged bleeding time.
CNS: *dizziness, somnolence, insomnia, headache.*
EENT: *tinnitus.*

Italicized side effects are common or life-threatening.
∗Liquid form contains alcohol.   ∗∗May contain tartrazine.

GI: *nausea, dyspepsia, gastrointestinal pain, diarrhea,* vomiting, constipation, flatulence.
Skin: *rash,* pruritus, sweating, dry mucous membranes, stomatitis.

INTERACTIONS
Aspirin, antacids: decreased diflunisal blood levels. Monitor for possible decreased therapeutic effect.

NURSING CONSIDERATIONS
• Contraindicated for patients in whom acute asthmatic attacks, urticaria, or rhinitis are precipitated by aspirin or other nonsteroidal anti-inflammatory drugs.
• Use cautiously in patients with active gastrointestinal bleeding or history of peptic ulcer disease; renal impairment; compromised cardiac function; or those taking anticoagulants.
• Similar to aspirin, diflunisal is a salicylic acid derivative but is metabolized differently.
• May be administered with water, milk, or meals.

ethoheptazine citrate
Zactane

INDICATIONS & DOSAGE
Mild pain—
Adults: 75 to 150 mg P.O. t.i.d. or q.i.d.

SIDE EFFECTS
CNS: dizziness, headache, syncope, nervousness.
EENT: visual disturbances.
GI: nausea, vomiting.
Skin: pruritus.

INTERACTIONS
None significant.

NURSING CONSIDERATIONS
• May use with aspirin for arthritic pain.

• Doesn't lower fever; may use alone when fever is valuable for diagnosis.
• Side effects other than GI distress and pruritus usually occur only when recommended is dosage exceeded.

ethoxazene hydrochloride
Serenium

INDICATIONS & DOSAGE
Pain with urinary tract irritation or infection—
Adults: 100 mg a.c. P.O. t.i.d.

SIDE EFFECTS
GI: nausea, vomiting.

INTERACTIONS
None significant.

NURSING CONSIDERATIONS
• Contraindicated in hepatic and renal disease. Use cautiously in GI disorders.
• Colors urine reddish-orange. May stain fabrics.
• Use only as analgesic. Use with antibiotic to treat urinary tract infection.

magnesium salicylate
Analate, Arthrin, Magan, Mobidin, MSG-600

INDICATIONS & DOSAGE
Adults:
*Arthritis—*up to 9.6 g daily in divided doses.
*Mild pain or fever—*600 mg P.O. t.i.d. or q.i.d.

SIDE EFFECTS
Blood: *prolonged bleeding time.*
EENT: *tinnitus and hearing loss (first signs of toxicity).*
GI: *nausea, vomiting, GI distress, occult bleeding.*
Hepatic: abnormal liver function studies, hepatitis.
Skin: *rash,* bruising.

Other: *hypersensitivity manifested by anaphylaxis and/or asthma.*

INTERACTIONS

Ammonium chloride (and other urine acidifiers): increases blood levels of aspirin products. Monitor for aspirin toxicity.

Antacids in high doses (and other urine alkalinizers): decrease levels of aspirin products. Monitor for decreased aspirin effect.

Carbonic anhydrase inhibitors, cimetidine: may elevate salicylate levels. Monitor for toxicity.

Corticosteroids: enhance salicylate elimination. Monitor for decreased salicylate effect.

Oral anticoagulants and heparin: increase risk of bleeding. Avoid using together if possible.

NURSING CONSIDERATIONS

• Contraindicated in severe chronic renal insufficiency because of risk of magnesium toxicity; GI ulcer; GI bleeding; aspirin hypersensitivity. Use cautiously in hypoprothrombinemia, vitamin K deficiency, bleeding disorders, and Hodgkin's disease (may cause profound hypothermia).

• Because of epidemiologic association with Reye's syndrome, the Centers for Disease Control recommend that children with chicken pox or influenza-like illness should not be given salicylates.

• Febrile, dehydrated children can develop toxicity rapidly.

• Give with food, milk, antacid, or large glass of water to reduce GI side effects.

• Warn patient to check with doctor before taking over-the-counter combinations containing aspirin.

• Therapeutic blood salicylate level in arthritis is 20 to 30 mg/100 ml.

• Alcohol may increase gastrointestinal blood loss.

• May cause an increase in serum levels of SGOT, SGPT, alkaline phosphatase, and bilirubin. May produce false-negative test results for urine glucose by glucose oxidase methods (Clinistix, Tes-Tape) and false-positive results using Clinitest.

• Obtain hemoglobin and prothrombin tests periodically in patients receiving large doses over an extended period of time.

---

methotrimeprazine
Levoprome, Nozinan♦♦

INDICATIONS & DOSAGE

Moderate to severe pain in nonambulatory patients—
Adults: 10 to 20 mg deep I.M. into large muscle mass, q 4 to 6 hours, p.r.n. Maximum dose 40 mg.

SIDE EFFECTS

Blood: *agranulocytosis.*
CNS: confusion, dizziness, *sedation,* weakness, amnesia, slurred speech.
CV: *orthostatic hypotension.*
EENT: nasal congestion.
GI: dry mouth, nausea, vomiting.
GU: difficulties in urination.
Local: pain, inflammation at injection site.
Other: chills.

INTERACTIONS

All antihypertensive agents and MAO inhibitors: increased orthostatic hypotension. Select other analgesic.

NURSING CONSIDERATIONS

• Contraindicated in phenothiazine hypersensitivity; cardiac, renal or hepatic disease; hypotension; coma; convulsive disorders. Use with extreme caution in elderly or debilitated patients with cardiac disease or any patients who may suffer severe consequences from a sudden drop in blood pressure.

• Used mainly in nonambulatory patients because of hypotension. Keep patient in bed or assist when out of bed for at least 6 hours after initial dose. Tolerance to this effect usually devel-

---

Italicized side effects are common or life-threatening.
*Liquid form contains alcohol.   **May contain tartrazine.

ops, but watch patient closely after each dose.
• May mix with atropine or scopolamine. Do not mix with other drugs.

phenacetin

INDICATIONS & DOSAGE
Mild pain or fever—
Adults: 300 mg P.O. q 3 to 4 hours, p.r.n. Maximum 2.4 g daily.

SIDE EFFECTS
Blood: methemoglobinemia in toxic doses, hemolytic anemia in G-6-PD deficiency.
GI: nausea, vomiting.
GU: *papillary necrosis and chronic interstitial nephritis with long-term high doses.*
Skin: rash.

INTERACTIONS
None significant.

NURSING CONSIDERATIONS
• Repeated use is contraindicated in anemia; cardiac, pulmonary, hepatic, or renal disease.
• Contained in many analgesic combinations. Warn patient to check ingredients of combination over-the-counter products.

phenazopyridine hydrochloride
Azodine, Azogesic, Azo-Pyridon, Azo-Standard, Azo-Sulfizin, Baridium, Di-Azo, Diridone, Phenazo♦♦, Phen-Azo, Phenazodine, Pyridiate, Pyridium♦, Urodine

INDICATIONS & DOSAGE
Pain with urinary tract irritation or infection—
Adults: 100 to 200 mg P.O. t.i.d.
Children: 100 mg P.O. t.i.d.

SIDE EFFECTS
CNS: headache.
GI: nausea.

INTERACTIONS
None significant.

NURSING CONSIDERATIONS
• Contraindicated in renal and hepatic insufficiency.
• Colors urine red or orange. May stain fabrics.
• Use only as analgesic. Use with antibiotic to treat urinary tract infection.
• Drug may be stopped in 3 days if pain is relieved.
• May alter Clinistix or Tes-Tape results. Use Clinitest for accurate urine glucose test results.
• Stop drug if skin or sclera becomes yellow-tinged. May indicate accumulation due to impaired renal excretion.

salicylamide
Amid-Sal, Doldram, Salamide

INDICATIONS & DOSAGE
Mild pain or fever—
Adults: 650 mg P.O. q.i.d., p.r.n.
Children: 65 mg/kg daily divided into 6 doses.

SIDE EFFECTS
Blood: *prolonged bleeding time.*
EENT: *tinnitus and hearing loss (first signs of toxicity).*
GI: *nausea, vomiting, GI distress, occult bleeding.*
Hepatic: abnormal liver function studies, hepatitis.
Skin: *rash,* bruising.
Other: *hypersensitivity manifested by anaphylaxis and/or asthma.*

INTERACTIONS
Ammonium chloride (and other urine acidifiers): increases blood levels of aspirin products. Monitor for aspirin toxicity.
Antacids in high doses (and other urine

---

alkalinizers): decrease levels of aspirin products. Monitor for decreased aspirin effect.

Carbonic anhydrase inhibitors, cimetidine: may elevate salicylate levels. Monitor for toxicity.

Corticosteroids: enhance salicylate elimination. Monitor for decreased salicylate effect.

Oral anticoagulants and heparin: increase risk of bleeding. Avoid using together if possible.

NURSING CONSIDERATIONS

• Contraindicated in GI ulcer, GI bleeding, aspirin hypersensitivity. Use cautiously in hypoprothrombinemia, vitamin K deficiency, bleeding disorders, and Hodgkin's disease (may cause profound hypothermia).

• Because of epidemiologic association with Reye's syndrome, the Centers for Disease Control recommend that children with chicken pox or influenza-like illness should not be given salicylates.

• Give with food, milk, antacid, or large glass of water to reduce GI side effects.

• Warn patient to check with doctor before taking over-the-counter combinations containing aspirin.

• Alcohol may increase gastrointestinal blood loss.

• May increase serum alkaline phosphatase, bilirubin, SGOT, and SGPT levels. May produce false-negative results for urine glucose using glucose oxidase methods (Clinistix and Tes-Tape) and false-positive results using Clinitest.

• Advise patients receiving large doses for an extended period of time to watch for petechiae, bleeding gums, and signs of GI bleeding, and to maintain adequate fluid intake. Obtain hemoglobin and prothrombin tests periodically.

salsalate
Disalcid

INDICATIONS & DOSAGE
Minor pain or fever, arthritis—
Adults: 1 g P.O. b.i.d., t.i.d., or q.i.d., p.r.n.

SIDE EFFECTS
Blood: *prolonged bleeding time.*
EENT: *tinnitus and hearing loss (first signs of toxicity).*
GI: *nausea, vomiting, GI distress, occult bleeding.*
Hepatic: abnormal liver function studies, hepatitis.
Skin: *rash,* bruising.
Other: *hypersensitivity manifested by anaphylaxis and/or asthma.*

INTERACTIONS
Ammonium chloride (and other urine acidifiers): increases blood levels of aspirin products. Monitor for aspirin toxicity.

Antacids in high doses (and other urine alkalinizers): decrease levels of aspirin products. Monitor for decreased aspirin effect.

Carbonic anhydrase inhibitors, cimetidine: may elevate salicylate levels. Monitor for toxicity.

Corticosteroids: enhance salicylate elimination. Monitor for decreased salicylate effect.

Oral anticoagulants and heparin: increase risk of bleeding. Avoid using together if possible.

NURSING CONSIDERATIONS
• Contraindicated in GI ulcer, GI bleeding, aspirin hypersensitivity. Use cautiously in hypoprothrombinemia, vitamin K deficiency, bleeding disorders, and Hodgkin's disease (may cause profound hypothermia).

• Because of epidemiologic association with Reye's syndrome, the Centers for Disease Control recommend that chil-

---

Italicized side effects are common or life-threatening.
*Liquid form contains alcohol.   **May contain tartrazine.

dren with chicken pox or influenza-like illness should not be given salicylates.
• Give with food, milk, antacid, or large glass of water to reduce GI side effects.
• Warn patient to check with doctor before taking over-the-counter combinations containing aspirin.
• Therapeutic blood salicylate level in arthritis is 20 to 30 mg/100 ml.
• Alcohol may increase gastrointestinal blood loss.
• May increase serum alkaline phosphatase, bilirubin, SGOT, and SGPT levels. May produce false-negative results for urine glucose using glucose oxidase methods (Clinistix and Tes-Tape) and false-positive results using Clinitest.
• Advise patients receiving large doses for extended period of time to watch for petechiae, bleeding gums, and signs of GI bleeding, and to maintain adequate fluid intake. Obtain hemoglobin and prothrombin tests periodically.

sodium salicylate
Uracel

INDICATIONS & DOSAGE
Minor pain or fever—
Adults: 325 to 650 mg P.O. q 4 to 6 hours, p.r.n., or 500 mg slow I.V. infusion over 4 to 8 hours. Maximum dose 1 g daily.
Children: 40 to 100 mg/kg P.O. q 4 to 6 hours, p.r.n.

SIDE EFFECTS
Blood: *prolonged bleeding time.*
EENT: *tinnitus and hearing loss (first signs of toxicity).*
GI: *nausea, vomiting, GI distress, occult bleeding.*
Hepatic: abnormal liver function studies, hepatitis.
Skin: *rash,* bruising.
Other: *hypersensitivity manifested by anaphylaxis and/or asthma.*

INTERACTIONS
Ammonium chloride (and other urine acidifiers): increases blood levels of aspirin products. Monitor for aspirin toxicity.
Antacids in large doses (and other urine alkalinizers): decrease levels of aspirin products. Monitor for decreased aspirin effect.
Carbonic anhydrase inhibitors, cimetidine: may elevate salicylate levels. monitor for toxicity.
Corticosteroids: enhance salicylate elimination. Monitor for decreased salicylate effect.
Oral anticoagulants and heparin: increase risk of bleeding. Avoid using together if possible.

NURSING CONSIDERATIONS
• Contraindicated in GI ulcer, GI bleeding, aspirin hypersensitivity. Use cautiously in hypoprothrombinemia, vitamin K deficiency, bleeding disorders, asthma with nasal polyps (may cause severe bronchospasm), and Hodgkin's disease (may cause profound hypothermia).
• Use cautiously in congestive heart failure and hypertension, because of increased sodium load.
• Because of epidemiologic association with Reye's syndrome, the Centers for Disease Control recommend that children with chicken pox or influenza-like illness should not be given salicylates.
• Febrile, dehydrated children can develop toxicity rapidly.
• Give with food, milk, antacid, or large glass of water to reduce GI side effects.
• Warn patient to check with doctor before taking over-the-counter combinations containing aspirin.
• Therapeutic salicylate level in arthritis is 20 to 30 mg/100 ml.
• Tinnitus, headache, dizziness, confusion, fever, sweating, thirst, drowsiness, dim vision, hyperventilation, and tachycardia are signs of mild toxicity.

Unmarked trade names available in the United States only.
♦ Also available in Canada.　　♦♦ Available in Canada only.

• Alcohol may increase gastrointestinal blood loss.
• May increase serum alkaline phosphatase, bilirubin, SGOT, and SGPT levels. May produce false-negative results for urine glucose using glucose oxidase methods (Clinistix and Tes-Tape) and false-positive results using Clinitest.
• Advise patients receiving large doses for extended period of time to watch for petechiae, bleeding gums, and signs of GI bleeding, and to maintain adequate fluid intake. Obtain hemoglobin and prothrombin tests periodically.

sodium thiosalicylate
Arthrolate, Nalate, Osteolate, Thiodyne, Thiolate, Thiosal, TH Sal

INDICATIONS & DOSAGE
Mild pain—
Adults: 50 to 100 mg I.M. daily or every other day.
Arthritis—
Adults: 100 mg I.M. daily.
Rheumatic fever—
Adults: 100 to 150 mg I.M. b.i.d. until asymptomatic.

SIDE EFFECTS
Blood: *prolonged bleeding time.*
EENT: *tinnitus and hearing loss (first signs of toxicity).*
GI: *nausea, vomiting, GI distress, occult bleeding.*
Hepatic: abnormal liver function studies, hepatitis.
Skin: *rash,* bruising.
Other: *hypersensitivity manifested by anaphylaxis.*

INTERACTIONS
Ammonium chloride (and other urine acidifiers): increases blood levels of aspirin products. Monitor for aspirin toxicity.
Antacids in large doses (and other urine alkalinizers): decrease levels of aspirin

products. Monitor for decreased aspirin effect.
Carbonic anhydrase inhibitors, cimetidine: may elevate salicylate levels. Monitor for toxicity.
Corticosteriods: enhance salicylate elimination. Monitor for decreased salicylate effects.
Oral anticoagulants and heparin: increase risk of bleeding. Avoid using together if possible.

NURSING CONSIDERATIONS
• Contraindicated in GI ulcer, GI bleeding, aspirin hypersensitivity. Use cautiously in hypoprothrombinemia, vitamin K deficiency, bleeding disorders, asthma with nasal polyps (may cause severe bronchospasm), and Hodgkin's disease (may cause profound hypothermia).
• Because of epidemiologic association with Reye's syndrome, the Centers for Disease Control recommend that children with chicken pox or influenza-like illness should not be given salicylates.
• Tinnitus, headache, dizziness, confusion, fever, sweating, thirst, drowsiness, dim vision, hyperventilation, and tachycardia are signs of mild toxicity.
• Alcohol may increase blood loss.
• May increase serum alkaline phosphatase, bilirubin, SGOT, and SGPT levels. May produce false-negative results for urine glucose using glucose oxidase method (Clinistix and Tes-Tape) and false-positive results using Clinitest.
• Advise patients receiving large doses for extended period of time to watch for petechiae, bleeding gums, and signs of GI bleeding, and to maintain adequate fluid intake. Obtain hemoglobin and prothrombin tests periodically.

zomepirac sodium
Zomax

INDICATIONS & DOSAGE
Mild to moderately severe pain—

Adults: 100 mg P.O. q 4 to 6 hours as required p.r.n. In mild pain, 50 mg q 4 to 6 hours may be adequate. Don't exceed 600 mg per day. Not recommended for children.

SIDE EFFECTS
EENT: tinnitus, stomatitis.
CNS: *drowsiness, dizziness, insomnia,* paresthesia, nervousness.
CV: *edema, hypertension,* cardiac irregularity, palpitations.
GI: *nausea, vomiting, diarrhea, dyspepsia,* constipation, flatulence, anorexia, GI bleeding.
GU: urinary frequency, urinary tract infection, elevated BUN and creatinine, reversible renal failure, vaginitis.
Skin: rash, pruritus, urticaria.
Other: chills, alterations in sense of taste, bronchospasm.

INTERACTIONS
None significant.

NURSING CONSIDERATIONS
• Contraindicated in patients in whom aspirin and nonsteroidal anti-inflammatory drugs induce bronchospasm, rhinitis, urticaria, or other hypersensitivity reactions. Give cautiously to patients with a history of gastrointestinal bleeding, fluid retention, hypertension, and heart failure.
• A nonnarcotic analgesic with narcotic potency. In some studies has been shown to be as effective as morphine.
• No evidence of addiction with zomepirac.
• Give with food or antacids if gastrointestinal symptoms occur.
• Also prescribed as a nonsteroid anti-inflammatory agent.

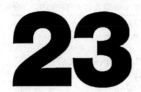

Nonsteroidal anti-inflammatory agents

fenoprofen calcium
ibuprofen
indomethacin
meclofenamate
mefenamic acid
naproxen
naproxen sodium
oxyphenbutazone
phenylbutazone
piroxicam
sulindac
tolmetin sodium

MECHANISM OF ACTION
Although their exact mechanism of action is unknown, these drugs probably inhibit prostaglandin synthesis.

COMBINATION PRODUCTS
None.

---

fenoprofen calcium
Nalfon♦

INDICATIONS & DOSAGE
Rheumatoid arthritis and osteoarthritis—
Adults: 300 to 600 mg P.O. q.i.d. Maximum 3.2 g daily.

SIDE EFFECTS
Blood: prolonged bleeding time, anemia.
CNS: headache, drowsiness, dizziness.
CV: peripheral edema.
GI: *epigastric distress, nausea, occult blood loss.*
GU: reversible renal failure.
Hepatic: elevated enzymes.
Skin: pruritus, rash, urticaria.

INTERACTIONS
None significant.

NURSING CONSIDERATIONS
• Contraindicated in asthmatics with nasal polyps. Use cautiously in patients with GI disorders, angioedema, cardiac disease, or allergy to other noncorticosteroid anti-inflammatory drugs.
• Use cautiously in patients with history of peptic ulcer disease.
• Tell patient that full therapeutic effect may be delayed for 2 to 4 weeks.
• Check renal, hepatic, and auditory function periodically in long-term therapy. Stop drug if abnormalities occur.
• Give dose 30 minutes before or 2 hours after meals. If GI side effects occur, give with milk or meals.
• Prothrombin time may be prolonged in patients receiving coumarin-type anticoagulants. Fenoprofen decreases platelet aggregation and may prolong bleeding time.

---

ibuprofen
Motrin♦ Rufen

INDICATIONS & DOSAGE
Arthritis, primary dysmenorrhea, gout, postextraction dental pain—
Adults: 300 to 600 mg P.O. q.i.d.

SIDE EFFECTS
Blood: prolonged bleeding time.
CNS: headache, drowsiness, dizziness.
CV: peripheral edema.
EENT: visual disturbances, tinnitus.

Italicized side effects are common or life-threatening.
∗Liquid form contains alcohol.   ∗∗May contain tartrazine.

GI: *epigastric distress, nausea, occult blood loss.*
GU: reversible renal failure.
Hepatic: elevated enzymes.
Skin: pruritus, rash, urticaria.
Other: aseptic meningitis, bronchospasm, edema.

INTERACTIONS
None significant.

NURSING CONSIDERATIONS
• Contraindicated in asthmatics with nasal polyps. Use cautiously in GI disorders, angioedema, allergy to other noncorticosteroid anti-inflammatory drugs, hepatic or renal disease, cardiac decompensation, or known intrinsic coagulation defects.
• Use cautiously in patients with history of peptic ulcer disease.
• Tell patient that full therapeutic effect may be delayed for 2 to 4 weeks.
• Check renal and hepatic function periodically in long-term therapy. Stop drug if abnormalities occur.
• Tell patient to report to doctor immediately any GI symptoms or signs of bleeding, visual disturbances, skin rashes, weight gain, or edema.
• Give with meals or milk to reduce GI side effects.

---

indomethacin
Indocid♦♦, Indocin, Indocin SR

INDICATIONS & DOSAGE
Moderate to severe arthritis, ankylosing spondylitis—
Adults: 25 mg P.O. b.i.d. or t.i.d. with food or antacids; may increase dose by 25 mg daily q 7 days up to 200 mg daily. Alternatively, sustained-release capsules (75 mg) may be given: 75 mg to start, in the morning or at bedtime, followed, if necessary, by 75 mg b.i.d.
*Acute gouty arthritis—*50 mg t.i.d. Reduce dose as soon as possible, then stop. Sustained-release capsules shouldn't be used for this condition

SIDE EFFECTS
Blood: *hemolytic anemia, aplastic anemia, agranulocytosis,* leukopenia, *thrombocytopenic purpura,* iron deficiency anemia.
CNS: *headache, dizziness,* depression, drowsiness, confusion, peripheral neuropathy, convulsions, psychic disturbances, syncope, *vertigo.*
CV: hypertension, edema.
EENT: *blurred vision, corneal and retinal damage,* hearing loss, tinnitus.
GI: *nausea, vomiting,* anorexia, *diarrhea, severe GI bleeding.*
GU: hematuria, hyperkalemia, acute renal failure.
Skin: pruritus, urticaria, *Stevens-Johnson syndrome.*
Other: hypersensitivity (shock-like symptoms, rash, respiratory distress, angioedema).

INTERACTIONS
Diflunisal, Probenecid: decreases indomethacin excretion; watch for increased incidence of indomethacin side effects.
Furosemide: impaired response to both drugs. Avoid if possible.
Triamterene: possible nephrotoxicity. Don't use together.

NURSING CONSIDERATIONS
• Contraindicated in aspirin allergy, GI disorders. Use cautiously in patients with epilepsy, parkinsonism, hepatic or renal disease, infection, history of mental illness, and in elderly patients.
• Severe headache may occur within 1 hour. Decrease dose if headache persists.
• Has an antipyretic effect.
• Tell patient to notify doctor immediately if any visual or hearing changes occur. Patients taking drug long-term should have regular eye examinations and hearing tests.
• Very irritating to GI tract. Give with meals. Advise patient to notify doctor of any GI side effects.

- CNS side effects are more common and serious in elderly patients.
- Monitor for bleeding in patients receiving anticoagulants.
- Causes sodium retention; monitor for increased blood pressure in patients with hypertension.
- Used investigationally as prophylaxis for gout when colchicine is not well tolerated. Also used investigationally to close patent ductus arteriosus in premature infants. The I.V. form used for this is available from the manufacturer.
- Patients taking drug long-term should receive periodic testing of CBC, renal function, and eye examinations.

meclofenamate
Meclomen

INDICATIONS & DOSAGE
Rheumatoid arthritis and osteoarthritis—
Adults: 200 to 400 mg/day P.O. in 3 or 4 equally divided doses.

SIDE EFFECTS
Blood: leukopenia, thrombocytopenia, *agranulocytosis, aplastic anemia.*
CNS: drowsiness, dizziness, nervousness, headache.
EENT: blurred vision, eye irritation.
GI: nausea, vomiting, *diarrhea,* hemorrhage.
GU: dysuria, hematuria, nephrotoxicity.
Hepatic: hepatotoxicity.
Skin: rash, urticaria.

INTERACTIONS
None significant.

NURSING CONSIDERATIONS
- Contraindicated in GI ulceration or inflammation. Use cautiously in patients with hepatic or renal disease, blood dyscrasias, diabetes mellitus, and in asthmatics with nasal polyps.
- Use cautiously in patients with history of peptic ulcer disease.

- Warn patient against activities that require alertness until CNS response to drug is determined.
- Stop drug if rash or diarrhea develops.
- Should not be administered for more than 1 week at a time, because incidence of toxicity increases.
- Administer with food to minimize GI side effects.
- Almost identical in chemical structure to mefenamic acid.
- Available as 50- and 100-mg capsules.
- False-positive reactions for urine bilirubin using the diazo tablet test have been reported.
- Patients taking drug long-term should receive periodic testing of CBC, renal and hepatic function.

mefenamic acid
Ponstan♦♦, Ponstel

INDICATIONS & DOSAGE
Mild to moderate pain, dysmenorrhea—
Adults and children over 14 years: 500 mg P.O. initially, then 250 mg q 4 hours, p.r.n.
Maximum therapy 1 week.

SIDE EFFECTS
Blood: leukopenia, thrombocytopenia, *agranulocytosis, aplastic anemia.*
CNS: drowsiness, dizziness, nervousness, headache.
EENT: blurred vision, eye irritation.
GI: nausea, vomiting, *diarrhea,* hemorrhage.
GU: dysuria, hematuria, nephrotoxicity.
Hepatic: hepatotoxicity.
Skin: rash, urticaria.

INTERACTIONS
None significant.

NURSING CONSIDERATIONS
- Contraindicated in GI ulceration or inflammation. Use cautiously in pa-

---

Italicized side effects are common or life-threatening.
*Liquid form contains alcohol.   **May contain tartrazine.

tients with hepatic or renal disease, blood dyscrasias, diabetes mellitus, and in asthmatics with nasal polyps.
• Use cautiously in patients with history of peptic ulcer disease.
• Warn patient against activities that require alertness until CNS response to drug is determined.
• Severe hemolytic anemia may occur with prolonged use.
• Stop drug if rash or diarrhea develops.
• Should not be administered for more than 1 week at a time, because incidence of toxicity increases.
• Administer with food to minimize GI side effects.
• False-positive reactions for urine bilirubin using the diazo tablet test have been reported.

naproxen
Naprosyn♦

naproxen sodium
Anaprox

INDICATIONS & DOSAGE
Arthritis, primary dysmenorrhea (free base)
Adults: 250 to 500 mg P.O. b.i.d. Maximum 1,000 mg daily.
Mild to moderate pain and for treatment of primary dysmenorrhea (naproxen sodium)—
Adults: 2 tablets (275 mg each tablet) to start, followed by 275 mg q 6 to 8 hours as needed. Maximum daily dose should not exceed 1,375 mg.

SIDE EFFECTS
Blood: prolonged bleeding time.
CNS: headache, drowsiness, dizziness.
CV: peripheral edema.
GI: *epigastric distress, occult blood loss, nausea.*
GU: reversible renal failure.
Hepatic: elevated enzymes.
Skin: pruritus, rash, urticaria.

INTERACTIONS
None significant.

NURSING CONSIDERATIONS
• Contraindicated in asthmatics with nasal polyps.
• Use cautiously in patients with renal disease, GI disorders, angioedema, and in those allergic to noncorticosteroid anti-inflammatory agents.
• Use cautiously in patients with history of peptic ulcer disease.
• Tell patient taking naproxen that full therapeutic effect may be delayed 2 to 4 weeks.
• Warn patient against taking both forms of naproxen at the same time because both circulate in the blood as the naproxen anion.
• Check renal and hepatic function periodically in long-term therapy. Stop drug if abnormalities occur.
• Monitor hemoglobin and bleeding time periodically.

oxyphenbutazone
Oxalid, Tandearil

INDICATIONS & DOSAGE
Pain, inflammation in arthritis, bursitis, superficial venous thrombosis—
Adults: 100 to 200 mg P.O. with food or milk t.i.d. or q.i.d.
Acute gouty arthritis—
Adults: 400 mg initially as single dose, then 100 mg q 4 hours for 4 days or until relief is obtained.

SIDE EFFECTS
Blood: *bone-marrow depression (fatal aplastic anemia, agranulocytosis, thrombocytopenia),* hemolytic anemia, leukopenia.
CNS: restlessness, confusion, lethargy.
CV: hypertension, pericarditis, myocarditis, *cardiac decompensation.*
EENT: optic neuritis, blurred vision, retinal hemorrhage or detachment, hearing loss.

GI: *nausea, vomiting, diarrhea,* ulceration, occult blood loss.
GU: proteinuria, hematuria, glomerulonephritis, nephrotic syndrome, *renal failure.*
Hepatic: *hepatitis.*
Metabolic: toxic and nontoxic goiter, respiratory alkalosis, and metabolic acidosis.
Skin: petechiae, pruritus, purpura, various dermatoses from rash to *toxic necrotizing epidermolysis.*

INTERACTIONS

Methandrostenolone: may increase oxyphenbutazone levels. Give together cautiously.

NURSING CONSIDERATIONS

• Contraindicated in children under 14 years; in patients with senility; GI ulcer; blood dyscrasias; renal, hepatic, cardiac, and thyroid disease. Should not be used in patients receiving long-term anticoagulant therapy.
• Tell patient to stop drug and notify doctor immediately if fever, sore throat, mouth ulcers, GI discomfort, black or tarry stools, bleeding, bruising, rash, or weight gain occurs.
• Give with food, milk, or antacids.
• Complete physical examination and laboratory evaluation are recommended before therapy. Warn patient to remain under close medical supervision and to keep all doctor and laboratory appointments.
• Monitor CBC every 2 weeks or weekly in elderly patients. Report any abnormality to doctor immediately.
• Record patient's weight, intake, and output daily. May cause sodium retention and edema.
• Response should be seen in 2 or 3 days. Drug should be stopped if no response seen within 1 week.
• Patient over age 60 should not receive drug for longer than 1 week.

phenylbutazone
Algoverine♦♦, Aneval♦♦, Azolid, Butagesic♦♦, Butazolidin♦, Intrabutazone♦♦, Malgesic♦♦, Nadozone♦♦, Neo-Zoline♦♦, Phenylbetazone♦♦

INDICATIONS & DOSAGE

Pain, inflammation in arthritis, bursitis, acute superficial thrombophlebitis—
Adults: initially, 100 to 200 mg P.O. t.i.d. or q.i.d. Maximum dose 600 mg per day. When improvement is obtained, decrease dose to 100 mg t.i.d. or q.i.d.
Acute, gouty arthritis—
Adults: 400 mg initially as single dose, then 100 mg q 4 hours for 4 days or until relief is obtained.

SIDE EFFECTS

Blood: *bone-marrow depression (fatal aplastic anemia, agranulocytosis,* thrombocytopenia), hemolytic anemia, leukopenia.
CNS: agitation, confusion, lethargy.
CV: hypertension, edema, pericarditis, myocarditis, *cardiac decompensation.*
EENT: optic neuritis, blurred vision, retinal hemorrhage or detachment, hearing loss.
GI: *nausea, vomiting, diarrhea,* ulceration, occult blood loss.
GU: proteinuria, hematuria, glomerulonephritis, nephrotic syndrome, *renal failure.*
Hepatic: *hepatitis.*
Metabolic: hyperglycemia, toxic and nontoxic goiter, respiratory alkalosis, and metabolic acidosis.
Skin: petechiae, pruritus, purpura, various dermatoses from rash to *toxic necrotizing epidermolysis.*

INTERACTIONS

Barbiturates, antidepressants: may impair phenylbutazone effect. Use together cautiously.
Cholestyramine: may alter phenylbuta-

Italicized side effects are common or life-threatening.
*Liquid form contains alcohol.   **May contain tartrazine.

zone absorption. Give 1 hour before cholestyramine.

NURSING CONSIDERATIONS
• Contraindicated in children under 14 years; in patients with senility; GI ulcer; blood dyscrasias; renal, hepatic, cardiac, and thyroid disease. Should not be used in patients receiving long-term anticoagulant therapy.
• Warn patient to stop drug and notify doctor immediately if fever, sore throat, mouth ulcers, GI discomfort, black or tarry stools, bleeding, bruising, rash, or weight gain occurs.
• Give with food, milk, or antacids.
• Complete physical examination and laboratory evaluation are recommended before therapy. Patient should remain under close medical supervision and keep all doctor and laboratory appointments.
• Monitor CBC every 2 weeks or weekly in elderly patients. Report any abnormalities to doctor right away.
• Record patient's weight, intake, and output daily. May cause sodium retention and edema.
• Response should be seen in 3 to 4 days. Stop drug if no response within 1 week.
• Patient over age 60 should not receive drug for longer than 1 week.

piroxicam
Feldene

INDICATIONS & DOSAGE
Osteoarthritis and rheumatoid arthritis—
Adults: 20 mg P.O. once daily. If desired, the dose may be divided.

SIDE EFFECTS
Blood: prolonged bleeding time, anemia.
CNS: headache, drowsiness, dizziness.
CV: peripheral edema.
GI: *epigastric distress, nausea, occult blood loss, severe gastrointestinal bleeding.*
GU: reversible renal failure.
Hepatic: elevated enzymes.
Skin: pruritus, rash, urticaria.

INTERACTIONS
None significant.

NURSING CONSIDERATIONS
• Contraindicated in asthmatics with nasal polyps. Use cautiously in patients with angioedema, GI disorders, cardiac disease, or allergy to other nonsteroidal anti-inflammatory drugs.
• Use cautiously in patients with history of peptic ulcer disease.
• Tell patient full therapeutic effect may be delayed for 2 to 4 weeks.
• Check renal, hepatic, and auditory function periodically during prolonged therapy. Drug should be discontinued if abnormalities occur.
• Give dose 30 minutes before or 2 hours after meals. If GI side effects occur, give with milk or meals.
• Prothrombin time may be prolonged in patients receiving coumarin-type anticoagulants. Piroxicam decreases platelet aggregation and may prolong bleeding time.
• The first nonsteroidal anti-inflammatory drug approved by the FDA for once-daily administration. Has a longer half-life and, hence, a longer duration of action than other similar drugs.

sulindac
Clinoril

INDICATIONS & DOSAGE
Osteoarthritis, rheumatoid arthritis, dysmenorrhea, ankylosing spondylitis—
Adults: 150 mg P.O. b.i.d. initially; may increase to 200 mg P.O. b.i.d.
Acute subacromial bursitis or supraspinatus tendinitis, acute gouty arthritis—
Adults: 200 mg P.O. b.i.d. for 7 to

---

14 days. Dose may be reduced as symptoms subside.

SIDE EFFECTS
Blood: prolonged bleeding time, *aplastic anemia*.
CNS: dizziness, headache, nervousness.
EENT: tinnitus, transient visual disturbances.
GI: *epigastric distress, occult blood loss, nausea*.
Skin: rash, pruritus.
Other: edema.

INTERACTIONS
None significant.

NURSING CONSIDERATIONS
• Contraindicated in acute asthmatics whose condition is precipitated by aspirin or other nonsteroidal anti-inflammatory agents; in patients who have active ulcers and GI bleeding. Use cautiously in patients with a history of ulcers and GI bleeding, renal dysfunction, compromised cardiac function, hypertension; or in those receiving oral anticoagulants or oral hypoglycemic agents.
• To reduce GI side effects, give with food, milk, or antacids.
• Patient should notify doctor and have complete visual examination if any visual disturbances occur.
• Tell patient to notify doctor immediately if prolonged bleeding occurs.
• Drug causes sodium retention. Patient should report edema and have blood pressure checked periodically.

tolmetin sodium
Tolectin♦, Tolectin DS**

INDICATIONS & DOSAGE
Rheumatoid arthritis and osteoarthritis, gout, dysmenorrhea, juvenile rheumatoid arthritis—
Adults: 400 mg P.O. t.i.d. or q.i.d. Maximum 2 g daily.
Children 2 years or older: 15 to 30 mg/kg daily in divided doses.

SIDE EFFECTS
Blood: prolonged bleeding time.
CNS: headache, dizziness, drowsiness.
GI: *epigastric distress, occult blood loss, nausea*.
GU: reversible renal failure.
Skin: rash, urticaria, pruritus.
Other: sodium retention, edema.

INTERACTIONS
None significant.

NURSING CONSIDERATIONS
• Contraindicated in asthmatics with nasal polyps. Use cautiously in cardiac and renal disease, and GI bleeding.
• Use cautiously in patients with history of peptic ulcer disease.
• Give with food, milk, or antacids to reduce GI side effects.
• Tell patient therapeutic effect should begin within 1 week, but full therapeutic effect may be delayed 2 to 4 weeks.
• Double-strength capsule (400 mg) is available.
• Extended therapy should be accompanied by periodic eye examinations and renal function studies.

Italicized side effects are common or life-threatening.
♦Liquid form contains alcohol.　**May contain tartrazine.

24

Narcotic and opioid analgesics

alphaprodine hydrochloride
Brompton's cocktail
butorphanol tartrate
codeine phosphate
codeine sulfate
fentanyl citrate
hydromorphone hydrochloride
levorphanol tartrate
meperidine hydrochloride
methadone hydrochloride
morphine sulfate
nalbuphine hydrochloride
oxycodone hydrochloride
oxymorphone hydrochloride
pentazocine hydrochloride
pentazocine lactate
propoxyphene hydrochloride
propoxyphene napsylate

MECHANISM OF ACTION

• Narcotic and opioid analgesics bind with opiate receptors at many sites in the central nervous system (brain, brain stem, and spinal cord), altering both perception of and emotional response to pain. The precise mechanism of action, however, is unknown.

COMBINATION PRODUCTS

B & O SUPPRETTES NO. 15A: powdered opium 30 mg and powdered belladonna extract 15 mg.
B & O SUPPRETTES NO. 16A: powdered opium 60 mg and powdered belladonna extract 15 mg.
EMPIRIN WITH CODEINE NO. 2: aspirin 325 mg and codeine phosphate 15 mg.
EMPIRIN WITH CODEINE NO. 3: aspirin 325 mg and codeine phosphate 30 mg.
EMPIRIN WITH CODEINE NO. 4: aspirin 325 mg and codeine phosphate 60 mg.

FIORINAL WITH CODEINE NO. 1: butalbital 50 mg, caffeine 40 mg, aspirin 200 mg, phenacetin 130 mg, and codeine phosphate 7.5 mg.
FIORINAL WITH CODEINE NO. 2♦: butalbital 50 mg, caffeine 40 mg, aspirin 200 mg, phenacetin 130 mg, and codeine phosphate 15 mg.
FIORINAL WITH CODEINE NO. 3♦: butalbital 50 mg, caffeine 40 mg, aspirin 200 mg, phenacetin 130 mg, and codeine 30 mg.
INNOVAR (INJECTION)♦: fentanyl (as the citrate) 0.05 mg and droperidol 2.5 mg per ml.
PANTOPON♦: hydrochlorides of opium alkaloids. 20 mg is therapeutically equivalent to 15 mg morphine.
PERCOCET-5: acetaminophen 325 mg and oxycodone hydrochloride 5 mg.
PERCODAN: oxycodone hydrochloride 4.5 mg, oxycodone terephthalate 0.38 mg, and aspirin 325 mg.
PERCODAN-DEMI: oxycodone hydrochloride 2.25 mg, oxycodone terephthalate 0.19 mg, and aspirin 325 mg.
TYLENOL WITH CODEINE NO 1: acetaminophen 300 mg and codeine phosphate 7.5 mg.
TYLENOL WITH CODEINE NO. 2: acetaminophen 300 mg and codeine phosphate 15 mg.
TYLENOL WITH CODEINE NO. 3: acetaminophen 300 mg and codeine phosphate 30 mg.
TYLENOL WITH CODEINE NO. 4: acetaminophen 300 mg and codeine phosphate 60 mg.
TYLOX: acetaminophen 500 mg, oxyco-

Unmarked trade names available in the United States only.
♦ Also available in Canada.   ♦♦ Available in Canada only.

done hydrochloride 4.5 mg, and oxycodone terephthalate 0.38 mg.
I.V.

alphaprodine hydrochloride
Controlled Substance Schedule II
Nisentil♦

INDICATIONS & DOSAGE
Moderate to severe pain—
Adults: 0.4 to 0.6 mg/kg I.V. or 0.4 to
1.2 mg/kg S.C. q 2 hours, p.r.n. Maximum 240 mg daily. Don't give I.M.

SIDE EFFECTS
CNS: *sedation, somnolence, clouded
sensorium, euphoria,* convulsions with
large doses.
CV: *hypotension,* bradycardia.
GI: *nausea, vomiting, constipation,*
ileus.
GU: *urinary retention.*
Other: *respiratory depression,* physical
dependence.

INTERACTIONS
Alcohol, CNS depressants: additive effects. Use together cautiously.

NURSING CONSIDERATIONS
• Use with extreme caution in head injury, increased intracranial pressure,
shock, elderly or debilitated patients,
increased cerebrospinal fluid pressure,
CNS depression, asthma, COPD, respiratory depression, seizures, hepatic or
renal disease, hypothyroidism, Addison's disease, alcoholism.
• Keep narcotic antagonist (naloxone)
available when giving drug I.V.
• Monitor respirations of newborns exposed to drug during labor.
• Rapid but short-lived effect makes
drug useful in minor surgery or in urologic procedures; not useful for relief of
chronic pain.
• Monitor respiratory and circulatory
status carefully.
• Related to meperidine.

• If used with other narcotic analgesics, general anesthetics, tranquilizers,
sedatives, hypnotics, alcohol, tricyclic
antidepressants, or MAO inhibitors, depressant effect is increased. Reduce
narcotic dose. Use together with extreme caution.
• For better analgesic effect, give before patient has intense pain.
• When used postoperatively, encourage turning, coughing, and deep
breathing to avoid atelectasis.

Brompton's cocktail
(Mixture containing varying
amounts of the following
ingredients: morphine or
methadone, cocaine or
amphetamine, syrup or honey,
alcohol [90% to 98%] or gin,
chloroform water)
Controlled Substance Schedule II

INDICATIONS & DOSAGE
*Severe chronic pain of terminal
cancer—*
Adults: 10 to 20 ml of standard phar-
macy-prepared mixture q 3 to 4 hours
(if morphine is used) or q 6 to 12 hours
(if methadone is used). Must be given
around the clock. Dosage titrations can
be made at 48- to 72-hour intervals.
Maximum dose totally dependent on
patient response.

SIDE EFFECTS
CNS: *sedation, somnolence, clouded
sensorium, euphoria,* convulsions with
large doses.
CV: *hypotension,* bradycardia.
GI: *nausea, vomiting, constipation,*
ileus.
GU: *urinary retention.*
Other: *respiratory depression,* physical
dependence.

INTERACTIONS
Alcohol, CNS depressants: additive effects. Use together cautiously.

Italicized side effects are common or life-threatening.
*Liquid form contains alcohol.   **May contain tartrazine.

NURSING CONSIDERATIONS
• Use with extreme caution in patients with head injury, increased intracranial pressure, shock, increased cerebrospinal fluid pressure, CNS depression, asthma, COPD, respiratory depression, seizures, hepatic or renal disease, hypothyroidism, Addison's disease, alcoholism, and in elderly or debilitated patients.
• Originated in Brompton Hospital in England to keep cancer patients in constant pain-free and euphoric state.
• Not commercially available—must be prepared by pharmacy.
• Has frequently proven to be effective when narcotic analgesics alone have failed to provide pain relief.
• Around-the-clock administration reduces patient's anticipation of pain and is major reason for effectiveness.
• If cocaine is ingredient in mixture— advise patient to swish mixture in mouth to aid absorption, as cocaine is absorbed only through oral mucosa.
• Phenothiazines are occasionally added to increase analgesic effect and prevent nausea.
• Most formulations are stable for up to 4 weeks at room temperature; storage in refrigerator may increase stability to 8 weeks.
• Not intended for mild to moderate pain.
• May worsen gallbladder pain.

butorphanol tartrate
Stadol

INDICATIONS & DOSAGE
Moderate to severe pain—
Adults: 1 to 4 mg I.M. q 3 to 4 hours, p.r.n.; or 0.5 to 2 mg I.V. q 3 to 4 hours, p.r.n.

SIDE EFFECTS
CNS: *sedation, headache, vertigo, floating sensation,* lethargy, confusion, nervousness, unusual dreams, agitation, euphoria, hallucinations, flushing.

CV: palpitations, fluctuation in blood pressure.
EENT: diplopia, blurred vision.
GI: *nausea,* vomiting, dry mouth.
Skin: rash, hives, *clamminess, excessive sweating.*
Other: *respiratory depression.*

INTERACTIONS
None significant.

NURSING CONSIDERATIONS
• Contraindicated in narcotic addiction; may precipitate narcotic abstinence syndrome. Use cautiously in head injury, increased intracranial pressure, acute MI, ventricular dysfunction, coronary insufficiency, respiratory disease or depression, renal or hepatic dysfunction.
• Psychological and physical addiction may occur.
• Possesses narcotic antagonist properties. May precipitate abstinence syndrome if given soon after other narcotics.
• Respiratory depression does not increase with increased dosage.
• Subcutaneous route not recommended.
• Also approved for use as a preoperative medication, as the analgesic component of balanced anesthesia, and for relief of postpartum pain.

codeine phosphate

codeine sulfate
Controlled Substance Schedule II

INDICATIONS & DOSAGE
Mild to moderate pain—
Adults: 15 to 60 mg P.O. or 15 to 60 mg (phosphate) S.C. or I.M. q 4 hours, p.r.n.
Children: 3 mg/kg daily P.O. divided q 4 hours, p.r.n.

SIDE EFFECTS
CNS: *sedation, clouded sensorium, euphoria,* convulsions with large doses.
CV: *hypotension,* bradycardia.
GI: *nausea, vomiting, constipation,* ileus.
GU: *urinary retention.*
Other: *respiratory depression,* physical dependence.

INTERACTIONS
Alcohol, CNS depressants: additive effects. Use together cautiously.

NURSING CONSIDERATIONS
• Use with extreme caution in patients with head injury, increased intracranial pressure, increased cerebrospinal fluid pressure, hepatic or renal disease, hypothyroidism, Addison's disease, acute alcoholism, seizures, severe CNS depression, bronchial asthma, COPD, respiratory depression, shock, and in elderly or debilitated patients.
• Warn ambulatory patient to avoid activities that require alertness.
• Monitor respiratory and circulatory status and bowel function.
• For full analgesic effect, give before patient has intense pain.
• Codeine and aspirin have additive effect. Give together for maximum pain relief.
• Do not administer discolored injection solution.
• If used with general anesthetics, other narcotic analgesics, tranquilizers, sedatives, hypnotics, alcohol, tricyclic antidepressants, or MAO inhibitors, CNS depression is increased. Use together with extreme caution. Monitor patient's response.

fentanyl citrate
Controlled Substance Schedule II
Sublimaze♦

INDICATIONS & DOSAGE
Adjunct to general anesthetic—
Adults: 0.05 to 0.1 mg I.V. repeated q 2 to 3 minutes, p.r.n. Dose should be reduced in elderly and poor-risk patients.
Postoperatively—
Adults: 0.05 to 0.1 mg I.M. q 1 to 2 hours, p.r.n.
Children 2 to 12 years: 0.02 to 0.03 mg per 9 kg.
Preoperatively—
Adults: 0.05 to 0.1 mg I.M. 30 to 60 minutes before surgery.

SIDE EFFECTS
CNS: *sedation, somnolence, clouded sensorium, euphoria,* convulsions with large doses.
CV: *hypotension,* bradycardia.
GI: *nausea, vomiting, constipation,* ileus.
GU: *urinary retention.*
Other: *respiratory depression,* physical dependence.

INTERACTIONS
Alcohol, CNS depressants: additive effects. Use together cautiously.

NURSING CONSIDERATIONS
• Contraindicated in patients who have received MAO inhibitors within 14 days and who have myasthenia gravis. Use cautiously in patients with head injury, increased cerebrospinal fluid pressure, asthma, COPD, respiratory depression, seizures, hepatic or renal disease, hypothyroidism, Addison's disease, alcoholism, increased intracranial pressure, CNS depression, shock, and in elderly or debilitated patients.
• Keep narcotic antagonist (naloxone) and resuscitative equipment available when giving drug I.V.
• Monitor respirations of newborns exposed to drug during labor.
• Use as postoperative analgesic only in recovery room. Make sure another analgesic is ordered for later use.
• Often used with droperidol (as Innovar) to produce neuroleptanalgesia.
• Monitor circulatory and respiratory status carefully.

Italicized side effects are common or life-threatening.
*Liquid form contains alcohol.   **May contain tartrazine.

• Respiratory depression, hypotension, profound sedation, and coma may result if used with other narcotic analgesics, general anesthetics, tranquilizers, alcohol, sedatives, hypnotics, tricyclic antidepressants, or MAO inhibitors. Fentanyl citrate dose should be reduced to ¼ to ⅓. Also give above drugs in reduced dosages.

• For better analgesic effect, give before patient has intense pain.

• When used postoperatively, encourage turning, coughing, and deep breathing to avoid atelectasis.

hydromorphone hydrochloride
Controlled Substance Schedule II
Dilaudid♦**

INDICATIONS & DOSAGE
Moderate to severe pain—
Adults: 1 to 6 mg P.O. q 4 to 6 hours, p.r.n.; or 2 to 4 mg I.M., S.C., or I.V. q 4 to 6 hours, p.r.n. (I.V. dose should be given over 3 to 5 minutes); or 3 mg rectal suppository at bedtime, p.r.n.

SIDE EFFECTS
CNS: *sedation, somnolence, clouded sensorium, euphoria,* convulsions with large doses.
CV: *hypotension,* bradycardia.
GI: *nausea, vomiting, constipation,* ileus.
GU: *urinary retention.*
Local: induration with repeated S.C. injection.
Other: *respiratory depression,* physical dependence.

INTERACTIONS
Alcohol, CNS depressants: additive effects. Use together cautiously.

NURSING CONSIDERATIONS
• Contraindicated in increased intracranial pressure and status asthmaticus. Use with extreme caution in patients with increased cerebrospinal fluid pres-

sure, respiratory depression, hepatic or renal disease, hypothyroidism, shock, Addison's disease, acute alcoholism, seizures, head injury, severe CNS depression, brain tumor, bronchial asthma, COPD, and in elderly or debilitated patients.

• Warn ambulatory patient to avoid activities that require alertness.
• Monitor respiratory and circulatory status and bowel function.
• Keep narcotic antagonist (naloxone) available.
• Respiratory depression and hypotension can occur with I.V. administration. Give very slowly and monitor constantly.
• Rotate injection sites to avoid induration with subcutaneous injection.
• Commonly abused narcotic.
• If used with general anesthetics, other narcotic analgesics, tranquilizers, sedatives, hypnotics, alcohol, tricyclic antidepressants, or MAO inhibitors, CNS depression is increased. Hydromorphone dose should be reduced. Use together with extreme caution. Monitor patient's response.
• Oral dosage form is particularly convenient for patients with chronic pain because tablets are available in 1 mg, 2 mg, 3 mg, and 4 mg. This enables these patients to titrate their own dose.
• For better analgesic effect, give before patient has intense pain.
• When used postoperatively, encourage turning, coughing, and deep breathing to avoid atelectasis.
• May worsen gallbladder pain.

levorphanol tartrate
Controlled Substance Schedule II
Levo-Dromoran♦

INDICATIONS & DOSAGE
Moderate to severe pain—
Adults: 2 to 3 mg P.O. or S.C. q 6 to 8 hours, p.r.n.

SIDE EFFECTS
CNS: *sedation, somnolence, clouded sensorium, euphoria,* convulsions with large doses.
CV: *hypotension,* bradycardia.
GI: *nausea, vomiting, constipation,* ileus.
GU: *urinary retention.*
Other: *respiratory depression,* physical dependence.

INTERACTIONS
None significant.

NURSING CONSIDERATIONS
• Contraindicated in patients with acute alcoholism, bronchial asthma, increased intracranial pressure, respiratory depression, and anoxia. Use with extreme caution in patients with hepatic or renal disease, hypothyroidism, Addison's disease, seizures, head injury, severe CNS depression, brain tumor, COPD, shock, and in elderly or debilitated patients.
• Warn ambulatory patient to avoid activities that require alertness.
• Monitor circulatory and respiratory status and bowel function.
• Warn patient drug has bitter taste.
• Protect from light.
• Keep narcotic antagonist (naloxone) available.
• If used with general anesthetics, other narcotic analgesics, tranquilizers, sedatives, hypnotics, alcohol, tricyclic antidepressants, or MAO inhibitors, CNS depression is increased. Reduce levorphanol dose. Use together with extreme caution. Monitor patient's response.
• For better analgesic effect, give before patient has intense pain.
• When used postoperatively, encourage turning, coughing, and deep breathing to avoid atelectasis.

meperidine hydrochloride
Controlled Substance Schedule II
Demer-Idine♦♦, Demerol♦,
Pethidine HCl B.P.♦♦

INDICATIONS & DOSAGE
Moderate to severe pain—
Adults: 50 to 150 mg P.O., I.M., or S.C. q 3 to 4 hours, p.r.n.
Children: 1 mg/kg P.O., I.M., or S.C. q 4 to 6 hours. Maximum—100 mg q 4 hours, p.r.n.
Preoperatively—
Adults: 50 to 100 mg I.M. or S.C. 30 to 90 minutes before surgery.
Children: 1 to 2.2 mg/kg I.M. or S.C. 30 to 90 minutes before surgery.

SIDE EFFECTS
CNS: *sedation, somnolence, clouded sensorium, euphoria,* convulsions with large doses.
CV: *hypotension,* bradycardia.
GI: *nausea, vomiting, constipation,* ileus.
GU: *urinary retention.*
Local: pain at injection site, local tissue irritation and induration after S.C. injection; phlebitis after I.V. injection.
Other: *respiratory depression,* physical dependence.

INTERACTIONS
MAO inhibitors, barbiturates, isoniazid: increased CNS excitation or depression can be severe or fatal. Don't use together.
Alcohol, CNS depressants: additive effects. Use together cautiously.
Phenytoin: decreased blood levels of meperidine. Monitor for decreased analgesia.

NURSING CONSIDERATIONS
• Contraindicated if patient has used MAO inhibitors within 14 days. Use with extreme caution in patients with increased intracranial pressure, increased cerebrospinal fluid pressure, shock, CNS depression, head injury,

---

Italicized side effects are common or life-threatening.
✱Liquid form contains alcohol. ✱✱May contain tartrazine.

asthma, COPD, respiratory depression, supraventricular tachycardias, seizures, acute abdominal conditions, hepatic or renal disease, hypothyroidism, Addison's disease, urethral stricture, prostatic hypertrophy, alcoholism, in children under 12 years, and in elderly or debilitated patients.
• May be used in patients allergic to morphine.
• Meperidine and active metabolite normeperidine accumulate in renal failure. Monitor for increased toxic effect in patients with poor renal function.
• Meperidine may be given slow I.V., preferably as a diluted solution. S.C. injection very painful.
• Keep narcotic antagonist (naloxone) available when giving this drug I.V.
• Warn ambulatory patient to avoid activities that require alertness.
• Monitor respirations of newborns exposed to drug during labor. Have resuscitation equipment available.
• P.O. dose less than half as effective as parenteral dose. Give I.M. if possible. When changing from parenteral to P.O. route, dose should be increased.
• Syrup has local anesthetic effect. Give with full glass of water.
• Chemically incompatible with barbiturates. Don't mix together.
• Monitor respiratory and cardiovascular status carefully. Don't give if respirations are below 12/minute or if change in pupils is noted.
• Watch for withdrawal symptoms if stopped abruptly after long-term use.
• If used with other narcotic analgesics, general anesthetics, phenothiazines, sedatives, hypnotics, tricyclic antidepressants, or alcohol, respiratory depression, hypotension, profound sedation, or coma may occur. Reduce meperidine dose. Use together with extreme caution.
• For better analgesic effect, give before patient has intense pain.
• When used postoperatively, encourage turning, coughing, and deep breathing to avoid atelectasis.

• May be the best narcotic for gallbladder spasm, because pain is not worsened.

methadone hydrochloride
Controlled Substance Schedule II
Dolophine, Methadone HCl Oral Solution

INDICATIONS & DOSAGE
Severe pain—
Adults: 2.5 to 10 mg P.O., I.M., or S.C. q 4 to 12 hours, p.r.n. or around the clock.
Narcotic abstinence syndrome—
Adults: 15 to 40 mg P.O. daily (highly individualized).
Maintenance: 20 to 120 mg P.O. daily. Adjust dose as needed. Daily doses greater than 120 mg require special state and federal approval.

SIDE EFFECTS
CNS: *sedation, somnolence, clouded sensorium, euphoria,* convulsions with large doses.
CV: *hypotension,* bradycardia.
GI: *nausea, vomiting, constipation,* ileus.
GU: *urinary retention.*
Local: pain at injection site, tissue irritation, induration following S.C. injection.
Other: *respiratory depression,* physical dependence.

INTERACTIONS
Rifampin: withdrawal symptoms; reduced blood levels of methadone. Use together cautiously.
Ammonium chloride and other urine acidifiers, phenytoin: may reduce methadone effect. Monitor for decreased pain control.
Alcohol, CNS depressants: additive effects. Use together cautiously.

NURSING CONSIDERATIONS
• Contraindicated in obstetric analgesia. Give with extreme caution in el-

derly or debilitated patients, or in patients with acute abdominal conditions, severe hepatic or renal impairment, hypothyroidism, Addison's disease, prostatic hypertrophy, urethral stricture, head injury, increased intracranial pressure, asthma, COPD, respiratory depression, CNS depression.
- Safe use in adolescents as maintenance drug not established.
- Oral dose is half as potent as injected dose.
- Rotate injection sites.
- Has cumulative effect; marked sedation can occur after repeated doses.
- Monitor circulatory and respiratory status and bowel function.
- Warn ambulatory patient to avoid activities that require alertness.
- One daily dose adequate for maintenance. No advantage to divided doses.
- Regimented scheduling (around the clock) beneficial in severe, chronic pain.
- Oral form legally required in maintenance programs.
- Give maintenance doses as oral liquid. Completely dissolve tablets in 120 ml of orange juice or powdered citrus drink.
- Constipation often severe with maintenance. Make sure stool softener or other laxative is ordered.
- Patient treated for narcotic abstinence syndrome will usually require an additional analgesic if pain control necessary.
- If used with general anesthetics, tranquilizers, sedatives, hypnotics, alcohol, tricyclic antidepressants or MAO inhibitors, respiratory depression, hypotension, profound sedation, or coma may occur. Use together with extreme caution. Monitor patient's response.
- Liquid form (1 mg/ml) available for patients who are unable to swallow tablets.

morphine sulfate✦
Controlled Substance Schedule II

INDICATIONS & DOSAGE
Severe pain—
Adults: 5 to 15 mg S.C. or I.M., or 30 to 60 mg P.O. q 4 hours, p.r.n. or around the clock. May be injected slow I.V. (over 4 to 5 minutes) diluted in 4 to 5 ml water for injection.
Children: 0.1 to 0.2 mg/kg dose S.C. Maximum 15 mg.

SIDE EFFECTS
CNS: *sedation, somnolence, clouded sensorium, euphoria,* convulsions with large doses.
CV: *hypotension,* bradycardia.
GI: *nausea, vomiting, constipation,* ileus.
GU: *urinary retention.*
Other: *respiratory depression, physical dependence.*

INTERACTIONS
Alcohol, CNS depressants: additional effects. Use together cautiously.

NURSING CONSIDERATIONS
- Use with extreme caution in patients with head injury, increased intracranial pressure, seizures, asthma, COPD, alcoholism, prostatic hypertrophy, severe hepatic or renal disease, acute abdominal conditions, hypothyroidism, Addison's disease, increased cerebrospinal fluid pressure, urethral stricture, cardiac arrhythmias, reduced blood volume, toxic psychosis, and in elderly or debilitated patients.
- Warn ambulatory patient to avoid activities that require alertness.
- Monitor circulatory and respiratory status and bowel function. Don't give if respirations are below 12/minute.
- Drug of choice in relieving pain of myocardial infarction. May cause transient decrease in blood pressure.
- Keep narcotic antagonist (naloxone) and resuscitative equipment available.

Italicized side effects are common or life-threatening.
✦Liquid form contains alcohol.   ✦✦May contain tartrazine.

• Constipation often severe with maintenance. Make sure stool softener or other laxative is ordered.

• Respiratory depression, hypotension, profound sedation, or coma may occur if used with general anesthetics, tranquilizers, sedatives, hypnotics, alcohol, tricyclic antidepressants, or MAO inhibitors. Reduce morphine dose. Use together with extreme caution. Monitor patient's response.

• Regimented scheduling (around the clock) beneficial in severe, chronic pain.

• When used postoperatively, encourage turning, coughing, and deep breathing to avoid atelectasis.

• Patients with very severe pain may receive up to 150 mg of morphine sulfate every 3 hours in some situations.

• Oral solution contains 10 mg/5 ml.

• May worsen gallbladder pain.

nalbuphine hydrochloride
Nubain

INDICATIONS & DOSAGE
Moderate to severe pain—
S.C., I.M., or I.V.
Adults: 10 to 20 mg q 3 to 6 hours
p.r.n. Maximum daily dose 160 mg.

SIDE EFFECTS
CNS: *sedation,* nervousness, depression, restlessness, crying, euphoria, hostility, unusual dreams, confusion, hallucinations, delusions.
GI: cramps, dyspepsia, bitter taste, nausea, vomiting.
GU: urinary urgency.
Skin: itching, burning, urticaria.
Other: *respiratory depression,* physical and psychological dependence.

INTERACTIONS
None significant.

NURSING CONSIDERATIONS
• Contraindicated in emotional instability, drug abuse, head injury, in-

creased intracranial pressure. Use cautiously in patients with hepatic and renal disease. These patients may overreact to customary doses.

• Causes respiratory depression which at 10 mg is equal to the respiratory depression produced by 10 mg of morphine.

• Psychological and physiologic dependence may occur.

• Respiratory depression can be reversed with naloxone.

• Also acts as a narcotic antagonist; may precipitate abstinence syndrome if given soon after other narcotics.

• Warn patient to avoid activities that require alertness until CNS response to drug is determined.

oxycodone hydrochloride
Controlled Substance Schedule II
Supeudol♦♦, Oxycodone Oral
Solution

Combinations:
Percocet♦♦, Percocet 5, Percocet-Demi♦, Percodan♦, Percodan-Demi♦, Tylox

INDICATIONS & DOSAGE
Moderate to severe pain—
Adults: available in combination with other drugs, such as aspirin, phenacetin, and caffeine (Percodan, Percodan-Demi), or acetaminophen (Percocet 5, Tylox). 1 to 2 tablets P.O. q 6 hours, p.r.n. Or 5 mg (5 ml) of Oxycodone Oral Solution P.O. q 6 hours, p.r.n.
Adults: (Supeudol) 1 to 3 suppositories rectally daily, p.r.n.
Children: (Percodan-Demi) ¼ to ½ tablet P.O. q 6 hours, p.r.n.

SIDE EFFECTS
CNS: *sedation, somnolence, clouded sensorium, euphoria,* convulsions with large doses.
CV: *hypotension,* bradycardia.
GI: *nausea, vomiting, constipation,* ileus.

GU: *urinary retention.*
Other: *respiratory depression,* physical dependence.

INTERACTIONS
Anticoagulants: oxycodone hydrochloride products containing aspirin may increase anticoagulant effect. Monitor clotting times. Use together cautiously.
Alcohol, CNS depressants: additive effects. Use together cautiously.

NURSING CONSIDERATIONS
• Use with extreme caution in patients with head injury, increased intracranial pressure, increased cerebrospinal fluid pressure, seizures, asthma, COPD, alcoholism, prostatic hypertrophy, severe hepatic or renal disease, acute abdominal conditions, urethral stricture, hypothyroidism, Addison's disease, cardiac arrhythmias, reduced blood volume, toxic psychosis, and in elderly or debilitated patients.
• Don't give to children, except for Percodan-Demi and Percocet-Demi.
• Warn ambulatory patient to avoid activities that require alertness.
• Monitor circulatory and respiratory status and bowel function. Do not give if respirations are below 12/minute.
• For full analgesic effect, give before patient has intense pain.
• High level of analgesia when given P.O., but poor choice due to high risk of addiction and presence of phenacetin in some combinations.
• Give after meals or with milk.
• If used with general anesthetics, other narcotic analgesics, tranquilizers, sedatives, hypnotics, alcohol, tricyclic antidepressants, or MAO inhibitors, CNS depression is increased. Reduce oxycodone dose. Use together with extreme caution. Monitor patient's response.
• Single-entity oxycodone solution, a new product, is especially good for patients who shouldn't take aspirin or acetominophen.

oxymorphone hydrochloride
Controlled Substance Schedule II
Numorphan◆

INDICATIONS & DOSAGE
Moderate to severe pain—
Adults: 1 to 1.5 mg I.M. or S.C. q 4 to 6 hours, p.r.n., or 0.5 mg I.V. q 4 to 6 hours, p.r.n., or 2.5 to 5 mg rectally q 4 to 6 hours, p.r.n.

SIDE EFFECTS
CNS: *sedation, somnolence, clouded sensorium, euphoria,* convulsions with large doses.
CV: *hypotension,* bradycardia.
GI: *nausea, vomiting, constipation,* ileus.
GU: *urinary retention.*
Other: *respiratory depression,* physical dependence.

INTERACTIONS
Alcohol, CNS depressants: additive effects. Use together cautiously.

NURSING CONSIDERATIONS
• Use with extreme caution in patients with head injury, increased intracranial pressure, seizures, asthma, COPD, alcoholism, increased cerebrospinal fluid pressure, acute abdominal conditions, prostatic hypertrophy, severe hepatic or renal disease, urethral stricture, CNS depression, respiratory depression, hypothyroidism, Addison's disease, cardiac arrhythmias, reduced blood volume, toxic psychosis, and in elderly or debilitated patients.
• Warn ambulatory patient to avoid activities that require alertness.
• Monitor cardiovascular and respiratory status. Don't give if respirations are below 12/minute.
• Well absorbed rectally. Alternative to narcotics with more limited dosage forms.
• Keep narcotic antagonist (naloxone) and resuscitative equipment available.

Italicized side effects are common or life-threatening.
∗Liquid form contains alcohol.   ∗∗May contain tartrazine.

• If used with general anesthetics, tranquilizers, sedatives, hypnotics, alcohol, tricyclic antidepressants, or MAO inhibitors, CNS depression is increased. Reduce oxymorphone dose. Use together with extreme caution. Monitor patient's response.

• For better analgesic effect, give before patient has intense pain.

• When used postoperatively, encourage turning, coughing, and deep breathing to avoid atelectasis.

• Not intended for mild to moderate pain. May worsen gallbladder pain.

cardial infarction with nausea, respiratory depression.

• Tablets not well absorbed.

• Possesses narcotic antagonist properties. May precipitate abstinence syndrome if given soon after other narcotics.

• Psychological and physiologic dependence may occur.

• Respiratory depression can be reversed with naloxone.

• Do not mix in same syringe with soluble barbiturates.

• Warn ambulatory patient to avoid activities that require alertness.

---

pentazocine hydrochloride

pentazocine lactate
Controlled Substance Schedule IV
Talwin♦

INDICATIONS & DOSAGE
Moderate to severe pain—
Adults: 50 to 100 mg P.O. q 3 to 4 hours, p.r.n. Maximum 600 mg daily or 30 mg I.M., I.V., or S.C. q 3 to 4 hours, p.r.n. Maximum 360 mg daily. Doses above 30 mg I.V. or 60 mg I.M. or S.C. not recommended.

SIDE EFFECTS
CNS: *sedation,* visual disturbances, hallucinations, drowsiness, dizziness, light-headedness, confusion, euphoria, headache.
GI: nausea, vomiting, dry mouth.
GU: urinary retention.
Local: induration, nodules, sloughing, and sclerosis of injection site.
Other: *respiratory depression,* physical and psychological dependence.

INTERACTIONS
None significant.

NURSING CONSIDERATIONS
• Contraindicated in emotional instability, drug abuse, head injury, increased intracranial pressure. Use cautiously in hepatic or renal disease, myo-

propoxyphene hydrochloride
Controlled Substance Schedule IV
Darvon, Dolene, Doraphen, Myospaz, Pargesic 65, Pro-Pox 65, Proxagesic, Ropoxy, Scrip-Dyne, SK-65, S-Pain-65, 642♦♦

propoxyphene napsylate
Controlled Substance Schedule IV
Darvocet-N, Darvon-N♦

INDICATIONS & DOSAGE
Mild to moderate pain—
Adults: 65 mg (hydrochloride) P.O. q 4 hours, p.r.n.
Mild to moderate pain—
Adults: 100 mg (napsylate) P.O. q 4 hours, p.r.n.

SIDE EFFECTS
CNS: dizziness, headache, sedation, euphoria, paradoxical excitement, insomnia.
GI: nausea, vomiting, constipation.
Other: psychological and physical dependence.

INTERACTIONS
None significant.

NURSING CONSIDERATIONS
• Not to be prescribed in narcotic addiction.

Unmarked trade names available in the United States only.
♦ Also available in Canada. ♦♦ Available in Canada only.

- Warn ambulatory patient to avoid activities that require alertness until CNS response to drug has been established.
- Warn patient not to exceed recommended dosage.
- Do not use caffeine or amphetamines to treat overdose: may cause fatal convulsions. Use narcotic antagonist instead.

- May cause false decreases in urinary steroid excretion tests.
- 65 mg propoxyphene HCl equals 100 mg propoxyphene napsylate.
- Can be considered a mild narcotic analgesic.
- Advise patients to limit their alcohol intake when taking this drug.

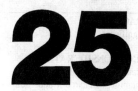

Narcotic antagonists

levallorphan tartrate
naloxone

MECHANISM OF ACTION
Although the precise mechanism of action of narcotic antagonists is unknown, levallorphan and naloxone apparently displace previously administered narcotic analgesics from their receptors (competitive antagonism).

• Levallorphan may have some narcotic *agonist* activity (narcotic analgesic effect), especially if administered alone, not as an antidote to narcotic analgesics.

• Naloxone—administered alone, not as an antidote to narcotic analgesics—has no pharmacologic activity.

COMBINATION PRODUCTS
None.

levallorphan tartrate
Lorfan

INDICATIONS & DOSAGE
Severe narcotic-induced respiratory depression—
Adults: 1 mg I.V., then 1 to 2 doses of 0.5 mg at 10- to 15-minute intervals, p.r.n. Maximum total dose 3 mg.
Children: 0.02 mg/kg I.V. May give 0.01 to 0.02 mg/kg in 10 to 15 minutes.

Neonates (asphyxia neonatorum): 0.05 to 0.1 mg I.V. into umbilical vein immediately after delivery. May repeat in 5 to 10 minutes.

SIDE EFFECTS
CNS: lethargy, dizziness, drowsiness, restlessness, sense of heaviness in limbs; with high doses: psychic disturbances (hallucinations, disorientation, weird dreams); in neonates: irritability, increased crying.
CV: pallor.
EENT: miosis, pseudoptosis.
GI: nausea.
Other: sweating, respiratory depression.

INTERACTIONS
None significant.

NURSING CONSIDERATIONS
• Contraindicated in mild respiratory depression and in narcotic addiction. (Violent withdrawal symptoms may occur.)
• Monitor respiratory depth and rate. Be prepared to provide oxygen, ventilation, and other resuscitative measures.
• May increase mild respiratory depression or that caused by nonnarcotic agents. Repeated doses may produce tolerance and increased respiratory depression.

naloxone
Narcan♦

INDICATIONS & DOSAGE
Narcotic-induced respiratory depression, including pentazocine and propoxyphene—
Adults: 0.4 mg I.V., S.C., or I.M. May repeat q 2 to 3 minutes, p.r.n., for 3 doses.

Postoperative narcotic depression—
Adults: 0.1 to 0.2 mg I.V. q 2 to 3 minutes, p.r.n. Adult concentration is 0.4 mg/ml.

Children: 0.01 mg/kg dose I.M., I.V., S.C. May repeat q 2 to 3 minutes for 3 doses.
Note: If initial dose 0.01 mg/kg does not result in clinical improvement, up to 10 times this dose (0.1 mg/kg) may be needed to be effective.

Neonates *(asphyxia neonatorum):* 0.01 mg/kg I.V. into umbilical vein. May repeat q 2 to 3 minutes for 3 doses. Neonatal concentration (for children also) is 0.02 mg/ml.

SIDE EFFECTS
With higher-than-recommended doses: nausea, vomiting.
In narcotic addicts: withdrawal symptoms.

INTERACTIONS
None significant.

NURSING CONSIDERATIONS
• Use cautiously in patients with cardiac irritability and narcotic addiction.
• Safest drug to use when cause of respiratory depression is uncertain.
• Monitor respiratory depth and rate. Be prepared to provide oxygen, ventilation, and other resuscitative measures.
• Although generally believed to be ineffective in respiratory depression caused by nonnarcotics, recent reports indicate that it may reverse coma induced by alcohol intoxication.
• May dilute adult concentration (0.4 mg) by mixing 0.5 ml with 9.5 ml sterile water or saline solution for injection to make neonatal concentration (0.02 mg/ml).

Italicized side effects are common or life-threatening.
*Liquid form contains alcohol.   **May contain tartrazine.

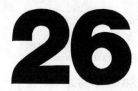

Sedatives and hypnotics

amobarbital
amobarbital sodium
aprobarbital
barbital
butabarbital
butabarbital sodium
chloral hydrate
ethchlorvynol
ethinamate
flurazepam hydrochloride
glutethimide
hexobarbital
mephobarbital
methaqualone
methaqualone hydrochloride
methotrimeprazine
   hydrochloride
methyprylon
paraldehyde
pentobarbital
pentobarbital sodium
phenobarbital
phenobarbital sodium
propiomazine hydrochloride
secobarbital
secobarbital sodium
talbutal
temazepam
triclofos sodium

MECHANISM OF ACTION
Although their mechanism of action is
not completely defined, barbiturates
probably interfere with transmission of
impulses from the thalamus to the cortex of the brain.
• Flurazepam and temezepam act on
the limbic system, thalamus, and hypothalamus of the central nervous system
to produce hypnotic effects.

COMBINATION PRODUCTS
Barbiturates
BUTATRAX CAPSULES: amobarbital 20
mg and butabarbital 30 mg.
CARBRITAL KAPSEALS: pentobarbital
sodium 97.5 mg and carbromal 260
mg.
ETHOBRAL CAPSULE: phenobarbital 50
mg, butabarbital sodium 30 mg, and
secobarbital sodium 50 mg.
HYPTRAN TABLET: secobarbital 60 mg
and phenyltoloxamine dihydrogen citrate 25 mg in outer layer (immediate
release), phenyltoloxamine dihydrogen
citrate 75 mg in core (delayed release).
NIDAR TABLET: phenobarbital sodium
7.5 mg, butabarbital sodium 7.5 mg,
secobarbital sodium 25 mg, and pentobarbital sodium 25 mg.
TRI-BARBS CAPSULE: phenobarbital 32
mg, butabarbital sodium 32 mg, and
secobarbital sodium 32 mg.
TUINAL 50 MG PULVULES: amobarbital
sodium 25 mg and secobarbital sodium
25 mg.
TUINAL 100 MG PULVULES♦: amobarbital sodium 50 mg and secobarbital sodium 50 mg.
TUINAL 200 MG PULVULES♦: amobarbital sodium 100 mg and secobarbital
sodium 100 mg.

amobarbital
Amytal♦, Isobec♦♦

amobarbital sodium
Controlled Substance Schedule II
Amytal Sodium♦

INDICATIONS & DOSAGE
Sedation—
Adults: usually 30 to 50 mg P.O. b.i.d.
or t.i.d. but may range from 15 to 120
mg b.i.d. to q.i.d.
Children: 3 to 6 mg/kg daily P.O. di-
vided into 4 equal doses.
Insomnia—
Adults: 65 to 200 mg P.O. or deep
I.M. at bedtime; I.M. injection not to
exceed 5 ml in any one site. Maximum
dose 500 mg.
Children: 3 to 5 mg/kg deep I.M. at
bedtime; I.M. injection not to exceed 5
ml in any one site.
Preanesthetic sedation—
Adults and children: 200 mg P.O. or
I.M. 1 to 2 hours before surgery.
*Manic reactions; as an adjunct in psy-
chotherapy; anticonvulsant—*
Adults and children over 6 years: 65
to 500 mg slow I.V.; rate not to exceed
100 mg/minute. Maximum dose 1 g.
Children under 6 years: 3 to 5 mg/kg
slow I.V. or I.M.

SIDE EFFECTS
CNS: *drowsiness, lethargy, hangover,*
paradoxical excitement in elderly pa-
tients.
GI: nausea, vomiting.
Skin: rash, urticaria.
Local: pain, irritation, sterile abscess
at injection site.
Other: *Stevens-Johnson syndrome,* an-
gioedema.

INTERACTIONS
*Alcohol or other CNS depressants, in-
cluding other narcotic analgesics:* excessive CNS and respiratory depression. Use together cautiously.
MAO inhibitors: inhibit metabolism of

barbiturates; may cause prolonged CNS
depression. Reduce barbiturate dosage.
Rifampin: may decrease barbiturate
levels. Monitor for decreased effect.

NURSING CONSIDERATIONS
• Contraindicated in patients with uncontrolled severe pain, respiratory disease with dyspnea or obstruction,
hypersensitivity to barbiturates, previous addiction to sedatives, porphyria.
Use with caution in hepatic or renal impairment.
• Use injection solution within
30 minutes after opening container to
minimize deterioration. Don't use
cloudy or precipitated solution. Don't
shake solution; mix with sterile water
only.
• Reserve I.V. injection for emergency
treatment. Give under close supervision. Be prepared to give artificial respiration. Administer slowly I.V.; not to
exceed 100 mg/minute.
• Administer I.M. injection deeply.
Superficial injection may cause pain,
sterile abscess, and sloughing.
• Because barbiturates potentiate narcotics, reduce dose when giving during
labor. Excessive dose may cause respiratory depression in neonate.
• Remove cigarettes of patient receiving hypnotic dose.
• Supervise walking; raise bed rails,
especially for elderly patients.
• Long-term high dosage may cause
drug dependence and severe withdrawal
symptoms. Withdraw barbiturates gradually.
• Prevent hoarding or self-overdosing
by patients who are depressed, suicidal,
or drug-dependent, or who have a history of drug abuse. Warn patient that
alcohol increases effects of drug, and
advise him not to perform activities requiring alertness or skill until CNS response is determined.
• Watch for signs of barbiturate toxicity: coma, pupillary constriction, cyanosis, clammy skin, hypotension. Overdose can be fatal.

Italicized side effects are common or life-threatening.
∗Liquid form contains alcohol.   ∗∗May contain tartrazine.

• Monitor prothrombin times carefully when patient on amobarbital starts or ends anticoagulant therapy. Anticoagulant dose may need to be adjusted.

aprobarbital
Controlled Substance Schedule III
Alurate*

INDICATIONS & DOSAGE
Sedation—
Adults: 15 to 40 mg P.O. t.i.d. or q.i.d.; usual dose 40 mg t.i.d.
Insomnia—
Adults: 40 to 160 mg P.O. at bedtime.

SIDE EFFECTS
CNS: *drowsiness, lethargy, hangover,* paradoxical excitement in elderly patients.
GI: nausea, vomiting.
Skin: rash, urticaria.
Other: *Stevens-Johnson syndrome,* angioedema.

INTERACTIONS
Alcohol or other CNS depressants, including narcotic analgesics: excessive CNS and respiratory depression. Use together cautiously.
MAO inhibitors: inhibit metabolism of barbiturates; may cause prolonged CNS depression. Reduce barbiturate dosage.
Rifampin: may decrease barbiturate levels. Monitor for decreased effect.

NURSING CONSIDERATIONS
• Contraindicated in patients with uncontrolled severe pain, respiratory disease with dyspnea or obstruction, hypersensitivity to barbiturates, previous addiction to sedatives, porphyria. Use with caution in hepatic or renal impairment.
• Remove cigarettes of patient receiving hypnotic dose.
• Supervise walking; raise bed rails, especially for elderly patients.
• Long-term high dosage may cause drug dependence and severe withdrawal symptoms. Withdraw barbiturates gradually.
• Prevent hoarding or self-overdosing by patients who are depressed, suicidal, or drug-dependent, or who have a history of drug abuse. Warn patient that alcohol increases effects of drug, and advise him not to perform activities requiring alertness or skill until CNS response is determined.
• Available as elixir only, with alcohol 20%.
• Monitor prothrombin times carefully when patient on aprobarbital starts or ends anticoagulant therapy. Anticoagulant dose may need to be adjusted.
• Watch for signs of barbiturate toxicity: coma, pupillary constriction, cyanosis, clammy skin, hypotension. Overdose can be fatal.

barbital
Controlled Substance Schedule IV
Barbital Sodium

INDICATIONS & DOSAGE
Insomnia—
Adults: 300 to 600 mg P.O. or I.M. 1 to 2 hours before bedtime.
Sedative—
Adults: 65 to 130 mg P.O. or I.M. b.i.d. or t.i.d.

SIDE EFFECTS
CNS: *drowsiness, lethargy, hangover,* paradoxical excitement in elderly patients.
GI: nausea, vomiting.
Skin: rash, urticaria.
Local: pain, swelling, thrombophlebitis.
Other: *Stevens-Johnson syndrome,* angioedema.

INTERACTIONS
Alcohol or other CNS depressants, including narcotic analgesics: excessive CNS and respiratory depression. Use together cautiously.
MAO inhibitors: inhibit metabolism of

barbiturates; may cause prolonged CNS depression. Reduce barbiturate dosage.
Rifampin: may decrease barbiturate levels. Monitor for decreased effect.

NURSING CONSIDERATIONS
• Contraindicated in patients with uncontrolled severe pain, respiratory disease with dyspnea or obstruction, hypersensitivity to barbiturates, previous addiction to sedatives, and porphyria. Use with caution in hepatic, renal, cardiac, or respiratory impairment.
• Use injection solution within 30 minutes after opening container to minimize deterioration. Don't use cloudy solution.
• Administer I.M. injection deeply. Superficial injection may cause pain, sterile abscess, and sloughing.
• Because barbiturates potentiate narcotics, reduce dose when giving during labor. Excessive dose may cause respiratory depression in neonate.
• Remove cigarettes of patient receiving hypnotic dose.
• Supervise walking; raise bed rails, especially for elderly patients.
• Long-term high dosage may cause drug dependence and severe withdrawal symptoms. Withdraw barbiturates gradually.
• Prevent hoarding or self-overdosing by patients who are depressed, suicidal, or drug-dependent, or who have a history of drug abuse. Warn patient that alcohol increases effects of drug, and advise him not to perform activities requiring alertness or skill until CNS response is determined.
• No analgesic action. May cause restlessness or delirium in presence of pain.
• Monitor prothrombin times carefully when patient on barbital starts or ends anticoagulant therapy. Anticoagulant dose may need to be adjusted.
• Watch for signs of barbiturate toxicity: coma, pupillary constriction, cyanosis, clammy skin, hypotension. Overdose can be fatal.

butabarbital
Buta-Barb♦♦, Butisol, Day-Barb♦♦, Medarsed, Neo-Barb♦♦

butabarbital sodium
Controlled Substance Schedule III
Butisol Sodium♦* **

INDICATIONS & DOSAGE
Sedation—
Adults: 15 to 30 mg P.O. t.i.d. or q.i.d.
Children: 6 mg/kg P.O. divided t.i.d. Dosage range 7.5 to 30 mg P.O. t.i.d.
Preoperatively—
Adults: 50 to 100 mg P.O. 60 to 90 minutes before surgery.
Insomnia—
Adults: 50 to 100 mg P.O. at bedtime.

SIDE EFFECTS
CNS: *drowsiness, lethargy, hangover,* paradoxical excitement in elderly patients.
GI: nausea, vomiting.
Skin: rash, urticaria.
Other: *Stevens-Johnson syndrome,* angioedema.

INTERACTIONS
Alcohol or other CNS depressants, including narcotic analgesics: excessive CNS and respiratory depression. Use together cautiously.
MAO inhibitors: inhibit the metabolism of barbiturates; may cause prolonged CNS depression. Reduce barbiturate dosage.
Rifampin: may decrease barbiturate levels. Monitor for decreased effect.

NURSING CONSIDERATIONS
• Contraindicated in patients with uncontrolled severe pain, respiratory disease with dyspnea or obstruction, hypersensitivity to barbiturates, previous addiction to sedatives, porphyria. Use with caution in hepatic or renal impairment.

Italicized side effects are common or life-threatening.
*Liquid form contains alcohol.   **May contain tartrazine.

- Remove cigarettes of patient receiving hypnotic dose.
- Supervise walking; raise bed rails, especially for elderly patients.
- Long-term high dosage may cause drug dependence and severe withdrawal symptoms. Withdraw barbiturates gradually.
- Prevent hoarding or self-overdosing by patients who are depressed, suicidal, or drug-dependent, or who have a history of drug abuse. Warn patient that alcohol increases effects of drug, and advise him not to perform activities requiring alertness or skill until CNS response is determined.
- Butisol sodium elixir is sugar-free.
- Monitor prothrombin times carefully when patient on butabarbital starts or ends anticoagulant therapy. Anticoagulant dose may need to be adjusted.
- Watch for signs of barbiturate toxicity: coma, pupillary constriction, cyanosis, clammy skin, hypotension. Overdose can be fatal.
- Prolonged administration is not recommended: drug not shown to be effective after 14 days. A drug-free interval of at least 1 week is advised.

chloral hydrate
Controlled Substance Schedule IV
Cohidrate, Noctec♦,
Novochlorhydrate♦♦, Oradrate, SK-Chloral Hydrate

INDICATIONS & DOSAGE
Sedation—
Adults: 250 mg P.O. or rectally t.i.d. after meals.
Children: 8 mg/kg P.O. t.i.d. Maximum 500 mg t.i.d.
Insomnia—
Adults: 500 mg to 1 g P.O. or rectally 15 to 30 minutes before bedtime.
Children: 50 mg/kg single dose. Maximum dose 1 g.
Premedication for EEG—
Children: 25 mg/kg single dose. Maximum dose 1 g.

SIDE EFFECTS
CNS: *hangover, drowsiness,* nightmares, dizziness, ataxia.
GI: *nausea,* vomiting, diarrhea, flatulence.
Skin: hypersensitivity reactions.

INTERACTIONS
Alcohol or other CNS depressants, including narcotic analgesics: excessive CNS depression or vasodilation reaction. Use together cautiously.
Furosemide I.V.: sweating, flushes, variable blood pressure, uneasiness. Use together cautiously. Use a different hypnotic drug.

NURSING CONSIDERATIONS
- Contraindicated in patients with marked hepatic or renal impairment, hypersensitivity to chloral hydrate or triclofos. Oral administration contraindicated in gastric disorders. Use with caution in severe cardiac disease, mental depression, suicidal tendencies.
- Dilute or administer with liquid to minimize unpleasant taste and stomach irritation. Administer after meals.
- Prevent hoarding by patients who are depressed, suicidal, or drug-dependent, or who have a history of drug abuse. Warn patient that alcohol increases effects of drug, and advise him not to perform activities requiring alertness or skill until CNS response is determined.
- Remove cigarettes of patient receiving hypnotic dose.
- Supervise walking; raise bed rails, especially for elderly patients.
- Large dosage may raise BUN level.
- May cause false-positive results in glycosuria tests using cupric sulfate as Benedict's solution. Use Clinitest, Clinistix, or Tes-Tape.
- May interfere with fluorometric tests for urine catecholamines and Reddy, Jenkins, Thorn test for urine 17-hydroxycorticosteroids. Do not administer drug for 48 hours before fluorometric test.

- Aqueous solutions incompatible with alkaline substances.
- Store in dark container. Store suppositories in refrigerator.
- If patient is given anticoagulant, monitor for increased prothrombin times during the first several days of therapy. Anticoagulant dose may need to be adjusted.

ethchlorvynol
Controlled Substance Schedule IV
Placidyl♦

INDICATIONS & DOSAGE
Sedation—
Adults: 100 to 200 mg P.O. b.i.d. or t.i.d.
Insomnia—
Adults: 500 mg to 1 g P.O. at bedtime. May repeat 100 to 200 mg if awakened in early a.m.

SIDE EFFECTS
Blood: thrombocytopenia.
CNS: facial numbness, drowsiness, fatigue, nightmares, dizziness, residual sedation, muscular weakness, syncope, ataxia.
CV: hypotension.
EENT: unpleasant aftertaste, blurred vision.
GI: distress, nausea, vomiting.
Skin: rashes, urticaria.

INTERACTIONS
Alcohol or other CNS depressants, including narcotic analgesics; MAO inhibitors: excessive CNS depression. Use together cautiously.

NURSING CONSIDERATIONS
- Contraindicated in patients with uncontrolled pain and porphyria. Use cautiously in hepatic or renal impairment; in elderly or debilitated patients; in mental depression with suicidal tendencies; if patient has previously overreacted to barbiturates or alcohol.
- Give with milk or food to minimize

transient dizziness or ataxia caused by rapid absorption.
- May cause dependence and severe withdrawal symptoms. Withdraw gradually.
- Prevent hoarding or self-overdosing by patients who are depressed, suicidal, or drug-dependent, or who have a history of drug abuse. Overdosage very difficult to treat and has a high mortality. Warn patient that alcohol increases effects of drug, and advise him not to perform activities requiring alertness or skill until CNS response is determined.
- Watch for signs of toxicity, such as poor muscle coordination, confusion, hypothermia, speech or vision disturbances, tremors, or weakness.
- 750-mg strength contains tartrazine dye. May cause allergic reactions in susceptible patients.
- Remove cigarettes of patient receiving hypnotic dose.
- Supervise walking; raise bed rails, especially for elderly patients.
- Slight darkening of liquid from exposure to air and light doesn't affect safety or potency, but store in tight, light-resistant container to avoid possible deterioration.
- Monitor prothrombin times carefully when patient on ethchlorvynol starts or ends anticoagulant therapy. Anticoagulant dose may need to be adjusted.
- Drug is effective for short-term use only; treatment period should not exceed 1 week.

ethinamate
Controlled Substance Schedule IV
Valmid

INDICATIONS & DOSAGE
Insomnia—
Adults: 500 mg to 1 g P.O. 20 minutes before bedtime. Starting dose may be 250 mg for elderly or debilitated patients.
Preanesthetic—

Italicized side effects are common or life-threatening.
*Liquid form contains alcohol.   **May contain tartrazine.

Adults: 500 mg to 1 g P.O. 2½ hours preoperatively.

SIDE EFFECTS
Blood: thrombocytopenia.
GI: mild upset.
Skin: rashes, purpura.
Other: fever (allergic reaction).

INTERACTIONS
None significant.

NURSING CONSIDERATIONS
• Contraindicated for uncontrolled pain. Use cautiously in patients with mental depression, suicidal tendencies, or history of drug abuse.
• Not usually given for daytime sedation because of short duration of effect.
• Long-term use may cause dependence and severe withdrawal symptoms. Withdraw gradually.
• Prevent hoarding or self-overdosing by patients who are depressed, suicidal, or drug-dependent, or who have a history of drug abuse. Warn patient that alcohol increases effects of drug, and advise him not to perform activities requiring alertness or skill until CNS response is determined.
• Abrupt withdrawal may cause blood pressure and pulse rate changes, sweating, and hallucinations.
• Remove cigarettes of patient receiving dose.
• Supervise walking; raise bed rails, especially for elderly patients.
• In overdosage, treat CNS and respiratory depression same as barbiturate intoxication; ethinamate is dialyzable.
• May cause falsely elevated urine 17-ketosteroid (modified Zimmerman reaction) and 17-hydroxycorticosteroid levels (Porter-Silber test).
• Prolonged therapy not recommended; drug is not effective for more than 7 days.

flurazepam hydrochloride
Controlled Substance Schedule IV
Dalmane♦

INDICATIONS & DOSAGE
Insomnia—
Adults: 15 to 30 mg P.O. at bedtime. May repeat dose once.

SIDE EFFECTS
Blood: leukopenia, granulocytopenia.
CNS: *daytime sedation, dizziness, drowsiness, disturbed coordination,* lethargy, confusion, *headache*.

INTERACTIONS
Cimetidine: increased sedation. Monitor carefully.
Alcohol or other CNS depressants, including narcotic analgesics: excessive CNS depression. Use together cautiously.

NURSING CONSIDERATIONS
• Use cautiously in patients with impaired hepatic or renal function, mental depression, suicidal tendencies, or history of drug abuse. Use caution and low end of dosage range for elderly or debilitated patients.
• Prevent hoarding or self-overdosing by patients who are depressed, suicidal, or drug-dependent, or who have a history of drug abuse. Warn patient that alcohol increases effects of drug, and advise him not to perform activities requiring alertness or skill until CNS response is determined.
• Remove cigarettes of patient receiving dose.
• Supervise walking; raise bed rails, especially for elderly patients.
• Dependence is possible with long-term use.

glutethimide
Controlled Substance Schedule III
Doriden♦, Rolathimide

INDICATIONS & DOSAGE
Insomnia—
Adults: 250 to 500 mg P.O. at bedtime.
May be repeated, but not less than 4
hours before intended awakening. Total
daily dose should not exceed 1 g.
Preoperatively—
Adults: 500 mg night before surgery;
500 mg to 1 g 1 hour before anesthesia.
First stage of labor—
500 mg at onset of labor; repeat once if
necessary.
Sedative—
Adults: 125 to 250 mg t.i.d. after
meals.

SIDE EFFECTS
CNS: *residual sedation,* paradoxical
excitation, headache, vertigo.
EENT: dry mouth, blurred vision.
GI: irritation, nausea, diarrhea.
GU: bladder atony.
Skin: rashes, urticaria.

INTERACTIONS
*Alcohol or other CNS depressants, in-
cluding narcotic analgesics:* excessive
CNS depression. Use together cautiously.

NURSING CONSIDERATIONS
• Contraindicated in uncontrolled
pain, severe renal impairment, porphyria. Use cautiously in patients with
mental depression, suicidal tendencies,
history of drug abuse, prostatic hypertrophy, stenosing peptic ulcer, pyloroduodenal or bladder-neck obstruction,
narrow-angle glaucoma, cardiac arrhythmias.
• Drug is effective for short-term use
only.
• Remove cigarettes of patient receiving dose.
• Supervise walking; raise bed rails,
especially for elderly patients.

• Prevent hoarding or self-overdosing
by patients who are depressed, suicidal,
or drug-dependent, or who have a history of drug abuse. Warn patient that
alcohol increases effects of drug, and
advise him not to perform activities requiring alertness or skill for 7 to 8
hours after receiving this drug.
• Abrupt withdrawal may produce nausea, vomiting, nervousness, tremors,
chills, fever, nightmares, insomnia,
tachycardia, delirium, numbness of extremities, hallucinations, dysphagia,
convulsions. Withdraw gradually.
• Monitor prothrombin times carefully
when patient on glutethimide starts or
ends anticoagulant therapy. Anticoagulant dose may need to be adjusted.

hexobarbital
Controlled Substance Schedule III
Sombulex

INDICATIONS & DOSAGE
Sedation—
Adults: 250 mg P.O., repeated as
needed, q 2 to 3 hours.
Insomnia—
Adults: 250 to 500 mg P.O. at bedtime.

SIDE EFFECTS
CNS: *drowsiness, lethargy, hangover,*
paradoxical excitement in elderly pa-
tients.
GI: nausea, vomiting.
Skin: rash, urticaria.
Other: *Stevens-Johnson syndrome,* an-
gioedema.

INTERACTIONS
*Alcohol or other CNS depressants, in-
cluding narcotic analgesics:* excessive
CNS and respiratory depression. Use
together cautiously.
MAO inhibitors: inhibit metabolism of
barbiturates; may cause prolonged CNS
depression. Reduce barbiturate dosage.
Rifampin: may decrease barbiturate
levels. Monitor for decreased effect.

Italicized side effects are common or life-threatening.
∗Liquid form contains alcohol.   ∗∗May contain tartrazine.

NURSING CONSIDERATIONS
• Contraindicated in patients with uncontrolled severe pain, respiratory disease with dyspnea or obstruction, hypersensitivity to barbiturates, previous addiction to sedatives, porphyria. Use with caution in hepatic or renal impairment.

• May be used preoperatively with atropine when morphine contraindicated.

• Because barbiturates potentiate narcotics, reduce dose when giving during labor. Excessive dose may cause respiratory depression in neonate.

• Remove cigarettes of patient receiving hypnotic dose.

• Supervise walking; raise bed rails, especially for elderly patients.

• Long-term high dosage may cause drug dependence and severe withdrawal symptoms. Withdraw barbiturates gradually.

• Prevent hoarding or self-overdosing by patients who are depressed, suicidal, or drug-dependent, or who have a history of drug abuse. Warn patient that alcohol increases effects of drug, and advise him not to perform activities requiring alertness or skill until CNS response is determined.

• Monitor prothrombin times carefully when patient on hexobarbital starts or ends anticoagulant therapy. Anticoagulant dose may need to be adjusted.

• Watch for signs of toxicity: coma, pupillary constriction (pupillary dilation with severe poisoning), clammy skin, hypotension. Overdose can be fatal.

---

mephobarbital
Controlled Substance Schedule IV
Mebaral♦

INDICATIONS & DOSAGE
Sedation—
Adults: 32 to 100 mg P.O. t.i.d. to q.i.d.

Children: 16 to 32 mg P.O. t.i.d. to q.i.d.
Incipient or active delirium tremens—
200 mg P.O. t.i.d.

SIDE EFFECTS
CNS: drowsiness, vertigo, headache, depression, residual sedation after hypnotic dose, paradoxical excitement.
GI: nausea, vomiting, diarrhea.
Skin: hypersensitivity reactions, jaundice.
Other: respiratory depression, apnea; discontinuance of hypnotic doses may induce nightmares or insomnia.

INTERACTIONS
Alcohol or other CNS depressants, including narcotic analgesics: excessive CNS and respiratory depression. Use together cautiously.
MAO inhibitors: inhibit metabolism of barbiturates; may cause prolonged CNS depression. Reduce barbiturate dosage.
Rifampin: may decrease barbiturate levels. Monitor for decreased effect.

NURSING CONSIDERATIONS
• Contraindicated in patients with uncontrolled severe pain, respiratory disease with dyspnea or obstruction, hypersensitivity to barbiturates, previous addiction to sedatives, porphyria. Use with caution in hepatic or renal impairment, impaired cardiac or respiratory function.

• Remove cigarettes of patient receiving hypnotic dose.

• Supervise walking; raise bed rails, especially for elderly patients.

• Long-term high dosage may cause drug dependence and severe withdrawal symptoms. Withdraw barbiturates gradually.

• Prevent hoarding or self-overdosing by patients who are depressed, suicidal, or drug-dependent, or who have a history of drug abuse. Warn patient that alcohol increases effects of drug, and advise him not to perform activities requiring alertness or skill until CNS response is determined.

• Mephobarbital is metabolized to phenobarbital, the active agent.

• Monitor prothrombin times carefully when patient on mephobarbital starts or ends anticoagulant therapy. Anticoagulant dose may need adjustment.

• Watch for signs of toxicity.

methaqualone
Mequin, Quaalude

methaqualone hydrochloride
Controlled Substance Schedule II
Parest, Parest 400, Rouqualone♦♦,
Somnafac, Somnafac Forte,
Tualone♦♦, Vitalone♦♦

INDICATIONS & DOSAGE
Sedation (methaqualone)—
Adults: 75 mg P.O. t.i.d. or q.i.d.
Insomnia (methaqualone)—
Adults: 150 to 300 P.O. at bedtime.
Insomnia (methaqualone hydrochloride)—
Adults: 200 to 400 mg P.O. at bedtime.

SIDE EFFECTS
CNS: headache, dizziness, fatigue, residual sedation, *transient paresthesias of extremities,* restlessness, anxiety, euphoria.
EENT: dry mouth.
GI: anorexia, *nausea, vomiting,* epigastric discomfort.

INTERACTIONS
Alcohol or other CNS depressants, including narcotic analgesics: excessive CNS depression. Use together cautiously.

NURSING CONSIDERATIONS
• Contraindicated in patients with history of drug abuse. Use cautiously in patients with hepatic impairment, mental depression, suicidal tendencies.

• Remove cigarettes of patient receiving hypnotic dose.

• Supervise walking; raise bed rails, especially for elderly patients.

• Warn patient that alcohol increases effects of drug, and advise him not to perform activities requiring alertness or skill until CNS response is determined.

• After switching from another hypnotic to methaqualone, onset of satisfactory hypnotic effect requires 5 to 7 consecutive nights of therapy.

• Prolonged administration of methaqualone is not recommended: drug not shown to be effective more than 14 days.

• One of major drugs of abuse "on the street." Because of high abuse potential, methaqualone is rarely clinically indicated.

methotrimeprazine hydrochloride
Levoprome, Nozinan♦♦

INDICATIONS & DOSAGE
Postoperative analgesia—
Adults and children over 12 years: initially, 2.5 to 7.5 mg I.M. q 4 to 6 hours, then adjust dose.
Preanesthetic medication—
Adults and children over 12 years: 2 to 20 mg I.M. 45 minutes to 3 hours before surgery.
Sedation, analgesia—
Adults and children over 12 years: 10 to 20 mg deep I.M. q 4 to 6 hours as required.
Elderly: 5 to 10 mg I.M. q 4 to 6 hours.

SIDE EFFECTS
Blood: agranulocytosis and other dyscrasias after long-term high dosage.
CNS: *orthostatic hypotension, fainting, weakness, dizziness,* drowsiness, excessive sedation, amnesia, disorientation, euphoria, headache, slurred speech.
CV: *drop in blood pressure,* palpitations.

Italicized side effects are common or life-threatening.
*Liquid form contains alcohol.   **May contain tartrazine.

EENT: dry mouth, nasal congestion.
GI: nausea, vomiting, abdominal discomfort.
GU: difficulty urinating.
Local: *pain, inflammation, swelling at injection site.*

INTERACTIONS
All antihypertensive agents: increased orthostatic hypotension. Don't use together.

NURSING CONSIDERATIONS
• Contraindicated in patients receiving concurrent antihypertensive drug therapy, including MAO inhibitors; also, in patients with history of convulsive disorders; hypersensitivity to phenothiazines; severe cardiac, hepatic, or renal disease; previous overdose of CNS depressant; coma. Use with extreme caution in elderly or debilitated patient with cardiac disease or in any patient who may suffer serious consequences from a sudden drop in blood pressure.
• Use low initial dose in susceptible patient; increase gradually while frequently checking pulse rate, blood pressure, and circulation.
• Expect drop in blood pressure 10 to 20 minutes after I.M. injection.
• Keep patient in bed or closely supervised for 6 to 12 hours after each of the first several injections because orthostatic hypotension may occur. If hypotension is severe, combat with phenylephrine, methoxamine, or levarterenol. Don't use epinephrine.
• Don't use for longer than 30 days except in terminal illness or when narcotics are contraindicated.
• In prolonged use, monitor liver function and blood studies periodically.
• Inject I.M. into large muscle masses. Rotate sites. Do not administer subcutaneously, as local irritation results. I.V. injection not recommended.
• May be mixed in same syringe with reduced dose of atropine and scopolamine. Do not mix with other drugs. Protect solution from light.

methyprylon
Controlled Substance Schedule III
Noludar♦

INDICATIONS & DOSAGE
Insomnia—
Adults: 200 to 400 mg P.O. 15 minutes before bedtime.
Children over 3 months: 50 mg P.O. at bedtime, increased to 200 mg, if necessary. Maximum 400 mg daily.

SIDE EFFECTS
CNS: morning drowsiness, dizziness, headache, paradoxical excitation.
GI: nausea, vomiting, diarrhea, esophagitis.
Skin: rash.

INTERACTIONS
Alcohol or other CNS depressants, including narcotic analgesics: excessive CNS and respiratory depression. Use together cautiously.

NURSING CONSIDERATIONS
• Contraindicated in intermittent porphyria. Use cautiously in patients with renal or hepatic impairment.
• Periodic blood counts are advisable during repeated or long-term use.
• Long-term high dosage may cause drug dependence and severe life-threatening withdrawal symptoms. Withdrawal should be gradual and closely monitored.
• Prevent hoarding or self-overdosing by patients who are depressed, suicidal, or drug-dependent, or who have a history of drug abuse. Warn patient that alcohol increases effect of drug, and advise him not to perform activities requiring alertness or skill until CNS response is determined.
• Remove cigarettes of patient receiving dose.
• Supervise walking; raise bed rails, especially for elderly patients.
• Value of this drug as a sedative has not been established.

Unmarked trade names available in the United States only.
♦ Also available in Canada.   ♦ ♦ Available in Canada only.

• Overdosage symptoms include somnolence, confusion, constricted pupils, respiratory depression, hypotension, coma. Hemodialysis is useful in severe intoxication.

---

paraldehyde
Controlled Substance Schedule IV
Paral

INDICATIONS & DOSAGE
Sedation—
Adults: 4 to 10 ml P.O. or rectally; or 5 ml deep I.M. in upper outer quadrant of buttock. 3 to 5 ml I.V. (in emergency only).
Children: 0.15 ml/kg P.O., rectally, or deep I.M.
Insomnia—
Adults: 10 to 30 ml P.O. or rectally; 10 ml I.M. or I.V.
Children: 0.3 ml/kg P.O., rectally, deep I.M.
Alcohol withdrawal syndrome—
Adults: 5 to 10 ml P.O. or rectally; or 5 ml deep I.M. q 4 to 6 hours for the first 24 hours, not to exceed a total of 60 ml P.O. or 30 ml I.M.; then q 6 hours on following days, not to exceed 40 ml P.O. or 20 ml I.M. per 24 hours.
Tetanus—
Adults: 4 to 5 ml I.V. (well diluted) or 12 ml (diluted 1:10) via gastric tube q 4 hours, p.r.n.; 5 to 10 ml I.M., p.r.n. to control seizures.

SIDE EFFECTS
CV: *I.V. administration may cause pulmonary edema or hemorrhage*, dilation of right side of heart, circulatory collapse.
GI: irritation, *foul breath odor*.
GU: nephrosis with prolonged use.
Skin: *erythematous rash*.
Local: *pain*, sterile abscesses, sloughing of skin, fat necrosis, muscular irritation, nerve damage at I.M. injection site (if injection is near nerve trunk).
Other: *respiratory depression*.

INTERACTIONS
Alcohol: excessive CNS depression. Use with caution.
Disulfiram (Antabuse): increase in paraldehyde and acetaldehyde blood levels. Use together cautiously. May produce toxic disulfiram reaction.

NURSING CONSIDERATIONS
• Contraindicated in bronchopulmonary disease or gastroenteritis with ulceration. Use cautiously in patients with hepatic impairment.
• Give rectal dose in olive oil or cottonseed oil as retention enema: 1 part paraldehyde, 2 parts oil, and 200 ml 0.9% sodium chloride solution.
• Dilute oral dose with iced juice or milk to mask taste and odor and to reduce GI distress.
• Use fresh supply; discard bottles opened more than 24 hours. Don't use if liquid has a brownish color or vinegary odor, or if it contains a precipitate.
• Drug reacts with plastic. Use glass syringe for parenteral dose, and don't put liquid in Styrofoam cup.
• Give I.M. injection deeply, away from nerve trunks, and massage injection site. Do not give more than 5 ml per injection site.
• Watch closely for respiratory depression, especially with repeated doses.
• Long-term high dosage may cause drug dependence and severe withdrawal symptoms. Withdraw gradually, with close monitoring.
• Remove cigarettes of patient receiving hypnotic dose.
• Supervise walking; raise bed rails, especially for elderly patients.
• Ventilate patient's room well to remove exhaled paraldehyde.
• No analgesic effect. May produce excitement or delirium in presence of pain.
• Oral or rectal administration of decomposed paraldehyde may cause severe corrosion of stomach or rectum.

Italicized side effects are common or life-threatening.
*Liquid form contains alcohol.   **May contain tartrazine.

pentobarbital
Controlled Substance Schedule II
Nebralin

pentobarbital sodium
Maso-Pent, Nembutal Sodium♦*,
Nova-Rectal♦♦, Penital,
Pentogen♦♦

INDICATIONS & DOSAGE
Sedation—
Adults: 20 to 40 mg P.O. b.i.d., t.i.d.,
or q.i.d.
Children: 6 mg/kg daily P.O. in divided doses.
Insomnia—
Adults: 100 to 200 mg P.O. at bedtime
or 150 to 200 mg deep I.M.; 100 mg
initially, I.V., then additional doses up
to 500 mg; 120 to 200 mg rectally.
Children: 3 to 5 mg/kg I.M.
Maximum dose: 100 mg. Rectal dosages: 2 months to 1 year, 30 mg; 1 to 4
years, 30 to 60 mg; 5 to 12 years,
60 mg; 12 to 14 years, 60 to 120 mg.
Preanesthetic medication—
Adults: 150 to 200 mg I.M. or P.O. in
2 divided doses.

SIDE EFFECTS
CNS: *drowsiness, lethargy, hangover,*
paradoxical excitement in elderly pa-
tients.
GI: nausea, vomiting.
Skin: rash, urticaria.
Other: *Stevens-Johnson syndrome,* an-
gioedema.

INTERACTIONS
*Alcohol or other CNS depressants, in-
cluding narcotic analgesics:* excessive
CNS and respiratory depression. Use
together cautiously.
MAO inhibitors: inhibit metabolism of
barbiturates; may cause prolonged CNS
depression. Reduce barbiturate dosage.
Rifampin: may decrease barbiturate
levels. Monitor for decreased effect.

NURSING CONSIDERATIONS
• Contraindicated in patients with uncontrolled severe pain, respiratory disease with dyspnea or obstruction,
hypersensitivity to barbiturates, previous addiction to sedatives, porphyria.
Use with caution in hepatic or renal impairment.
• Use injection solution within 30 minutes after opening container to minimize deterioration. Don't use cloudy
solution.
• Parenteral solution alkaline. Avoid
extravasation; may cause tissue necrosis.
• I.V. injection should be reserved for
emergency treatment and should be
given under close supervision. Be prepared to give artificial respiration.
• Administer I.M. injection deeply.
Superficial injection may cause pain,
sterile abscess, and slough.
• Do not mix with other medication.
• Because barbiturates potentiate narcotics, reduce dose when giving during
labor. Excessive dose may cause respiratory depression in neonate.
• Remove cigarettes of patient receiving hypnotic dose.
• Supervise walking; raise bed rails,
especially for elderly patients.
• Long-term high dosage may cause
drug dependence and severe withdrawal
symptoms. Withdraw barbiturates gradually.
• Prevent hoarding or self-overdosing
by patients who are depressed, suicidal,
or drug-dependent, or who have a history of drug abuse. Warn patient that
alcohol increases effects of drug, and
advise him not to perform activities requiring alertness or skill until CNS response is determined.
• No analgesic effect. May cause restlessness or delirium in presence of pain.
• Monitor prothrombin times carefully
when patient on pentobarbital starts or
ends anticoagulant therapy. Anticoagulant dose may need to be adjusted.
• Watch for signs of barbiturate toxicity: coma, pupillary constriction, cya-

---

nosis, clammy skin, hypotension. Overdose can be fatal.
• To ensure accurate dosage, don't divide rectal suppositories.
• Nembutal sodium contains tartrazine dye; may cause allergic reactions in susceptible persons.

---

phenobarbital
Barbipil, Barbita, Eskabarb♦, Gardenal♦, Henomint, Luminal♦, Orprine, PBR 12, SK-Phenobarbital, Solfoton, Solu-barb, Stental

phenobarbital sodium
Controlled Substance Schedule IV
Luminal Sodium♦

INDICATIONS & DOSAGE
Sedation—
Adults: 30 to 120 mg P.O. daily in 2 or 3 divided doses.
Children: 6 mg/kg P.O. divided t.i.d.
Insomnia—
Adults: 100 to 320 mg P.O. or I.M.
Children: 3 to 6 mg/kg.
Preoperative sedation—
Adults: 100 to 200 mg I.M. 60 to 90 minutes before surgery.
Children: 16 to 100 mg I.M. 60 to 90 minutes before surgery.
Hyperbilirubinemia—
Neonates: 7 mg/kg daily P.O. from first to fifth day of life, or 5 mg/kg daily I.M. on first day, repeated P.O. on second to seventh days.
Chronic cholestasis—
Adults: 90 to 180 mg P.O. daily in 2 or 3 divided doses.
Children under 12 years: 3 to 12 mg/kg daily P.O. in 2 or 3 divided doses.

SIDE EFFECTS
CNS: *drowsiness, lethargy, hangover,* paradoxical excitement in elderly patients.
GI: nausea, vomiting.
Skin: rash, urticaria.

Local: pain, swelling, thrombophlebitis, necrosis, nerve injury.
Other: *Stevens-Johnson syndrome,* angioedema.

INTERACTIONS
Alcohol or other CNS depressants, including narcotic analgesics: excessive CNS and respiratory depression. Use together cautiously.
MAO inhibitors: inhibit metabolism of barbiturates; may cause prolonged CNS depression. Reduce barbiturate dosage.
Rifampin: may decrease barbiturate levels. Monitor for decreased effect.
Primidone: monitor for excessive phenobarbital blood levels.

NURSING CONSIDERATIONS
• Contraindicated in patients with uncontrolled severe pain, respiratory disease with dyspnea or obstruction, hypersensitivity to barbiturates, previous addiction to sedatives, porphyria. Use with caution in patients with impaired hepatic, renal, cardiac, or respiratory function; hyperthyroidism; diabetes mellitus; anemia; and in elderly or debilitated patients.
• Use injection solution within 30 minutes after opening container to minimize deterioration. Don't use cloudy solution.
• I.V. injection should be reserved for emergency treatment and should be given under close supervision. Be prepared to give artificial respiration.
• When administering I.V., do not give more than 60 mg/minute.
• Give I.M. injection deeply. Superficial injection may cause pain, sterile abscess, and tissue sloughing.
• Because barbiturates potentiate narcotics, reduce dose when giving during labor. Excessive dose may cause respiratory depression in neonate.
• Remove cigarettes of patient receiving hypnotic dose.
• Supervise walking; raise bed rails, especially for elderly patients.
• Long-term high dosage may cause

Italicized side effects are common or life-threatening.
♦Liquid form contains alcohol.   ♦♦May contain tartrazine.

drug dependence and severe withdrawal symptoms. Withdraw barbiturates gradually.
• Prevent hoarding or self-overdosing by patients who are depressed, suicidal, or drug-dependent, or who have a history of drug abuse. Warn patient that alcohol increases effects of drug, and advise him not to perform activities requiring alertness or skill until CNS response is determined.
• No analgesic action. May cause restlessness or delirium in presence of pain.
• Monitor prothrombin times carefully when patient on phenobarbital starts or ends anticoagulant therapy. Anticoagulant dose may need to be adjusted.
• Watch for signs of barbiturate toxicity: coma, pupillary constriction, cyanosis, clammy skin, hypotension. Overdose can be fatal.

propiomazine hydrochloride
Largon

INDICATIONS & DOSAGE
Sedation—
Adults: 20 to 40 mg I.M. or I.V.
Preoperatively; during surgery; in conjunction with local, nerve block, or spinal anesthetic—
Adults: 10 to 20 mg I.M. or I.V.
Obstetrics—
Adults: 20 to 40 mg I.M. or I.V. during early stages of labor, repeated q 3 hours, if necessary.
Sedation the night before surgery as a preanesthetic, or postoperatively—
Children under 27 kg: 0.55 to 1.1 mg/kg I.M. or I.V.
Children 6 to 12 years: 25 mg I.M. or I.V. in a single dose.
Children 4 to 6 years: 15 mg I.M. or I.V. in a single dose.

SIDE EFFECTS
CNS: dizziness, confusion, amnesia (primarily in the elderly), restlessness.
CV: tachycardia, rise in blood pressure, transient hypotension with rapid I.V. infusion.
EENT: dry mouth.
GI: distress.
Skin: rashes.
Local: vein irritation and thrombophlebitis after I.V. injection.
Other: respiratory depression.

INTERACTIONS
None significant.

NURSING CONSIDERATIONS
• Contraindicated if patients have received large doses of other CNS depressants or are comatose. Use extreme caution in patients with hypertensive crisis.
• Give I.V. injection slowly to avoid transient fall in blood pressure.
• Inject in large, undamaged vein to minimize irritation. Avoid extravasation. Don't inject into artery; irritation may cause severe arteriospasm, impaired circulation, and gangrene.
• Do not give subcutaneously.
• Do not use solution for injection if it is cloudy or contains a precipitate.
• Antiemetic effect may mask signs of drug overdose or other disorders.
• Warn about increased effects of alcohol, tranquilizers, antihistamines, and other CNS depressants and against performing hazardous activities requiring alertness or skill.
• Supervise walking; raise bed rails, especially in elderly patients.
• Propiomazine reverses vasopressor effect of epinephrine. Use norepinephrine when vasopressor effect needed.

secobarbital
Seconal*

secobarbital sodium
Controlled Substance Schedule II
Secogen Sodium♦♦, Seconal
Sodium♦, Seral♦♦

INDICATIONS & DOSAGE
Sedation, preoperatively—
Adults: 200 to 300 mg P.O. 1 to
2 hours before surgery.
Children: 50 to 100 mg P.O. or 4 to
5 mg/kg rectally 1 to 2 hours before
surgery.
Insomnia—
Adults: 100 to 200 mg P.O. or I.M.
Children: 3 to 5 mg/kg I.M., not to exceed 100 mg, with no more than 5 ml
injected in any one site. 4 to 5 mg/kg
rectally.
Acute tetanus convulsion—
Adults and children: 5.5 mg/kg I.M.
or slow I.V., repeated q 3 to 4 hours, if
needed; I.V. injection rate not to exceed
50 mg per 15 seconds.
Acute psychotic agitation—
Adults: 50 mg/minute I.V. up to
250 mg I.V. initially, additional doses
given cautiously after 5 minutes if desired response is not obtained. Not to
exceed 500 mg total.
Status epilepticus—
Adults and children: 250 to 350 mg
I.M. or I.V.

SIDE EFFECTS
CNS: *drowsiness, lethargy, hangover,*
paradoxical excitement in elderly pa-
tients.
GI: nausea, vomiting.
Skin: rash, urticaria.
Other: *Stevens-Johnson syndrome,* an-
gioedema.

INTERACTIONS
*Alcohol or other CNS depressants, in-
cluding narcotic analgesics:* excessive
CNS and respiratory depression. Use
together cautiously.

MAO inhibitors: inhibit metabolism of
barbiturates; may cause prolonged CNS
depression. Reduce barbiturate dosage.
Rifampin: may decrease barbiturate
levels. Monitor for decreased effect.

NURSING CONSIDERATIONS
• Contraindicated in uncontrolled severe pain, respiratory disease with dyspnea or obstruction, hypersensitivity to
barbiturates, previous addiction to sedatives, porphyria. Use with caution in
patients with hepatic or renal impairment; also, in pregnant women with
toxemia or history of bleeding.
• Use injection solution within
30 minutes after opening container to
minimize deterioration. Don't use
cloudy solution.
• I.V. injection should be reserved for
emergency treatment and should be
given under close supervision. Be prepared to give artificial respiration.
• Give I.M. injection deeply. Superficial injection may cause pain, sterile
abscess, and slough.
• Because barbiturates potentiate narcotics, reduce dose when giving during
labor. Excessive dose may cause respiratory depression in neonate.
• Remove cigarettes of patient receiving hypnotic dose.
• Supervise walking; raise bed rails,
especially for elderly patients.
• Long-term high dosage may cause
drug dependence and severe withdrawal
symptoms. Withdraw barbiturates gradually.
• Prevent hoarding or self-overdosing
by patients who are depressed, suicidal,
or drug-dependent, or who have a history of drug abuse. Warn patient that
alcohol increases effects of drug, and
advise him not to perform activities requiring alertness or skill until CNS response is determined.
• If patient has renal insufficiency, use
sterile drug reconstituted with sterile
water for injection. Avoid commercial
solution containing polyethylene glycol;
it may irritate kidneys.

Italicized side effects are common or life-threatening.
*Liquid form contains alcohol.   **May contain tartrazine.

- Secobarbital in polyethylene glycol must be refrigerated.
- Secobarbital sodium injection not compatible with lactated Ringer's solution.
- Sterile secobarbital sodium compatible with Ringer's injection and normal saline solution. Don't mix with acidic solutions.
- To reconstitute, rotate ampul. Do not shake.
- Monitor prothrombin times carefully when patient on secobarbital starts or ends anticoagulant therapy. Anticoagulant dose may need to be adjusted.
- Watch for signs of barbiturate toxicity: coma, pupillary construction, cyanosis, clammy skin, hypotension. Overdose can be fatal.

talbutal
Controlled Substance Schedule III
Lotusate

INDICATIONS & DOSAGE
Insomnia—
Adults: 120 mg P.O. at bedtime.

SIDE EFFECTS
CNS: *drowsiness, lethargy, hangover,* paradoxical excitement in elderly patients.
GI: nausea, vomiting.
Skin: rash, urticaria.
Other: *Stevens-Johnson syndrome,* angioedema.

INTERACTIONS
Alcohol or other CNS depressants, including narcotic analgesics: excessive CNS and respiratory depression. Use together cautiously.
MAO inhibitors: inhibit the metabolism of barbiturates; may cause prolonged CNS depression. Reduce barbiturate dosage.
Rifampin: may decrease barbiturate levels. Monitor for decreased effect.

NURSING CONSIDERATIONS
- Contraindicated in patients with uncontrolled severe pain, respiratory disease with dyspnea or obstruction, hypersensitivity to barbiturates, previous addiction to sedatives, porphyria. Use with caution in hepatic or renal impairment.
- Remove cigarettes of patient receiving hypnotic dose.
- Supervise walking; raise bed rails, especially for elderly patients.
- Long-term high dosage may cause drug dependence and severe withdrawal symptoms. Withdraw barbiturates gradually.
- Prevent hoarding or self-overdosing by patients who are depressed, suicidal, or drug-dependent, or who have a history of drug abuse. Warn patient that alcohol increases effects of drug, and advise him not to perform activities requiring alertness or skill until CNS response is determined.
- Monitor prothrombin times carefully when patient on talbutal starts or ends anticoagulant therapy. Anticoagulant dose may need to be adjusted.
- Watch for signs of barbiturate toxicity: coma, pupillary constriction, cyanosis, clammy skin, hypotension. Overdose can be fatal.

temazepam
Controlled Substance Schedule IV
Restoril

INDICATIONS & DOSAGE
Insomnia—
Adults: 15 to 30 mg P.O. at bedtime.

SIDE EFFECTS
CNS: *drowsiness, dizziness, lethargy,* disturbed coordination, daytime sedation, confusion.
GI: anorexia, diarrhea.

INTERACTIONS
Cimetidine: increased sedation. Monitor carefully.

NURSING CONSIDERATIONS
• Use cautiously in patients with impaired hepatic or renal function; in patients with mental depression or suicidal tendencies; and in patients with history of drug abuse. Use caution and low end of dosage range for elderly or debilitated patients.
• Prevent hoarding or self-overdosing by patients who are depressed, suicidal, or drug-dependent, or who have a history of drug abuse. Warn about increased alcohol effects and against hazardous activity requiring alertness or skill.
• Remove cigarettes of patient receiving drug.
• Supervise walking; raise bed rails, especially for elderly patients
• May have less residual sedative effects ("hangover") the next day than flurazepam and diazepam. Relatively short acting.
• May take as long as 2 to 2½ hours for onset of action.

triclofos sodium
Triclos

INDICATIONS & DOSAGE
Insomnia—
Adults: 1.5 g P.O. 15 to 20 minutes before bedtime.
To induce sleep in EEG—
Children under 12 years: 22 mg/kg P.O.

SIDE EFFECTS
CNS: light-headedness, dizziness, hangover, *drowsiness,* headache, ataxia.
GI: *nausea,* vomiting, flatulence, bad taste in mouth.
Skin: hypersensitivity reactions.

INTERACTIONS
*Alcohol or other CNS depressants, in-*cluding *narcotic analgesics:* excessive CNS depression or vasodilation. Use together cautiously.
Furosemide I.V.: possible sweating, flushes, variable blood pressure, uneasiness. Use together cautiously.

NURSING CONSIDERATIONS
• Contraindicated in patients with hepatic or renal impairment, hypersensitivity to triclofos sodium or chloral hydrate; and in women in labor. Use with caution in patients with cardiac arrhythmias, severe cardiac disease, mental depression, suicidal tendencies, or drug dependency.
• In prolonged use, monitor liver function and blood studies periodically.
• Withdraw slowly after prolonged use to avoid delirium, tremors, hallucinations.
• Prevent hoarding or self-overdosing by patients who are depressed, suicidal, or drug-dependent, or who have a history of drug abuse. Warn patient that alcohol increases effects of drug, and advise him not to perform activities requiring alertness or skill until CNS response is determined.
• Supervise walking; raise bed rails, especially for elderly patients.
• May cause false-positive results in glycosuria tests using cupric sulfate as Benedict's or Fehling's solution. Use Clinitest, Clinistix, or Tes-Tape.
• May interfere with fluorometric tests for urine catecholamines and Reddy, Jenkins, Thorn test for urine 17-hydroxycorticosteroids. Don't administer drug for 48 hours before fluorometric test.
• Monitor prothrombin times carefully when patient on triclofos starts or ends anticoagulant therapy. Anticoagulant dose may need to be adjusted.

Italicized side effects are common or life-threatening.
∗Liquid form contains alcohol.   ∗∗May contain tartrazine.

27

Anticonvulsants

acetazolamide
acetazolamide sodium
bromides
carbamazepine
clonazepam
diazepam
ethosuximide
ethotoin
magnesium sulfate
mephenytoin
mephobarbital
metharbital
methsuximide
paraldehyde
paramethadione
phenacemide
phenobarbital
phenobarbital sodium
phensuximide
phenytoin sodium (extended)
phenytoin sodium (prompt)
primidone
trimethadione
valproic acid
valproate sodium

MECHANISM OF ACTION

- Acetazolamide may inhibit carbonic anhydrase in the central nervous system (CNS) and decrease abnormal paroxysmal or excessive neuronal discharge.
- Barbiturate derivatives depress monosynaptic and polysynaptic transmission in the CNS and increase the threshold for seizure activity in the motor cortex.
- Benzodiazepine derivatives appear to act on the limbic system, thalamus, and hypothalamus to produce anticonvulsant effects.
- Bromides depress all nerve tissue, but their exact mechanism of CNS depression is unknown.
- Hydantoin derivatives and carbamazepine stabilize neuronal membranes and limit seizure activity by either increasing efflux or decreasing influx of sodium ions across cell membranes in the motor cortex during generation of nerve impulses.
- Magnesium sulfate may decrease acetylcholine released by nerve impulse, but its anticonvulsant mechanism is unknown.
- Oxazolidone derivatives raise the threshold for cortical seizure but do not modify seizure pattern. They decrease projection of focal activity and reduce both repetitive spinal-cord transmission and spike-and-wave patterns of absence (petit mal) seizures.
- Paraldehyde's mechanism of action is unknown.
- Succinimide derivatives increase seizure threshold. They reduce the paroxysmal spike-and-wave pattern of absence seizures by depressing nerve transmisson in the motor cortex.
- Valproic acid may increase brain levels of gamma-aminobutyric acid, which transmits inhibitory nerve impulses in the CNS.

COMBINATION PRODUCTS

DILANTIN WITH PHENOBARBITAL♦: phenytoin sodium 100 mg and phenobarbital 16 mg.
DILANTIN WITH PHENOBARBITAL♦: phenytoin sodium 100 mg and phenobarbital 32 mg.
PHELANTIN KAPSEALS♦: phenytoin 100 mg, phenobarbital 30 mg, and

Unmarked trade names available in the United States only.
♦ Also available in Canada. ♦♦ Available in Canada only.

methamphetamine hydrochloride
2.5 mg.

acetazolamide
Acetazolam♦♦, Diamox♦, Hydrazol,
Roxolamide

acetazolamide sodium
Diamox♦

INDICATIONS & DOSAGE
*Myoclonic seizures, refractory grand
mal or petit mal, mixed seizures—*
Adults: 375 mg P.O., I.M., or I.V.
daily up to 250 mg q.i.d. Or, Diamox
Sequels 250 to 500 mg daily or b.i.d.
Initial dose when used with other anticonvulsants usually 250 mg daily.
Children: 8 to 30 mg/kg daily, divided
t.i.d. or q.i.d. Maximum dose 1.5 g
daily, or 300 to 900 mg/m^2 daily.

SIDE EFFECTS
Blood: leukopenia, *aplastic anemia.*
CNS: paresthesias, drowsiness.
EENT: transient myopia.
GI: anorexia, nausea, vomiting.
GU: crystalluria, renal calculi.
Metabolic: *hyperchloremic acidosis.*
Skin: rash.
Local: *pain at injection site,* sterile ab-
scesses.

INTERACTIONS
Methenamine: antagonized methenamine effect. If used together, urine
must be kept at pH 5.5 or lower.

NURSING CONSIDERATIONS
• Contraindicated in sulfonamide sensitivity, chronic pulmonary disease,
renal or hepatic dysfunction, Addison's
disease (adrenocortical insufficiency),
hyponatremia, hypokalemia, hyperchloremic acidosis, chronic noncongee-
tive narrow-angle glaucoma. Use cautiously in hypercalciuria, diabetes mellitus, gout, and respiratory acidosis.
• Obtain CBC and serum electrolytes

every 3 months; serum calcium every 6
months.
• Don't withdraw drug suddenly. Call
doctor if side effects develop.
• Warn patient to avoid activities that
require alertness and good psychomotor coordination until CNS response
to drug has been determined.
• This drug is also a diuretic. Use diuretic precautions.
• Chronic use may result in tolerance
to drug.
• Reconstitute 500-mg vial with 5 ml
sterile water for injection. Provides 100
mg/ml. Refrigerate reconstituted solution. Discard after 24 hours.
• Oral liquid: soften 1 tablet in 2 teaspoonfuls of very warm water and add
to 2 teaspoonfuls honey or syrup (chocolate, cherry). Don't use fruit juice.
• May cause hyperglycemia in predi-
abetics or diabetics on insulin or oral
drugs. Monitor patients carefully.
• Observe and report signs of hypokalemia or metabolic acidosis.
• Rarely used alone. Usually given
with other anticonvulsants.
• Has been successfully used to treat
and prevent "mountain sickness."

bromides
Bromide, Calcium Bromide,
Lanabrom, Peacock's Bromides,
Potassium Bromide, Sodium
Bromide

INDICATIONS & DOSAGE
Major motor and myoclonic seizures—
Adults: 1 to 2 g t.i.d.
Children: 50 to 100 mg/kg daily, di-
vided equally t.i.d. Or, 1.5 to 3 g/m^2
daily in divided doses t.i.d.

SIDE EFFECTS
CNS: *drowsiness,* mental dullness,
toxic psychosis.
Skin: *rashes* (acneiform, morbilliform,
granulomatous), *Stevens-Johnson syndrome.*

Italicized side effects are common or life-threatening.
∗Liquid form contains alcohol.　　∗∗May contain tartrazine.

INTERACTIONS
None significant.

NURSING CONSIDERATIONS
• Contraindicated in debilitated, dehydrated, or alcoholic patients, or in those with cerebral arteriosclerosis, organic brain damage, impaired renal function, severe depression, neurologic or psychological disorders, tuberculosis or skin disorders (acne, dermatitis herpetiformis). Especially in adults, use may lead to chronic toxicity (mental, psychic, GI, and neurologic disturbances; skin eruptions). May be mistaken for acute alcohol intoxication, tabes dorsalis, cerebral tumor, uremia, or multiple sclerosis.
• Watch closely for toxicity. In adults, blood levels above 5 mEq/liter may cause toxicity.
• Bromides are better tolerated in children than in adults. Therapeutic blood level in children usually 20 to 25 mEq/liter (200 mg/100 ml), but range is 10 to 35 mEq/liter.
• Effect may not be seen for 2 to 3 weeks.
• Patients should follow a low chloride diet.
• Notify doctor if side effects develop.
• Rarely used; considered a drug of last resort.

carbamazepine
Tegretol♦

INDICATIONS & DOSAGE
Psychomotor, temporal lobe, grand mal, mixed seizure patterns—
Adults and children over 12 years: 200 mg P.O. b.i.d. on day 1. May increase by 200 mg P.O. per day, in divided doses at 6- to 8-hour intervals. Adjust to minimum effective level when control achieved. Usual maintenance 800 to 1,200 mg daily. Don't exceed 1 g total daily dose in 12- to 15-year-olds and 1,200 mg P.O. daily in patients over 15 years.

Children under 12 years: 10 to 20 mg/kg P.O daily in 2 to 4 divided doses.
Trigeminal neuralgia—
Adults: 100 mg P.O. b.i.d. with meals on day 1. Increase by 100 mg q 12 hours until pain relieved. Don't exceed 1.2 g daily. Maintenance dose 200 to 400 mg P.O. b.i.d.

SIDE EFFECTS
Blood: *aplastic anemia, agranulocytosis,* eosinophilia, leukocytosis, *thrombocytopenia.*
CNS: dizziness, *vertigo, drowsiness,* fatigue, *ataxia.*
CV: congestive heart failure, hypertension, hypotension, aggravation of coronary artery disease.
EENT: conjunctivitis, dry mouth and pharynx, blurred vision, diplopia, nystagmus.
GI: *nausea,* vomiting, abdominal pain, diarrhea, anorexia, *stomatitis,* glossitis, *dry mouth.*
GU: urinary frequency or retention, impotence, albuminuria, glycosuria, elevated BUN.
Hepatic: abnormal liver function tests, hepatitis.
Metabolic: water intoxication.
Skin: *rash,* urticaria, erythema multiforme, *Stevens-Johnson syndrome.*
Other: diaphoresis, fever, chills, pulmonary hypersensitivity.

INTERACTIONS
Troleandomycin, erythromycin, isoniazid: may increase carbamazepine blood levels. Use cautiously.
Propoxyphene: may raise carbamazepine levels. Use another analgesic.

NURSING CONSIDERATIONS
• Contraindicated in patients with bone-marrow depression, hypersensitivity to carbamazepine or tricyclic antidepressants. Use cautiously in cardiac, renal, or hepatic damage, or increased intraocular pressure.
• Warn patient to avoid activities that

require alertness and good psycho-motor coordination until CNS response to drug has been determined.
• Never stop the drug suddenly when treating seizures or status epilepticus. Notify doctor immediately if side effects occur.
• Obtain CBC, platelet and reticulo-cyte counts, and serum iron levels weekly for first 3 months, then monthly. If bone-marrow depression develops, stop drug. Obtain urinalysis, BUN, and liver function tests every 3 months. Periodic eye examinations are recommended.
• Tell patient to notify doctor immediately if fever, sore throat, mouth ulcers, or easy bruising occurs.
• Therapeutic anticonvulsant blood level is 3 to 9 mcg/ml.
• When used for trigeminal neuralgia, an attempt should be made every 3 months to decrease dose or stop drug.

---

clonazepam
Controlled Substance Schedule IV
Clonopin, Rivotril♦

INDICATIONS & DOSAGE
Petit mal and petit mal variant (Lennox syndrome); akinetic and myoclonic seizures—
Adults: initial dose should not exceed 1.5 mg P.O. per day, divided into 3 doses. May be increased by 0.5 to 1 mg q 3 days until seizures controlled. Maximum recommended daily dose is 20 mg.
Children up to 10 years or 30 kg: 0.01 to 0.03 mg/kg P.O. daily (not to exceed 0.05 mg/kg daily), divided q 8 hours. Increase dosage by 0.25 to 0.5 mg q third day to a maximum maintenance dose of 0.1 mg to 0.2 mg/kg daily.

SIDE EFFECTS
Blood: leukopenia, thrombocytopenia, eosinophilia.
CNS: *drowsiness, ataxia, behavioral*

disturbances (especially in children), slurred speech, tremor, confusion.
EENT: *increased salivation,* diplopia, nystagmus, abnormal eye movements.
GI: constipation, gastritis, change in appetite, nausea, abnormal thirst, sore gums.
GU: dysuria, enuresis, nocturia, urinary retention.
Skin: rash.
Other: respiratory depression.

INTERACTIONS
None significant.

NURSING CONSIDERATIONS
• Contraindicated in hepatic disease; chlordiazepoxide, diazepam, or other benzodiazepine sensitivity; acute narrow-angle glaucoma. Use with caution in chronic respiratory disease, impaired renal function, open-angle glaucoma.
• Warn patient to avoid activities that require alertness and good psycho-motor coordination until CNS response to drug has been determined.
• Never withdraw drug suddenly. Call doctor at once if side effects develop.
• Obtain periodic CBC and liver function tests.
• Monitor patient for oversedation.
• Withdrawal symptoms similar to barbiturates.

---

diazepam
Controlled Substance Schedule IV
Valium♦

INDICATIONS & DOSAGE
Status epilepticus—
Adults: 5 to 20 mg slow I.V. push 5 mg/minute; may repeat 5 to 10 minutes up to maximum total dose of 60 mg. Use 2 to 5 mg in elderly or debilitated patients. May repeat therapy in 20 to 30 minutes with caution if seizures recur.
Children: 0.1 to 0.3 mg/kg slow I.V. push (1 mg/minute over 3 minutes). May repeat q 15 minutes for 2 doses.

Italicized side effects are common or life-threatening.
∗Liquid form contains alcohol.   ∗∗May contain tartrazine.

Maximum single dose: children under 5 years—5 mg; children over 5 years—10 mg.

Adjunctive use in convulsive disorders—
Adults and children: 2 to 10 mg P.O. b.i.d., t.i.d., or q.i.d. Or, 15 to 30 mg of extended-release capsule once daily.

SIDE EFFECTS
CNS: fatigue, *drowsiness, ataxia*, dizziness, headache, dysarthria, slurred speech, tremor.
CV: hypotension, bradycardia, *cardiovascular collapse*.
EENT: diplopia, blurred vision, nystagmus.
GI: nausea, constipation, change in salivation.
GU: incontinence, urinary retention.
Local: *pain, phlebitis at injection site*.
Skin: rash, urticaria.

INTERACTIONS
None significant.

NURSING CONSIDERATIONS
• Contraindicated in shock, psychosis, coma, acute alcohol intoxication with depression of vital signs, acute narrow-angle glaucoma. Use cautiously in elderly or debilitated patients; those with limited pulmonary reserve; those in whom blood pressure drop might cause cardiovascular complications; and also those with history of anxiety states with suicidal tendencies, blood dyscrasias, hepatic or renal damage, open-angle glaucoma, or alcoholism.
• Monitor respirations every 5 to 15 minutes and before each I.V. repeated dose. Have emergency resuscitative equipment and oxygen at bedside.
• Do not mix with other drugs or I.V. fluids.
• Do not use small veins such as those on dorsum of hand or wrist.
• Avoid extravasation.
• Give slowly I.V. at rate not exceeding 5 mg/minute. Watch for phlebitis at injection site.

• Do not infuse drug through plastic tubing. Do not store in plastic syringe.
• Drug should not be withdrawn abruptly.
• Tell patient to avoid heavy use of alcohol or other CNS depressants.
• Effectiveness poor when administered I.M.
• Seizures may recur within 20 to 30 minutes of initial control, because of redistribution of the drug.
• Continuous infusions of 1 to 10 mg hourly have been used to prevent seizure recurrence.

ethosuximide
Zarontin♦

INDICATIONS & DOSAGE
Petit mal—
Adults and children over 6 years: initially, 250 mg P.O. b.i.d. May increase by 250 mg q 4 to 7 days up to 1.5 g daily.
Children 3 to 6 years: 250 mg P.O. daily or 125 mg P.O. b.i.d. May increase by 250 mg q 4 to 7 days up to 1.5 g daily.

SIDE EFFECTS
Blood: leukopenia, eosinophilia, *agranulocytosis,* pancytopenia, *aplastic anemia*.
CNS: *drowsiness,* headache, *fatigue, dizziness,* ataxia, irritability, hiccups, *euphoria, lethargy*.
EENT: myopia.
GI: *nausea, vomiting,* diarrhea, gum hypertrophy, weight loss, cramps, tongue swelling, *anorexia, epigastric and abdominal pain*.
GU: vaginal bleeding.
Skin: urticaria, pruritic and erythematous rashes, hirsutism.

INTERACTIONS
None significant.

NURSING CONSIDERATIONS
• Contraindicated in hypersensitivity

---

to succinimide derivatives. Use cautiously in hepatic or renal disease.
• Never withdraw drug suddenly. Abrupt withdrawal may precipitate petit mal seizures. Call doctor immediately if side effects develop.
• Warn patient to avoid activities that require alertness and good psychomotor coordination until CNS response to drug has been determined.
• Obtain CBC every 3 months.
• Therapeutic blood levels 40 to 80 mcg/ml.
• May increase frequency of grand mal seizures when used alone in patients who have mixed types of seizures.
• May cause positive direct Coombs' test.

ethotoin
Peganone

INDICATIONS & DOSAGE
Grand mal or psychomotor seizures—
Adults: initially, 250 mg P.O. q.i.d. after meals. May increase slowly over several days to 3 g daily divided q.i.d.
Children: initially, 250 mg P.O. b.i.d. May increase up to 250 mg P.O. q.i.d.

SIDE EFFECTS
Blood: thrombocytopenia, leukopenia, *agranulocytosis,* pancytopenia, megaloblastic anemia.
CNS: fatigue, insomnia, dizziness, headache, numbness.
CV: chest pain.
EENT: diplopia, nystagmus.
GI: nausea, vomiting, diarrhea, gingival hyperplasia (rare).
Skin: rash.
Other: fever, lymphadenopathy.

INTERACTIONS
Alcohol; folic acid, loxapine succinate: monitor for decreased ethotoin activity.
Oral anticoagulants, antihistamines, chloramphenicol, diazepam, diazoxide, disulfiram, isoniazid, phenylbutazone, phenyramidol, salicylates, sulfamethi-

zole, valproate: monitor for increased ethotoin activity and toxicity.

NURSING CONSIDERATIONS
• Contraindicated in patients with hydantoin hypersensitivity and in hepatic or hematologic disorders. Use cautiously in patients receiving other hydantoin derivatives.
• Never withdraw drug suddenly. Call doctor at once if side effects develop.
• Warn patient to avoid activities that require alertness and good psychomotor coordination until CNS response to drug has been determined.
• Obtain CBC and urinalysis when therapy starts and monthly thereafter.
• Give after meals. Schedule doses as evenly as possible over 24 hours.
• Stop at once if lymphadenopathy or lupus-like syndrome develops.
• Heavy use of alcohol may diminish benefits of drug.
• Hydantoin derivative of choice in young adults who are prone to gingival hyperplasia caused by phenytoin.

magnesium sulfate

INDICATIONS & DOSAGE
Hypomagnesemic seizures—
Adults: 1 to 2 g (as 10% solution) I.V. over 15 minutes, then 1 g I.M. q 4 to 6 hours, based on patient's response and magnesium blood levels.
Children: seizures secondary to hypomagnesemia in acute nephritis—0.2 ml/kg of 50% solution I.M. q 4 to 6 hours, p.r.n. or 100 mg/kg of 10% solution I.V. very slowly. Titrate dosage according to magnesium blood levels and seizure response.
Prevention or control of seizures in preeclampsia or eclampsia—
Women: initially, 4 g I.V. in 250 ml 5% dextrose in water and 4 g deep I.M. each buttock; then 4 g deep I.M. into alternate buttock q 4 hours, p.r.n. Alternatively, 4 g I.V. loading dose fol-

lowed by 1 to 4 g hourly as an I.V. infusion.

SIDE EFFECTS
CNS: *sweating,* drowsiness, *depressed reflexes,* flaccid paralysis, hypothermia.
CV: *hypotension, flushing, circulatory collapse,* depressed cardiac function, *heart block.*
Other: *respiratory paralysis,* hypocalcemia.

INTERACTIONS
Neuromuscular blocking agents: may cause increased neuromuscular blockade. Use cautiously.

NURSING CONSIDERATIONS
• Use cautiously in patients with impaired renal function, myocardial damage, heart block, and in women in labor.
• Magnesium sulfate can decrease the frequency and force of uterine contractions.
• Keep I.V. calcium gluconate available to reverse magnesium intoxication; however, use cautiously in patient undergoing digitalization due to danger of arrhythmias.
• Monitor vital signs every 15 minutes when giving drug I.V.
• Watch for respiratory depression and signs of heart block. Respirations should be approximately 16 per minute before each dose given.
• Monitor intake and output. Urinary output should be 100 ml or more in 4-hour period before each dose.
• Check magnesium blood levels after repeated doses. Disappearance of knee jerk and patellar reflexes is a sign of pending magnesium toxicity.
• Maximum infusion rate is 150 mg per minute. Rapid drip will induce uncomfortable feeling of heat.
• Especially when given I.V. to toxemic mothers within 24 hours before delivery, observe newborn for signs of magnesium toxicity, including neuromuscular or respiratory depression.
• Signs of hypermagnesemia begin to appear at blood levels of 4 mEq/liter.
• I.V. infusion should not be faster than 150 mg/minute.

mephenytoin
Mesantoin♦

INDICATIONS & DOSAGE
Refractory grand mal, focal, or psychomotor seizures—
Adults: 50 to 100 mg P.O. daily. May increase by 50 to 100 mg at weekly intervals up to 200 mg P.O. t.i.d.
Children: initial dose 50 to 100 mg P.O. daily or 100 to 450 mg/m² P.O. daily in 3 divided doses. May increase slowly by 50 to 100 mg at weekly intervals up to 200 mg P.O. t.i.d., divided q 8 hours. Dosage must be adjusted individually.

SIDE EFFECTS
Blood: *leukopenia,* neutropenia, *agranulocytosis,* thrombocytopenia, pancytopenia, eosinophilia.
CNS: ataxia, *drowsiness,* fatigue, irritability, choreiform movements, depression, tremor, sleeplessness, dizziness (usually transient).
EENT: photophobia, conjunctivitis, diplopia, nystagmus.
GI: gingival hyperplasia, nausea and vomiting (with prolonged use).
Skin: *rashes, exfoliative dermatitis.*
Other: hypertrichosis, edema, dysarthria, lymphadenopathy, polyarthropathy, pulmonary fibrosis.

INTERACTIONS
Alcohol (chronic abuse), folic acid, loxapine succinate: monitor for decreased mephenytoin activity.
Alcohol (acute intoxication), oral anticoagulants, antihistamines, chloramphenicol, diazepam, diazoxide, disulfiram, isoniazid, phenylbutazone, phenyramidol, salicylates, sulfamethizole,

valproate: monitor for increased me-phenytoin activity and toxicity.

NURSING CONSIDERATIONS
• Contraindicated in hydantoin hyper-sensitivity. Use cautiously in patients receiving other hydantoin derivatives.
• Tell patient to notify doctor if fever, sore throat, bleeding, or rash occurs.
• Check CBC and platelet count initially and every 2 weeks thereafter, up to 2 weeks after full dose attained; then monthly for first year and every 3 months thereafter. Stop drug if neutrophil count becomes less than 1,600/mm^3.
• Never withdraw drug suddenly. Call doctor if side effects develop.
• Warn patient to avoid activities that require alertness and good psychomotor coordination until CNS response to drug has been determined.
• Therapeutic blood level is 5 to 20 mcg/ml.
• Heavy use of alcohol may diminish benefit of drug.

mephobarbital
Controlled Substance Schedule IV
Mebaral♦, Mentabal, Mephoral

INDICATIONS & DOSAGE
Grand or petit mal—
Adults: 400 to 600 mg P.O. daily or in divided doses.
Children: 6 to 12 mg/kg P.O. daily, divided q 6 to 8 hours (smaller doses are given initially and increased over 4 to 5 days as needed).

SIDE EFFECTS
Blood: megaloblastic anemia, agranulocytosis, thrombocytopenia.
CNS: dizziness, headache, hangover, confusion, paradoxical excitation, exacerbation of existing pain, drowsiness.
CV: hypotension.
GI: nausea, vomiting, epigastric pain.
Skin: urticaria, morbilliform rash,

blisters, purpura, erythema multiforme.
Other: allergic reactions (facial edema).

INTERACTIONS
Alcohol and other CNS depressants, including narcotic analgesics: excessive CNS depression. Use cautiously.
MAO inhibitors: potentiated barbiturate effect. Monitor patient for increased CNS and respiratory depression.
Rifampin: may decrease barbiturate levels. Monitor for decreased effect.

NURSING CONSIDERATIONS
• Contraindicated in barbiturate hypersensitivity, porphyria, and respiratory disease with dyspnea or obstruction. Use cautiously in hepatic, renal, cardiac, or respiratory function impairment, and in myasthenia gravis and myxedema.
• Never withdraw drug suddenly. Call doctor at once if side effects develop.
• Warn patient to avoid activities that require alertness and good psychomotor coordination until CNS response to drug has been determined.
• Store in light-resistant container.
• In adults, give total or largest dose at night if seizures occur then.
• Three quarters of drug metabolized to phenobarbital; therapeutic blood levels as phenobarbital are 15 to 40 mcg/ml.
• Monitor prothrombin times carefully when patient on mephobarbital starts or ends anticoagulant therapy. Anticoagulant dose may need to be adjusted.

metharbital
Controlled Substance Schedule III
Gemonil

INDICATIONS & DOSAGE
Grand or petit mal; myoclonic or mixed seizures—
Adults: initially, 100 mg P.O. daily to

Italicized side effects are common or life-threatening.
✴Liquid form contains alcohol.   ✴✴May contain tartrazine.

t.i.d. May increase to 800 mg daily in divided doses.
Children: 5 to 15 mg/kg P.O. daily, divided t.i.d. May increase to 50 to 100 mg P.O. daily, b.i.d., or t.i.d.

SIDE EFFECTS
Blood: megaloblastic anemia, *agranulocytosis,* thrombocytopenia.
CNS: dizziness, irritability, drowsiness, headache, confusion, excitation.
CV: hypotension.
GI: nausea, vomiting, discomfort.
Skin: rash, urticaria, purpura, erythema multiforme.

INTERACTIONS
Alcohol and other CNS depressants, including narcotic analgesics: excessive CNS depression. Use cautiously.
MAO inhibitors: potentiated barbiturate effect. Monitor patient for increased CNS and respiratory depression.
Rifampin: may decrease barbiturate levels. Monitor for decreased effect.

NURSING CONSIDERATIONS
• Contraindicated in barbiturate hypersensitivity, in manifest or latent porphyria, and in respiratory disease with dyspnea or obstruction. Use cautiously in hepatic, cardiac, or renal impairment.
• Don't stop drug abruptly. Call doctor at once if side effects develop.
• Warn patient to avoid activities that require alertness and good psychomotor coordination until response to drug is determined.
• Monitor prothrombin times carefully when patient on metharbital starts or ends anticoagulant therapy. Anticoagulant dose may need to be adjusted.

methsuximide
Celontin♦

INDICATIONS & DOSAGE
Refractory petit mal—
Adults and children: initially, 300 mg P.O. daily. May increase by 300 mg

weekly. Maximum daily dosage of 1.2 g in divided doses.

SIDE EFFECTS
Blood: eosinophilia, leukopenia, monocytosis, pancytopenia.
CNS: *drowsiness, ataxia, dizziness,* irritability, nervousness, headache, insomnia, confusion, depression, aggressiveness.
EENT: blurred vision, photophobia, periorbital edema.
GI: *nausea, vomiting, anorexia,* diarrhea, weight loss, abdominal or epigastric pain.
Skin: urticaria, pruritic and erythematous rashes.

INTERACTIONS
None significant.

NURSING CONSIDERATIONS
• Contraindicated in hypersensitivity to succinimide derivatives. Use cautiously in hepatic or renal dysfunction.
• Never change or withdraw drug suddenly. Abrupt withdrawal may precipitate petit mal seizures. Call doctor immediately if side effects develop.
• Warn patient to avoid activities that require alertness and good psychomotor coordination until CNS response to drug has been determined.
• Obtain CBC every 3 months; urinalysis and liver function tests every 6 months.
• May color urine pink or brown.
• Therapeutic blood levels 40 to 100 mcg/ml.

paraldehyde
Controlled Substance Schedule IV
Paral

INDICATIONS & DOSAGE
Refractory grand mal seizures, status epilepticus—
Adults: 5 to 10 ml I.M. (divide 10 ml

dose into 2 injections); 0.2 to 0.4 ml/kg in 0.9% saline injection I.V.

Children: 0.15 ml/kg dose deep I.M. q 4 to 6 hours, p.r.n.; or 0.3 ml/kg rectally in olive oil q 4 to 6 hours; or 1 ml per year of age not to exceed 5 ml, repeated in 1 hour, p.r.n.; or dilute 5 ml in 95 ml 0.9% saline injection for I.V. infusion and titrate dose beginning at 5 ml/hour.

SIDE EFFECTS
CV: *I.V. administration may cause pulmonary edema or hemorrhage*, dilatation of right side of heart, *circulatory collapse*.
GI: irritation, *foul breath odor*.
GU: nephrosis with prolonged use.
Skin: *erythematous rash*.
Local: *pain*, sterile abscesses, sloughing of skin, fat necrosis, muscular irritation, nerve damage (if injection is near nerve trunk) at I.M. injection site.
Other: respiratory depression.

INTERACTIONS
Alcohol: increased CNS depression. Use with caution.
Disulfiram: increased paraldehyde and acetaldehyde blood levels; possible toxic disulfiram reaction. Use together cautiously.

NURSING CONSIDERATIONS
• Contraindicated in gastroenteritis with ulceration. Use cautiously in impaired hepatic function or in asthma or other pulmonary disease.
• Use fresh supply. Don't expose to air. Don't use if liquid is brown, has a vinegary odor, or if container has been open longer than 24 hours.
• Watch closely for respiratory depression, especially in repeated doses.
• Drug reacts with plastic. Use glass syringe and bottle for parenteral dose. Prepare fresh I.V. solution every 4 hours. I.V. administration very hazardous.
• Give I.M. dose deeply, away from nerve trunks; massage injection site.

• Dilute paraldehyde in olive oil or cottonseed oil 1:2 for rectal administration. Give as retention enema. May also use 200 ml normal saline solution to prepare enema.
• Keep patient's room well ventilated to remove exhaled paraldehyde.
• Long-term high dosage may cause drug dependence and severe withdrawal symptoms.
• Oral or rectal administration of decomposed paraldehyde may cause severe corrosion of stomach or rectum.

paramethadione
Paradione* **

INDICATIONS & DOSAGE
Refractory petit mal—
Adults: initially, 300 mg P.O. t.i.d. May increase by 300 mg weekly, up to 600 mg q.i.d., if needed.
Children over 6 years: 0.9 g P.O. daily in divided doses t.i.d. or q.i.d.
Children 2 to 6 years: 0.6 g P.O. daily in divided doses t.i.d. or q.i.d.
Children under 2 years: 0.3 g P.O. daily in divided doses b.i.d.

SIDE EFFECTS
Blood: neutropenia, leukopenia, eosinophilia, thrombocytopenia, pancytopenia, *agranulocytosis, hypoplastic and aplastic anemia*.
CNS: *drowsiness*, fatigue, vertigo, headache, paresthesias, irritability.
CV: hypertension, hypotension.
EENT: hemeralopia, photophobia, diplopia, epistaxis, retinal hemorrhage.
GI: nausea, vomiting, abdominal pain, weight loss, bleeding gums.
GU: albuminuria, vaginal bleeding.
Hepatic: abnormal liver function tests.
Skin: acneiform or morbilliform rash, *exfoliative dermatitis*, erythema multiforme, petechiae, alopecia.
Other: lymphadenopathy, lupus erythematosus.

Italicized side effects are common or life-threatening.
*Liquid form contains alcohol.   **May contain tartrazine.

INTERACTIONS
None significant.

NURSING CONSIDERATIONS
• Contraindicated in renal and hepatic dysfunction, severe blood dyscrasias. Use cautiously in retinal or optic nerve diseases.
• Never withdraw drug suddenly. Call doctor at once if side effects develop.
• Therapeutic blood levels 6 to 71 mcg/ml.
• Stop drug if scotomata or signs of hepatitis, systemic lupus erythematosus, lymphadenopathy, skin rash, nephrosis, hair loss, or grand mal seizures appear.
• Tell patient to report sore throat, fever, malaise, bruises, petechiae, or epistaxis to doctor immediately. Advise patient to wear dark glasses if photophobia occurs. Warn him not to drive car or operate machinery until CNS response to drug has been determined.
• Obtain liver function studies and urinalysis before therapy; then monthly.
• Dilute oral solution with water before giving.
• Monitor CBC. Discontinue drug if neutrophil count falls below 2,500/mm³.

phenacemide
Phenurone

INDICATIONS & DOSAGE
Refractory, mixed psychomotor, grand mal, petit mal, and petit mal variant seizures—
Adults: 500 mg P.O. t.i.d. May increase by 500 mg weekly up to 5 g daily, p.r.n.
Children 5 to 10 years: 250 mg P.O. t.i.d. May increase by 250 mg weekly, up to 1.5 g daily, p.r.n.

SIDE EFFECTS
Blood: *aplastic anemia, agranulocytosis,* leukopenia.
CNS: drowsiness, dizziness, insomnia, headaches, paresthesias, *depression, suicidal tendencies,* aggressiveness.
GI: anorexia, weight loss.
GU: nephritis with marked albuminuria.
Hepatic: hepatitis, jaundice.
Skin: rashes.

INTERACTIONS
None significant.

NURSING CONSIDERATIONS
• Contraindicated in patients with preexisting personality disturbances. Use with caution in patients with hepatic dysfunction, history of allergy, and when a hydantoin is used concomitantly.
• Obtain liver function tests, CBCs, and urinalyses before and at monthly intervals during therapy.
• Tell patient to report sore throat or fever to doctor immediately.
• Warn patient to avoid activities that require alertness or good psychomotor coordination until CNS response to drug has been determined.
• Never withdraw drug suddenly. Call doctor at once if side effects develop.
• Tell patient's family to watch for personality or psychological changes and report them to doctor at once.
• Extremely toxic. Use drug only when other anticonvulsants are ineffective.
• Notify doctor if patient develops jaundice or other signs of hepatitis, abnormal urinary findings, or WBC below 4,000/mm³.

phenobarbital
Bar, Barbipil, Barbita, Eskabarb♦,
Floramine, Gardenal♦♦, Henomint,
Luminal♦, Nova-Pheno♦♦, Orprine,
PB, PBR, Solfoton, Solu-Barb,
Stental

phenobarbital sodium
Controlled Substance Schedule IV
Luminal Sodium♦

INDICATIONS & DOSAGE
All forms of epilepsy, febrile seizures in children—
Adults: 100 to 200 mg P.O. daily, divided t.i.d. or given as single dose at bedtime.
Children: 4 to 6 mg/kg P.O. daily, usually divided q 12 hours. It can, however, be administered once daily.
Status epilepticus—
Adults: 90 to 120 mg I.V., followed by 30 to 60 mg q 10 to 15 minutes, as needed, up to 500 mg total.
Children: 5 to 10 mg/kg I.V. May repeat q 10 to 15 minutes up to total of 20 mg/kg. I.V. injection rate should not exceed 60 mg/minute.

SIDE EFFECTS
CNS: *drowsiness, lethargy, hangover,* paradoxical excitement in elderly patients.
GI: nausea, vomiting.
Skin: rash, *Stevens-Johnson syndrome,* urticaria.
Other: angioedema.

INTERACTIONS
Alcohol and other CNS depressants, including narcotic analgesics: excessive CNS depression. Use cautiously.
MAO inhibitors: potentiated barbiturate effect. Monitor for increased CNS and respiratory depression.
Rifampin: may decrease barbiturate levels. Monitor for decreased effect.
Primidone: monitor for excessive phenobarbital blood levels.
Valproic acid: increased phenobarbital levels. Monitor for toxicity.

NURSING CONSIDERATIONS
● Contraindicated in patients with barbiturate hypersensitivity, porphyria, hepatic dysfunction, respiratory disease with dyspnea or obstruction, nephritis, and in lactating women. Use cautiously in patients with hyperthyroidism, diabetes mellitus, anemia, and in elderly or debilitated patients.
● I.V. injection should be reserved for emergency treatment and should be given slowly under close supervision. Monitor respirations closely.
● Watch for barbiturate toxicity signs, such as coma, asthmatic breathing, cyanosis, clammy skin, hypotension. Overdose can be fatal.
● Warn patient to avoid activities that require alertness and good psychomotor coordination until CNS response to drug is determined.
● Don't stop drug abruptly. Call doctor immediately if side effects develop.
● Full therapeutic effects not seen for 2 to 3 weeks, except when loading dose is used.
● Do not use injection solution if it contains a precipitate.
● Therapeutic blood levels are 15 to 40 mg/ml.
● Monitor prothrombin times carefully when patient on phenobarbital starts or ends anticoagulant therapy. Anticoagulant dose may need to be adjusted.
● Do not mix parenteral form with acidic solutions: precipitation may result.

phensuximide
Milontin♦

INDICATIONS & DOSAGE
Petit mal—
Adults and children: 500 mg to 1 g P.O. b.i.d. to t.i.d.

Italicized side effects are common or life-threatening.
♦Liquid form contains alcohol.   ♦♦May contain tartrazine.

SIDE EFFECTS
Blood: transient leukopenia, pancytopenia, *agranulocytosis.*
CNS: muscular weakness, *drowsiness,* dizziness, ataxia, headache.
GI: nausea, vomiting, anorexia.
GU: urinary frequency, renal damage, hematuria.
Skin: pruritus, eruptions, erythema.

INTERACTIONS
None significant.

NURSING CONSIDERATIONS
• Contraindicated in hypersensitivity to succinimide derivatives. Use cautiously in patients with hepatic or renal disease.
• Never withdraw drug suddenly. Abrupt withdrawal may precipitate petit mal seizures. Call doctor immediately if side effects develop.
• Obtain CBCs every 3 months; urinalyses and liver function tests every 6 months.
• May color urine pink or red to reddish brown.
• Therapeutic blood level 40 to 80 mcg/ml.
• May increase incidence of grand mal seizures if used alone to treat patients with mixed seizure types.

---

phenytoin sodium (extended)
Dilantin♦

phenytoin sodium (prompt)
Di-Phen, Diphenylan, Ditan

INDICATIONS & DOSAGE
Grand mal and psychomotor seizures, status epilepticus, nonepileptic seizures (post-head trauma, Reye's syndrome)—
Adults: loading dose 900 mg to 1.5 g I.V. at 50 mg/minute or P.O. divided t.i.d., then start maintenance dose of 300 mg P.O. daily (extended only) or divided t.i.d. (extended and prompt).
Children: loading dose 15 mg/kg I.V.

at 50 mg/minute or P.O. divided q 8 to 12 hours, then start maintenance dose of 5 to 7 mg/kg P.O. or I.V. daily, divided q 12 hours.
A loading dose is given if patient has not taken phenytoin in the past or has no detectable status epilepticus. If patient has not received phenytoin previously or has no detectable blood level, use loading dose—
Adults: 900 mg to 1.5 g I.V. divided into t.i.d. at 50 mg/minute. Do not exceed 500 mg each dose.
Children: 15 mg/kg I.V. at 50 mg/minute.
If patient has been receiving phenytoin but has missed one or more doses and has subtherapeutic levels—
Adults: 100 to 300 mg I.V. at 50 mg/minute.
Children: 5 to 7 mg/kg I.V. at 50 mg/minute. May repeat lower dose in 30 minutes if needed.
Neuritic pain (migraine, trigeminal neuralgia, Bell's palsy)—
Adults: 200 to 400 mg P.O. daily.

SIDE EFFECTS
Blood: thrombocytopenia, leukopenia, *agranulocytosis,* pancytopenia, macrocytosis, megaloblastic anemia.
CNS: *ataxia, slurred speech, confusion,* dizziness, insomnia, nervousness, twitching, headache.
CV: hypotension, *ventricular fibrillation.*
EENT: *nystagmus, diplopia,* blurred vision.
GI: *nausea, vomiting, gingival hyperplasia (especially children).*
Hepatic: *toxic hepatitis.*
Skin: scarlatiniform or morbilliform rash; bullous, *exfoliative,* or purpuric *dermatitis;* Stevens-Johnson syndrome; lupus erythematosus; *hirsutism; toxic epidermal necrolysis,* photosensitivity.
Local: pain, necrosis, and inflammation at injection site.
Other: periarteritis nodosa, lymphadenopathy, hyperglycemia, osteomalacia, hypertrichosis.

INTERACTIONS

Alcohol, folic acid, loxapine: monitor for decreased phenytoin activity.
Oral anticoagulants, antihistamines, chloramphenicol, cimetidine, diazepam, diazoxide, disulfiram, isoniazid, phenylbutazone, phenyramidol, salicylates, sulfamethizole, thioridazine, valproate: monitor for increased phenytoin activity and toxicity.

NURSING CONSIDERATIONS

• Contraindicated in phenacemide or hydantoin hypersensitivity, bradycardia, SA and AV block, Stokes-Adams syndrome. Use cautiously in patients with hepatic or renal dysfunction, hypotension, myocardial insuffiency, respiratory depression, and in elderly or debilitated patients, or patients receiving other hydantoin derivatives.
• Don't withdraw drug suddenly. Call doctor at once if side effects develop.
• Warn patient to avoid activities that require alertness and good psychomotor coordination until CNS response to drug is determined.
• Don't mix drug with 5% dextrose in water because it will precipitate. Clear I.V. tubing first with normal saline solution. Never use cloudy solution. May mix with normal saline solution at a concentration of 50 mg/50 ml if necessary.
• Do not give I.M. unless dosage adjustments are made. Drug may precipitate at injection site, cause pain, and give erratic blood levels.
• Obtain CBC and serum calcium every 6 months. Doctor may order folic acid and vitamin B_{12} if megaloblastic anemia is evident.
• Drug may color urine pink or red to reddish brown.
• Tell patient to carry identification stating that he's taking phenytoin.
• Stress importance of good oral hygiene and regular dental examinations. Gingivectomy may be necessary periodically.

• Drug should be stopped if rash appears. If rash is scarlet or measles-like, drug may be resumed after rash clears. If rash reappears, therapy should be stopped. If rash is exfoliative, purpuric, or bullous, don't resume drug.
• Use only clear solution for injection. Slight yellow color acceptable. Don't refrigerate.
• Divided doses given with or after meals may decrease GI side effects.
• Available as suspension. Shake well before each dose. Use solid form (chewable tablets or capsules) if possible.
• Therapeutic blood level is 10 to 20 mcg/ml.
• Heavy use of alcohol may diminish benefits of drug.
• Phenytoin levels may be decreased in mononucleosis. Monitor for increased seizure activity.
• Dilantin brand is the only oral form that can be given on a once-daily basis. Toxic levels may result if any other brand is given once daily.
• Advise patient not to change brands once stabilized on therapy.
• Suspension available as 30 mg/5 ml or 125 mg/5 ml. Read label carefully.
• The drug was formerly known as diphenylhydantoin.
• Also used to treat neuralgia and migraine headache.

primidone
Mysoline♦, Sertan♦♦

INDICATIONS & DOSAGE

Grand mal, psychomotor, and focal seizures—
Adults and children over 8 years: 250 mg P.O. daily. Increase by 250 mg weekly, up to maximum 2 g daily, divided q.i.d.
Children under 8 years: 125 mg P.O. daily. Increase by 125 mg weekly, up to maximum 1 g daily, divided q.i.d.

SIDE EFFECTS
Blood: leukopenia, eosinophilia.
CNS: *drowsiness, ataxia,* emotional disturbances, vertigo, hyperirritability, fatigue.
EENT: *diplopia,* nystagmus, edema of the eyelids.
GI: anorexia, *nausea, vomiting.*
GU: impotence, polyuria.
Skin: morbilliform rash, alopecia.
Other: edema, thirst.

INTERACTIONS
Phenytoin: stimulated conversion of primidone to phenobarbital. Observe for increased phenobarbital effect.

NURSING CONSIDERATIONS
• Contraindicated in phenobarbital hypersensitivity, porphyria.
• Don't withdraw drug suddenly. Call doctor at once if side effects develop.
• Warn patient to avoid activities that require alertness and good psychomotor coordination until CNS response to drug has been determined.
• Therapeutic blood levels of primidone 7 to 15 mcg/ml. Therapeutic blood levels of phenobarbital 15 to 40 mcg/ml.
• CBC and routine blood chemistry should be done every 6 months.
• Partially converted to phenobarbital; use cautiously with phenobarbital.
• Shake liquid suspension well.

trimethadione
Tridione

INDICATIONS & DOSAGE
Refractory petit mal—
Adults: initially, 300 mg P.O. t.i.d. May increase by 300 mg weekly up to 600 mg P.O. q.i.d.
Children: 20 to 50 mg/kg P.O. daily, divided q 6 to 8 hours. May increase by 150 to 300 mg. Usual maintenance 40 mg/kg or 1 g/m^2 P.O. daily in divided doses t.i.d. or q.i.d.

SIDE EFFECTS
Blood: neutropenia, leukopenia, eosinophilia, thrombocytopenia, pancytopenia, *agranulocytosis, hypoplastic and aplastic anemia.*
CNS: *drowsiness,* fatigue, *malaise,* insomnia, dizziness, headache, paresthesias, irritability.
CV: hypertension, hypotension.
EENT: *hemeralopia,* diplopia, photophobia, epistaxis, retinal hemorrhage.
GI: nausea, vomiting, anorexia, abdominal pain, bleeding gums.
GU: nephrosis, albuminuria, vaginal bleeding.
Hepatic: abnormal liver function tests.
Skin: acneiform and morbilliform rash, *exfoliative dermatitis,* erythema multiforme, petechiae, alopecia.
Other: lymphadenopathy.

INTERACTIONS
None significant.

NURSING CONSIDERATIONS
• Contraindicated in paramethadione and trimethadione hypersensitivity, severe blood dyscrasias, severe hepatic dysfunction. Use with extreme caution in retinal and optic nerve diseases.
• Don't withdraw drug suddenly. Abrupt withdrawal may precipitate petit mal seizures. Call doctor immediately if side effects develop.
• Check CBC, hepatic function, and urinalysis before starting therapy and monthly thereafter. Drug should be stopped if neutrophil count falls below 2,500/mm^3.
• Watch for impending toxicity; may precipitate grand mal seizure.
• Warn patient to report skin rash, alopecia, sore throat, fever, bruises, or epistaxis to doctor immediately.
• Warn patient to avoid activities requiring alertness and good psychomotor coordination until CNS response to drug has been determined.
• Suggest sunglasses if vision blurs in bright light. Notify doctor.

Unmarked trade names available in the United States only.
♦ Also available in Canada.   ♦ ♦ Available in Canada only.

- If scotomata or rash occurs, drug should be stopped.
- Therapeutic blood levels 20 to 40 mcg/ml.
- May increase incidence of grand mal seizures if used alone to treat patients who have mixed types of seizures.

valproic acid
Depakene

valproate sodium
Depakene Syrup

INDICATIONS & DOSAGE
Simple and complex absence seizures (including petit mal), mixed seizure types (including absence seizures), investigationally in major motor (grand mal, tonic clonic) seizures—
Adults and children: initially, 15 mg/kg P.O. daily divided b.i.d. or t.i.d.; then may increase by 5 to 10 mg/kg daily at weekly intervals up to maximum of 30 mg/kg daily, divided b.i.d. or t.i.d.

SIDE EFFECTS
Because drug usually used in combination with other anticonvulsants, side effects reported may not be caused by valproic acid alone.
Blood: *inhibited platelet aggregation, thrombocytopenia, increased bleeding time.*
CNS: *sedation,* emotional upset, depression, psychosis, aggression, hyperactivity, behavioral deterioration, muscle weakness, tremors.
EENT: stomatitis.
GI: *nausea, vomiting,* indigestion, diarrhea, abdominal cramps, constipation, increased appetite and weight gain, *anorexia, pancreatitis.*
Hepatic: *enzyme elevations, toxic hepatitis.*
Metabolic: *elevated serum ammonia levels.*
Other: alopecia.

INTERACTIONS
Antacids, aspirin: May cause valproic acid toxicity. Use together cautiously and monitor blood levels.

NURSING CONSIDERATIONS
- Use cautiously in hepatic dysfunction.
- Don't withdraw suddenly. Call doctor at once if side effects develop.
- Obtain liver function studies, platelet counts, and prothrombin time before starting drug and every month thereafter.This is especially important during the first 6 months of therapy.
- Warn patient to avoid activities that require alertness and good psychomotor coordination until response to drug is determined.
- May give drug with food or milk to reduce GI side effects. Advise against chewing capsules; causes irritation of mouth and throat.
- Tremors may indicate the need for dosage reduction.
- May produce false-positive test for ketones in urine.
- Available as tasty red syrup. Keep out of reach of children.
- Syrup is more rapidly absorbed. Peak effect within 15 minutes.
- Syrup shouldn't be mixed with carbonated beverages; may be irritating to mouth and throat.

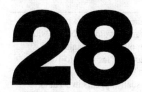

Antidepressants

amitriptyline hydrochloride
amoxapine
desipramine hydrochloride
doxepin hydrochloride
imipramine hydrochloride
isocarboxazid
maprotiline hydrochloride
nortriptyline hydrochloride
phenelzine sulfate
protriptyline hydrochloride
tranylcypromine sulfate
trazodone hydrochloride
trimipramine maleate

MECHANISM OF ACTION
• Tricyclic and tetracylic antidepressants are thought to increase the amount of norepinephrine or serotonin, or both, in the central nervous system by blocking their reuptake by the presynaptic neurons. This action allows these neurotransmitters to accumulate.
• Monoamine oxidose (MAO) inhibitors block MAO (which helps metabolize neurotransmitters at synapse), causing buildup of certain neurotransmitters and probably resulting in antidepressant action.
• Trazodone is believed to inhibit serotonin uptake in the brain.

COMBINATION PRODUCTS
ETRAFON 2-10♦: perphenazine 2 mg and amitripyline HCl 10 mg.
ETRAFON: perphenazine 2 mg and amitriptyline HCl 25 mg.
ETRAFON-A: perphenazine 4 mg and amitriptyline 10 mg.
ETRAFON-FORTE: perphenazine 4 mg and amitriptyline 25 mg.

LIMBITROL 10-25: chlordiazepoxide 10 mg and amitriptyline (as HCl) 25 mg.
LIMBITROL 5-12.5: chlordiazepoxide 5 mg and amitriptyline (as HCl) 12.5 mg.
TRIAVIL-2-10, TRIAVIL-4-10, TRIAVIL-2-25, TRIAVIL-4-25 are products identical to the Etrafon products listed above. Triavil is also available as TRIAVIL-4-50 (perphenazine 4 mg and amitriptyline HCl 50 mg).

amitriptyline hydrochloride
Amitid, Amitril, Deprex♦♦, Elavil♦, Endep, Enovil, Levate♦♦, Meravil♦♦, Novotriptyn♦♦, Rolavil

INDICATIONS & DOSAGE
Treatment of depression—
Adults: 50 to 100 mg P.O. h.s., increasing to 200 mg daily; maximum 300 mg daily if needed; or 20 to 30 mg I.M. q.i.d. Alternatively, the entire dosage can be given at bedtime.
Elderly and adolescents: 30 mg P.O. daily in divided doses. May be increased to 150 mg.

SIDE EFFECTS
CNS: *drowsiness, dizziness,* excitation, tremors, weakness, confusion, headache, nervousness.
CV: *orthostatic hypotension, tachycardia, EKG changes,* hypertension.
EENT: *blurred vision,* tinnitus, mydriasis.
GI: *dry mouth, constipation,* nausea, vomiting, anorexia, paralytic ileus.
GU: *urinary retention.*
Skin: rash, urticaria.

Other: *sweating,* allergy.
Abrupt cessation after long-term therapy: nausea, headache, malaise. (Does not indicate addiction.)

INTERACTIONS
MAO inhibitors: may cause severe excitation, hyperpyrexia, convulsions, usually with high dose. Use together cautiously.
Epinephrine, levarterenol: increase hypertensive effect. Use with caution.
Barbiturates: decrease TCA blood levels. Monitor for decreased antidepressant effect.
Methylphenidate: increases TCA blood levels. Monitor for enhanced antidepressant effect.

NURSING CONSIDERATIONS
• Contraindicated during acute recovery phase of myocardial infarction, and in patients with prostatic hypertrophy. Use with caution in patients who are suicide risks or who have a history of seizures; in patients with urinary retention, narrow-angle glaucoma, increased intraocular pressure, cardiovascular disease, impaired hepatic function, hyperthyroidism; and in patients receiving thyroid medications, electroshock therapy, or elective surgery.
• Reduce dose in elderly or debilitated persons and adolescents.
• Do not withdraw abruptly.
• If psychotic signs increase, dose should be reduced. Chart mood changes. Watch for suicidal tendencies. Allow minimum supply of tablets to lessen suicide risk.
• Check for urinary retention and constipation. Increase fluids to lessen constipation. Suggest stool softener, if needed.
• Warn patient to avoid activities that require alertness and good psychomotor coordination until CNS response to drug is determined. Drowsiness and dizziness usually subside after first few weeks.
• Has strong anticholinergic effects;

one of the most sedating tricyclic antidepressants. Avoid combining with alcohol or other depressants.
• Expect time lag of up to 10 to 14 days before noticeable effect. Full effect usually appears in 30 days.
• Dry mouth may be relieved with sugarless hard candy or gum.
• Advise the patient not to take any other drugs (prescription or over-the-counter) without first consulting the doctor.
• Whenever possible, patient should take full dose at bedtime.
• Has been used successfully to treat chronic pain associated with post-herpetic neuralgia.

amoxapine
Asendin

INDICATIONS & DOSAGE
Treatment of depression—
Adults: initial dose 50 mg P.O. t.i.d. May increase to 100 mg t.i.d. on third day of treatment. Increases above 300 mg daily should be made only if 300 mg daily has been ineffective during a trial period of at least 2 weeks. When effective dosage is established, entire dosage (not exceeding 300 mg) may be given at bedtime. Maximum 600 mg in hospitalized patients.

SIDE EFFECTS
CNS: *drowsiness, dizziness,* excitation, tremors, weakness, confusion, headache, nervousness.
CV: *orthostatic hypotension, tachycardia, EKG changes,* hypertension.
EENT: *blurred vision,* tinnitus, mydriasis.
GI: *dry mouth, constipation,* nausea, vomiting, anorexia, paralytic ileus.
GU: *urinary retention.*
Skin: rash, urticaria.
Other: *sweating, weight gain and craving for sweets,* allergy.
Abrupt cessation after long-term

Italicized side effects are common or life-threatening.
*Liquid form contains alcohol.   **May contain tartrazine.

therapy: nausea, headache, malaise. (Does not indicate addiction.)

INTERACTIONS
MAO inhibitors: may cause severe excitation, hyperpyrexia, convulsions, usually with high dose. Use together cautiously.
Epinephrine, levarterenol: increase hypertensive effect. Use with caution.
Barbiturates: decrease TCA blood levels. Monitor for decreased antidepressant effect.
Methylphenidate: increases TCA blood levels. Monitor for enhanced antidepressant effect.

NURSING CONSIDERATIONS
• Contraindicated in acute recovery phase of myocardial infarction, and in prostatic hypertrophy. Use with caution in patients who are suicide risks or who have a history of seizures; in patients with urinary retention, narrow-angle glaucoma, increased intraocular pressure, cardiovascular disease, impaired hepatic function, hyperthyroidism; and in patients receiving thyroid medications, electroshock therapy, or elective surgery.
• Reduce dose in elderly or debilitated persons and adolescents.
• Do not withdraw abruptly.
• If psychotic signs increase, reduce dose. Chart mood changes. Watch for suicidal tendencies. Allow minimum supply of tablets to lessen suicide risk.
• Check for urinary retention and constipation. Increase fluids to lessen constipation. Suggest stool softener, if needed.
• Warn patient to avoid activities that require alertness and good psychomotor coordination until CNS response to drug is determined. Drowsiness and dizziness usually subside after first few weeks.
• Dry mouth may be relieved with sugarless hard candy or gum.
• Beneficial response may occur within 4 to 7 days.

• Whenever possible, patient should take full dose at bedtime.

desipramine hydrochloride
Norpramin♦**, Pertofrane♦

INDICATIONS & DOSAGE
Treatment of depression—
Adults: 75 to 150 mg P.O. daily in divided doses, increasing to maximum 300 mg daily. Alternatively, the entire dosage can be given at bedtime.
Elderly and adolescents: 25 to 50 mg P.O. daily, increasing gradually to maximum 100 mg daily.

SIDE EFFECTS
CNS: *drowsiness, dizziness,* excitation, tremors, weakness, confusion, headache, nervousness.
CV: *orthostatic hypotension, tachycardia, EKG changes,* hypertension.
EENT: *blurred vision,* tinnitus, mydriasis.
GI: *dry mouth, constipation,* nausea, vomiting, anorexia, paralytic ileus.
GU: *urinary retention.*
Skin: rash, urticaria.
Other: *sweating,* allergy.
Abrupt cessation after long-term therapy: nausea, headache, malaise. (Does not indicate addiction.)

INTERACTIONS
MAO inhibitors: may cause severe excitation, hyperpyrexia, convulsions, usually with high dose. Use together cautiously.
Epinephrine, levarterenol: increase hypertensive effect. Use with caution.
Barbiturates: decrease TCA blood levels. Monitor for decreased antidepressant effect.
Methylphenidate: increases TCA blood levels. Monitor for enhanced antidepressant effect.

NURSING CONSIDERATIONS
• Contraindicated during acute recovery phase of myocardial infarction, in

---

patients with prostatic hypertrophy. Use with caution in patients with cardiovascular disease, urinary retention, narrow-angle glaucoma, thyroid disease, seizure disorders, blood dyscrasias, impaired hepatic function; in patients who are suicide risks; and in those receiving electroshock therapy, thyroid medication, or elective surgery.

• Reduce dose in elderly or debilitated persons, and adolescents.

• Do not withdraw abruptly.

• Orthostatic hypotension not as severe with this drug compared to that with other tricyclics.

• If psychotic signs increase, dose should be decreased. Chart mood changes. Watch for suicidal tendencies. To lessen suicide risk, allow minimum supply of tablets.

• Check for urinary retention and constipation. Increase fluids to lessen constipation. Suggest stool softener, if needed.

• Warn patient to avoid activities that require alertness and good psychomotor coordination until response to drug is determined. Drowsiness and dizziness usually subside after a few weeks.

• Dry mouth may be relieved with sugarless hard candy or gum.

• Drug has anticholinergic effect, is a metabolite of imipramine, and produces less sedation than amitriptyline or doxepin. Alcohol may antagonize effects of desipramine.

• Because it produces less tachycardia and other anticholinergic effects compared with other tricyclics, desipramine is often prescribed for cardiac patients.

• Expect time lag of 10 to 14 days before noticeable effects. Full effect usually appears in 30 days.

• Advise patient not to take any other drugs (prescription or over-the-counter) without first consulting the doctor.

• Whenever possible, patient should take full dose at bedtime.

doxepin hydrochloride
Adapin∗∗, Sinequan♦

INDICATIONS & DOSAGE
Treatment of depression—
Adults: initially, 50 to 75 mg P.O. daily in divided doses, to maximum 300 mg daily. Alternatively, entire dosage may be given at bedtime.

SIDE EFFECTS
CNS: *drowsiness, dizziness,* excitation, tremors, weakness, confusion, headache, nervousness.
CV: *orthostatic hypotension, tachycardia, EKG changes,* hypertension.
EENT: *blurred vision,* tinnitus, glossitis, mydriasis.
GI: *dry mouth, constipation,* nausea, vomiting, anorexia, paralytic ileus.
GU: *urinary retention.*
Skin: rash, urticaria.
Other: *sweating,* allergy.
Abrupt cessation after long-term therapy: nausea, headache, malaise. (Does not indicate addiction.)

INTERACTIONS
MAO inhibitors: may cause severe excitation, hyperpyrexia, convulsions, usually with high dose. Use together cautiously.
Barbiturates: decrease TCA blood levels. Monitor for decreased antidepressant effect.
Methylphenidate: increases TCA blood levels. Monitor for enhanced antidepressant effect.

NURSING CONSIDERATIONS
• Contraindicated in patients with urinary retention, narrow-angle glaucoma, or prostatic hypertrophy. Use with caution in suicide risks.

• Reduce dose in elderly or debilitated persons, adolescents, and those receiving other medications (especially anticholinergics).

• Dilute oral concentrate with 120 ml water, milk, or juice (orange, grape-

---

Italicized side effects are common or life-threatening.
∗Liquid form contains alcohol.   ∗∗May contain tartrazine.

fruit, tomato, prune, or pineapple). Avoid carbonated beverages.
• If psychotic symptoms increase, dose should be decreased. Chart mood changes. Watch for suicidal tendencies.
• Check for urinary retention and constipation. Increase fluids to lessen constipation. Suggest stool softener, if needed.
• Warn patient to avoid activities that require alertness and good psychomotor coordination until CNS response to drug is determined. Drowsiness and dizziness usually subside after a few weeks.
• Expect time lag of 10 to 14 days before effect is noticeable. Full effect usually appears within 30 days.
• Dry mouth may be relieved with sugarless hard candy or gum.
• Has strong anticholinergic effects; one of the most sedating tricyclic antidepressants. Avoid combining with alcohol or other depressants.
• Advise patient not to take any other drugs (over-the-counter or prescription) without first consulting the doctor.
• Liquid formulation available.
• Whenever possible, patient should take full dose at bedtime.

---

imipramine hydrochloride
Antipress, Impril♦♦, Janimine, Novopramine♦♦, Praminil♦♦ Presamine, Ropramine, SK-Pramine, Tofranil♦

INDICATIONS & DOSAGE
Treatment of depression—
Adults: 75 to 100 mg P.O. or I.M. daily in divided doses, with 25- to 50-mg increments up to 200 mg. Maximum 300 mg daily. Alternatively, the entire dosage may be given at bedtime. (I.M. route rarely used.)
Childhood enuresis—
25 to 75 mg P.O. daily.

SIDE EFFECTS
CNS: *drowsiness, dizziness,* excitation, tremors, weakness, confusion, headache, nervousness.
CV: *orthostatic hypotension, tachycardia, EKG changes,* hypertension.
EENT: *blurred vision,* tinnitus, mydriasis.
GI: *dry mouth, constipation,* nausea, vomiting, anorexia, paralytic ileus.
GU: *urinary retention.*
Skin: rash, urticaria.
Other: *sweating,* allergy.
Abrupt cessation after long-term therapy: nausea, headache, malaise. (Does not indicate addiction.)

INTERACTIONS
MAO inhibitors: may cause severe excitation, hyperpyrexia, convulsions, usually with high dose. Use together cautiously.
Epinephrine, levarterenol: increase hypertensive effect. Use with caution.
Barbiturates: decrease TCA blood levels. Monitor for decreased antidepressant effect.
Methylphenidate: increases TCA blood levels. Monitor for enhanced antidepressant effect.

NURSING CONSIDERATIONS
• Contraindicated during acute recovery phase of myocardial infarction; in patients with prostatic hypertrophy. Use with extreme caution in patients with cardiovascular disease, urinary retention, narrow-angle glaucoma or increased intraocular pressure, thyroid disease, seizure disorders, blood dyscrasias, impaired hepatic function; in patients who are suicide risks; and in those receiving electroshock therapy, thyroid medication, or elective surgery.
• Reduce dose in elderly or debilitated persons, adolescents, and patients with aggravated psychotic symptoms.
• Do not withdraw abruptly.
• If psychotic signs increase, dose should be reduced. Chart mood changes. Watch for suicidal tendencies. To lessen suicide risk, allow minimum tablet supply.

Unmarked trade names available in the United States only.
♦ Also available in Canada.   ♦ ♦ Available in Canada only.

• Check for urinary retention and constipation. Increase fluids to lessen constipation. Suggest stool softener, if needed.

• Warn patient to avoid activities that require alertness and good psychomotor coordination until CNS response to drug is determined. Drowsiness and dizziness usually subside after a few weeks.

• Expect time lag of 10 to 14 days before noticeable effect. Full effect usually appears in 30 days.

• Dry mouth may be relieved with sugarless hard candy or gum.

• Avoid combining with alcohol or other depressants.

• Advise patient not to take any other drugs (prescription or over-the-counter) without first consulting the doctor.

• Whenever possible, patient should take full dose at bedtime.

isocarboxazid
Marplan♦

INDICATIONS & DOSAGE
Treatment of depression—
Adults: 30 mg P.O. daily in divided doses. Reduce to 10 to 20 mg daily when condition improves. Not recommended for children under 16 years.

SIDE EFFECTS
CNS: dizziness, vertigo, weakness, headache, overactivity, hyperreflexia, tremors, muscle twitching, mania, *insomnia,* confusion, memory impairment, fatigue.
CV: *orthostatic hypotension,* arrhythmias, paradoxical hypertension.
EENT: blurred vision.
GI: dry mouth, *anorexia,* nausea, diarrhea, constipation.
GU: altered libido.
Skin: rash.
Other: peripheral edema, sweating, weight changes.

INTERACTIONS
Amphetamines, ephedrine, levodopa, meperidine, metaraminol, methotrimeprazine, methylphenidate, phenylephrine, phenylpropanolamine: pressor effects of these drugs are enhanced by isocarboxazid. Use together very cautiously.
Alcohol, barbiturates, and other sedatives; tranquilizers; narcotics; dextromethorphan; tricyclic antidepressants: unpredictable interaction. Use with caution and in reduced dosage.

NURSING CONSIDERATIONS
• Contraindicated in elderly or debilitated patients, and in patients with severe hepatic or renal impairment; congestive heart failure; pheochromocytoma; hypertensive, cardiovascular, or cerebrovascular disease; severe or frequent headaches. Also contraindicated with foods containing tryptophan or tyramine. Also during therapy with other MAO inhibitor (including pargyline HCl, phenelzine sulfate, tranylcypromine sulfate) or within 10 days of such therapy; within 10 days of elective surgery requiring general anesthetic, cocaine, or local anesthetic containing sympathomimetic vasoconstrictors. Use cautiously with other psychotropic drugs or with spinal anesthetic; in hyperactive, agitated, or schizophrenic patients; in suicide risks; and in patients with diabetes or epilepsy.

• Recommended only when TCA or electroshock therapy is ineffective or contraindicated.

• If patient develops symptoms of overdosage (palpitations or frequent headaches, or severe orthostatic hypotension), hold dose and notify doctor.

• Watch for suicidal tendencies.

• Dose is usually reduced to maintenance level as soon as possible.

• Do not withdraw drug abruptly.

• Weigh patient biweekly; check for edema and urinary retention.

• Warn patient to avoid foods high in tyramine or tryptophan; large amounts

---

Italicized side effects are common or life-threatening.
*Liquid form contains alcohol.   **May contain tartrazine.

of caffeine; and self-medication with over-the-counter cold, hay fever, or diet preparations.
• Incidence of orthostatic hypotension is high. Supervise walking. Tell patient to get out of bed slowly, sitting up first for 1 minute.
• Have phentolamine (Regitine) available to counteract severe hypertension.
• Continue precautions 10 days after stopping drug; long-lasting effects.
• Expect time lag of 1 to 4 weeks before noticeable effect.
• Drug is MAO inhibitor and is generally less effective than tricyclic antidepressant. Avoid combining with alcohol or other depressant.
• Obtain baseline blood pressure readings, CBC, and liver function tests before beginning therapy, and continue to monitor throughout treatment.

maprotiline hydrochloride
Ludiomil

INDICATIONS & DOSAGE
Treatment of depression—
Adults: initial dose of 75 mg daily for patients with mild-to-moderate depression. The dosage may be increased as required to a dose of 150 mg daily. Maximum dose is 225 mg in patients who are not hospitalized. More severely depressed, hospitalized patients may receive up to 300 mg daily.

SIDE EFFECTS
CNS: *drowsiness, dizziness,* excitation, seizures, tremors, weakness, confusion, headache, nervousness.
CV: *orthostatic hypotension, tachycardia, EKG changes,* hypertension.
EENT: *blurred vision,* tinnitus, mydriasis.
GI: *dry mouth, constipation,* nausea, vomiting, anorexia, paralytic ileus.
GU: *urinary retention.*
Skin: rash, urticaria.
Other: *sweating,* allergy.
Abrupt cessation after long-term

therapy: nausea, headache, malaise. (Does not indicate addiction.)

INTERACTIONS
MAO inhibitors: may cause severe excitation, hyperpyrexia, convulsions, usually with high dose. Use together cautiously.
Epinephrine, levarterenol: increase hypertensive effect. Use with caution.
Barbiturates: decrease maprotiline blood levels. Monitor for decreased antidepressant effect.
Methylphenidate: increases maprotiline blood levels. Monitor for enhanced antidepressant effect.

NURSING CONSIDERATIONS
• Contraindicated during acute recovery phase of myocardial infarction, in patients with prostatic hypertrophy. Use with caution in cardiovascular disease, urinary retention, narrow-angle glaucoma, thyroid disease or medication, seizure disorders, blood dyscrasias, impaired hepatic functon; in patients who are suicide risks; and in those receiving electroshock therapy or elective surgery.
• Reduce dose in elderly or debilitated persons, and adolescents.
• Do not withdraw abruptly.
• If psychotic signs increase, reduce dose. Chart mood changes. Watch for suicidal tendencies. To lessen suicide risk, allow minimum supply of tablets.
• Check for urinary retention and constipation. Increase fluids to lessen constipation. Suggest stool softener, if needed.
• Warn patient to avoid activities that require alertness and good psychomotor coordination until CNS response to drug is determined. Drowsiness and dizziness usually subside after a few weeks.
• Dry mouth may be relieved with sugarless hard candy or gum.
• Beneficial response may occur within 4 to 7 days.

• Whenever possible, patient should take full dose at bedtime.
• The first "tetracyclic" antidepressant.

nortriptyline hydrochloride
Aventyl♦*, Pamelor

INDICATIONS & DOSAGE
Treatment of depression—
Adults: 25 mg P.O. t.i.d. or q.i.d., gradually increasing to maximum 150 mg daily. Alternatively, entire dose may be given at bedtime.

SIDE EFFECTS
CNS: *drowsiness, dizziness,* excitation, seizures, tremors, weakness, confusion, headache, nervousness.
CV: *tachycardia, EKG changes,* hypertension.
EENT: *blurred vision,* tinnitus, mydriasis.
GI: *dry mouth, constipation,* nausea, vomiting, anorexia, paralytic ileus.
GU: *urinary retention.*
Skin: rash, urticaria.
Other: *sweating,* allergy.
Abrupt cessation after long-term therapy: nausea, headache, malaise. (Does not indicate addiction.)

INTERACTIONS
MAO inhibitors: may cause severe excitation, hyperpyrexia, convulsions, usually with high dose. Use together cautiously.
Epinephrine, levarterenol: increase hypertensive effect. Use with caution.
Barbiturates: decrease TCA blood levels. Monitor for decreased antidepressant effect.
Methylphenidate: increases TCA blood levels. Monitor for enhanced antidepressant effect.

NURSING CONSIDERATIONS
• Contraindicated during acute recovery phase of myocardial infarction and in patients with prostatic hypertrophy.
Use with caution in patients with cardiovascular disease, urinary retention, glaucoma, thyroid disease, seizure disorders, impaired hepatic function, blood dyscrasias; in patients who are suicide risks; or in those receiving electroshock therapy, thyroid medicaton, or elective surgery.
• Reduce dose in elderly or debilitated persons, and adolescents.
• Do not withdraw abruptly.
• If psychotic signs increase, dose should be reduced. Chart mood changes. Watch for suicidal tendencies. To lessen suicide risk, allow minimum tablet supply.
• Check for urinary retention and constipation. Increase fluids to lessen constipation. Suggest stool softener, if needed.
• Warn patient to avoid activities that require alertness and good psychomotor coordination until CNS response to drug is determined. Drowsiness and dizziness usually subside after a few weeks.
• Expect time lag of 10 to 14 days before noticeable effects. Full effect usually appears in 30 days.
• Dry mouth may be relieved with sugarless hard candy or gum.
• Drug is tricyclic antidepressant, similar in anticholinergic effects to other tricyclics. Avoid combining with alcohol or other depressants.
• Advise patient not to use other drugs (prescription or over-the-counter) without first consulting the doctor.
• Liquid formulation available.
• Whenever possible, patient should take full dose at bedtime.

phenelzine sulfate
Nardil♦

INDICATIONS & DOSAGE
Treatment of depression—
Adults: 45 mg P.O. daily in divided doses, increasing rapidly to 60 mg

---

daily. Maximum 90 mg daily. Not recommended for children under 16 years.

SIDE EFFECTS
CNS: dizziness, vertigo, headache, overactivity, hyperreflexia, tremors, muscle twitching, mania, jitters, *insomnia,* confusion, memory impairment, drowsiness, weakness, fatigue.
CV: paradoxical hypertension, *orthostatic hypotension,* arrhythmias.
GI: dry mouth, *anorexia,* nausea, constipation.
Other: peripheral edema, sweating, weight changes.

INTERACTIONS
Amphetamines, ephedrine, levodopa, meperidine, metaraminol, methotrimeprazine, methylphenidate, phenylephrine, phenylpropanolamine: enhance pressor effects. Use together cautiously.
Alcohol, barbiturates, and other sedatives; tranquilizers; narcotics; dextromethorphan; tricyclic antidepressants: unpredictable interaction. Use with caution and in reduced dosage.

NURSING CONSIDERATIONS
• Contraindicated elderly or debilitated patients, and in patients with hepatic impairment, congestive heart failure, pheochromocytoma, hypertension, cardiovascular or cerebrovascular disease, severe or frequent headaches; also contraindicated with foods containing tryptophan (broad beans) or tyramine. Also contraindicated during therapy with other MAO inhibitor, including pargyline HCl, isocarboxazid, tranylcypromine sulfate, or within 10 days of such therapy; within 10 days of elective surgery requiring general anesthetic, cocaine, or local anesthetic containing sympathomimetic vasoconstrictors; in hyperactive, agitated, or schizophrenic patients. Use cautiously with antihypertensive drugs containing thiazide diuretics or with spinal anesthetic; in suicide risk, diabetes, epilepsy.

• Use only when TCA or electroshock therapy is ineffective or contraindicated.
• If patient develops symptoms of overdose (severe hypotension, palpitations, or frequent headaches), hold dose and notify doctor.
• Watch for suicidal tendencies.
• Dose is usually reduced to maintenance level as soon as possible.
• Store drug in tight container, away from heat and light.
• Have phentolamine (Regitine) available to counteract severe hypertension.
• Warn patient to avoid foods high in tyramine or tryptophan, and self-medication with over-the-counter cold, hay fever, or diet preparations.
• Incidence of orthostatic hypotension is high. Supervise walking. Tell patient to get out of bed slowly, sitting up first for 1 minute.
• Continue precautions 10 days after stopping drug; long-lasting effects.
• Expect time lag of 1 to 4 weeks before noticeable effect.
• Drug is MAO inhibitor and is generally less effective than tricyclic antidepressant. Avoid combining with alcohol or other depressants.
• Obtain baseline blood pressure readings, CBC, and liver function tests before beginning therapy, and continue to monitor throughout treatment.

---

protriptyline hydrochloride
Triptil♦♦, Vivactil

INDICATIONS & DOSAGE
Treatment of depression—
Adults: 15 to 40 mg P.O. daily in divided doses, increasing gradually to maximum 60 mg daily.

SIDE EFFECTS
CNS: excitation, seizures, tremors, weakness, confusion, headache, nervousness.
CV: *orthostatic hypotension, tachycardia, EKG changes,* hypertension.

Unmarked trade names available in the United States only.
♦ Also available in Canada. ♦ ♦ Available in Canada only.

EENT: *blurred vision,* tinnitus, mydriasis.
GI: *dry mouth, constipation,* nausea, vomiting, anorexia, paralytic ileus.
GU: *urinary retention.*
Skin: rash, urticaria.
Other: *sweating,* allergy.
Abrupt cessation after long-term therapy: nausea, headache, malaise. (Does not indicate addiction.)

INTERACTIONS

MAO inhibitors: may cause severe excitation, hyperpyrexia, convulsions, and death, usually with high dose. Use together cautiously.
Epinephrine, levarterenol: increase hypertensive effect. Use with caution.
Barbiturates: decrease TCA blood levels. Monitor for decreased antidepressant effect.
Methylphenidate: increases TCA blood levels. Monitor for enhanced antidepressant effect.

NURSING CONSIDERATIONS

• Contraindicated during acute recovery phase of myocardial infarction and in patients with prostatic hypertrophy. Use with caution in the elderly and in patients with cardiovascular disease, urinary retention, increased intraocular tension, thyroid disease, seizure disorders, blood dyscrasias; in suicide risks; and in those receiving electroshock therapy, thyroid medication, or elective surgery.
• Reduce dose in elderly or debilitated persons, and adolescents.
• Do not withdraw abruptly.
• Watch for increased psychotic signs, anxiety, agitation, or cardiovascular reactions; dose should be reduced if they occur. Chart mood changes. Watch for suicidal tendencies. To lessen suicide risk, allow minimum supply of tablets.
• Check for urinary retention and constipation. Increase fluids to lessen constipation. Suggest stool softener, if needed.
• Warn patient to avoid activities that

require alertness and good psychomotor coordination until CNS response to drug is determined. Drowsiness and dizziness usually subside after a few weeks.
• Dry mouth may be relieved with sugarless hard candy or gum.
• Expect time lag of 7 to 14 days before effect is noticeable.
• Drug is possibly the most rapid-acting but least sedating tricyclic antidepressant. May even have an amphetamine-like effect. Avoid combining with alcohol or other depressants.
• Do not give entire dose at bedtime as patient may develop insomnia.
• Advise patient not to use other drugs (prescription or over-the-counter) without first consulting the doctor.

tranylcypromine sulfate
Parnate♦

INDICATIONS & DOSAGE

Treatment of depression—
Adults: 10 mg P.O. b.i.d. Increase to maximum 30 mg daily, if necessary, after 2 weeks. Not recommended for children under 16 years.

SIDE EFFECTS

CNS: dizziness, vertigo, headache, overactivity, hyperreflexia, tremors, muscle twitching, mania, jitters, confusion, memory impairment, fatigue.
CV: *orthostatic hypotension,* arrhythmias, paradoxical hypertension.
EENT: blurred vision.
GI: dry mouth, *anorexia,* nausea, diarrhea, constipation, abdominal pain.
GU: changed libido, impotence.
Skin: rash.
Other: peripheral edema, sweating, weight changes, chills.

INTERACTIONS

Amphetamines, ephedrine, levodopa, meperidine, metaraminol, methotrimeprazine, methylphenidate, phenyl-

---

Italicized side effects are common or life-threatening.
*Liquid form contains alcohol.   **May contain tartrazine.

ephrine, phenylpropanolamine: pressor effects of these drugs are enhanced by tranylcypromine. Use together cautiously.

Alcohol, barbiturates, and other sedatives; tranquilizers; narcotics; dextromethorphan; tricyclic antidepressants: use with caution and in reduced dosage.

NURSING CONSIDERATIONS

• Contraindicated in patients with severe hepatic or renal impairment; congestive heart failure; pheochromocytoma, hypertension, or cardiovascular or cerebrovascular disease; severe or frequent headaches; in patients taking antihypertensive drugs or diuretics; in elderly or debilitated patients; in patients for whom close supervision is not possible; and in hyperactive, agitated, or schizophrenic patients. Also contraindicated with foods containing tryptophan or tyramine. Also contraindicated during therapy with other MAO inhibitor (including pargyline HCl, phenelzine sulfate, isocarboxazid) or within 7 days of such therapy; within 7 days of elective surgery requiring general anesthetic, cocaine, or local anesthetic containing sympathomimetic vasoconstrictors. Use cautiously with anti-Parkinson drugs, spinal anesthetic; in renal disease, diabetes, epilepsy, hyperthyroidism; and in suicide risks.

• Use only when TCA or electroshock therapy is ineffective or contraindicated.

• If patient develops symptoms of overdose (palpitations, severe orthostatic hypotension), hold dose and notify doctor.

• Watch for suicidal tendencies.

• Dose is usually reduced to maintenance level as soon as possible.

• Do not withdraw drug abruptly.

• Have phentolamine (Regitine) available to counteract severe hypertension.

• Warn patient to avoid foods high in tyramine or trytophan, and self-medication with over-the-counter cold, hay fever, or reducing preparations.

• Tell patient to get out of bed slowly, sitting up for 1 minute.

• Continue precautions for 7 days after stopping drug; effects last that long.

• Expect time lag of 1 to 3 weeks before effect is noticeable.

• More rapid onset of action than isocarboxazid or phenelzine sulfate.

• MAO inhibitor most often reported to cause hypertensive crisis in presence of high-tyramine ingestion. Generally less effective than a tricyclic antidepressant. Avoid combining with alcohol or other depressants.

• Obtain baseline blood pressure readings, CBC, and liver function tests before beginning therapy, and continue to monitor throughout treatment.

---

trazodone hydrochloride
Desyrel

INDICATIONS & DOSAGE
Treatment of depression—
Adults: Initial dosage is 150 mg daily in divided doses, which can be increased by 50 mg per day q 3 to 4 days. Average dose ranges from 150 mg to 400 mg daily. Maximum dose 600 mg.

SIDE EFFECTS
CNS: *drowsiness, dizziness,* nervousness, fatigue, confusion, tremors, weakness.
CV: orthostatic hypotension, tachycardia.
EENT: blurred vision, tinnitus.
GI: dry mouth, constipation, nausea, vomiting, anorexia.
GU: urinary retention.
Skin: rash, urticaria.
Other: sweating.

INTERACTIONS
Antihypertensives: added hypotensive effect of trazodone. Dose of antihypertensive drug may have to be decreased.
MAO inhibitors: No clinical experience. Use together very cautiously.

Unmarked trade names available in the United States only.
♦ Also available in Canada.   ♦ ♦ Available in Canada only.

NURSING CONSIDERATIONS
- Should not be used during initial recovery phase of myocardial infarction. Avoid concurrent administration with electroshock therapy.
- Watch for suicidal tendencies and chart mood changes. Allow minimum amount of tablets to lessen suicide risk.
- Warn patient to avoid activities that require alertness and good psychomotor coordination until CNS response to drug is determined. Drowsiness and dizziness usually subside after the first few weeks.
- Administer after meals or a light snack for optimal absorption and to decrease incidence of dizziness.
- Not chemically related to tricyclic antidepressants or MAO inhibitors.
- Anticholinergic and adverse cardiac effects are minimal.
- Expect similar lag time as with tricyclic antidepressants. Expect lag time of up to 10 to 14 days before noticeable effect. Full effect appears in 30 days.
- Avoid combining with alcohol or other depressants.

---

trimipramine maleate
Surmontil

INDICATIONS & DOSAGE
Treatment of depression—
Adults: 75 mg daily in divided doses, increased to 200 mg per day. Dosages over 300 mg per day not recommended.
Enuresis—
Children over 6 years: initial dose 25 mg P.O. 1 hour before bedtime; if no response, increase dose to 50 mg in children under 12 years, and to 75 mg in children over 12 years.

SIDE EFFECTS
CNS: *drowsiness, dizziness,* excitation, seizures, tremors, weakness, confusion, headache, nervousness.
CV: *orthostatic hypotension, tachycardia, EKG changes,* hypertension.

EENT: *blurred vision,* tinnitus, mydriasis.
GI: *dry mouth, constipation,* nausea, vomiting, anorexia, paralytic ileus.
GU: *urinary retention.*
Skin: rash, urticaria.
Other: *sweating,* allergy.
Abrupt cessation after long-term therapy: nausea, headache, malaise. (Does not indicate addiction.)

INTERACTIONS
MAO inhibitors: may cause severe excitation, hyperpyrexia, convulsions, usually with high dose. Use together cautiously.
Epinephrine, levarterenol: increase hypertensive effect. Use with caution.
Barbiturates: decrease TCA blood levels. Monitor for decreased antidepressant effect.
Methylphenidate: increases TCA blood levels. Monitor for enhanced antidepressant effects.

NURSING CONSIDERATIONS
- Contraindicated during acute recovery phase of myocardial infarction; in patients with prostatic hypertrophy. Use with extreme caution in patients with cardiovascular disease, urinary retention, narrow-angle glaucoma or increased intraocular pressure, thyroid disease, seizure disorders, blood dyscrasias, impaired hepatic function. Also contraindicated in patients who are suicide risks and in those receiving electroshock therapy, thyroid medication, or elective surgery.
- Reduce dose in elderly or debilitated persons, and adolescents.
- Do not withdraw abruptly.
- Watch for increased psychotic signs; dose should be reduced if they occur. Chart mood changes. Watch for suicidal tendencies. Allow only minimum supply of tablets to lessen suicide risk.
- Check for urinary retention and constipation. Increase fluids to lessen constipation. Suggest stool softener, if necessary.

Italicized side effects are common or life-threatening.
*Liquid form contains alcohol.   **May contain tartrazine.

- Warn patient to avoid activities that require alertness and good psychomotor coordination until CNS response to drug has been determined. Drowsiness and dizziness usually subside after a few weeks.
- Don't combine with alcohol or other depressants.
- Expect time lag of 10 to 14 days before noticeable effect. Full effect usually appears in 30 days.

- Dry mouth may be relieved with sugarless hard candy or gum.
- Effectiveness in enuresis may decrease over time. Similar in anticholinergic effects to other tricyclics.
- Advise patient not to use other drugs (prescription or over-the-counter) without first consulting the doctor.
- Whenever possible, patient should take full dose at bedtime.

29

Antianxiety agents

alprazolam
chlordiazepoxide hydrochloride
chlormezanone
clorazepate dipotassium
diazepam
halazepam
hydroxyzine hydrochloride
hydroxyzine pamoate
lorazepam
meprobamate
oxazepam
prazepam
tybamate

MECHANISM OF ACTION
• Benzodiazepines (alprazolam, chlordiazepoxide, clorazepate, diazepam, halazepam, lorazepam, oxazepam, and prazepam) appear to depress the CNS at the limbic and subcortical levels of the brain, with sedative, skeletal-muscle relaxant, and anticonvulsant effects. They can produce physical and psychological dependence.
• The mechanisms of the other tranquilizers are still unclear.

COMBINATION PRODUCTS
DEPROL**: meprobamate 400 mg and benactyzine HCl 1 mg.
EQUAGESIC: meprobamate 150 mg, ethoheptazine citrate 75 mg, and aspirin 250 mg.
EQUANITRATE 10•**: meprobamate 200 mg and pentaerythritol tetranitate 10 mg.
EQUANITRATE 20•**: meprobamate 200 mg and pentaerythritol tetranitrate 20 mg.

LIBRAX CAPSULES: chlordiazepoxide hydrochloride 5 mg and clidinium bromide 2.5 mg.
LIMBITROL 5-12.5: chlordiazepoxide 5 mg and amitriptyline (as HCl) 12.5 mg.
LIMBITROL 10-25: chlordiazepoxide 10 mg and amitriptyline (as HCl) 25 mg.
MENRIUM 5-2: chlordiazepoxide 5 mg and esterified estrogens 0.2 mg.
MENRIUM 5-4: chlordiazepoxide 5 mg and esterified estrogens 0.4 mg.
MENRIUM 10-4: chlordiazepoxide 10 mg and esterified estrogens 0.4 mg.
MILPATH-200: meprobamate 200 mg and tridihexethyl chloride 25 mg.
MILPATH-400: meprobamate 400 mg and tridihexethyl chloride 25 mg.
MILPREM-200: meprobamate 200 mg and conjugated estrogens 0.45 mg.
MILPREM-400: meprobamate 400 mg and conjugated estrogens 0.45 mg.
MILTRATE-10: meprobamate 200 mg and pentaerythritol tetranitrate 10 mg.
PATHIBAMATE-200 AND PATHIBAMATE-400• are identical to above Milpath products.
PMB 200: meprobamate 200 mg and conjugated estrogens 0.45 mg.
PMB 400: meprobamate 400 mg and conjugated estrogens 0.45 mg.

Italicized side effects are common or life-threatening.
*Liquid form contains alcohol.   **May contain tartrazine.

alprazolam
Xanax
Controlled Substance
Schedule IV

INDICATIONS & DOSAGE
Anxiety and tension—
Adults: Usual starting dose is 0.25 to
0.5 mg t.i.d. Maximum total daily dosage is 4 mg in divided doses. In elderly
or debilitated patients, usual starting
dose is 0.25 mg b.i.d. or t.i.d.

SIDE EFFECTS
CNS: *drowsiness, lightheadedness,*
headache, confusion, hostility.
CV: transient hypotension.
EENT: dry mouth.
GI: nausea, vomiting, discomfort.

INTERACTIONS
Cimetidine: possible increased sedation. Monitor patient carefully if used
together.

NURSING CONSIDERATIONS
• Contraindicated in acute narrow-
angle glaucoma, psychosis, and
anxiety-free psychiatric disorders.
• Reduce dosage in elderly or debilitated patients.
• Do not withdraw drug abruptly.
Abuse or addiction is possible. Withdrawal symptoms may occur.
• Warn patient not to combine drug
with alcohol or other depressants, and
also to avoid activities that require
alertness and psychomotor coordination
until response to drug is determined.
• Caution patient against giving medication to others.
• Drug should not be prescribed for everyday stress.
• Drug is not for long-term use (more
than 4 months).
• Warn patient not to continue drug
without doctor's approval.
• Alprazolam is the first of a new type
of benzodiazepine, known as a triazolo-
benzodiazepine. It's more rapidly metabolized and excreted than most of the
other drugs in the benzodiazepine class
and has a lower incidence of lethargy
than other drugs of this class.
• May also be effective for treatment
of depression.

chlordiazepoxide hydrochloride
Controlled Substance Schedule IV
A-poxide, Chlordiazachel,
C-Tran♦♦, J-Liberty, Libritabs,
Librium♦, Medilium♦♦,
Novopoxide♦♦, Protensin♦♦,
Relaxil♦♦, Sereen,
SK-Lygen, Solium♦♦, Tenax, Zetran

INDICATIONS & DOSAGE
Mild to moderate anxiety and tension—
Adults: 5 to 10 mg t.i.d. or q.i.d.
Children over 6 years: 5 mg P.O.
b.i.d. to q.i.d. Maximum 10 mg P.O.
b.i.d. to t.i.d.
Severe anxiety and tension—
Adults: 20 to 25 mg t.i.d. or q.i.d.
*Withdrawal symptoms of acute alcohol-
ism—*
Adults: 50 to 100 mg P.O., I.M., or
I.V. Maximum 300 mg daily.
*Preoperative apprehension and anx-
iety—*
Adults: 5 to 10 mg P.O. t.i.d. or q.i.d.
on day preceding surgery; or 50 to 100
mg I.M. 1 hour before surgery.
Note: parenteral form not recom-
mended in children under 12 years.

SIDE EFFECTS
CNS: *drowsiness, lethargy, hangover,*
fainting.
CV: transient hypotension.
GI: nausea, vomiting, abdominal dis-
comfort.
Local: *pain at injection site.*

INTERACTIONS
Cimetidine: increased sedation. Monitor carefully.

Unmarked trade names available in the United States only.
♦ Also available in Canada.   ♦♦ Available in Canada only.

NURSING CONSIDERATIONS

• Use with caution in patients with mental depression, blood dyscrasias, hepatic or renal disease, or in those undergoing anticoagulant therapy.
• Dosage should be reduced in elderly or debilitated patients.
• Possibility of abuse and addiction. Do not withdraw drug abruptly; withdrawal symptoms may occur.
• Warn patient to avoid activities that require alertness and good psychomotor coordination until CNS response to drug is determined.
• Warn patient not to combine drug with alcohol or other depressants.
• Although package recommends I.M. use only, this drug may be given I.V.
• Injectable form (as hydrochloride) comes as two ampuls—diluent and powdered drug. Read directions carefully. For I.M., add 2 ml of diluent to powder and agitate gently until clear. Use immediately. I.M. form may be erratically absorbed.
• For I.V., use 5 ml of saline injection or sterile water for injection as diluent; do not give packaged diluent I.V. Give slowly over 1 minute.
• Keep powder away from light; mix just before use; discard remainder.
• Do not mix injectable form with any other parenteral drug.
• Caution patient against giving medication to others.
• Drug should not be prescribed regularly for everyday stress.

chlormezanone
Fenarol, Trancopal♦

INDICATIONS & DOSAGE

Mild anxiety and tension, muscle relaxation—
Adults: 100 to 200 mg P.O. t.i.d. or q.i.d.
Children 5 to 12 years: 50 to 100 mg P.O. t.i.d. or q.i.d.

SIDE EFFECTS

CNS: *drowsiness,* mental depression, headache, dizziness, ataxia, lethargy, muscular weakness.
CV: edema.
GI: nausea, anorexia, dry mouth.
GU: urinary retention.
Skin: rash.

INTERACTIONS
None significant.

NURSING CONSIDERATIONS

• Use with caution in hepatic or renal disease.
• Dosage should be reduced in elderly or debilitated patients.
• Possibility of abuse and addiction exists. Do not withdraw drug abruptly; withdrawal symptoms may occur.
• Warn patient to avoid activities that require alertness and good psychomotor coordination until CNS response to drug is determined.
• Warn patient not to combine drug with alcohol or other depressants.
• Rapid onset of action (15 to 30 minutes), with effects lasting 4 to 6 hours.
• Chemically unrelated to other antianxiety agents.
• Suggest sugarless chewing gum or hard candy to relieve dry mouth.

clorazepate dipotassium
Controlled Substance Schedule IV
Tranxene♦

INDICATIONS & DOSAGE

Acute alcohol withdrawal—
Adults: Day 1—30 mg P.O. initially, followed by 30 to 60 mg P.O. in divided doses; Day 2—45 to 90 mg P.O. in divided doses; Day 3—22.5 to 45 mg P.O. in divided doses; Day 4—15 to 30 mg P.O. in divided doses; gradually reduce daily dose to 7.5 to 15 mg.
Anxiety—
Adults: 15 to 60 mg P.O. daily.
As an adjunct in epilepsy—

Adults and children over 12 years:
Maximum recommended initial dosage
is 7.5 mg P.O. t.i.d. Dosage increases
should be no greater than 7.5 mg/week.
Maximum daily dosage should not exceed 90 mg daily.
Children between 9 and 12 years:
Maximum recommended initial dosage
is 7.5 mg P.O. b.i.d. Dosage increases
should be no greater than 7.5 mg/
week. Maximum daily dosage should
not exceed 60 mg/day.

SIDE EFFECTS
CNS: *drowsiness, lethargy, hangover,*
fainting.
CV: transient hypotension.
GI: nausea, vomiting, abdominal dis-
comfort.

INTERACTIONS
Cimetidine: increased sedation. Monitor carefully.

NURSING CONSIDERATIONS
• Contraindicated in patients with
acute narrow-angle glaucoma, depressive neuroses, psychotic reactions, and
in children under 18 years. Use with
caution when hepatic or renal damage
is present.
• Dosage should be reduced in elderly
or debilitated patients.
• Possibility of abuse and addiction exists. Do not withdraw drug abruptly;
withdrawal symptoms may occur.
• Warn patient to avoid activities requiring alertness and good psychomotor coordination until CNS response
to drug is determined.
• Warn patient not to combine drug
with alcohol or other depressants.
• Suggest sugarless chewing gum or
hard candy to relieve dry mouth.
• Caution patient against giving medication to others.
• Drug should not be prescribed regularly for everyday stress.

diazepam
Controlled Substance Schedule IV
D-Tran♦♦, E-Pam♦♦, Erital♦♦,
Meval♦♦, NeoCalme♦♦,
Novodipam♦♦, Stress-Pam♦♦,
Valium♦, Valrelease, Vivol♦♦

INDICATIONS & DOSAGE
*Tension, anxiety, adjunct in convulsive
disorders or skeletal-muscle spasm—*
Adults: 2 to 10 mg P.O. t.i.d. or q.i.d.
Or, 15 to 30 mg of extended-release
capsule once daily.
Children over 6 months: 1 to 2.5 mg
P.O. t.i.d. or q.i.d.
*Tension, anxiety, muscle spasm, endos-
copic procedures, seizures—*
Adults: 5 to 10 mg I.V. initially, up to
30 mg in 1 hour or possibly more for
cardioversion or status epilepticus, de-
pending on response.
Children 5 years and over: 1 mg I.V.
or I.M. slowly q 2 to 5 minutes to maximum 10 mg. Repeat q 2 to 4 hours.
Children 30 days to 5 years: 0.2 to
0.5 mg I.V. or I.M. slowly q 2 to
5 minutes to maximum 5 mg. Repeat q
2 to 4 hours.
Tetanic muscle spasms—
Children over 5 years: 5 to 10 mg
I.M. or I.V. q 3 to 4 hours, p.r.n.
Infants over 30 days: 1 to 2 mg I.M.
or I.V. q 3 to 4 hours, p.r.n.

SIDE EFFECTS
CNS: *drowsiness, lethargy, hangover,*
fainting.
CV: transient hypotension.
GI: nausea, vomiting, abdominal dis-
comfort.
Local: desquamation, pain, phlebitis at
injection site.

INTERACTIONS
Cimetidine: increased sedation. Monitor carefully.

NURSING CONSIDERATIONS
• Contraindicated in shock, coma,
acute alcohol intoxication, acute

narrow-angle glaucoma, psychosis; in oral form for children under 6 months. Use with caution in patients with blood dyscrasias, hepatic or renal damage, depression, open-angle glaucoma; in elderly and debilitated patients; and in those with limited pulmonary reserve.

- Dosage should be reduced in elderly or debilitated patients.
- Possibility of abuse and addiction exists. Do not withdraw drug abruptly; withdrawal symptoms may occur.
- Warn patient to avoid activities that require alertness and good psychomotor coordination until CNS response to drug is determined.
- Warn patient not to combine drug with alcohol or other depressants.
- Do not dilute with solutions or mix with other drugs: incompatible.
- Avoid extravasation. Do not inject into small veins.
- Watch daily for phlebitis at injection site.
- Give I.V. slowly, at rate not exceeding 5 mg per minute.
- I.V. route is more reliable; I.M. absorption is variable, to be discouraged.
- Drug of choice (I.V. form) for status epilepticus.
- Do not store diazepam in plastic syringes.
- Caution patient against giving medication to others.
- Drug should not be prescribed regularly for everyday stress.

halazepam
Paxipam
Controlled Substance
Schedule IV

INDICATIONS & DOSAGE
Relief of anxiety and tension—
Adults: Usual dose is 20 to 40 mg P.O. t.i.d. or q.i.d.
Optimal daily dosage is generally 80 to 160 mg. Daily doses up to 600 mg have been given. In elderly or debilitated pa-

tients, initial dosage is 20 mg once or twice daily.
CNS: *drowsiness, lethargy, hangover,* fainting
CV: transient hypotension.
EENT: dry mouth.
GI: nausea and vomiting, discomfort.

INTERACTIONS
Cimetidine: possible increased sedation. Monitor carefully.

NURSING CONSIDERATIONS
- Contraindicated in acute narrow-angle glaucoma, psychosis, and anxiety-free psychiatric disorders. Use with caution in hepatorenal impairment.
- Reduce dosage in elderly or debilitated patients.
- Do not withdraw drug abruptly.
- Abuse and addiction are possible. Withdrawal symptoms may occur.
- Warn patient not to combine drug with alcohol or other depressants, and also to avoid activities that require alertness and psychomotor coordination until response to drug is determined.
- Caution patient against giving medication to others.
- Drug should not be prescribed for everyday stress.
- Halazepam is not for long-term use (more than 4 months).
- Warn patient not to continue the drug without the doctor's approval.

hydroxyzine hydrochloride
Atarax♦*, Hyzine-50, Orgatrax, Quiess, Vistaril (parenteral)

hydroxyzine pamoate
Vistaril (oral)

INDICATIONS & DOSAGE
Anxiety and tension—
Adults: 25 to 100 mg P.O. t.i.d. or q.i.d.
Anxiety, tension, hyperkinesia—
Children over 6 years: 50 to 100 mg P.O. daily in divided doses.

Italicized side effects are common or life-threatening.
*Liquid form contains alcohol.   **May contain tartrazine.

Children under 6 years: 50 mg P.O. daily in divided doses.
Preoperative and postoperative adjunctive therapy—
Adults: 25 to 100 mg I.M. q 4 to 6 hours.
Children: 1.1 mg/kg I.M. q 4 to 6 hours.

SIDE EFFECTS
CNS: *drowsiness,* involuntary motor activity.
GI: *dry mouth.*
Local: marked discomfort at site of I.M. injection.

INTERACTIONS
None significant.

NURSING CONSIDERATIONS
• Contraindicated in patients in shock or comatose states.
• Dosage should be reduced in elderly or debilitated patients.
• Possibility of abuse and addiction exists. Do not withdraw drug abruptly; withdrawal symptoms may occur.
• Warn patient to avoid activities that require alertness and good psychomotor coordination until CNS response to drug is determined.
• Warn patient not to combine drug with alcohol or other depressants.
• Observe for excessive sedation due to potentiation with other CNS drugs.
• Used as an antiemetic and antianxiety drug.
• Used in psychogenically induced allergic conditions, such as chronic urticaria and pruritus.
• Parenteral form (hydroxyzine HCl) for I.M. use only, never I.V.
• Aspirate injection carefully to prevent inadvertent intravascular injection. Inject deep into a large muscle.
• Suggest sugarless hard candy or gum to relieve dry mouth.

lorazepam
Controlled Substance Schedule IV
Ativan♦

INDICATIONS & DOSAGE
Anxiety, tension, agitation, irritability, especially in anxiety neuroses or organic (especially GI or CV) disorders—
Adults: 2 to 6 mg P.O. daily in divided doses. Maximum 10 mg daily.
Insomnia—
Adults: 2 to 4 mg P.O. h.s.
Premedication before operative procedure—
Adults: 2 to 4 mg I.M. or I.V.

SIDE EFFECTS
CNS: *drowsiness, lethargy, hangover,* fainting.
CV: transient hypotension.
GI: abdominal discomfort.

INTERACTIONS
None significant.

NURSING CONSIDERATIONS
• Contraindicated in myasthenia gravis, acute narrow-angle glaucoma, psychosis, mental depression. Use with caution in organic brain syndrome, renal or hepatic impairment.
• Dosage should be reduced in elderly or debilitated patients.
• Possibility of abuse and addiction exists. Do not withdraw drug abruptly; withdrawal symptoms may occur.
• When administering I.M., inject deep into muscle mass. Don't dilute.
• When administering I.V., dilute with an equal volume of sterile water for injection, sodium chloride injection, or 5% dextrose injection.
• Warn patient to avoid activities that require alertness or good psychomotor coordination until CNS response to drug is determined.
• Warn patient not to combine drug with alcohol or other depressants.
• Caution patient against giving medication to others.

- Drug should not be prescribed regularly for everyday stress.
- Fewer cumulative effects than other benzodiazepines, due to short half-life.

meprobamate
Controlled Substance Schedule IV
Arcoban, Bamate, Equanil**,
Kalmm, Maso-Bamate, Meditran,
Mep-E, Mepriam**, Meprocon,
Meprotabs, Meribam, Miltown♦,
Neo-Tran♦♦, Novomepro♦♦, Pax-
400, Quietal♦♦, Saronil,
Sedabamate, SK-Bamate, Tranmep

INDICATIONS & DOSAGE
Anxiety and tension—
Adults: 1.2 to 1.6 g P.O. in 3 or
4 equally divided doses. Maximum
2.4 g daily.
Children 6 to 12 years: 100 to 200 mg
P.O. b.i.d. or t.i.d. Not recommended
for children under 6 years.

SIDE EFFECTS
Blood: *thrombocytopenia, leukopenia,*
eosinophilia.
CNS: *drowsiness,* ataxia, dizziness,
slurred speech, headache, vertigo.
CV: palpitation, tachycardia, hypotension.
GI: anorexia, nausea, vomiting, diarrhea, stomatitis.
Skin: pruritus, urticaria, erythematous
maculopapular rash.

INTERACTIONS
None significant.

NURSING CONSIDERATIONS
- Contraindicated in patients with
hypersensitivity to meprobamate, carisoprodol, mebutamate, tybamate, carbromal; and in those with renal insufficiency or porphyria. Use with caution
in patients with impaired hepatic or
renal function, in lactating women, and
in patients with suicidal tendencies.
- Dosage should be reduced in elderly
or debilitated patients.

- Possibility of abuse and addiction exists. Withdraw drug gradually (over
2 weeks) or withdrawal symptoms may
occur.
- Warn patient to avoid activities that
require alertness or good psychomotor
coordination until CNS response to
drug is determined.
- Warn patient not to combine drug
with alcohol or other depressants.
- Give I.M. deep into muscle.
- Give P.O. with meals to reduce gastric distress.
- Therapeutic blood levels 0.5 to
2 mg/100 ml; levels above 20 mg/
100 ml may cause coma and death.
- Periodic evaluation of CBC and liver
function tests are indicated in patients
receiving high doses.

oxazepam
Controlled Substance Schedule IV
Serax♦**

INDICATIONS & DOSAGE
Alcohol withdrawal—
Adults: 15 to 30 mg P.O. t.i.d. or
q.i.d.
Severe anxiety—
Adults: 15 to 30 mg P.O. t.i.d. or
q.i.d.
Tension, mild to moderate anxiety—
Adults: 10 to 15 mg P.O. t.i.d. or
q.i.d.

SIDE EFFECTS
CNS: *drowsiness, lethargy, hangover,*
fainting.
CV: transient hypotension.
GI: nausea, vomiting, abdominal discomfort.

INTERACTIONS
None significant.

NURSING CONSIDERATIONS
- Contraindicated in psychoses. Use
cautiously in patients with history of
convulsive disorders, drug allergies,

Italicized side effects are common or life-threatening.
*Liquid form contains alcohol.   **May contain tartrazine.

blood dyscrasias, renal disease, depression.
- Dose should be reduced in elderly or debilitated patients.
- Possibility of abuse and addiction exists. Do not withdraw drug abruptly; withdrawal symptoms may occur.
- Warn patient to avoid activities that require alertness or good psychomotor coordination until CNS response to drug is determined.
- Warn patient not to combine drug with alcohol or other depressants.
- Fewer cumulative effects than most other benzodiazepines due to short half-life.
- Caution patient against giving medication to others.
- Drug should not be prescribed for everyday stress.

prazepam
Controlled Substance Schedule IV
Centrax

INDICATIONS & DOSAGE
Anxiety—
Adults: 30 mg P.O. in divided doses. Range 20 to 60 mg daily. May be administered as single daily dose at bedtime. Start with 20 mg.

SIDE EFFECTS
CNS: *drowsiness, lethargy, hangover,* fainting.
CV: transient hypotension.
GI: nausea, vomiting, abdominal discomfort.

INTERACTIONS
Cimetidine: increased sedation. Monitor carefully.

NURSING CONSIDERATIONS
- Contraindicated in patients with acute narrow-angle glaucoma, psychosis, and psychiatric disorders not showing anxiety. Use with caution in renal or hepatic impairment.

- Dosage should be reduced in elderly or debilitated patients.
- Possibility of abuse, addiction exists. Do not withdraw drug abruptly; withdrawal symptoms may occur.
- Warn patient to avoid activities that require alertness and good psychomotor coordination until CNS response to drug is determined.
- Warn patient not to combine drug with alcohol or other depressants.
- Caution patient against giving medication to others.
- Drug should not be prescribed for everyday stress.

tybamate
Controlled Substance Schedule IV
Tybatran**

INDICATIONS & DOSAGE
Anxiety and tension—
Adults: 750 mg to 2 g P.O. daily in divided doses; maximum 3 g daily.
Children 6 to 12 years: 20 to 25 mg/kg daily, divided into 3 or 4 doses.

SIDE EFFECTS
Blood: dyscrasias.
CNS: *drowsiness,* dizziness, fatigue, weakness, ataxia, depressive or panic reactions, paradoxical irritability, excitement, confusion, euphoria, insomnia, headache, paresthesias.
CV: flushing, light-headedness, hypotension, palpitation, tachycardia, fainting.
GI: nausea, anorexia, dry mouth, glossitis.
Skin: urticaria, pruritus, pruritus ani, rash.

INTERACTIONS
None significant.

NURSING CONSIDERATIONS
- Contraindicated in patients with history of hypersensitivity to tybamate or related compounds, such as meprobamate, carisoprodol, or mebutamate; in

---

Unmarked trade names available in the United States only.
♦ Also available in Canada.   ♦ ♦ Available in Canada only.

patients with convulsive disorders, drug allergies, blood dyscrasias, or porphyria; and in lactating women. Use with caution in hepatic or renal dysfunction.

• Dosage should be reduced in elderly or debilitated patients.

• Possibility of abuse and addiction exists. Do not withdraw drug abruptly; withdrawal symptoms may occur.

• Warn patient to avoid activities that require alertness and good psychomotor coordination until CNS response to drug is determined.

• Warn patient not to combine drug with alcohol or other depressants.

• Shorter acting than meprobamate.

• Periodic evaluation of CBC, liver and renal function tests are advised in patients receiving high doses or prolonged therapy.

• Suggest sugarless hard candy or gum to relieve dry mouth.

• This drug is rarely prescribed.

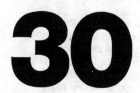

Antipsychotics

acetophenazine maleate
carphenazine maleate
chlorpromazine hydrochloride
chlorprothixene
droperidol
fluphenazine decanoate
fluphenazine enanthate
fluphenazine hydrochloride
haloperidol
loxapine succinate
mesoridazine besylate
molindone hydrochloride
perphenazine
piperacetazine
prochlorperazine edisylate
prochlorperazine maleate
promazine hydrochloride
thioridazine hydrochloride
thiothixene
thiothixene hydrochloride
trifluoperazine hydrochloride
triflupromazine hydrochloride

MECHANISM OF ACTION
• As antipsychotics, these drugs block postsynaptic dopamine receptors in the brain.
• As antiemetics, the drugs inhibit the medullary chemoreceptor trigger zone.

COMBINATION PRODUCTS
COMBID: prochlorperazine maleate 10 mg and isopropamide iodide 5 mg.
ESKATROL: prochlorperazine maleate 7.5 mg and dextroamphetamine sulfate 15 mg.
ETRAFON 2-10: perphenazine 2 mg and amitriptyline HCl 10 mg.
ETRAFON A: perphenazine 2 mg and amitriptyline HCl 25 mg.
ETRAFON-FORTE: perphenazine 4 mg and amitriptyline HCl 25 mg.
LIMBITROL 10-25: chlordiazepoxide 10 mg and amitriptyline (as HCl) 25 mg.
LIMBITROL 5-12.5: chlordiazepoxide 5 mg and amitriptyline (as HCl) 12.5 mg.
TRIAVIL 2-10, TRIAVIL 4-10, TRIAVIL 2-25 are identical to Etrafon products listed above; TRIAVIL 4-50: perphenazine 4 mg and amitriptyline HCl 50 mg.

acetophenazine maleate
Tindal

INDICATIONS & DOSAGE
Psychotic disorders—
Adults: initially, 20 mg P.O. t.i.d. or q.i.d. Daily dosage ranges from 40 to 80 mg in outpatients, or 80 to 120 mg in hospitalized patients, but in severe psychotic states up to 600 mg daily has been safely administered. Smallest effective dose should be used at all times.

SIDE EFFECTS
Blood: *transient leukopenia, agranulocytosis.*
CNS: *extrapyramidal reactions (high incidence),* sedation (low incidence), pseudoparkinsonism, EEG changes, dizziness.
CV: *orthostatic hypotension,* tachycardia, EKG changes.
EENT: *ocular changes, blurred vision.*
GI: *dry mouth, constipation.*
GU: *urinary retention,* dark urine, menstrual irregularities, gynecomastia, inhibited ejaculation.

Hepatic: *cholestatic jaundice, abnormal liver function tests.*
Metabolic: hyperprolactinemia.
Skin: *mild photosensitivity,* dermal allergic reactions, *exfoliative dermatitis.*
Other: weight gain, increased appetite.
After abrupt withdrawal of long-term therapy: gastritis, nausea, vomiting, dizziness, tremors, feeling of warmth or cold, sweating, tachycardia, headache, insomnia.

INTERACTIONS
Antacids: inhibit absorption of oral phenothiazines. Separate antacid and phenothiazine doses by at least 2 hours.
Barbiturates: may decrease phenothiazine effect. Observe patient.

NURSING CONSIDERATIONS
• Contraindicated in CNS depression, bone-marrow depression, subcortical damage, and coma; also with use of spinal or epidural anesthetic, or adrenergic blocking agents. Use cautiously with other CNS depressants, anticholinergics; in elderly or debilitated patients; and in patients with hepatic disease, arteriosclerosis or cardiovascular disease (may cause sudden drop in blood pressure), exposure to extreme heat or cold (including antipyretic therapy), respiratory disorders, hypocalcemia, convulsive disorders (may lower seizure threshold), severe reactions to insulin or electroshock therapy, suspected brain tumor or intestinal obstruction, glaucoma, or prostatic hypertrophy.
• Hold dose and notify doctor if patient develops symptoms of blood dyscrasias (fever, sore throat, infection, cellulitis, weakness), persistent (longer than a few hours) extrapyramidal reactions, or any such reaction during pregnancy.
• Dose of 20 mg is therapeutic equivalent of 100 mg chlorpromazine.
• Monitor therapy by weekly bilirubin tests during first month; periodic blood tests (CBC, liver function); and ophthalmic tests (long-term use).

• Check intake/output for urinary retention or constipation.
• Tell patient to use sunscreening agents and protective clothing to avoid photosensitivity reactions.
• Warn against activities requiring alertness or good psychomotor coordination until CNS response to drug is determined.
• Obtain baseline measures of blood pressure before starting therapy and monitor routinely. Watch for orthostatic hypotension. Advise patient to get up slowly.
• Dry mouth may be relieved with sugarless gum, sour hard candy, or rinsing with mouthwash.
• Avoid combining with alcohol or other depressants.
• Do not withdraw drug abruptly unless required by severe side effects.
• Patient on maintenance may take medication at bedtime to facilitate sleep and decrease sedation during daytime.

carphenazine maleate
Proketazine**

INDICATIONS & DOSAGE
Psychotic disorders—
Adults: initially, 12.5 to 50 mg P.O., b.i.d. or t.i.d. Increase gradually to maximum 100 mg daily.

SIDE EFFECTS
Blood: *transient leukopenia, agranulocytosis.*
CNS: *extrapyramidal reactions (high incidence),* sedation (low incidence), pseudoparkinsonism, EEG changes, dizziness.
CV: *orthostatic hypotension,* tachycardia, EKG changes.
EENT: *ocular changes, blurred vision.*
GI: *dry mouth, constipation.*
GU: *urinary retention,* dark urine, menstrual irregularities, gynecomastia, inhibited ejaculation.
Hepatic: *cholestatic jaundice, abnormal liver function tests.*

Italicized side effects are common or life-threatening.
∗Liquid form contains alcohol.   ∗∗May contain tartrazine.

Metabolic: hyperprolactinemia.
Skin: *mild photosensitivity,* dermal allergic reactions, *exfoliative dermatitis.*
Other: weight gain, increased appetite.
After abrupt withdrawal of long-term therapy: gastritis, nausea, vomiting, dizziness, tremors, feeling of warmth or cold, sweating, tachycardia, headache, insomnia.

INTERACTIONS

Antacids: inhibit absorption of oral phenothiazines. Separate antacid and phenothiazine doses by at least 2 hours.
Barbiturates: may decrease phenothiazine effect. Observe patient.

NURSING CONSIDERATIONS

• Contraindicated in CNS depression, bone-marrow depression, subcortical damage, and coma; also contraindicated with use of spinal or epidural anesthetic, or adrenergic blocking agents. Use cautiously with other CNS depressants, anticholinergics; in elderly or debilitated patients; in patients with hepatic disease, arteriosclerosis or cardiovascular disease (may cause sudden drop in blood pressure), exposure to extreme heat or cold (including antipyretic therapy), respiratory disorders, hypocalcemia, convulsive disorders (may lower seizure threshold), severe reactions to insulin or electroshock therapy, suspected brain tumor or intestinal obstruction, glaucoma, or prostatic hypertrophy; and in acutely ill or dehydrated children.
• Hold dose and notify doctor if patient develops symptoms of jaundice, blood dyscrasias (fever, sore throat, infection, cellulitis, weakness) or persistent (longer than a few hours) extrapyramidal reactions.
• Monitor therapy by weekly bilirubin tests during first month; periodic blood tests (CBC, liver function); and ophthalmic tests (long-term use).
• Check intake/output for urinary retention or constipation.
• Tell patient to use sunscreening agents and protective clothing to avoid photosensitivity reactions.
• Warn against activities that require alertness or good psychomotor coordination until CNS response to drug is determined. Drowsiness and dizziness usually subside after a few weeks.
• Obtain baseline measures of blood pressure before starting therapy and monitor regularly. Watch for orthostatic hypotension. Advise patient to get up slowly.
• Avoid combining with alcohol or other depressants.
• Do not withdraw drug abruptly unless required by severe side effects.
• Dry mouth may be relieved by sugarless gum, sour hard candy, or rinsing with mouthwash.
• Dose of 25 mg is therapeutic equivalent of 100 mg chlorpromazine.

chlorpromazine hydrochloride

Chlorprom♦♦, Chlor-Promanyl♦♦, Chlorzine, Klorazine, Largactil♦♦, Ormazine, Promachlor, Promapar, Promaz, Sonazine, Terpium, Thoradex, Thorazine

INDICATIONS & DOSAGE

Intractable hiccups—
Adults: 25 to 50 mg P.O. or I.M. t.i.d. or q.i.d.
Mild alcohol withdrawal, acute intermittent porphyria, and tetanus—
Adults: 25 to 50 mg I.M. t.i.d. or q.i.d.
Nausea and vomiting—
Adults: 10 to 25 mg P.O. or I.M. q 4 to 6 hours, p.r.n.; or 50 to 100 mg rectally q 6 to 8 hours, p.r.n.
Children: 0.25 mg/kg P.O. q 4 to 6 hours; or 0.25 mg/kg I.M. q 6 to 8 hours; or 0.5 mg/kg rectally q 6 to 8 hours.
Psychosis—
Adults: 500 mg P.O. daily in divided doses, increasing gradually to 2 g; or 25 to 50 mg I.M. q 1 to 4 hours, p.r.n.

Children: 0.25 mg/kg P.O. q 4 to 6 hours; or 0.25 mg/kg I.M. q 6 to 8 hours; or 0.5 mg/kg rectally q 6 to 8 hours. Maximum dose is 40 mg in children under 5 years, and 75 mg in children 5 to 12 years.

SIDE EFFECTS
Blood: *transient leukopenia, agranulocytosis.*
CNS: *extrapyramidal reactions (moderate incidence), sedation (high incidence),* pseudoparkinsonism, EEG changes, dizziness.
CV: *orthostatic hypotension,* tachycardia, EKG changes.
EENT: *ocular changes, blurred vision.*
GI: *dry mouth, constipation.*
GU: *urinary retention,* dark urine, menstrual irregularities, gynecomastia, inhibited ejaculation.
Hepatic: *cholestatic jaundice, abnormal liver function tests.*
Metabolic: hyperprolactinemia.
Skin: *mild photosensitivity,* dermal allergic reactions, *exfoliative dermatitis.*
Local: pain on I.M. injection, sterile abscess.
Other: weight gain, increased appetite.
After abrupt withdrawal of long-term therapy: gastritis, nausea, vomiting, dizziness, tremors, feeling of warmth or cold, sweating, tachycardia, headache, insomnia.

INTERACTIONS
Antacids: inhibit absorption of oral phenothiazines. Separate antacid and phenothiazine doses by at least 2 hours.
Anticholinergics (including antidepressant and antiparkinson agents): increased anticholinergic activity, aggravated parkinson-like symptoms. Use with caution.
Barbiturates: may decrease phenothiazine effect. Observe patient.
Lithium: possible decreased response to chlorpromazine. Observe patient.

NURSING CONSIDERATIONS
• Contraindicated in CNS depression, bone-marrow depression, subcortical damage, Reye's syndrome, and coma; also contraindicated with use of spinal or epidural anesthetic, or adrenergic blocking agents. Use cautiously with other CNS depressants, anticholinergics; in elderly or debilitated patients; in patients with hepatic disease, arteriosclerosis or cardiovascular disease (may cause sudden drop in blood pressure), exposure to extreme heat or cold (including antipyretic therapy), respiratory disorders, hypocalcemia, convulsive disorders (may lower seizure threshold), severe reactions to insulin or electroshock therapy, suspected brain tumor or intestinal obstruction, glaucoma, or prostatic hypertrophy; and in acutely ill or dehydrated children.
• Hold dose and notify doctor if patient develops jaundice, symptoms of blood dyscrasias (fever, sore throat, infection, cellulitis, weakness), persistent (longer than a few hours) extrapyramidal reactions, or any such reaction in pregnancy or in children.
• Monitor therapy by weekly bilirubin tests during first month; periodic blood tests (CBC, liver function); and ophthalmic tests (long-term use).
• Check intake/output for urinary retention or constipation.
• Tell patient to use sunscreening agents and protective clothing to avoid photosensitivity reactions.
• Warn against activities that require alertness or good psychomotor coordination until CNS response to drug is determined. Drowsiness and dizziness usually subside after first few weeks.
• Obtain baseline measures of blood pressure before starting therapy and monitor regularly. Watch for orthostatic hypotension, especially with parenteral administration. Monitor blood pressure before and after I.M. administration. Keep patient supine for 1 hour afterward. Advise patient to get up slowly.
• Avoid combining with alcohol or other depressants.

Italicized side effects are common or life-threatening.
*Liquid form contains alcohol.   **May contain tartrazine.

• Give deep I.M. only in upper outer quadrant of buttocks. Massage slowly afterward to prevent sterile abscess. Injection stings.

• Prevent contact dermatitis by keeping drug off patient's skin and clothes.

• Protect liquid concentrate from light. Dilute with fruit juice, milk, or semisolid food just before administration.

• Slight yellowing of injection or concentrate is common; does not affect potency. Discard markedly discolored solutions.

• Do not withdraw drug abruptly unless required by severe side effects.

• Dry mouth may be relieved by sugarless gum, sour hard candy, or rinsing with mouthwash.

• An aliphatic; has greater tendency to cause anticholinergic side effects than other phenothiazines.

---

chlorprothixene
Taractan**, Tarasan♦♦

INDICATIONS & DOSAGE
Psychotic disorders—
Adults: initially, 10 mg P.O. t.i.d. or q.i.d. Increase gradually to maximum 600 mg daily.
Children over 6 years: 10 to 25 mg P.O. t.i.d. or q.i.d.
Agitation of severe neurosis, depression, schizophrenia—
Adults: 25 to 50 mg P.O. or I.M. t.i.d. or q.i.d. Increase as needed up to maximum 600 mg.

SIDE EFFECTS
Blood: *transient leukopenia, agranulocytosis.*
CNS: extrapyramidal reactions (low incidence), sedation (low incidence), pseudoparkinsonism, EEG changes, dizziness.
CV: *orthostatic hypotension,* tachycardia, EKG changes.
EENT: *ocular changes, blurred vision.*
GI: *dry mouth, constipation.*
GU: *urinary retention,* dark urine,

menstrual irregularities, gynecomastia, inhibited ejaculation.
Hepatic: *cholestatic jaundice, abnormal liver function tests.*
Metabolic: hyperprolactinemia.
Skin: *mild photosensitivity,* dermal allergic reactions, *exfoliative dermatitis.*
Local: pain on I.M. injection, sterile abscess.
Other: weight gain, increased appetite.
After abrupt withdrawal of long-term therapy: gastritis, nausea, vomiting, dizziness, tremors, feeling of warmth or cold, sweating, tachycardia, headache, insomnia.

INTERACTIONS
None significant.

NURSING CONSIDERATIONS
• Contraindicated in coma, CNS depression, bone-marrow depression, circulatory collapse, congestive heart failure, cardiac decompensation, coronary artery or cerebral vascular disorders, subcortical damage; with use of spinal or epidural anesthetic, or adrenergic blocking agents. Use cautiously with other CNS depressants, anticholinergics; in elderly or debilitated patients; in patients with hepatic or renal disease, arteriosclerosis or cardiovascular disease (may cause sudden drop in blood pressure), exposure to extreme heat or cold (including antipyretic therapy), respiratory disorders, hypocalcemia, convulsive disorders (may lower seizure threshold), severe reactions to insulin or electroshock therapy, suspected brain tumor or intestinal obstruction, glaucoma, or prostatic hypertrophy; and in acutely ill or dehydrated children.

• Hold dose and notify doctor if patient develops symptoms of blood dyscrasias (fever, sore throat, infection, cellulitis, weakness), jaundice, persistent (longer than a few hours) extrapyramidal reactions, or any such reactions in children.

• Monitor therapy by weekly bilirubin tests during first month; periodic blood

---

tests (CBC, liver function) before and during therapy; and ophthalmic tests (long-term therapy).

• Check intake/output for urinary retention or constipation.

• Tell patient to use sunscreening agents and protective clothing to avoid photosensitivity reactions.

• Warn against activities that require alertness or good psychomotor coordination until CNS response to drug is determined. Drowsiness and dizziness usually subside after first few weeks.

• Obtain baseline measures of blood pressure before starting therapy and monitor regularly. Watch for orthostatic hypotension, especially with parenteral administration, since adrenergic blockage is high. Keep patient in a supine position for 1 hour afterward. Advise patient to change positions slowly.

• Avoid combining with alcohol or other depressants.

• Give deep I.M. only in upper outer quadrant of buttocks or midlateral thigh. Massage slowly afterward to prevent sterile abscess. Injection stings.

• Dilute liquid concentrate with fruit juice, milk, or semisolid food just before administration.

• Protect medication from light. Slight yellowing of injection or concentrate is common; does not affect potency. Discard markedly discolored solutions.

• Do not withdraw drug abruptly unless required by severe side effects.

• Prevent contact dermatitis by keeping drug off patient's skin and clothes.

• Dry mouth may be relieved by sugarless gum, sour hard candy, or rinsing with mouthwash.

• Dose of 100 mg is the therapeutic equivalent of 100 mg chlorpromazine.

droperidol
Inapsine♦

INDICATIONS & DOSAGE
Premedication—

Adults: 2.5 to 10 mg (1 to 4 ml) I.M. 30 to 60 minutes preoperatively.
Children 2 to 12 years: 1 to 1.5 mg (0.4 to 0.6 ml) per 20 to 25 lbs of body weight I.M..
As induction agent—
Adults: 2.5 mg (1 ml) per 20 to 25 lbs I.V. with analgesic and/or general anesthetic.
Children 2 to 12 years: 1 to 1.5 mg (0.4 to 0.6 ml) per 20 to 25 lbs. I.V. Dose should be titrated.
Elderly, debilitated patients: initial dose should be decreased.
*Maintenance dose in general anesthesia—*1.25 to 2.5 mg (0.5 to 1 ml) I.V.

SIDE EFFECTS
CNS: extrapyramidal reactions (dystonia, akathisia), upward rotation of eyes and oculogyric crises, extended neck, flexed arms, fine tremor of limbs, dizziness, chills or shivering, facial sweating, restlessness.
CV: hypotension, tachycardia.

INTERACTIONS
None significant.

NURSING CONSIDERATIONS
• Use cautiously in elderly or debilitated patients; and in patients with hypotension or other cardiovascular disease, impaired hepatic or renal function, Parkinson's disease.

• Watch for extrapyramidal reactions. Call doctor at once if any occur.

• Approved by FDA *only* for use preoperatively and during induction and maintenance of anesthesia.

• A butyrophenone compound, related to haloperidol; has greater tendency to cause extrapyramidal reactions than other antipsychotics.

• Keep intravenous fluids and vasopressors handy for hypotension.

• If used with a narcotic analgesic such as fentanyl (Sublimaze), be familiar with the special properties of each drug, particularly the widely differing

---

Italicized side effects are common or life-threatening.
✦Liquid form contains alcohol.   ✦✦May contain tartrazine.

10

45678910

durations of action. Watch for respiratory depression, apnea, and muscular rigidity, which could lead to respiratory arrest if untreated. Have narcotic antagonist and CPR equipment on hand.
• Monitor vital signs frequently; notify doctor of any changes immediately.
• Give intravenous injections slowly.
• Do not place patient in Trendelenburg position (that is, shock position); severe hypotension and deeper anesthesia may result, causing respiratory arrest.
• Has been used to prevent cisplatin-associated nausea and vomiting.

fluphenazine decanoate
Modecate Decanoate♦♦, Prolixin Decanoate

fluphenazine enanthate
Moditen Enanthate♦♦, Prolixin Enanthate

fluphenazine hydrochloride
Moditen Hydrochloride♦♦, Permitil Hydrochloride* **, Prolixin Hydrochloride* **

INDICATIONS & DOSAGE
Psychotic disorders—
Adults: initially, 0.5 to 10 mg fluphenazine HCl P.O. daily in divided doses q 6 to 8 hours; may increase cautiously to 20 mg. Higher doses (50 to 100 mg) have been given. Maintenance: 1 to 5 mg P.O. daily. I.M. doses are ⅓ to ½ oral doses. Lower doses for geriatric patients (1 to 2.5 mg daily).
Children: 0.25 to 3.5 mg fluphenazine HCl P.O. daily in divided doses q 4 to 6 hours; or ⅓ to ½ of oral dose I.M.; maximum 10 mg daily.
Adults, and children over 12 years: 12.5 to 25 mg of long-acting esters (fluphenazine decanoate and enanthate) I.M. or S.C. q 1 to 6 weeks. Maintenance: 25 to 100 mg, p.r.n.

SIDE EFFECTS
Blood: *transient leukopenia, agranulocytosis.*
CNS: *extrapyramidal reactions (high incidence),* sedation (low incidence), pseudoparkinsonism, EEG changes, dizziness.
CV: orthostatic hypotension, tachycardia, EKG changes.
EENT: *ocular changes, blurred vision.*
GI: *dry mouth, constipation.*
GU: *urinary retention,* dark urine, menstrual irregularities, gynecomastia, inhibited ejaculation.
Hepatic: *cholestatic jaundice, abnormal liver function tests.*
Metabolic: hyperprolactinemia.
Skin: *mild photosensitivity,* dermal allergic reactions, *exfoliative dermatitis.*
Other: weight gain, increased appetite.
After abrupt withdrawal of long-term therapy: gastritis, nausea, vomiting, dizziness, tremors, feeling of warmth or cold, sweating, tachycardia, headache, insomnia.

INTERACTIONS
Antacids: inhibit absorption of oral phenothiazines. Separate antacid and phenothiazine doses by at least 2 hours. *Barbiturates:* may decrease phenothiazine effect. Observe patient.

NURSING CONSIDERATIONS
• Contraindicated in coma, CNS depression, bone-marrow depression or other blood dyscrasia, subcortical damage, hepatic damage, renal insufficiency; and with use of spinal or epidural anesthetic, or adrenergic blocking agents. Use cautiously with other CNS depressants, anticholinergics; in elderly or debilitated patients; in acutely ill or dehydrated children; and in patients with hepatic disease, pheochromocytoma, arteriosclerotic, cerebrovascular, or cardiovascular disease (may cause sudden drop in blood pressure), peptic ulcer, exposure to extreme heat or cold (including antipyretic therapy), respiratory disorders, hypocalcemia, convul-

sive disorders (may lower seizure threshold), severe reactions to insulin or electroshock therapy, suspected brain tumor or intestinal obstruction, glaucoma, or prostatic hypertrophy.

• Hold dose and notify doctor if patient develops symptoms of blood dyscrasias (fever, sore throat, infection, cellulitis, weakness), persistent (longer than a few hours) extrapyramidal reactions, or any such reactions in pregnancy or in children.

• Monitor therapy by weekly bilirubin tests during first month; periodic blood tests (CBC, liver function); periodic renal function and ophthalmic tests (long-term use).

• Check intake/output for urinary retention or constipation.

• Tell patient to use sunscreening agents and protective clothing to avoid photosensitivity reactions.

• Warn against activities that require alertness and good psychomotor coordination until CNS response to drug is determined. Drowsiness and dizziness usually subside after first few weeks.

• Avoid combining with alcohol or other depressants.

• Decanoate and enanthate may be given subcutaneously.

• For long-acting forms (decanoate and enanthate), which are oil preparations, use a dry needle of at least 21 gauge. Allow 24 to 96 hours for onset of action. Important: note and report adverse side effects in patients taking the long-acting drug forms.

• Prevent contact dermatitis by keeping drug off patient's skin and clothes.

• Dilute liquid concentrate with water, fruit juice, milk, or semisolid food just before administration.

• Protect medication from light. Slight yellowing of injection or concentrate is common; does not affect potency. Discard markedly discolored solutions.

• Dry mouth may be relieved by sugarless gum, sour hard candy, or rinsing with mouthwash.

• Do not withdraw drug abruptly unless required by severe side effects.

• Dose of 2 mg is therapeutic equivalent of 100 mg chlorpromazine.

• Note that Permitil Concentrate is 10 times more concentrated than Prolixin Elixir (5 mg/ml vs. 0.5 mg/ml).

haloperidol
Haldol♦**

INDICATIONS & DOSAGE
Psychotic disorders—
Adults: dosage varies for each patient. Initial range is 0.5 to 5 mg P.O. b.i.d. or t.i.d.; or 2 to 5 mg I.M. q 4 to 8 hours, increasing rapidly if necessary for prompt control. Maximum 100 mg P.O. daily. Doses over 100 mg have been used for patients with severely resistant conditions.
Control of tics, vocal utterances in Gilles de la Tourette's syndrome—
Adults: 0.5 to 5 mg P.O. b.i.d. or t.i.d., increasing p.r.n.

SIDE EFFECTS
Blood: transient leukopenia and leukocytosis.
CNS: *high incidence of severe extrapyramidal reactions,* low incidence of sedation.
CV: low incidence of cardiovascular effects with therapeutic dosages.
EENT: blurred vision, dry mouth.
GU: urinary retention, menstrual irregularities, gynecomastia.
Skin: rash.

INTERACTIONS
Lithium: lethargy and confusion with high doses. Observe patient.
Methyldopa: possible symptoms of dementia. Observe patient.

NURSING CONSIDERATIONS
• Contraindicated in parkinsonism, coma, or CNS depression. Use with caution in elderly and debilitated patients; in severe cardiovascular disor-

---

Italicized side effects are common or life-threatening.
*Liquid form contains alcohol.   **May contain tartrazine.

ders, allergies, glaucoma, urinary retention; and in conjunction with anticonvulsant, anticoagulant, antiparkinson, or lithium medications.

• Warn patient against activities that require alertness and good psychomotor coordination until CNS response to drug is determined. Drowsiness and dizziness usually subside after a few weeks.

• Avoid combining with alcohol or other depressants.

• Protect medication from light. Slight yellowing of injection or concentrate is common; does not affect potency. Discard markedly discolored solutions.

• Do not withdraw drug abruptly unless required by severe side effects.

• Dry mouth may be relieved by sugarless gum, sour hard candy, and rinsing with mouthwash.

• Dose of 2 mg is therapeutic equivalent of 100 mg chlorpromazine.

• Only butyrophenone compound used as an antipsychotic in the United States.

loxapine succinate
Loxapac♦♦, Loxitane, Loxitane-C

INDICATIONS & DOSAGE
Psychotic disorders—
Adults: 10 mg P.O. or I.M. b.i.d. to q.i.d., rapidly increasing to 60 to 100 mg P.O. daily for most patients; dose varies from patient to patient.

SIDE EFFECTS
Blood: *transient leukopenia.*
CNS: *extrapyramidal reactions (moderate incidence), sedation (moderate incidence),* pseudoparkinsonism, EEG changes, dizziness.
CV: *orthostatic hypotension,* tachycardia, EKG changes.
EENT: *blurred vision.*
GI: *dry mouth, constipation.*
GU: *urinary retention,* dark urine, menstrual irregularities, gynecomastia.
Skin: *mild photosensitivity,* dermal allergic reactions, *exfoliative dermatitis.*

Other: weight gain, increased appetite.

INTERACTIONS
None significant.

NURSING CONSIDERATIONS
• Contraindicated in coma, severe CNS depression, drug-induced depressed states. Use with caution in epilepsy, cardiovascular disorders, glaucoma, urinary retention, suspected intestinal obstruction or brain tumor, renal damage.

• Warn against activities that require alertness and good psychomotor coordination until CNS response to drug is determined. Drowsiness and dizziness usually subside after first few weeks.

• Avoid combining with alcohol or other depressants.

• Obtain baseline measures of blood pressure before starting therapy and monitor regularly. Advise patient to get up slowly to avoid orthostatic hypotension.

• Dilute liquid concentrate with orange or grapefruit juice just before giving.

• Dry mouth may be relieved by sugarless gum, sour hard candy, or rinsing with mouthwash.

• Periodic ophthalmic tests recommended.

• Tricyclic dibenzoxazepine; the only dibenzoxazepine derivative.

• Dose of 10 mg is therapeutic equivalent of 100 mg chlorpromazine.

mesoridazine besylate
Serentil♦* **

INDICATIONS & DOSAGE
Alcoholism—
Adults and children over 12 years: 25 mg P.O. b.i.d. up to maximum 200 mg daily.
Behavioral problems associated with chronic brain syndrome—
Adults and children over 12 years: 25 mg P.O. t.i.d. up to maximum of 300 mg daily.

Unmarked trade names available in the United States only.
♦ Also available in Canada.   ♦ ♦ Available in Canada only.

Psychoneurotic manifestations (anxiety)—
Adults and children over 12 years: 10 mg P.O. t.i.d. up to maximum 150 mg daily.
Schizophrenia—
Adults and children over 12 years: initially, 50 mg P.O. t.i.d. or 25 mg I.M. repeated in 30 to 60 minutes, p.r.n.

SIDE EFFECTS
Blood: *transient leukopenia, agranulocytosis.*
CNS: extrapyramidal reactions (low incidence), *sedation (high incidence),* EEG changes, dizziness.
CV: *orthostatic hypotension,* tachycardia, EKG changes.
EENT: *ocular changes, blurred vision,* pigmentary retinopathy.
GI: *dry mouth, constipation.*
GU: *urinary retention,* dark urine, menstrual irregularities, gynecomastia, inhibited ejaculation.
Hepatic: *cholestatic jaundice, abnormal liver function tests.*
Metabolic: hyperprolactinemia.
Skin: *mild photosensitivity,* dermal allergic reactions, *exfoliative dermatitis.*
Local: pain at I.M. injection site, sterile abscess.
Other: weight gain, increased appetite.
After abrupt withdrawal of long-term therapy: gastritis, nausea, vomiting, dizziness, tremors, feeling of warmth or cold, sweating, tachycardia, headache, insomnia.

INTERACTIONS
Antacids: inhibit absorption of oral phenothiazines. Separate antacid and phenothiazine doses by at least 2 hours.
Barbiturates: may decrease phenothiazine effect. Observe patient.

NURSING CONSIDERATIONS
• Contraindicated in coma, CNS depression, bone-marrow depression, subcortical damage, and with use of spinal or epidural anesthetic or adrenergic blocking agents. Use cautiously with other CNS depressants, anticholinergics; in elderly or debilitated patients; in acutely ill or dehydrated children; and in patients with hepatic disease, arteriosclerosis or cardiovascular disease (may cause sudden drop in blood pressure), exposure to extreme heat or cold (including antipyretic therapy), respiratory disorders, hypocalcemia, convulsive disorders, severe reactions to insulin or electroshock therapy, suspected brain tumor or intestinal obstruction, glaucoma, or prostatic hypertrophy.
• Hold dose and notify doctor if patient develops jaundice, symptoms of blood dyscrasias (fever, sore throat, infection, cellulitis, weakness), persistent (longer than a few hours) extrapyramidal reactions, or any such reactions in pregnancy or in children over 12 years.
• Monitor therapy by weekly bilirubin tests during first month; periodic blood tests (CBC, liver function); and ophthalmic tests (long-term use).
• Check intake/output for urinary retention or constipation.
• Tell patient to use sunscreening agents and protective clothing to avoid photosensitivity reactions.
• Warn against activities that require alertness and good psychomotor coordination until CNS response to drug is determined. Drowsiness and dizziness usually subside after a few weeks.
• Avoid combining with alcohol or other depressants.
• Obtain baseline measures of blood pressure before starting therapy and monitor regularly. Watch for orthostatic hypotension, especially with parenteral administration. Advise patient to change positions slowly.
• Give deep I.M. only in upper outer quadrant of buttocks. Massage slowly afterward to prevent sterile abscess. Injection may sting.
• Protect medication from light. Slight yellowing of injection or concentrate is

---

Italicized side effects are common or life-threatening.
*Liquid form contains alcohol.   **May contain tartrazine.

common; does not affect potency. Discard markedly discolored solutions.
• Prevent contact dermatitis by keeping drug off patient's skin and clothes.
• Dry mouth may be relieved with sugarless gum, sour hard candy, or rinsing with mouthwash.
• Do not withdraw drug abruptly unless required by severe side effects.
• Drug is a piperidine phenothiazine (a metabolite of thioridazine).
• Dose of 50 mg is therapeutic equivalent of 100 mg chlorpromazine.

molindone hydrochloride
Lidone, Moban

INDICATIONS & DOSAGE
Psychotic disorders—
Adults: 50 to 75 mg P.O. daily, increasing to maximum 225 mg daily. Doses up to 400 mg may be required.

SIDE EFFECTS
Blood: *transient leukopenia.*
CNS: *extrapyramidal reactions (moderate incidence), sedation (moderate incidence),* pseudoparkinsonism, EEG changes, dizziness.
CV: *orthostatic hypotension,* tachycardia, EKG changes.
EENT: *blurred vision.*
GI: *dry mouth, constipation.*
GU: *urinary retention,* dark urine, menstrual irregularities, gynecomastia, inhibited ejaculation.
Hepatic: *cholestatic jaundice, abnormal liver function tests.*
Metabolic: hyperprolactinemia.
Skin: *mild photosensitivity,* dermal allergic reactions, *exfoliative dermatitis.*

INTERACTIONS
None significant.

NURSING CONSIDERATIONS
• Contraindicated in coma or severe CNS depression. Use with caution when increased physical activity would be harmful, as this agent increases activity; in seizures (may lower seizure threshold), suicide risk, suspected brain tumor, or intestinal obstruction.
• Warn against activities that require alertness or good psychomotor coordination until CNS response to drug is determined. Drowsiness and dizziness usually subside after first few weeks.
• Avoid combining with alcohol or other depressants.
• Dry mouth may be relieved with sugarless gum, sour hard candy, or rinsing with mouthwash.
• Drug is the only dihydroindolone derivative.
• Dose of 20 mg is therapeutic equivalent of 100 mg chlorpromazine.
• No injection available.
• Liquid oral concentrate is available.
• Lidone capsules contain tartrazine dye. May cause allergy in susceptible patients.
• May be administered in a single daily dose.

perphenazine
Phenazine♦♦, Trilafon♦

INDICATIONS & DOSAGE
Hospitalized psychiatric patients—
Adults: initially, 8 to 16 mg P.O. b.i.d., t.i.d., or q.i.d., increasing to 64 mg daily.
Children over 12 years: 6 to 12 mg P.O. daily in divided doses.
Mental disturbances, acute alcoholism, nausea, vomiting, hiccups—
Adults and children over 12 years: 5 to 10 mg I.M., p.r.n. Maximum 15 mg daily in ambulatory patients, 30 mg daily in hospitalized patients.

SIDE EFFECTS
Blood: *transient leukopenia, agranulocytosis.*
CNS: *extrapyramidal reactions (high incidence),* sedation (low incidence), pseudoparkinsonism, EEG changes, dizziness.

CV: *orthostatic hypotension,* tachycardia, EKG changes.
EENT: *ocular changes, blurred vision.*
GI: *dry mouth, constipation.*
GU: *urinary retention,* dark urine, menstrual irregularities, gynecomastia, inhibited ejaculation.
Hepatic: *cholestatic jaundice, abnormal liver function tests.*
Metabolic: hyperprolactinemia.
Skin: *mild photosensitivity,* dermal allergic reactions, *exfoliative dermatitis.*
Local: pain at I.M. injection site, sterile abscess.
Other: weight gain, increased appetite.
After abrupt withdrawal of long-term therapy: gastritis, nausea, vomiting, dizziness, tremors, feeling of warmth or cold, sweating, tachycardia, headache, insomnia.

INTERACTIONS

Antacids: inhibit absorption of oral phenothiazines. Separate antacid and phenothiazine doses by at least 2 hours.
Barbiturates: may decrease phenothiazine effect. Observe patient.

NURSING CONSIDERATIONS

• Contraindicated in coma, CNS depression, bone-marrow depression, subcortical damage, use of spinal or epidural anesthetic or adrenergic blocking agents. Use cautiously with other CNS depressants, anticholinergics; in elderly or debilitated patients; in acutely ill or dehydrated children; and in patients with hepatic disease, arteriosclerosis or cardiovascular disease (may cause sudden drop in blood pressure), exposure to extreme heat or cold (including antipyretic therapy), respiratory disorders, hypocalcemia, convulsive disorders (may lower seizure threshold), severe reactions to insulin or electroshock therapy, suspected brain tumor or intestinal obstruction, glaucoma, prostatic hypertrophy.
• Hold dose and notify doctor if patient develops jaundice, symptoms of blood dyscrasias (fever, sore throat, infection,

cellulitis, weakness), persistent (longer than a few hours) extrapyramidal reactions, or any such reactions in pregnancy or in children.
• Monitor therapy by weekly bilirubin tests during first month; periodic blood tests (CBC, liver function); and ophthalmic tests (long-term use).
• Check intake/output for urinary retention or constipation.
• Tell patient to use sunscreening agents and protective clothing to avoid photosensitivity reactions.
• Warn against activities that require alertness or good psychomotor coordination until CNS response to drug is determined. Drowsiness and dizziness usually subside after a few weeks.
• Avoid combining with alcohol or other depressants.
• Obtain baseline measures of blood pressure before starting therapy and monitor regularly. Watch for orthostatic hypotension, especially with parenteral administration. Keep patient supine for 1 hour afterward. Advise patient to change positions slowly.
• Give deep I.M. only in upper outer quadrant of buttocks. Massage slowly afterward to prevent sterile abscess. Injection may sting.
• Do not withdraw drug abruptly unless required by severe side effects.
• Protect drug from light. Slight yellowing of injection or concentrate is common; does not affect potency. Discard markedly discolored solutions.
• Prevent contact dermatitis by keeping drug off patient's skin and clothes.
• Dilute liquid concentrate with fruit juice, milk, carbonated beverage, or semisolid food just before giving. Exceptions: oral concentrate causes turbidity or precipitation in colas, black coffee, grape or apple juice, or tea. Do not mix with these liquids.
• Dry mouth may be relieved with sugarless gum, sour hard candy, or rinsing with mouthwash.
• Dose of 8 mg is therapeutic equivalent of 100 mg chlorpromazine.

Italicized side effects are common or life-threatening.
*Liquid form contains alcohol.   **May contain tartrazine.

piperacetazine
Quide♦**

INDICATIONS & DOSAGE
Psychotic disorders—
Adults: initially, 10 mg P.O. b.i.d. to
q.i.d. Dosage may be gradually increased to 160 mg daily if necessary.

SIDE EFFECTS
Blood: *transient leukopenia, agranulo-
cytosis.*
CNS: extrapyramidal reactions (low in-
cidence), *sedation (high incidence),*
EEG changes, dizziness.
CV: *orthostatic hypotension,* tachycar-
dia, EKG changes.
EENT: *ocular changes, blurred vision,*
pigmentary retinopathy.
GI: *dry mouth, constipation.*
GU: *urinary retention,* dark urine,
menstrual irregularities, gynecomastia,
inhibited ejaculation.
Hepatic: *cholestatic jaundice, abnormal liver function tests.*
Metabolic: hyperprolactinemia.
Skin: *mild photosensitivity,* dermal allergic reactions, *exfoliative dermatitis.*
Other: weight gain, increased appetite.
**After abrupt withdrawal of long-
term therapy:** gastritis, nausea, vomiting, dizziness, tremors, feeling of
warmth or cold, sweating, tachycardia,
headache, insomnia.

INTERACTIONS
Antacids: inhibit absorption of oral
phenothiazines. Separate antacid and
phenothiazine doses by at least 2 hours.
Barbiturates: may decrease phenothiazine effect. Observe patient.

NURSING CONSIDERATIONS
• Contraindicated in coma, CNS
depression, bone-marrow depression,
thrombocytopenia and other blood dyscrasias, subcortical damage, and with
use of spinal or epidural anesthetic or
adrenergic blocking agents. Use cautiously with other CNS depressants,

anticholinergics; in elderly or debilitated patients; in patients with hepatic
disease, arteriosclerosis or cardiovascular disease (may cause sudden drop in
blood pressure), exposure to extreme
heat or cold (including antipyretic therapy), respiratory disorders, hypocalcemia, convulsive disorders (may lower
seizure threshold), severe reactions to
insulin or electroshock therapy, suspected brain tumor or intestinal obstruction, glaucoma, or prostatic hypertrophy.
• Hold dose and notify doctor if patient
develops jaundice, symptoms of blood
dyscrasias (fever, sore throat, infection,
cellulitis, weakness), persistent (longer
than a few hours) extrapyramidal reactions, or any such reactions during
pregnancy.
• Monitor therapy by weekly bilirubin
tests during first month; periodic blood
tests (CBC, liver function); and
ophthalmic tests (long-term use).
• Check intake/output for urinary retention or constipation.
• Tell patient to use sunscreening
agents and protective clothing to avoid
photosensitivity reactions.
• Monitor blood pressure. Obtain baseline measures of blood pressure before
starting therapy. Watch for orthostatic
hypotension.
• Warn against activities that require
alertness or good psychomotor coordination until CNS response to drug is determined. Drowsiness and dizziness
usually subside after a few weeks.
• Avoid combining with alcohol or
other depressants.
• Protect tablets from light.
• Do not withdraw drug abruptly unless required by severe side effects.
• Dry mouth may be relieved with sugarless gum, sour hard candy, or rinsing
with mouthwash.
• Drug is a piperidine phenothiazine.
• Dose of 10 mg is therapeutic equivalent of 100 mg chlorpromazine.

prochlorperazine edisylate

prochlorperazine maleate

Compazine**, Stemetil◆◆

INDICATIONS & DOSAGE

Mild to moderate emotional disturbances—
Adults: 5 to 10 mg P.O. t.i.d. or q.i.d.; extended-release 15 mg P.O. in a.m. or 10 mg q 12 hours; 25 mg rectally b.i.d.; 5 to 10 mg I.M. q 3 to 4 hours.
Children weighing 18 to 38.5 kg:
5 mg P.O. or rectally b.i.d., to maximum of 15 mg daily.
Children weighing 13.5 to 17.5 kg:
2.5 mg P.O. or rectally b.i.d. or t.i.d., up to maximum 10 mg daily.
Children weighing 9 to 13 kg: 2.5 mg P.O. or rectally daily or b.i.d. to maximum 7.5 mg daily. I.M. dose 0.13 mg/kg; repeat if necessary. Not recommended in children under 9 kg.
Psychomotor agitation in schizophrenia; manic phase of manic-depressive psychosis; involutional toxic and senile psychoses—
Adults: initially, 10 mg P.O. t.i.d. to q.i.d., increasing up to 50 to 150 mg daily; or 10 to 20 mg I.M. q 1 to 4 hours, p.r.n., up to 100 mg daily, until symptoms are controlled. Prolonged I.M. dosage 10 to 20 mg q 4 to 6 hours.

SIDE EFFECTS

Blood: *transient leukopenia, agranulocytosis.*
CNS: *extrapyramidal reactions (high incidence),* sedation (low incidence), pseudoparkinsonism, EEG changes, dizziness.
CV: *orthostatic hypotension,* tachycardia, EKG changes.
EENT: *ocular changes, blurred vision.*
GI: dry mouth, constipation.
GU: *urinary retention,* dark urine, menstrual irregularities, gynecomastia, inhibited ejaculation.

Hepatic: *cholestatic jaundice, abnormal liver function tests.*
Metabolic: hyperprolactinemia.
Skin: *mild photosensitivity,* dermal allergic reactions, *exfoliative dermatitis.*
Local: pain at I.M. injection site, sterile abscess.
Other: weight gain, increased appetite.
After abrupt withdrawal of long-term therapy: gastritis, nausea, vomiting, dizziness, tremors, feeling of warmth or cold, sweating, tachycardia, headache, insomnia.

INTERACTIONS

Antacids: inhibit absorption of oral phenothiazines. Separate antacid and phenothiazine doses by at least 2 hours.
Barbiturates: may decrease phenothiazine effect. Observe patient.

NURSING CONSIDERATIONS

• Contraindicated in coma, depression, CNS depression, bone-marrow depression, subcortical damage, pediatric surgery, and with use of spinal or epidural anesthetic, adrenergic blocking agents, or alcohol. Use cautiously with other CNS depressants, anticholinergics; in elderly or debilitated patients; in patients with hepatic disease, arteriosclerosis or cardiovascular disease (may cause sudden drop in blood pressure), exposure to extreme heat or cold (including antipyretic therapy), respiratory disorders, hypocalcemia, vomiting in children, convulsive disorders (may lower seizure threshold) or severe reactions to insulin or electroshock therapy, suspected brain tumor or intestinal obstruction, glaucoma, or prostatic hypertrophy; and in acutely ill or dehydrated children.
• Hold dose and notify doctor if patient develops jaundice, symptoms of blood dyscrasias (fever, sore throat, infection, cellulitis, weakness), persistent (longer than a few hours) extrapyramidal reactions, or any such reactions during pregnancy or in children.
• Monitor therapy by weekly bilirubin

Italicized side effects are common or life-threatening.
∗Liquid form contains alcohol.　　∗∗May contain tartrazine.

tests during first month; periodic blood tests (CBC, liver function); and ophthalmic tests (long-term use).
- Check intake/output for urinary retention or constipation.
- Tell patient to use sunscreening agents and protective clothing to avoid photosensitivity reactions.
- Warn against activities that require alertness or good psychomotor coordination until CNS response to drug is determined. Drowsiness and dizziness usually subside after a few weeks.
- Avoid combining with alcohol or other depressants.
- Obtain baseline measures of blood pressure. Monitor blood pressure and heart rate regularly. Watch for orthostatic hypotension, especially with parenteral administration. Advise patient to change positions slowly.
- Give deep I.M. only in upper outer quadrant of buttocks. Massage slowly afterward to prevent sterile abscess. Injection may sting.
- Do not mix in same syringe with another drug.
- Do not give subcutaneously.
- Protect from light. Slight yellowing of injection or concentrate is common; does not affect potency. Discard markedly discolored solutions.
- Prevent contact dermatitis by keeping drug off patient's skin and clothes.
- Dilute liquid concentrate with at least 60 ml fruit juice, milk, coffee, tea, carbonated beverages, or semisolid food just before giving.
- Do not withdraw drug abruptly unless required by severe side effects.
- Dry mouth may be relieved with sugarless gum, sour hard candy, or rinsing with mouthwash.
- Piperazine phenothiazine; most commonly used as an antiemetic.
- If more than 4 doses are needed in 24-hour period, notify doctor.
- Injectable form may be mixed with solutions of 5% dextrose, 10% dextrose, 10% fructose, 5% invert sugar, 10% invert sugar, normal saline, Ring-

er's injection, lactated Ringer's I.V. infusion, and dextrose-saline combinations.

promazine hydrochloride
Promabec◆◆, Promanyl◆◆, Promazettes◆◆, Sparine◆**

INDICATIONS & DOSAGE
Psychosis—
Adults: 25 to 200 mg P.O. or I.M. q 4 to 6 hours, up to 1 g daily. I.V. dose in concentrations no greater than 25 mg/ml for acutely agitated patients. Initial dose 50 to 150 mg; repeat within 5 to 10 minutes if necessary.
Children over 12 years: 10 to 25 mg P.O. or I.M. q 4 to 6 hours.

SIDE EFFECTS
Blood: *transient leukopenia, agranulocytosis.*
CNS: *extrapyramidal reactions (moderate incidence), sedation (high incidence),* pseudoparkinsonism, EEG changes, dizziness.
CV: *orthostatic hypotension,* tachycardia, EKG changes.
EENT: *ocular changes, blurred vision.*
GI: *dry mouth, constipation.*
GU: *urinary retention,* dark urine, menstrual irregularities, gynecomastia, inhibited ejaculation.
Hepatic: *cholestatic jaundice, abnormal liver function tests.*
Metabolic: hyperprolactinemia.
Skin: *mild photosensitivity,* dermal allergic reactions, *exfoliative dermatitis.*
Local: pain at I.M. injection site, sterile abscess.
Other: weight gain, increased appetite.
After abrupt withdrawal of long-term therapy: gastritis, nausea, vomiting, dizziness, tremors, feeling of warmth or cold, sweating, tachycardia, headache, insomnia.

INTERACTIONS
Antacids: inhibit absorption of oral

phenothiazines. Separate antacid and phenothiazine doses by at least 2 hours.
Anticholinergics (including antidepressant and antiparkinson agents): increased anticholinergic activity, aggravated parkinson-like symptoms. Use with caution.
Barbiturates: may decrease phenothiazine effect. Observe patient.

NURSING CONSIDERATIONS
• Contraindicated in coma, CNS depression, bone-marrow depression, subcortical damage, and with use of spinal or epidural anesthetic or adrenergic blocking agents. Use cautiously with other CNS depressants, anticholinergics; in elderly or debilitated patients; in patients with hepatic disease, arteriosclerosis or cardiovascular disease (may cause sudden drop in blood pressure), exposure to extreme heat or cold (including antipyretic therapy), respiratory disorders, hypocalcemia, convulsive disorders (may lower seizure threshold), severe reactions to insulin or electroshock therapy, suspected brain tumor or intestinal obstruction, glaucoma, prostatic hypertrophy; and in acutely ill or dehydrated children.
• Hold dose and notify doctor if patient develops jaundice, symptoms of blood dyscrasias (fever, sore throat, infection, cellulitis, weakness), persistent (longer than a few hours) extrapyramidal reactions, or such reactions during pregnancy or in children.
• Monitor therapy by weekly bilirubin tests during first month; periodic blood tests (CBC, liver function); and ophthalmic tests (long-term use).
• Check intake/output for urinary retention or constipation.
• Tell patient to use sunscreening agents and protective clothing to avoid photosensitivity reactions.
• Warn against activities that require alertness or good psychomotor coordination until CNS response to drug is de-

termined. Drowsiness and dizziness usually subside after a few weeks.
• Avoid combining with alcohol or other depressants.
• Monitor blood pressure with patient lying and standing before starting therapy, and routinely throughout course of treatment.
• Watch for orthostatic hypotension, especially with parenteral administration. Keep patient supine for 1 hour afterward. Advise patient to change positions slowly.
• Give deep I.M. only in upper outer quadrant of buttocks. Massage slowly afterward to prevent sterile abscess. Injection may sting.
• Protect drug from light. Slight yellowing of injection or concentrate is common; does not affect potency. Discard markedly discolored solutions.
• Prevent contact dermatitis by keeping drug off patient's skin and clothes.
• Dilute liquid concentrate with fruit juice, milk, semisolid food, or chocolate-flavored drinks just before giving. For best taste, use at least 10 ml diluent per 25 mg drug.
• Do not withdraw drug abruptly unless required by severe side effects.
• Dry mouth may be relieved with sugarless gum, sour hard candy, or rinsing with mouthwash.
• Drug is an aliphatic phenothiazine; it's seldom prescribed for psychiatric treatment.

thioridazine hydrochloride
Mellaril♦*, Novoridazine♦♦

INDICATIONS & DOSAGE
Psychosis—
Adults: initially, 50 to 100 mg P.O. t.i.d., with gradual increments up to 800 mg daily in divided doses, if needed. Dosage varies. Dose above 800 mg may be associated with ocular toxicity (pigmentary retinopathy).
Depressive neurosis, alcohol with-

---

drawal, dementia in geriatric patients, behavioral problems in children—
Adults: initially, 25 mg P.O. t.i.d. Maintenance dose is 20 to 200 mg daily.
Children over 2 years: 0.5 to 3 mg/kg daily in divided doses.

SIDE EFFECTS
Blood: *transient leukopenias, agranulocytosis.*
CNS: extrapyramidal reactions (low incidence), *sedation (high incidence),* EEG changes, dizziness.
CV: *orthostatic hypotension,* tachycardia, EKG changes.
EENT: *ocular changes, blurred vision,* pigmentary retinopathy.
GI: *dry mouth, constipation.*
GU: *urinary retention,* dark urine, menstrual irregularities, gynecomastia, inhibited ejaculation.
Hepatic: *cholestatic jaundice.*
Metabolic: hyperprolactinemia.
Skin: *mild photosensitivity,* dermal allergic reactions, *exfoliative dermatitis.*
Other: weight gain, increased appetite.
After abrupt withdrawal of long-term therapy: gastritis, nausea, vomiting, dizziness, tremors, feeling of warmth or cold, sweating, tachycardia, headache, insomnia.

INTERACTIONS
Antacids: inhibit absorption of oral phenothiazines. Separate antacid and phenothiazine doses by at least 2 hours.
Barbiturates: may decrease phenothiazine effect. Observe patient.

NURSING CONSIDERATIONS
• Contraindicated in coma, CNS depression, bone-marrow depression, hypertensive or hypotensive cardiac disease, subcortical damage, and with use of spinal or epidural anesthetic or adrenergic blocking agents. Use cautiously with other CNS depressants, anticholinergics; in elderly or debilitated patients; in patients with hepatic disease, arteriosclerosis or cardiovascular disease (may cause sudden drop in blood pressure), exposure to extreme heat or cold (including antipyretic therapy), respiratory disorders, hypocalcemia, convulsive disorders, severe reactions to insulin or electroshock therapy, suspected brain tumor or intestinal obstruction, glaucoma, or prostatic hypertrophy; and in acutely ill or dehydrated children.
• Hold dose and notify doctor if patient develops jaundice, symptoms of blood dyscrasias (fever, sore throat, infection, cellulitis, weakness), persistent (longer than a few hours) extrapyramidal reactions, or such reactions during pregnancy or in children.
• Monitor therapy by weekly bilirubin tests during first month; periodic blood tests (CBC, liver function); and ophthalmic tests (long-term therapy).
• Check intake/output for urinary retention or constipation.
• Watch for blurred vision, dry mouth; high incidence of anticholinergic effects.
• Tell patient to use sunscreening agents and protective clothing to avoid photosensitivity reactions.
• Monitor blood pressure.
• Warn against activities that require alertness or good psychomotor coordination until response to drug is determined. Drowsiness and dizziness usually subside after a few weeks.
• Avoid combining with alcohol or other depressants.
• Watch for orthostatic hypotension, especially with parenteral administration. Advise patient to change positions slowly.
• Prevent contact dermatitis by keeping drug off patient's skin and clothes.
• Caution: There are four different liquid formulations available (two concentrates and two suspensions).
• Dilute liquid concentrate with water or fruit juice just before giving.
• Do not withdraw abruptly unless required by severe side effects.
• Dry mouth may be relieved with sug-

arless gum, sour hard candy, or rinsing with mouthwash.
• A piperidine phenothiazine.
• Dose of 100 mg is the therapeutic equivalent of 100 mg chlorpromazine.

thiothixene

thiothixene hydrochloride
Navane♦*

INDICATIONS & DOSAGE
Acute agitation—
Adults: 4 mg I.M. b.i.d. to q.i.d. Maximum 30 mg daily I.M. Change to P.O. as soon as possible.
Mild to moderate psychosis—
Adults: initially, 2 mg P.O. t.i.d. May increase gradually to 15 mg daily.
Severe psychosis—
Adults: initially, 5 mg P.O. b.i.d. May increase gradually to 15 to 30 mg daily. Maximum recommended daily dose 60 mg. Not recommended in children under 12 years.

SIDE EFFECTS
Blood: *transient leukopenia, agranulocytosis.*
CNS: *extrapyramidal reactions (high incidence),* sedation (low incidence), pseudoparkinsonism, EEG changes, dizziness.
CV: *orthostatic hypotension,* tachycardia, EKG changes.
EENT: *ocular changes, blurred vision.*
GI: *dry mouth,* constipation.
GU: *urinary retention,* dark urine, menstrual irregularities, gynecomastia, inhibited ejaculation.
Hepatic: *cholestatic jaundice.*
Metabolic: hyperprolactinemia.
Skin: *mild photosensitivity,* dermal allergic reactions, *exfoliative dermatitis.*
Local: pain at I.M. injection site, sterile abscess.
Other: weight gain, increased appetite.
After abrupt withdrawal of long-term therapy: gastritis, nausea, vomiting, dizziness, tremors, feeling of warmth or cold, sweating, tachycardia, headache, insomnia.

INTERACTIONS
None significant.

NURSING CONSIDERATIONS
• Contraindicated in convulsive seizures, circulatory collapse, coma, CNS depression, blood dyscrasias, bone-marrow depression, alcohol withdrawal, akathisia or restlessness, subcortical damage, and with use of spinal or epidural anesthetic or adrenergic blocking agents. Use cautiously with other CNS depressants, anticholinergics; in elderly or debilitated patients; and in patients with hepatic disease, arteriosclerosis or cardiovascular disease (may cause sudden drop in blood pressure), exposure to extreme heat or cold (including antipyretic therapy) or undue sunlight, respiratory disorders, hypocalcemia, severe reactions to insulin or electroshock therapy, suspected brain tumor or intestinal obstruction, glaucoma, or prostatic hypertrophy.
• Hold dose and notify doctor if patient develops jaundice, symptoms of blood dyscrasias (fever, sore throat, infection, cellulitis, weakness), persistent (longer than a few hours) extrapyramidal reactions, or any such reactions during pregnancy.
• Monitor therapy by weekly bilirubin tests during first month; periodic blood tests (CBC, liver function); and ophthalmic tests (long-term therapy).
• Check intake/output for urinary retention or constipation.
• Tell patient to use sunscreening agents and protective clothing to avoid photosensitivity reactions.
• Warn against activities that require alertness or good psychomotor coordination until CNS response to drug is determined. Drowsiness and dizziness usually subside after a few weeks.
• Avoid combining with alcohol or other depressants.

Italicized side effects are common or life-threatening.
*Liquid form contains alcohol.   **May contain tartrazine.

• Watch for orthostatic hypotension, especially with parenteral administration. Keep patient in a supine position for 1 hour afterward. Advise patient to change positions slowly.

• Give I.M. only in upper outer quadrant of buttocks or midlateral thigh. Massage slowly afterward to prevent sterile abscess. Injection may sting.

• I.M. form must be stored in refrigerator.

• Slight yellowing of injection or concentrate is common; does not affect potency. Discard markedly discolored solutions.

• Prevent contact dermatitis by keeping drug off patient's skin and clothes.

• Dilute liquid concentrate with fruit juice, milk, or semisolid food just before giving.

• Do not withdraw abruptly unless required by severe side effects.

• Dry mouth may be relieved with sugarless gum, sour hard candy, or rinsing with mouthwash.

• Drug is a thioxanthene derivative but produces responses similar to phenothiazines and butyrophenones.

• Dose of 4 mg is therapeutic equivalent of 100 mg chlorpromazine.

trifluoperazine hydrochloride
Novoflurazine♦♦, Solazine♦♦, Stelazine♦, Terfluzine♦♦, Triflurin♦♦

INDICATIONS & DOSAGE
Anxiety states—
Adults: 1 to 2 mg P.O. b.i.d.
Schizophrenia and other psychotic disorders—
Adults: outpatients—1 to 2 mg P.O. b.i.d., up to 4 mg daily; hospitalized—2 to 5 mg P.O. b.i.d.; may gradually increase to 40 mg daily. 1 to 2 mg I.M. q 4 to 6 hours, p.r.n.
Children 6 to 12 years (hospitalized or under close supervision): 1 mg P.O. daily or b.i.d.; may increase gradually to 15 mg daily.

SIDE EFFECTS
Blood: *transient leukopenia, agranulocytosis.*
CNS: *extrapyramidal reactions (high incidence),* sedation (low incidence), pseudoparkinsonism, EEG changes, dizziness.
CV: *orthostatic hypotension,* tachycardia, EKG changes.
EENT: *ocular changes, blurred vision.*
GI: *dry mouth, constipation.*
GU: *urinary retention,* dark urine, menstrual irregularities, gynecomastia, inhibited ejaculation.
Hepatic: *cholestatic jaundice.*
Metabolic: hyperprolactinemia.
Skin: *mild photosensitivity,* dermal allergic reactions, *exfoliative dermatitis.*
Local: pain at I.M. injection site, sterile abscess.
Other: weight gain, increased appetite.
After abrupt withdrawal of long-term therapy: gastritis, nausea, vomiting, dizziness, tremors, feeling of warmth or cold, sweating, tachycardia, headache, insomnia.

INTERACTIONS
Antacids: inhibit absorption of oral phenothiazines. Separate antacid and phenothiazine doses by at least 2 hours.
Barbiturates: may decrease phenothiazine effect. Observe patient.

NURSING CONSIDERATIONS
• Contraindicated in coma, CNS depression, bone-marrow depression, subcortical damage, and with use of spinal or epidural anesthetic or adrenergic blocking agents. Use cautiously with other CNS depressants, anticholinergics; in elderly or debilitated patients; in patients with hepatic disease, arteriosclerosis or cardiovascular disease (may cause drop in blood pressure), exposure to extreme heat or cold (including antipyretic therapy), respiratory disorders, hypocalcemia, convulsive disorders, severe reactions to insulin or electroshock therapy, suspected brain tumor or intestinal obstruction,

---

Unmarked trade names available in the United States only.
♦ Also available in Canada.   ♦♦ Available in Canada only.

glaucoma, or prostatic hypertrophy; and in acutely ill or dehydrated children.

• Hold dose and notify doctor if patient develops jaundice, symptoms of blood dyscrasias (fever, sore throat, infection, cellulitis, weakness), persistent (longer than a few hours) extrapyramidal reactions, or any such reactions during pregnancy or in children.

• Monitor therapy by weekly bilirubin tests during first month; periodic blood tests (CBC, liver function); and ophthalmic tests (long-term therapy).

• Check intake/output for urinary retention or constipation.

• Tell patient to use sunscreening agents and protective clothing to avoid photosensitivity reactions.

• Warn against activities that require alertness or good psychomotor coordination until CNS response to drug is determined. Drowsiness and dizziness usually subside after a few weeks.

• Avoid combining with alcohol or other depressants.

• Watch for orthostatic hypotension, especially with parenteral administration. Keep patient supine for 1 hour afterward. Advise patient to change positions slowly.

• Give deep I.M. only in upper outer quadrant of buttocks. Massage slowly afterward to prevent sterile abscess. Injection may sting.

• Protect drug from light. Slight yellowing of injection or concentrate is common; does not affect potency. Discard markedly discolored solutions.

• Prevent contact dermatitis by keeping drug off patient's skin and clothes.

• Dilute liquid concentrate with 60 ml tomato or fruit juice, carbonated beverages, coffee, tea, milk, water, or semisolid food just before giving.

• Do not withdraw abruptly unless required by severe side effects.

• Dry mouth may be relieved with sugarless gum, sour hard candy, or rinsing with mouthwash.

• Drug is a prototype piperazine phenothiazine.

• Dose of 5 mg is therapeutic equivalent of 100 mg chlorpromazine.

triflupromazine hydrochloride
Vesprin**

INDICATIONS & DOSAGE
Acute, severe agitation—
Adults: 60 to 150 mg I.M. in 2 or 3 divided doses.
Children over 2½ years: 0.2 to 0.25 mg/kg in divided doses. Maximum dose 10 mg daily.
Nausea and vomiting—
Adults: 20 to 30 mg P.O. daily; or 1 to 3 mg I.V. daily; or 5 to 15 mg I.M. daily up to maximum 60 mg daily.
Children: 0.2 mg/kg P.O. or I.M. up to maximum 10 mg daily.
Psychotic disorders (mild to moderate symptoms)—
Adults: 10 to 25 mg P.O. b.i.d.
Children over 2½ years: 10 mg P.O. t.i.d.
Elderly or debilitated patients: 10 mg b.i.d. or t.i.d.; increase gradually to desired effect.
Severe symptoms—
Adults: 50 mg P.O. b.i.d. or t.i.d.
Children over 2½ years: 2 mg/kg P.O. in 3 divided doses; may increase gradually to 150 mg daily.

SIDE EFFECTS
Blood: *transient leukopenia, agranulocytosis.*
CNS: *extrapyramidal reactions (moderate incidence), sedation (high incidence),* pseudoparkinsonism, EEG changes, dizziness.
CV: *orthostatic hypotension,* tachycardia, EKG changes.
EENT: *ocular changes, blurred vision.*
GI: *dry mouth, constipation.*
GU: *urinary retention,* dark urine, menstrual irregularities, gynecomastia, inhibited ejaculation.

Italicized side effects are common or life-threatening.
*Liquid form contains alcohol.   **May contain tartrazine.

Hepatic: *cholestatic jaundice.*
Metabolic: hyperprolactinemia.
Skin: *mild photosensitivity,* dermal allergic reactions, *exfoliative dermatitis.*
Local: pain at I.M. injection site, sterile abscess.
Other: weight gain, increased appetite.
After abrupt withdrawal of long-term therapy: gastritis, nausea, vomiting, dizziness, tremors, feeling of warmth or cold, sweating, tachycardia, headache, insomnia.

INTERACTIONS

Antacids: inhibit absorption of oral phenothiazines. Separate antacid and phenothiazine doses by at least 2 hours.
Anticholinergics (including antidepressant and antiparkinson agents): increased anticholinergic activity, aggravated parkinson-like symptoms. Use with caution.
Barbiturates: may decrease phenothiazine effect. Observe patient.

NURSING CONSIDERATIONS

• Contraindicated in coma, CNS depression, blood dyscrasias, bone-marrow depression, subcortical brain damage, and with use of spinal or epidural anesthetic or adrenergic blocking agents. Use cautiously with other CNS depressants, anticholinergics; in elderly or debilitated patients; in patients with hepatic disease, arteriosclerosis or cardiovascular disease (may cause sudden drop in blood pressure), exposure to extreme heat or cold (including antipyretic therapy), respiratory disorders, pheochromocytoma, hypocalcemia, convulsive disorders, severe reactions to insulin or electroshock therapy, suspected brain tumor or intestinal obstruction, glaucoma, prostatic hypertrophy; and in acutely ill or dehydrated children.
• Hold dose and notify doctor if patient develops jaundice, symptoms of blood dyscrasias (fever, sore throat, infection, cellulitis, weakness), persistent (longer than a few hours) extrapyramidal reactions, or any such reactions during pregnancy or in children.
• Monitor therapy by weekly bilirubin tests during first month; periodic blood tests (CBC, liver function); and ophthalmic tests in long-term therapy.
• Check intake/output for urinary retention or constipation.
• Tell patient to use sunscreening agents and protective clothing to avoid photosensitivity reactions.
• Warn against activities that require alertness or good psychomotor coordination until response to drug is determined. Drowsiness and dizziness usually subside after a few weeks.
• Avoid combining with alcohol or other depressants.
• Watch for orthostatic hypotension, especially with parenteral administration. Keep patient supine for 1 hour afterward. Advise patient to change positions slowly.
• Give I.M. only in upper outer quadrant of buttocks. Massage slowly afterward to prevent sterile abscess. Injection may sting.
• Protect drug from light. Slight yellowing of injection or concentrate is common; does not affect potency. Discard markedly discolored solutions.
• Keep liquid suspension tightly closed.
• Prevent contact dermatitis by keeping drug off patient's skin and clothes.
• Do not withdraw abruptly unless required by severe side effects.
• Dry mouth may be relieved with sugarless gum, sour hard candy, or rinsing with mouthwash.
• Drug is an aliphatic phenothiazine.
• Dose of 25 mg is therapeutic equivalent of 10 mg chlorpromazine.

31

Miscellaneous psychotherapeutics

lithium carbonate
lithium citrate

MECHANISM OF ACTION
Lithium alters chemical transmitters in the central nervous system, possibly by interfering with ionic pump mechanisms in brain cells. Its exact mechanism of action in mania, however, is unknown.

COMBINATION PRODUCTS
None.

lithium carbonate
Carbolith♦♦, Eskalith, Eskalith CR, Lithane♦**, Lithizine♦♦, Lithobid, Lithonate, Lithotabs, Pfi-Lith

lithium citrate
Cibalith-S

INDICATIONS & DOSAGE
Prevention or control of mania—
Adults: 300 to 600 mg P.O. up to 4 times daily, increasing on the basis of blood levels to achieve optimal dosage. Recommended therapeutic lithium blood levels: 1 to 1.5 mEq/liter for acute mania; 0.6 to 1.2 mEq/liter for maintenance therapy; and 2 mEq/liter as maximum.
Adults: 5 ml lithium citrate (liquid) contains 8 mEq lithium equal to 300 mg lithium carbonate.

SIDE EFFECTS
Blood: *leukocytosis of 14,000 to 18,000 (reversible).*
CNS: tremors, drowsiness, headache, confusion, restlessness, dizziness, psychomotor retardation, stupor, lethargy, coma, blackouts, epileptiform seizures, EEG changes, worsened organic brain syndrome, impaired speech, ataxia, muscle weakness, incoordination, hyperexcitability.
CV: *reversible EKG changes,* arrhythmia, hypotension, peripheral circulatory collapse, allergic vasculitis, ankle and wrist edema.
EENT: tinnitus, impaired vision.
GI: nausea, vomiting, anorexia, diarrhea, dry mouth, thirst, metallic taste.
GU: *polyuria,* glycosuria, incontinence, renal toxicity with long-term use.
Metabolic: transient hyperglycemia, goiter, hypothyroidism (lowered T_3, T_4, and PBI, but elevated ^{131}I uptake), hyponatremia.
Skin: pruritus, rash, diminished or lost sensation, drying and thinning of hair.

INTERACTIONS
Diuretics: increased reabsorption of lithium by kidneys, with possible toxic effect. Use with extreme caution, and monitor lithium and electrolyte levels (especially sodium).
Haloperidol and thioridazine: encephalopathic syndrome (lethargy, tremors, extrapyramidal symptoms). Watch for syndrome, and stop drug if it occurs.
Aminophylline, sodium bicarbonate, and sodium chloride: ingestion of these salts increases lithium excretion. Avoid salt loads and monitor lithium levels.
Probenecid, indomethacin, methyl-

Italicized side effects are common or life-threatening.
*Liquid form contains alcohol.   **May contain tartrazine.

dopa: increased effect of lithium. Monitor for lithium toxicity.

NURSING CONSIDERATIONS
• Contraindicated if therapy cannot be closely monitored. Use with caution with haloperidol, other antipsychotics, neuromuscular blocking agents, and diuretics; in elderly or debilitated persons; and in thyroid disease, epilepsy, renal or cardiovascular disease, brain damage, severe debilitation or dehydration, and sodium depletion.
• Monitor baseline EKG, thyroid, and renal studies, and electrolyte levels. Monitor lithium blood levels 8 to 12 hours after first dose, usually before morning dose, two or three times weekly first month, then weekly to monthly on maintenance.
• When blood levels of lithium are below 1.5 mEq/liter, side effects generally remain mild.
• Check fluid intake and output, especially when surgery is scheduled.
• Warn patient and family to watch for signs of toxicity (diarrhea, vomiting, drowsiness, muscular weakness, ataxia) and to expect transient nausea, polyuria, thirst, and discomfort during first few days. Patient should withhold one dose and call doctor if toxic symptoms appear, but not stop drug abruptly.
• Expect lag of 1 to 3 weeks before drug's beneficial effects are noticed.
• Weigh patient daily; check for signs of edema or sudden weight gain.

• Adjust fluid and salt ingestion to compensate if excessive loss occurs through protracted sweating or diarrhea. Under normal conditions, patients should have fluid intake of 2,500 to 3,000 ml daily and a balanced diet with adequate salt intake.
• Have outpatient follow-up of thyroid and renal functions every 6 to 12 months. Palpate thyroid to check for enlargement.
• Patient should carry identification/instruction card (available from pharmacy) with toxicity and emergency information.
• Warn ambulatory patient to avoid activities that require alertness and good psychomotor coordination until CNS response to drug is determined.
• Administer with plenty of water, and after meals to minimize GI upset.
• Check urine for specific gravity and report level below 1.015, which may indicate diabetes insipidus syndrome.
• Has been used to treat syndrome of inappropriate ADH.
• Tell patient not to switch brands of lithium or to take other drugs (prescription or over-the-counter) without doctor's guidance.
• Investigationally used to increase white cells in patients undergoing cancer chemotherapy.
• Also used investigationally for treatment of cluster headaches, aggression, organic brain syndrome, and tardive dyskinesia.

32

Cerebral stimulants

amphetamine hydrochloride
amphetamine phosphate
amphetamine sulfate
benzphetamine hydrochloride
caffeine
caffeine, citrated
caffeine sodium benzoate injection
chlorphentermine hydrochloride
clortermine hydrochloride
deanol acetamidobenzoate
dextroamphetamine phosphate
dextroamphetamine sulfate
diethylpropion hydrochloride
fenfluramine hydrochloride
mazindol
methamphetamine hydrochloride
methylphenidate hydrochloride
pemoline
phendimetrazine tartrate
phenmetrazine hydrochloride
phentermine hydrochloride

MECHANISM OF ACTION

• Amphetamines and amphetamine-like drugs, caffeine, methylphenidate, and pemoline are sympathomimetics whose main sites of activity appear to be the cerebral cortex and the reticular activating system. They probably promote nerve impulse transmission by releasing stored norepinephrine from nerve terminals in the brain.

• In children with hyperkinesia, amphetamines have a paradoxical calming effect that is probably related to the actions of the drug on CNS neurotransmitters. The mechanism by which amphetamines produce mental and behavioral effects in children, however, has not been established.

• Deanol probably elicits a CNS-stimulating effect by increasing brain levels of choline—a precursor of acetylcholine.

COMBINATION PRODUCTS

AMPHAPLEX-10/OBETROL-10: dextroamphetamine saccharate 2.5 mg, amphetamine aspartate 2.5 mg, amphetamine sulfate 2.5 mg, dextroamphetamine sulfate 2.5 mg.
AMPHAPLEX-20/OBETROL-20: dextroamphetamine saccharate 5 mg, amphetamine aspartate 5 mg, amphetamine sulfate 5 mg, dextroamphetamine sulfate 5 mg.
BIPHETAMINE 12½: dextroamphetamine 6.25 mg and amphetamine 6.25 mg.
BIPHETAMINE 20: dextroamphetamine 10 mg and amphetamine 10 mg.
ESKATROL: dextroamphetamine sulfate 15 mg and prochlorperazine maleate 7.5 mg.

amphetamine hydrochloride

amphetamine phosphate

amphetamine sulfate

Controlled Substance Schedule II
Benzedrine♦

INDICATIONS & DOSAGE

Minimal brain dysfunction—
Children 6 years and older: 5 mg P.O. daily, with 5-mg increments weekly, p.r.n.
Children 3 to 5 years: 2.5 mg P.O.

Italicized side effects are common or life-threatening.
*Liquid form contains alcohol. **May contain tartrazine.

daily, with 2.5-mg increments weekly, p.r.n.
Narcolepsy—
Adults: 5 to 60 mg P.O. daily in divided doses.
Children over 12 years: 10 mg P.O. daily, with 10-mg increments weekly, p.r.n.
Children 6 to 12 years: 5 mg P.O. daily, with 5-mg increments weekly, p.r.n.
Short-term adjunct in exogenous obesity—
Adults: single 10- or 15-mg long-acting capsule daily, or 2 if needed, up to 30 mg daily; or 5 to 30 mg daily in divided doses 30 to 60 minutes before meals. Not recommended for children under 12 years old.

SIDE EFFECTS
CNS: *restlessness,* tremor, *hyperactivity, talkativeness, insomnia,* irritability, dizziness, headache, chills, overstimulation, dysphoria.
CV: *tachycardia, palpitations,* hypertension, hypotension.
GI: nausea, vomiting, cramps, dry mouth, diarrhea, constipation, metallic taste, anorexia, weight loss.
Other: urticaria, impotence, changes in libido.

INTERACTIONS
MAO inhibitors: severe hypertension; possible hypertensive crisis. Don't use together.
Sodium bicarbonate, acetazolamide: increased renal reabsorption. Monitor for enhanced effect.
Ammonium chloride, ascorbic acid: observe for decreased amphetamine effect.
Phenothiazines, haloperidol: observe for decreased amphetamine effect.

NURSING CONSIDERATIONS
• Contraindicated in symptomatic cardiovascular diseases, hyperthyroidism, nephritis, angina pectoris, moderate to severe hypertension, parkinsonism due to arteriosclerosis, certain types of glaucoma, advanced arteriosclerosis, agitated states, or patients with history of drug abuse. Use with caution in patients with diabetes mellitus and in elderly, debilitated, or hyperexcitable patients.
• Psychic dependence or habituation may occur, especially in patients with history of drug addiction. Avoid prolonged administration. When used long-term, lower dosage gradually to prevent acute rebound depression.
• When used for obesity, make sure patient is also on a weight-reduction program. Give drug 30 to 60 minutes before meals.
• Fatigue may result as drug effects wear off. Patient will need more rest.
• Tell patient to avoid drinks containing caffeine, which increase the effects of amphetamines and related amines.
• Check vital signs regularly for signs of excessive stimulation.
• Urinary acidification enhances renal excretion; urinary alkalinization enhances renal reabsorption and recycling.
• When tolerance to anorexigenic effect develops, dosage should not be increased, but drug discontinued.
• Discourage use to combat fatigue.
• Warn patient to avoid activities that require alertness or good psychomotor coordination until CNS response to drug is determined.
• May alter daily insulin needs in patients with diabetes. Monitor blood and urine sugars.
• Use as analeptic is usually discouraged, since CNS stimulation superimposed on CNS depression can lead to neuronal instability and seizures.
• May reverse beneficial effect of antihypertensives. Monitor blood pressure.

benzphetamine hydrochloride
Controlled Substance Schedule III
Didrex**

INDICATIONS & DOSAGE
Short-term adjunct in exogenous obesity—
Adults: 25 to 50 mg P.O. daily, b.i.d., or t.i.d.

SIDE EFFECTS
CNS: *restlessness*, tremor, *hyperactivity, talkativeness, insomnia*, irritability, dizziness, headache, chills, overstimulation, dysphoria.
CV: *tachycardia, palpitations*, hypertension, hypotension.
GI: nausea, vomiting, cramps, dry mouth, diarrhea, constipation, metallic taste, anorexia, weight loss.
Skin: urticaria.
Other: impotence, changes in libido.

INTERACTIONS
MAO inhibitors: severe hypertension; possible hypertensive crisis. Don't use together.
Sodium bicarbonate, acetazolamide: increased renal reabsorption. Monitor for enhanced effects.
Ammonium chloride, ascorbic acid: observe for decreased benzphetamine effects.
Phenothiazines, haloperidol: observe for decreased benzphetamine effects.

NURSING CONSIDERATIONS
• Contraindicated in symptomatic cardiovascular diseases, hyperthyroidism, nephritis, angina pectoris, moderate to severe hypertension, parkinsonism due to arteriosclerosis, certain types of glaucoma, advanced arteriosclerosis, agitated states, or patients with history of drug abuse. Use with caution in patients with diabetes mellitus and in elderly, debilitated, or hyperexcitable patients.
• Psychic dependence or habituation may occur, especially in patients with history of drug addiction. Avoid prolonged administration. When used long-term, lower dosage gradually to prevent acute rebound depression.
• Use in conjunction with weight-reduction program. Give 30 to 60 minutes before meals.
• Fatigue may result as drug effects wear off. Patient will need more rest.
• Tell patient to avoid caffeine-containing drinks, which increase the effects of amphetamines and related amines.
• Check vital signs regularly for signs of excessive stimulation.
• Urinary acidification enhances renal excretion; urinary alkalinization enhances renal reabsorption and recycling.
• When tolerance to anorexigenic effect develops, dosage should not be increased, but drug discontinued.
• Warn patient to avoid activities that require alertness or good psychomotor coordination until CNS response to drug is determined.
• May alter daily insulin needs in patients with diabetes. Monitor blood and urine sugars.

caffeine
Ban-Drowz, Kirkaffeine, Nodoz, Tirend, Vivarin

caffeine, citrated

caffeine sodium benzoate injection

INDICATIONS & DOSAGE
Respiratory and central nervous system stimulant—
Adults: 100 to 200 mg anhydrous caffeine P.O.; 500 mg to 1 g caffeine sodium benzoate I.M. or I.V. in emergency only.

SIDE EFFECTS
CNS: *stimulation, insomnia*, restless-

ness, nervousness, mild delirium, headache, excitement, agitation, muscle tremors, twitches.
CV: *tachycardia.*
GI: nausea, vomiting.
GU: *diuresis.*
Skin: hyperesthesia.

INTERACTIONS
None significant.

NURSING CONSIDERATIONS
• Contraindicated in patients with gastric or duodenal ulcer.
• Tolerance or psychological dependence may develop.
• Be alert for signs of overdose: GI pain, mild delirium, insomnia, diuresis, dehydration, and fever. Treat with short-acting barbiturates, gastric emesis, or lavage.
• Single dose should not exceed 1 g.
• Caffeine content in cola beverages, 17 to 55 mg/180 ml; tea, 40 to 100 mg/180 ml; instant coffee, 60 to 180 mg/180 ml; brewed coffee, 100 to 150 mg/180 ml.
• Caffeine does not reverse alcohol intoxication or depressant effects of alcohol. Overvigorous therapy with caffeine may aggravate depression in an already depressed patient.
• Use as analeptic is discouraged.

---

chlorphentermine hydrochloride
Controlled Substance Schedule III
Chlorophen, Pre-Sate♦

INDICATIONS & DOSAGE
Short-term adjunct in exogenous obesity—
Adults— 65 mg P.O. taken after breakfast.

SIDE EFFECTS
CNS: *insomnia,* overstimulation, nervousness, dizziness, paradoxical sedation, headache.

CV: *tachycardia, palpitations,* increased blood pressure.
GI: nausea, dry mouth, constipation.
Skin: urticaria.

INTERACTIONS
MAO inhibitors: severe hypertension; possible hypertensive crisis. Don't use together.
Sodium bicarbonate, acetazolamide: increased renal reabsorption. Monitor for enhanced effects.
Ammonium chloride, ascorbic acid: observe for decreased chlorphentermine effects.

NURSING CONSIDERATIONS
• Contraindicated in hyperexcitability states, hyperthyroidism, hypertension, angina pectoris, severe cardiovascular disease, glaucoma, or patients with history of drug abuse.
• Psychic dependence and habituation may occur. When tolerance to anorexigenic effect develops, dose should not be increased, but drug discontinued.
• May alter daily insulin needs in patients with diabetes. Monitor blood and urine sugars.
• Teach patient a good dietary plan and exercise program.
• Withdraw drug gradually.
• Fatigue may result as drug effects wear off. Patient will need more rest.
• Tell patient to avoid caffeine-containing drinks, which increase the effects of amphetamines and related amines.
• Check vital signs regularly. Observe for signs of excessive stimulation.
• Urinary acidification enhances renal excretion; urinary alkalinization enhances renal reabsorption and recycling.

---

clortermine hydrochloride
Controlled Substance Schedule III
Voranil**

INDICATIONS & DOSAGE
Short-term adjunct in exogenous obesity—
Adults: 50 mg P.O. taken at midmorning.

SIDE EFFECTS
CNS: *restlessness,* dizziness, *insomnia,* euphoria, tremor, headache.
CV: *tachycardia, palpitations,* arrhythmias, increased blood pressure.
GI: dry mouth, diarrhea, constipation.
Skin: urticaria.
Other: impotence, libido changes.

INTERACTIONS
MAO inhibitors: severe hypertension; possible hypertensive crisis. Don't use together.
Sodium bicarbonate, acetazolamide: increased renal reabsorption. Monitor for enhanced effects.
Ammonium chloride, ascorbic acid: observe for decreased clortermine effects.

NURSING CONSIDERATIONS
• Contraindicated in hyperthyroidism, glaucoma, severe hypertension, cardiovascular diseases, agitated states, and patients with history of drug abuse. Use with caution in diabetes mellitus. Insulin requirements may be altered. Monitor blood and urine sugars.
• Warn patient to avoid activities that require alertness or good psychomotor coordination until CNS response to drug is determined.
• Be sure patient is following a sensible dietary regimen.
• Drug should be discontinued when tolerance develops.
• Fatigue may result as drug effects wear off. Patient will need more rest.
• Tell patient to avoid drinks containing caffeine, which increase the effects of amphetamines and related amines.
• Check vital signs regularly. Observe for signs of excessive stimulation.
• Urinary acidification enhances renal excretion; urinary alkalinization enhances renal reabsorption and recycling.

deanol acetamidobenzoate
Deaner, Deaner-100♦♦, Deaner-250

INDICATIONS & DOSAGE
Minimal brain dysfunction—
Children over 6 years: initially, 500 mg P.O. daily after breakfast; may reduce to maintenance 250 to 500 mg daily. Dose adjusted to patient's needs and response.
Dyskinesia, blepharospasm—
Adults: 600 mg to 1.6 g P.O. daily.

SIDE EFFECTS
CNS: insomnia, mild overstimulation, irritability, headache, muscle twitching, tenseness.
CV: postural hypotension.
EENT: increased nasal and oral secretions.
GI: constipation.
Skin: transient rash.
Other: dyspnea.

INTERACTIONS
None significant.

NURSING CONSIDERATIONS
• Contraindicated in patients with grand mal epilepsy.
• In long-term use, monitor child closely for signs of growth suppression.
• Beneficial effects may not appear until after several weeks of therapy.
• Used with some success in treatment of tardive dyskinesia.

Italicized side effects are common or life-threatening.
*Liquid form contains alcohol.   **May contain tartrazine.

dextroamphetamine phosphate

dextroamphetamine sulfate
Controlled Substance Schedule II
Dexampex**, Dexedrine♦* **,
Ferndex, Robese, Spancap #1 and
#4, Tidex

INDICATIONS & DOSAGE
Narcolepsy—
Adults: 5 to 60 mg P.O. daily in divided doses.
Children over 12 years: 10 mg P.O. daily, with 10-mg increments weekly, p.r.n.
Children 6 to 12 years: 5 mg P.O. daily, with 5-mg increments weekly, p.r.n.
Short-term adjunct in exogenous obesity—
Adults: single 10- to 15-mg long-acting capsule, up to 30 mg daily; or in divided doses, 5 to 10 mg ½ hour before meals.
Minimal brain dysfunction—
Children 6 years and over: 5 mg once daily or b.i.d., with 5-mg increments weekly, p.r.n.
Children 3 to 5 years: 2.5 mg P.O. daily, with 2.5-mg increments weekly, p.r.n.

SIDE EFFECTS
CNS: *restlessness,* tremor, *hyperactivity, talkativeness, insomnia,* irritability, dizziness, headache, chills, overstimulation, dysphoria.
CV: *tachycardia, palpitations,* hypertension, hypotension.
GI: nausea, vomiting, cramps, dry mouth, diarrhea, constipation, metallic taste, anorexia, weight loss.
Skin: urticaria.
Other: impotence, changes in libido.

INTERACTIONS
MAO inhibitors: severe hypertension; possible hypertensive crisis. Don't use together.

Sodium bicarbonate, acetazolamide: increased renal reabsorption. Monitor for enhanced amphetamine effects.
Ammonium chloride, ascorbic acid: observe for decreased amphetamine effects.
Phenothiazines, haloperidol: observe for decreased amphetamine effects.

NURSING CONSIDERATIONS
• Contraindicated in patients with hyperthyroidism, nephritis, severe hypertension, angina pectoris or other severe cardiovascular disease, some types of glaucoma, or history of drug abuse. Use with caution in patients with diabetes mellitus and in elderly, debilitated, or hyperexcitable patients.
• Psychic dependence or habituation may occur, especially in patients with history of drug addiction. Avoid prolonged administration. When used long-term, lower dosage gradually to prevent acute rebound depression.
• When used for obesity, be sure patient is also on a weight-reduction program. Give 30 to 60 minutes before meals. Avoid giving within 6 hours of bedtime.
• Fatigue may result as drug effects wear off. Patient will need more rest.
• Tell patient to avoid drinks containing caffeine, which increase the effects of amphetamines and related amines.
• Check vital signs regularly. Observe for signs of excessive stimulation.
• Urinary acidification enhances renal excretion; urinary alkalinization enhances renal reabsorption and recycling.
• When tolerance to anorexigenic effect develops, dosage should not be increased, but drug discontinued.
• Discourage use to combat fatigue.
• Warn patient to avoid activities that require alertness or good psychomotor coordination until CNS response to drug is determined.
• May alter daily insulin needs in patients with diabetes. Monitor blood and urine sugars.

• Use as analeptic is usually discouraged, since CNS stimulation superimposed on CNS depression can lead to neuronal instability and seizures.

diethylpropion hydrochloride
Controlled Substance Schedule IV
Dietec◆◆, Nobesine◆◆, Nu-Dispoz, Regibon◆◆, Ro-Diet, Tenuate◆, Tepanil

INDICATIONS & DOSAGE
Short-term adjunct in exogenous obesity—
Adults: 25 mg P.O. before meals, t.i.d.; or 75 mg controlled-release tablet P.O. in midmorning.

SIDE EFFECTS
CNS: headache, *nervousness*, dizziness.
CV: *tachycardia*, *palpitations*, rise in blood pressure.
EENT: blurred vision.
GI: nausea, abdominal cramps, dry mouth, diarrhea, constipation.
Skin: urticaria.
Other: impotence, libido changes, menstrual upset.

INTERACTIONS
MAO inhibitors: hypertension; possible hypertensive crisis. Don't use together.

NURSING CONSIDERATIONS
• Contraindicated in patients with hyperthyroidism, hypertension, angina pectoris, severe cardiovascular disease, glaucoma, or history of drug abuse. Use with caution in epilepsy, diabetes mellitus, or hyperexcitability states. May alter insulin requirements. Monitor blood and urine sugars.
• When tolerance to anorexigenic effect develops, dosage should not be increased, but drug discontinued.
• Habituation or psychic dependence may occur.

• Be sure patient is also on a weight-reduction program.
• Can be used to stop nighttime eating. Rarely causes insomnia.
• Fatigue may result as drug effects wear off. Patient will need more rest.
• Tell patient to avoid drinks containing caffeine, which increase the effects of amphetamines and related amines.
• Check vital signs regularly. Observe for signs of excessive stimulation.
• Urinary acidification enhances renal excretion; urinary alkalinization enhances renal reabsorption and recycling.
• Use as analeptic is usually discouraged, since CNS stimulation superimposed on CNS depression can lead to neuronal instability and seizures.

fenfluramine hydrochloride
Controlled Substance Schedule IV
Pondimin◆

INDICATIONS & DOSAGE
Short-term adjunct in exogenous obesity—
Adults: initially, 20 mg P.O. t.i.d. before meals. Maximum 40 mg t.i.d. Adjust dosage according to patient's response.

SIDE EFFECTS
CNS: dizziness, incoordination, headache, euphoria or depression, anxiety, *insomnia*, weakness or fatigue, agitation.
CV: *palpitations*, hypotension, hypertension, chest pain.
EENT: eye irritation, blurred vision.
GI: diarrhea, dry mouth, nausea, vomiting, abdominal pain, constipation.
GU: dysuria, increased urinary frequency, impotence, increased libido.
Skin: rashes, urticaria, burning sensation.
Other: sweating, chills, fever.

INTERACTIONS
MAO inhibitors: severe hypertension;

Italicized side effects are common or life-threatening.
*Liquid form contains alcohol. **May contain tartrazine.

possible hypertensive crisis. Don't use together.

NURSING CONSIDERATIONS
• Contraindicated in patients with glaucoma, hypersensitivity to sympathomimetic amines, symptomatic cardiovascular disease, alcoholism, or history of drug abuse. Use with caution in patients with hypertension, history of mental depression, diabetes mellitus.
• Because of possible hypoglycemia, patients with diabetes may have altered insulin or sulfonylurea requirements. Monitor blood and urine sugars.
• Check vital signs regularly. Observe patient for signs of excessive sedation, depression, or excessive stimulation. Closely monitor blood pressure.
• Be sure patient is on a weight-reduction program.
• Tolerance or dependence may occur. Avoid prolonged administration.
• Fatigue may result as drug effects wear off. Patient will need more rest.
• Tell patient to avoid drinks containing caffeine, which increase the effects of amphetamines and related amines.
• Fenfluramine should not be discontinued abruptly; may precipitate an acute depressive reaction.

---

mazindol
Controlled Substance Schedule IV
Mazanor, Sanorex♦

INDICATIONS & DOSAGE
Short-term adjunct in exogenous obesity—
Adults: 1 mg t.i.d. 1 hour before meals, or 2 mg daily 1 hour before lunch. Use lowest effective dose.

SIDE EFFECTS
CNS: *nervousness,* restlessness, dizziness, *insomnia,* dysphoria, headache, depression, drowsiness, weakness, tremors.
CV: *palpitations, tachycardia.*

GI: dry mouth, nausea, constipation, diarrhea, unpleasant taste.
GU: difficulty initiating micturition, impotence, libido changes.
Skin: rash, clamminess, pallor.
Other: shivering, excessive sweating.

INTERACTIONS
MAO inhibitors: severe hypertension; possible hypertensive crisis. Don't use together.

NURSING CONSIDERATIONS
• Contraindicated in patients with glaucoma, cardiovascular disease including arrhythmias, agitated states, and history of drug abuse. Use with caution in diabetes mellitus, hypertension, hyperexcitability states.
• Warn patient to avoid activities that require alertness or good psychomotor coordination until CNS response to drug has been determined.
• Fatigue may result as drug effects wear off. Patient will need more rest.
• Tell patient to avoid caffeine-containing drinks, which increase the effects of amphetamines and related amines.
• Check vital signs regularly. Observe for signs of excessive stimulation.
• Tolerance or dependence may develop. Avoid prolonged use.
• Be sure patient is also on a weight-reduction program.
• May alter insulin needs in patients with diabetes. Monitor blood and urine sugars.

---

methamphetamine hydrochloride
Controlled Substance Schedule II
Desoxyn, Methampex

INDICATIONS & DOSAGE
Minimal brain dysfunction—
Children 6 years and over: 2.5 to 5 mg P.O. once daily or b.i.d., with 5-mg increments weekly, p.r.n. Usual effective dosage is 20 to 25 mg daily.

Unmarked trade names available in the United States only.
♦ Also available in Canada.   ♦♦ Available in Canada only.

Short-term adjunct in exogenous obesity—
Adults: 2.5 to 5 mg P.O. once to t.i.d. 30 minutes before meals; or 1 long-acting 5- to 15-mg tablet daily before breakfast.

SIDE EFFECTS
CNS: *nervousness, insomnia,* irritability, *talkativeness,* dizziness, headache, hyperexcitability, tremor.
CV: hypertension or hypotension, *tachycardia, palpitations,* cardiac arrhythmias.
EENT: blurred vision, mydriasis.
GI: nausea, vomiting, abdominal cramps, diarrhea or constipation, dry mouth, anorexia, metallic taste.
Skin: urticaria.
Other: impotence, libido changes.

INTERACTIONS
MAO inhibitors: severe hypertension; possible hypertensive crisis. Don't use together.
Sodium bicarbonate, acetazolamide: increased renal reabsorption. Monitor for enhanced effects.
Ammonium chloride, ascorbic acid: observe for decreased amphetamine effects.
Phenothiazines, haloperidol: observe for decreased amphetamine effects.

NURSING CONSIDERATIONS
• Contraindicated in patients with hypertension, hyperthyroidism, nephritis, angina pectoris or other severe cardiovascular disease, glaucoma, parkinsonism due to arteriosclerosis, agitated states, or history of drug abuse. Use with caution in patients with diabetes mellitus; and in patients who are elderly, debilitated, asthenic, psychopathic, or who have a history of suicidal or homicidal tendencies.
• Warn that potential for abuse is high. Discourage use to combat fatigue.
• May alter insulin needs in patients with diabetes. Monitor blood and urine sugars.

• When used for obesity, be sure patient is on a weight-reduction program.
• Tell patient to avoid caffeinic drinks, which increase the effects of amphetamines and related amines.
• Check vital signs regularly. Observe for signs of excessive stimulation.
• Urinary acidification enhances renal excretion; urinary alkalinization enhances renal reabsorption and recycling.
• When tolerance to anorexigenic effect develops, dosage should not be increased, but drug discontinued.
• Warn patient to avoid activities that require alertness or good psychomotor coordination until CNS response to drug is determined.

methylphenidate hydrochloride
Controlled Substance Schedule II
Methidate◆◆, Ritalin◆, Ritalin SR

INDICATIONS & DOSAGE
Minimal brain dysfunction (hyperkinetic behavior disorders)—
Children 6 years and over: initial dose 5 to 10 mg P.O. daily before breakfast and lunch, with 5- to 10-mg increments weekly as needed, up to 60 mg daily.
Narcolepsy—
Adults: 10 mg P.O. b.i.d. or t.i.d. ½ hour before meals. Dosage varies with patient needs. Dosage range is 5 to 50 mg daily.

SIDE EFFECTS
CNS: *nervousness, insomnia,* dizziness, headache, akathisia, dyskinesia.
CV: *palpitations,* angina, *tachycardia,* changes in blood pressure and pulse rate.
EENT: difficulty with accommodation and blurring of vision.
GI: nausea, dry throat, abdominal pain, anorexia, weight loss.
Skin: rash, urticaria, *exfoliative dermatitis,* erythema multiforme.

Italicized side effects are common or life-threatening.
*Liquid form contains alcohol.   **May contain tartrazine.

INTERACTIONS

MAO inhibitors: severe hypertension; possible hypertensive crisis. Don't use together.

NURSING CONSIDERATIONS

• Contraindicated in patients with symptomatic cardiac disease; hyperthyroidism; moderate to severe hypertension; angina pectoris; advanced arteriosclerosis; severe depression of either endogenous or exogenous form; glaucoma; parkinsonism; history of drug abuse or dependency; history of marked anxiety, tension, or agitation. Use with caution in elderly, debilitated, or hyperexcitable patients and those with history of cardiovascular disease, diabetes, or seizures.

• Closely monitor blood pressure. Observe for signs of excessive stimulation.

• Discourage use to combat fatigue.

• Observe for interactions, as treatment of other disease states may be affected. May alter daily insulin needs in patients with diabetes. Monitor blood and urine sugars. May decrease seizure threshold in patients with seizure disorders.

• Drug of choice for minimal brain dysfunction. Usually stopped postpuberty.

• Periodic CBC, differential, and platelet counts advised with long-term use.

• Tolerance, psychic dependence, or habituation may develop, especially in patients with history of drug addiction. High abuse potential. Avoid prolonged administration. When used long-term, lower dosage gradually to prevent acute rebound depression.

• Fatigue may result as drug effects wear off. Patient will need more rest.

• Tell patient to avoid drinks containing caffeine, which increase the effects of amphetamines and related amines.

• Warn patient to avoid activities that require alertness or good psychomotor coordination until CNS response to drug is determined.

• Monitor height and weight in children on prolonged therapy.

• Now available in a sustained-release form.

pemoline
Controlled Substance Schedule IV
Cylert

INDICATIONS & DOSAGE

Minimal brain dysfunction—
Children 6 years and over: initially, 37.5 mg P.O. given in the morning. Daily dose can be raised by 18.75 mg weekly. Effective dosage range 56.25 to 75 mg daily; maximum is 112.5 mg daily.

SIDE EFFECTS

CNS: *insomnia,* malaise, irritability, fatigue, mild depression, dizziness, headache, drowsiness, hallucinations, nervousness (large doses), seizures.
CV: tachycardia (large doses).
GI: anorexia, abdominal pain, nausea, diarrhea.
Hepatic: liver enzyme elevations.
Skin: rash.

INTERACTIONS

None significant.

NURSING CONSIDERATIONS

• Use with caution in patients with impaired renal function. Drug may accumulate.

• Safety and efficacy for more than 2 years of administration has not been established. Closely monitor patients on long-term therapy for possible hepatic function abnormalities and for growth suppression.

• Structurally dissimilar to amphetamines or methylphenidate.

• Therapeutic effects may not be evident for 2 to 3 weeks.

Unmarked trade names available in the United States only.
♦ Also available in Canada. ♦ ♦ Available in Canada only.

phendimetrazine tartrate
Controlled Substance Schedule IV
Anorex, Bacarate, Bontril PDM,
Delcozine, Di-Ap-Trol, Limit, Metra,
Obalan, Obepar, Obeval,
Obezine**, Phenazine♦, Phenzine,
Plegine, Sprx 1, Sprx-105,
Statobex**, Trimstat, Trimtabs

INDICATIONS & DOSAGE
Short-term adjunct in exogenous obesity—
Adults: 35 mg P.O. 2 to 3 times daily 1 hour before meals. Maximum dosage is 70 mg t.i.d. Use lowest effective dosage. Adjust dose to individual response.

SIDE EFFECTS
CNS: *nervousness,* dizziness, *insomnia,* tremor, headache.
CV: *tachycardia, palpitations,* rise in blood pressure.
EENT: blurred vision.
GI: dry mouth, nausea, abdominal cramps, diarrhea or constipation.
GU: dysuria.

INTERACTIONS
MAO inhibitors: severe hypertension; possible hypertensive crisis. Don't use together.
Sodium bicarbonate, acetazolamide: increased renal reabsorption. Monitor for enhanced effects.
Ammonium chloride, ascorbic acid: observe for decreased phendimetrazine effects.
Phenothiazines, haloperidol: observe for decreased effect.

NURSING CONSIDERATIONS
• Contraindicated in hyperthyroidism, hypertension, angina pectoris or other severe cardiovascular disease, glaucoma. Use with caution in hyperexcitability states or patients with history of addiction.
• Warn patient to avoid activities that require alertness or good psychomotor coordination until CNS response to drug has been determined.
• Be sure patient is following weight-reduction program.
• Tolerance or dependence can develop. Not advised for prolonged use.
• Fatigue may result as drug effects wear off. Patient will need more rest.
• Tell patient to avoid caffeine-containing drinks, which increase the effects of amphetamines and related amines.
• Check vital signs regularly. Observe for signs of excessive stimulation.
• Urinary acidification enhances renal excretion; urinary alkalinization enhances renal reabsorption and recycling.
• May alter daily insulin needs in patients with diabetes. Monitor blood and urine sugars.

phenmetrazine hydrochloride
Controlled Substance Schedule II
Preludin**

INDICATIONS & DOSAGE
Short-term adjunct in exogenous obesity—
Adults: 25 mg P.O. b.i.d. or t.i.d. 1 hour before meals, up to 75 mg daily; or single 50- to 75-mg extended-release tablet daily in midmorning.

SIDE EFFECTS
CNS: *nervousness,* dizziness, *insomnia,* headache.
CV: *tachycardia, palpitations,* increased blood pressure.
EENT: blurred vision.
GI: dry mouth, nausea, abdominal cramps, constipation.
Skin: urticaria.
Other: libido changes, impotence.

INTERACTIONS
MAO inhibitors: severe hypertension; possible hypertensive crisis. Don't use together.

Italicized side effects are common or life-threatening.
*Liquid form contains alcohol.   **May contain tartrazine.

Sodium bicarbonate, acetazolamide: increased renal reabsorption. Monitor for enhanced effects.
Ammonium chloride, ascorbic acid: observe for decreased phenmetrazine effects.
Phenothiazines, haloperidol: observe for decreased effect.

NURSING CONSIDERATIONS
• Contraindicated in patients with hyperthyroidism, hypertension, angina pectoris or other cardiovascular disease, glaucoma, or history of drug abuse. Use with caution in hyperexcitability states.
• Tolerance or dependence may develop. High abuse potential. Not advised for prolonged use.
• Be sure patient is also following weight-reduction program.
• Fatigue may result as drug effects wear off. Patient will need more rest.
• Tell patient to avoid drinks containing caffeine, which increase the effects of amphetamines and related amines.
• Check vital signs regularly. Observe for signs of excessive stimulation.
• Urinary acidification enhances renal excretion; urinary alkalinization enhances renal reabsorption and recycling.

---

phentermine hydrochloride
Controlled Substance Schedule IV
Anoxine, Fastin, Ionamin♦,
Parmine, Phentrol, Rolaphent,
Wilpowr

INDICATIONS & DOSAGE
Short-term adjunct in exogenous obesity—
Adults: 8 mg P.O. t.i.d. ½ hour before meals; or 15 to 30 mg daily before breakfast (resin complex).

SIDE EFFECTS
CNS: *nervousness,* dizziness, *insomnia.*
CV: *palpitations, tachycardia,* increased blood pressure.
GI: dry mouth, unpleasant taste, nausea, constipation, diarrhea.
Skin: urticaria.
Other: libido changes, impotence.

INTERACTIONS
MAO inhibitors: severe hypertension; possible hypertensive crisis. Don't use together.
Sodium bicarbonate, acetazolamide: increased renal reabsorption. Monitor for enhanced effects.
Ammonium chloride, ascorbic acid: observe for decreased phentermine effects.
Phenothiazines, haloperidol: observe for decreased effect.

NURSING CONSIDERATIONS
• Contraindicated in hyperthyroidism, hypertension, angina pectoris or other severe cardiovascular disease, glaucoma. Use with caution in hyperexcitability states or patients with history of drug addiction.
• Tolerance or dependence may develop. Avoid prolonged administration.
• Use with weight-reduction program. Give 30 minutes before meals.
• Fatigue may result as drug effects wear off. Patient will need more rest.
• Tell patient to avoid caffeine drinks, which increase the effects of amphetamines and related amines.
• Check vital signs regularly. Observe for signs of excessive stimulation.
• Urinary acidification enhances renal excretion; urinary alkalinization enhances renal reabsorption and recycling.

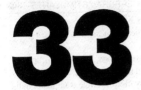

Respiratory stimulants

ammonia, aromatic spirits
doxapram hydrochloride
nikethamide
pentylenetetrazol

MECHANISM OF ACTION
Respiratory stimulants act either directly on the central respiratory centers in the medulla or indirectly on the chemoreceptors.
• Ammonia causes irritation of the sensory receptors in the nasal membranes, producing reflex stimulation of the respiratory centers.

COMBINATION PRODUCTS
NICO-METRAZOL*: pentylenetetrazol 100 mg and niacin 50 mg.

---

ammonia, aromatic spirits

INDICATIONS & DOSAGE
Fainting—
Adults and children: inhale as needed.

SIDE EFFECTS
None reported.

INTERACTIONS
None significant.

NURSING CONSIDERATIONS
• Stimulates mucous membranes of upper respiratory tract.

---

doxapram hydrochloride
Dopram♦

INDICATIONS & DOSAGE
Postanesthesia respiratory stimulant, drug-induced central nervous system depression, and chronic pulmonary disease associated with acute hypercapnia—
Adults: 0.5 to 1 mg/kg of body weight (up to 2 mg/kg in CNS depression), I.V. injection or infusion. Maximum 4 mg/kg, up to 3 g in 1 day. Infusion rate 1 to 3 mg/minute (initial: 5 mg/minute for postanesthesia).
Chronic obstructive pulmonary disease—
Adults: infusion, 1 to 2 mg/minute. Maximum 3 mg/minute for a maximum duration of 2 hours.

SIDE EFFECTS
CNS: seizures, headache, dizziness, apprehension, disorientation, pupillary dilation, bilateral Babinski's signs, flushing, sweating, paresthesias.
CV: chest pain and tightness, variations in heart rate, hypertension, lowered T waves.
GI: nausea, vomiting, diarrhea.
GU: urinary retention, or stimulation of the bladder with incontinence.
Other: sneezing, coughing, laryngospasm, bronchospasm, hiccups, rebound hypoventilation, pruritus.

INTERACTIONS
MAO inhibitors: potentiate adverse cardiovascular effects. Use together cautiously.

Italicized side effects are common or life-threatening.
*Liquid form contains alcohol.   **May contain tartrazine.

NURSING CONSIDERATIONS

• Contraindicated in convulsive disorders; head injury; cardiovascular disorders; frank uncompensated heart failure; severe hypertension; cerebrovascular accidents; respiratory failure or incompetence secondary to neuromuscular disorders, muscle paresis, flail chest, obstructed airway, pulmonary embolism, pneumothorax, restrictive respiratory disease, acute bronchial asthma, extreme dyspnea; hypoxia not associated with hypercapnia. Use with caution in bronchial asthma, severe tachycardia or cardiac arrhythmias, cerebral edema or increased cerebrospinal fluid pressure, hyperthyroidism, pheochromocytoma, or profound metabolic disorders.

• Establish adequate airway before administering drug. Prevent patient from aspirating vomitus by placing him on his side.

• Monitor blood pressure, heart rate, deep tendon reflexes, and arterial blood gases before giving drug and every 30 minutes afterward to avoid overdosage.

• Be alert for signs of overdosage: hypertension, tachycardia, arrhythmias, skeletal muscle hyperactivity, dyspnea. Discontinue if patient shows signs of increased arterial carbon dioxide or oxygen tension, or if mechanical ventilation is started. May give I.V. injection of anticonvulsant for convulsions.

• Use only in surgical or emergency room situations.

• Do not combine with alkaline solutions such as thiopental sodium; doxapram is acidic.

nikethamide
Coramine♦

INDICATIONS & DOSAGE

Acute alcoholism—
Adults: 1.25 to 5 g I.V.; repeat as necessary.
Carbon monoxide poisoning—

Adults: 1.25 to 2.5 g I.V. initially, then 1.25 g q 5 minutes for first hour, depending on response.
Cardiac arrest associated with anesthetic overdose—
Adults: 125 to 250 mg intracardially.
Combat respiratory paralysis—
Adults: 3.75 g I.V.; repeat as required.
Overcome respiratory depression—
Adults: 1.25 to 2.5 g I.V.
Shock—
Adults: 2.5 to 3.75 g I.V. or I.M. initially; repeat as indicated.
Shorten narcosis—
Adults: 1 g I.V. or I.M.
Adjunct in neonatal asphyxia—
Neonates: 375 mg injected into umbilical vein.
Oral maintenance:
Adults and children: 3 to 5 ml oral solution q 4 to 6 hours.

SIDE EFFECTS

CNS: seizure, restlessness, muscle twitching or fasciculations, fear.
CV: increased heart rate and blood pressure.
EENT: unpleasant burning or itching at back of nose, sneezing, coughing.
GI: nausea, vomiting.
Other: increased respiratory rate, flushing, feeling of warmth, sweating.

INTERACTIONS
None significant.

NURSING CONSIDERATIONS

• Monitor patient's respiratory rate and volume frequently during therapy.
• Mechanical support of breathing is often preferred over nikethamide.
• Don't inject intra-arterially; arterial spasm and thrombosis may result.
• Watch for signs of overdosage: muscle tremors or spasm, retching, tachycardia, arrhythmias, hyperpyrexia, hyperpnea, convulsions, psychotic reactions, postictal depression. May give I.V. injection of diazepam or barbiturate such as thiopental sodium for con-

vulsions. Induced emesis and gastric lavage aren't effective.
- Marketed as 25% solution, 1.5 ml ampuls. Be extra careful with calculations to avoid error.

pentylenetetrazol
Metrazol, Nioric, Petrazole

INDICATIONS & DOSAGE
Overdose of CNS depressants—
Adults: 100 to 500 mg I.V. Repeat, if necessary, followed by 100 to 200 mg I.M., p.r.n.
In depression from barbiturates—
5 ml of 10% solution I.V. within 3 to 5 seconds. If necessary, may be repeated until patient awakens.
To improve mental and physical activity in elderly patients—
Adults: 100 to 200 mg P.O. t.i.d.

SIDE EFFECTS
Few side effects with oral administration; narrow margin of safety with parenteral administration.
Signs of overdose:
CNS: fasciculations, clonic convulsions.
CV: slight increases in blood pressure, bradycardia.
GI: nausea, vomiting.
Other: hypersalivation, coughing, hyperthermia.

INTERACTIONS
None significant.

NURSING CONSIDERATIONS
- Use with caution in patients with a history of seizures or focal brain lesion. If dosage is high, use with caution in patients with cardiac disease.
- Analeptic use is not recommended.
- May cause false-positive response to HCG pregnancy test.
- Rarely used.

34

Cholinergics (parasympathomimetics)

ambenonium chloride
bethanechol chloride
edrophonium chloride
neostigmine bromide
neostigmine methylsulfate
physostigmine salicylate
pyridostigmine bromide

MECHANISM OF ACTION
• Ambenonium, edrophonium, neostigmine, physostigmine, and pyridostigmine inhibit the destruction of acetylcholine released from the parasympathetic nerves. Acetylcholine accumu-
lates, promoting increased stimulation
of the receptor.
• Bethanechol and neostigmine directly bind to muscarinic receptors,
mimicking the action of acetylcholine.

COMBINATION PRODUCTS
None.

---

ambenonium chloride
Mytelase♦

INDICATIONS & DOSAGE
*Symptomatic treatment of myasthenia
gravis in patients who cannot take neostigmine bromide and pyridostigmine
bromide—*
Adults: dose must be individualized for
each patient, but usually ranges from 5
to 25 mg P.O. q 3 to 4 hours while
awake. Starting dose usually 5 mg P.O.
q 3 to 4 hours. Increase gradually and
adjust at 1- to 2-day intervals to avoid
drug accumulation and overdosage.
May range from 5 mg to as much as
75 mg per dose.

SIDE EFFECTS
CNS: headache, dizziness, muscle
weakness, convulsions, mental confu-
sion, jitters, sweating, respiratory
depression.
CV: bradycardia, hypotension.
EENT: miosis.
GI: *nausea, vomiting, diarrhea, ab-
dominal cramps,* increased salivation.
GU: urinary frequency, incontinence.
Other: bronchospasm, *muscle cramps,*
bronchoconstriction.

INTERACTIONS
*Procainamide, aminoglycoside antibiot-
ics, quinidine:* may reverse cholinergic
effect on muscle. Observe for lack of
drug effect.

NURSING CONSIDERATIONS
• Contraindicated in patients with mechanical obstruction of intestine or urinary tract, bradycardia, hypotension.
• Use with extreme caution in patients
with bronchial asthma.
• Use cautiously in patients with epilepsy, recent coronary occlusion, vagotonia, hyperthyroidism, cardiac arrhythmias, peptic ulcer.
• Avoid large dose in patients with decreased gastrointestinal motility or
megacolon.
• Discontinue all other cholinergics
before administering this drug.
• Watch patient very closely for side
effects, particularly if total dose is
greater than 200 mg daily. Side effects
may indicate drug toxicity. Notify doctor immediately if they develop.
• Monitor and document vital signs
frequently, being especially careful to

---

check respirations. Always have atropine injection readily available and be prepared to give atropine 0.5 mg subcutaneously or slow I.V. push as ordered, and provide respiratory support as needed.
• Administer each dose exactly as ordered, on time. Amount and frequency of dosage should vary with patient's activity level. The doctor will probably order larger doses to be given when patient is fatigued, for example, in the afternoon and at mealtime.
• If muscle weakness is severe, doctor must determine if this is caused by drug toxicity or exacerbation of myasthenia gravis. A test dose of edrophonium I.V. will aggravate drug-induced weakness but will temporarily relieve weakness that results from the disease.
• Observe and record the patient's variations in muscle strength. Show him how to do it himself.
• When given for myasthenia gravis, explain to patient that this drug will relieve symptoms of ptosis, double vision, difficulty in chewing and swallowing, trunk and limb weakness. Stress the importance of taking this drug exactly as ordered. Explain to patient and his family that he must take this drug for the rest of his life. Teach them about the disease and the drug's effect on symptoms.
• Monitor intake and output.
• Patient may develop resistance to drug.
• Seek approval when indicated for hospitalized patient to have bedside supply of tablets to take himself. Patients with long-standing disease often insist on this.
• Give with milk or food to produce fewer muscarinic side effects.
• Advise patient to wear identification tag indicating he has myasthenia gravis.

bethanechol chloride
Duvoid, Myotonachol, Urecholine♦, Vesicholine

INDICATIONS & DOSAGE
Acute postoperative and postpartum nonobstructive (functional) urinary retention, neurogenic atony of urinary bladder with retention, abdominal distention, megacolon—
Adults: 10 to 30 mg P.O. t.i.d. to q.i.d. Never give I.M. or I.V. When used for urinary retention, some patients may require 50 to 100 mg P.O. per dose. Use such doses with extreme caution.
Test dose: 2.5 mg S.C. repeated at 15- to 30-minute intervals to total of 4 doses to determine the minimal effective dose; then use minimal effective dose q 6 to 8 hours. All doses must be adjusted individually.

SIDE EFFECTS
Dose-related:
CNS: headache, malaise.
CV: bradycardia, hypotension, *cardiac arrest*, tachycardia.
EENT: lacrimation, miosis.
GI: *abdominal cramps, diarrhea*, salivation, nausea, vomiting, belching, borborygmus.
GU: urinary urgency.
Skin: flushing, sweating.
Other: bronchoconstriction.

INTERACTIONS
Procainamide, aminoglycoside antibiotics, quinidine: may reverse cholinergic effects on muscle. Observe for lack of drug effect.

NURSING CONSIDERATIONS
• Contraindicated in patients with uncertain strength or integrity of bladder wall; when increased muscular activity of GI or urinary tract is harmful; in mechanical obstructions of GI or urinary tract; in hyperthyroidism, peptic ulcer, latent or active bronchial asthma, car-

---

Italicized side effects are common or life-threatening.
*Liquid form contains alcohol.   **May contain tartrazine.

diac or coronary artery disease, vagotonia, epilepsy, Parkinson's disease,
bradycardia, chronic obstructive pulmonary disease, hypotension. Use cautiously in hypertension, vasomotor instability, peritonitis, or other acute inflammatory conditions of GI tract.

• *Never* give I.M. or I.V.; could cause
circulatory collapse, hypotension, severe abdominal cramping, bloody diarrhea, shock, cardiac arrest.

• Should stop all other cholinergics before giving this drug.

• Watch closely for side effects that
may indicate drug toxicity, especially
with subcutaneous administration.

• Monitor vital signs frequently, being
especially careful to check respirations.
Always have atropine injection readily
available and be prepared to give atropine 0.5 mg subcutaneously or slow
I.V. push as ordered, and provide respiratory support if needed.

• If used to treat urinary retention,
make sure bedpan is readily available.
Monitor intake and output.

• When used to prevent abdominal distention and GI distress, the doctor may
also order a rectal tube inserted to help
passage of gas.

• Poor and variable oral absorption requires larger oral doses. Oral and subcutaneous doses are *not* interchangeable.

• Drug usually effective 5 to 15 minutes after injection and 30 to 90 minutes after oral use.

• Give on empty stomach; if taken
after meals, may cause nausea and
vomiting.

---

edrophonium chloride
Tensilon♦

INDICATIONS & DOSAGE
*As a curare antagonist (to reverse neu-
romuscular blocking action)—*
Adults: 10 mg I.V. given over 30 to 45
seconds. Dose may be repeated as necessary to 40 mg maximum dose. Larger

doses may potentiate rather than antagonize effect of curare.
*Diagnostic aid in myasthenia gravis (the
Tensilon test)—*
Adults: 1 to 2 mg I.V. within 15 to
30 seconds, then 8 mg if no response
(increase in muscular strength).
Children over 34 kg: 2 mg I.V. If no
response within 45 seconds, give 1 mg
q 45 seconds to maximum of 10 mg.
Children up to 34 kg: 1 mg I.V. If no
response within 45 seconds, give 1 mg
q 45 seconds to maximum of 5 mg.
Infants: 0.5 mg I.V.
*To differentiate myasthenic crisis from
cholinergic crisis—*
Adults: 1 mg I.V. If no response in
1 minute, repeat dose once. Increased
muscular strength confirms myasthenic
crisis; no increase or exaggerated weakness confirms cholinergic crisis.
*Paroxysmal supraventricular tachycar-
dia—*
Adults: 10 mg I.V. given over 1 minute
or less.

SIDE EFFECTS
CNS: weakness, respiratory paralysis,
sweating.
CV: hypotension, bradycardia.
EENT: miosis.
GI: nausea, vomiting, *diarrhea, ab-
dominal cramps,* excessive salivation.
Other: increased bronchial secretions,
bronchospasm, muscle cramps, muscle
fasciculation.

INTERACTIONS
*Procainamide, aminoglycoside antibiot-
ics, quinidine:* may reverse cholinergic
effects on muscle. Observe for lack of
drug effect.

NURSING CONSIDERATIONS
• Contraindicated in mechanical obstruction of intestine or urinary tract,
bradycardia, hypotension. Use cautiously in hyperthyroidism, cardiac disease, peptic ulcer, bronchial asthma.
• Should stop all other cholinergics before giving this drug.

• Watch closely for side effects; may indicate toxicity.

• Monitor vital signs frequently, being especially careful to check respirations. Always have atropine injection readily available and be prepared to give atropine 0.5 mg subcutaneously or slow I.V. push as ordered, and provide respiratory support as needed.

• When giving drug to differentiate myasthenic crisis from cholinergic crisis, observe patient's muscle strength closely.

• Edrophonium not effective against muscle relaxation induced by decamethonium bromide and succinylcholine chloride.

• This cholinergic has the most rapid onset but shortest duration; therefore not used for treatment of myasthenia gravis.

• For easier parenteral administration, use a tuberculin syringe with an I.V. needle.

• I.M. route may be used in children due to difficulty with I.V. route: for children under 34 kg, inject 2 mg I.M.; children over 34 kg, 5 mg I.M. Expect same reactions as with I.V. test, but these appear after 2- to 10-minute delay.

---

neostigmine bromide
Prostigmin Bromide◆

neostigmine methylsulfate
Prostigmin◆

INDICATIONS & DOSAGE
Antidote for tubocurarine—
Adults: 0.5 to 2 mg I.V. slowly. Repeat p.r.n. Give 0.6 to 1.2 mg atropine sulfate I.V. before antidote dose.
Functional amenorrhea— 1 mg I.M. or S.C. daily for 3 days.
Postoperative abdominal distention and bladder atony—
Adults: 0.5 to 1 mg I.M. or S.C. q 4 to 6 hours.
Postoperative ileus—

Adults: 0.25 to 1 mg I.M. or S.C. q 4 to 6 hours.
Treatment of myasthenia gravis—
Adults: 15 to 30 mg t.i.d. (range 15 to 375 mg daily); or 0.5 to 2 mg I.M. or I.V. q 1 to 3 hours. Dose must be individualized, depending on response and tolerance of side effects. Therapy may be required day and night.
Children: 7.5 to 15 mg P.O. t.i.d. to q.i.d.
Note: 1:1,000 solution of injectable solution contains 1 mg/1 ml; 1:2,000 solution contains 0.5 mg/ml.

SIDE EFFECTS
CNS: dizziness, muscle weakness, mental confusion, jitters, sweating, respiratory depression.
CV: bradycardia, hypotension.
EENT: miosis.
GI: *nausea, vomiting, diarrhea, abdominal cramps,* excessive salivation.
Skin: rash (bromide).
Other: bronchospasm, *muscle cramps,* bronchoconstriction.

INTERACTIONS
Procainamide, quinidine: may reverse cholinergic effect on muscle. Observe for lack of drug effect.

NURSING CONSIDERATIONS
• Contraindicated in hypersensitivity to cholinergics or to bromide, mechanical obstruction of the intestine or urinary tract, bradycardia, hypotension. Use with extreme caution in bronchial asthma. Use cautiously in epilepsy, recent coronary occlusion, peritonitis, vagotonia, hyperthyroidism, cardiac arrhythmias, or peptic ulcer.

• Should stop all other cholinergics before giving this drug.

• Watch closely for side effects; may indicate toxicity.

• Monitor vital signs frequently, being especially careful to check respirations. Always have atropine injection readily available and be prepared to give atropine 0.5 mg subcutaneously or slow

---

I.V. push as ordered, and provide respiratory support as needed.
• Difficult to judge optimum dose. Help doctor by documenting patient's response after each dose. Show patient how to observe and record variations in muscle strength.
• When using for myasthenia gravis, explain that this drug will relieve ptosis, double vision, difficulty in chewing and swallowing, trunk and limb weakness. Stress importance of taking drug exactly as ordered. Explain that drug may have to be taken for life. Explain drug's effect on myasthenic symptoms.
• If patient has dysphagia, schedule dose 30 minutes before each meal.
• When used to prevent abdominal distention and GI distress, the doctor may order a rectal tube inserted to help passage of gas.
• Patients sometimes develop a resistance to neostigmine.
• When used for functional amenorrhea, check for vaginal bleeding and instruct patient to report any vaginal bleeding. If no bleeding in 72 hours after third injection, patient has nonfunctional amenorrhea.
• If muscle weakness is severe, doctor determines if it is caused by drug-induced toxicity or exacerbation of myasthenia gravis. Test dose of edrophonium I.V. will aggravate drug-induced weakness but will temporarily relieve weakness caused by disease.
• Hospitalized patients with longstanding myasthenia may request bedside supply of tablets. This will enable patient to take each dose precisely as ordered. Seek approval for self-medication program according to hospital policy, but continue to oversee medication regimen.
• GI side effects may be reduced by taking drug with milk or food.
• Advise patient to wear an identification tag indicating that he has myasthenia gravis.

physostigmine salicylate
Antilirium♦

INDICATIONS & DOSAGE
Anticholinergic poisoning—
Adults: 0.5 to 4 mg P.O., I.M., or I.V. q 2 hours.
Tricyclic antidepressant and anticholingeric poisoning—
Adults: 0.5 to 3 mg P.O., I.M., or I.V. (1 mg per minute I.V.) repeated as necessary if life-threatening signs recur (coma, convulsions, arrhythmias).

SIDE EFFECTS
CNS: hallucinations, muscular twitching, muscle weakness, ataxia, *restlessness, excitability, sweating.*
CV: irregular pulse, palpitations.
EENT: miosis.
GI: nausea, vomiting, epigastric pain, *diarrhea, excessive salivation.*
Other: bronchospasm, bronchial constriction, dyspnea.

INTERACTIONS
Procainamide, aminoglycoside antibiotics, quinidine: may reverse cholinergic effects on muscle. Observe for lack of drug effect.

NURSING CONSIDERATIONS
• Use cautiously in preexisting conditions: mechanical obstruction of intestine or urogenital tract, bronchial asthma, gangrene, diabetes, cardiovascular disease, vagotonia, bradycardia, hypotension, epilepsy, Parkinson's disease, hyperthyroidism, peptic ulcer.
• Watch closely for side effects, particularly CNS disturbances. Use side rails if patient becomes restless or hallucinates. Side effects may indicate drug toxicity.
• Monitor vital signs frequently, being especially careful to check respirations. Position patient to make breathing easier. Always have atropine injection readily available and be prepared to give atropine 0.5 mg subcutaneously or

slow I.V. push as ordered, and provide respiratory support as needed. Best administered in presence of doctor.
• Use only clear solution. Darkening may indicate loss of potency.
• Give I.V. at controlled rate; use slow, direct injection at no more than 1 mg/minute.
• Only cholinergic that crosses blood/brain barrier; therefore the only one useful for treating CNS effects of anticholinergic or tricyclic antidepressant toxicity.
• Effectiveness often immediate and dramatic but may be transient and may require repeat dose.

pyridostigmine bromide
Mestinon◆*, Regonol◆

INDICATIONS & DOSAGE
Curariform antagonist—
Adults: 10 to 30 mg I.V. preceded by atropine sulfate 0.6 to 1.2 mg I.V.
Myasthenia gravis—
Adults: 60 to 180 mg P.O. b.i.d. or q.i.d. Usual dose 600 mg daily but higher doses may be needed (up to 1,500 mg daily). Give 1/30 of oral dose I.M. or I.V. Dose must be adjusted for each patient, depending on response and tolerance of side effects.

SIDE EFFECTS
CNS: headache (with high doses), weakness, sweating, convulsions.
CV: bradycardia, hypotension.
EENT: miosis.
GI: abdominal cramps, nausea, vomiting, diarrhea, excessive salivation.
Skin: rash.
Local: thrombophlebitis.
Other: bronchospasm, bronchoconstriction, increased bronchial secretions, muscle cramps.

INTERACTIONS
Procainamide, aminoglycoside antibiotics, quinidine: may reverse cholinergic

effects on muscle. Observe for lack of drug effect.

NURSING CONSIDERATIONS
• Contraindicated in mechanical obstruction of intestine or urinary tract, bradycardia, hypotension. Use with extreme caution in bronchial asthma. Use cautiously in epilepsy, recent coronary occlusion, vagotonia, hyperthyroidism, cardiac arrhythmias, peptic ulcer. Avoid large doses in decreased gastrointestinal motility or megacolon.
• Difficult to judge optimum dosage. Help doctor by recording patient's response after each dose.
• Should stop all other cholinergics before giving this drug.
• Watch closely for side effects; may indicate toxicity.
• Monitor vital signs frequently, being especially careful to check respirations. Position patient to make breathing easier. Always have atropine injection readily available and be prepared to give atropine 0.5 mg subcutaneously or slow I.V. push as ordered, and provide respiratory support as needed.
• If muscle weakness is severe, doctor determines if it is caused by drug-induced toxicity or exacerbation of myasthenia gravis. Test dose of edrophonium I.V. will aggravate drug-induced weakness but will temporarily relieve weakness caused by disease.
• When using for myasthenia gravis, stress importance of taking drug exactly as ordered, on time, in evenly spaced doses. If doctor has ordered extended-release tablets, explain how these work. Patient must take them at the same time each day, at least 6 hours apart. Explain that he may have to take this drug for life. Tell about drug's effect on myasthenic symptoms.
• Has longest duration of the cholinergics used for myasthenia gravis.
• Available in 60-mg tablets, sustained-release (180-mg) tablets, injection, and syrup.

Italicized side effects are common or life-threatening.
*Liquid form contains alcohol.   **May contain tartrazine.

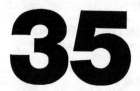

Cholinergic blockers (parasympatholytics)

atropine sulfate
benztropine mesylate
biperiden hydrochloride
biperiden lactate
chlorphenoxamine
  hydrochloride
cycrimine hydrochloride
glycopyrrolate
procyclidine hydrochloride
scopolamine hydrobromide
trihexyphenidyl hydrochloride

MECHANISM OF ACTION
Cholinergic blockers inhibit the effect of acetylcholine—as the neurotransmitter for impulses in the parasympathetic nervous system—at the junction between postganglionic nerve endings and effector organs.

COMBINATION PRODUCTS
Cholinergic blocking agents are available in tablets and capsules, combined with varying amounts of sedatives.

---

atropine sulfate

INDICATIONS & DOSAGE
Antidote for anticholinesterase insecticide poisoning—
Adults and children: 2 mg I.M. or I.V. repeated at hourly intervals until muscarinic symptoms disappear. Severe cases may require up to 6 mg I.M. or I.V. q 1 hour.
Preoperatively for diminishing secretions and blocking cardiac vagal reflexes—
Adults: 0.4 to 0.6 mg I.M. 45 to 60 minutes before anesthesia.

Children: 0.01 mg/kg I.M. up to a maximum dose of 0.4 mg 45 to 60 minutes before anesthesia.

SIDE EFFECTS
With usual doses of 0.4 to 0.6 mg, there are few side effects other than dry mouth. However, individual tolerance varies greatly.
CNS: disorientation, restlessness, irritability, incoherence, hallucinations, headache.
CV: palpitations, tachycardia, paradoxical bradycardia with doses less than 0.4 mg.
EENT: *dilated pupils, blurred vision,* photophobia, increased intraocular pressure, eye pain, dysphagia.
GI: *constipation, mouth dryness,* nausea, vomiting.
GU: *urinary hesitancy or retention.*
Skin: flushing, dryness.
Other: bronchial plugging, fever.
Side effects above may be due to pending atropine toxicity and are dose-related.

INTERACTIONS
None significant.

NURSING CONSIDERATIONS
● Contraindicated in narrow-angle glaucoma, obstructive uropathy, obstructive disease of GI tract, myasthenia gravis, paralytic ileus, intestinal atony, unstable cardiovascular status in acute hemorrhage, and toxic megacolon. Use with caution in autonomic neuropathy, hyperthyroidism, coronary artery disease, cardiac arrhythmias, congestive heart failure, hypertension,

---

hiatal hernia associated with reflux esophagitis, hepatic or renal disease, ulcerative colitis; in patients over 40 years because of the increased incidence of glaucoma; and in children under 6 years. Use with caution in hot or humid environments. Drug-induced heatstroke possible.
• Check all dosages carefully. Even slight overdose could lead to toxicity.
• Monitor vital signs carefully. Watch closely for side effects, especially in elderly or debilitated patients. Call doctor promptly.
• When given I.V., may cause paradoxical initial bradycardia. Usually disappears within 2 minutes.
• Monitor intake/output. Drug causes urinary retention and hesitancy; have patient void before receiving the drug.
• Many of the side effects (such as dry mouth and constipation) are an extension of the drug's pharmacologic activity and may be expected.

benztropine mesylate
Cogentin♦

INDICATIONS & DOSAGE
Acute dystonic reaction—
Adults: 2 mg I.V. or I.M. followed by 1 to 2 mg P.O. b.i.d. to prevent recurrence.
Parkinsonism—
Adults: 0.5 to 6 mg P.O. daily. Initial dose 0.5 mg to 1 mg. Increase 0.5 mg every 5 to 6 days. Adjust dosage to meet individual requirements.

SIDE EFFECTS
CNS: disorientation, restlessness, irritability, incoherence, hallucinations, headache, sedation, depression, muscular weakness.
CV: palpitations, tachycardia, paradoxical bradycardia.
EENT: dilated pupils, blurred vision, photophobia, difficulty swallowing.
GI: *constipation, mouth dryness,* nausea, vomiting, epigastric distress.

GU: urinary hesitancy or retention. Some side effects may be due to pending atropine-like toxicity and are dose related.

INTERACTIONS
Amantadine: anticholinergic side effects, such as confusion and hallucinations. Reduce dosage before administering amantadine.

NURSING CONSIDERATIONS
• Contraindicated in narrow-angle glaucoma. Use cautiously in patients with prostatic hypertrophy, tendency to tachycardia, and in elderly or debilitated patients; produces atropine-like side effects.
• Monitor vital signs carefully. Watch closely for side effects, especially in elderly or debilitated patients. Call doctor promptly.
• Never discontinue this drug abruptly. Dosage must be reduced gradually.
• Warn patient to avoid activities that require alertness until CNS response to drug is determined. If patient is to receive single daily dose, give at bedtime.
• Explain that drug may take 2 to 3 days to exert full effect.
• Monitor intake/output; urinary hesitancy and retention may develop.
• Watch for intermittent constipation, distention, abdominal pain; may be onset of paralytic ileus.
• Relieve dry mouth with cool drinks, ice chips, sugarless gum, or hard candy.
• To help prevent gastric irritation, administer after meals.

biperiden hydrochloride
Akineton♦

biperiden lactate
Akineton Lactate♦

INDICATIONS & DOSAGE
Extrapyramidal disorders—
Adults: 2 to 6 mg P.O. daily, b.i.d., or

Italicized side effects are common or life-threatening.
*Liquid form contains alcohol.   **May contain tartrazine.

t.i.d., depending on severity. Usual dose is 2 mg daily, or 2 mg I.M. or I.V. q ½ hour, not to exceed 4 doses or 8 mg total daily.

Parkinsonism—
Adults: 2 mg P.O. t.i.d. to q.i.d.

SIDE EFFECTS
CNS: disorientation, euphoria, restlessness, irritability, incoherence, dizziness, increased tremor.
CV: transient postural hypotension.
EENT: blurred vision.
GI: *constipation, mouth dryness,* nausea, vomiting, epigastric distress.
GU: urinary hesitancy or retention.
Side effects are dose-related and may resemble atropine toxicity.

INTERACTIONS
None significant.

NURSING CONSIDERATIONS
• Use with caution in prostatism, cardiac arrhythmias, narrow-angle glaucoma.
• Monitor vital signs carefully. Watch closely for side effects, especially in elderly or debilitated patients. Call doctor promptly.
• Give oral doses with or after meals to decrease GI side effects.
• When giving parenterally, keep patient in a supine position. Parenteral administration may cause transient postural hypotension and coordination disturbances.
• I.V. injections should be made very slowly.
• Because of possible dizziness, help patient when he gets out of bed.
• Tolerance may develop, requiring increased dosage.
• In severe parkinsonism, tremors may increase as spasticity is relieved.
• Warn patient to avoid activities that require alertness until CNS response to drug is determined.
• Monitor intake/output; urinary hesitancy and retention may develop.
• Relieve dry mouth with cool drinks, ice chips, sugarless gum, or hard candy.

chlorphenoxamine hydrochloride
Phenoxene♦

INDICATIONS & DOSAGE
Parkinsonism—
Adults: 50 mg P.O. t.i.d.; in severe cases, 300 to 400 mg daily, 100 mg t.i.d. to q.i.d.

SIDE EFFECTS
CNS: drowsiness, sedation, increased tremors.
EENT: blurred vision.
GI: *constipation, dry mouth,* nausea, vomiting, epigastric distress.

INTERACTIONS
None significant.

NURSING CONSIDERATIONS
• Use cautiously in narrow-angle glaucoma, tachycardia, or prostatic hypertrophy.
• Monitor vital signs carefully. Watch closely for side effects, especially in elderly or debilitated patients. Call doctor promptly.
• Warn patient to avoid activities that require alertness until CNS response to drug is determined.
• Administer doses with milk after meals to decrease GI side effects.
• In severe parkinsonism, tremors may increase as spasticity is relieved.
• Tolerance may develop, requiring increased dosage.
• Relieve dry mouth with cool drinks, ice chips, sugarless gum, or hard candy.

cycrimine hydrochloride
Pagitane Hydrochloride

INDICATIONS & DOSAGE
Idiopathic and arteriosclerotic parkinsonism—
Adults: initially, 1.25 to 2.5 mg P.O. t.i.d.; gradually increase dosage to 5 mg q.i.d.
Postencephalitic parkinsonism—
Adults: 5 mg t.i.d. or up to 5 mg q 2 hours while awake.

SIDE EFFECTS
CNS: disorientation, incoherence, weakness, drowsiness, dizziness.
EENT: blurred vision.
GI: epigastric distress, sore mouth and tongue, *constipation, mouth dryness.* Also transient nausea and anorexia 30 minutes to 1 hour after administration.
Skin: flushing, dryness, rash.
Other: fever.

INTERACTIONS
None significant.

NURSING CONSIDERATIONS
• Use with caution in narrow-angle glaucoma; in the elderly with arteriosclerotic changes; in tachycardia or tendency toward urinary retention.
• Monitor vital signs carefully.
• Watch closely for side effects, especially vertigo, disorientation, and weakness. Call doctor promptly if these develop; he may want to stop drug or reduce dosage.
• Explain that mild side effects, such as dry mouth, blurred vision, epigastric distress, disappear with continued administration.
• Administer doses with milk or after meals to decrease GI side effects.
• Relieve dry mouth with cool drinks, ice chips, sugarless gum, or hard candy.

glycopyrrolate
Robinul

INDICATIONS & DOSAGE
To reverse neuromuscular blockade—
Adults: 0.2 mg I.V. for each 1 mg neostigmine or equivalent dose of pyridostigmine. May be given intravenously without dilution or may be added to dextrose injection and given by infusion.
Preoperatively to diminish secretions and block cardiac vagal reflexes—
Adults: 0.002 mg/lb of body weight I.M. 30 to 60 minutes before anesthesia.

SIDE EFFECTS
CNS: disorientation, irritability, incoherence, weakness, nervousness, drowsiness, dizziness, headache.
CV: palpitations, tachycardia, paradoxical bradycardia.
EENT: *dilated pupils, blurred vision,* photophobia, increased intraocular pressure, difficulty swallowing.
GI: *constipation, mouth dryness,* nausea, vomiting, epigastric distress.
GU: urinary hesitancy or retention.
Skin: flushing, dryness, rash.
Local: burning at injection site.
Other: bronchial plugging, fever.

INTERACTIONS
None significant.

NURSING CONSIDERATIONS
• Contraindicated in narrow-angle glaucoma, obstructive uropathy, obstructive disease of the GI tract, myasthenia gravis, paralytic ileus, intestinal atony, unstable cardiovascular status in acute hemorrhage, toxic megacolon. Use with caution in patients with autonomic neuropathy, hyperthyroidism, coronary artery disease, cardiac arrhythmias, congestive heart failure, hypertension, hiatal hernia associated with reflux esophagitis, hepatic or renal disease, ulcerative colitis, and in pa-

---

Italicized side effects are common or life-threatening.
*Liquid form contains alcohol.   **May contain tartrazine.

tients over 40 years because of increased incidence of glaucoma. Use with caution in hot or humid environments. Drug-induced heatstroke possible.
• Check all dosages carefully. Even slight overdose could lead to toxicity.
• Don't mix with I.V. solution containing sodium chloride or bicarbonate.
• Monitor vital signs carefully. Watch closely for side effects, especially in elderly or debilitated patients. Call doctor promptly.
• Monitor intake/output. Causes urinary retention or hesitancy.
• Warn patient to avoid activities that require alertness until CNS response to drug is determined.
• Side effects less likely than with other parasympatholytics, unless dosages are excessive.

procyclidine hydrochloride
Kemadrin♦, Procyclid♦♦

INDICATIONS & DOSAGE
Parkinsonism, muscle rigidity—
Adults: initially, 2 to 2.5 mg P.O. t.i.d., after meals. Increase as needed to maximum 60 mg daily.
Also used to relieve extrapyramidal dysfunction that accompanies treatment with phenothiazines and rauwolfia derivatives. Also controls sialorrhea from neuroleptic medications.

SIDE EFFECTS
CNS: light-headedness, giddiness.
EENT: blurred vision, mydriasis.
GI: *constipation, mouth dryness,* nausea, vomiting, epigastric distress.
Skin: rash.

INTERACTIONS
None significant.

NURSING CONSIDERATIONS
• Contraindicated in narrow-angle glaucoma. Use cautiously in tachycar-

dia, hypotension, urinary retention, or prostatic hypertrophy.
• Watch closely for mental confusion, disorientation, agitation, hallucinations, and psychotic symptoms, especially in elderly. Call doctor promptly if these occur.
• In severe parkinsonism, tremors may increase as spasticity is relieved.
• Give after meals to minimize GI distress.
• Warn patient to avoid activities that require alertness until CNS response to drug is determined.
• Relieve dry mouth with cool drinks, ice chips, sugarless gum, or hard candy.

scopolamine hydrobromide

INDICATIONS & DOSAGE
Postencephalitic parkinsonism and other spastic states—
Adults: 0.5 to 1 mg P.O. t.i.d. to q.i.d.; 0.3 to 0.6 mg S.C., I.M., or I.V. (with suitable dilution) t.i.d. to q.i.d.
Children: 0.006 mg/kg P.O. or S.C. t.i.d. to q.i.d.; or 0.2 mg/m².
Preoperatively to reduce secretions—
Adults: 0.4 to 0.6 mg S.C.

SIDE EFFECTS
CNS: disorientation, restlessness, irritability, incoherence, headache.
CV: palpitations, tachycardia, paradoxical bradycardia.
EENT: dilated pupils, blurred vision, photophobia, increased intraocular pressure, difficulty swallowing.
GI: *constipation, mouth dryness, nausea, vomiting, epigastric distress.*
GU: urinary hesitancy or retention.
Skin: flushing, dryness.
Other: bronchial plugging, fever, depressed respirations.
Side effects may be due to pending atropine-like toxicity and are dose related. Individual tolerance varies greatly.

INTERACTIONS
None significant.

NURSING CONSIDERATIONS
• Contraindicated in narrow-angle glaucoma, obstructive uropathy, obstructive disease of the GI tract, asthma, chronic pulmonary disease, myasthenia gravis, paralytic ileus, intestinal atony, unstable cardiovascular status in acute hemorrhage, or toxic megacolon. Use with caution in patients with autonomic neuropathy, hyperthyroidism, coronary artery disease, cardiac arrhythmias, congestive heart failure, hypertension, hiatal hernia associated with reflux esophagitis, hepatic or renal disease, ulcerative colitis; in patients over 40 years because of the increased incidence of glaucoma; and in children under 6 years. Use with caution in hot or humid environments. Drug-induced heatstroke possible.
• Some patients become temporarily excited or disoriented. Symptoms disappear when sedative effect is complete. Use bed rails as precaution.
• Warn patients to avoid activities requiring alertness until CNS response to drug is determined.
• Monitor intake/output; urinary hesitancy or retention may develop.
• Tolerance may develop when given over a long period of time.
• Many of the side effects (such as dry mouth, constipation) are an extension of the drug's pharmacologic activity and may be expected.

---

trihexyphenidyl hydrochloride
Aparkane◆◆, Artane◆*, Hexaphen, Novohexidyl◆◆, T.H.P., Tremin, Trihexane, Trihexidyl, Trihexy◆◆, Trixyl◆◆

INDICATIONS & DOSAGE
Drug-induced parkinsonism—
Adults: 1 mg P.O. 1st day, 2 mg 2nd day, then increase 2 mg every 3 to 5 days until total of 6 to 10 mg given daily. Usually given t.i.d. with meals and, if needed, q.i.d. (last dose should be before bedtime). Postencephalitic parkinsonism may require 12 to 15 mg total daily dose.

SIDE EFFECTS
CNS: nervousness, dizziness, headache, restlessness, agitation, hallucinations, euphoria, delusion, amnesia.
CV: tachycardia.
EENT: blurred vision, mydriasis, increased intraocular pressure.
GI: constipation, *dry mouth, nausea*.
GU: urinary hesitancy or retention.
Side effects are dose related.

INTERACTIONS
Amantadine: anticholinergic side effects, such as confusion and hallucinations. Reduce dosage before administering amantadine.

NURSING CONSIDERATIONS
• Use cautiously in patients with narrow-angle glaucoma; cardiac, hepatic, or renal disorders; hypertension; obstructive disease of the gastrointestinal and the genitourinary tracts; possible prostatic hypertrophy; patients over 60 years; and those with arteriosclerosis or history of drug hypersensitivities.
• Warn patient to avoid activities that require alertness until CNS response to drug is determined.
• Causes nausea if given before meals.
• Relieve dry mouth with cool drinks, ice chips, sugarless gum, or hard candy.
• Patient may develop a tolerance to this drug.
• Monitor intake/output; urinary hesitancy or retention may develop.
• Gonioscopic evaluation and close monitoring of intraocular pressures advised, especially in patients over 40 years.

Italicized side effects are common or life-threatening.
*Liquid form contains alcohol.   **May contain tartrazine.

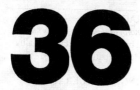

36

Adrenergics (sympathomimetics)

albuterol
dobutamine hydrochloride
dopamine hydrochloride
ephedrine sulfate
epinephrine
epinephrine bitartrate
epinephrine hydrochloride
ethylnorepinephrine
  hydrochloride
isoetharine hydrochloride 1%
isoetharine mesylate
isoproterenol hydrochloride
isoproterenol sulfate
mephentermine sulfate
metaproterenol sulfate
metaraminol bitartrate
norepinephrine injection
  (formerly levarterenol
  bitartrate)
pseudoephedrine hydrochloride
pseudoephedrine sulfate
terbutaline sulfate

MECHANISM OF ACTION
Adrenergics simulate or increase the effect of epinephrine and norepinephrine on alpha- and beta-adrenergic receptors within the sympathetic nervous system. Effects vary and include bronchodilation, release of glucose from the liver, increase in heart rate and ventricular contractility, central nervous system excitation, dilation (beta effect) of blood vessels in skeletal muscles, and constriction (alpha effect) of blood vessels in cutaneous areas.

COMBINATION PRODUCTS
Only a few of the many combinations are included here as examples of this group.

Inhalants
DUO-MEDIHALER: isoproterenol hydrochloride 0.16 mg and phenylephrine bitartrate 0.24 mg per dose.
Oral bronchodilators
AMESEC♦: aminophylline 130 mg, ephedrine HCl 25 mg, and amobarbital 25 mg.
BRONCHOBID DURACAPS: theophylline 260 mg and ephedrine HCl 35 mg.
MARAX♦*: theophylline 130 mg, ephedrine sulfate 25 mg, and hydroxyzine HCl 10 mg.
QUADRINAL♦: theophylline calcium salicylate 65 mg, ephedrine hydrochloride 24 mg, potassium iodide 320 mg, and phenobarbital 24 mg.
QUIBRON PLUS*: theophylline 150 mg, ephedrine hydrochloride 25 mg, guaifenesin 100 mg, and butabarbital 20 mg.
TEDRAL SA♦: theophylline 180 mg, ephedrine hydrochloride 48 mg, and phenobarbital 25 mg.
(OTC) ASMA-LIEF: theophylline 130 mg, ephedrine hydrochloride 24 mg, and phenobarbital 8 mg.
(OTC) TEDRAL: theophylline 130 mg, ephedrine hydrochloride 24 mg, and phenobarbital 8 mg.
(OTC) THALFED: theophylline 120 mg, ephedrine hydrochloride 25 mg, and phenobarbital 8 mg.
Decongestants
ACTIFED: pseudoephedrine hydrochloride 60 mg and triprolidine hydrochloride 2.5 mg.
CONGESPRIN: phenylephrine hydrochloride 1.25 mg and aspirin 81 mg.
DRISTAN: phenylephrine hydrochloride

Unmarked trade names available in the United States only.
♦ Also available in Canada.   ♦♦ Available in Canada only.

5 mg, chlorpheniramine maleate 2 mg, aspirin 325 mg, and caffeine 16.2 mg.
HISTASPAN-PLUS: phenylephrine hydrochloride 20 mg and chlorpheniramine maleate 8 mg.
NALDECON: phenylpropanolamine hydrochloride 40 mg, phenylephrine hydrochloride 10 mg, chlorpheniramine maleate 5 mg, and phenyltoloxamine citrate 15 mg.
ORNEX: phenylpropanolamine hydrochloride 18 mg and acetaminophen 325 mg.
PHENERGAN-D: pseudoephedrine hydrochloride 60 mg and promethazine hydrochloride 6.25 mg.
SINUTAB-II: phenylpropanolamine hydrochloride 25 mg and acetaminophen 325 mg.
TRIAMINIC: phenylpropanolamine hydrochloride 50 mg, pyrilamine maleate 25 mg, and pheniramine maleate 25 mg.

albuterol
Proventil, Ventolin

INDICATIONS & DOSAGE
Relief of bronchospasm in patients with reversible obstructive airway disease—
Adults and children 12 years or older: 1 to 2 inhalations q 4 to 6 hours. More frequent administration or a greater number of inhalations is not recommended.
Oral tablets—2 to 4 mg t.i.d. or q.i.d. Maximum 8 mg.
Not recommended for children under age 12.

SIDE EFFECTS
CNS: *tremor, nervousness,* dizziness, insomnia, headache.
CV: tachycardia, palpitations, hypertension.
EENT: drying and irritation of nose and throat (with inhaled form).
GI: heartburn, nausea, vomiting.
Other: muscle cramps.

INTERACTIONS
Propranolol and other beta blockers: blocked bronchodilating effect of albuterol. Monitor patient carefully.

NURSING CONSIDERATIONS
• Use cautiously in patients with cardiovascular disorders, including coronary insufficiency and hypertension; in patients with hyperthyroidism or diabetes mellitus; and in patients who are unusually responsive to adrenergics.
• Warn patient about the possibility of paradoxical bronchospasm. If this occurs, the drug should be discontinued immediately.
• Patients may use tablets and aerosol concomitantly. Monitor closely for toxicity.
• Albuterol reportedly produces less cardiac stimulation than other sympthomimetics, especially isoproterenol.
• Elderly patients usually require a lower dose.
• Albuterol is also known by the generic name of salbutamol.
• Teach patient how to administer metered dose correctly. Have him shake container; exhale through nose; administer aerosol while inhaling deeply on mouthpiece of inhaler; hold breath for a few seconds, then exhale slowly. Tell him to allow 2 minutes between inhalations.
• Store drug in light-resistant container.

dobutamine hydrochloride
Dobutrex

INDICATIONS & DOSAGE
Refractory heart failure and as adjunct in cardiac surgery—
Adults: 2.5 to 10 mcg/kg/minute as an I.V. infusion. Rarely, infusion rates up to 40 mcg/kg/minute have been required. May be reconstituted with 5% dextrose in water, normal saline solution, or lactated Ringer's solution.

Italicized side effects are common or life-threatening.
*Liquid form contains alcohol.   **May contain tartrazine.

SIDE EFFECTS
CNS: headache.
CV: *increased heart rate, hypertension, premature ventricular beats,* angina, nonspecific chest pain.
GI: nausea, vomiting.
Other: shortness of breath.

INTERACTIONS
Propranolol, metoprolol: These beta blockers may make dobutamine ineffective. Do not use together.

NURSING CONSIDERATIONS
• Contraindicated in idiopathic hypertrophic subaortic stenosis.
• A unique agent. Increases contractility of failing heart without inducing marked tachycardia, except at high doses.
• Dobutamine is chemical modification of isoproterenol.
• Often used with nitroprusside for additive effects.
• EKG, blood pressure, pulmonary wedge pressure, and cardiac output should be monitored continuously. Also monitor urinary output.
• Incompatible with alkaline solutions. Do not mix with sodium bicarbonate injection.
• Infusions of up to 72 hours produce no more adverse effects than shorter infusions.
• Oxidation of drug may slightly discolor admixtures containing dobutamine. This does not indicate a significant loss of potency.
• Intravenous solutions remain stable for 24 hours.

dopamine hydrochloride
Intropin♦, Dopastat

INDICATIONS & DOSAGE
To treat shock and correct hemodynamic imbalances; to improve perfusion to vital organs, increase cardiac output; to correct hypotension—

Adults: 2 to 5 mcg/kg/minute I.V. infusion, up to 50 mcg/kg/minute.
Titrate the dosage to the desired hemodynamic and/or renal response.

SIDE EFFECTS
CNS: headache.
CV: ectopic beats, tachycardia, anginal pain, palpitations, *hypotension.* Less frequently, bradycardia, widening of QRS complex, conduction disturbances, vasoconstriction.
GI: nausea, vomiting.
Local: necrosis and tissue sloughing with extravasation.
Other: piloerection, dyspnea.

INTERACTIONS
Ergot alkaloids: extreme elevations in blood pressure. Don't use together.
Phenytoin: may lower blood pressure of dopamine-stabilized patients. Monitor carefully.

NURSING CONSIDERATIONS
• Contraindicated in uncorrected tachyarrhythmias, pheochromocytoma, ventricular fibrillation. Use cautiously in patients with occlusive vascular disease, cold injuries, diabetic endarteritis, arterial embolism; also, in pregnant patients and those taking MAO inhibitors.
• Not a substitute for blood or fluid volume deficit. If volume deficit exists, it should be replaced before vasopressors are administered.
• Use large vein, as in antecubital fossa, to minimize risk of extravasation. Watch site carefully for signs of extravasation. If it occurs, stop infusion immediately and call doctor. He may want to counteract effect by infiltrating the area with 5 to 10 mg phentolamine and 10 to 15 ml normal saline solution.
• Check blood pressure, pulse rate, urinary output, and extremity color and temperature often during infusion. Titrate infusion rate according to findings, using doctor's guidelines. Use a

microdrip or infusion pump to regulate flow rate.
• Observe patient closely for side effects. If adverse effects develop, dosage may need to be adjusted or discontinued.
• If a disproportionate rise in the diastolic pressure (a marked decrease in pulse pressure) is observed in patients receiving dopamine, decrease infusion rate and observe carefully for further evidence of predominant vasoconstrictor activity, unless such an effect is desired.
• Most patients satisfactorily maintained on less than 20 mcg/kg/minute.
• If doses exceed 50 mcg/kg/minute, check urinary output often. If urine flow decreases without hypotension, consider reducing dose.
• If drug is stopped, watch closely for sudden drop in blood pressure.
• Don't mix with alkaline solutions. Use 5% dextrose in water, normal saline solution, or combination of 5% dextrose in water and saline solution. Mix just before use.
• Dopamine solutions deteriorate after 24 hours. Discard at that time or earlier if solution is discolored.
• Do not mix other drugs in bottle containing dopamine.
• Do not give alkaline drugs (sodium bicarbonate, phenytoin sodium) through I.V. line containing dopamine.

ephedrine sulfate

INDICATIONS & DOSAGE
To correct hypotensive states; to support ventricular rate in Adams-Stokes syndrome—
Adults: 25 to 50 mg I.M. or S.C., or 10 to 25 mg I.V. p.r.n. to maximum 150 mg/24 hours.
Children: 3 mg/kg S.C. or I.V. daily, divided into 4 to 6 doses.
Bronchodilator or nasal decongestant—
Adults: 12.5 to 50 mg P.O. b.i.d.,

t.i.d., or q.i.d. Maximum 400 mg daily in 6 to 8 divided doses.
Children: 2 to 3 mg/kg P.O. daily in 4 to 6 divided doses.

SIDE EFFECTS
CNS: *insomnia, nervousness,* dizziness, headache, muscle weakness, sweating, euphoria, confusion, delirium.
CV: *palpitations,* tachycardia, hypertension.
EENT: dryness of nose and throat.
GI: nausea, vomiting, anorexia.
GU: urinary retention, painful urination due to visceral sphincter spasm.

INTERACTIONS
MAO inhibitors and tricyclic antidepressants: when given with sympathomimetics, may cause severe hypertension (hypertensive crisis). Don't use together.
Methyldopa: may inhibit effect of ephedrine. Give together cautiously.

NURSING CONSIDERATIONS
• Contraindicated in patients with porphyria, severe coronary artery disease, cardiac arrhythmias, narrow-angle glaucoma, psychoneurosis, and in patients on MAO-inhibitor therapy. Use with caution in elderly patients and those with hypertension, hyperthyroidism, nervous or excitable states, cardiovascular disease, prostatic hypertrophy.
• Not a substitute for blood or fluid volume deficit. Volume deficit should be replaced before vasopressors are administered.
• Give I.V. injection slowly.
• Hypoxia, hypercapnia, and acidosis, which may reduce effectiveness or increase the incidence of adverse effects, must be identified and corrected before or during ephedrine administration.
• Effectiveness decreases after 2 to 3 weeks. Then increased dosage may be needed. Tolerance develops, but drug is not known to cause addiction.

Italicized side effects are common or life-threatening.
*Liquid form contains alcohol.   **May contain tartrazine.

- To prevent insomnia, avoid giving within 2 hours before bedtime.
- Warn patient not to take over-the-counter drugs that contain ephedrine without informing doctor.

epinephrine
Inhalants:
Bronkaid Mist♦, Primatene Mist

epinephrine bitartrate
Inhalants:
AsthmaHaler, Medihaler-Epi♦

epinephrine hydrochloride
Adrenalin Chloride, Asmolin, Sus-Phrine♦

INDICATIONS & DOSAGE
Bronchospasm, hypersensitivity reactions, and anaphylaxis—
Adults: 0.1 to 0.5 ml of 1:1,000 S.C. or I.M. Repeat q 10 to 15 minutes, p.r.n. Or 0.1 to 0.25 ml 1:1,000 I.V.
Children: 0.01 ml (10 mcg) of 1:1,000/kg S.C. Repeat q 20 minutes to 4 hours, p.r.n.; 0.005 ml/kg of 1:200 (Sus-Phrine). Repeat q 8 to 12 hours, p.r.n.
Hemostatic—
Adults: 1:50,000 to 1:1,000, applied topically.
Acute asthmatic attacks (inhalation)—
Adults and children: 1 or 2 inhalations of 1:100 or 2.25% racemic, p.r.n.; 0.2 mg/dose usual content.
To prolong local anesthetic effect—
Adults and children: 0.2 to 0.4 ml of 1:1,000 intraspinal; 1:500,000 to 1:50,000 local mixed with local anesthetic.
To restore cardiac rhythm in cardiac arrest—
Adults: 0.5 to 1 mg I.V. or into endotracheal tube. May be given intracardiac if no I.V. route or intratracheal route available.
Children: 10 mcg/kg I.V. or 5 to 10 mcg (0.05 to 0.1 ml of 1:10,000)/kg intracardiac.

Note: 1 mg = 1 ml of 1:1,000 or 10 ml of 1:10,000.

SIDE EFFECTS
CNS: *nervousness,* tremor, euphoria, anxiety, coldness of extremities, vertigo, *headache,* sweating, cerebral hemorrhage, disorientation, agitation. In patients with Parkinson's disease, the drug increases rigidity and tremor.
CV: *palpitations;* widened pulse pressure; hypertension; *tachycardia; ventricular fibrillation; CVA;* anginal pain; EKG changes, including a decrease in the T-wave amplitude.
Metabolic: *hyperglycemia,* glycosuria.
Other: pulmonary edema, dyspnea, *pallor.*

INTERACTIONS
Tricyclic antidepressants: when given with sympathomimetics, may cause severe hypertension (hypertensive crisis). Don't give together.
Propranolol: vasoconstriction and reflex bradycardia. Monitor patient carefully.

NURSING CONSIDERATIONS
- Contraindicated in narrow-angle glaucoma, shock (other than anaphylactic shock), organic brain damage, cardiac dilatation, and coronary insufficiency. Also during general anesthesia with halogenated hydrocarbons or cyclopropane and in labor (may delay second stage). Use with extreme caution in patients with long-standing bronchial asthma and emphysema who have developed degenerative heart disease. Use with caution in elderly patients, and those with hyperthyroidism, angina, hypertension, psychoneurosis, diabetes.
- Don't mix with alkaline solutions. Use 5% dextrose in water, normal saline solution, or a combination of 5% dextrose in water and saline solution. Mix just before use.
- Epinephrine is rapidly destroyed by oxidizing agents, such as iodine, chromates, nitrates, nitrites, oxygen, and

salts of easily reducible metals such as iron.

• Epinephrine solutions deteriorate after 24 hours. Discard after that time or before if solution is discolored or contains precipitate. Keep solution in light-resistant container, and don't remove before use.

• Massage site after injection to counteract possible vasoconstriction. Repeated local injection can cause necrosis at site due to vasoconstriction.

• Avoid intramuscular administration of oil injection into buttocks. Gas gangrene may occur because epinephrine reduces oxygen tension of the tissues, encouraging the growth of contaminating organisms.

• This drug may widen patient's pulse pressure.

• In the event of a sharp blood pressure rise, rapid-acting vasodilators, such as the nitrites or alpha-adrenergic blocking agents, can be given to counteract the marked pressor effect of large doses of epinephrine.

• Observe patient closely for side effects. If adverse effects develop, dosage may need to be adjusted or discontinued.

• If patient has acute hypersensitivity reactions, it may be necessary to instruct him to self-inject epinephrine at home.

• Drug of choice in emergency treatment of acute anaphylactic reactions, including anaphylactic shock.

ethylnorepinephrine hydrochloride
Bronkephrine

INDICATIONS & DOSAGE
To relieve bronchospasm due to asthma—
Adults: 0.5 to 1 ml S.C. or I.M.
Children: 0.1 to 0.5 ml S.C. or I.M.

SIDE EFFECTS
CNS: *headache*, dizziness.

CV: changes in blood pressure, *elevation in pulse rate*, palpitations.
GI: nausea.

INTERACTIONS
None significant.

NURSING CONSIDERATIONS
• Use with caution in patients with cardiovascular disease or history of stroke.
• Safer than epinephrine for use in hypertensive or severely ill patients in whom significant pressor effects are undesirable.
• Valuable when used in children due to low incidence of adverse effects; may be useful in diabetic asthmatics due to low glycogenolytic activity.
• Choose anatomic injection site carefully to avoid inadvertent intraneural or intravascular injection.

isoetharine hydrochloride 1%
Beta-Z Solution, Bronkosol

isoetharine mesylate
Bronkometer

INDICATIONS & DOSAGE
Bronchial asthma and reversible bronchospasm that may occur with bronchitis and emphysema—
Adults: (hydrochloride): administered by hand nebulizer, oxygen aerosolization, or IPPB.

Method	Dose	Dilution
Hand	3 to 7 inhalations	undiluted
Oxygen aerosolization	0.5 ml	1:3 with saline
IPPB	0.5 ml	1:3 with saline

Adults: (mesylate): 1 to 2 inhalations. Occasionally, more may be required.

SIDE EFFECTS
CNS: *tremor, headache,* dizziness, excitement.
CV: *palpitations,* increased heart rate.

Italicized side effects are common or life-threatening.
∗Liquid form contains alcohol.   ∗∗May contain tartrazine.

GI: nausea, vomiting.

INTERACTIONS
Propranolol and other beta blockers: blocked bronchodilating effect of isoetharine. Monitor patient carefully if used together.

NURSING CONSIDERATIONS
• Use cautiously in patients with hyperthyroidism, hypertension, coronary disease, or those with sensitivity to sympathomimetics.
• Excessive use can lead to decreased effectiveness.
• Monitor for severe paradoxical bronchoconstriction after excessive use. Discontinue immediately if bronchoconstriction occurs.
• Although isoetharine has minimal effects on the heart, use cautiously in patients receiving general anesthetics that sensitize the myocardium to sympathomimetic drugs.
• Instruct patient in the use of aerosol and mouthpiece.

---

isoproterenol hydrochloride
Isuprel♦*, Proternol (tabs)
Inhalants: Norisodrine, Vapo-Iso

isoproterenol sulfate
Iso-Autohaler, Luf-Iso Inhalation, Medihaler-Iso♦, Norisodrine

---

INDICATIONS & DOSAGE
Bronchial asthma and reversible bronchospasm (hydrochloride)—
Adults: 10 to 20 mg S.L. q 6 to 8 hours.
Children: 5 to 10 mg S.L. q 6 to 8 hours. Not recommended for children under 6 years.
Bronchospasm (sulfate)—
Adults and children: acute dyspneic episodes: 1 inhalation initially. May repeat if needed after 2 to 5 minutes. Maintenance: 1 to 2 inhalations q.i.d. to 6 times daily. May repeat once more 10 minutes after second dose. Not more

than 3 doses should be administered for each attack.
Heart block and ventricular arrhythmias (sulfate)—
Adults: initially, 0.02 to 0.06 mg I.V. Subsequent doses 0.01 to 0.2 mg I.V. or 5 mcg/minute I.V.; or 0.2 mg I.M. initially, then 0.02 to 1 mg, p.r.n.
Children: may give ½ of initial adult dose.
Maintenance for Stokes-Adams disease or AV block (sulfate)—
Adults: 30 to 180 mg timed-release tablets P.O. daily swallowed whole.
Shock (sulfate)—
Adults and children: 0.5 to 5 mcg/minute by continuous I.V. infusion. Usual concentration: 1 mg (5 ml) in 500 ml 5% dextrose in water. Adjust rate according to heart rate, central venous pressure, blood pressure, and urine flow.

SIDE EFFECTS
CNS: *headache,* mild tremor, weakness, dizziness, nervousness, insomnia.
CV: *palpitations,* tachycardia, anginal pain; blood pressure may be elevated and then fall.
GI: nausea, vomiting.
Metabolic: hyperglycemia.
Other: sweating, flushing of face, bronchial edema and inflammation.

INTERACTIONS
Propranolol and other beta blockers: blocked bronchodilating effect of isoproterenol. Monitor patient carefully if used together.

NURSING CONSIDERATIONS
• Contraindicated in tachycardia caused by digitalis intoxication and in patients with preexisting arrhythmias, especially tachycardia, because chronotropic effect on the heart may aggravate such disorders. Contraindicated in recent myocardial infarction. Use cautiously in coronary insufficiency, diabetes, hyperthyroidism.
• Not a substitute for blood or fluid

volume deficit. If deficit exists, it should be replaced before vasopressors are administered.

• If heart rate exceeds 110 beats/minute, it may be advisable to decrease infusion rate or temporarily stop infusion. Doses sufficient to increase the heart rate to more than 130 beats per minute (bpm) may induce ventricular arrhythmias.

• If precordial distress or anginal pain occurs, stop drug immediately.

• When administering I.V. isoproterenol for shock, closely monitor blood pressure, CVP, EKG, arterial blood gas measurements, and urinary output. Carefully adjust infusion rate according to these measurements.

• Oral and sublingual tablets are poorly and erratically absorbed.

• Teach patient how to take sublingual tablet properly. Tell him to hold tablet under tongue until it dissolves and is absorbed and not to swallow saliva until that time. Prolonged use of sublingual tablets can cause tooth decay. Instruct patient to rinse mouth with water between doses. Will also help prevent dryness of oropharynx.

• If possible, don't give at bedtime because it interrupts sleep patterns.

• Oral tablets not for sublingual use; must be swallowed whole, not broken. Store in cool, dry place in airtight, light-resistant container. Keep bottle tightly capped after opening.

• This drug may cause slight rise in systolic blood pressure and slight to marked drop in diastolic blood pressure.

• Use a microdrip or infusion pump to regulate infusion flow rate.

• Observe patient closely for side effects. Dosage may need to be adjusted or discontinued.

• Teach patient to perform oral inhalation correctly. Give the following instructions for using a metered-dose nebulizer:

—Clear nasal passages and throat.

—Breathe out, expelling as much air from lungs as possible.

—Place mouthpiece well into mouth as dose from nebulizer is released, and inhale deeply.

—Hold breath for several seconds, remove mouthpiece, and exhale slowly.

• Instructions for metered powder nebulizer are the same, except that deep inhalation is not necessary.

• Patient may develop a tolerance to this drug. Warn against overuse.

• Warn patient using oral inhalant that drug may turn sputum and saliva pink.

• May aggravate ventilation perfusion abnormalities; even while ease of breathing is improved, arterial oxygen tension may fall paradoxically.

• Discard inhalation solution if it is discolored or contains precipitate.

---

mephentermine sulfate
Wyamine•

INDICATIONS & DOSAGE

Hypotension following spinal anesthesia—
Adults: 30 to 45 mg I.V. in a single injection, then 30 mg I.V. repeated p.r.n. Maintenance of blood pressure: continuous I.V. infusion of 0.1% solution of mephentermine in 5% dextrose in water.
Hypotension following spinal anesthesia during obstetric procedures—
Adults: initially, 15 mg I.V., p.r.n.
Prevention of hypotension during spinal anesthesia—
Adults: 30 to 40 mg I.M. 10 to 20 minutes prior to anesthesia.
Treatment of shock and hypotension—
Adults: 0.5 mg/kg I.V.
Children: 0.4 mg/kg I.V.

SIDE EFFECTS

CNS: euphoria, nervousness, anxiety, tremor, incoherence, drowsiness, convulsions.

Italicized side effects are common or life-threatening.
*Liquid form contains alcohol.　　**May contain tartrazine.

CV: arrhythmias, marked elevation of blood pressure (with large doses).

INTERACTIONS

Propranolol and other beta blockers: blocked bronchodilating effect of metaproterenol. Monitor patient carefully if used together.

NURSING CONSIDERATIONS

• Contraindicated in concealed hemorrhage or hypotension from hemorrhage, except in emergencies; also in patients receiving phenothiazines, or who have received MAO inhibitors within 2 weeks. Use cautiously in arteriosclerosis, cardiovascular disease, hyperthyroidism, hypertension, chronic illness.

• Not a substitute for blood or fluid volume deficit. If deficit exists, it should be replaced before vasopressors are administered.

• During infusion, check blood pressure every 5 minutes until stabilized; then every 15 minutes.

• Observe patient closely for side effects. If adverse effects develop, dosage may need to be adjusted or discontinued.

• Monitor blood pressure even after stopping drug.

• I.M. route may be used since drug is not irritating to tissue.

• I.V. drug is not irritating to tissue, and extravasation is not dangerous. To prepare 0.1% I.V. solution: add 16.6 ml mephentermine (30 mg/ml) to 500 ml 5% dextrose in water.

• Can be given I.V. undiluted.

• May increase uterine contractions during third trimester of pregnancy.

• Hypercapnia, hypoxia, and acidosis may reduce effectiveness or increase adverse effects. Identify and correct before and during administration.

metaproterenol sulfate
Alupent♦, Metaprel

INDICATIONS & DOSAGE

Acute episodes of bronchial asthma—
Adults and children: 2 to 3 inhalations. Should not repeat inhalations more often than q 3 to 4 hours. Should not exceed 12 inhalations daily.
Bronchial asthma and reversible bronchospasm—
Adults: 20 mg P.O. q 6 to 8 hours.
Children over 9 years or over 27 kg: 20 mg P.O. q 6 to 8 hours. (0.4 mg to 0.9 mg/kg/dose t.i.d.)
Children 6 to 9 years or less than 27 kg: 10 mg P.O. q 6 to 8 hours. (0.4 mg to 0.9 mg/kg/dose t.i.d.)
Not recommended for children under 6 years.

SIDE EFFECTS

CNS: nervousness, weakness, drowsiness, tremor.
CV: tachycardia, hypertension, palpitations; *with excessive use, cardiac arrest.*
GI: vomiting, nausea, bad taste in mouth.
Other: paradoxical bronchiolar constriction with excessive use.

INTERACTIONS

Propranolol and other beta blockers: blocked bronchodilating effect of metaproterenol. Monitor patient carefully if used together.

NURSING CONSIDERATIONS

• Contraindicated in tachycardia, and in arrhythmias associated with tachycardia. Use with caution in hypertension, coronary artery disease, hyperthyroidism, diabetes.

• Safe use of inhalant in children under 12 years not established.

• Teach patient how to administer metered dose correctly. Instructions: shake container; exhale through nose; administer aerosol while inhaling deeply on

mouthpiece of inhaler; hold breath for a few seconds, then exhale slowly. Allow 2 minutes between inhalations. Store drug in light-resistant container.
• Inhalant solution can be administered by IPPB diluted in saline solution or via a hand nebulizer at full strength.
• Tell patient to notify doctor if no response is derived from dosage. Warn against changing dose without calling doctor.

metaraminol bitartrate
Aramine

INDICATIONS & DOSAGE
Prevention of hypotension—
Adults: 2 to 10 mg I.M. or S.C.
Severe shock—
Adults: 0.5 to 5 mg direct I.V. followed by I.V. infusion.
Treatment of hypotension due to shock—
Adults: 15 to 100 mg in 500 ml normal saline solution or 5% dextrose in water I.V. infusion. Adjust rate to maintain blood pressure.
All indications—
Children: 0.01 mg/kg as single I.V. injection; 1 mg/25 ml 5% dextrose in water as I.V. infusion. Adjust rate to maintain blood pressure in normal range. 0.1 mg/kg I.M. as single dose, p.r.n. Allow at least 10 minutes to elapse before increasing dose because maximum effect is not immediately apparent.

SIDE EFFECTS
CNS: apprehension, restlessness, dizziness, headache, tremor, weakness; with excessive use, *convulsions.*
CV: *hypertension;* hypotension; precordial pain; *palpitations; arrhythmias, including sinus or ventricular tachycardia; bradycardia;* premature supraventricular beats; atrioventricular dissociation.
GI: nausea, vomiting.
GU: decreased urinary output.
Metabolic: hyperglycemia.

Skin: flushing, pallor, sweating.
Local: *irritation upon extravasation.*
Other: *metabolic acidosis in hypovolemia, increased body temperature, respiratory distress.*

INTERACTIONS
MAO inhibitors: may cause severe hypertension (hypertensive crisis). Don't use together.

NURSING CONSIDERATIONS
• Contraindicated in peripheral or mesenteric thrombosis, pulmonary edema, hypercarbia, and acidosis; also during anesthesia with cyclopropane and halogenated hydrocarbon anesthetics. Use cautiously in patients with hypertension, thyroid disease, diabetes, cirrhosis, or malaria, and those receiving digitalis.
• Not a substitute for blood or fluid volume deficit. Fluid deficit should be replaced before vasopressors are administered.
• Keep solution in light-resistant container, away from heat.
• Use large veins, as in antecubital fossa, to minimize risk of extravasation. Watch infusion site carefully for signs of extravasation. If it occurs, stop infusion immediately and call doctor.
• During infusion, check blood pressure every 5 minutes until stabilized; then every 15 minutes. Check pulse rates, urinary output, and color and temperature of extremities. Titrate infusion rate according to findings, using doctor's guidelines.
• Use a microdrip or infusion pump to regulate infusion flow rate.
• Observe patient closely for side effects. If adverse effects develop, dosage may need to be adjusted or discontinued.
• For I.V. therapy, use 2-bottle setup so I.V. can continue if this drug is stopped.
• Blood pressure should be raised to slightly less than the patient's normal level. Be careful to avoid excessive

---

Italicized side effects are common or life-threatening.
*Liquid form contains alcohol.   **May contain tartrazine.

blood pressure response. Rapidly induced hypertensive response can cause acute pulmonary edema, arrhythmias, and cardiac arrest.
• Because of prolonged action, a cumulative effect is possible. With an excessive vasopressor response, elevated blood pressure may persist after the drug is stopped.
• Urinary output may decrease initially, then increase as blood pressure reaches normal level. Report persistent decreased urinary output.
• When discontinuing therapy with this drug, slow infusion rate gradually. Continue monitoring vital signs, watching for possible severe drop in blood pressure. Keep equipment nearby to start drug again, if necessary. Pressor therapy should not be reinstated until the systolic blood pressure falls below 70 to 80 mmHg.
• Keep emergency drugs on hand to reverse effects of metaraminol: atropine for reflex bradycardia; phentolamine to decrease vasopressor effects; propranolol for arrhythmias.
• Closely monitor patients with diabetes. Adjustment in insulin dose may be needed.
• Metaraminol should not be mixed with other drugs.

norepinephrine injection (formerly levarterenol bitartrate)
Levophed♦

INDICATIONS & DOSAGE
To restore blood pressure in acute hypotensive states—
Adults: initially, 8 to 12 mcg/minute I.V. infusion, then adjust to maintain normal blood pressure. Average maintenance dose 2 to 4 mcg/minute.

SIDE EFFECTS
CNS: *headache,* anxiety, weakness, dizziness, tremor, restlessness, insomnia.

CV: bradycardia, severe hypertension, marked increase in peripheral resistance, decreased cardiac output, arrhythmias, *ventricular tachycardia, fibrillation,* bigeminal rhythm, atrioventricular dissociation, precordial pain.
GU: *decreased urinary output.*
Metabolic: *metabolic acidosis,* hyperglycemia, increased glycogenolysis.
Local: irritation with extravasation.
Other: fever, respiratory difficulty.

INTERACTIONS
Tricyclic antidepressants: when given with sympathomimetics, may cause severe hypertension (hypertensive crisis). Don't give together.

NURSING CONSIDERATIONS
• Contraindicated in mesenteric or peripheral vascular thrombosis, pregnancy, profound hypoxia, hypercarbia, hypotension from blood volume deficits, or during cyclopropane and halothane anesthesia. Use cautiously in hypertension, hyperthyroidism, severe cardiac disease. Use with extreme caution in patients receiving MAO inhibitors or tricyclic antidepressants.
• Not a substitute for blood or fluid volume deficit. If deficit exists, it should be replaced before vasopressors are administered.
• Norepinephrine solutions deteriorate after 24 hours. Discard after that time.
• Use large vein, as in antecubital fossa, to minimize risk of extravasation. Check site frequently for signs of extravasation. If it occurs, stop infusion immediately and call doctor. He may counteract effect by infiltrating area with 5 to 10 mg phentolamine and 10 to 15 ml normal saline solution. Also check for blanching along course of infused vein; may progress to superficial slough. During infusion, check blood pressure every 2 minutes until stabilized; then every 5 minutes. Also check pulse rates, urinary output, and color and temperature of extremities. Titrate infusion rate according to findings, us-

ing doctor's guidelines. In previously hypertensive patients, blood pressure should be raised no more than 40 mm Hg below preexisting systolic pressure.
• Never leave patient unattended during infusion.
• Use a microdrip or infusion pump to regulate infusion flow rate.
• For I.V. therapy, use two-bottle setup with Y-port so I.V. can continue if norepinephrine is stopped.
• Report decreased urinary output to doctor immediately.
• If prolonged I.V. therapy is necessary, change injection site frequently.
• When stopping drug, slow infusion rate gradually. Monitor vital signs, even after drug is stopped. Watch for possible severe drop in blood pressure.
• Keep emergency drugs on hand to reverse effects of norepinephrine: atropine for reflex bradycardia; propranolol for arrhythmias; phentolamine for increased vasopressor effects.
• Administer in dextrose and saline solution; saline solution alone is not recommended.

---

pseudoephedrine hydrochloride
Besan, Cenafed, Eltor♦♦, First Sign, Gyrocaps, Neo-Synephrinol Day Relief, Novafed, Robidrine♦♦, Ro-Fedrin, Sudabid, Sudafed♦, Sudafed SA

pseudoephedrine sulfate
Afrinol Repetabs

INDICATIONS & DOSAGE
Nasal and eustachian tube decongestant—
Adults: 60 mg P.O. q 4 hours.
Children 6 to 12 years: 30 mg P.O. q 4 hours. Maximum 120 mg daily.
Children 2 to 6 years: 15 mg P.O. q 4 hours. Maximum 60 mg/day.
Extended-relief tablets and capsules:
Adults and children over 12 years: 60 to 120 mg P.O. q 12 hours. This form

contraindicated for children under 12 years.
Relief of nasal congestion—
Adults: 120 mg every 12 hours.

SIDE EFFECTS
CNS: *anxiety,* transient stimulation, tremors, dizziness, headache, insomnia, *nervousness.*
CV: arrhythmias, *palpitations,* tachycardia.
GI: anorexia, nausea, vomiting, dry mouth.
GU: difficulty in urination.
Skin: pallor.

INTERACTIONS
MAO inhibitors: may cause severe hypertension (hypertensive crisis). Don't use together.

NURSING CONSIDERATIONS
• Contraindicated in patients with severe hypertension or severe coronary artery disease; in those receiving MAO inhibitors; and in breast-feeding mothers. Use cautiously in hypertension, cardiac disease, glaucoma, hyperthyroidism, or prostatic hypertrophy.
• Tell patient to stop drug if he becomes unusually restless and to notify doctor promptly.
• Warn against using over-the-counter products containing ephedrine or other sympathomimetic amines.
• Tell patient not to take drug within 2 hours of bedtime because it can cause insomnia.
• Tell patient he can relieve dry mouth with sugarless gum or sour hard candy.

---

terbutaline sulfate
Brethine, Bricanyl ♦

INDICATIONS & DOSAGE
Bronchodilator—
Adults: 2.5 to 5 mg P.O. q 8 hours; or 0.25 mg S.C. If no improvement in 15 to 30 minutes, repeat dose. Do not exceed 0.5 mg in 4 hours.

Children 12 to 15 years: 2.5 mg P.O. t.i.d. Not recommended for children under 12 years.

SIDE EFFECTS
CNS: *nervousness, tremors, headache,* drowsiness, sweating.
CV: palpitations, increased heart rate.
GI: vomiting, nausea.

INTERACTIONS
MAO inhibitors: when given with sympathomimetics, may cause severe hypertension (hypertensive crisis). Don't use together.
Propranolol and other beta blockers: blocked bronchodilating effects of ter-

butaline. Monitor patient carefully if used together.

NURSING CONSIDERATIONS
• Use cautiously in patients with diabetes, hypertension, hyperthyroidism, severe cardiac disease, or cardiac arrhythmias.
• Protect injection from light. Do not use if discolored.
• Make sure patient and his family understand why drug is necessary.
• Give subcutaneous injections in lateral deltoid area.
• Tolerance may develop with prolonged use.

37

Adrenergic blockers (sympatholytics)

dihydroergotamine mesylate
ergotamine tartrate
methysergide maleate
phenoxybenzamine
hydrochloride
phentolamine hydrochloride
phentolamine mesylate
propranolol hydrochloride

MECHANISM OF ACTION
• Alpha blockers inhibit the effects of epinephrine, norepinephrine, and other sympathomimetic amines on both smooth muscle and exocrine glands, preventing sympathetic stimulation.
• Methysergide specifically blocks serotonin (a neurotransmitter); other alpha blockers may also have some antiserotonin effects.
• Propranolol's beta-blocking action prevents vasodilation of the cerebral arteries.

COMBINATION PRODUCTS
CAFERGOT: ergotamine tartrate 1 mg and caffeine 100 mg.
CAFERGOT SUPPOSITORIES: ergotamine tartrate 2 mg and caffeine 100 mg.
CAFERGOT P-B (SUPPOSITORIES): ergotamine tartrate 2 mg, caffeine 100 mg, pentobarbital 30 mg, and levorotatory belladonna alkaloids 0.125 mg.
ERGOCAF: ergotamine tartrate 1 mg and caffeine 100 mg.
MIGRAL: ergotamine tartrate 1 mg, caffeine 50 mg, and cyclizine HCl 25 mg.
WIGRAINE♦: ergotamine tartrate 1 mg, caffeine 100 mg, levorotatory belladonna alkaloids 0.1 mg, and phenacetin 130 mg.
WIGRAINE SUPPOSITORIES: ergotamine

tartrate 1 mg, caffeine 100 mg, levorotatory belladonna alkaloids 0.1 mg, and phenacetin 130 mg.

---

dihydroergotamine mesylate
D.H.E. 45

INDICATIONS & DOSAGE
Vascular or migraine headache—
Adults: 1 mg I.M. or I.V. May repeat q 1 to 2 hours, p.r.n., up to total of 3 mg. Maximum weekly dose is 6 mg.

SIDE EFFECTS
CV: numbness and tingling in fingers and toes, *transient tachycardia or bradycardia,* precordial distress and pain, increased arterial pressure.
GI: nausea, vomiting.
Skin: itching.
Other: weakness in legs, muscle pains in extremities, localized edema.

INTERACTIONS
Propranolol and other beta blockers: blocked natural pathway for vasodilation in patients receiving ergot alkaloids and thus could result in excessive vasoconstriction. Watch closely if drugs are used together.

NURSING CONSIDERATIONS
• Contraindicated in patients with peripheral and occlusive vascular disease, coronary artery disease, hypertension, hepatic or renal dysfunction, sepsis.
• Avoid prolonged administration; don't exceed recommended dosage.
• Tell patient to report any feeling of

Italicized side effects are common or life-threatening.
∗Liquid form contains alcohol.   ∗∗May contain tartrazine.

coldness in extremities or tingling of fingers and toes due to vasoconstriction. Severe vasoconstriction may result in tissue damage.

• Most effective when used to prevent migraine or soon after onset. Provide a quiet, low-light environment to help patient relax.

• Help patient evaluate underlying causes of stress.

• Protect ampuls from heat and light. Discard if solution is discolored.

• Best results are obtained by adjusting the dose in order to determine the most effective, minimal dose.

• Ergotamine rebound, or an increase in frequency and duration of headache, may occur if the drug is stopped.

ergotamine tartrate
Ergomar♦, Ergostat, Gynergen♦, Medihaler-Ergotamine♦

INDICATIONS & DOSAGE
Vascular or migraine headache—
Adults: initially, 2 mg P.O. S.L., then 1 to 2 mg P.O. q hour or S.L. q ½ hour, to maximum 6 mg daily and 10 mg weekly; or initially, 0.25 mg I.M. or S.C.; repeat in 40 minutes if needed. Maximum dose 0.5 mg/24 hours and 1 mg/week; or 1 inhalation initially, if not relieved in 5 minutes, use another inhalation. May repeat inhalations at least 5 minutes apart up to maximum of 6 per 24 hours.

SIDE EFFECTS
CV: numbness and tingling in fingers and toes, transient tachycardia or bradycardia, precordial distress and pain, increased arterial pressure, angina pectoris.
GI: nausea, vomiting, diarrhea, abdominal cramps.
Skin: itching.
Other: weakness in legs, muscle pains in extremities, localized edema.

INTERACTIONS
Propranolol and other beta blockers: blocked natural pathway for vasodilation in patients receiving ergot alkaloids and thus could result in excessive vasoconstriction. Watch closely if drugs are used together.

NURSING CONSIDERATIONS
• Contraindicated in patients with peripheral and occlusive vascular diseases, coronary artery disease, hypertension, hepatic or renal dysfunction, sepsis.

• Avoid prolonged administration; don't exceed recommended dosage.

• Most effective when used to during prodromal stage or as soon after onset as possible.

• Provide a quiet, low-light environment to help patient relax.

• Help patient evaluate underlying causes of physical or emotional stress, which may precipitate attacks.

• Instruct patient on long-term therapy to check for and report feeling of coldness in extremities or tingling of fingers and toes due to vasoconstriction. Severe vasoconstriction may result in tissue damage.

• Store drug in light-resistant container.

• Sublingual tablet is preferred during early stage of attack because of its rapid absorption.

• Warn patient not to increase dosage without first consulting the doctor.

• Obtain an accurate dietary history from patient to determine if a relationship exists between certain foods and onset of headache.

• Ergotamine rebound, or an increase in frequency and duration of headache, may occur if the drug is stopped.

methysergide maleate
Sansert♦**

INDICATIONS & DOSAGE
Prevention of frequent, severe, uncon-

---

trollable, or disabling migraine or vas-cular headache—
Adults: 2 to 4 mg P.O. b.i.d. with meals.

SIDE EFFECTS
Blood: neutropenia, eosinophilia.
CNS: insomnia, drowsiness, *euphoria, vertigo,* ataxia, *light-headedness,* hyperesthesia, weakness, *hallucinations or feelings of dissociation.*
CV: *fibrotic thickening of cardiac valves and aorta, inferior vena cava, and common iliac branches (retroperitoneal fibrosis);* vasoconstriction, causing chest pain, abdominal pain, vascular insufficiency of lower limbs; cold, numb, painful extremities with or without paresthesias and diminished or absent pulses; postural hypotension; tachycardia; peripheral edema; murmurs; bruits.
EENT: nasal stuffiness.
GI: nausea, vomiting, diarrhea, constipation, epigastric pain.
Skin: hair loss, dermatitis, sweating, flushing, rash.
Other: *retroperitoneal fibrosis,* causing general malaise, fatigue, weight gain, backache, low-grade fever, urinary obstruction; *pulmonary fibrosis,* causing dyspnea, tightness and pain in chest, pleural friction rubs and effusion, arthralgia, myalgia.

INTERACTIONS
None significant.

NURSING CONSIDERATIONS
• Contraindicated in patients with severe hypertension, arteriosclerosis, peripheral vascular insufficiency, renal or hepatic disease, severe coronary artery diseases, thromboembolic disorders, phlebitis or cellulitis of lower limbs, fibrotic processes, valvular heart disease; and in debilitated patients. Use cautiously in patients with peptic ulcers or suspected coronary artery disease. EKG and cardiac status evaluation ad-

visable before giving to patients over 40 years.
• GI effects may be prevented by gradual introduction of medication and by administering with meals.
• Obtain laboratory studies of cardiac and renal function, blood count, and sedimentation rate before and during therapy.
• Stop drug every 6 months; then restart after at least 3 or 4 weeks.
• Tell patient not to stop drug abruptly; may cause rebound headaches. Stop gradually over 2 to 3 weeks.
• Patient should keep daily weight record and report unusually rapid weight gain. Teach him to check for peripheral edema. Explain and suggest low-salt diet if necessary.
• Give drug for 3 weeks before evaluating effectiveness.
• Tell patient to report to doctor promptly if he experiences cold, numb, or painful hands and feet; leg cramps when walking; pelvic, chest, or flank pain.
• Not for treatment of migraine or vascular headache in progress, or for treatment of tension (muscle contraction) headaches.
• Indicated only for patients who are unresponsive to other drugs and who can be kept under close medical supervision.

phenoxybenzamine hydrochloride
Dibenzyline

INDICATIONS & DOSAGE
To control or prevent hypertension and sweating associated with pheochromocytoma; Raynaud's syndrome; frostbite; acrocyanosis—
Adults: initially, 10 mg P.O., then increase by 10 mg q 4 days to a maximum of 60 mg daily.

SIDE EFFECTS
CNS: sedation, fatigue, lassitude.

CV: tachycardia, *postural hypotension with dizziness.*
EENT: miosis, nasal congestion.
GI: irritation.
GU: inhibition of ejaculation.

INTERACTIONS
None significant.

NURSING CONSIDERATIONS
• Contraindicated whenever a fall in blood pressure is undesirable. Use cautiously in cerebral or coronary arteriosclerosis, renal damage, or respiratory disease.
• May aggravate symptoms of respiratory infections.
• Safe use in pregnancy has not been established, but drug has been used during the third trimester to treat hypertension caused by pheochromocytoma without apparent harm to mother or fetus.
• Reduce gastric irritation by giving with milk or in divided doses.
• Instruct patient to change position slowly to prevent possible hypotension. Advise him to dangle his legs for a few minutes before standing if he has been lying down.
• Place overdosed patient in Trendelenburg position. Treat hypotension with I.V. infusion of norepinephrine.
• Full therapeutic effect may not be seen for several weeks.
• Store drug in airtight containers, protected from light.

phentolamine hydrochloride
Regitine, Rogitine♦♦

phentolamine mesylate

INDICATIONS & DOSAGE
To control or prevent hypertension before or during pheochromocytomectomy—
Adults: 50 to 100 mg P.O. 4 to 6 times daily; or 5 mg I.M. or I.V. 1 to 2 hours

preoperatively. May repeat if needed. During surgery, 5 mg I.V. may be given as needed.
Children: 25 mg P.O. daily, divided q 4 to 6 hours; or 1 mg I.M. or I.V. 1 to 2 hours preoperatively. May repeat if needed. During surgery, 1 mg I.V. may be given as needed.
To treat extravasation—infiltrate area with 5 to 10 mg phentolamine in 10 ml normal saline solution. Must be done within 12 hours.

SIDE EFFECTS
CV: acute and prolonged hypotension, tachycardia, cardiac arrhythmia, angina, orthostatic hypotension, flushing.
EENT: nasal congestion.
GI: nausea, vomiting, diarrhea, exacerbation of peptic ulcer.

INTERACTIONS
None significant.

NURSING CONSIDERATIONS
• Contraindicated in angina, coronary artery disease, or in history of myocardial infarction. Use with caution in gastritis or peptic ulcer.
• If cardiac arrhythmias occur, don't give cardiotonic glycosides until cardiac rhythm returns to normal.
• Place overdosed patient in Trendelenburg position. Treat hypotension with I.V. infusion of norepinephrine.
• Monitor blood pressure closely, especially after parenteral administration. Patient should be in supine position when receiving drug parenterally.
• To reconstitute injection, add 1 ml sterile water for injection to 5-mg vial of drug. Use immediately after reconstitution.

propranolol hydrochloride
Inderal♦

INDICATIONS & DOSAGE
Prevention of frequent, severe, uncon-

trollable, or disabling migraine or vascular headache—
Adults: initially, 80 mg daily in divided doses. Usual maintenance dose: 160 to 240 mg daily, divided t.i.d. or q.i.d.

SIDE EFFECTS

CNS: *fatigue, lethargy,* vivid dreams, hallucinations.
CV: *bradycardia, hypotension, congestive heart failure,* peripheral vascular disease.
GI: nausea, vomiting, diarrhea.
Metabolic: hypoglycemia without symptoms.
Skin: rash.
Other: *increased airway resistance,* fever.

INTERACTIONS

Insulin, hypoglycemic drugs (oral): can alter requirements for these drugs in previously stabilized diabetics. Monitor for hypoglycemia.
Cardiotonic glycosides: excessive bradycardia and increased depressant effect on myocardium. Monitor pulse rate.
Aminophylline: antagonized beta-blocking effects of propranolol. Use together cautiously.
Isoproterenol, glucagon: antagonized propranolol effect. May be used therapeutically and in emergencies.
Cimetidine: inhibits propranolol's metabolism. Monitor for greater beta-blocking effect.
Epinephrine: severe vasoconstriction.

Monitor blood pressure and observe patient carefully.

NURSING CONSIDERATIONS

• Contraindicated in diabetes mellitus, asthma, or allergic rhinitis; during ethyl ether anesthesia; in sinus bradycardia and in heart block greater than first degree; in cardiogenic shock; in right ventricular failure secondary to pulmonary hypertension. Use with caution in congestive heart failure or respiratory disease.
• Withdraw drug slowly in patients with coronary artery disease. Abrupt withdrawal might precipitate myocardial infarction or aggravate angina or pheochromocytoma. Abrupt withdrawal in thyrotoxicosis may exacerbate hyperthyroidism or precipitate thyroid storm. In thyrotoxicosis, propranolol may mask clinical signs of hyperthyroidism.
• Don't stop before surgery for pheochromocytoma. Before any surgical procedure, notify anesthesiologist that patient is receiving propranolol.
• Monitor blood pressure frequently. If patient develops excessive hypotension, notify doctor. Tell patient that orthostatic hypotension can be minimized by rising slowly and avoiding sudden position changes.
• Drug masks common signs of shock and hypoglycemia.
• Has been used successfully to treat familial tremor.

Italicized side effects are common or life-threatening.
*Liquid form contains alcohol.   **May contain tartrazine.

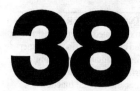

Skeletal muscle relaxants

baclofen
carisoprodol
chlorphenesin carbamate
chlorzoxazone
cyclobenzaprine
dantrolene sodium
metaxalone
methocarbamol
orphenadrine citrate

MECHANISM OF ACTION
• Baclofen's mechanism of action is unclear.
• Carisoprodol, chlorphenesin, chlorzoxazone, cyclobenzaprine, metaxalone, methocarbamol, and orphenadrine reduce transmission of impulses from the spinal cord to skeletal muscle.
• Dantrolene acts directly on skeletal muscle to interfere with intracellular calcium movement.

COMBINATION PRODUCTS
NORGESIC: orphenadrine citrate 25 mg, aspirin 385 mg, and caffeine 30 mg.
NORGESIC FORTE: orphenadrine citrate 50 mg, aspirin 770 mg, and caffeine 60 mg.
PARAFON FORTE♦**: chlorzoxazone 250 mg and acetaminophen 300 mg.
ROBAXISAL♦: methocarbamol 400 mg and aspirin 325 mg.
SOMA COMPOUND♦: carisoprodol 200 mg, phenacetin 160 mg, and caffeine 32 mg.
SOMA COMPOUND WITH CODEINE: carisoprodol 200 mg, phenacetin 160 mg, caffeine 32 mg, and codeine phosphate 16 mg.

baclofen
Lioresal, Lioresal DS

INDICATIONS & DOSAGE
Spasticity in multiple sclerosis, spinal cord injury—
Adults: initially, 5 mg t.i.d. for 3 days, 10 mg t.i.d. for 3 days, 15 mg t.i.d. for 3 days, 20 mg t.i.d. for 3 days. Increase according to response up to maximum 80 mg daily.

SIDE EFFECTS
CNS: *drowsiness, dizziness,* headache, *weakness, fatigue,* confusion, insomnia.
CV: hypotension.
EENT: nasal congestion.
GI: *nausea,* constipation.
GU: urinary frequency.
Hepatic: increased SGOT, alkaline phosphatase.
Metabolic: hyperglycemia.
Skin: rash, pruritus.
Other: ankle edema, excessive perspiration, weight gain.

INTERACTIONS
None significant.

NURSING CONSIDERATIONS
• Use cautiously in patients with impaired renal function, stroke (minimal benefit, poor tolerance), epilepsy, and when spasticity is used to maintain motor function.
• Give with meals or milk to prevent gastric distress.
• Amount of relief determines if dosage (and drowsiness) can be reduced.

Unmarked trade names available in the United States only.
♦ Also available in Canada.   ♦ ♦ Available in Canada only.

• Tell patient to avoid activities that require alertness until CNS response to drug is determined. Drowsiness is usually transient.
• Watch for increased incidence of seizures in epileptics.
• Watch for sensitivity reactions such as fever, skin eruptions, respiratory distress.
• Advise patient to follow doctor's orders regarding rest, physical therapy.
• Do not withdraw abruptly unless required by severe side effects; may precipitate hallucinations or rebound spasticity.
• Overdosage treatment is supportive only; do not induce emesis or use a respiratory stimulant in obtunded patients.
• Used investigationally for treatment of unstable bladder.

carisoprodol
Rela◆, Soma◆

INDICATIONS & DOSAGE
As an adjunct in acute, painful musculoskeletal conditions—
Adults and children over 12 years: 350 mg P.O. t.i.d. and at bedtime. Not recommended for children under 12 years.

SIDE EFFECTS
CNS: *drowsiness, dizziness,* vertigo, ataxia, tremor, agitation, irritability, headache, depressive reactions, insomnia.
CV: orthostatic hypotension, tachycardia, facial flushing.
GI: nausea, vomiting, hiccups, increased bowel activity, epigastric distress.
Skin: rash, *erythema multiforme,* pruritus.
Other: asthmatic episodes, fever, angioneurotic edema, *anaphylaxis.*

INTERACTIONS
None significant.

NURSING CONSIDERATIONS
• Contraindicated in hypersensitivity to related compounds (including meprobamate, tybamate); or intermittent porphyria. Use with caution in impaired hepatic or renal function.
• Watch for idiosyncratic reactions after first to fourth dose (weakness, ataxia, visual and speech difficulties, fever, skin eruptions, mental changes) or severe reactions, including bronchospasm, hypotension, anaphylactic shock. Hold dose and notify doctor immediately of any unusual reactions.
• Record amount of relief to determine whether dosage can be reduced.
• Warn patient to avoid activities that require alertness until CNS response to drug is determined. Drowsiness is transient.
• Avoid combining with alcohol or other depressants.
• Advise patient to follow doctor's orders regarding rest, physical therapy.
• Do not stop drug abruptly; mild withdrawal effects such as insomnia, headache, nausea, abdominal cramps may result.

chlorphenesin carbamate
Maolate**

INDICATIONS & DOSAGE
As an adjunct in short-term, acute, painful musculoskeletal conditions—
Adults: initial dose 800 mg P.O. t.i.d. Maintenance 400 mg P.O. q.i.d. for maximum of 8 weeks.

SIDE EFFECTS
Blood: blood dyscrasia.
CNS: *drowsiness, dizziness,* confusion, headache, weakness. Dose-related side effects include paradoxical stimulation, agitation, insomnia, nervousness, headache.
GI: *nausea, epigastric distress.*
Other: *anaphylaxis.*

Italicized side effects are common or life-threatening.
*Liquid form contains alcohol.   **May contain tartrazine.

INTERACTIONS
None significant.

NURSING CONSIDERATIONS
• Use cautiously in hepatic disease or impaired renal function.
• Safe use for periods over 8 weeks not established.
• Take with meals or milk to prevent gastric distress.
• Amount of relief determines if dosage (and drowsiness) can be reduced.
• Watch for sensitivity reactions such as fever, skin eruptions, and respiratory distress. Hold dose and notify doctor of unusual reactions.
• Monitor blood studies.
• Watch for unusual bleeding and infections that may indicate blood dyscrasia.

---

chlorzoxazone
Paraflex**

INDICATIONS & DOSAGE
As an adjunct in acute, painful musculoskeletal conditions—
Adults: 250 to 750 mg t.i.d. or q.i.d.
Children: 20 mg/kg daily divided t.i.d. or q.i.d.

SIDE EFFECTS
CNS: *drowsiness, dizziness, light-headedness,* malaise, headache, overstimulation.
GI: anorexia, nausea, vomiting, heartburn, abdominal distress, constipation, diarrhea.
GU: urine discoloration (orange or purple-red).
Hepatic: hepatic dysfunction.
Skin: urticaria, redness, itching, petechiae, bruising.

INTERACTIONS
None significant.

NURSING CONSIDERATIONS
• Contraindicated in impaired hepatic function. Use cautiously in patients with a history of drug allergies.
• Record amount of relief to determine whether dosage can be reduced.
• Watch for signs of hepatic dysfunction. Hold dose and notify doctor.
• Warn patient to avoid activities that require alertness until CNS response to drug is determined. Drowsiness is transient.
• Avoid combining with alcohol or other depressants.
• Expect urine color to change.
• Advise patient to follow doctor's orders regarding rest, physical therapy.
• Give with meals or milk to prevent gastric distress.

---

cyclobenzaprine
Flexeril♦

INDICATIONS & DOSAGE
Short-term treatment of muscle spasm—
Adults: 10 mg P.O. t.i.d. for 7 days. Maximum: 60 mg daily for 2 to 3 weeks.

SIDE EFFECTS
CNS: *drowsiness,* euphoria, weakness, headache, insomnia, nightmares, paresthesias, dizziness.
CV: tachycardia.
EENT: blurred vision.
GI: abdominal pain, dyspepsia, peculiar taste, constipation, dry mouth.
GU: urinary retention.
Skin: rash, urticaria, pruritus.
Other: in high doses, watch for side effects like those of other tricyclic drugs (amitriptyline, imipramine).

INTERACTIONS
None significant.

NURSING CONSIDERATIONS
• Contraindicated in patients who have received MAO inhibitors within 14 days; during acute recovery phase of myocardial infarction; in heart block, arrhythmias, conduction disturbances,

---

or congestive heart failure. Use cautiously in patients with urinary retention, narrow-angle glaucoma, increased intraocular pressure, cardiovascular disease, impaired hepatic function, seizures; and in elderly or debilitated patients.

• Withdrawal symptoms (nausea, headache, malaise) may occur if drug is stopped abruptly after long-term use.

• Watch for symptoms of overdose, including possible cardiotoxicity. Notify doctor immediately and have physostigmine available.

• Check intake and output. Be alert for urinary retention. If constipation is a problem, increase fluid intake and get an order for a stool softener.

• Warn patient to avoid activities that require alertness until CNS response to drug is determined. Drowsiness and dizziness usually subside after 2 weeks.

• Avoid combining alcohol or other depressants with cyclobenzaprine.

• Tell patient that dry mouth may be relieved with sugarless candy or gum.

---

dantrolene sodium
Dantrium♦, Dantrium I.V.

INDICATIONS & DOSAGE
Spasticity and sequelae secondary to severe chronic disorders (multiple sclerosis, cerebral palsy, spinal cord injury, stroke)—
Adults: 25 mg P.O. daily. Increase gradually in increments of 25 mg, up to 100 mg b.i.d. to q.i.d. to maximum of 400 mg daily for 4 to 7 days.
Children: 1 mg/kg daily P.O. b.i.d. to q.i.d. Increase gradually as needed by 1 mg/kg daily to maximum of 100 mg q.i.d.
Management of malignant hyperthermia—
Adults and children: 1 mg/kg I.V. initially; may repeat dose up to cumulative dose of 10 mg/kg.

SIDE EFFECTS
Blood: eosinophilia.
CNS: *muscle weakness, drowsiness,* dizziness, light-headedness, malaise, headache, confusion, nervousness, insomnia.
CV: tachycardia, blood pressure changes.
EENT: excessive tearing, visual disturbances.
GI: anorexia, constipation, cramping, dysphagia, *severe diarrhea.*
GU: urinary frequency, incontinence, nocturia, dysuria, crystalluria, difficulty achieving erection.
Hepatic: *hepatitis.*
Skin: eczematoid eruption, pruritus, urticaria, photosensitivity.
Other: abnormal hair growth, drooling, sweating, pleural effusion, myalgia, chills, fever.

INTERACTIONS
None significant.

NURSING CONSIDERATIONS
The following are considerations for the P.O. form only:
• Contraindicated when spasticity is used to maintain motor function; in spasms in rheumatic disorders; lactation. Use with caution in patients with severely impaired cardiac or pulmonary function or preexisting hepatic disease; in females; and in patients over 35 years.

• Safety and efficacy in long-term use not established; value may be determined by therapeutic trial. Do not give more than 45 days if no benefits obtained.

• Give with meals or milk to prevent gastric distress.

• Prepare oral suspension for single dose by dissolving capsule contents in juice or other suitable liquid. For multiple dose, use acid vehicle, such as citric acid in USP Syrup; refrigerate. Use in several days.

• Record amount of relief to determine whether dosage can be reduced.

Italicized side effects are common or life-threatening.
∗Liquid form contains alcohol.   ∗∗May contain tartrazine.

• Liver function tests should be performed at the beginning of therapy
• Watch for hepatitis (fever, jaundice), severe diarrhea or weakness, or sensitivity reactions (fever, skin eruptions). Hold dose and notify doctor.
• Warn patient to avoid driving and other hazardous activities until CNS response to drug is determined. Side effects should subside after 4 days.
• Tell patient to avoid combining with alcohol or other depressants; to avoid photosensitivity reactions by using sunscreening agents and protective clothing; to report abdominal discomfort or GI problems immediately; and to follow doctor's orders regarding rest, physical therapy.
The following are considerations for the I.V. form only:
• Administer as soon as malignant hyperthermia reaction is recognized.
• Reconstitute each vial by adding 60 ml of sterile water for injection and shaking vial until clear.
• Protect contents from light and use within 6 hours.

metaxalone
Skelaxin

INDICATIONS & DOSAGE
As an adjunct in acute, painful musculoskeletal conditions—
Adults and children over 12 years: 800 mg P.O. t.i.d. or q.i.d.

SIDE EFFECTS
Blood: leukopenia, hemolytic anemia.
CNS: *drowsiness,* dizziness, headache, nervousness, irritability, exacerbation of grand mal epilepsy.
GI: *nausea, vomiting.*
Hepatic: jaundice.
Skin: light rash with or without pruritus.

INTERACTIONS
None significant.

NURSING CONSIDERATIONS
• Contraindicated in patients with impaired hepatic or renal function, and in those with a history of drug-induced hemolytic or other anemias.
• Test hepatic function periodically. May cause abnormalities in liver function studies; repeat tests after drug is discontinued.
• Record amount of relief to determine if dosage can be reduced.
• Watch for sensitivity reactions such as rash with pruritus.
• Warn patient to avoid combining with alcohol or other depressants.
• Advise patient to follow doctor's orders regarding rest, physical therapy.
• Give with meals or milk to prevent gastric distress.
• False-positive results in glucose tests if cupric sulfate is used. Use glucose oxidase instead.
• Rarely used clinically.

methocarbamol
Delaxin, Forbaxin, Metho-500, Robamol, Robaxin♦, Romethocarb, SK-Methocarbamol, Spenaxin

INDICATIONS & DOSAGE
As an adjunct in acute, painful musculoskeletal conditions—
Adults: 1.5 g P.O. for 2 to 3 days, then 1 g P.O. q.i.d., or not more than 500 mg (5 ml) I.M. into each gluteal region. May repeat q 8 hours. Or 1 to 3 g daily (10 to 30 ml) I.V. directly into vein at 3 ml/minute, or 10 ml may be added to no more than 250 ml of 5% dextrose in water or normal saline solution. Maximum dose 3 g daily.
Supportive therapy in tetanus management—
Adults: 1 to 2 g into tubing of running I.V. or 1 to 3 g in infusion bottle q 6 hours.
Children: 15 mg/kg I.V. q 6 hours.

SIDE EFFECTS
Blood: hemolysis, increased hemoglobin (I.V. only).
CNS: drowsiness, dizziness, light-headedness, headache, vertigo, mild muscular incoordination (I.M. or I.V. only), convulsions (I.V. only).
CV: hypotension, bradycardia (I.M. or I.V. only).
GI: *nausea, anorexia, GI upset.*
GU: red blood cells in urine (I.V. only), discoloration of urine.
Skin: urticaria, pruritus, rash.
Local: thrombophlebitis, extravasation (I.V. only).
Other: fever, metallic taste, flushing, *anaphylactic reactions (I.M. or I.V. only).*

INTERACTIONS
None significant.

NURSING CONSIDERATIONS
• Contraindicated in patients with impaired renal function (injectable form), myasthenia gravis, epilepsy (injectable form); in children under 12 years (except in tetanus); and in patients receiving anticholinesterase agents.
• I.V. irritates veins, may cause phlebitis, aggravates seizures, may cause fainting if injected rapidly.
• In tetanus management, use methocarbamol with tetanus antitoxin, penicillin, tracheotomy, and aggressive supportive care. Long course of I.V. methocarbamol required.
• Watch for sensitivity reactions such as fever, skin eruptions.
• Warn patient to avoid activities that require alertness until CNS response to drug is determined. Drowsiness subsides.
• Avoid combining with alcohol or other depressants.
• Advise patient to follow doctor's orders regarding rest, physical therapy.
• Tell patient urine may turn green, black, or brown.
• Give with meals or milk to prevent gastric distress.

• Watch for orthostatic hypotension, especially with parenteral administration. Keep patient supine for 15 minutes afterward, and supervise ambulation. Advise patient to get up slowly.
• Give I.V. slowly. Maximum rate 300 mg (3 ml)/minute. Give I.M. deeply, only in upper outer quadrant of buttocks, with maximum of 5 ml in each buttock, and inject slowly. Do not give subcutaneously.
• Have epinephrine, antihistamines, corticosteroids available.
• Prepare liquid by crushing tablets into water or saline solution. Give through nasogastric tube.
• Obtain WBC count periodically during prolonged therapy.

orphenadrine citrate
Banflex, Flexon, Myolin, Norflex♦, Ro-Orphena, X-Otag

INDICATIONS & DOSAGE
Adjunctive treatment in painful, acute musculoskeletal conditions—
Adults: 100 mg P.O. b.i.d., or 60 mg I.V. or I.M. q 12 hours, p.r.n.

SIDE EFFECTS
CNS: disorientation, restlessness, irritability, weakness, *drowsiness,* headache.
CV: palpitations, tachycardia.
EENT: dilated pupils, blurred vision, difficulty swallowing.
GI: constipation, *dry mouth,* nausea, vomiting, paralytic ileus, epigastric distress.
GU: urinary hesitancy or retention.

INTERACTIONS
None significant.

NURSING CONSIDERATIONS
• Contraindicated in patients with narrow-angle glaucoma; prostatic hypertrophy; pyloric, duodenal, or bladder-neck obstruction; myasthenia gravis; tachycardia; severe hepatic or renal dis-

ease; ulcerative colitis. Use cautiously in elderly or debilitated patients with cardiac disease, arrhythmias; and in those exposed to high temperatures.
• Check all dosages carefully. Even a slight overdose can lead to toxicity. Early signs are excessive dry mouth, dilated pupils, blurred vision, skin flushing, fever.
• Monitor vital signs carefully.
• When given I.V., may cause paradox-

ical initial bradycardia. Usually disappears in 2 minutes.
• Monitor intake and output. Causes urinary retention and hesitancy; have patient void before taking the drug.
• Relieve dry mouth with cool drinks, ice chips, sugarless gum, or hard candy.
• Patient may develop a tolerance to this drug.

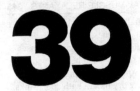

Neuromuscular blockers

gallamine triethiodide
hexafluorenium bromide
metocurine iodide
pancuronium bromide
succinylcholine chloride
tubocurarine chloride

MECHANISM OF ACTION
These agents block transmission of
nerve impulses at the skeletal neuromuscular junction by one of two mechanisms:
• Succinylcholine (depolarizing
agents) prolongs depolarization of the
muscle end-plate. (Hexafluorenium inhibits the enzymatic breakdown of succinylcholine, prolonging its duration.)
• Gallamine, metocurine, pancuronium, and tubocurarine (nondepolariz-
ing agents) prevent acetylcholine from
binding to the receptors on the muscle
end-plate, thus blocking depolarization.

COMBINATION PRODUCTS
None.

gallamine triethiodide
Flaxedil♦

INDICATIONS & DOSAGE
*Adjunct to anesthesia to induce skeletal
muscle relaxation; facilitate intubation;
reduction of fractures and dislocations;
lessen muscle contractions in pharmacologically or electrically induced convulsions; assist with mechanical ventilation—*
Dose depends on anesthetic used, individual needs, and response. Doses are
representative and must be adjusted.

Adults and children over 1 month:
initially, 1 mg/kg I.V. to maximum of
100 mg, regardless of patient's weight;
then 0.5 mg to 1 mg/kg q 30 to 40 minutes.
**Children under 1 month but over
5 kg (11 lbs):** initially, 0.25 to 0.75
mg/kg I.V., then 0.01 to 0.05 mg/kg q
30 to 40 minutes.

SIDE EFFECTS
CV: tachycardia.
Other: *respiratory paralysis, dose-
related prolonged apnea,* residual muscle weakness, increased oropharyngeal
secretions, allergic or idiosyncratic
hypersensitivity reactions.

INTERACTIONS
*Aminoglycoside antibiotics (amikacin,
gentamicin, kanamycin, neomycin,
streptomycin); polymyxin antibiotics
(polymyxin B sulfate, colistin); clindamycin; quinidine; local anesthetics:* potentiated neuromuscular blockade,
leading to increased skeletal muscle relaxation and possible respiratory paralysis. Use cautiously during surgical and
postoperative periods.
Narcotic analgesics: potentiated neuromuscular blockade, leading to increased skeletal muscle relaxation and
possible respiratory paralysis. Use with
extreme caution, and reduce dose of
gallamine.

NURSING CONSIDERATIONS
• Contraindicated in patients with
hypersensitivity to iodides, impaired
renal function, myasthenia gravis; patients in shock; and patients in whom

---

Italicized side effects are common or life-threatening.
*Liquid form contains alcohol.   **May contain tartrazine.

tachycardia may be hazardous. Use cautiously in elderly or debilitated patients; those with hepatic or pulmonary impairment, respiratory depression, myasthenic syndrome of lung cancer, dehydration, thyroid disorders, collagen diseases, porphyria, electrolyte disturbances, fractures, muscle spasms; and patients undergoing cesarean section.

• Monitor baseline electrolyte determinations (electrolyte imbalance can potentiate neuromuscular effects).

• Watch respirations for early symptoms of paralysis, inability to keep eyelids open and eyes focused, difficulty in swallowing and speaking. Notify doctor immediately.

• Take vital signs every 15 minutes, especially for developing tachycardia. Notify doctor immediately of significant changes.

• Measure intake/output (renal dysfunction prolongs duration of action, since drug is unchanged before excretion).

• Keep airway clear. Have emergency respiratory support (endotracheal equipment, ventilator, oxygen, atropine, neostigmine) on hand.

• Reassure patient that postoperative stiffness is normal and will soon subside.

• Determine whether patient has iodide allergy.

• Protect drug from light or excessive heat; use only fresh solutions.

• Do not mix solution with meperidine HCl or barbiturate solutions.

• Give I.V. slowly (over 30 to 90 seconds).

• Do not give without direct supervision of doctor.

• May be preferred in patients who have bradycardia.

hexafluorenium bromide
Mylaxen

INDICATIONS & DOSAGE
Adjunct for use with succinylcholine to prolong neuromuscular blockade and reduce muscular fasciculations—
Dose depends on individual needs and response. Doses are representative and must be adjusted.
Adults and children: use in ratio of 2 mg/1 mg succinylcholine. Maximum hexafluorenium bromide 10 to 36 mg; should not be administered more frequently than q 15 to 30 minutes.

SIDE EFFECTS
CNS: *prolonged neuromuscular blockade.*
CV: hypotension, hypertension, tachycardia, bradycardia.
EENT: increased intraocular pressure.
Other: increased bronchial tone, *bronchospasm.*

INTERACTIONS
None reported for this drug alone; always used with succinylcholine. See succinylcholine.

NURSING CONSIDERATIONS
• Contraindicated in hypersensitivity to bromides, in bronchial asthma. Use cautiously in elderly or debilitated patients; in renal, hepatic, or pulmonary impairment, respiratory depression, myasthenia gravis, myasthenic syndrome of lung cancer, dehydration, thyroid disorders, collagen diseases, porphyria, electrolyte disturbances, and glaucoma; and during ocular surgery and (in large doses) cesarean section.
• Not used extensively in clinical practice.
• Monitor baseline electrolyte determinations (electrolyte imbalance potentiates neuromuscular effects) and vital signs (watch respirations closely).
• Keep airway clear. Have emergency respiratory support (endotracheal

equipment, ventilator, oxygen, atropine, neostigmine) on hand.
● Reassure patient that postoperative stiffness is normal and will soon subside.
● Determine whether patient has bromide allergy.
● Use only fresh solutions; do not give without direct supervision of doctor.

---

metocurine iodide
Metubine

INDICATIONS & DOSAGE
Adjunct to anesthesia to induce skeletal muscle relaxation; facilitate intubation, reduction of fractures and dislocations—
Dose depends on anesthetic used, individual needs, and response. Doses are representative and must be adjusted. Administer as sustained injection over 30 to 60 seconds.
Adults: given cyclopropane: 2 to 4 mg I.V. (2.68 mg average).
Given ether: 1.5 to 3 mg I.V. (2.1 mg average).
Given nitrous oxide: 4 to 7 mg I.V. (4.79 mg average). Supplemental injections of 0.5 to 1 mg in 25 to 90 minutes, repeated p.r.n.
Lessen muscle contractions in pharmacologically or electrically induced convulsions—
Adults: 1.75 to 5.5 mg I.V.

SIDE EFFECTS
CV: hypotension secondary to histamine release, ganglionic blockade in rapid dose or overdose.
Other: *dose-related prolonged apnea,* residual muscle weakness, increased oropharyngeal secretions, allergic or idiosyncratic hypersensitivity reactions, *bronchospasm.*

INTERACTIONS
Aminoglycoside antibiotics (including amikacin, gentamicin, kanamycin, neomycin, streptomycin); polymyxin antibiotics (polymyxin B sulfate, colistin); clindamycin; quinidine; local anesthetics: potentiated neuromuscular blockade, leading to increased skeletal muscle relaxation and possible respiratory paralysis. Use cautiously during surgical and postoperative periods.
Narcotic analgesics: potentiated neuromuscular blockade, leading to increased skeletal muscle relaxation and possible respiratory paralysis. Use with extreme caution, and reduce dose of metocurine iodide.

NURSING CONSIDERATIONS
● Contraindicated in patients with hypersensitivity to iodides; and in whom histamine release is a hazard (asthmatic or atopic patients). Use cautiously in elderly or debilitated patients; and in renal, hepatic, or pulmonary impairment, respiratory depression, myasthenia gravis, myasthenic syndrome of lung cancer, dehydration, thyroid disorders, collagen diseases, porphyria, electrolyte disturbances, hyperthermia, and (in large doses) cesarean section.
● Neostigmine, edrophonium, and epinephrine may be used to reverse effects of metocurine because of their anticurare effects.
● Dose of 1 mg is the therapeutic equivalent of 3 mg *d*-tubocurarine chloride.
● Monitor baseline electrolyte determinations (electrolyte imbalance, especially potassium, calcium, and magnesium, can potentiate neuromuscular effects) and vital signs, especially respiration.
● Measure intake and output (renal dysfunction prolongs duration of action, since drug is mainly unchanged before excretion).
● Keep airway clear. Have emergency respiratory support (endotracheal equipment, ventilator, oxygen, atropine, edrophonium, epinephrine, and neostigmine) on hand.
● Reassure patient that postoperative

Italicized side effects are common or life-threatening.
*Liquid form contains alcohol.   **May contain tartrazine.

stiffness is normal and will soon subside.
- Determine whether patient has iodide allergy.
- Store solution away from heat, sunlight; do not mix with barbiturates, methohexital, or thiopental (precipitate will form). Use fresh solutions only.
- Do not give without direct supervision of doctor.

pancuronium bromide
Pavulon♦

INDICATIONS & DOSAGE
Adjunct to anesthesia to induce skeletal muscle relaxation; facilitate intubation, lessen muscle contractions in pharmacologically or electrically induced convulsions; assist with mechanical ventilation—
Dose depends on anesthetic used, individual needs, and response. Doses are representative and must be adjusted.
Adults: initially, 0.04 to 0.1 mg/kg I.V.; then 0.01 mg/kg q 30 to 60 minutes.
Children over 10 years: initially, 0.04 to 0.1 mg/kg I.V., then ⅕ initial dose q 30 to 60 minutes.

SIDE EFFECTS
CV: tachycardia, increased blood pressure.
Local: burning sensation.
Skin: transient rashes.
Other: excessive sweating and salivation, *prolonged dose-related apnea,* residual muscle weakness, allergic or idiosyncratic hypersensitivity reactions.

INTERACTIONS
Aminoglycoside antibiotics (including amikacin, gentamicin, kanamycin, neomycin, streptomycin); polymyxin antibiotics (polymyxin B sulfate, colistin); clindamycin; quinidine; local anesthetics: potentiated neuromuscular blockade, leading to increased skeletal muscle relaxation and possible respiratory paralysis. Use cautiously during surgical and postoperative periods.
Lithium, narcotic analgesics: potentiated neuromuscular blockade, leading to increased skeletal muscle relaxation and possible respiratory paralysis. Use with extreme caution, and reduce dose of pancuronium.

NURSING CONSIDERATIONS
- Contraindicated in hypersensitivity to bromides; preexisting tachycardia; and in patients for whom even a minor increase in heart rate is undesirable. Use cautiously in elderly or debilitated patients; renal, hepatic, or pulmonary impairment, respiratory depression, myasthenia gravis, myasthenic syndrome of lung cancer, dehydration, thyroid disorders, collagen diseases, porphyria, electrolyte disturbances, hyperthermia, toxemic states, and (in large doses) cesarean section.
- Causes no histamine release or hypotension.
- Dose of 1 mg is the approximate therapeutic equivalent of 5 mg *d*-tubocurarine chloride.
- Monitor baseline electrolyte determinations (electrolyte imbalance can potentiate neuromuscular effects) and vital signs (watch respiration and heart rate closely).
- Measure intake and output (renal dysfunction may prolong duration of action, since 25% of the drug is unchanged before excretion).
- Have emergency respiratory support (endotracheal equipment, ventilator, oxygen, atropine, neostigmine) on hand.
- Allow succinylcholine effects to subside before giving pancuronium.
- Store in refrigerator. Do not store in plastic containers or syringes, although plastic syringes may be used for administration.
- Do not mix with barbiturate solutions; use only fresh solutions.

• Do not give without direct supervision of doctor.

---

succinylcholine chloride
Anectine♦, Anectine Flo-Pack Powder, Sux-Cert

INDICATIONS & DOSAGE
Adjunct to anesthesia to induce skeletal muscle relaxation; facilitate intubation and assist with mechanical ventilation or orthopedic manipulations (drug of choice); lessen muscle contractions in pharmacologically or electrically induced convulsions—
Dose depends on anesthetic used, individual needs, and response. Doses are representative and must be adjusted.
Adults: 25 to 75 mg I.V., then 2.5 mg/minute, p.r.n., or 2.5 mg/kg I.M. up to maximum 150 mg I.M. in deltoid muscle.
Children: 1 to 2 mg/kg I.M. or I.V. Maximum I.M. dose 150 mg. (Children may be less sensitive to succinylcholine than adults.)

SIDE EFFECTS
CV: bradycardia, tachycardia, hypertension, hypotension, arrhythmias.
EENT: increased intraocular pressure.
Other: *prolonged respiratory depression, apnea, malignant hyperthermia,* muscle fasciculation, *postoperative muscle pain,* myoglobinemia, excessive salivation, allergic or idiosyncratic hypersensitivity reactions.

INTERACTIONS
Aminoglycoside antibiotics (including amikacin, gentamicin, kanamycin, neomycin, paromomycin, streptomycin); polymyxin antibiotics (polymyxin B sulfate, colistin); echothiophate; local anesthetics: potentiated neuromuscular blockade, leading to increased skeletal muscle relaxation and possible respiratory paralysis. Use cautiously during surgical and postoperative periods.
Narcotic analgesics, methotrimepra-

zine: potentiated neuromuscular blockade, leading to increased skeletal muscle relaxation and possible respiratory paralysis. Use with extreme caution.
MAO inhibitors, lithium, cyclophosphamide: prolonged apnea. Use with caution.
Magnesium sulfate (parenterally): potentiated neuromuscular blockade, increased skeletal muscle relaxation, and possible respiratory paralysis. Use with caution, preferably with reduced doses.
Cardiotonic glycosides: possible cardiac arrhythmias. Use together cautiously.

NURSING CONSIDERATIONS
• Contraindicated in abnormally low plasma pseudocholinesterase levels. Use with caution in patients with personal or family history of malignant hypertension or hyperthermia; elderly or debilitated patients; and in hepatic, renal, or pulmonary impairment, respiratory depression, severe burns or trauma, electrolyte imbalances, quinidine or digitalis therapy, hyperkalemia, paraplegia, spinal neuraxis injury, degenerative or dystrophic neuromuscular disease, myasthenia gravis, myasthenic syndrome of lung cancer, dehydration, thyroid disorders, collagen diseases, porphyria, fractures, muscle spasms, glaucoma, eye surgery or penetrating eye wounds, pheochromocytoma, and (in large doses) cesarean section.
• Drug of choice for short procedures (less than 3 minutes) and for orthopedic manipulations; use caution in fractures or dislocations.
• Duration of action prolonged to 20 minutes by continuous I.V. infusion or single-dose administration, along with hexafluorenium bromide.
• Repeated or continuous infusions of succinylcholine alone not advised; may cause reduced response or prolonged apnea.
• Monitor baseline electrolyte determinations and vital signs (check respira-

---

tion every 5 to 10 minutes during infusion).
• Keep airway clear. Have emergency respiratory support (endotracheal equipment, ventilator, oxygen, atropine, neostigmine) on hand.
• Reassure patient that postoperative stiffness is normal and will soon subside.
• Store injectable form in refrigerator. Store powder form at room temperature, tightly closed. Use immediately after reconstitution. Do not mix with alkaline solutions (thiopental, sodium bicarbonate, barbiturates).
• Give test dose (10 mg I.M. or I.V.) after patient has been anesthetized. Normal response (no respiratory depression or transient depression lasting less than 5 minutes) indicates drug may be given. Do not give if patient develops respiratory paralysis sufficient to permit endotracheal intubation. (Recovery within 30 to 60 minutes.)
• Do not give without direct supervision of doctor.
• Give deep I.M., preferably high into the deltoid muscle.

---

tubocurarine chloride
Tubarine♦♦

INDICATIONS & DOSAGE

Adjunct to anesthesia to induce skeletal muscle relaxation; facilitate intubation, orthopedic manipulations—
Dose depends on anesthetic used, individual needs, and response. Doses listed are representative and must be adjusted.
Adults: 1 unit/kg or 0.15 mg/kg I.V. slowly over 60 to 90 seconds. Average, initially, 40 to 60 units I.V. May give 20 to 30 units in 3 to 5 minutes. For longer procedures, give 20 units, p.r.n.
Children: 1 unit/kg or 0.15 mg/kg.
Assist with mechanical ventilation—
Adults and children: initially, 0.0165 mg/kg I.V. (average 1 mg or

7 units), then adjust subsequent doses to patient's response.
Diagnose myasthenia gravis—
Adults and children: 0.0041 to 0.033 mg/kg I.V. or ¹/₁₅ to ¹/₅ normal adult dose for electroshock. Positive result: profound exaggeration of myasthenic symptoms. Dose may also be given I.M. when necessary.
Lessen muscle contractions in pharmacologically or electrically induced convulsions—
Adults and children: 1 unit/kg or 0.15 mg/kg slowly over 60 to 90 seconds. Initial dose 20 units (3 mg) less than calculated dose.

SIDE EFFECTS

CV: hypotension, circulatory depression.
Other: profound and prolonged muscle relaxation, *respiratory depression to the point of apnea,* hypersensitivity, idiosyncrasy, residual muscle weakness, *bronchospasm.*

INTERACTIONS

Aminoglycoside antibiotics (including amikacin, gentamicin, kanamycin, neomycin, paromomycin, streptomycin); polymyxin antibiotics (polymyxin B sulfate, colistin); local anesthetics: potentiated neuromuscular blockade, leading to increased skeletal muscle relaxation and possible respiratory paralysis. Use cautiously during surgical and postoperative periods.
Quinidine: prolonged neuromuscular blockade. Use together with caution. Monitor closely.
Thiazide diuretics, furosemide, ethacrynic acid, amphotericin B, propranolol, methotrimeprazine, narcotic analgesics: potentiated neuromuscular blockade, leading to increased respiratory paralysis. Use with extreme caution during surgical and postoperative periods.

NURSING CONSIDERATIONS

• Contraindicated in patients for whom

---

histamine release is a hazard (asthmatics). Use cautiously in elderly or debilitated patients; in hepatic or pulmonary impairment, respiratory depression, myasthenia gravis, myasthenic syndrome of lung cancer, dehydration, thyroid disorders, collagen diseases, porphyria, electrolyte disturbances, fractures, muscle spasms, and (in large doses) cesarean section.

• Small margin of safety between therapeutic dose and dose causing respiratory paralysis.

• Used to diagnose myasthenia gravis, but procedure is hazardous.

• Allow succinylcholine effects to subside before giving tubocurarine.

• Monitor baseline electrolyte determinations (electrolyte imbalance can potentiate neuromuscular effects).

• Watch respirations closely for early symptoms of paralysis—inability to keep eyelids open and eyes focused, or difficulty in swallowing and speaking;

notify doctor immediately.

• Check vital signs every 15 minutes. Notify doctor at once of changes.

• Measure intake and output (renal dysfunction prolongs duration of action, since much of drug is unchanged before excretion).

• Keep airway clear. Have emergency respiratory support (endotracheal equipment, ventilator, oxygen, atropine, edrophonium, epinephrine, and neostigmine) on hand.

• Reassure patient that postoperative stiffness is normal and will soon subside.

• Decrease dose if inhalation anesthetics are used.

• Do not mix with barbiturates. Use only fresh solutions and discard if discolored.

• Give I.V. slowly (60 to 90 seconds); give deep I.M. in deltoid muscle.

• Do not give without direct supervision of doctor.

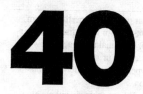

40

Antihistamines

azatadine maleate
brompheniramine maleate
carbinoxamine maleate
chlorpheniramine maleate
clemastine fumarate
cyproheptadine hydrochloride
dexchlorpheniramine maleate
dimethindene maleate
diphenhydramine hydrochloride
diphenylpyraline hydrochloride
doxylamine succinate
methdilazine hydrochloride
promethazine hydrochloride
trimeprazine tartrate
tripelennamine hydrochloride
triprolidine hydrochloride

MECHANISM OF ACTION
● Antihistamines compete with histamine for H_1-receptor sites on effector cells. They can prevent but not reverse histamine-mediated responses, particularly histamine's effects on the smooth muscle of the bronchial tubes, gastrointestinal tract, uterus, and blood vessels.
● Anticholinergic actions of antihistamines dry the nasal mucosa and also relieve vertigo and motion sickness.
● Diphenhydramine, structurally related to local anesthetics, provides anesthesia by preventing initiation and transmission of nerve impulses.

COMBINATION PRODUCTS
ALLEREST: phenylpropanolamine hydrochloride 18.7 mg and chlorpheniramine maleate 2 mg.
BENDECTIN: doxylamine succinate 10 mg and pyridoxine hydrochloride 10 mg.
CHLOR-TRIMETON DECONGESTANT: chlorpheniramine maleate 4 mg and pseudoephedrine sulfate 60 mg.
CHLOR-TRIMETON DECONGESTANT REPETABS: chlorpheniramine maleate 8 mg and pseudoephedrine sulfate 120 mg.
CODIMAL DH*: hydrocodone bitartrate 1.66 mg, phenylephrine hydrochloride 5 mg, pyrilamine maleate 8.33 mg, potassium guaiacolsulfonate 83.3 mg, sodium citrate 216 mg, and citric acid 50 mg.
DIMETAPP EXTENTABS: brompheniramine maleate 12 mg, phenylephrine hydrochloride 15 mg, and phenylpropanolamine hydrochloride 15 mg.
DISOPHROL CHRONOTAB: dexbrompheniramine maleate 6 mg and pseudoephedrine sulfate 120 mg.
DRIXORAL♦: dexbrompheniramine maleate 6 mg and pseudoephedrine sulfate 120 mg.
HISTASPAN-D: chlorpheniramine maleate 8 mg, phenylephrine hydrochloride 20 mg, and methscopolamine nitrate 2.5 mg.
NALDECON: phenylephrine hydrochloride 10 mg, phenylpropanolamine hydrochloride 40 mg, phenyltoloxamine citrate 15 mg, and chlorpheniramine maleate 5 mg.
NEOTEP: chlorpheniramine maleate 9 mg and phenylephrine hydrochloride 21 mg.
NOLAMINE: chlorpheniramine maleate 4 mg, phenindamine tartrate 24 mg, and phenylpropanolamine hydrochloride 50 mg.
NOVAFED A: pseudoephedrine hydrochloride 120 mg and chlorpheniramine maleate 8 mg.

NOVAHISTINE ELIXIR*: phenylpropanolamine hydrochloride 18.7 mg, chlorpheniramine maleate 2 mg, and alcohol 5%/5 ml.

ORNADE: phenylpropanolamine hydrochloride 75 mg and chlorpheniramine maleate 12 mg.

RHINEX D-LAY: acetaminophen 300 mg, salicylamide 300 mg, phenylpropanolamine hydrochloride 60 mg, and chlorpheniramine maleate 4 mg.

RONDEC: carbinoxamine maleate 4 mg and pseudoephedrine hydrochloride 60 mg.

TRIAMINIC TABLETS: phenylpropanolamine hydrochloride 50 mg, pheniramine maleate 25 mg, and pyrilamine maleate 25 mg.

azatadine maleate
Optimine♦

INDICATIONS & DOSAGE
Rhinitis, allergy symptoms, chronic urticaria—
Adults: 1 to 2 mg P.O. b.i.d. Maximum 4 mg daily.
Not intended for children under 12 years.

SIDE EFFECTS
Blood: thrombocytopenia.
CNS (especially in the elderly): *drowsiness, dizziness,* vertigo, disturbed coordination.
CV: hypotension, palpitations.
GI: anorexia, *nausea,* vomiting, *dry mouth and throat.*
GU: urinary retention.
Skin: urticaria, rash.
Other: thickening of bronchial secretions.

INTERACTIONS
None significant.

NURSING CONSIDERATIONS
• Contraindicated in acute asthmatic attack. Use cautiously in elderly patients, and in patients with increased in-

traocular pressure, hyperthyroidism, cardiovascular or renal disease, hypertension, bronchial asthma, narrow-angle glaucoma, urinary retention, prostatic hypertrophy, bladder-neck obstruction.
• Warn patient against drinking alcoholic beverages during therapy and against activities that require alertness until CNS response to drug is determined.
• Reduce GI distress by giving with food or milk.
• Coffee or tea may reduce drowsiness. Sugarless gum, sour hard candy, or ice chips may relieve dry mouth.
• Titrate each patient's dose; response to drug varies.
• If tolerance develops, another antihistamine may be substituted.
• Warn patient to stop taking drug 4 days before allergy skin tests; otherwise, accuracy of tests may be affected.
• Monitor blood counts during long-term therapy; watch for signs of blood dyscrasias.

brompheniramine maleate
Dimetane*♦, Dimetane-Ten, Rolabromophen, Spentane, Veltane

INDICATIONS & DOSAGE
Rhinitis, allergy symptoms—
Adults: 4 to 8 mg P.O. t.i.d. or q.i.d.; or (timed-release) 8 to 12 mg P.O. b.i.d. or t.i.d.; or 5 to 20 mg q 6 to 12 hours I.M., I.V., or S.C. Maximum 40 mg daily.
Children over 6 years: 2 to 4 mg t.i.d. or q.i.d.; or (timed-release) 8 to 12 mg q 12 hours; or 0.5 mg/kg daily I.M., I.V., or S.C. divided t.i.d. or q.i.d.
Children under 6 years: 0.5 mg/kg daily P.O., I.M., I.V., or S.C. divided t.i.d. or q.i.d.

SIDE EFFECTS
Blood: thrombocytopenia, *agranulocytosis.*
CNS (especially in the elderly): dizzi-

Italicized side effects are common or life-threatening.
*Liquid form contains alcohol.   **May contain tartrazine.

ness, tremors, irritability, insomnia, *drowsiness, stimulation*.
CV: hypotension, palpitations.
GI: anorexia, nausea, vomiting, *dry mouth and throat*.
GU: urinary retention.
Skin: urticaria, rash.
After parenteral administration: local reaction, sweating, syncope.

INTERACTIONS
None significant.

NURSING CONSIDERATIONS
• Contraindicated in acute asthmatic attack. Use cautiously in elderly patients, and in patients with increased intraocular pressure, hyperthyroidism, cardiovascular or renal disease, hypertension, bronchial asthma, narrow-angle glaucoma, urinary retention, prostatic hypertrophy, bladder-neck obstruction.
• Warn patient against drinking alcoholic beverages during therapy and against activities that require alertness until CNS response to drug is determined.
• Reduce GI distress by giving with food or milk.
• Causes less drowsiness than some other antihistamines.
• Coffee or tea may reduce drowsiness. Sugarless gum, sour hard candy, or ice chips may relieve dry mouth.
• Titrate each patient's dose; response to drug varies.
• If tolerance develops, another antihistamine may be substituted.
• Warn patient to stop taking drug 4 days before allergy skin tests; otherwise, accuracy of tests may be affected.
• Injectable form containing 10 mg/ml can be given diluted or undiluted very slowly I.V. The 100 mg/ml injection should not be given I.V.
• Monitor blood count during long-term therapy; observe for signs of blood dyscrasias.

carbinoxamine maleate
Clistin*, Clistin RA**

INDICATIONS & DOSAGE
Rhinitis, allergy symptoms—
Adults: 4 to 8 mg P.O. t.i.d. to q.i.d., or (timed-release) 8 to 12 mg q 8 to 12 hours.
Children over 6 years: 4 to 6 mg P.O. t.i.d. to q.i.d.
Children 3 to 6 years: 2 to 4 mg P.O. t.i.d. to q.i.d.
Children 1 to 3 years: 2 mg P.O. t.i.d. to q.i.d.

SIDE EFFECTS
CNS (especially in the elderly): *drowsiness, dizziness*.
GI: anorexia, nausea, vomiting, *dry mouth*.

INTERACTIONS
None significant.

NURSING CONSIDERATIONS
• Contraindicated in acute asthmatic attack. Use cautiously in elderly patients, and in patients with increased intraocular pressure, hyperthyroidism, cardiovascular or renal disease, hypertension, bronchial asthma, narrow-angle glaucoma, urinary retention, prostatic hypertrophy, bladder-neck obstruction.
• Warn patient against drinking alcoholic beverages during therapy and against driving or other activities that require alertness until CNS response to drug is determined.
• Reduce GI distress by giving with food or milk.
• Coffee or tea may reduce drowsiness. Sugarless gum, sour hard candy, or ice chips may relieve dry mouth.
• Titrate each patient's dose; response to drug varies.
• If tolerance develops, another antihistamine may be substituted.
• Warn patient to stop taking drug

4 days before allergy skin tests; otherwise, accuracy of tests may be affected.

chlorpheniramine maleate
Allerid-O.D., AL-R, Chloramate, Chlormene, Chlortab, Chlor-Trimeton*, Chlor-Tripolon♦♦, Histaspan, Histex, Novopheniram♦♦, Pyranistan, Teldrin

INDICATIONS & DOSAGE
Rhinitis, allergy symptoms—
Adults: 2 to 4 mg P.O. t.i.d. or q.i.d.; or (timed-release) 8 to 12 mg P.O. b.i.d. or t.i.d.; or 5 to 40 mg I.M., I.V., or S.C. daily. Give I.V. injection over 1 minute.
Not recommended for children under 12 years, except under medical supervision.

SIDE EFFECTS
CNS: *stimulation,* sedation, *drowsiness* (especially in the elderly), excitability (in children).
CV: hypotension, palpitations.
GI: epigastric distress, *dry mouth.*
GU: urinary retention.
Other: thickening of bronchial secretions.
After parenteral administration: local stinging, burning sensation, pallor, weak pulse, transient hypotension.

INTERACTIONS
None significant.

NURSING CONSIDERATIONS
• Contraindicated in acute asthmatic attack. Use cautiously in elderly patients, and in patients with increased intraocular pressure, hyperthyroidism, cardiovascular or renal disease, hypertension, bronchial asthma, narrow-angle glaucoma, urinary retention, prostatic hypertrophy, bladder-neck obstruction.
• Warn patient against drinking alcoholic beverages and using other CNS depressants during therapy and against driving or other activities that require alertness until CNS response to drug is determined.
• Causes less drowsiness than some other antihistamines.
• Coffee or tea may reduce drowsiness. Sugarless gum, sour hard candy, or ice chips may relieve dry mouth.
• Titrate each patient's dose; response to drug varies.
• If tolerance develops, another antihistamine may be substituted.
• Warn patient to stop taking drug 4 days before allergy skin tests; otherwise, accuracy of tests may be affected.
• Only injectable forms *without* preservatives can be given I.V. Give *slowly.*
• If symptoms occur after parenteral dose, stop drug. Notify doctor.

clemastine fumarate
Tavist, Tavist-1

INDICATIONS & DOSAGE
Rhinitis, allergy symptoms—
Adults: 1.34 to 2.68 mg once daily. Maximum recommended daily dosage is 8.04 mg; or (timed-release) 1.34 mg (long-acting tablet) b.i.d., not to exceed 8.04 mg (six long-acting tablets) per day.
Allergic skin manifestation of urticaria and angioedema—
Adults: 2.68 mg up to t.i.d. maximum.

SIDE EFFECTS
Blood: hemolytic anemia, thrombocytopenia, *agranulocytosis.*
CNS (especially in the elderly): *sedation, drowsiness.*
CV: hypotension, palpitations, tachycardia.
GI: epigastric distress, anorexia, nausea, vomiting, constipation, *dry mouth.*
GU: urinary retention.
Skin: rash, urticaria.
Other: thickening of bronchial secretions.

INTERACTIONS
None significant.

NURSING CONSIDERATIONS
• Contraindicated in acute asthmatic attack. Use cautiously in elderly patients, and in patients with increased intraocular pressure, hyperthyroidism, cardiovascular or renal disease, hypertension, bronchial asthma, narrow-angle glaucoma, urinary retention, prostatic hypertrophy, bladder-neck obstruction.
• Warn patient against drinking alcoholic beverages during therapy and against driving or other activities that require alertness until CNS response to drug is determined.
• Coffee or tea may reduce drowsiness. Sugarless gum, sour hard candy, or ice chips may relieve dry mouth.
• Titrate each patient's dose; response to drug varies.
• If tolerance develops, another antihistamine may be substituted.
• Warn patient to stop taking drug 4 days before allergy skin tests; otherwise, accuracy of tests may be affected.
• Tablets are available as 1.34 and 2.68 mg. Long-acting tablets are 1.34 mg.
• Monitor blood counts during long-term therapy; observe for signs of blood dyscrasias.

cyproheptadine hydrochloride
Periactin♦, Vimicon♦♦

INDICATIONS & DOSAGE
Allergy symptoms, pruritus—
Adults: 4 mg P.O. t.i.d. or q.i.d. Maximum 0.5 mg/kg daily.
Children 7 to 14 years: 4 mg P.O. b.i.d. or t.i.d. Maximum 16 mg daily.
Children 2 to 6 years: 2 mg P.O. b.i.d. or t.i.d. Maximum 12 mg daily.

SIDE EFFECTS
CNS (especially in the elderly):
drowsiness, dizziness, headache, fatigue.
GI: nausea, vomiting, *dry mouth*.
Skin: rash.
Other: weight gain.

INTERACTIONS
None significant.

NURSING CONSIDERATIONS
• Contraindicated in acute asthmatic attack. Use cautiously in elderly patients, and in patients with increased intraocular pressure, hyperthyroidism, cardiovascular or renal disease, hypertension, bronchial asthma, narrow-angle glaucoma, urinary retention, prostatic hypertrophy, bladder-neck obstruction.
• Warn patient against drinking alcoholic beverages during therapy and against driving or other activities that require alertness until CNS response to drug is determined.
• Reduce GI distress by giving with food or milk.
• Coffee or tea may reduce drowsiness. Sugarless gum, sour hard candy, or ice chips may relieve dry mouth.
• Titrate each patient's dose; response to drug varies.
• If tolerance develops, another antihistamine may be substituted.
• Warn patient to stop taking drug 4 days before allergy skin tests; otherwise, accuracy of tests may be affected.
• Used experimentally to stimulate appetite and increase weight gain in children.

dexchlorpheniramine maleate
Polaramine♦

INDICATIONS & DOSAGE
Rhinitis, allergy symptoms, contact dermatitis, pruritus—
Adults: 1 to 2 mg P.O. t.i.d. or q.i.d.; or (timed-release) 4 to 6 mg b.i.d. or t.i.d.

Children under 12 years: 0.15 mg/kg P.O. daily divided into 4 doses.
Do not use timed-release tablets for children younger than 6 years.

SIDE EFFECTS
CNS (especially in the elderly):
drowsiness, dizziness, *stimulation.*
GI: nausea, *dry mouth.*
GU: polyuria, dysuria.

INTERACTIONS
None significant.

NURSING CONSIDERATIONS
● Contraindicated in acute asthmatic attack. Use cautiously in elderly patients, and in patients with increased intraocular pressure, hyperthyroidism, cardiovascular or renal disease, hypertension, bronchial asthma, narrow-angle glaucoma, urinary retention, prostatic hypertrophy, bladder-neck obstruction.
● Warn patient against drinking alcoholic beverages during therapy and against driving or other activities that require alertness until CNS response to drug is determined.
● Causes less drowsiness than some other antihistamines.
● Coffee or tea may reduce drowsiness. Sugarless gum, sour hard candy, or ice chips may relieve dry mouth.
● Titrate each patient's dose; response to drug varies.
● If tolerance develops, another antihistamine may be substituted.
● Warn patient to stop taking drug 4 days before allergy skin tests; otherwise, accuracy of tests may be affected.

SIDE EFFECTS
CNS (especially in the elderly):
drowsiness, dizziness, insomnia, irritability, headache, *stimulation.*
GI: anorexia, nausea, vomiting, *dry mouth,* diarrhea.
GU: urinary frequency.

INTERACTIONS
None significant.

NURSING CONSIDERATIONS
● Contraindicated in acute asthmatic attack. Use cautiously in elderly patients, and in patients with increased intraocular pressure, hyperthyroidism, cardiovascular or renal disease, hypertension, bronchial asthma, narrow-angle glaucoma, urinary retention, prostatic hypertrophy, bladder-neck obstruction.
● Warn patient against drinking alcoholic beverages during therapy and against driving or other activities that require alertness until CNS response to drug is determined.
● Reduce GI distress by giving with food or milk.
● Causes less drowsiness than some other antihistamines.
● Coffee or tea may reduce drowsiness. Sugarless gum, sour hard candy, or ice chips may relieve dry mouth.
● Titrate each patient's dose; response to drug varies.
● If tolerance develops, another antihistamine may be substituted.
● Warn patient to stop taking drug 4 days before allergy skin tests; otherwise, accuracy of tests may be affected.

dimethindene maleate
Triten**

INDICATIONS & DOSAGE
Allergy symptoms—
Adults and children over 6 years:
(timed-release) 2.5 mg P.O. daily b.i.d.

Italicized side effects are common or life-threatening.
*Liquid form contains alcohol.   **May contain tartrazine.

diphenhydramine hydrochloride

Allerdryl, Baramine, Bax*, Benachlor, Benadryl♦*, Benahist, Ben-Allergin, Bendylate, Bentrac, Bonyl, Compoz, Eldadryl, Fenylhist, Nordryl, Nytol with DPH,Phen-Amin 50, Phenamine, Rodryl, Rohydra, SK-Diphenhydramine*, Sominex Formula 2, Span-Lanin, Valdrene, Wehdryl

INDICATIONS & DOSAGE

Rhinitis, allergy symptoms, motion sickness, antiparkinsonism—
Adults: 25 to 50 mg P.O. t.i.d. to q.i.d.; or 10 to 50 mg deep I.M. or I.V. Maximum 400 mg daily.
Children under 12 years: 5 mg/kg daily P.O., deep I.M., or I.V. divided q.i.d. Maximum 300 mg daily.
Sedation—
Adults: 25 to 50 mg P.O., deep I.M., p.r.n.

SIDE EFFECTS

CNS (especially in the elderly): *drowsiness,* confusion, insomnia, headache, vertigo.
CV: palpitations.
EENT: photosensitivity, diplopia, nasal stuffiness.
GI: *nausea,* vomiting, diarrhea, *dry mouth,* constipation.
GU: dysuria.
Skin: urticaria.

INTERACTIONS

None significant.

NURSING CONSIDERATIONS

• Contraindicated in acute asthmatic attack. Use cautiously in narrow-angle glaucoma, prostatic hypertrophy, peptic ulcer, pyloroduodenal and bladder-neck obstruction; in newborns, and in asthmatic, hypertensive, or cardiac patients.
• Alternate injection sites to prevent irritation. Administer deep I.M. into large muscle.
• Warn patient against drinking alcoholic beverages during therapy and against driving or other hazardous activities until CNS response to drug is determined.
• Reduce GI distress by giving with food or milk.
• Coffee or tea may reduce drowsiness. Sugarless gum, sour hard candy, or ice chips may relieve dry mouth.
• Titrate each patient's dose; response to drug varies.
• If tolerance develops, another antihistamine may be substituted.
• Warn patient to stop taking drug 4 days before allergy skin tests; otherwise, accuracy of tests may be affected.
• Used with epinephrine in anaphylaxis.
• One of most sedating antihistamines; often used as a nighttime sedative.

diphenylpyraline hydrochloride

Diafen, Hispril

INDICATIONS & DOSAGE

Rhinitis, allergy symptoms—
Adults: 2 mg P.O. q 4 hours, p.r.n.; or (timed-release) 5 mg P.O. q 12 hours.
Children over 6 years: 2 mg P.O. q 6 hours, p.r.n.; or (timed-release) 5 mg P.O. daily.
Children 2 to 6 years: 1 to 2 mg P.O. q 8 hours, p.r.n.

SIDE EFFECTS

CNS (especially in the elderly): *drowsiness,* dizziness, headache.
EENT: nasal congestion.
GI: *dry mouth and throat,* epigastric distress.
Skin: flushing.

INTERACTIONS

None significant.

NURSING CONSIDERATIONS

• Contraindicated in acute asthmatic attack. Use cautiously in elderly patients, and in patients with increased intraocular pressure, hyperthyroidism, cardiovascular or renal disease, hypertension, diabetes mellitus, bronchial asthma, narrow-angle glaucoma, urinary retention, prostatic hypertrophy, bladder-neck obstruction.

• Warn patient against drinking alcoholic beverages during therapy and against driving or other activities that require alertness until CNS response to drug is determined.

• Reduce GI distress by giving with food or milk.

• Coffee or tea may reduce drowsiness. Sugarless gum, sour hard candy, or ice chips may relieve dry mouth.

• Titrate each patient's dose; response to drug varies.

• If tolerance develops, another antihistamine may be substituted.

• Warn patient to stop taking drug 4 days before allergy skin tests; otherwise, accuracy of tests may be affected.

---

doxylamine succinate
Bendectin, Decapryn**, Unisom

INDICATIONS & DOSAGE
Rhinitis, allergy symptoms—
Adults: 12.5 to 25 mg P.O. q 4 to 6 hours, p.r.n. Maximum 150 mg daily.
Children 6 to 12 years: 6.25 to 12.5 mg P.O. q 4 to 6 hours, p.r.n.
Nausea and vomiting of pregnancy—
Adults: 2 Bendectin tablets at bedtime. Maximum 4 tablets daily.

SIDE EFFECTS
CNS (especially in the elderly):
drowsiness, dizziness, insomnia, disorientation, confusion, tremor, irritability, vertigo.
CV: palpitations.
GI: *dry mouth and throat.*

INTERACTIONS
None significant.

NURSING CONSIDERATIONS

• Contraindicated in acute asthmatic attack. Use cautiously in elderly patients, and in patients with increased intraocular pressure, hyperthyroidism, cardiovascular or renal disease, hypertension, bronchial asthma, narrow-angle glaucoma, urinary retention, prostatic hypertrophy, bladder-neck obstruction.

• Warn patient against drinking alcoholic beverages during therapy and against driving or other activities that require alertness until CNS response to drug is determined.

• Coffee or tea may reduce drowsiness. Sugarless gum, sour hard candy, or ice chips may relieve dry mouth.

• Titrate each patient's dose; response to drug varies.

• If tolerance develops, another antihistamine may be substituted.

• Warn patient to stop taking drug 4 days before allergy skin tests; otherwise, accuracy of tests may be affected.

• Although Bendectin is indicated in the treatment of nausea and vomiting of pregnancy, it should only be used in extreme cases. Advise your patient to request Bendectin only if other measures, such as eating crackers or toast or drinking hot or cold liquids, have proven unsuccessful.

• Tell patient to request the patient package insert for Bendectin, which is available from the doctor or pharmacist.

---

methdilazine hydrochloride
Dilosyn◆◆, Tacaryl

INDICATIONS & DOSAGE
Pruritus—
Adults: 8 mg P.O. b.i.d. to q.i.d. or (chewable tablets) 7.2 mg P.O. b.i.d. to q.i.d.
Children over 3 years: 4 mg P.O.

Italicized side effects are common or life-threatening.
*Liquid form contains alcohol.   **May contain tartrazine.

b.i.d. to q.i.d. or (chewable tablets)
3.6 mg P.O. b.i.d. to q.i.d.

SIDE EFFECTS
CNS (especially in the elderly):
drowsiness, dizziness, headache.
GI: nausea, *dry mouth and throat*.
Hepatic: cholestatic jaundice.
Skin: rash.

INTERACTIONS
Phenothiazines: increased effects.
Don't use together.

NURSING CONSIDERATIONS
• Contraindicated in acute asthmatic
attack. Use cautiously in elderly or debilitated patients; acutely ill or dehydrated children; and in patients with
pulmonary, hepatic, or cardiovascular
disease, asthma, hypertension, narrow-
angle glaucoma, peptic ulcer, prostatic
hypertrophy, bladder-neck obstruction,
CNS depression.
• Warn patient against drinking alcoholic beverages during therapy and
against driving or other activities that
require alertness until CNS response to
drug is determined.
• Reduce GI distress by giving with
food or milk.
• Coffee or tea may reduce drowsiness.
Sugarless gum, sour hard candy, or ice
chips may relieve dry mouth.
• Titrate each patient's dose; response
to drug varies.
• If tolerance develops, another antihistamine may be substituted.
• Available as chewable tablet for children. Instruct child to chew completely
and swallow promptly; may cause local
anesthetic effect in mouth.
• Warn patient to stop taking drug
4 days before allergy skin tests; otherwise, accuracy of tests may be affected.

promethazine hydrochloride
Ganphen, K-Phen, Methazine,
Pentazine,
Phencen-50, Phenergan♦*,
Promethamead, Promethazine,
Prorex, Provigan, Remsed,
Rolamethazine*, Sigazine

INDICATIONS & DOSAGE
Motion sickness—
Adults: 25 mg P.O. b.i.d.
Children: 12.5 to 25 mg P.O., I.M., or
rectally b.i.d.
Nausea—
Adults: 12.5 to 25 mg P.O., I.M., or
rectally q 4 to 6 hours, p.r.n.
Children: 0.25 to 0.5 mg/kg I.M. or
rectally q 4 to 6 hours, p.r.n.
Rhinitis, allergy symptoms—
Adults: 12.5 mg P.O. q.i.d.; or 25 mg
P.O. at bedtime.
Children: 6.25 to 12.5 mg P.O. t.i.d.
or 25 mg P.O. or rectally at bedtime.
Sedation—
Adults: 25 to 50 mg P.O., I.M. at bed-
time or p.r.n.
Children: 12.5 to 25 mg P.O., I.M., or
rectally at bedtime.
Preoperative sedation—
Adults: 50 mg P.O. or I.M. on the
night preceding surgery.
Children: 12.5 to 25 mg P.O. or I.M.
on the night preceding surgery.
CNS (especially in the elderly):
sedation, confusion, restlessness, trem-
ors, *drowsiness*.
CV: hypotension.
EENT: transient myopia, nasal conges-
tion.
GI: anorexia, nausea, vomiting, consti-
pation, *dry mouth*.
Other: *photosensitivity*.

INTERACTIONS
Phenothiazines: increased effects.
Don't give together.

NURSING CONSIDERATIONS
• Contraindicated in narrow-angle

glaucoma, peptic ulcer, intestinal obstruction, prostatic hypertrophy, bladder-neck obstruction, epilepsy, bone-marrow depression, coma, CNS depression, pregnancy (except during labor), lactation; in newborns and acutely ill or dehydrated children. Use cautiously in pulmonary, hepatic, or cardiovascular disease; asthma; hypertension; and in elderly or debilitated patients.

• Warn patient against drinking alcoholic beverages during therapy and against driving or other activities that require alertness until CNS response to drug is determined.

• Reduce GI distress by giving with food or milk.

• Coffee or tea may reduce drowsiness. Sugarless gum, sour hard candy, or ice chips may relieve dry mouth.

• Titrate each patient's dose; response to drug varies.

• If tolerance develops, another antihistamine may be substituted.

• Warn patient to stop taking drug 4 days before allergy skin tests; otherwise, accuracy of tests may be affected.

• Pronounced sedative effect limits use in many ambulatory patients.

• May cause false-positive immunologic urine pregnancy test (Gravindex). Also may interfere with blood grouping in ABO system.

• When treating motion sickness, tell patient to take first dose 30 to 60 minutes before travel. On succeeding days of travel, he should take dose upon arising and with evening meal.

• Inject deep I.M. into large muscle mass.

• Warn patient about possible photosensitivity reaction and precautions he should take to avoid it.

trimeprazine tartrate
Panectyl♦♦, Temaril

INDICATIONS & DOSAGE
Pruritus—

Adults: 2.5 mg P.O. q.i.d.; or (timed-release) 5 mg P.O. b.i.d.
Children 3 to 12 years: 2.5 mg P.O. h.s. or t.i.d., p.r.n.
Children 6 months to 3 years: 1.25 mg P.O. h.s. or t.i.d., p.r.n.

SIDE EFFECTS
Blood: *agranulocytosis,* leukopenia.
CNS: *drowsiness,* dizziness, confusion, headache, restlessness, tremors, irritability, insomnia (especially in the elderly). Paradoxical excitation (in children).
CV: hypotension, palpitations, tachycardia.
GI: anorexia, nausea, vomiting, *dry mouth and throat.*
GU: urinary frequency or retention.
Skin: urticaria, rash.

INTERACTIONS
Phenothiazines: increased effects. Don't use together.

NURSING CONSIDERATIONS
• Contraindicated in acute asthmatic attack. Use cautiously in pulmonary, hepatic, or cardiovascular disease; asthma; hypertension; narrow-angle glaucoma; peptic ulcer; intestinal obstruction; prostatic hypertrophy; previously detected breast cancer; bladder-neck obstruction; epilepsy; bone-marrow depression; coma; CNS depression; in elderly or debilitated patients, and acutely ill or dehydrated children.

• Warn patient against drinking alcoholic beverages during therapy and against driving or other activities that require alertness until CNS response to drug is determined.

• Reduce GI distress by giving with food or milk.

• Coffee or tea may reduce drowsiness. Sugarless gum, sour hard candy, or ice chips may relieve dry mouth.

• Titrate each patient's dose; response to drug varies.

• If tolerance develops, another antihistamine may be substituted.

Italicized side effects are common or life-threatening.
*Liquid form contains alcohol.   **May contain tartrazine.

• Warn patient to stop taking drug 4 days before allergy skin tests; otherwise, accuracy of tests may be affected.
• Monitor blood counts during long-term therapy.

tripelennamine hydrochloride
PBZ-SR, Pyribenzamine♦,Ro-Hist

INDICATIONS & DOSAGE
Rhinitis, allergy symptoms—
Adults: 25 to 50 mg P.O. q 4 to 6 hours; or (timed-release) 100 mg b.i.d. to t.i.d. Maximum 600 mg daily.
Children over 5 years: 50 mg P.O. q 8 to 12 hours (timed-release).
Children under 5 years: 5 mg/kg daily P.O. in 4 to 6 divided doses. Maximum 300 mg daily.

SIDE EFFECTS
CNS (especially in the elderly): *drowsiness,* dizziness, confusion, restlessness, tremors, irritability, insomnia.
CV: palpitations.
GI: anorexia, diarrhea or constipation, *nausea, vomiting, dry mouth.*
GU: urinary frequency or retention.
Skin: urticaria, rash.
Other: thickening of bronchial secretions.

INTERACTIONS
None significant.

NURSING CONSIDERATIONS
• Contraindicated in acute asthmatic attack. Use cautiously in elderly patients, and in patients with increased intraocular pressure, hyperthyroidism, cardiovascular or renal disease, hypertension, or bronchial asthma, narrow-angle glaucoma, urinary retention, prostatic hypertrophy, bladder-neck obstruction.
• Warn patient against drinking alcoholic beverages during therapy and against driving or other activities that require alertness until CNS response to drug is determined.
• Reduce GI distress by giving with food or milk.
• Coffee or tea may reduce drowsiness. Sugarless gum, sour hard candy, or ice chips may relieve dry mouth.
• Titrate each patient's dose; response to drug varies.
• If tolerance develops, another antihistamine may be substituted.
• Warn patient to stop taking drug 4 days before allergy skin tests; otherwise, accuracy of tests may be affected.

triprolidine hydrochloride
Actidil♦

INDICATIONS & DOSAGE
Colds and allergy symptoms—
Adults: 2.5 mg P.O. t.i.d. or q.i.d.
Children over 6 years: 1.25 mg t.i.d. or q.i.d.
Children 4 to 6 years: 0.9 mg t.i.d. or q.i.d.
Children 2 to 4 years: 0.6 mg t.i.d. or q.i.d.
Children 4 months to 2 years: 0.3 mg t.i.d. or q.i.d.

SIDE EFFECTS
CNS (especially in the elderly): *drowsiness,* dizziness, confusion, restlessness, insomnia, *stimulation.*
GI: anorexia, diarrhea or constipation, nausea, vomiting, *dry mouth.*
GU: urinary frequency or retention.
Skin: urticaria, rash.

INTERACTIONS
None significant.

NURSING CONSIDERATIONS
• Contraindicated in acute asthma. Use cautiously in elderly patients, and in patients with increased intraocular pressure, hyperthyroidism, cardiovascular or renal disease, hypertension, diabetes mellitus, bronchial asthma, narrow-angle glaucoma, urinary reten-

---

Unmarked trade names available in the United States only.
♦ Also available in Canada.   ♦♦ Available in Canada only.

tion, prostatic hypertrophy, bladder-neck obstruction.
• Warn patient against drinking alcoholic beverages during therapy and against driving or other activities that require alertness until CNS response to drug is determined.
• Reduce GI distress by giving with food or milk.
• Causes less drowsiness than some other antihistamines.
• Coffee or tea may reduce drowsiness. Sugarless gum, sour hard candy, or ice chips may relieve dry mouth.
• Titrate each patient's dose; response to drug varies.
• Warn patient to stop taking drug 4 days before allergy skin tests; otherwise, accuracy of tests may be affected.

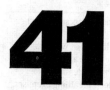

Expectorants and antitussives

acetylcysteine
ammonium chloride
benzonatate
chlophedianol hydrochloride
codeine
codeine phosphate
codeine sulfate
dextromethorphan
  hydrobromide
diphenhydramine hydrochloride
guaifenesin (formerly glyceryl
  guaiacolate)
hydriodic acid
hydrocodone bitartrate
hydromorphone hydrochloride
iodinated glycerol
levopropoxyphene napsylate
noscapine hydrochloride
potassium iodide (SSKI)
terpin hydrate

MECHANISM OF ACTION

• Expectorants may increase production of respiratory tract fluids to help liquefy and reduce the viscosity of thick, tenacious secretions.
• Antitussives suppress the cough reflex by direct action on the cough center in the medulla (brain) or by peripheral action on sensory nerve endings.

Benzonatate, chlophedianol, and diphenhydramine also act as local anesthetics.

COMBINATION PRODUCTS

Preparations are available in the following combinations:

• expectorants with decongestants or antihistamines, or both
• antitussives with decongestants or antihistamines, or both
• expectorants and antitussives
• expectorants and antitussives with decongestants or antihistamines, or both.

acetylcysteine
Airbron♦♦, Mucomyst♦, NAC♦♦

INDICATIONS & DOSAGE
Pneumonia, bronchitis, tuberculosis, cystic fibrosis, emphysema, atelectasis (adjunct), complications of thoracic surgery and CV surgery—
Adults and children: 1 to 2 ml 10% to 20% solution by direct instillation into trachea as often as every hour; or 3 to 5 ml 20% solution, or 6 to 10 ml 10% solution, by mouthpiece t.i.d. or q.i.d.
Acetaminophen toxicity—
140 mg/kg initially P.O., followed by 70 mg/kg q 4 hours for 17 doses (a total of 1,330 mg/kg).

SIDE EFFECTS
EENT: *rhinorrhea, hemoptysis.*
GI: *stomatitis, nausea.*
Other: *bronchospasm (especially in asthmatics).*

INTERACTIONS
None significant.

NURSING CONSIDERATIONS
• Use cautiously in patients with asthma or severe respiratory insufficiency; in elderly or debilitated patients.
• Classified as a mucolytic.

• Use plastic, glass, stainless steel, or another nonreactive metal when administering by nebulization. Handbulb nebulizers not recommended because output too small and particle size too large.

• After opening, store in refrigerator; use within 96 hours.

• Incompatible with oxytetracycline, tetracycline, erythromycin lactobionate, amphotericin B, ampicillin, iodized oil, chymotrypsin, trypsin, and hydrogen peroxide.

• Monitor cough type and frequency. For maximum effect, instruct patient to clear his airway by coughing before aerosol administration.

• Available in combination with isoproterenol in a 4-ml vial.

• Large doses are used P.O. to treat acetaminophen overdose.

ammonium chloride

INDICATIONS & DOSAGE
As expectorant—
Adults: 250 to 500 mg P.O. q 2 to 4 hours.

SIDE EFFECTS
CNS: headache, drowsiness, confusion, excitation alternating with coma, twitching, hyperreflexia, EEG abnormalities.
CV: bradycardia.
GI: *anorexia, nausea, vomiting*.
GU: renal impairment, glycosuria.
Metabolic: *acidosis, hypokalemia*, hypocalcemic tetany, hyperglycemia.
Skin: rash.
Other: thirst, hyperventilation.

INTERACTIONS
Spironolactone: systemic acidosis. Use cautiously.

NURSING CONSIDERATIONS
• Contraindicated in hepatic or renal impairment. Use cautiously in pulmonary insufficiency, congestive heart failure.

• Give with full glass of water.
• Monitor cough type and frequency.
• Monitor for hypokalemia.
• Encourage deep-breathing exercises.
• Watch for potentiated diuresis when used with diuretics.
• Also used to acidify urine.
• Most authorities feel that the benefits of this drug are outweighed by the potential risks.

benzonatate
Tessalon♦

INDICATIONS & DOSAGE
Nonproductive cough—
Adults and children over 10 years: 100 mg P.O. t.i.d.; up to 600 mg daily.
Children under 10 years: 8 mg/kg P.O. in 3 to 6 divided doses.

SIDE EFFECTS
CNS: dizziness, drowsiness, headache.
EENT: nasal congestion, sensation of burning in eyes.
GI: nausea, constipation.
Skin: rash.

INTERACTIONS
None significant.

NURSING CONSIDERATIONS
• Patient should not chew capsules or leave in mouth to dissolve; local anesthesia will result. If capsules dissolve in mouth, CNS stimulation may cause restlessness, tremors, and possibly convulsions.

• A cough suppressant; don't use when cough is valuable as diagnostic sign or is beneficial (as after thoracic surgery).

• Monitor cough type and frequency.
• Use with percussion and chest vibration.
• Maintain fluid intake to help liquefy sputum.

Italicized side effects are common or life-threatening.
*Liquid form contains alcohol.   **May contain tartrazine.

chlophedianol hydrochloride
Ulo, Ulone♦♦

INDICATIONS & DOSAGE
Nonproductive cough—
Adults and children over 12 years: 25 mg P.O. t.i.d. or q.i.d.
Children 6 to 12 years: 12.5 to 25 mg P.O. t.i.d. or q.i.d.
Children 2 to 6 years: 12.5 mg P.O. t.i.d. or q.i.d.

SIDE EFFECTS
CNS: *drowsiness,* dizziness, excitation, irritability, nightmares, hallucinations, vertigo, visual disturbances.
GI: *nausea,* vomiting, dry mouth.
Skin: uticaria.

INTERACTIONS
None significant.

NURSING CONSIDERATIONS
• An antitussive; don't use when cough is valuable diagnostic sign or beneficial (as after thoracic surgery).
• Monitor cough type and frequency.
• Use with percussion and chest vibration.
• CNS side effects disappear when drug is stopped.

codeine

codeine phosphate

codeine sulfate
Controlled Substance Schedule II

INDICATIONS & DOSAGE
Nonproductive cough—
Adults: 8 to 20 mg P.O. q 4 to 6 hours. Maximum 120 mg/24 hours.
Children: 1 to 1.5 mg/kg P.O. daily in 4 divided doses. Maximum 60 mg/24 hours.

SIDE EFFECTS
CNS: *dizziness, sedation,* respiratory depression, disorientation.
CV: palpitations.
GI: *nausea,* vomiting; with repeated doses, *constipation, dry mouth.*
GU: urinary retention and hesitancy.
Skin: pruritus, sweating.
Other: tolerance and physical dependence.

INTERACTIONS
None significant.

NURSING CONSIDERATIONS
• Contraindicated in increased intracranial or CSF pressure. Use cautiously in debilitated patients; in dehydrated postoperative patients; in those with asthma, emphysema, head injury, history of drug abuse, hepatic or renal disease, hypothyroidism, Addison's disease, acute alcoholism, seizures, severe CNS depression, chronic obstructive pulmonary disease, psychosis; after thoracotomies or laparotomies; and when other CNS depressants are given. Monitor patient carefully.
• Use with percussion and chest vibration.
• Warn patient against driving or other activities that require alertness until CNS response to drug is determined.
• An antitussive; don't use when cough is a valuable diagnostic sign or beneficial (as after thoracic surgery).
• Monitor cough type and frequency.

dextromethorphan hydrobromide

Balminil DM♦♦, Broncho-Grippol-DM♦♦, Contratuss♦♦, Pertussin 8-hour, Romilar Chewable Tablets for Children, St. Joseph's Cough Syrup for Children, Silence Is Golden. More commonly available in combination products such as Benylin-DM, Coryban-D Cough Syrup*, Dimacol*, Naldetuss, Novahistine DMX, Ornacol, Phenergan Expectorant with Dextromethorphan*, Robitussin DM*, Romilar CF*, Rondec-DM*, Triaminicol, Trind-DM*, Tussi-Organidin-DM*, 2G-DM

INDICATIONS & DOSAGE
Nonproductive cough—
Adults: 10 to 20 mg q 4 hours, or 30 mg q 6 to 8 hours. Maximum 120 mg daily.
Children 6 to 12 years: 5 to 10 mg q 4 hours, or 15 mg q 6 to 8 hours. Maximum 60 mg daily.
Children 2 to 6 years: 2.5 to 5 mg q 4 hours, or 7.5 mg q 6 to 8 hours. Maximum 30 mg daily.

SIDE EFFECTS
CNS: drowsiness, dizziness.
GI: nausea.

INTERACTIONS
MAO inhibitors: hypotension, coma, hyperpyrexia, and death have occurred. Do not use together.

NURSING CONSIDERATIONS
• Contraindicated in patients currently taking or within 2 weeks of stopping MAO inhibitors.
• Produces no analgesia or addiction and little or no CNS depression.
• An antitussive; don't use when cough is valuable diagnostic sign or beneficial (as after thoracic surgery).
• Instruct patient not to take fluids immediately after taking drug.

• Use with percussion and chest vibration.
• Monitor cough type and frequency.
• Available in most over-the-counter cough medicines.

diphenhydramine hydrochloride

Allerdryl, Baramine, Bax*, Benachlor, Benadryl♦*, Benahist, Ben-Allergin, Bendylate, Bentrac, Benylin Cough Syrup♦*, Eldadryl, Fenylhist, Hyrexin, Nordryl, Phen-Amin 50, Phenamine, Rodryl, Rohydra, Valdrene*, Wehdryl

INDICATIONS & DOSAGE
Nonproductive cough—
Adults: 25 mg P.O. q 4 hours (not to exceed 100 mg daily).
Children 6 to 12 years: 12.5 mg P.O. q 4 hours (not to exceed 50 mg daily).
Children 2 to 6 years: 6.25 mg P.O. q 4 hours (not to exceed 25 mg daily).

SIDE EFFECTS
CNS: *sedation,* confusion, restlessness, insomnia, headache.
CV: palpitations.
EENT: diplopia, blurred vision, nasal congestion.
GI: *dry mouth and throat,* nausea, vomiting, diarrhea, constipation.
GU: dysuria.
Skin: urticaria.

INTERACTIONS
None significant.

NURSING CONSIDERATIONS
• Contraindicated in acute asthma, narrow-angle glaucoma, prostatic hypertrophy, peptic ulcer, pyloroduodenal and bladder-neck obstruction. Use cautiously in asthmatic, hypertensive, or cardiac patients.
• Warn patient against drinking alcoholic beverages during therapy and against driving or other activities that

---

Italicized side effects are common or life-threatening.
*Liquid form contains alcohol.   **May contain tartrazine.

require alertness until CNS response to drug is determined.
- Liquid preparations are recommended for antitussive effect.
- Instruct patient not to take fluids immediately after taking drug.
- Coffee and tea may reduce drowsiness. Sugarless gum, sour hard candy, or ice chips may relieve dry mouth.
- If tolerance develops, another antihistamine may be substituted.
- Warn patient to stop taking drug 4 days before allergy skin tests; otherwise, accuracy of tests may be affected.

guaifenesin (formerly glyceryl guaiacolate)

Anti-Tuss, Balminil♦♦, Bowtussin, Breonesin, Colrex*, Cosin-GG, Dilyn, 2/G, G-100, G-200, GG-CEN, Glycotuss, Gly-O-Tussin, Glytuss, G-Tussin, Guaiatussin*, Hytuss, Malotuss, Motussin♦♦, Nortussin, Proco, Recsei-Tuss, Resyl♦♦, Robitussin♦*, Tursen, Wal-Tussin DM

INDICATIONS & DOSAGE
Productive and nonproductive cough—
Adults: 100 to 200 mg P.O. q 2 to 4 hours. Maximum 800 mg daily.
Children: 12 mg/kg P.O. daily in 6 divided doses.

SIDE EFFECTS
CNS: drowsiness.
GI: vomiting and nausea occur with large doses.

INTERACTIONS
None significant.

NURSING CONSIDERATIONS
- May interfere with certain laboratory tests for 5-hydroxyindoleacetic acid and vanillylmandelic acid.
- Watch for bleeding gums, hematuria, and bruising if given to patients on hep-

arin. Should such symptoms appear, guaifenesin should be discontinued.
- Liquefies thick, tenacious sputum; maintain fluid intake. Advise patient to take with a glass of water whenever possible.
- Monitor cough type and frequency.
- An expectorant.
- Encourage deep-breathing exercises.
- Although a very popular expectorant, many medical authorities doubt its efficacy.

hydriodic acid

INDICATIONS & DOSAGE
Chronic bronchitis, bronchial asthma—
Adults: 1.25 to 5 ml syrup well diluted in water P.O. b.i.d. or t.i.d.
Children over 1 year: 1 to 10 drops, well diluted in water, daily or t.i.d. after meals.

SIDE EFFECTS
EENT: tooth damage.
Other: iodism, drug fever.

INTERACTIONS
None significant.

NURSING CONSIDERATIONS
- Dilute well. Use straw to avoid injuring teeth; syrup is very acidic.
- Liquefies thick, tenacious sputum; maintain fluid intake. Advise patient to take with a glass of water whenever possible.
- Don't use if syrup is deep brown color.
- Monitor cough type and frequency.
- Encourage deep-breathing exercises.
- An expectorant.

Unmarked trade names available in the United States only.
♦ Also available in Canada.   ♦♦ Available in Canada only.

hydrocodone bitartrate
Controlled Substance Schedule II
Coditrate, Corutol DH♦♦,
Dicodethal, Dicodid, Hycodan♦,
Robidone♦♦

INDICATIONS & DOSAGE
Nonproductive cough—
Adults: 5 to 10 mg P.O. t.i.d. or q.i.d.,
p.r.n. Maximum single dose 15 mg.
Children: 0.6 mg/kg or 20 mg/m² P.O.
daily in 3 or 4 divided doses.

SIDE EFFECTS
CNS: *drowsiness, dizziness.*
EENT: dryness of throat.
GI: *nausea, constipation,* vomiting.
Skin: pruritis, sweating.
Other: tolerance and physical dependence after long-term use.

INTERACTIONS
None significant.

NURSING CONSIDERATIONS
• Contraindicated in glaucoma. Use cautiously in asthma, emphysema, drug dependence; after thoracotomy or laparotomy; in debilitated or dehydrated patients.
• Warn patient against driving or other activities that require alertness until CNS response to drug is determined.
• Evaluate patient's need for drug, which is addictive.
• An antitussive; don't use when cough is valuable diagnostic sign or beneficial (as after thoracic surgery).
• Use with percussion and chest vibration.
• Monitor cough type and frequency.

hydromorphone hydrochloride
Controlled Substance Schedule II
Dilaudid Cough Syrup♦

INDICATIONS & DOSAGE
Cough—
Adults: 1 mg P.O. q 3 to 4 hours, p.r.n.
Children 6 to 12 years: 0.5 mg P.O. q
3 to 4 hours, p.r.n.

SIDE EFFECTS
CNS: *dizziness, somnolence,* respiratory depression.
CV: hypotension.
GI: *nausea,* vomiting, anorexia, constipation.

INTERACTIONS
CNS depressants: increased sedation.
Use together cautiously.

NURSING CONSIDERATIONS
• Contraindicated in increased intracranial pressure, status asthmaticus. Use cautiously in hepatic or renal disease, hypothyroidism, Addison's disease, acute alcoholism, seizures, head injury, severe CNS depression, brain tumor, bronchial asthma, chronic obstructive pulmonary disease, or psychosis.
• Warn patient against driving and other activities that require alertness until CNS response to drug is determined.
• Monitor respirations, pupil size, bowel function during therapy.
• An antitussive; don't use when cough is valuable diagnostic sign or beneficial (as after thoracic surgery).
• Use with percussion or chest vibration.
• Monitor cough type and frequency.
• Considered more addictive than codeine.

iodinated glycerol
Organidin♦*

INDICATIONS & DOSAGE
Bronchial asthma, bronchitis, emphysema (adjunct)—
Adults: 60 mg P.O. q.i.d. (tablets), or 20 drops (solution) P.O. q.i.d. with fluids, or 5 ml (elixir) P.O. q.i.d.

Italicized side effects are common or life-threatening.
*Liquid form contains alcohol.   **May contain tartrazine.

Children: up to ½ adult dose based on child's weight.

SIDE EFFECTS
After long-term use:
GI: *nausea*, gastrointestinal distress.
Skin: *eruptions*.
Other: acute parotitis, thyroid enlargement.

INTERACTIONS
None significant.

NURSING CONSIDERATIONS
• Contraindicated in hypothyroidism, iodine sensitivity.
• Skin rash or other hypersensitivity reaction may require stopping drug.
• May liquefy thick, tenacious sputum; maintain fluid intake.
• Monitor cough type and frequency.
• Encourage deep-breathing exercises.
• An expectorant.

levopropoxyphene napsylate
Novrad

INDICATIONS & DOSAGE
Nonproductive cough—
Adults: 50 to 100 mg q 4 hours. Maximum dose 600 mg daily.
Children 23 to 45 kg: 50 mg q 4 hours. Maximum dose 200 mg daily.
Children 11 to 23 kg: 25 mg q 4 hours. Maximum dose 150 mg daily.
Children up to 11 kg: 12.5 mg q 4 hours. Maximum dose 75 mg daily.

SIDE EFFECTS
CNS: *drowsiness,* nervousness, *dizziness,* headache, sedation.
EENT: visual disturbances, dry mouth.
GI: *nausea,* vomiting, diarrhea, *epigastric burning.*
GU: urinary frequency or urgency.
Skin: rash, urticaria.

INTERACTIONS
None significant.

NURSING CONSIDERATIONS
• If CNS stimulation or sedation occurs, lower dose or stop drug. Report to doctor.
• An antitussive; don't use when cough is valuable diagnostic sign or beneficial (as after thoracic surgery).
• Tell patient not to take fluids just after liquid preparation.
• Use with percussion or chest vibration.
• Monitor cough type and frequency.
• Warn patient against driving or other activities that require mental alertness until CNS response to drug is determined.
• Narcotic antagonist of no value in overdose.

noscapine hydrochloride
Noscatuss♦♦, Tusscapine

INDICATIONS & DOSAGE
Nonproductive cough—
Adults: 15 to 30 mg P.O. q 4 to 6 hours as chewable tablet or syrup. Maximum dose 120 mg daily.
Children 6 to 12 years: 7.5 to 15 mg P.O. t.i.d. or q.i.d. as syrup. Maximum dose 60 mg daily.
Children 2 to 6 years: 5 to 10 mg P.O. t.i.d. or q.i.d. as syrup. Maximum dose 40 mg daily.

SIDE EFFECTS
CNS: slight drowsiness.
EENT: acute vasomotor rhinitis, conjunctivitis.
GI: nausea.

INTERACTIONS
None significant.

NURSING CONSIDERATIONS
• An antitussive; don't use when cough is valuable diagnostic sign or is beneficial (as after thoracic surgery). Use

cautiously in sedated or debilitated patients.
- Tell patient not to take fluids just after liquid preparation.
- Use with percussion and chest vibration.
- Monitor cough type and frequency.

potassium iodide (SSKI)

INDICATIONS & DOSAGE
Chronic bronchitis, bronchial asthma—
Adults: 300 to 600 mg P.O. q 4 to 6 hours.
Children: 0.25 to 1 ml of saturated solution (1 g/ml) b.i.d., t.i.d., or q.i.d.
Nuclear radiation protection—
Adults and children: 0.13 ml P.O. of SSKI immediately before or after initial exposure will block 90% of radioactive iodine. Same dose given 3 to 4 hours after exposure will provide 50% block. Should be administered for up to 10 days under medical supervision.
Infants under 1 year: ½ adult dose.

SIDE EFFECTS
GI: nonspecific small bowel lesions, *nausea*, vomiting, *epigastric pain*, metallic taste.
Metabolic: goiter, hyperthyroid adenoma, hypothyroidism (with excessive use), collagen disease-like syndrome.
Skin: rash.
Other: drug fever.
Prolonged use: chronic iodine poisoning, soreness of mouth, coryza, sneezing, swelling of eyelids.

INTERACTIONS
Lithium carbonate: may cause hypothyroidism. Don't use together.

NURSING CONSIDERATIONS
- Contraindicated in iodine hypersensitivity, tuberculosis, hyperkalemia, acute bronchitis, hyperthyroidism.
- Maintain fluid intake to help liquefy sputum.
- Has strong, salty, metallic taste. Dilute with milk or fruit juice to reduce GI distress and disguise taste.
- If given over long period, sudden withdrawal may precipitate thyroid storm.
- Monitor cough type and frequency.
- Encourage deep-breathing exercises.
- If skin rash appears, discontinue use. Contact doctor.
- An expectorant.
- Warn patient not to use any over-the-counter drugs without first consulting doctor.

terpin hydrate

INDICATIONS & DOSAGE
Excessive bronchial secretions—
Adults: 5 to 10 ml P.O. of elixir q 4 to 6 hours.

SIDE EFFECTS
GI: nausea, vomiting.

INTERACTIONS
None significant.

NURSING CONSIDERATIONS
- Contraindicated on empty stomach, in peptic ulcer or severe diabetes mellitus. Use cautiously in patients with history of alcohol or drug abuse.
- Don't give in large doses; high alcoholic content of elixir (86 proof).
- Monitor cough type and frequency.

Italicized side effects are common or life-threatening.
∗Liquid form contains alcohol. ∗∗May contain tartrazine.

42

Antacids, adsorbents, and antiflatulents

activated charcoal
aluminum carbonate
aluminum hydroxide
aluminum phosphate
calcium carbonate
dihydroxyaluminum aminoacetate
dihydroxyaluminum sodium carbonate
magaldrate
magnesia magma (MOM)
magnesium carbonate
magnesium oxide
magnesium trisilicate
oxethazaine
simethicone
sodium bicarbonate

MECHANISM OF ACTION

- Antacids reduce total acid load in the GI tract and elevate gastric pH to reduce pepsin activity. They also strengthen the gastric mucosal barrier and increase esophageal sphincter tone. They don't seem to have a coating effect on ulcers.
- Oxethazaine is a potent local anesthetic that may adhere to receptor sites, producing a prolonged topical anesthetic effect on the gastric mucosa.
- Adsorbents adhere to many drugs and chemicals, inhibiting their absorption from the GI tract.
- Antiflatulents, by the defoaming action of simethicone, disperse or prevent formation of mucus-surrounded gas pockets in the GI tract. These preparations form a film in the GI tract that causes gas bubbles to collapse.

COMBINATION PRODUCTS

ALUDROX TABLETS: aluminum hydroxide 233 mg, magnesium hydroxide 83 mg, and sodium 1.6 mg.
ALUDROX SUSPENSION: aluminum hydroxide 307 mg, magnesium hydroxide 103 mg, and sodium 1.1 mg per 5 ml.
A-M-T: aluminum hydroxide 162 mg and magnesium trisilicate 250 mg.
CAMALOX♦: aluminum hydroxide 225 mg, magnesium hydroxide 200 mg, and calcium carbonate 250 mg.
DELCID SUSPENSION: aluminum hydroxide 600 mg, magnesium hydroxide 665 mg, and sodium < 15 mg/5 ml.
DI-GEL: aluminum hydroxide and magnesium carbonate 282 mg, magnesium hydroxide 85 mg, simethicone 25 mg, and sodium 10.6 mg.
FLACID: aluminum hydroxide and magnesium carbonate 282 mg, magnesium hydroxide 85 mg, and simethicone 25 mg.
GAVISCON♦: aluminum hydroxide 80 mg, magnesium trisilicate 20 mg, sodium bicarbonate 70 mg, alginic acid 200 mg, and approximately 0.8 mEq sodium.
GELUSIL♦: aluminum hydroxide 200 mg, magnesium hydroxide 200 mg, simethicone 25 mg, and sodium 1.4 mg.
GELUSIL-II: aluminum hydroxide 400 mg, magnesium hydroxide 400 mg, simethicone 30 mg, and sodium 2.7 mg.
GELUSIL-M: aluminum hydroxide 300 mg, magnesium hydroxide 200 mg, simethicone 25 mg, and sodium 3 mg.
KOLANTYL TABLETS: aluminum hy-

Unmarked trade names available in the United States only.
♦ Also available in Canada. ♦♦ Available in Canada only.

droxide 300 mg, magnesium oxide 185 mg, and sodium < 15 mg.

KOLANTYL WAFERS♦: aluminum hydroxide 180 mg and magnesium hydroxide 170 mg.

MAALOX NO. 1: aluminum hydroxide 200 mg and magnesium hydroxide 200 mg.

MAALOX NO. 2: aluminum hydroxide 400 mg and magnesium hydroxide 400 mg.

MAALOX PLUS♦: aluminum hydroxide 200 mg, magnesium hydroxide 200 mg, simethicone 25 mg, and sodium 1.6 mg.

MAALOX THERAPEUTIC CONCENTRATE: aluminum hydroxide 600 mg, magnesium hydroxide 300 mg, and sodium 1.25 mg.

MAGNATRIL: aluminum hydroxide 260 mg, magnesium hydroxide 130 mg, and magnesium trisilicate 455 mg.

MYLANTA♦: aluminum hydroxide 200 mg, magnesium hydroxide 200 mg, simethicone 20 mg, and sodium 0.5 mg.

MYLANTA-II♦: aluminum hydroxide 400 mg, magnesium hydroxide 400 mg, simethicone 30 mg, and sodium 1 mg.

NEUTRALOX: aluminum hydroxide 300 mg and magnesium hydroxide 150 mg.

RIOPAN PLUS CHEW TABLETS: magaldrate 480 mg, simethicone 20 mg, and sodium < 0.65 mg.

RIOPAN PLUS SUSPENSION; magaldrate 400 mg, simethicone 20 mg, and sodium < 0.65 mg per 5 ml.

SILAIN-GEL: aluminum hydroxide 282 mg, magnesium hydroxide 285 mg, simethicone 25 mg, and sodium 4.8 mg.

SIMECO SUSPENSION: aluminum hydroxide 365 mg, magnesium hydroxide 300 mg, simethicone 30 mg, and sodium 0.3 to 0.6 mEq per 5 ml.

TITRALAC LIQUID: calcium carbonate 1,000 mg, glycine 300 mg, and sodium 11 mg per 5 ml.

TITRALAC TABLETS: calcium carbonate 420 mg, glycine 180 mg, and sodium 0.3 mg.

TRISOGEL: aluminum hydroxide 98 mg and magnesium trisilicate 293 mg.

UNIVOL♦♦: aluminum hydroxide and magnesium carbonate co-dried gel 300 mg and magnesium hydroxide 100 mg.

WINGEL: aluminum hydroxide 180 mg, magnesium hydroxide 160 mg, and sodium < 2.5 mg.

activated charcoal
Charcocaps, Charcodote, Charcotabs, Digestalin

INDICATIONS & DOSAGE
Flatulence or dyspepsia—
Adults: 600 mg to 5 g P.O. t.i.d. or q.i.d.
Poisoning—
Adults and children: 5 to 10 times estimated weight of drug or chemical ingested. Minimum dose 30 g in 250 ml water to make a slurry.

Give orally, preferably within 30 minutes of poisoning. Larger doses are necessary if food is in the stomach. For treatment of poisoning or overdosage with acetaminophen, amphetamines, aspirin, antimony, atropine, arsenic, barbiturates, camphor, cocaine, cardiotonic glycosides, glutethimide, ipecac, malathion, morphine, poisonous mushrooms, opium, oxalic acid, parathion, phenol, phenothiazines, potassium permanganate, propoxyphene, quinine, strychnine, sulfonamides, tricyclic antidepressants.

SIDE EFFECTS
GI: black stools.

INTERACTIONS
None significant.

NURSING CONSIDERATIONS
• Because activated charcoal absorbs and inactivates syrup of ipecac, give after emesis.
• Don't give in ice cream. Ice cream decreases absorptive capacity.
• Powder form most effective. Mix

Italicized side effects are common or life-threatening.
★Liquid form contains alcohol.   **★★**May contain tartrazine.

with tap water to form consistency of thick syrup. May add small amount of fruit juice or flavoring to make more palatable.
• Space doses at least 1 hour apart from other drugs if activated charcoal is being used for any indication other than poisoning.
• Warn patient that feces will be black.

aluminum carbonate
Basaljel♦*

INDICATIONS & DOSAGE
As antacid—
Adults: suspension: 5 to 10 ml, p.r.n. Extra-strength suspension: 2.5 to 5 ml, p.r.n. Tablets: 1 to 2, p.r.n. Capsules: 1 to 2, p.r.n.
To prevent formation of urinary phosphate stones (with low-phosphate diet)—
Adults: suspension: 15 to 30 ml suspension in water or juice 1 hour after meals and h.s.; 5 to 15 ml extra-strength in water or juice 1 hour after meals and h.s.; 2 to 6 tablets or capsules 1 hour after meals and h.s.

SIDE EFFECTS
GI: anorexia, *constipation,* intestinal obstruction.
Metabolic: hypophosphatemia.

INTERACTIONS
None significant.

NURSING CONSIDERATIONS
• Use cautiously in elderly patients, especially those with decreased bowel motility (those receiving antidiarrheals, antispasmodics, or anticholinergics), dehydration, fluid restriction, chronic renal disease, and suspected intestinal obstruction.
• Record amount and consistency of stools. Manage constipation with laxatives or stool softeners; alternate with magnesium-containing antacids (if patient does not have renal disease).

• Shake suspension well; give with small amount of water or fruit juice to assure passage to stomach. When administering through nasogastric tube, be sure tube is placed correctly and is patent; follow antacid with water to clear tube.
• Watch long-term, high-dose use in patient on restricted sodium intake.
• Warn patient not to take aluminum carbonate indiscriminately and not to switch antacids without doctor's advice.
• Because it contains aluminum, it is used in patients with renal failure to help control hyperphosphatemia. Binds phosphate in GI tract.
• Monitor serum phosphate levels.
• Watch for symptoms of hypophosphatemia with prolonged use (anorexia, malaise, muscle weakness); can also lead to resorption of calcium and bone demineralization.
• Make patient responsible for taking his own antacid while hospitalized, if he is able.
• May cause enteric-coated drugs to be released prematurely in stomach. Separate doses by 1 hour.
• Basaljel liquid contains no sugar.

aluminum hydroxide
ALternaGel, Alu-Cap, Al-U-Creme, Aluminett, Amphojel♦, Basaljel♦♦, Dialume, Hydroxal, No-Co-Gel, Nutrajel

INDICATIONS & DOSAGE
Antacid—
Adults: 600 mg P.O. (5 to 10 ml of most products) 1 hour after meals and h.s.; 300- or 600-mg tablet, chewed before swallowing, taken with milk or water 5 to 6 times daily after meals and h.s.
Hyperphosphatemia in renal failure—
Adults: 500 mg to 2 g b.i.d. to q.i.d.

SIDE EFFECTS
GI: anorexia, *constipation,* intestinal obstruction.
Metabolic: hypophosphatemia.

INTERACTIONS
None significant.

NURSING CONSIDERATIONS
• Use cautiously in elderly patients, especially those with decreased bowel motility (those receiving antidiarrheals, antispasmodics, or anticholinergics), dehydration, fluid restriction, chronic renal disease, and suspected intestinal obstruction.
• Record amount and consistency of stools. Manage constipation with laxatives or stool softeners; alternate with magnesium-containing antacids (if not patient with renal disease.)
• Shake suspension well; give with small amount of milk or water to assure passage to stomach. When administering through nasogastric tube, be sure tube is placed correctly and is patent. After instilling antacid, flush tube with water.
• Watch long-term, high-dose use in patient on restricted sodium intake.
• Warn patient not to take aluminum hydroxide indiscriminately and not to switch antacids without doctor's advice.
• Because it contains aluminum, it is used in patients with renal failure to help control hyperphosphatemia. Binds phosphate in the GI tract.
• Monitor serum phosphate levels.
• Watch for symptoms of hypophosphatemia with prolonged use (anorexia, malaise, muscle weakness); can also lead to resorption of calcium and bone demineralization.
• Make patient responsible for taking his own antacid while hospitalized, if he is able.
• May cause enteric-coated drugs to be released prematurely in stomach. Separate doses by 1 hour.

aluminum phosphate
Phosphaljel

INDICATIONS & DOSAGE
Antacid—
Adults: 15 to 30 ml undiluted q 2 hours between meals and h.s.

SIDE EFFECTS
GI: *constipation,* intestinal obstruction.

INTERACTIONS
None significant.

NURSING CONSIDERATIONS
• Use cautiously in elderly patients, especially those with decreased bowel motility (those receiving antidiarrheals, antispasmodics, or anticholinergics), dehydration, fluid restriction, chronic renal disease, and suspected intestinal obstruction.
• Record amount and consistency of stools. Manage constipation with laxatives or stool softeners; alternate with magnesium-containing antacids (if patient does not have renal disease.)
• Shake well; give alone or with small amount of milk or water. When administering through nasogastric tube, be sure tube is placed correctly and is patent; after instilling, flush tube with water to facilitate passage to stomach and maintain tube patency.
• Watch long-term, high-dose use in patient on restricted sodium intake.
• Warn patient not to take aluminum phosphate indiscriminately and not to switch antacids without doctor's advice.
• This drug is a very weak antacid.
• Can reverse hypophosphatemia induced by aluminum hydroxide.
• Make patient responsible for taking his own antacid while hospitalized, if he is able.
• May cause enteric-coated drugs to be released prematurely in stomach. Separate doses by 1 hour.
• Phosphaljel contains no sugar.

ANTACIDS, ABSORBENTS, AND ANTIFLATULENTS 375

calcium carbonate
Alka-2, Amitone, Calcilac, Calglycine, Dicarbosil, El-Da-Mint, Equilet, Gustalac, Mallamint, P.H. Tablets, Titracid, Titralac, Trialea, Tums

INDICATIONS & DOSAGE
Antacid—
Adults: 1-g tablet, 4 to 6 times daily, chewed well and taken with water; or 1 g of suspension (5 ml of most products) 1 hour after meals and h.s.

SIDE EFFECTS
GI: *constipation*, gastric distention, flatulence, acid-rebound, *nausea*.
Metabolic: *hypercalcemia;* if taken with milk—milk-alkali syndrome.

INTERACTIONS
None significant.

NURSING CONSIDERATIONS
• Contraindicated in severe renal disease. Use cautiously in elderly patients, especially those with decreased bowel motility (those receiving antidiarrheals, antispasmodics, anticholinergics), dehydration, fluid restriction, chronic renal disease, and suspected intestinal obstruction.
• Do not administer with milk or other foods high in vitamin D. Can cause milk-alkali syndrome (headache, confusion, distaste for food, nausea, vomiting, hypercalcemia, hypercalciuria, calcinosis, hyperphosphatemia).
• Record amount and consistency of stools. Manage constipation with laxatives or stool softeners.
• Watch for symptoms of hypercalcemia (nausea, vomiting, headache, mental confusion, anorexia).
• Monitor serum calcium levels, especially in mild renal impairment.
• Warn patient not to take calcium carbonate indiscriminately and not to switch antacids without doctor's advice.

• Make patient responsible for taking his own antacid while hospitalized if he is able.
• Has been known to cause rebound hyperacidity.
• Emphasize that it is *not* candy.
• May cause enteric-coated tablets to be released prematurely in stomach. Separate doses by 1 hour.

dihydroxyaluminum aminoacetate
Alkam, Hyperacid, Robalate♦

INDICATIONS & DOSAGE
Antacid—
Adults: 0.5 to 1 g (1 to 2 tablets) after meals and h.s., chewed before swallowing and taken with milk or water.

SIDE EFFECTS
GI: anorexia, *constipation*, intestinal obstruction.
Metabolic: hypophosphatemia.

INTERACTIONS
None significant.

NURSING CONSIDERATIONS
• Use cautiously in elderly patients, especially those with decreased bowel motility (those receiving antidiarrheals, antispasmodics, or anticholinergics), dehydration, fluid restriction, chronic renal disease, and suspected intestinal obstruction.
• Record amount and consistency of stools. Less constipating than aluminum hydroxide. Manage constipation with laxatives or stool softeners; alternate with magnesium-containing antacids (if not patient with renal disease).
• Watch for symptoms of hypophosphatemia with prolonged use (anorexia, malaise, muscle weakness); can also lead to resorption of calcium and bone demineralization.
• Monitor serum phosphate levels.
• Watch long-term, high-dose use in patient on restricted sodium intake.

• Warn patient not to take dihydroxy-aluminum aminoacetate indiscriminately and not to switch antacids without doctor's advice.

• Make patient responsible for taking his own antacid while hospitalized, if he is able.

• May cause enteric-coated drugs to be released prematurely in stomach. Separate doses by 1 hour.

---

dihydroxyaluminum sodium carbonate
Rolaids

INDICATIONS & DOSAGE
Antacid—
Adults: chew 1 to 2 tablets (334 to 668 mg), p.r.n.

SIDE EFFECTS
GI: anorexia, *constipation,* intestinal obstruction.

INTERACTIONS
None significant.

NURSING CONSIDERATIONS
• Use cautiously in elderly patients, especially those with decreased bowel motility (those receiving antidiarrheals, antispasmodics, or anticholinergics), dehydration, fluid restriction, chronic renal disease, and suspected intestinal obstruction.

• Has high sodium content and may increase sodium and water retention.

• Record amount and consistency of stools. Manage constipation with laxatives or stool softeners; alternate with magnesium-containing antacids (if patient does not have renal disease).

• Watch long-term, high-dose use in patient on restricted sodium intake.

• Warn patient not to take dihydroxy-aluminum sodium carbonate indiscriminately.

• Make patient responsible for taking his own antacid while hospitalized if he is able.

• Emphasize that it is *not* candy.

• May cause enteric-coated drugs to be released prematurely in stomach. Separate doses by 1 hour.

---

magaldrate (aluminum-magnesium complex)
Riopan♦

INDICATIONS & DOSAGE
Antacid—
Adults: suspension: 400 to 800 mg (5 to 10 ml) between meals and h.s. with water. Tablet: 400 to 800 mg (1 to 2 tablets) P.O. with water between meals and h.s. Chewable tablet: 400 to 800 mg (1 to 2 tablets) chewed before swallowing, between meals and h.s.

SIDE EFFECTS
GI: mild constipation or diarrhea.

INTERACTIONS
None significant.

NURSING CONSIDERATIONS
• Contraindicated in severe renal disease. Use cautiously in elderly patients, especially those with decreased bowel motility (those receiving antidiarrheals, antispasmodics, or anticholinergics), dehydration, fluid restriction, and mild renal impairment.

• Record amount and consistency of stools.

• Shake suspension well; give with small amount of water to assure passage to stomach. When administering through nasogastric tube, be sure tube is placed properly and is patent. After instilling, flush tube with water to assure passage to stomach and maintain tube patency.

• Monitor serum magnesium in patients with mild renal impairment. Symptomatic hypermagnesemia usually occurs only in severe renal failure.

• Not usually used in patients with renal failure (although it contains

---

Italicized side effects are common or life-threatening.
*Liquid form contains alcohol.   **May contain tartrazine.

aluminum) to help control hypophos-phatemia, since it contains magnesium, which may accumulate in renal failure.
• Good for patient on restricted sodium intake; very low sodium content.
• Warn patient not to take magaldrate indiscriminately and not to switch antacids without doctor's advice.
• Make patient responsible for taking his own antacid while hospitalized, if he is able.
• May cause enteric-coated drugs to be released prematurely in stomach. Separate doses by 1 hour.
• Riopan and Riopan Plus liquid, and Riopan swallow tablet contain no sugar. Chewable tablets contain sugar.

magnesia magma (MOM) (magnesium hydroxide)
Milk of Magnesia, Mint-O-mag

INDICATIONS & DOSAGE
Antacid—
Adults: 5 to 10 ml or 1 to 2 tablets chewed before swallowing q.i.d., usually after meals and h.s.
Oral replacement therapy in mild hypomagnesemia—
Adults: 5 to 10 ml q.i.d., usually after meals and h.s. Monitor serum magnesium response.

SIDE EFFECTS
GI: *diarrhea,* abdominal pain, nausea.
Metabolic: hypermagnesemia.

INTERACTIONS
None significant.

NURSING CONSIDERATIONS
• Contraindicated in severe renal disease. Use cautiously in elderly patients and in patients with mild renal impairment.
• Usually not used as antacid, even though it is very effective and potent, due to increased frequency of stools. Usually used as laxative.

• Record amount and consistency of stools.
• Shake suspension well; give with small amount of water when used as antacid. When administering through nasogastric tube, be sure tube is placed properly and is patent. After instilling, flush tube with water to assure passage to stomach and maintain tube patency.
• With prolonged use and some degree of renal impairment, watch for symptoms of hypermagnesemia (hypotension, nausea, vomiting, depressed reflexes, respiratory depression, coma). Monitor serum magnesium levels.
• May cause enteric-coated drugs to be released prematurely in stomach. Separate doses by 1 hour.
• If diarrhea occurs with antacid doses, suggest alternative preparation.
• Subcathartic doses also used as oral magnesium replacement therapy in hypomagnesemia.
• Warn patient not to take magnesia magma indiscriminately and not to switch antacids without doctor's advice.
• Make patient responsible for taking his own antacid while hospitalized, if he is able.
• Phillips Milk of Magnesia (flavored) contains no sugar.

magnesium carbonate

INDICATIONS & DOSAGE
Antacid—
Adults: 0.5 to 2 g of powder product or chewable tablets between meals with ½ glass of water.
Laxative—
Adults: 8 g of powder product or chewable tablets with water h.s.

SIDE EFFECTS
GI: *diarrhea,* gastric distention, flatulence, abdominal pain, nausea.
Metabolic: hypermagnesemia.

INTERACTIONS
None significant.

NURSING CONSIDERATIONS
• Contraindicated in severe renal disease. Use cautiously in elderly patients, and in patients with mild renal impairment.
• With prolonged use and some degree of renal impairment, watch for symptoms of hypermagnesemia (hypotension, nausea, vomiting, depressed reflexes, respiratory depression, coma). Monitor serum magnesium levels.
• When used as laxative, do not give other oral drugs 1 to 2 hours before or after.
• Record amount and consistency of stools.
• Warn patient not to take magnesium carbonate indiscriminately and not to switch antacids without doctor's advice.
• Make patient responsible for taking his own antacid while hospitalized if he is able.
• May cause enteric-coated drugs to be released prematurely in stomach. Separate doses by 1 hour.

magnesium oxide
Mag-Ox, Maox, Niko-Mag, Oxabid, Par-Mag, Uro-Mag

INDICATIONS & DOSAGE
Antacid—
Adults: 250 mg to 1 g with water or milk after meals and h.s.
Laxative—
Adults: 4 g with water or milk, usually h.s.
Oral replacement therapy in mild hypomagnesemia—
Adults: 650-mg to 1.3-g tablet or capsule daily. Monitor serum magnesium response.

SIDE EFFECTS
GI: *diarrhea,* nausea, abdominal pain.
Metabolic: hypermagnesemia.

INTERACTIONS
None significant.

NURSING CONSIDERATIONS
• Contraindicated in severe renal disease. Use cautiously in elderly patients, and in patients with mild renal impairment.
• With prolonged use and some degree of renal impairment, watch for symptoms of hypermagnesemia (hypotension, nausea, vomiting, depressed reflexes, respiratory depression, coma). Monitor serum magnesium levels.
• When used as laxative, do not give other oral drugs 1 to 2 hours before or after.
• If diarrhea occurs on antacid doses, suggest alternate preparation.
• Warn patient not to take magnesium oxide indiscriminately and not to switch antacids without doctor's advice.
• Make patient responsible for taking his own antacid while hospitalized if he is able.
• May cause enteric-coated drugs to be released prematurely in stomach. Separate doses by 1 hour.

magnesium trisilicate
Trisomin

INDICATIONS & DOSAGE
Antacid—
Adults: 1- to 4-g tablet t.i.d. chewed well and taken with ½ glass of water.

SIDE EFFECTS
GI: *diarrhea,* gastric distention, flatulence, nausea, abdominal pain.
GU: possible formation of silica renal calculi with prolonged use.
Metabolic: hypermagnesemia.

INTERACTIONS
None significant.

NURSING CONSIDERATIONS
• Contraindicated in severe renal disease. Use cautiously in elderly patients,

and in patients with mild renal impairment.

• With prolonged use and some degree of renal impairment, watch for symptoms of hypermagnesemia (hypotension, nausea, vomiting, depressed reflexes, respiratory depression, coma). Monitor serum magnesium levels.

• If diarrhea occurs on antacid doses, suggest alternate preparation.

• Warn patient not to take magnesium trisilicate indiscriminately and not to switch antacids without doctor's advice.

• Make patient responsible for taking his own antacid while hospitalized, if he is able.

• May cause enteric-coated drugs to be released prematurely in stomach. Separate doses by 1 hour.

oxethazaine
Oxaine M (oxethazaine in aluminum hydroxide gel)

INDICATIONS & DOSAGE
Adjunctive therapy for hyperacidity—
Adults: 10 to 20 mg suspended in 5 to 10 ml aluminum hydroxide gel (equivalent to 5 to 10 ml of commercial product) q.i.d. 15 minutes before meals and h.s.

SIDE EFFECTS
CNS: with high doses (120 mg oxethazaine daily): dizziness, faintness, drowsiness.
GI: anorexia, *constipation*, intestinal obstruction.

INTERACTIONS
None significant.

NURSING CONSIDERATIONS
• Use cautiously in elderly patients, especially those with decreased bowel motility (those receiving antidiarrheals, antispasmodics, or anticholinergics), dehydration, fluid restriction, chronic renal disease, suspected intestinal obstruction.

• Record amount and consistency of stools. Manage constipation with laxatives or stool softeners.

• Shake suspension well; give with small amount of water to assure passage to stomach. When administering antacids through nasogastric tube, be sure tube is placed correctly and is patent; after instilling, flush tube with water to assure passage to stomach and maintain tube patency.

• Caution: Local anesthetic can affect gastric mucosa for up to 6 hours. Prolonged use may mask extension of ulcerative disease and may lead to perforation. May also mask symptoms of gastric neoplasm.

• Warn patient not to take oxethazaine indiscriminately and not to switch antacids without doctor's advice.

• Make patient responsible for taking his own antacid while hospitalized if he is able.

• May cause enteric-coated drugs to be released prematurely in stomach. Separate doses by 1 hour.

simethicone
Mylicon, Silain, Ovol♦♦

INDICATIONS & DOSAGE
Flatulence, functional gastric bloating—
Adults and children over 12 years: 40 to 100 mg after each meal and h.s.

SIDE EFFECTS
GI: expulsion of excessive liberated gas as belching, rectal flatus.

INTERACTIONS
None significant.

NURSING CONSIDERATIONS
• Observe patient for drug effectiveness.

• Warn patient not to take simethicone indiscriminately.

• Tablets should be chewed, not swallowed whole.

sodium bicarbonate
Bell-ans, Soda Mint

INDICATIONS & DOSAGE
Antacid—
Adults: 300 mg to 2 g tablets chewed well and taken with full glass of water, p.r.n.

SIDE EFFECTS
GI: *gastric distention, belching, flatulence.*
GU: renal calculi or crystals.
Metabolic: systemic alkalosis (prolonged use), sodium and water retention; if taken with milk—milk-alkali syndrome.

INTERACTIONS
None significant.

NURSING CONSIDERATIONS
■ Contraindicated in congestive heart failure, hypertension, advanced renal disease, sodium restrictions, tendency toward edema; in patients losing chloride from continuous GI suction, and patients receiving diuretics that cause hypochloremic alkalosis. Also contraindicated for long-term use. Use cautiously in elderly patients and in patients with mild renal impairment.
• Discourage use as antacid. Offer nonabsorbable alternative antacid if it is to be used repeatedly.
• Make patient responsible for taking his own antacid while hospitalized if he is able.
• Do not administer with milk; can cause milk-alkali syndrome (headache, confusion, distaste for food, nausea, vomiting, hypercalcemia, hypercalciuria, calcinosis, hyperphosphatemia).
• May be used with caution to treat chronic metabolic acidosis.

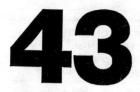

Digestants

bile salts
dehydrocholic acid
glutamic acid hydrochloride
hydrochloric acid, diluted
ketocholanic acids
pancreatin
pancrelipase

MECHANISM OF ACTION

• Bile salts, dehydrocholic acid, and ketocholanic acid stimulate bile flow from the liver, promoting normal digestion and absorption of fats, fat-soluble vitamins, and cholesterol.

• Glutamic and hydrochloric acids replace gastric acid.

• Pancreatin and pancrelipase replace endogenous exocrine pancreatic enzymes and aid intestinal digestion of starches, fats, and proteins.

COMBINATION PRODUCTS

ACCELERASE-PB CAPSULES: lipase 4,000 units, amylase 15,000 units, protease 15,000 units, cellulase 2 mg, mixed conjugated bile salts 65 mg, calcium carbonate 20 mg, l-alkaloids of belladonna 0.2 mg, and phenobarbital 16 mg.

BILOGEN TABLETS: pancreatin 250 mg, ox bile extract 120 mg, oxidized mixed ox bile acids 75 mg, and desoxycholic acid 30 mg.

BILRON♦: bile salts and iron.

BUTIBEL-ZYME TABLETS: proteolytic enzyme 10 mg, amylolytic enzyme 20 mg, lipolytic enzyme 100 mg, cellulolytic enzyme 5 mg, iron ox bile 30 mg, belladonna extract 15 mg, and sodium butabarbital 15 mg.

CHOLAN-HMB TABLETS: dehydrocholic acid 250 mg, homatropine methylbromide 2.5 mg, and phenobarbital 8 mg.

COTAZYM-B TABLETS: lipase 4,000 units, amylase 15,000 units, protease 15,000 units, cellulase 2 mg, and mixed conjugated bile salts 65 mg.

DONNAZYME TABLETS: pancreatin 300 mg, pepsin 150 mg, bile salts 150 mg, hyoscyamine sulfate 0.0518 mg, atropine sulfate 0.0097 mg, hyoscine hydrobromide 0.0033 mg, and phenobarbital 8.1 mg.

ENTOZYME TABLETS♦: pancreatin 300 mg, pepsin 250 mg, and bile salts 150 mg.

ENZYPAN TABLETS: pancreatin (sufficient to digest 19 g protein, 43 g starch, 10 g fat), pepsin 9 mg, and desiccated ox bile 56 mg.

FESTAL ENTERIC-COATED TABLETS: protease 17 units, amylase 10 units, lipase 10 units, bile constituents 25 mg, and hemicellulase 50 mg.

FESTALAN TABLETS: protease 17 units, amylase 10 units, lipase 10 units, lipase 10 units, bile constituents 25 mg, hemicellulase 50 mg, and atropine methylnitrate 1 mg.

KANULASE TABLETS: pancreatin 500 mg, pepsin 150 mg, ox bile extract 100 mg, cellulase 9 mg, and glutamic acid hydrochloride 200 mg.

MURIPSIN TABLETS: glutamic acid hydrochloride 500 mg and pepsin 35 mg.

PHAZYME TABLETS (enteric-coated): pancreatin 240 mg and simethicone 60 mg.

PHAZYME-95 TABLETS (enteric-coated): pancreatin 240 mg and simethicone 95 mg.

PHAZYME-PB TABLETS (enteric-coated): pancreatin 240 mg, phenobarbital 15 mg, and simethicone 60 mg.
PROBILAGOL LIQUID: d-sorbitol 4.5 g and homatropine methylbromide 1 mg/5 ml.
RO-BILE TABLETS (enteric-coated): enzyme concentrate 75 mg (lipase equivalent to 750 mg pancreatin, amylase and protease equivalent to 300 mg pancreatin), ox bile extract 100 mg, dehydrocholic acid 30 mg, belladonna extract 8 mg, and pepsin 260 mg.

bile salts
Biso, Chobile, Ox-Bile Extract
Enseals, Bilron◆

INDICATIONS & DOSAGE
Uncomplicated constipation—
Adults and children: 300 to 500 mg (enteric-coated tablets) b.i.d. or t.i.d. after meals; or 150 to 450 mg capsules with or after meals.

SIDE EFFECTS
GI: loose stools and mild cramping (with large doses).

INTERACTIONS
None significant.

NURSING CONSIDERATIONS
• Contraindicated in marked hepatic dysfunction and complete biliary obstruction, except in malnutrition with steatorrhea and vitamin K deficiency with hypoprothrombinemia.
• Use Ox-Bile Extract cautiously in obstructive jaundice.
• Don't use Ox-Bile Extract if other preparations are available, since it doesn't provide an adequate amount of conjugated bile salts.
• Has not been shown to effectively treat bile salt deficiency.

dehydrocholic acid
Cholan-DH, Decholin, Dycholium◆◆, Hepahydrin, Idrocrine◆◆, Neocholan**

INDICATIONS & DOSAGE
Constipation, biliary tract conditions—
Adults: 250 to 500 mg P.O. b.i.d. to t.i.d. after meals for 4 to 6 weeks.

SIDE EFFECTS
GI: diarrhea with weakness (in large doses).

INTERACTIONS
None significant.

NURSING CONSIDERATIONS
• Contraindicated in complete mechanical biliary obstruction. Use cautiously in prostatic hypertrophy, acute hepatitis, asthmatic bronchitis, elderly patients, partial GI or GU tract obstruction.
• Do not use when patient is nauseated or vomiting, or has abdominal pain.
• Simultaneous administration of bile salts may be needed in biliary fistula.
• Used to prevent bacterial accumulation after biliary tract surgery.
• Probably much less effective than natural bile salts in lowering surface tension and promoting absorption.
• Don't use dehydrocholic acid to accelerate rate of healing in patients with jaundice.
• Frequent use may result in dependence on laxatives.

glutamic acid hydrochloride
Acidulin◆

INDICATIONS & DOSAGE
Hypoacidity—
Adults: 1 to 3 capsules P.O. t.i.d. before meals.

Italicized side effects are common or life-threatening.
*Liquid form contains alcohol.   **May contain tartrazine.

SIDE EFFECTS
Metabolic: systemic acidosis in massive overdose.

INTERACTIONS
None significant.

NURSING CONSIDERATIONS
• Contraindicated in gastric hyperacidity or peptic ulcer.
• Use instead of hydrochloric acid so tooth enamel won't be damaged; however, glutamic acid HCl is not as effective in decreasing gastric pH.
• Gastric acidifier.

hydrochloric acid, diluted

INDICATIONS & DOSAGE
Hypoacidity—
Adults: 2 to 8 ml P.O. well diluted in 25 to 50 ml water.

SIDE EFFECTS
Metabolic: systemic acidosis in massive overdose.
Other: *tooth enamel damage.*

INTERACTIONS
None significant.

NURSING CONSIDERATIONS
• Contraindicated in gastric hyperacidity or peptic ulcer.
• Sip, during meal, through glass straw to protect tooth enamel.
• Alleviates primary functional hypoacidity or hypoacidity caused by organic disease such as pernicious anemia, certain allergies, chronic gastritis, other chronic debilitating diseases, or gastric resection.
• Gastric acidifier; usual dose not sufficient to release free acid in stomach; no evidence that even larger doses are beneficial for this.

ketocholanic acids
Ketochol

INDICATIONS & DOSAGE
Constipation, biliary tract conditions—
Adults: 250 mg to 500 mg P.O. t.i.d. with meals.

SIDE EFFECTS
None reported.

INTERACTIONS
None significant.

NURSING CONSIDERATIONS
• Use cautiously in elderly patients and in those with prostatic hypertrophy, acute hepatitis, asthmatic bronchitis, partial GI or GU tract obstruction.
• Bile salt; derived from beef bile.
• Approximately equivalent to 250 mg dehydrocholic acid.
• Do not use when patient is nauseated or vomiting, or has abdominal pain.
• Frequent use may result in dependence on laxatives.

pancreatin
Elzyme, Viokase

INDICATIONS & DOSAGE
Exocrine pancreatic secretion insufficiency, digestive aid in cystic fibrosis—
Adults and children: 325 mg to 1 g P.O. before or with meals.

SIDE EFFECTS
GI: nausea, diarrhea with high doses.
Other: hyperuricosuria (with high doses).

INTERACTIONS
None significant.

NURSING CONSIDERATIONS
• Use cautiously in patients who are hypersensitive to pork. Bovine preparations are available for these patients, but are less effective.

- Balance fat, protein, and starch intake properly to avoid indigestion. Dosage varies according to degree of maldigestion and malabsorption, amount of fat in diet, and enzyme activity of individual preparations.
- Pancreatin therapy shouldn't delay or replace treatment of primary disorder.
- Adequate replacement decreases number of bowel movements and improves stool consistency.
- Use only after confirmed diagnosis of exocrine pancreatic insufficiency. Not effective in GI disorders unrelated to pancreatic enzyme deficiency.
- For infants, mix powder with applesauce and give with meals. Avoid inhalation of powder. Older children may swallow capsules with food.
- Enteric coating on some products may reduce availability of enzyme in upper portion of jejunum where it is primarily required.
- Store in tight containers at room temperature.

pancrelipase
Cotazym♦, Ilozyme, Ku-Zyme HP, Pancrease

INDICATIONS & DOSAGE
Dose must be titrated to patient's response. Exocrine pancreatic secretion insufficiency, cystic fibrosis in adults and children, steatorrhea and other disorders of fat metabolism secondary to insufficient pancreatic enzymes—
Adults and children: dosage range 1 to 3 capsules or tablets P.O. before or with meals and 1 capsule or tablet with snack; or 1 to 2 powder packets before meals or snacks.

SIDE EFFECTS
GI: *nausea,* diarrhea with high doses.

INTERACTIONS
None significant.

NURSING CONSIDERATIONS
- Contraindicated in patients with severe pork hypersensitivity.
- Pancrelipase therapy shouldn't delay or replace treatment of primary disorder.
- Use only after confirmed diagnosis of exocrine pancreatic insufficiency. Not effective in GI disorders unrelated to enzyme deficiency.
- Lipase activity greater than with other pancreatic enzymes.
- For infants, mix powder from capsules with applesauce and give at mealtime. Avoid inhalation of powder. Older children may swallow capsules with food.
- Dosage varies with degree of maldigestion and malabsorption, amount of fat in diet, and enzyme activity of individual preparations.
- Adequate replacement decreases number of bowel movements and improves stool consistency.
- Enteric coating on some products may reduce availability of enzyme in upper portion of jejunum where it is primarily required.
- Crushing or chewing of capsule interferes with the enteric coating.

Italicized side effects are common or life-threatening.
∗Liquid form contains alcohol.   ∗∗May contain tartrazine.

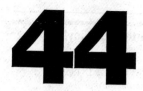

Antidiarrheals

bismuth subcarbonate
bismuth subgallate
bismuth subsalicylate
calcium polycarbophil
diphenoxylate hydrochloride
   (with atropine sulfate)
kaolin and pectin mixtures
lactobacillus
loperamide
opium tincture
opium tincture, camphorated

MECHANISM OF ACTION

• Bismuth subcarbonate, subgallate, and subsalicylate have a mild water-binding capacity; they also may adsorb toxins and provide protective coating for intestinal mucosa.

• Calcium polycarbophil absorbs free fecal water, thereby producing formed stools.

• Diphenoxylate hydrochloride and opium tinctures increase smooth-muscle tone in the GI tract, inhibit motility and propulsion, and diminish digestive secretions.

• Kaolin and pectin decrease the stool's fluid content, although *total* water loss seems to remain the same.

• Lactobacillus cultures may suppress the growth of pathogenic microorganisms to help reestablish normal intestinal flora.

• Loperamide inhibits peristaltic activity, prolonging transit of intestinal contents.

COMBINATION PRODUCTS

CORRECTIVE MIXTURE*: zinc sulfocarbolate 10 mg, phenyl salicylate 22 mg, bismuth subsalicylate 85 mg, pepsin 45 mg, and alcohol 1.5% in 5-ml suspension.

CORRECTIVE MIXTURE WITH PAREGORIC*: paregoric 0.6 ml, zinc sulfocarbolate 10 mg, phenyl salicylate 22 mg, bismuth subsalicylate 85 mg, pepsin 45 mg, and alcohol 2% in 5-ml suspension.

DONNAGEL SUSPENSION♦*: kaolin 6 g, pectin 142.8 mg, hyoscyamine sulfate 0.1037 mg, atropine sulfate 0.0194 mg, hyoscine hydrobromide 0.0065 mg, and alcohol 3.8% in 30-ml suspension.

DONNAGEL-MB♦♦*: kaolin 6 g, pectin 142.8 mg, and alcohol 3.8% in 30-ml suspension.

DONNAGEL-PG*: powdered opium 24 mg, kaolin 6 g, pectin 142.8 mg, hyoscyamine sulfate 0.1037 mg, atropine sulfate 0.0194 mg, hyoscine hydrobromide 0.0065 mg, and alcohol 5% in 30-ml suspension.

KENPECTIN-P*: opium 16.27 mg (equivalent to 3.7 ml paregoric), kaolin 5.85 g, pectin 195 mg, alcohol 6%, and aluminum hydroxide 650 mg in 30-ml suspension.

PARELIXIR*: tincture opium 0.2 ml, pectin 145 mg, and alcohol 18% in 30-ml suspension.

PAREPECTOLIN*: opium 15 mg (equivalent to paregoric 3.7 ml), kaolin 5.85 g, pectin 162 mg, and alcohol 0.69% in 30-ml suspension.

PECTOCEL: kaolin 5.85 g, pectin 292.5 mg, and zinc phenolsulfonate 73.13 mg in 30-ml suspension.

PEKTAMALT: kaolin 6.5 g, pectin 600 mg, potassium gluconate 1.1 g,

---

and sodium citrate 318 mg in 30-ml suspension.
POLYMAGMA PLAIN: activated attapulgite 500 mg, pectin 45 mg, and hydrated alumina powder 50 mg.

bismuth subcarbonate

bismuth subgallate
Devrom

INDICATIONS & DOSAGE
Deodorize fecal odors in colostomy and ileostomy (subcarbonate)—
Adults: 600 mg P.O. t.i.d. after each meal.
Mild, nonspecific diarrhea (subgallate)—
Adults: 1 to 2 tablets chewed or swallowed whole t.i.d.

SIDE EFFECTS
CNS: personality changes. Prolonged use (especially in colostomy and ileostomy patients) may lead to reversible deterioration of mental ability, confusion, tremors, and impaired coordination.
GI: *transient darkened tongue and stool* (both with subgallate); fecal impaction or ulceration (in infants, elderly, or debilitated patients) after chronic use; *constipation.*

INTERACTIONS
None significant.

NURSING CONSIDERATIONS
• GI adsorbent.
• Don't use in place of specific therapy for underlying cause.
• May reduce absorption of other P.O. drugs, requiring dosage adjustment.
• Store in tight, light-resistant containers.

bismuth subsalicylate
Pepto-Bismol

INDICATIONS & DOSAGE
Mild, nonspecific diarrhea—
Adults: 30 ml or 2 tablets q ½ to 1 hour up to a maximum of 8 doses and for no longer than 2 days.
Children 10 to 14 years: 20 ml.
Children 6 to 10 years: 10 ml.
Children 3 to 6 years: 5 ml.

SIDE EFFECTS
GI: temporary darkening of tongue and stools.
Other: salicylism (high doses).

INTERACTIONS
None significant.

NURSING CONSIDERATIONS
• Has been used successfully to treat turista (traveler's diarrhea).
• Warn patient that this drug contains a large amount of salicylate. Should be used cautiously in patients already taking aspirin products.

calcium polycarbophil
Mitrolan

INDICATIONS & DOSAGE
Diarrhea associated with irritable bowel syndrome, as well as acute nonspecific diarrhea (tablets must be chewed before swallowing)—
Adults: 1 g P.O. q.i.d. as required. Maximum 6 g in 24-hour period.
Children 6 to 12 years: 500 mg P.O. t.i.d. as required. Maximum 3 g in 24-hour period.
Children 3 to 6 years: 500 mg P.O. b.i.d. as required. Maximum 1.5 g in 24-hour period.

SIDE EFFECTS
GI: abdominal fullness and increased flatus, intestinal obstruction.

INTERACTIONS
None significant.

NURSING CONSIDERATIONS
• Contraindicated in patients with signs of GI obstruction.
• Don't use for more than 2 days.
• Don't use in place of specific therapy for underlying cause of the diarrhea.
• Advise patient to chew tablets thoroughly before swallowing. When used as an antidiarrheal, tell patient *not* to drink a glass of water afterward.
• For episodes of severe diarrhea, the dose may be repeated every half hour, but maximum daily dosage should not be exceeded.
• Also used as a bulk laxative.

---

diphenoxylate hydrochloride (with atropine sulfate)
Controlled Substance Schedule V
Colonaid, Lofene, Loflo, Lomo-Plus, Lomotil♦*, Lotrol, Ro-Diphen-Atro, SK-Diphenoxylate

INDICATIONS & DOSAGE
Acute, nonspecific diarrhea—
Adults: initially, 5 mg P.O. q.i.d., then adjust dose to individual response.
Children 2 to 12 years: 0.3 to 0.4 mg/kg P.O. daily in divided doses, using liquid form only.
Don't use in children under 2 years.

SIDE EFFECTS
CNS: *sedation, dizziness,* headache, drowsiness, lethargy, restlessness, depression, euphoria.
CV: tachycardia.
EENT: mydriasis.
GI: *dry mouth,* nausea, vomiting, abdominal discomfort or distention, *paralytic ileus,* anorexia, fluid retention in bowel (may mask depletion of extracellular fluid and electrolytes, especially in young children treated for acute gastroenteritis).
GU: urinary retention.

Skin: pruritus, giant urticaria, rash.
Other: possibly physical dependence in long-term use, angioedema, respiratory depression.

INTERACTIONS
None significant.

NURSING CONSIDERATIONS
• Contraindicated in acute diarrhea resulting from poison until toxic material is eliminated from GI tract; in acute diarrhea caused by organisms that penetrate intestinal mucosa; in diarrhea resulting from antibiotic-induced pseudomembranous enterocolitis; and in jaundiced patients. Use cautiously in children, and in hepatic disease, narcotic dependence, and pregnancy. Use cautiously in acute ulcerative colitis. Stop therapy immediately if abdominal distention or other signs of toxic megacolon develop.
• Risk of physical dependence increases with high dosage and long-term use. Discourage long-term or unsupervised use. Atropine sulfate is included to discourage abuse.
• Don't use for more than 2 days when treating acute diarrhea.
• Warn patient not to exceed recommended dosage.
• Dehydration, especially in young children, may increase risk of delayed toxicity. Correct fluid and electrolyte disturbances before starting drug.
• Dose of 2.5 mg as effective as 5 ml camphorated tincture of opium.
• Not indicated in treatment of antibiotic-induced diarrhea.
• Not likely to be effective if there is no response within 48 hours.

---

kaolin and pectin mixtures
Baropectin, Kaoparin, Kaopectate♦, Kapectin, Keotin, Pectokay

INDICATIONS & DOSAGE
Mild, nonspecific diarrhea—

Adults: 60 to 120 ml after each bowel movement.
Children over 12 years: 60 ml after each bowel movement.
Children 6 to 12 years: 30 to 60 ml after each bowel movement.
Children 3 to 6 years: 15 to 30 ml after each bowel movement.

SIDE EFFECTS
GI: drug absorbs nutrients and enzymes; fecal impaction or ulceration in infants, elderly, debilitated patients after chronic use; constipation.

INTERACTIONS
None significant.

NURSING CONSIDERATIONS
• Contraindicated in suspected obstructive bowel lesions.
• Don't use for more than 2 days.
• Don't use in place of specific therapy for underlying cause.
• May reduce absorption of other P.O. drugs, requiring dosage adjustments.
• GI absorbent.

lactobacillus
Bacid♦, DoFUS, Lactinex♦

INDICATIONS & DOSAGE
Diarrhea, especially that caused by antibiotics—
Adults: 2 capsules (Bacid) P.O. b.i.d., t.i.d., or q.i.d., preferably with milk; or 4 tablets or 1 packet (Lactinex) P.O. t.i.d. or q.i.d., preferably with food, milk, or juice; or 1 tablet (DoFUS) P.O. daily before meals.

SIDE EFFECTS
GI: (with Bacid and DoFUS) increased intestinal flatus at beginning of therapy; subsides with continued therapy.

INTERACTIONS
None significant.

NURSING CONSIDERATIONS
• Bacid and DoFUS contraindicated in fever.
• Don't use Bacid for more than 2 days.
• Store in refrigerator.
• Diet containing large amounts of carbohydrate (up to 400 g), such as lactose, lactulose, and dextrin, may be more effective than lactobacillus in reestablishing normal flora after antibiotic therapy.
• Controversial form of diarrhea treatment.
• May be used prophylactically in patients with history of antibiotic-induced diarrhea.

loperamide
Controlled Substance Schedule V
Imodium♦

INDICATIONS & DOSAGE
Acute, nonspecific diarrhea—
Adults: initially, 4 mg P.O., then 2 mg after each unformed stool. Maximum 16 mg daily.
Chronic diarrhea—
Adults: initially, 4 mg P.O., then 2 mg after each unformed stool until diarrhea subsides. Adjust dose to individual response.

SIDE EFFECTS
CNS: drowsiness, fatigue, dizziness.
GI: dry mouth; abdominal pain, distention, or discomfort; *constipation;* nausea; vomiting.
Skin: rash.

INTERACTIONS
None significant.

NURSING CONSIDERATIONS
• Contraindicated in acute diarrhea resulting from poison until toxic material is removed from GI tract, when constipation must be avoided, and in acute diarrhea caused by organisms that penetrate intestinal mucosa. Use cautiously

---

Italicized side effects are common or life-threatening.
♦Liquid form contains alcohol.   **♦♦**May contain tartrazine.

in patients with severe prostatic hypertrophy, hepatic disease, and history of narcotic dependence.
• Stop drug immediately if abdominal distention or other symptoms develop in patients with acute ulcerative colitis.
• In acute diarrhea, stop drug if no improvement within 48 hours; in chronic diarrhea, stop drug if no improvement after giving 16 mg daily for at least 10 days.
• Appears to have low potential for abuse.
• Warn patient not to exceed recommended dosage.
• Produces antidiarrheal action similar to diphenoxylate HCl but without as many CNS side effects; three times more potent than diphenoxylate HCl.

opium tincture

opium tincture, camphorated
Controlled Substance Schedule III
Paregoric♦

INDICATIONS & DOSAGE
Acute, nonspecific diarrhea—
Adults: 0.6 ml opium tincture (range 0.3 to 1 ml) P.O. q.i.d. Maximum dose 6 ml daily; or 5 to 10 ml camphorated opium tincture daily b.i.d., t.i.d., or q.i.d. until diarrhea subsides.
Children: 0.25 to 0.5 ml/kg camphorated opium tincture daily, b.i.d., t.i.d., or q.i.d. until diarrhea subsides.

SIDE EFFECTS
GI: nausea, vomiting.

Other: physical dependence after long-term use.

INTERACTIONS
None significant.

NURSING CONSIDERATIONS
• Contraindicated in acute diarrhea resulting from poisons until toxic material is removed from GI tract, and in acute diarrhea caused by organisms that penetrate intestinal mucosa. Use cautiously in asthma, severe prostatic hypertrophy, hepatic disease, narcotic dependence.
• Risk of physical dependence increases with long-term use. Discourage long-term or unsupervised use.
• Don't use for more than 2 days.
• An effective and prompt-acting antidiarrheal.
• Opium content of opium tincture 25 times greater than camphorated tincture of opium. Camphorated opium tincture is more dilute, and teaspoonful doses easier to measure than dropper quantities of opium tincture.
• Not used as widely today as in past, but unique because dose can be adjusted precisely to patient's needs.
• Milky fluid forms when camphorated opium tincture is added to water.
• Camphorated opium tincture 0.06 to 0.5 ml daily has been used to treat infants with mild narcotic physical dependence.
• Narcotic antagonist naloxone can reverse the respiratory depression resulting from overdose.

45

Laxatives

barley-malt extract
bisacodyl
calcium polycarbophil
cascara sagrada
castor oil
danthron
docusate calcium (formerly dioctyl calcium sulfosuccinate)
docusate potassium (formerly dioctyl potassium sulfosuccinate)
docusate sodium (formerly dioctyl sodium sulfosuccinate)
glycerin
lactulose
magnesium salts
methylcellulose
mineral oil
phenolphthalein
psyllium
senna
sodium biphosphate
sodium phosphate

MECHANISM OF ACTION

- Bulk-forming laxatives absorb water and expand to increase bulk and moisture content of the stool. The increased bulk encourages peristalsis and bowel movement.
- Emollient laxatives, or stool softeners, reduce surface tension of interfacing liquid contents of the bowel. This mechanism, or detergent activity, promotes incorporation of additional liquid into the stool, forming a softer mass.
- Among the hyperosmolar laxatives, glycerin draws water from the tissues into the feces and thus stimulates evacuation.

  Lactulose produces an osmotic effect in the colon and is biodegraded by the intestinal flora into lactic, formic, and acetic acids. Distention of the bowel from fluid accumulation promotes peristalsis and bowel movement.

  The saline agents (magnesium salts, sodium biphosphate, and sodium phosphate) produce an osmotic effect in the small intestine by drawing water into the intestinal lumen. Fluid accumulation produces distention, which then encourages peristalsis and bowel movement. Saline laxatives also promote cholecystokinin secretion, stimulating intestinal motility and inhibiting fluid and electrolyte absorption from the jejunum and ileum.
- Lubricant laxatives increase water retention in the stool by creating a barrier between colon wall and feces that prevents colonic reabsorption of fecal water.
- Stimulant laxatives may increase peristalsis by direct effect on the smooth muscle of the intestine. Although the precise mechanism is unknown, stimulant laxatives are thought either to irritate the musculature or to stimulate the colonic intramural plexus. These drugs also promote fluid accumulation in the colon and small intestine, increasing the laxative effect.

COMBINATION PRODUCTS

AGORAL: mineral oil 28% and white phenolphthalein 1.3% in emulsion, with tragacanth, agar, egg albumin, acacia, and glycerin.
CASYLLIUM: psyllium husk powder 4.1

Italicized side effects are common or life-threatening.
*Liquid form contains alcohol. **May contain tartrazine.

g, debittered fluidextract cascara 3 ml, and prune powder 1.2 g per 6 g.

COMFOLAX-PLUS: docusate sodium 100 mg and casanthranol 30 mg.

CORRECTOL: yellow phenolphthalein 64.8 mg and docusate sodium 100 mg.

DIALOSE: docusate sodium 100 mg and sodium carboxymethylcellulose 400 mg.

DIALOSE-PLUS: docusate sodium 100 mg and casanthranol 30 mg.

DORBANTYL: docusate sodium 50 mg and danthron 25 mg.

DORBANTYL FORTE: docusate sodium 100 mg and danthron 50 mg.

DOXAN-TABLETS: docusate sodium 60 mg and danthron 50 mg.

DOXIDAN♦: docusate calcium 60 mg and danthron 50 mg.

D-S-S PLUS: docusate sodium 100 mg and casanthranol 30 mg.

HALEY'S M-O: mineral oil (25%) and magnesium hydroxide.

HYDROCIL, FORTIFIED: blond psyllium coating 50% and casanthranol (with dextrose) 30 mg per 6 g.

KONDREMUL WITH CASCARA♦: heavy mineral oil 55%, cascara sagrada extract 660 mg per 15 ml, and Irish moss as emulsifier.

KONDREMUL WITH PHENOLPHTHALEIN♦: heavy mineral oil 55%, white phenolphthalein 147 mg per 15 ml, and Irish moss as emulsifier.

OXIPHEN: phenolphthalein 32.4 mg, cascara sagrada extract 32.4 mg, aloin 8.1 mg, sodium glycocholate 16.2 mg, and sodium taurocholate 16.2 mg.

PERI-COLACE♦ (capsules): docusate sodium 100 mg and casanthranol 30 mg.

PERI-COLACE (syrup): docusate sodium 60 mg and casanthranol 30 mg per 15 ml.

PETROGALAR WITH PHENOLPHTHALEIN: mineral oil 65% and phenolphthalein 0.3%.

SENOKOT-S♦: docusate sodium 50 mg and standardized senna concentrate 187 mg.

SENOKOT WITH PSYLLIUM: psyllium 1 g and standardized senna concentrate 326 mg per teaspoon.

SYLLAMALT: malt soup extract 3.5 g and powdered psyllium seed husks 3.5 g per rounded teaspoon.

SYLLAMALT EFFERVESCENT: malt-soup extract 1.75 g, powdered psyllium seed husks 1.75 g, sodium bicarbonate, and citric acid per rounded teaspoon.

barley-malt extract
Maltsupex

INDICATIONS & DOSAGE
Constipation—
Adults: 4 tablets P.O. with meals and at bedtime for 4 days, then 2 to 4 tablets at bedtime; or 2 tablespoonfuls powder or liquid b.i.d. for 3 to 4 days, until stools become soft, then 1 to 2 tablespoonfuls at bedtime.

Children over 2 months: ½ to 2 tablespoonfuls in milk or on cereal daily or b.i.d.

Infants 1 or 2 months: ½ tablespoonful daily with milk or cereal. To prevent constipation, may add 1 to 2 teaspoonfuls to each day's feeding.

SIDE EFFECTS
GI: loose stools.
Other: laxative dependence with frequent or long-term use.

INTERACTIONS
None significant.

NURSING CONSIDERATIONS
• Contraindicated in abdominal pain, nausea, vomiting, or other symptoms of appendicitis or acute surgical abdomen, and in intestinal obstruction or ulceration, disabling adhesion, or difficulty swallowing.
• In patients with diabetes, allow for carbohydrate content of approximately 14 g/tablespoon of liquid, 13 g/tablespoon of powder, and 0.6 g/tablet.
• Tell patient to take with at least 8 oz (240 ml) liquid.

• For short-term use. Before giving, determine if patient has adequate fluid intake, exercise, and diet. Tell him that dietary sources of bulk include bran and other cereals, fresh fruit, and vegetables.

• Infants usually need diet change to increase bulk in addition to laxative.

• Laxative effect usually takes 12 to 24 hours; may be delayed 3 days.

• Bulk laxative; increases bulk and water content of stool.

• Not absorbed systemically; nontoxic.

• Reduces fecal pH. Especially useful in constipated postpartum mothers, debilitated patients, infants, patients with chronic laxative abuse, irritable bowel syndrome, diverticular disease, and to clear the colon before barium enema examination.

bisacodyl
Biscolax♦**, Codylax, Dulcolax♦, Dulcolax Micro-enema♦♦, Fleet Bisacodyl, Rolax

INDICATIONS & DOSAGE
Chronic constipation; preparation for delivery, surgery, or rectal or bowel examination—
Adults: 10 to 15 mg P.O. in evening or before breakfast. Up to 30 mg may be used for thorough evacuation needed for examinations or surgery.
Children over 3 years: 5 to 10 mg P.O.
Rectal: **Adults, and children over 2 years:** 10 mg.
Under 2 years: 5 mg.
Enema: **Adults:** 1.25 oz.
Children under 6 years: approximately ½ contents of micro enema.

SIDE EFFECTS
CNS: muscle weakness in excessive use.
GI: *nausea, vomiting, abdominal cramps,* diarrhea in high doses, *burning sensation in rectum with suppositories.*
Metabolic: alkalosis, hypokalemia, tet-

any, protein-losing enteropathy in excessive use, fluid and electrolyte imbalance.
Other: laxative dependence in long-term or excessive use.

INTERACTIONS
None significant.

NURSING CONSIDERATIONS
• Contraindicated in patients with abdominal pain, nausea, vomiting, or other symptoms of appendicitis or acute surgical abdomen, or in rectal fissures or ulcerated hemorrhoids.

• Tell patient to swallow enteric-coated tablet whole to avoid GI irritation. Don't give with milk or antacids. Begins to act 6 to 12 hours after oral administration.

• Soft, formed stool usually produced 15 to 60 minutes after rectal administration. Time administration of drug so as not to interfere with scheduled activities or sleep.

• Tablets and suppositories may be used together to cleanse colon before and after surgery and before barium enema.

• Use for short-term treatment. Stimulant laxative, class of laxative most abused. Discourage excessive use.

• Before giving for constipation, determine if patient has adequate fluid intake, exercise, and diet. Tell him that dietary sources of bulk include bran and other cereals, fresh fruit, and vegetables.

• Store tablets and suppositories at temperature below 30° C. (86° F.).

• Tell patient to report adverse side effects to the doctor.

calcium polycarbophil
Mitrolan

INDICATIONS & DOSAGE
Constipation (tablets must be chewed before swallowing)—

Italicized side effects are common or life-threatening.
*Liquid form contains alcohol.   **May contain tartrazine.

Adults: 1 g P.O. q.i.d. as required. Maximum 6 g in 24-hour period.
Children 6 to 12 years: 500 mg P.O. t.i.d. as required. Maximum 3 g in 24-hour period.
Children 3 to 6 years: 500 mg P.O. b.i.d. as required. Maximum 1.5 g in 24-hour period.

SIDE EFFECTS
GI: abdominal fullness and increased flatus, intestinal obstruction.
Other: laxative dependence in long-term or excessive use.

INTERACTIONS
None significant.

NURSING CONSIDERATIONS
• Contraindicated in patients with signs of GI obstruction.
• Rectal bleeding or failure to respond to therapy may indicate need for surgery.
• Use for short-term treatment.
• Before giving for constipation, determine if patient has adequate fluid intake, sufficient exercise, and proper diet. Tell him that dietary sources of bulk include bran and other cereals, fresh fruit, and vegetables.
• Advise patient to chew the tablets thoroughly and drink a full glass of water with each dose.
• Not absorbed systemically; nontoxic.
• Bulk laxative; increases bulk and water content of stool.
• Also used to treat diarrhea because it absorbs fecal water.

cascara sagrada

cascara sagrada aromatic fluidextract

cascara sagrada fluidextract

INDICATIONS & DOSAGE
Acute constipation; preparation for bowel or rectal examination—
Adults: 325 mg cascara sagrada tablets P.O. h.s.; or 1 ml fluidextract daily; or 5 ml aromatic fluidextract daily.
Children 2 to 12 years: ½ adult dose.
Children under 2 years: ¼ adult dose.

SIDE EFFECTS
GI: *nausea;* vomiting; diarrhea; loss of normal bowel function with excessive use; *abdominal cramps,* especially in severe constipation; malabsorption of nutrients; "cathartic colon" (syndrome resembling ulcerative colitis radiologically and pathologically) after chronic misuse; discoloration of rectal mucosa after long-term use.
Metabolic: hypokalemia, protein enteropathy, electrolyte imbalance in excessive use.
Other: laxative dependence in long-term or excessive use.

INTERACTIONS
None significant.

NURSING CONSIDERATIONS
• Contraindicated in abdominal pain, nausea, vomiting, or other symptoms of appendicitis or acute surgical abdomen; in acute surgical delirium, fecal impaction, intestinal obstruction or perforation. Use cautiously when rectal bleeding is present.
• Aromatic cascara fluidextract is less active and less bitter than nonaromatic fluidextract.
• Liquid preparations more reliable than solid dosage forms.

Unmarked trade names available in the United States only.
♦ Also available in Canada.   ♦ ♦ Available in Canada only.

• Drug of choice among stimulant laxatives. Use for short-term treatment.
• Before giving for constipation, determine if patient has adequate fluid intake, exercise, and diet. Tell him that dietary sources of bulk include bran and other cereals, fresh fruit, and vegetables.
• May turn alkaline urine red-pink and acidic urine yellow-brown.
• Monitor serum electrolytes during prolonged use.

castor oil
Alphamul, Neoloid♦, Purge

INDICATIONS & DOSAGE
Preparation for rectal or bowel examination, or surgery; acute constipation (rarely)—
Adults: 15 to 60 ml P.O. as liquid or 1.25 to 3.7 mg P.O. as tablet.
Children over 2 years: 5 to 15 ml P.O.
Children under 2 years: 1.25 to 7.5 ml P.O.
Infants: up to 4 ml P.O. Increased dose produces no greater effect.

SIDE EFFECTS
GI: *nausea;* vomiting; diarrhea; loss of normal bowel function with excessive use; *abdominal cramps,* especially in severe constipation; malabsorption of nutrients; "cathartic colon" (syndrome resembling ulcerative colitis radiologically and pathologically) in chronic misuse. May cause constipation after catharsis.
GU: pelvic congestion in menstruating women.
Metabolic: hypokalemia, protein enteropathy, other electrolyte imbalance in excessive use.
Other: laxative dependence in long-term or excessive use.

INTERACTIONS
None significant.

NURSING CONSIDERATIONS
• Contraindicated in ulcerative bowel lesions; during menstruation; in abdominal pain, nausea, vomiting, or other symptoms of appendicitis or acute surgical abdomen; in anal or rectal fissures; fecal impaction; intestinal obstruction or perforation. Use cautiously in rectal bleeding.
• Failure to respond may indicate acute condition requiring surgery.
• Give with juice or carbonated beverage to mask oily taste. Ice held in mouth before taking drug will help prevent tasting it.
• Shake emulsion well. Store below 4.4° C. (40° F.). Don't freeze.
• Give on empty stomach for best results.
• Produces complete evacuation after 3 hours. Tell patient that after castor oil has emptied bowel, he will not have bowel movement for 1 to 2 days.
• Time drug administration so that it doesn't interfere with scheduled activities or sleep.
• Monitor serum electrolytes during prolonged use.
• Generally used before diagnostic testing or therapy requiring thorough evacuation of GI tract.
• Use for short-term treatment. Not recommended for routine use; useful for acute constipation not responsive to milder laxatives.
• Before giving for constipation, determine if patient has adequate fluid intake, exercise, and diet. Tell him that dietary sources of bulk include bran and other cereals, fresh fruit, and vegetables.
• Stimulant laxative.
• Increased intestinal motility lessens absorption of concomitantly administered P.O. drugs. Reschedule dose.
• Castor oil affects the small intestine. Regular use may cause excessive loss of water and salt.

Italicized side effects are common or life-threatening.
*Liquid form contains alcohol.   **May contain tartrazine.

danthron
Dorbane♦, Duolax, Modane♦*,
Modane Mild♦

INDICATIONS & DOSAGE
Acute constipation, preparation for rectal or bowel examination, postsurgical and postpartum constipation—
Adults and children: 37.5 to 150 mg P.O. after or with evening meal.

SIDE EFFECTS
GI: *nausea;* vomiting; diarrhea; loss of normal bowel function in excessive use; *abdominal cramps,* especially in severe constipation; malabsorption of nutrients; "cathartic colon" (syndrome resembling ulcerative colitis radiologically and pathologically) in chronic misuse; discoloration of rectal mucosa in long-term use.
Metabolic: hypokalemia, protein enteropathy, electrolyte imbalance in excessive use.
Other: laxative dependence in long-term or excessive use.

INTERACTIONS
None significant.

NURSING CONSIDERATIONS
• Contraindicated in abdominal pain, nausea, vomiting, or other symptoms of appendicitis or acute surgical abdomen; in intestinal obstruction or perforation; and in hepatic dysfunction. Use cautiously in rectal bleeding or fecal impaction.
• Give with fruit juice or carbonated beverage to mask oily taste.
• Give on empty stomach for best results.
• Produces complete evacuation of bowel in 6 to 24 hours. Tell patient that he will not have another bowel movement for 1 to 2 days. Time drug administration so that it doesn't interfere with scheduled activities or sleep.
• Generally used before diagnostic testing or therapy requiring thorough evacuation of GI tract.
• Agent of choice for cardiac patients; reduces strain of evacuation.
• Use for short-term treatment. Not recommended for routine use; useful for acute constipation not responsive to milder laxatives.
• Before giving for constipation, determine if patient has adequate fluid intake, exercise, and diet. Tell him that dietary sources of bulk include bran and other cereals, fresh fruit, and vegetables.
• May discolor alkaline urine red-pink and acidic urine yellow-brown.
• Stimulant laxative.
• Monitor serum electrolytes during prolonged use.

docusate calcium (formerly dioctyl calcium sulfosuccinate)
Surfak♦

docusate potassium (formerly dioctyl potassium sulfosuccinate)
Kasof

docusate sodium (formerly dioctyl sodium sulfosuccinate)
Bu-Lax, Colace*, Comfolax**, Disonate, Doctate, Doxinate, D.S.S., Laxinate, Regutol, Roctate

INDICATIONS & DOSAGE
Stool softener—
Adults and older children: 50 to 300 mg (docusate sodium) P.O. daily or 240 mg (docusate calcium and docusate potassium) P.O. daily until bowel movements are normal; or 5 ml (250 mg) (docusate potassium) enema.
Children over 12 years: 2 ml (100 mg) (docusate potassium) enema.
Children 6 to 12 years: 40 to 120 mg (docusate sodium) P.O. daily.

Children 3 to 6 years: 20 to 60 mg (docusate sodium) P.O. daily.
Children under 3 years: 10 to 40 mg (docusate sodium) P.O. daily.
Higher doses are for initial therapy. Adjust dose to individual response. Usual dose in children and adults with minimal needs: 50 to 150 mg (docusate calcium) P.O. daily.

SIDE EFFECTS
EENT: throat irritation.
GI: bitter taste, mild abdominal cramping, diarrhea.
Other: laxative dependence in long-term or excessive use.

INTERACTIONS
None significant.

NURSING CONSIDERATIONS
• Sodium salts: use cautiously in patients on sodium-restricted diets, or with edema, congestive heart failure, renal dysfunction.
• Should only be used occasionally. Don't use for more than 1 week without doctor's knowledge.
• Docusate sodium contains 5.17 mg sodium/100 mg capsule.
• Potassium salts: contraindicated in renal dysfunction.
• Give liquid in milk, fruit juice, or infant formula to mask bitter taste.
• Not for use in treating existing constipation, but prevents constipation from developing.
• Laxative of choice in patients who should not strain during defecation, such as those recovering from myocardial infarction or rectal surgery; in disease of rectum and anus that makes passage of firm stool difficult; or postpartum constipation.
• Acts within 24 to 48 hours to produce firm, semisolid stool.
• Instruct patient that dietary sources of bulk include bran and other cereals, fresh fruit, and vegetables.
• Emollient laxative or stool softener;

doesn't stimulate intestinal peristaltic movements.
• Store at 15° to 30° C. (59° to 86° F.). Protect liquid from light.

glycerin

INDICATIONS & DOSAGE
Constipation—
Adults and children over 6 years: 3 g as a suppository; or 5 to 15 ml as an enema.
Children under 6 years: 1 to 1.5 g as a suppository; or 2 to 5 ml as an enema.

SIDE EFFECTS
GI: *cramping pain,* rectal discomfort, hyperemia of rectal mucosa.

INTERACTIONS
None significant.

NURSING CONSIDERATIONS
• A hyperosmolar laxative used mainly to reestablish proper toilet habits in laxative-dependent patients.

lactulose
Cephulac♦, Chronulac♦

INDICATIONS & DOSAGE
Treatment of constipation—
Adults: 15 to 30 ml P.O. daily.
To prevent and treat portal-systemic encephalopathy, including hepatic precoma and coma in patients with severe hepatic disease—
Adults: initially, 20 to 30 g P.O. (30 to 45 ml) t.i.d. or q.i.d., until two or three soft stools are produced daily. Usual dose is 60 to 100 g daily in divided doses. Can also be given by retention enema in at least 100 ml of fluid.

SIDE EFFECTS
GI: abdominal cramps, belching, diarrhea, gaseous distention, flatulence.

INTERACTIONS
None significant.

NURSING CONSIDERATIONS
• Contraindicated in patients who need low-galactose diet. Use cautiously in diabetes mellitus.
• Reduce dosage if diarrhea occurs. Replace fluid loss.
• If desired, minimize drug's sweet taste by diluting with water or fruit juice or giving with food.
• Store at room temperature, preferably below 30° C. (86° F.). Don't freeze.

magnesium salts
Concentrated Milk of Magnesia, Magnesium Citrate, Magnesium Sulfate, Milk of Magnesia

INDICATIONS & DOSAGE
Constipation, to evacuate bowel before surgery—
Adults and children over 6 years: 15 g magnesium sulfate P.O. in glass of water; 10 to 20 ml concentrated milk of magnesia P.O.; or 15 to 60 ml milk of magnesia P.O.; or 5 to 10 oz magnesium citrate at bedtime.
Laxative—
Adults: 30 to 60 ml, usually h.s., Milk of Magnesia P.O.
Children 6 to 12 years: 15 to 30 ml P.O. Milk of Magnesia.
Children 2 to 6 years: 5 to 15 ml P.O. Milk of Magnesia.

SIDE EFFECTS
GI: *abdominal cramping, nausea.*
Metabolic: fluid and electrolyte disturbances if used daily.
Other: laxative dependence in long-term or excessive use.

INTERACTIONS
None significant.

NURSING CONSIDERATIONS
• Contraindicated in abdominal pain, nausea, vomiting, or other symptoms of appendicitis or acute surgical abdomen; in myocardial damage, heart block, imminent delivery, fecal impaction, rectal fissures, intestinal obstruction or perforation, renal disease. Use cautiously in rectal bleeding.
• Shake suspension well; give with large amount of water when used as laxative. When administering through nasogastric tube, be sure tube is placed properly and is patent. After instilling, flush tube with water to assure passage to stomach and maintain tube patency.
• For short-term therapy; don't use longer than 1 week.
• When used as laxative, don't give oral drugs 1 to 2 hours before or after.
• Saline laxative; produces watery stool in 3 to 6 hours. Time drug administration so that it doesn't interfere with scheduled activities or sleep.
• Magnesium sulfate is more potent than other saline laxatives.
• Before giving for constipation, determine if patient has adequate fluid intake, exercise, and diet. Tell him that dietary sources of bulk include bran and other cereals, fresh fruit, and vegetables.
• Magnesium may accumulate in renal insufficiency.
• Chilling before use may make magnesium citrate more palatable.
• Monitor serum electrolytes during prolonged use.
• Frequent or prolonged use as a laxative may cause dependence.

methylcellulose
Cellothyl, Cologel, Hydrolose, Syncelose

INDICATIONS & DOSAGE
Chronic constipation—
Adults: 5 to 20 ml liquid P.O. t.i.d. with a glass of water; or 15 ml syrup P.O. morning and evening.
Children: 5 to 10 ml P.O. daily or b.i.d.

SIDE EFFECTS

GI: *nausea,* vomiting, diarrhea (all after excessive use); esophageal, gastric, small intestinal, or colonic strictures when drug is chewed or taken in dry form; *abdominal cramps,* especially in severe constipation.
Other: laxative dependence in long-term or excessive use.

INTERACTIONS
None significant.

NURSING CONSIDERATIONS

• Contraindicated in abdominal pain, nausea, vomiting, or other symptoms of appendicitis or acute surgical abdomen; and in intestinal obstruction or ulceration, disabling adhesion, or difficulty swallowing.
• Laxative effect usually takes 12 to 24 hours, but may be delayed 3 days.
• Tell patient to take drug with at least 8 oz (240 ml) of pleasant-tasting liquid to mask grittiness.
• Especially useful in postpartum constipation, debilitated patients, chronic laxative abuse, irritable bowel syndrome, diverticular disease, colostomies, and to empty colon before barium enema examinations.
• Use for short-term treatment.
• Before giving for constipation, determine if patient has adequate fluid intake, exercise, and diet. Tell him that dietary sources of bulk include bran and other cereals, fresh fruit, and vegetables.
• Not absorbed systemically; nontoxic.
• Bulk laxative; increases bulk and water content of stool.
• Instruct patient to notify doctor in 1 week about response to therapy.

mineral oil

Agoral Plain, Fleet Mineral Oil Enema, Kondremul Plain♦, Neo-Cultol, Petrogalar Plain, Saf-Tip Oil Retention Enema

INDICATIONS & DOSAGE
Constipation; preparation for bowel studies or surgery—
Adults: 15 to 30 ml P.O. h.s.; or 4 oz enema.
Children: 5 to 15 ml P.O. h.s.; or 1 to 2 oz enema.

SIDE EFFECTS
GI: *nausea;* vomiting; diarrhea in excessive use; *abdominal cramps,* especially in severe constipation; decreased absorption of nutrients and fat-soluble vitamins, resulting in deficiency; slowed healing after hemorrhoidectomy; and increased risk of rectal infections due to seepage from rectum.
Other: laxative dependence in long-term or excessive use.

INTERACTIONS
None significant.

NURSING CONSIDERATIONS
• Contraindicated in abdominal pain, nausea, vomiting, or other symptoms of appendicitis or acute surgical abdomen; in fecal impaction, intestinal obstruction or perforation. Use cautiously in young children; in elderly or debilitated patients due to susceptibility to lipid pneumonitis through aspiration, absorption, and transport from intestinal mucosa; in rectal bleeding. Enema contraindicated in children under 2 years.
• Don't give drug with meals or immediately after, as it delays passage of food from stomach. More active on an empty stomach.
• To be taken only at bedtime. Warn patients not to take for more than 1 week.
• A lubricant laxative.

- Give with fruit juices or carbonated drinks to disguise taste.
- Use when patient needs to ease the strain of evacuation.
- Before giving for constipation, determine if patient has adequate fluid intake, exercise, and diet. Tell him that dietary sources of bulk include bran and other cereals, fresh fruit, and vegetables.

phenolphthalein
Alophen**, Espotabs, Evac-U-Lac, Ex-Lax, Feen-A-Mint, Phenolax, Evac-U-Gen

INDICATIONS & DOSAGE
Constipation—
Adults: 60 to 200 mg P.O., preferably h.s.

SIDE EFFECTS
GI: diarrhea; *colic in large doses;* factitious nausea; vomiting; loss of normal bowel function in excessive use; *abdominal cramps,* especially in severe constipation; malabsorption of nutrients; "cathartic colon" (syndrome resembling ulcerative colitis radiologically and pathologically) in chronic misuse; reddish discoloration in alkaline feces.
Skin: dermatitis, pruritus, rash, pigmentation.
Other: laxative dependence in long-term or excessive use, *hypersensitivity.*

INTERACTIONS
None significant.

NURSING CONSIDERATIONS
- Contraindicated in abdominal pain, nausea, vomiting, or other symptoms of appendicitis or acute surgical abdomen; in fecal impaction, intestinal obstruction or perforation. Use cautiously in rectal bleeding.
- Laxative effect may last up to 3 to 4 days.
- Produces semisolid stool within 6 to

8 hours, with little or no griping. Time drug administration so that it doesn't interfere with scheduled activities or sleep.
- Warn patient with rash to avoid sun and discontinue use. Don't use any other product containing phenolphthalein.
- Before giving for constipation, determine if patient has adequate fluid intake, exercise, and diet. Tell him that dietary sources of bulk include bran and other cereals, fresh fruit, and vegetables.
- May discolor alkaline urine red-pink and acidic urine yellow-brown.
- Drug is available in many dosage forms. Most popular over-the-counter laxative; a frequent constituent of chewing gum and chocolate laxatives. Stimulant laxative, class of laxative most abused.

psyllium
Effersyllium Instant Mix, Hydrocil Instant Powder, Konsyl, L.A. Formula, Metamucil◆, Metamucil Instant Mix◆, Modane Bulk, Mucillium, Mucilose, Plain Hydrocil, Siblin◆, Syllact

INDICATIONS & DOSAGE
Constipation; bowel management—
Adults: 1 to 2 rounded teaspoonfuls P.O. in full glass of liquid daily, b.i.d., or t.i.d., followed by second glass of liquid; or 1 packet P.O. dissolved in water daily, b.i.d., or t.i.d.
Children over 6 years: 1 level teaspoonful P.O. in ½ glass of liquid h.s.

SIDE EFFECTS
GI: nausea, vomiting, diarrhea, all after excessive use; esophageal, gastric, small intestinal, or colonic strictures when drug taken in dry form; abdominal cramps, especially in severe constipation.

INTERACTIONS
None significant.

NURSING CONSIDERATIONS
• Contraindicated in abdominal pain, nausea, vomiting, or other symptoms of appendicitis; and in intestinal obstruction or ulceration, disabling adhesion, or difficulty swallowing.
• Metamucil Instant Mix (effervescent form) contains a significant amount of sodium and should not be used for patients on sodium-restricted diets.
• All forms of Metamucil brand contain sugar. Use different brands of psyllium in diabetic patients.
• Mix with at least 8 oz (240 ml) of cold, pleasant-tasting liquid to mask grittiness, and stir only a few seconds. Patient should drink it immediately or mixture will congeal. Follow with additional glass of liquid.
• Use for short-term treatment. Don't use for maintenance.
• Frequent use of laxatives can cause drug dependence for evacuation.
• Before giving for constipation, determine if patient has adequate fluid intake, exercise, and diet. Tell him that dietary sources of bulk include bran and other cereals, fresh fruit, and vegetables.
• Laxative effect usually seen in 12 to 24 hours, but may be delayed 3 days.
• Popular bulk laxative; increases bulk and water content of stool.
• Highly refined, purified vegetable mucilloid; from seeds of plantago plant.
• Not absorbed systemically; nontoxic. Especially useful in postpartum constipation, debilitated patients, chronic laxative abuse, irritable bowel syndrome, diverticular disease, and in combination with other laxatives to empty colon before barium enema examinations.

senna
Black Draught, Glysennid, Senokot, X-Prep*

INDICATIONS & DOSAGE
Acute constipation, preparation for bowel or rectal examination—
Adults: Dosage range for Senokot: 1 to 8 tablets P.O.; ½ to 4 teaspoonfuls of granules added to liquid; 1 to 2 suppositories h.s.; 1 to 4 teaspoonfuls syrup h.s. Black Draught: 7.5 to 15 ml.
Children over 27 kg: ½ adult dose of tablets, granules, or syrup (except Black Draught tablets and granules not recommended for children).
Children 1 month to 1 year: 1.25 to 2.5 ml Senokot syrup P.O. h.s.
X-Prep used solely as single dose for preradiographic bowel evacuation. Give ¾ oz powder dissolved in juice or 2.5 oz liquid between 2 and 4 p.m. on day before X-ray procedure. May be given in divided doses for elderly or debilitated patients.

SIDE EFFECTS
GI: *nausea;* vomiting; diarrhea; loss of normal bowel function in excessive use; *abdominal cramps,* especially in severe constipation; malabsorption of nutrients; "cathartic colon" (syndrome resembling ulcerative colitis radiologically in chronic misuse; may cause constipation after catharsis); yellow, yellow-green cast feces, diarrhea in nursing infants of mothers on senna; darkened pigmentation of rectal mucosa in long-term use, which is usually reversible within 4 to 12 months after stopping drug.
GU: red-pink discoloration in alkaline urine; yellow-brown color to acid urine.
Metabolic: hypokalemia, protein enteropathy, electrolyte imbalance with excessive use.
Other: laxative dependence in long-term or excessive use.

Italicized side effects are common or life-threatening.
*Liquid form contains alcohol.   **May contain tartrazine.

INTERACTIONS
None significant.

NURSING CONSIDERATIONS
• Contraindicated in ulcerative bowel lesions; in nausea, vomiting, abdominal pain, or other symptoms of appendicitis or acute surgical abdomen; and in fecal impaction, intestinal obstruction, or perforation.
• Use for short-term treatment.
• More potent than cascara sagrada. Acts in 6 to 10 hours. X-Prep gives thorough, strong bowel action beginning in 6 hours.
• Most recommended stimulant laxative.
• Before giving for constipation, determine if patient has adequate fluid intake, exercise, and diet. Tell him that dietary sources of bulk include bran and other cereals, fresh fruit, and vegetables.
• After X-Prep liquid is taken, diet should be confined to clear liquids.
• Senna is one of the most effective laxatives for counteracting constipation caused by narcotic analgesics.

---

sodium biphosphate
Enemeez, Fleet Enema♦, Phospho-Soda**, Saf-Tip Phosphate Enema

sodium phosphate
Sal-Hepatica

INDICATIONS & DOSAGE
Constipation—
Adults: 5 to 20 ml liquid P.O. with water; or 4 g powder P.O. dissolved in warm water; or 20 to 46 ml solution mixed with 4 oz cold water; or 2 to 4.5 oz enema.

SIDE EFFECTS
GI: *abdominal cramping.*
Metabolic: fluid and electrolyte disturbances (hypernatremia, hyperphosphatemia) if used daily.
Other: laxative dependence in long-term or excessive use.

INTERACTIONS
None significant.

NURSING CONSIDERATIONS
• Contraindicated in abdominal pain, nausea, vomiting, or other symptoms of appendicitis or acute surgical abdomen; in intestinal obstruction or perforation; edema; congestive heart failure; megacolon; impaired renal function; and in patients on salt-restricted diets.
• Available in oral and rectal forms.
• Before giving for constipation, determine if patient has adequate fluid intake, exercise, and diet. Tell him that dietary sources of bulk include bran and other cereals, fresh fruit, and vegetables.
• Saline laxative; up to 10% of sodium content may be absorbed.
• Enema form elicits response in 5 to 10 minutes.
• Used in preparation for barium enema and for fecal impaction.

46

Emetics and antiemetics

apomorphine hydrochloride
benzquinamide hydrochloride
buclizine hydrochloride
cyclizine hydrochloride
cyclizine lactate
dimenhydrinate
diphenidol
ipecac syrup
meclizine hydrochloride
prochlorperazine edisylate
prochlorperazine maleate
scopolamine
thiethylperazine maleate
trimethobenzamide
   hydrochloride

MECHANISM OF ACTION
• Apomorphine acts directly on the
chemoreceptor trigger zone in the medulla oblongata to induce vomiting.
• Ipecac syrup induces vomiting by
acting locally on the gastric mucosa
and centrally on the chemoreceptor
trigger zone.
• Benzquinamide and trimethobenzamide may act on the chemoreceptor
trigger zone to inhibit nausea and vomiting, but this mechanism is not certain.
• Buclizine, cyclizine, dimenhydrinate, meclizine (antihistamine antiemetics), and scopolamine may affect
neural pathways originating in the labyrinth to inhibit nausea and vomiting,
but the exact mechanism of action is
unknown.
• Diphenidol influences the chemoreceptor trigger zone to inhibit nausea
and vomiting.
• Prochlorperazine and thiethylperazine (phenothiazine antiemetics) also
act on the chemoreceptor trigger zone

to inhibit nausea and vomiting, and in
larger doses partially depress the vomiting center as well.

COMBINATION PRODUCTS
None.

apomorphine hydrochloride
Controlled Substance Schedule II

INDICATIONS & DOSAGE
To induce vomiting in poisoning—
Adults: 2 to 10 mg S.C. or I.M. pre-
ceded by 200 to 300 ml water or, pref-
erably, evaporated milk. Don't repeat.
Children over 1 year: 0.07 mg/kg
S.C. or I.M. preceded by up to 2 glasses
of water or, preferably, evaporated
milk.
Children under 1 year: 0.07 mg/kg
S.C. preceded by ½ to 1 glass of water
or, preferably, evaporated milk.

SIDE EFFECTS
CNS: *depression, euphoria,* restlessness, tremors.
CV: *acute circulatory failure in elderly
or debilitated patients,* tachycardia.
Other: *depressed respiratory center in
large or repeated doses.*

INTERACTIONS
None significant.

NURSING CONSIDERATIONS
• Contraindicated in patients with
hypersensitivity to narcotics; impending shock; corrosive poisoning; narcosis resulting from opiates, barbiturates, alcohol, or other CNS depres-

sants; and in patients too inebriated to stand unaided. Use cautiously in children and in patients who are debilitated, have cardiac decompensation, or are predisposed to nausea and vomiting.

• Don't give after ingestion of petroleum distillates (for example, kerosene, gasoline) or volatile oils; retching and vomiting may cause aspiration and lead to bronchospasm, pulmonary edema, or aspiration pneumonitis. Vegetable oil will delay absorption of these substances.

• Emetic action is increased if dose is followed immediately by water or evaporated milk. Evaporated milk is preferred because studies show that water may increase absorption of toxic substances.

• Don't give after ingestion of caustic substances, such as lye; additional injury to the esophagus and mediastinum can occur.

• Keep narcotic antagonists, such as naloxone, available to help stop vomiting and to alleviate drowsiness.

• If delay in giving emetic is expected, give activated charcoal P.O. immediately. When absorbable poison is ingested, give activated charcoal P.O. immediately after apomorphine hydrochloride.

• Vomiting occurs in 5 to 10 minutes in adults. If vomiting doesn't occur within 15 minutes, gastric lavage should begin. Apomorphine HCl is emetic of choice when rapid removal of poisons is necessary, and when identification of enteric-coated tablets or other ingested toxic material in vomitus is important. Stomach contents are usually expelled completely; vomitus may also contain material from upper portion of intestinal tract.

• Don't administer if solution for injection is discolored green, or if precipitate is present.

benzquinamide hydrochloride
Emete-Con

INDICATIONS & DOSAGE
Nausea and vomiting associated with anesthesia and surgery—
Adults: 50 mg I.M. (0.5 mg/kg to 1 mg/kg). May repeat in 1 hour, and thereafter q 3 to 4 hours, p.r.n.; or 25 mg (0.2 mg/kg to 0.4 mg/kg) I.V. as single dose, administered slowly.

SIDE EFFECTS
CNS: *drowsiness,* fatigue, insomnia, restlessness, headache, excitation, tremors, twitching, dizziness.
CV: sudden rise in blood pressure and transient arrhythmias (premature atrial and ventricular contractions, atrial fibrillation) after I.V. administration; hypertension; hypotension.
EENT: dry mouth, salivation, blurred vision.
GI: anorexia, nausea.
Skin: urticaria, rash.
Other: muscle weakness, flushing, hiccups, sweating, chills, fever. May mask signs of overdose of toxic agents or underlying conditions (intestinal obstruction, brain tumor).

INTERACTIONS
None significant.

NURSING CONSIDERATIONS
• I.V. use contraindicated in cardiovascular disease. Don't give I.V. within 15 minutes of preanesthetic or cardiovascular drugs.
• Give I.M. injections in large muscle mass. Use deltoid area only if well developed. Be sure to aspirate syringe for I.M. injection to avoid inadvertent intravenous injection.
• Reconstituted solution stable for 14 days at room temperature. Store dry powder and reconstituted solution in light-resistant container.

- Precipitation occurs if reconstituted with 0.9% sodium chloride injection.
- Monitor blood pressure frequently.
- Excellent antiemetic if prochlorperazine (Compazine) is contraindicated.

buclizine hydrochloride
Bucladin-S**, Softran

INDICATIONS & DOSAGE
Motion sickness (prevention)—
Adults: 50 mg P.O. at least ½ hour before beginning travel. If needed, may repeat another 50 mg P.O. after 4 to 6 hours.
Vertigo—
Adults: 50 mg P.O., up to 150 mg P.O. daily in severe cases. Maintenance dose is 50 mg b.i.d.

SIDE EFFECTS
CNS: *drowsiness,* headache, dizziness, jitters.
EENT: blurred vision, dry mouth.
GU: urinary retention.
Other: may mask symptoms of ototoxicity, intestinal obstruction, or brain tumor.

INTERACTIONS
None significant.

NURSING CONSIDERATIONS
- Use cautiously in patients with glaucoma, GU or GI obstruction, and in elderly males with possible prostatic hypertrophy.
- Warn patient against driving and other activities that require alertness until CNS response to drug is established.
- Tablets may be placed in mouth and allowed to dissolve without water. May also be chewed or swallowed whole.
- Classified as an antihistamine.

cyclizine hydrochloride

cyclizine lactate
Marezine, Marzine♦♦

INDICATIONS & DOSAGE
Motion sickness (prevention and treatment)—
Adults: 50 mg P.O. (hydrochloride) ½ hour before travel, then q 4 to 6 hours, p.r.n., to maximum of 200 mg daily; or 50 mg I.M. (lactate) q 4 to 6 hours, p.r.n.
Postoperative vomiting (prevention)—
Adults: 50 mg I.M. (lactate) preoperatively or 20 to 30 minutes before expected termination of surgery; then postoperatively 50 mg I.M. (lactate) q 4 to 6 hours, p.r.n.
Motion sickness and postoperative vomiting—
Children 6 to 12 years: 3 mg/kg (lactate) I.M. divided t.i.d., or 25 mg (hydrochloride) P.O. q 4 to 6 hours p.r.n. to a maximum of 75 mg daily.

SIDE EFFECTS
CNS: *drowsiness,* dizziness, auditory and visual hallucinations.
CV: hypotension.
EENT: blurred vision, dry mouth.
GI: constipation.
GU: urinary retention.
Other: may mask symptoms of ototoxicity, brain tumor, or intestinal obstruction.

INTERACTIONS
None significant.

NURSING CONSIDERATIONS
- Use cautiously in patients with glaucoma, in patients with GU or GI obstruction, and in elderly males with possible prostatic hypertrophy.
- Warn patient against driving and other activities that require alertness until CNS response to drug is determined.
- Classified as an antihistamine.

• Store in cool place. When stored at room temperature, injection may turn slightly yellow, but this color change does not indicate loss of potency.

---

dimenhydrinate
Dimate, Dimen, Dimentabs, Dipendrate, Dramaject, Dramamine♦*, Dramamine Junior, Dramocen, Dymenate, Gravol♦♦, Hydrate, Hypo-emesis, Marmine, Nauseal♦♦, Nauseatol♦♦, Novodimenate♦♦, Ram, Reidamine, Signate, Travamine♦♦, Trav-Arex, Traveltabs, Vertiban, Wehamine

INDICATIONS & DOSAGE
Nausea, vomiting, dizziness of motion sickness (treatment and prevention)—
Adults: 50 mg P.O. q 4 hours, or 100 mg q 4 hours if drowsiness is not objectionable; or 100 mg rectally daily or b.i.d. if oral route is not practical; or 50 mg I.M., p.r.n.; or 50 mg I.V. diluted in 10 ml NaCl solution, injected over 2 minutes.
Children: 5 mg/kg P.O. or I.M., divided q.i.d. Maximum 300 mg daily. Don't use in children less than 2 years old.

SIDE EFFECTS
CNS: *drowsiness,* headache, incoordination, dizziness.
CV: palpitations, hypotension.
EENT: blurred vision, tinnitus, dry mouth and respiratory passages.
Other: may mask symptoms of ototoxicity, brain tumor, or intestinal obstruction.

INTERACTIONS
None significant.

NURSING CONSIDERATIONS
• Use cautiously in seizures, narrow-angle glaucoma, enlargement of prostate gland.
• Undiluted solution is irritating to veins; may cause sclerosis.

• Classified as an antihistamine.
• Warn patient against driving and other activities that require alertness until CNS response to drug is determined.
• May mask ototoxicity of aminoglycoside antibiotics.
• Avoid mixing parenteral preparation with other drugs; incompatible with many solutions.

---

diphenidol
Vontrol♦

INDICATIONS & DOSAGE
Peripheral (labyrinthine) dizziness; nausea and vomiting—
Adults: 25 to 50 mg P.O. q 4 hours, p.r.n., or 20 to 40 mg deep I.M. injection (for rapid control of acute symptoms), then another 20 mg I.M. after 1 hour if symptoms persist. Thereafter 20 to 40 mg I.M. q 4 hours, p.r.n., or 20 mg I.V. injected directly or through venoclysis already in operation (for rapid control of acute symptoms). May inject another 20 mg I.V. after 1 hour if symptoms persist, then switch to P.O. or I.M. route. Total daily dosage should not exceed 300 mg.
Nausea and vomiting—
Children: 0.9 mg/kg P.O. or rectally, or 0.4 mg/kg I.M. Give children's doses no more frequently than q 4 hours unless symptoms persist after 1 dose. Then, an oral or I.M. dose may be repeated after 1 hour. Thereafter, doses may be given q 4 hours p.r.n. Maximum children's dose 5.5 mg/kg P.O. daily; or 3.3 mg/kg I.M. daily.

SIDE EFFECTS
CNS: drowsiness, dizziness, sleep disturbances, *confusion;* auditory and visual hallucinations, disorientation occur within 3 days of starting drug; subside within 3 days after stopping drug.
CV: transient hypotension.
GI: dry mouth, nausea, indigestion, heartburn.

Skin: urticaria.
Other: antiemetic effect may mask signs of overdose of drugs, or may obscure diagnosis of intestinal obstruction, brain tumor, or other conditions.

INTERACTIONS
None significant.

NURSING CONSIDERATIONS
• Contraindicated in anuria. Use cautiously in glaucoma, pyloric stenosis, pylorospasm, obstructive lesions of GI or GU tract, prostatic hypertrophy, or organic cardiospasm.
• Don't use in children under 6 months or less than 11 kg.
• I.V. use contraindicated in children and in patients with sinus tachycardia.
• Don't give subcutaneously. Administer deep I.M.
• Drug should be stopped if auditory or visual hallucinations, or disorientation or confusion occurs.
• Closely supervise patient. Patients are usually hospitalized when receiving this drug. Monitor intake and output; report any changes.
• Treatment of toxicity is symptomatic and supportive.
• Used in Ménière's disease, following middle and inner ear surgery, labyrinthine disturbances, and to control nausea and vomiting associated with infectious disease, malignancies, radiation sickness, general anesthetics, and antineoplastic agents.

---

ipecac syrup

INDICATIONS & DOSAGE
To induce vomiting in poisoning—
Adults: 15 ml P.O., followed by 200 to 300 ml of water.
Children 1 year or older: 15 ml P.O., followed by about 200 ml of water or milk.
Children under 1 year: 5 to 10 ml P.O., followed by 100 to 200 ml of water or milk. May repeat dose once after 20 minutes, if necessary.

SIDE EFFECTS
CNS: depression.
CV: *cardiac arrhythmias, bradycardia, hypotension, atrial fibrillation, or fatal myocarditis* if drug is absorbed (e.g., if patient doesn't vomit within 30 minutes) or after ingestion of excessive dose.
GI: *diarrhea.*

INTERACTIONS
Activated charcoal: neutralized emetic effect. Don't give together but may give activated charcoal after vomiting has occurred.

NURSING CONSIDERATIONS
• Contraindicated in semicomatose or unconscious patients, or those with severe inebriation, convulsions, shock, loss of gag reflex.
• Don't give after ingestion of petroleum distillates (for example, kerosene, gasoline) or volatile oils; retching and vomiting may cause aspiration and lead to bronchospasm, pulmonary edema, or aspiration pneumonitis. Vegetable oil will delay absorption of these substances.
• Don't give after ingestion of caustic substances, such as lye; additional injury to the esophagus and mediastinum can occur.
• Clearly indicate ipecac *syrup*, not single word "ipecac," to avoid confusion with fluidextract. Fluidextract is 14 times more concentrated and, if inadvertently used instead of syrup, may cause death.
• Induces vomiting within 30 minutes in more than 90% of patients; average time usually less than 20 minutes.
• Stomach is usually emptied completely; vomitus may contain some intestinal material as well.
• In antiemetic toxicity, ipecac syrup is usually effective if less than 1 hour has passed since ingestion of antiemetic.

Italicized side effects are common or life-threatening.
∗Liquid form contains alcohol.   ∗∗May contain tartrazine.

- Recommend that 1 ounce of syrup be readily available in the home when child becomes 1 year old for immediate use in case of emergency.
- No systemic toxicity with doses of 30 ml or less.
- If two doses do not induce vomiting, gastric lavage is necessary.

meclizine hydrochloride
Antivert♦, Bonamine♦♦, Bonine, Lamine, Roclizine, Vertrol, Whevert

INDICATIONS & DOSAGE
Dizziness—
Adults: 25 to 100 mg P.O. daily in divided doses. Dose varies with patient response.
Motion sickness—
Adults: 25 to 50 mg P.O. 1 hour before travel, repeated daily for duration of journey.

SIDE EFFECTS
CNS: *drowsiness,* fatigue.
EENT: dry mouth, blurred vision.
Other: may mask symptoms of ototoxicity, brain tumor, or intestinal obstruction.

INTERACTIONS
None significant.

NURSING CONSIDERATIONS
- Use cautiously in patients with glaucoma, GU or GI obstruction, and in elderly males with possible prostatic hypertrophy.
- Warn patient against driving and other activities that require alertness until CNS response to drug is deterned.
- Antihistamine with a slower onset and longer duration of action than other antihistamine antiemetics.

prochlorperazine edisylate

prochlorperazine maleate
Compazine**, Stemetil♦♦

INDICATIONS & DOSAGE
Preoperative nausea control—
Adults: 5 to 10 mg I.M. 1 to 2 hours before induction of anesthetic, repeat once in 30 minutes, if necessary; or 5 to 10 mg I.V. 15 to 30 minutes before induction of anesthetic (repeat once if necessary); or 20 mg/liter dextrose 5% and sodium chloride 0.9% solution by I.V. infusion, added to infusion 15 to 30 minutes before induction. Maximum parenteral dose 40 mg daily.
Severe nausea, vomiting—
Adults: 5 to 10 mg P.O. t.i.d. or q.i.d.; or 15 mg sustained-release form P.O. on arising; or 10 mg sustained-release form P.O. q 12 hours; or 25 mg rectally b.i.d. or 5 to 10 mg I.M. injected deeply into upper outer quadrant of gluteal region. Repeat q 3 to 4 hours, p.r.n. Maximum I.M. dose 40 mg daily.
Children 18 to 39 kg: 2.5 mg P.O. or rectally t.i.d.; or 5 mg P.O. or rectally b.i.d. Maximum 15 mg daily; or 0.132 mg/kg deep I.M. injection. (Control usually obtained with 1 dose.)
Children 14 to 17 kg: 2.5 mg P.O. or rectally b.i.d. or t.i.d. Maximum 10 mg daily; or 0.132 mg/kg deep I.M. injection. (Control usually obtained with 1 dose.)
Children 9 to 13 kg: 2.5 mg P.O. or rectally daily or b.i.d. Maximum 7.5 mg daily; or 0.132 mg/kg deep I.M. injection. (Control usually obtained with 1 dose.)

SIDE EFFECTS
Blood: *transient leukopenia, agranulocytosis.*
CNS: *extrapyramidal reactions (high incidence),* sedation (low incidence), pseudoparkinsonism, EEG changes, dizziness.

CV: *orthostatic hypotension,* tachycardia, EKG changes.
EENT: *ocular changes, blurred vision.*
GI: *dry mouth, constipation.*
GU: *urinary retention,* dark urine, menstrual irregularities, gynecomastia, inhibited ejaculation.
Hepatic: *cholestatic jaundice.*
Metabolic: hyperprolactinemia.
Skin: *mild photosensitivity,* dermal allergic reactions, *exfoliative dermatitis.*
Other: weight gain, increased appetite.

INTERACTIONS

Anticholinergics, including antidepressant and antiparkinson agents: increased anticholinergic activity, aggravated parkinson-like symptoms. Use together cautiously.
Antacids: inhibited absorption of oral phenothiazines. Separate antacid and phenothiazine dosage by at least 2 hours.
Barbiturates: may decrease phenothiazine effect. Monitor patient for decreased antiemetic effect.

NURSING CONSIDERATIONS

• Contraindicated in phenothiazine hypersensitivity, coma, depression, CNS depression, bone-marrow depression, subcortical damage; during pediatric surgery, use of spinal or epidural anesthetic or adrenergic blocking agents, alcohol usage. Use with caution in combination with other CNS depressants; in hepatic disease, arteriosclerosis or cardiovascular disease (may cause sudden drop in blood pressure), exposure to extreme heat or cold (including antipyretic therapy), respiratory disorders, hypocalcemia, vomiting in children, convulsive disorders or severe reactions to insulin or electroshock therapy, suspected brain tumor or intestinal obstruction, glaucoma, or prostatic hypertrophy; in acutely ill or dehydrated children; and in elderly or debilitated patients.
• Store in light-resistant container. Slight yellowing does not affect potency; discard very discolored solutions.
• Since drug has a very long duration of action, timed-release capsules have no significant advantage over ordinary oral dosage forms.
• Use only when vomiting can't be controlled by other measures, or when only a few doses are required. If more than 4 doses needed in 24-hour period, notify doctor.
• Not effective in motion sickness.
• To prevent contact dermatitis, avoid getting concentrate or injection solution on hands or clothing.
• Dilute oral concentrate with tomato or fruit juice, milk, coffee, carbonated beverage, tea, water, soup, or pudding.
• Monitor CBC and liver function studies during prolonged therapy. Warn patients to wear protective clothing when exposed to sunlight.
• Watch for orthostatic hypotension, especially when giving I.V.
• Do not give subcutaneously or mix in syringe with another drug. Give deep I.M.

scopolamine
Transderm-Scop

INDICATIONS & DOSAGE

Prevention of nausea and vomiting associated with motion sickness—
Adults: One Transderm-Scop system (a circular flat unit) programmed to deliver 0.5 mg scopolamine over 3 days (72 hours), applied to the skin behind the ear several hours before the antiemetic is required.
Not recommended for children.

SIDE EFFECTS

CNS: *drowsiness,* restlessness, disorientation, confusion
EENT: *dry mouth,* transient impairment of eye accommodation.

INTERACTIONS

None significant.

Italicized side effects are common or life-threatening.
*Liquid form contains alcohol.   **May contain tartrazine.

NURSING CONSIDERATIONS

• Use cautiously in patients with glaucoma, pyloric obstruction, or urinary bladder-neck obstruction.
• Wash and dry hands thoroughly before applying the system on dry skin behind the ear. After removing the system, discard it, then wash both the hands and application site thoroughly.
• If the system becomes displaced, remove and replace it with another system on a fresh skin site in the postauricular area.
• A patient brochure is available with this product; tell patient to request it from the pharmacist.
• Warn patient against driving and other activities that require alertness until response to drug is determined.
• Sugarless hard candy may be helpful in minimizing dry mouth.
• Transderm-Scop is effective if applied 2 to 3 hours before experiencing motion, but more effective if used 12 hours before. Therefore, advise patient to apply system the night before a planned trip.
• Transdermal method of administration releases a controlled therapeutic amount of scopolamine.

thiethylperazine maleate
Torecan♦

INDICATIONS & DOSAGE
Nausea, vomiting—
Adults: 10 mg P.O., I.M., or rectally daily, b.i.d. or t.i.d.

SIDE EFFECTS
Blood: *transient leukopenia, agranulocytosis.*
CNS: *extrapyramidal reactions (high incidence)*, sedation (low incidence), pseudoparkinsonism, EEG changes, dizziness.
CV: *orthostatic hypotension*, tachycardia, EKG changes.
EENT: *ocular changes, blurred vision.*
GI: *dry mouth, constipation.*

GU: *urinary retention*, dark urine, menstrual irregularities, gynecomastia, inhibited ejaculation.
Hepatic: *cholestatic jaundice.*
Metabolic: hyperprolactinemia.
Skin: *mild photosensitivity*, dermal allergic reactions, *exfoliative dermatitis.*
Other: weight gain, increased appetite.

INTERACTIONS
Anticholinergics, including antidepressants and antiparkinson agents: increased anticholinergic activity, aggravated parkinson-like symptoms. Use together cautiously.
Antacids: inhibited absorption of oral phenothiazines. Separate antacid and phenothiazine dosage by at least 2 hours.
Barbiturates: may decrease phenothiazine effect. Monitor for decreased antiemetic effect.

NURSING CONSIDERATIONS
• Contraindicated in severe CNS depression, hepatic disease, coma, phenothiazine hypersensitivity.
• Don't give I.V.
• For nausea and vomiting associated with anesthesia and surgery, give deep I.M. injection on or shortly before terminating anesthesia.
• Possibly effective in dizziness; not effective in motion sickness.
• Use only when vomiting can't be controlled by other measures, or when only a few doses are required.
• Warn patient about hypotension. Advise him to stay in bed for 1 hour after receiving the drug.
• If drug gets on skin, wash off at once to prevent contact dermatitis.

trimethobenzamide hydrochloride
Tigan♦, Spengan, Ticon

INDICATIONS & DOSAGE
Nausea and vomiting (treatment)—

Adults: 250 mg P.O. t.i.d. or q.i.d.; or 200 mg I.M. or rectally t.i.d. or q.i.d.
Postoperative nausea and vomiting (prevention)—
Adults: 200 mg I.M. or rectally (single dose) before or during surgery; may repeat 3 hours after termination of anesthesia, p.r.n.
Children 13 to 40 kg: 100 to 200 mg P.O. or rectally t.i.d. or q.i.d.
Children under 13 kg: 100 mg rectally t.i.d. or q.i.d. Limited to prolonged vomiting of known etiology.

SIDE EFFECTS
CNS: drowsiness, dizziness (in large doses).
CV: hypotension.
GI: diarrhea, exaggeration of pre-existing nausea (in large doses).
Hepatic: *liver toxicity.*
Local: pain, stinging, burning, redness, swelling at I.M. injection site.
Skin: skin hypersensitivity reactions.
Other: antiemetic effect may mask signs of overdosage of toxic agents, or intestinal obstruction, brain tumor, or other conditions.

INTERACTIONS
None significant.

NURSING CONSIDERATIONS
• Contraindicated in children with viral illness (a possible cause of vomiting in children); may contribute to the development of Reye's syndrome, a potentially fatal acute childhood encephalopathy, characterized by fatty degeneration of the liver.
• Suppositories contraindicated in hypersensitivity to benzocaine hydrochloride or similar local anesthetic.
• Stop drug if allergic skin reaction occurs.
• Give I.M. dose by deep injection into upper outer quadrant of gluteal region to reduce pain and local irritation.
• Warn patient of the possibility of drowsiness and dizziness, and caution him against driving or other activities requiring alertness until CNS response to drug is determined.
• Store suppositories in refrigerator.
• Has little or no value in preventing motion sickness; limited value as antiemetic.

Italicized side effects are common or life-threatening.
*Liquid form contains alcohol.   **May contain tartrazine.

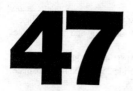

Gastrointestinal anticholinergics

Belladonna alkaloids
atropine sulfate
belladonna leaf
levorotatory alkaloids of
belladonna
l-hyoscyamine sulfate

Quaternary anticholinergics
anisotropine methylbromide
clidinium bromide
diphemanil methylsulfate
glycopyrrolate
hexocyclium methylsulfate
homatropine methylbromide
isopropamide iodide
mepenzolate bromide
methantheline bromide
methscopolamine bromide
oxyphenonium bromide
propantheline bromide
tridihexethyl chloride

Tertiary synthetics
(antispasmodics)
dicyclomine hydrochloride
methixene hydrochloride
oxyphencyclimine hydrochloride
thiphenamil hydrochloride

MECHANISM OF ACTION
• Quaternary anticholinergics block the actions of acetylcholine on the vagus nerve. (This blocking mechanism is known as competitive inhibition.) They decrease GI motility and inhibit gastric acid secretion.
• Tertiary synthetics exert a nonspecific direct spasmolytic action on smooth muscle. They also possess local anesthetic properties that may be partly responsible for the spasmolysis.

COMBINATION PRODUCTS
BARBIDONNA ELIXIR*: atropine sulfate 0.034 mg/5 ml, phenobarbital 21.6 mg/5 ml, hyoscyamine hydrobromide or sulfate 0.174 mg/5 ml, hyoscine hydrobromide 0.01 mg/5 ml, and alcohol 15%.
BARBIDONNA TABLETS: atropine sulfate 0.025 mg, hyoscine hydrobromide 0.0074 mg, hyoscyamine hydrobromide or sulfate 0.1286 mg, and phenobarbital 16 mg.
BARBIDONNA #2 TABLETS: atropine sulfate 0.025 mg, hyoscine hydrobromide 0.0074 mg, hyoscyamine hydrobromide or sulfate 0.1286 mg, and phenobarbital 32 mg.
BELLADENAL TABLETS♦: L-alkaloids of belladonna 0.25 mg and phenobarbital 50 mg.
BENTYL WITH PHENOBARBITAL SYRUP*: dicyclomine hydrochloride 10 mg/5 ml, phenobarbital 15 mg/5 ml, and alcohol 19%.
BENTYL 10 MG WITH PHENOBARBITAL CAPSULES: dicyclomine hydrochloride 10 mg and phenobarbital 15 mg.
BENTYL 20 MG WITH PHENOBARBITAL TABLETS: dicyclomine hydrochloride 20 mg and phenobarbital 15 mg.
BUTIBEL ELIXIR*: belladonna extract 15 mg/5 ml, butabarbital sodium 15 mg/5 ml, and alcohol 7%.
BUTIBEL TABLETS: belladonna extract 15 mg and butabarbital sodium 15 mg.
CANTIL WITH PHENOBARBITAL TABLETS: mepenzolate bromide 25 mg and phenobarbital 16 mg.
CHARDONNA-2: belladonna extract 15 mg and phenobarbital 15 mg.
COMBID SPANSULES♦: isopropamide

iodide 5 mg and prochlorperazine maleate 10 mg.

DARICON PB TABLETS: oxyphencyclimine hydrochloride 5 mg and phenobarbital 15 mg.

DONNATAL ELIXIR♦*: atropine sulfate 0.0194 mg/5 ml, hyoscine hydrobromide 0.0065 mg/5 ml, alcohol 23%, hyoscyamine hydrobromide or sulfate 0.1037 mg/5 ml and phenobarbital 16 mg/5 ml.

DONNATAL EXTENTABS♦: atropine sulfate 0.0582 mg, hyoscine hydrobromide 0.0195 mg, hyoscyamine sulfate 0.3111 mg, and phenobarbital 48.6 mg.

DONNATAL TABLETS AND CAPSULES♦: atropine sulfate 0.0194 mg, hyoscine hydrobromide 0.0065 mg, hyoscyamine hydrobromide or sulfate 0.1037 mg, and phenobarbital 16 mg.

DONNATAL #2 TABLETS: atropine sulfate 0.0194 mg, hyoscine hydrobromide 0.0065 mg, hyoscyamine hydrobromide or sulfate 0.1037 mg, and phenobarbital 32.4 mg.

ENARAX 5 TABLETS: oxyphencyclimine hydrochloride 5 mg and hydroxyzine hydrochloride 25 mg.

ENARAX 10 TABLETS: oxyphencyclimine hydrochloride 10 mg and hydroxyzine hydrochloride 25 mg.

HYBEPHEN ELIXIR*: atropine sulfate 0.0233 mg/5 ml, hyoscine hydrobromide 0.0094 mg/5 ml, hyoscyamine hydrobromide or sulfate 0.1277 mg/5 ml, phenobarbital 15 mg/5 ml, and alcohol 16.5%.

KINESED TABLETS: atropine sulfate 0.02 mg, hyoscine hydrobromide 0.007 mg, hyoscyamine hydrobromide or sulfate 0.1 mg, and phenobarbital 16 mg.

LIBRAX CAPSULES: clidinium bromide 2.5 mg and chlordiazepoxide hydrochloride 5 mg.

MILPATH 200 TABLETS: tridihexethyl chloride 25 mg and meprobamate 200 mg.

MILPATH 400 TABLETS: tridihexethyl chloride 25 mg and meprobamate 400 mg.

PATHIBAMATE 200 TABLETS: tridihexethyl chloride 25 mg and meprobamate 200 mg.

PATHIBAMATE 400 TABLETS: tridihexethyl chloride 25 mg and meprobamate 400 mg.

PATHILON WITH PHENOBARBITAL TABLETS: tridihexethyl chloride 25 mg and phenobarbital 15 mg.

PRO-BANTHINE WITH PHENOBARBITAL TABLETS♦: propantheline bromide 15 mg and phenobarbital 15 mg.

ROBINUL PH TABLETS♦: glycopyrrolate 1 mg and phenobarbital 16.2 mg.

ROBINUL PH FORTE TABLETS♦: glycopyrrolate 2 mg and phenobarbital 16.2 mg.

VALPIN 50-PB TABLETS: anisotropine methylbromide 50 mg and phenobarbital 15 mg.

VISTRAX 10 TABLETS: oxyphencyclimine hydrochloride 10 mg and hydroxyzine hydrochloride 25 mg.

anisotropine methylbromide
Valpin 50

INDICATIONS & DOSAGE
Adjunctive treatment of peptic ulcer—
Adults: 50 mg P.O. t.i.d. To be effective should be titrated to individual patient needs.

SIDE EFFECTS
CNS: headache, insomnia, drowsiness, dizziness, *confusion or excitement in elderly patients,* nervousness, weakness.
CV: *palpitations,* tachycardia.
EENT: *blurred vision,* mydriasis, increased ocular tension, cycloplegia, photophobia.
GI: *dry mouth,* dysphagia, heartburn, loss of taste, nausea, vomiting, *paralytic ileus, constipation.*
GU: *urinary hesitancy and retention,* impotence.
Skin: urticaria, decreased sweating and possible anhidrosis, other dermal manifestations.

Italicized side effects are common or life-threatening.
*Liquid form contains alcohol.   **May contain tartrazine.

Other: fever, allergic reactions. Overdosage may cause curare-like symptoms.

INTERACTIONS
None significant.

NURSING CONSIDERATIONS
• Contraindicated in narrow-angle glaucoma, obstructive uropathy, obstructive disease of the GI tract, severe ulcerative colitis, myasthenia gravis, hypersensitivity to anticholinergics, paralytic ileus, intestinal atony, unstable cardiovascular status in acute hemorrhage, and toxic megacolon. Use cautiously in autonomic neuropathy, hyperthyroidism, coronary artery disease, cardiac arrhythmias, congestive heart failure, hypertension, hiatal hernia associated with reflux esophagitis, hepatic or renal disease, ulcerative colitis, or in patients over 40 years because of increased incidence of glaucoma.
• Use with caution in hot or humid environments. Drug-induced heatstroke can develop.
• Give 30 minutes to 1 hour before meals.
• Administer smaller doses to the elderly.
• Monitor patient's vital signs and urinary output carefully.
• Instruct patient to avoid driving and other hazardous activities if he is drowsy, dizzy, or has blurred vision; to drink plenty of fluids to help prevent constipation; to report any skin rash or local eruption.
• Gum or sugarless hard candy may relieve mouth dryness.

atropine sulfate

INDICATIONS & DOSAGE
Adjunctive therapy in peptic ulcers, irritable bowel syndrome, neurogenic bowel disturbances, and functional gastrointestinal disorders—

Adults: 0.25 to 0.6 mg P.O. q 4 to 6 hours.
Children 3 to 7 kg: 0.1 mg ($\frac{1}{600}$ gr) P.O. q 4 to 6 hours.
Children 8 to 11 kg: 0.15 mg ($\frac{1}{400}$ gr) P.O. q 4 to 6 hours.
Children 11 to 18 kg: 0.2 mg ($\frac{1}{300}$ gr) P.O. q 4 to 6 hours.
Children 18 to 30 kg: 0.3 mg ($\frac{1}{200}$ gr) P.O. q 4 to 6 hours.
Children 30 to 41 kg: 0.4 mg ($\frac{1}{150}$ gr) P.O. q 4 to 6 hours.
Children over 41 kg: 0.4 to 0.6 mg ($\frac{1}{150}$ to $\frac{1}{100}$ gr) P.O. q 4 to 6 hours.

SIDE EFFECTS
CNS: headache, insomnia, drowsiness, dizziness, *confusion or excitement in elderly patients,* nervousness, weakness.
CV: *palpitations,* tachycardia.
EENT: *blurred vision,* mydriasis, increased ocular tension, cycloplegia, photophobia.
GI: *dry mouth,* dysphagia, heartburn, loss of taste, nausea, vomiting, paralytic ileus.
GU: *urinary hesitancy and retention,* impotence.
Skin: urticaria, decreased sweating or anhidrosis, other dermal manifestations.
Other: fever, allergic reactions. Overdosage may cause curare-like symptoms.

INTERACTIONS
None significant

NURSING CONSIDERATIONS
• Contraindicated in narrow-angle glaucoma, obstructive uropathy, obstructive disease of GI tract, severe ulcerative colitis, myasthenia gravis, hypersensitivity to anticholinergics, paralytic ileus, intestinal atony, unstable cardiovascular status in acute hemorrhage, toxic megacolon. Use cautiously in autonomic neuropathy, hyperthyroidism, coronary artery disease, cardiac arrhythmias, congestive heart failure, hypertension, hiatal her-

nia associated with reflux esophagitis, hepatic or renal disease, ulcerative colitis, or in patients over 40 years, because of increased incidence of glaucoma.

• Use with caution in hot or humid environments. Drug-induced heatstroke can develop.

• Give 30 minutes to 1 hour before meals and at bedtime. Bedtime dose can be larger and should be given at least 2 hours after last meal of day.

• Administer smaller doses to the elderly.

• Monitor patient's vital signs and urinary output carefully.

• Instruct patient to avoid driving and other hazardous activities if he is drowsy, dizzy, or has blurred vision; to drink plenty of fluids to help prevent constipation; to report any skin rash.

• Gum, sugarless hard candy, or pilocarpine syrup may relieve mouth dryness.

• Other anticholinergic drugs may increase vagal blockage.

belladonna leaf
(used to prepare extract and tincture)
Belladonna Tincture USP

INDICATIONS & DOSAGE
Adjunctive therapy for peptic ulcer, irritable bowel syndrome, functional gastrointestinal disorders, and neurogenic bowel disturbances—
Adults: 10.8 to 21.6 mg P.O. t.i.d. or q.i.d. of the extract; 0.3 to 1 ml t.i.d. or q.i.d. of tincture.

SIDE EFFECTS
CNS: headache, insomnia, drowsiness, dizziness, *confusion or excitement in elderly patients,* nervousness, weakness.
CV: *palpitations,* tachycardia.
EENT: *blurred vision,* mydriasis, increased ocular tension, cycloplegia, photophobia.
GI: *dry mouth,* dysphagia, heartburn, loss of taste, *constipation,* nausea, vomiting.
GU: *urinary hesitancy and retention,* impotence.
Skin: urticaria, decreased sweating or anhidrosis, other dermal manifestations.
Other: fever, allergic reactions.
Overdosage may cause curare-like symptoms.

INTERACTIONS
None significant.

NURSING CONSIDERATIONS
• Contraindicated in narrow-angle glaucoma, obstructive uropathy, obstructive disease of GI tract, severe ulcerative colitis, myasthenia gravis, hypersensitivity to anticholinergics, paralytic ileus, intestinal atony, unstable cardiovascular status in acute hemorrhage, and toxic megacolon. Use cautiously in autonomic neuropathy, hyperthyroidism, coronary artery disease, cardiac arrhythmias, congestive heart failure, hypertension, hiatal hernia associated with reflux esophagitis, hepatic or renal disease, ulcerative colitis, or in patients over 40 years because of increased incidence of glaucoma.

• Give 30 minutes to 1 hour before meals and at bedtime. Bedtime dose can be larger and should be given at least 2 hours after last meal of day.

• Administer smaller doses to the elderly.

• Use with caution in hot or humid environments. Drug-induced heatstroke can develop.

• Monitor patient's vital signs and urinary output carefully.

• Instruct patient to avoid driving and other hazardous activities if he is drowsy, dizzy, or has blurred vision; to drink plenty of fluids to help prevent constipation; to report any skin rash.

• Gum or sugarless hard candy may relieve mouth dryness.

clidinium bromide
Quarzan

INDICATIONS & DOSAGE
Adjunctive therapy for peptic ulcers—
Dosage should be individualized according to severity of symptoms and occurrence of side effects.
Adults: 2.5 to 5 mg P.O. t.i.d. or q.i.d. before meals and at bedtime.
Geriatric or debilitated patients: 2.5 mg P.O. t.i.d. before meals.

SIDE EFFECTS
CNS: headache, insomnia, drowsiness, dizziness, *confusion or excitement in elderly patients,* nervousness, weakness.
CV: *palpitations,* tachycardia.
EENT: *blurred vision,* mydriasis, increased ocular tension, cycloplegia, photophobia.
GI: *dry mouth,* dysphagia, heartburn, loss of taste, nausea, vomiting, *paralytic ileus, constipation.*
GU: *urinary hesitancy and retention,* impotence.
Skin: urticaria, decreased sweating or anhidrosis, other dermal manifestations.
Other: fever, allergic reactions. Overdosage may cause curare-like symptoms.

INTERACTIONS
None significant.

NURSING CONSIDERATIONS
• Contraindicated in narrow-angle glaucoma, obstructive uropathy, obstructive disease of GI tract, severe ulcerative colitis, myasthenia gravis, hypersensitivity to anticholinergics, paralytic ileus, intestinal atony, unstable cardiovascular status in acute hemorrhage, and toxic megacolon. Use cautiously in autonomic neuropathy, hyperthyroidism, coronary artery disease, cardiac arrhythmias, congestive heart failure, hypertension, hiatal hernia associated with reflux esophagitis,

hepatic or renal disease, ulcerative colitis, or in patients over 40 years, because of increased incidence of glaucoma.
• Give 30 minutes to 1 hour before meals and at bedtime. Bedtime dose can be larger and should be given at least 2 hours after last meal of day.
• Administer smaller doses to the elderly.
• Use with caution in hot or humid environments. Drug-induced heatstroke may develop.
• Monitor patient's vital signs and urinary output carefully.
• Instruct patient to avoid driving and other hazardous activities if he is drowsy, dizzy, or has blurred vision; to drink plenty of fluids to help prevent constipation; and to report any skin rash or local eruption.
• Gum or sugarless hard candy may relieve mouth dryness.
• There is no conclusive evidence that clidinium aids in healing, decreases recurrence of, or prevents complications of peptic ulcers.

dicyclomine hydrochloride
Antispas, Bentyl, Bentylol♦♦, Cyclobec♦♦, Dibent, Dicen, Formulex♦♦, Menospasm♦♦, Nospaz, Or-Tyl, Rocyclo, Rotyl HCl, Stannitol, Viscerol♦♦, Neoquess

INDICATIONS & DOSAGE
Adjunctive therapy for peptic ulcers and other functional gastrointestinal disorders—
Adults: 10 to 20 mg P.O. t.i.d. or q.i.d.; 20 mg I.M. q 4 to 6 hours.
Children: 10 mg P.O. t.i.d. or q.i.d.
Infant colic—
Infants: 5 mg P.O. t.i.d. or q.i.d.
Always adjust dosage according to patient's needs and response.

SIDE EFFECTS
CNS: *headache,* insomnia, drowsiness, *dizziness.*

CV: *palpitations,* tachycardia.
GI: nausea, *constipation,* vomiting, *paralytic ileus.*
GU: urinary hesitancy and retention, impotence.
Skin: urticaria, decreased sweating or anhidrosis, other dermal manifestations.
Other: fever, allergic reactions. Overdosage may cause curare-like symptoms.

INTERACTIONS
None significant.

NURSING CONSIDERATIONS
• Contraindicated in obstructive uropathy, obstructive disease of GI tract, severe ulcerative colitis, myasthenia gravis, hypersensitivity to anticholinergics, paralytic ileus, intestinal atony, unstable cardiovascular status in acute hemorrhage, and toxic megacolon. Use cautiously in autonomic neuropathy, narrow-angle glaucoma, hyperthyroidism, coronary artery disease, cardiac arrhythmias, congestive heart failure, hypertension, hiatal hernia associated with reflux esophagitis, hepatic or renal disease, ulcerative colitis.
• Use with caution in hot or humid environments. Drug-induced heatstroke can develop.
• Give 30 minutes to 1 hour before meals and at bedtime. Bedtime dose can be larger and should be given at least 2 hours after last meal of day.
• Administer smaller doses to the elderly.
• Monitor patient's vital signs and urinary output carefully.
• Instruct patient to avoid driving and other hazardous activities if he is drowsy, dizzy, or has blurred vision; to drink plenty of fluids to help prevent constipation; and to report any skin rash.
• Gum or sugarless hard candy may relieve mouth dryness.
• A synthetic tertiary derivative that is

relatively free of atropine-like side effects.
• Not for I.V. use.

diphemanil methylsulfate
Prantal

INDICATIONS & DOSAGE
Adjunctive therapy in gastric hypersecretion associated with duodenal ulcer—
Adults: 100 to 200 mg P.O. q 4 to 6 hours, between meals (initial dose). Daily dosage should be adjusted according to response and tolerance. Maintenance dose: 50 to 100 mg q 4 to 6 hours.

SIDE EFFECTS
CNS: headache, insomnia, drowsiness, dizziness, *confusion or excitement in elderly patients,* nervousness, weakness.
CV: *palpitations,* tachycardia.
EENT: *blurred vision,* mydriasis, increased ocular tension, cycloplegia, photophobia.
GI: *dry mouth,* dysphagia, *constipation,* heartburn, loss of taste, nausea, vomiting, *paralytic ileus.*
GU: *urinary hesitancy and retention,* impotence.
Skin: urticaria, decreased sweating or anhidrosis, other dermal manifestations.
Other: fever, allergic reactions. Overdosage may cause curare-like symptoms.

INTERACTIONS
None significant.

NURSING CONSIDERATIONS
• Contraindicated in narrow-angle glaucoma, obstructive uropathy, obstructive disease of GI tract, severe ulcerative colitis, myasthenia gravis, hypersensitivity to anticholinergics, paralytic ileus, intestinal atony, unstable cardiovascular status in acute hemorrhage, and toxic megacolon. Use

cautiously in autonomic neuropathy, hyperthyroidism, coronary artery disease, cardiac arrhythmias, congestive heart failure, hypertension, hiatal hernia associated with reflux esophagitis, hepatic or renal disease, ulcerative colitis, or in patients over 40 years because of increased incidence of glaucoma.

• Use with caution in hot or humid environments. Drug-induced heatstroke can develop.

• Give 30 minutes to 1 hour before meals and at bedtime. Bedtime dose can be larger and should be given at least 2 hours after last meal of day.

• Administer smaller doses to the elderly.

• Monitor patient's vital signs and urinary output carefully.

• Instruct patient to avoid driving and other hazardous activities if he is drowsy, dizzy, or has blurred vision; to drink plenty of fluids to help prevent constipation; and to report any skin rash.

• Gum or sugarless hard candy may relieve mouth dryness.

---

glycopyrrolate
Robinul♦, Robinul Forte♦

INDICATIONS & DOSAGE
Adjunctive therapy in peptic ulcers and other gastrointestinal disorders—
Adults: 1 to 2 mg P.O. t.i.d. or 0.1 mg I.M. t.i.d. or q.i.d. Dosage should be individualized.

SIDE EFFECTS
CNS: headache, insomnia, drowsiness, dizziness, *confusion or excitement in elderly patients,* nervousness, weakness.
CV: *palpitations,* tachycardia.
EENT: *blurred vision,* mydriasis, increased ocular tension, cycloplegia, photophobia.
GI: *dry mouth,* dysphagia, *constipation,* heartburn, loss of taste, nausea, vomiting, *paralytic ileus.*

GU: *urinary hesitancy and retention,* impotence.
Skin: urticaria, decreased sweating or anhidrosis, other dermal manifestations.
Other: fever, allergic reactions. Overdosage may cause curare-like symptoms.

INTERACTIONS
None significant.

NURSING CONSIDERATIONS
• Contraindicated in narrow-angle glaucoma, obstructive uropathy, obstructive disease of GI tract, severe ulcerative colitis, myasthenia gravis, hypersensitivity to anticholinergics, paralytic ileus, intestinal atony, unstable cardiovascular status in acute hemorrhage, and toxic megacolon. Use cautiously in autonomic neuropathy, hyperthyroidism, coronary artery disease, cardiac arrhythmias, congestive heart failure, hypertension, hiatal hernia associated with reflux esophagitis, hepatic or renal disease, ulcerative colitis, or in patients over 40 years because of increased incidence of glaucoma.

• Use with caution in hot or humid environments. Drug-induced heatstroke can develop.

• Administer 30 minutes to 1 hour before meals.

• Administer smaller doses to the elderly.

• Monitor patient's vital signs and urinary output carefully.

• Instruct patient to avoid driving and other hazardous activities if he is drowsy, dizzy, or has blurred vision; to drink plenty of fluids to help prevent constipation; to report any skin rash.

• Gum or sugarless hard candy may relieve mouth dryness.

---

hexocyclium methylsulfate
Tral

INDICATIONS & DOSAGE
Adjunctive therapy in peptic ulcer and other gastrointestinal disorders—
Adults: 25 mg q.i.d. before meals and h.s.; 50 mg (timed release) daily, in the morning or b.i.d.

SIDE EFFECTS
CNS: headache, insomnia, drowsiness, dizziness, *confusion or excitement in elderly patients,* nervousness, weakness.
CV: *palpitations,* tachycardia.
EENT: *blurred vision,* mydriasis, increased ocular tension, cycloplegia, photophobia.
GI: *dry mouth,* dysphagia, heartburn, loss of taste, nausea, *constipation,* vomiting, *paralytic ileus.*
GU: *urinary hesitancy and retention,* impotence.
Skin: urticaria, decreased sweating or anhidrosis, other dermal manifestations.
Other: fever, allergic reactions. Overdosage may cause curare-like symptoms.

INTERACTIONS
None significant.

NURSING CONSIDERATIONS
• Contraindicated in narrow-angle glaucoma, obstructive uropathy, obstructive disease of GI tract, severe ulcerative colitis, myasthenia gravis, hypersensitivity to anticholinergics, paralytic ileus, intestinal atony, unstable cardiovascular status in acute hemorrhage, toxic megacolon. Use cautiously in autonomic neuropathy, hyperthyroidism, coronary artery disease, cardiac arrhythmias, congestive heart failure, hypertension, hiatal hernia associated with reflux esophagitis, hepatic or renal disease, ulcerative colitis, or in patients over 40 years because of increased incidence of glaucoma.

• Use with caution in hot or humid environments. Drug-induced heatstroke can develop.
• Give 30 minutes to 1 hour before meals and at bedtime. Bedtime dose can be larger and should be given at least 2 hours after last meal of day.
• Administer smaller doses to the elderly.
• Monitor patient's vital signs and urinary output carefully.
• Instruct patient to avoid driving and other hazardous activities if he is drowsy, dizzy, or has blurred vision; to drink plenty of fluids to help prevent constipation; and to report any skin rash.
• Gum or sugarless hard candy may relieve mouth dryness.
• Tablets contain tartrazine dye. May cause allergy in susceptible patients.

homatropine methylbromide
Ru-Spas No. 2

INDICATIONS & DOSAGE
Treatment of gastrointestinal spasm, hyperchlorhydria, and other mild spastic conditions of the bile ducts and gallbladder—
Adults: 10 mg t.i.d. to q.i.d. before meals and h.s.

SIDE EFFECTS
CNS: headache, insomnia, drowsiness, dizziness, *confusion or excitement in elderly patients,* nervousness, weakness.
CV: *palpitations,* tachycardia.
EENT: *blurred vision,* mydriasis, increased ocular tension, cycloplegia, photophobia.
GI: *dry mouth,* dysphagia, *constipation,* heartburn, loss of taste, nausea, vomiting, *paralytic ileus.*
GU: *urinary hesitancy and retention,* impotence.
Skin: urticaria, decreased sweating or anhidrosis, other dermal manifestations.

Italicized side effects are common or life-threatening.
*Liquid form contains alcohol.   **May contain tartrazine.

Other: fever, allergic reactions. Overdosage may cause curare-like symptoms.

INTERACTIONS
None significant.

NURSING CONSIDERATIONS
• Contraindicated in narrow-angle glaucoma, obstructive uropathy, obstructive disease of GI tract, severe ulcerative colitis, myasthenia gravis, hypersensitivity to anticholinergics, paralytic ileus, intestinal atony, unstable cardiovascular status in acute hemorrhage, and toxic megacolon. Use cautiously in autonomic neuropathy, hyperthyroidism, coronary artery disease, cardiac arrhythmias, congestive heart failure, hypertension, hiatal hernia associated with reflux esophagitis, hepatic or renal disease, ulcerative colitis, or in patients over 40 years because of increased incidence of glaucoma.
• Use with caution in hot or humid environments. Drug-induced heatstroke can develop.
• Give 30 minutes to 1 hour before meals and at bedtime. Bedtime dose can be larger and should be given at least 2 hours after last meal of day.
• Administer smaller doses to the elderly.
• Monitor patient's vital signs and urinary output carefully.
• Instruct patient to avoid driving and other hazardous activities if he is drowsy, dizzy, or has blurred vision; to drink plenty of fluids to help prevent constipation; and to report any skin rash.
• Gum or sugarless hard candy may relieve mouth dryness.

isopropamide iodide
Darbid♦

INDICATIONS & DOSAGE
Adjunctive therapy for peptic ulcer, irritable bowel syndrome—

Adults and children over 12 years: 5 mg P.O. q 12 hours. Some patients may require 10 mg or more b.i.d. Dose should be individualized to patient's need.

SIDE EFFECTS
CNS: headache, insomnia, drowsiness, dizziness, *confusion or excitement in elderly patients,* nervousness, weakness.
CV: *palpitations,* tachycardia.
EENT: *blurred vision,* mydriasis, increased ocular tension, cycloplegia, photophobia.
GI: *dry mouth,* dysphagia, heartburn, loss of taste, nausea, vomiting, *constipation, paralytic ileus.*
GU: *urinary hesitancy and retention,* impotence.
Skin: urticaria, decreased sweating or anhidrosis, other dermal manifestations, iodine skin rash.
Other: fever, allergic reactions. Overdosage may cause curare-like symptoms.

INTERACTIONS
None significant.

NURSING CONSIDERATIONS
• Contraindicated in narrow-angle glaucoma, obstructive uropathy, obstructive disease of GI tract, severe ulcerative colitis, myasthenia gravis, hypersensitivity to anticholinergics, paralytic ileus, intestinal atony, unstable cardiovascular status in acute hemorrhage, toxic megacolon. Use cautiously in autonomic neuropathy, hyperthyroidism, coronary artery disease, cardiac arrhythmias, congestive heart failure, hypertension, hiatal hernia associated with reflux esophagitis, hepatic or renal disease, ulcerative colitis, or in patients over 40 years because of increased incidence of glaucoma.
• Use with caution in hot or humid environments. Drug-induced heatstroke can develop.
• Give 30 minutes to 1 hour before meals and at bedtime. Bedtime dose

can be larger and should be given at least 2 hours after the last meal of the day.

• Administer smaller doses to the elderly.

• Monitor patient's vital signs and urinary output carefully.

• Instruct patient to avoid driving and other hazardous activities if he is drowsy, dizzy, or has blurred vision; to drink plenty of fluids to help prevent constipation; and to report any skin rash.

• Gum or sugarless hard candy may relieve mouth dryness.

• Single dose produces 10- to 12-hour antisecretory effect and gastrointestinal antispasmodic effect.

• Discontinue 1 week before thyroid function tests.

levorotatory alkaloids of belladonna
(as maleate salts)
Bellafoline

INDICATIONS & DOSAGE
Adjunctive therapy for peptic ulcer, irritable bowel syndrome, and functional gastrointestinal disorders—
Adults: 0.25 to 0.5 mg P.O. t.i.d.; or 0.125 to 0.5 mg S.C. daily or b.i.d.
Children over 6 years: 0.125 to 0.25 mg P.O. t.i.d.

SIDE EFFECTS
CNS: headache, insomnia, drowsiness, dizziness, *confusion or excitement in elderly patients,* nervousness, weakness.
CV: *palpitations,* tachycardia.
EENT: *blurred vision,* mydriasis, increased ocular tension, cycloplegia, photophobia.
GI: *dry mouth,* dysphagia, heartburn, loss of taste, *constipation, paralytic ileus.*
GU: *urinary hesitancy and retention,* impotence.
Skin: urticaria, decreased sweating or anhidrosis, other dermal manifestations.
Other: fever, allergic reactions. Overdosage may cause curare-like symptoms.

INTERACTIONS
None significant.

NURSING CONSIDERATIONS
• Contraindicated in narrow-angle glaucoma, obstructive uropathy, obstructive disease of GI tract, severe ulcerative colitis, myasthenia gravis, hypersensitivity to anticholinergics, paralytic ileus, intestinal atony, unstable cardiovascular status in acute hemorrhage, and toxic megacolon. Use cautiously in autonomic neuropathy, hyperthyroidism, coronary artery disease, cardiac arrhythmias, congestive heart failure, hypertension, hiatal hernia associated with reflux esophagitis, hepatic or renal disease, ulcerative colitis, or in patients over 40 years, because of increased incidence of glaucoma.

• Use with caution in hot or humid environments. Drug-induced heatstroke can develop.

• Administer 30 minutes to 1 hour before meals.

• Administer smaller doses to the elderly.

• Monitor patient's vital signs and urinary output carefully.

• Instruct patient to avoid driving and other hazardous activities if he is drowsy, dizzy, or has blurred vision; to drink plenty of fluids to help prevent constipation; to report any skin rash.

• Gum or sugarless hard candy may relieve mouth dryness.

l-hyoscyamine sulfate
Anaspaz, Levsinex, Levsinex Time Caps, Levsin

INDICATIONS & DOSAGE
Treatment of gastrointestinal tract dis-

*orders due to spasm; adjunctive therapy
for peptic ulcers—*
Adults: 0.125 to 0.25 mg P.O. or S.L.
t.i.d. or q.i.d. before meals and at bed-
time; sustained-release form 0.375 mg
P.O. q 12 hours; or 0.25 to 0.5 mg (1 or
2 ml) I.M., I.V., or S.C. q 6 hours.
(Substitute oral medication when symp-
toms are controlled.)
Children 2 to 10 years: ½ adult dose
P.O.
Children under 2 years: ¼ adult dose
P.O.

SIDE EFFECTS
CNS: headache, insomnia, drowsiness,
dizziness, *confusion or excitement in elderly patients,* nervousness, weakness.
CV: *palpitations,* tachycardia.
EENT: *blurred vision,* mydriasis, increased ocular tension, cycloplegia,
photophobia.
GI: *dry mouth,* dysphagia, *constipation,* heartburn, loss of taste, nausea,
vomiting, *paralytic ileus.*
GU: *urinary hesitancy and retention,*
impotence.
Skin: urticaria, decreased sweating or
anhidrosis, other dermal manifestations.
Other: fever, allergic reactions.
Overdosage may cause curare-like
symptoms.

INTERACTIONS
None significant.

NURSING CONSIDERATIONS
• Contraindicated in narrow-angle
glaucoma, obstructive uropathy, obstructive disease of GI tract, severe ulcerative colitis, myasthenia gravis,
hypersensitivity to anticholinergics,
paralytic ileus, intestinal atony, unstable cardiovascular status in acute
hemorrhage, toxic megacolon. Use cautiously in autonomic neuropathy,
hyperthyroidism, coronary artery disease, cardiac arrhythmias, congestive
heart failure, hypertension, hiatal hernia associated with reflux esophagitis,

hepatic or renal disease, ulcerative colitis, or in patients over 40 years, because of the increased incidence of
glaucoma.
• Use with caution in hot or humid environments. Drug-induced heatstroke
can develop.
• Give 30 minutes to 1 hour before
meals and at bedtime. Bedtime dose
can be larger and should be given at
least 2 hours after the last meal of the
day.
• Administer smaller doses to the
elderly.
• Monitor patient's vital signs and urinary output carefully.
• Instruct patient to avoid driving and
other hazardous activities if he is
drowsy, dizzy, or has blurred vision; to
drink plenty of fluids to help prevent
constipation; and to report any skin
rash.
• Gum or sugarless hard candy may relieve mouth dryness.

---

mepenzolate bromide
Cantil**

INDICATIONS & DOSAGE
*Adjunctive therapy in treating peptic ul-
cer, irritable bowel syndrome, and neurologic bowel disturbances—*
Adults: 25 to 50 mg P.O. q.i.d. with
meals and at bedtime. Adjust dosage to
individual patient's needs.

SIDE EFFECTS
CNS: headache, insomnia, drowsiness,
dizziness, *confusion or excitement in elderly patients,* nervousness, weakness.
CV: *palpitations,* tachycardia.
EENT: *blurred vision,* mydriasis, increased ocular tension, cycloplegia,
photophobia.
GI: *dry mouth,* dysphagia, heartburn,
loss of taste, nausea, *constipation,* vomiting, *paralytic ileus.*
GU: *urinary hesitancy and retention,*
impotence.
Skin: urticaria, decreased sweating or

anhidrosis, other dermal manifestations.
Other: fever, allergic reactions.
Overdosage may cause curare-like symptoms.

INTERACTIONS
None significant.

NURSING CONSIDERATIONS
• Contraindicated in narrow-angle glaucoma, obstructive uropathy, obstructive disease of GI tract, severe ulcerative colitis, myasthenia gravis, hypersensitivity to anticholinergics, paralytic ileus, intestinal atony, unstable cardiovascular status in acute hemorrhage, toxic megacolon. Use cautiously in autonomic neuropathy, hyperthyroidism, coronary artery disease, cardiac arrhythmias, congestive heart failure, hypertension, hiatal hernia associated with reflux esophagitis, hepatic or renal disease, ulcerative colitis, or in patients over 40 years, because of increased incidence of glaucoma.
• Use with caution in hot or humid environments. Drug-induced heatstroke can develop.
• Give with meals and at bedtime.
• Administer smaller doses to the elderly.
• Monitor patient's vital signs and urinary output carefully.
• Instruct patient to avoid driving and other hazardous activities if he is drowsy, dizzy, or has blurred vision; to drink plenty of fluids to help prevent constipation; and to report any skin rash.
• Gum or sugarless hard candy may relieve mouth dryness.

---

methantheline bromide
Banthine

INDICATIONS & DOSAGE
Adjunctive therapy in peptic ulcer, pylorospasm, spastic colon, biliary dyskinesia, pancreatitis, and certain forms of gastritis—
Adults: 50 to 100 mg P.O. q 6 hours.
Children over 1 year: 12.5 to 50 mg q.i.d.
Children under 1 year: 12.5 to 25 mg q.i.d.
Neonates: 12.5 mg b.i.d., then t.i.d.

SIDE EFFECTS
CNS: headache, insomnia, drowsiness, dizziness, *confusion or excitement in elderly patients,* nervousness, weakness.
CV: *palpitations,* tachycardia.
EENT: *blurred vision,* mydriasis, increased ocular tension, cycloplegia, photophobia.
GI: *dry mouth,* dysphagia, *constipation,* heartburn, loss of taste, nausea, vomiting, *paralytic ileus.*
GU: *urinary hesitancy and retention,* impotence.
Skin: urticaria, decreased sweating or anhidrosis, other dermal manifestations.
Other: fever, allergic reactions.
Overdosage may cause curare-like symptoms.

INTERACTIONS
None significant.

NURSING CONSIDERATIONS
• Contraindicated in narrow-angle glaucoma, obstructive uropathy, obstructive disease of GI tract, severe ulcerative colitis, myasthenia gravis, hypersensitivity to anticholinergics, paralytic ileus, intestinal atony, unstable cardiovascular status in acute hemorrhage, toxic megacolon. Use cautiously in autonomic neuropathy, hyperthyroidism, coronary artery disease, cardiac arrhythmias, congestive heart failure, hypertension, hiatal hernia associated with reflux esophagitis, hepatic or renal disease, ulcerative colitis, or in patients over 40 years, because of the increased incidence of glaucoma.
• Use with caution in hot or humid en-

vironments. Drug-induced heatstroke can develop.

• Give 30 minutes to 1 hour before meals and at bedtime. Bedtime dose can be larger and should be given at least 2 hours after the last meal of the day.

• Administer smaller doses to the elderly.

• If patient is also taking antihistamines, he may experience increased dryness of mouth.

• Monitor patient's vital signs and urinary output carefully.

• Instruct patient to avoid driving and other hazardous activities if he is drowsy, dizzy, or has blurred vision; to drink plenty of fluids to help prevent constipation; and to report any skin rash.

• Gum or sugarless hard candy may relieve mouth dryness.

• Therapeutic effects appear in 30 to 45 minutes; persist for 4 to 6 hours after oral administration.

methixene hydrochloride
Trest♦

INDICATIONS & DOSAGE
Adjunctive treatment of gastrointestinal disorders associated with hypermotility or spasm—
Adults: 1 or 2 mg P.O. t.i.d.

SIDE EFFECTS
CNS: *headache,* insomnia, drowsiness, *dizziness.*
CV: *palpitations,* tachycardia.
EENT: *blurred vision,* mydriasis, increased ocular tension, cycloplegia, photophobia.
GI: *constipation,* nausea, vomiting, *paralytic ileus.*
GU: urinary hesitancy and retention, impotence.
Skin: urticaria, decreased sweating or anhidrosis, other dermal manifestations.
Other: fever, allergic reactions.

Overdosage may cause curare-like symptoms.

INTERACTIONS
None significant.

NURSING CONSIDERATIONS
• Contraindicated in narrow-angle glaucoma, obstructive uropathy, obstructive disease of GI tract, severe ulcerative colitis, myasthenia gravis, hypersensitivity to anticholinergics, paralytic ileus, intestinal atony, unstable cardiovascular status in acute hemorrhage, toxic megacolon. Use cautiously in autonomic neuropathy, hyperthyroidism, coronary artery disease, cardiac arrhythmias, congestive heart failure, hypertension, hiatal hernia associated with reflux esophagitis, hepatic or renal disease, ulcerative colitis, or in patients over 40 years, because of the increased incidence of glaucoma.

• Use with caution in hot or humid environment. Drug-induced heatstroke could develop.

• Administer 30 minutes to 1 hour before meals.

• Administer smaller doses to the elderly.

• Monitor patient's vital signs and urinary output.

• Instruct patient to avoid driving and other hazardous activities if he is drowsy, dizzy, or has blurred vision; to drink plenty of fluids to help prevent constipation; and to report any skin rash.

• Gum or sugarless hard candy may relieve mouth dryness.

• Synthetic tertiary derivative that is relatively free of atropine-like side effects.

methscopolamine bromide
Pamine, Scoline

INDICATIONS & DOSAGE
Adjunctive therapy in peptic ulcer—

Adults: 2.5 to 5 mg ½ hour before meals and h.s.

SIDE EFFECTS
CNS: headache, insomnia, dizziness, *confusion or excitement in elderly patients,* nervousness, weakness.
CV: *palpitations,* tachycardia.
EENT: *blurred vision,* mydriasis, increased ocular tension, cycloplegia, photophobia.
GI: *dry mouth,* dysphagia, *constipation,* heartburn, loss of taste, nausea, vomiting, *paralytic ileus.*
GU: *urinary hesitancy and retention,* impotence.
Skin: urticaria, decreased sweating or anhidrosis, other dermal manifestations.
Other: fever, allergic reactions. Overdosage may cause curare-like symptoms.

INTERACTIONS
None significant.

NURSING CONSIDERATIONS
• Contraindicated in narrow-angle glaucoma, obstructive uropathy, obstructive disease of GI tract, severe ulcerative colitis, myasthenia gravis, hypersensitivity to anticholinergics, paralytic ileus, intestinal atony, unstable cardiovascular status in acute hemorrhage, toxic megacolon. Use cautiously in autonomic neuropathy, hyperthyroidism, coronary artery disease, cardiac arrhythmias, congestive heart failure, hypertension, hiatal hernia associated with reflux esophagitis, hepatic or renal disease, ulcerative colitis, or in patients over 40 years, because of increased incidence of glaucoma.
• Use with caution in hot or humid environments. Drug-induced heatstroke can develop.
• Give 30 minutes to 1 hour before meals and at bedtime. Bedtime dose can be larger and should be given at least 2 hours after the last meal of the day.
• Administer smaller doses to the elderly.
• Monitor patient's vital signs and urinary output carefully.
• Instruct patient to avoid driving and other hazardous activities if he is drowsy, dizzy, or has blurred vision; to drink plenty of fluids to help prevent constipation; and to report any skin rash.
• Gum or sugarless hard candy may relieve mouth dryness.

oxyphencyclimine hydrochloride
Daricon♦

INDICATIONS & DOSAGE
Adjunctive treatment of peptic ulcer—
Adults: 10 mg b.i.d. in the morning and h.s., or 5 mg b.i.d. or t.i.d.

SIDE EFFECTS
CNS: *headache,* insomnia, drowsiness, *dizziness.*
CV: *palpitations,* tachycardia.
EENT: *blurred vision,* mydriasis, increased ocular tension, cycloplegia, photophobia.
GI: *constipation,* nausea, vomiting, *paralytic ileus.*
GU: urinary hesitancy and retention, impotence.
Skin: urticaria, decreased sweating or anhidrosis, other dermal manifestations.
Other: fever, allergic reactions. Overdosage may cause curare-like symptoms.

INTERACTIONS
None significant.

NURSING CONSIDERATIONS
• Contraindicated in narrow-angle glaucoma, obstructive uropathy, obstructive disease of GI tract, severe ulcerative colitis, myasthenia gravis,

hypersensitivity to anticholinergics, paralytic ileus, intestinal atony, unstable cardiovascular status in acute hemorrhage, toxic megacolon. Use cautiously in autonomic neuropathy, hyperthyroidism, coronary artery disease, cardiac arrhythmias, congestive heart failure, hypertension, hiatal hernia associated with reflux esophagitis, hepatic or renal disease, ulcerative colitis, or in patients over 40 years, because of increased incidence of glaucoma.

• Use with caution in hot or humid environments. Drug-induced heatstroke can develop.

• Give 30 minutes to 1 hour before breakfast and at bedtime.

• Administer smaller doses to the elderly.

• Monitor patient's vital signs and urinary output carefully.

• Instruct patient to avoid driving and other hazardous activities if he is drowsy, dizzy, or has blurred vision; to drink plenty of fluids to help prevent constipation; and to report any skin rash.

• Gum or sugarless hard candy may relieve mouth dryness.

• Synthetic tertiary derivative that is relatively free of atropine-like side effects.

oxyphenonium bromide
Antrenyl

INDICATIONS & DOSAGE
Adjunctive treatment of peptic ulcer—
Adults: 10 mg P.O. q.i.d. for several days, then reduced according to patient response.

SIDE EFFECTS
CNS: headache, insomnia, drowsiness, dizziness, *confusion or excitement in elderly patients,* nervousness, weakness.
CV: *palpitations,* tachycardia.
EENT: *blurred vision,* mydriasis, in-

creased ocular tension, cycloplegia, photophobia.
GI: *dry mouth,* dysphagia, *constipation,* heartburn, loss of taste, nausea, vomiting, *paralytic ileus.*
GU: *urinary hesitancy and retention,* impotence.
Skin: urticaria, decreased sweating or anhidrosis, other dermal manifestations.
Other: fever, allergic reactions. Overdosage may cause curare-like symptoms.

INTERACTIONS
None significant.

NURSING CONSIDERATIONS
• Contraindicated in narrow-angle glaucoma, obstructive uropathy, obstructive disease of GI tract, severe ulcerative colitis, myasthenia gravis, hypersensitivity to anticholinergics, paralytic ileus, intestinal atony, unstable cardiovascular status in acute hemorrhage, toxic megacolon. Use cautiously in autonomic neuropathy, hyperthyroidism, coronary artery disease, cardiac arrhythmias, congestive heart failure, hypertension, hiatal hernia associated with reflux esophagitis, hepatic or renal disease, ulcerative colitis, or in patients over 40 years, because of increased incidence of glaucoma.

• Use with caution in hot or humid environments. Drug-induced heatstroke can develop.

• Give 30 minutes to 1 hour before meals and at bedtime. Bedtime dose can be larger and should be given at least 2 hours after the last meal of the day.

• Administer smaller doses to the elderly.

• Monitor patient's vital signs and urinary output.

• Instruct patient to avoid driving and other hazardous activities if he is drowsy, dizzy, or has blurred vision; to drink plenty of fluids to help prevent constipation; and to report any skin rash.

• Gum or sugarless hard candy may relieve mouth dryness.

---

propantheline bromide
Banlin◆◆, Norpanth, Pro-Banthine◆, Propanthel◆◆, Robantaline, SK-Propantheline Bromide

INDICATIONS & DOSAGE
Adjunctive treatment of peptic ulcer, irritable bowel syndrome, and other gastrointestinal disorders; to reduce duodenal motility during diagnostic radiologic procedures—
Adults: 15 mg P.O. t.i.d. before meals, and 30 mg at bedtime up to 60 mg q.i.d. For elderly patients, 7.5 mg P.O. t.i.d. before meals.
When oral dosage not possible, or if prompt action is needed, 30 mg I.M. or I.V. q 6 hours, depending on individual response. Maintenance dose 15 mg I.M. q 6 hours.

SIDE EFFECTS
CNS: headache, insomnia, drowsiness, dizziness, *confusion or excitement in elderly patients,* nervousness, weakness.
CV: *palpitations,* tachycardia.
EENT: *blurred vision,* mydriasis, increased ocular tension, cycloplegia, photophobia.
GI: *dry mouth,* dysphagia, constipation, heartburn, loss of taste, nausea, vomiting, paralytic ileus.
GU: *urinary hesitancy and retention,* impotence.
Skin: urticaria, decreased sweating or anhidrosis, other dermal manifestations.
Other: fever, allergic reactions.
Overdosage may cause curare-like symptoms.

INTERACTIONS
None significant.

NURSING CONSIDERATIONS
• Contraindicated in narrow-angle glaucoma, obstructive uropathy, obstructive disease of GI tract, severe ulcerative colitis, myasthenia gravis, hypersensitivity to anticholinergics, paralytic ileus, intestinal atony, unstable cardiovascular status in acute hemorrhage, toxic megacolon. Use cautiously in autonomic neuropathy, hyperthyroidism, coronary artery disease, cardiac arrhythmias, congestive heart failure, hypertension, hiatal hernia associated with reflux esophagitis, hepatic or renal disease, ulcerative colitis, or in patients over 40 years, because of the increased incidence of glaucoma.
• Use with caution in hot or humid environments. Drug-induced heatstroke can develop.
• Give 30 minutes to 1 hour before meals and at bedtime. Bedtime dose can be larger and should be given at least 2 hours after the last meal of the day.
• Administer smaller doses to the elderly.
• Monitor patient's vital signs and urinary output carefully.
• Instruct patient to avoid driving and other hazardous activities if he is drowsy, dizzy, or has blurred vision; to drink plenty of fluids to help prevent constipation; and to report any skin rash.
• Gum or sugarless hard candy may relieve mouth dryness.

---

thiphenamil hydrochloride
Trocinate

INDICATIONS & DOSAGE
Hypermotility and spasm of the gastrointestinal tract—
Adults: initially, 400 mg P.O. repeated in 4 hours, usually to maximum of 4 doses. Maintenance dose may be given at a reduced frequency of dosage.

SIDE EFFECTS
CNS: headache, insomnia, drowsiness, dizziness, *confusion or excitement in elderly patients,* nervousness, weakness.
CV: *palpitations,* tachycardia.
EENT: *blurred vision,* mydriasis, increased ocular tension, cycloplegia, photophobia.
GI: *dry mouth,* dysphagia, *constipation,* heartburn, loss of taste, nausea, vomiting, *paralytic ileus.*
GU: *urinary hesitancy and retention,* impotence.
Skin: urticaria, decreased sweating or anhidrosis, other dermal manifestations.
Other: fever, allergic reactions. Overdosage may cause curare-like symptoms.

INTERACTIONS
None significant.

NURSING CONSIDERATIONS
• Contraindicated in narrow-angle glaucoma, obstructive uropathy, obstructive disease of GI tract, severe ulcerative colitis, myasthenia gravis, hypersensitivity to anticholinergics, paralytic ileus, intestinal atony, unstable cardiovascular status in acute hemorrhage, toxic megacolon. Use cautiously in autonomic neuropathy, hyperthyroidism, coronary artery disease, cardiac arrhythmias, congestive heart failure, hypertension, hiatal hernia associated with reflux esophagitis, hepatic or renal disease, ulcerative colitis, or in patients over 40 years, because of increased incidence of glaucoma.
• Use with caution in hot or humid environments. Drug-induced heatstroke can develop.
• Administer smaller doses to the elderly.
• Monitor patient's vital signs and urinary output carefully.
• Instruct patient to avoid driving and other hazardous activities if he is drowsy, dizzy, or has blurred vision; to

drink plenty of fluids to help prevent constipation; and to report any skin rash.
• Gum or sugarless hard candy may relieve mouth dryness.

tridihexethyl chloride
Pathilon

INDICATIONS & DOSAGE
Adjunctive treatment of peptic ulcer, irritable bowel syndrome, and other gastrointestinal disorders—
Adults: initially, 25 to 50 mg P.O. t.i.d. before meals, and 50 mg h.s., increased to 75 mg q.i.d., if needed. With sustained-release capsules, 75 mg q 12 or q 6 hours. Maintenance dose usually half the therapeutic dose. Parenteral use: 10 to 20 mg I.V., I.M., or S.C. q 6 hours. Change to oral as soon as possible.

SIDE EFFECTS
CNS: headache, insomnia, drowsiness, dizziness, *confusion or excitement in elderly patients,* nervousness, weakness.
CV: *palpitations,* tachycardia.
EENT: *blurred vision,* mydriasis, increased ocular tension, cycloplegia, photophobia.
GI: *dry mouth,* dysphagia, *constipation,* heartburn, loss of taste, nausea, vomiting, *paralytic ileus.*
GU: *urinary hesitancy and retention,* impotence.
Skin: urticaria, decreased sweating or anhidrosis, other dermal manifestations.
Other: fever, allergic reactions. Overdosage may cause curare-like symptoms.

INTERACTIONS
None significant.

NURSING CONSIDERATIONS
• Contraindicated in narrow-angle glaucoma, obstructive uropathy, obstructive disease of GI tract, severe ul-

cerative colitis, myasthenia gravis, hypersensitivity to anticholinergics, paralytic ileus, intestinal atony, unstable cardiovascular status in acute hemorrhage, toxic megacolon. Use cautiously in autonomic neuropathy, hyperthyroidism, coronary artery disease, cardiac arrhythmias, congestive heart failure, hypertension, hiatal hernia associated with reflux esophagitis, hepatic or renal disease, ulcerative colitis, or in patients over 40 years, because of increased incidence of glaucoma.

• Use with caution in hot or humid environments. Drug-induced heatstroke can develop.

• Give 30 minutes to 1 hour before meals and at bedtime. Bedtime dose can be larger and should be given at least 2 hours after the last meal of the day.

• Administer smaller doses to the elderly.

• Monitor patient's vital signs and urinary output carefully.

• Instruct patient to avoid driving and other hazardous activities if he is drowsy, dizzy, or has blurred vision; to drink plenty of fluids to help prevent constipation; and to report any skin rash.

• Gum or sugarless hard candy may relieve mouth dryness.

Italicized side effects are common or life-threatening.
*Liquid form contains alcohol.   **May contain tartrazine.

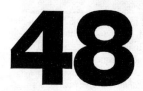

Miscellaneous gastrointestinal drugs

choline
cimetidine
dexpanthenol
metoclopramide hydrochloride
sucralfate

MECHANISM OF ACTION

• Choline promotes phospholipid turn-over and enhances fat transport from the liver to the tissues, decreasing the liver's fat content.

• Cimetidine competitively inhibits the action of histamine at receptor sites of the parietal cells, decreasing gastric acid secretion.

• Dexpanthenol both stimulates and restores tone to intestinal smooth muscles.

• Metoclopramide stimulates motility of the upper GI tract by antagonizing dopamine's action. It also blocks dopamine receptors at the chemoreceptor trigger zone.

• Sucralfate adheres to and protects the ulcer surface by forming a barrier.

COMBINATION PRODUCTS

GERIPLEX: choline 20 mg, vitamin A 5,000 units, vitamin E 5 units, vitamin B_1 5 mg, vitamin B_2 5 mg, vitamin B_3 15 mg, vitamin B_{12} 2 mcg, vitamin C 50 mg, iron 6 mg, calcium 59 mg, and phosphorus 46 mg.

GERIZYME*: inositol 100 mg, l-lysine 100 mg, vitamin B_1 3.3 mg, vitamin B_2 3.3 mg, vitamin B_3 33 mg, vitamin B_5 3.3 mg, vitamin B_6 1 mg, vitamin B_{12} 3.3 mcg, iron 5 mg, calcium 19 mg, phosphorus 15 mg, liver concentrate 75 mg, copper, potassium, manganese, magnesium, and alcohol 18% per 15 ml.

ILOPAN CHOLINE: dexpanthenol 50 mg and choline bitartrate 25 mg.

LIPOFLAVONOID: choline 111 mg, inositol 111 mg, vitamin B_1 0.3 mg, vitamin B_2 0.3 mg, vitamin B_3 3.3 mg, vitamin B_5 0.3 mg, vitamin B_6 0.3 mg, vitamin C 100 mg, and vitamin B_{12} 1.7 mcg.

LUFA: choline 111 mg, inositol 40 mg, methionine 66 mg, vitamin E 4 units, vitamin B_1 2 mg, vitamin B_2 2 mg, vitamin B_3 5 mg, vitamin B_5 1 mg, vitamin B_6 2 mg, vitamin B_{12} 1 mcg, desiccated liver 87 mg, and unsaturated fatty acids 423 mg.

METHISCHOL: choline 115 mg, inositol 83 mg, methionine 110 mg, vitamin B_1 3 mg, vitamin B_2 3 mg, vitamin B_3 10 mg, vitamin B_5 2 mg, vitamin B_6 2 mg, vitamin B_{12} 2 mcg, desicated liver 56 mg, and liver concentrate 30 mg.

---

choline

INDICATIONS & DOSAGE

Hepatic disorders and disturbed fat metabolism—

Adults and children: 650 to 750 mg P.O. daily.

SIDE EFFECTS

CNS: dizziness.

GI: irritation if taken on an empty stomach, nausea.

Metabolic: ketosis after excessive dosages.

Other: breath and body odor smelling like dead fish.

INTERACTIONS
None significant.

NURSING CONSIDERATIONS
- Foods supplying choline include egg yolk, beef liver, legumes, vegetables, and milk. Average diet contains from 500 to 900 mg per day.
- Lipotropic agent.
- Used in many multivitamin preparations, but there is no evidence supplemental choline intake is more beneficial for long periods than an adequate diet.
- Synthesized by the body from serine, with methionine acting as a methyl-donor in the reaction.
- Choline is no longer considered effective in treatment of hepatic disorders or disorders of lipid transport or metabolism.
- Investigative use in treatment of tardive dyskinesia: restores cholinergic tone and decreases choreic movements. Oral choline elevates brain choline and acetylcholine (the cholinergic neurotransmitter of the cholinergic nervous system) levels and restores cholinergic tone.
- Lecithin (available in health food stores) is a source of choline.

---

cimetidine
Tagamet♦

INDICATIONS & DOSAGE
Duodenal ulcer (short-term treatment)—
Adults and children over 16 years:
300 mg P.O. q.i.d. with meals and h.s. for maximum therapy of 8 weeks. When healing occurs, stop treatment or give bedtime dose only to control nocturnal hypersecretion. Parenteral: 300 mg diluted to 20 ml with 0.9% normal saline solution or other compatible I.V. solution by I.V. push over 1 to 2 minutes q 6 hours. Or 300 mg diluted in 100 ml 5% dextrose solution or other compatible I.V. solution by I.V. infusion

over 15 to 20 minutes q 6 hours. Or 300 mg I.M. q 6 hours (no dilution necessary). To increase dose, give 300 mg doses more frequently to maximum daily dose of 2,400 mg.
Duodenal ulcer prophylaxis—
Adults and children over 16 years:
400 mg P.O. h.s.
Pathologic hypersecretory conditions (such as Zollinger-Ellison syndrome, systemic mastocytosis, and multiple endocrine adenomas)—
Adults and children over 16 years:
300 mg P.O. q.i.d. with meals and h.s.; adjust to individual needs. Maximum daily dose 2,400 mg.
Parenteral: 300 mg diluted to 20 ml with 0.9% normal saline solution or other compatible I.V. solutions by I.V. push over 1 to 2 minutes q 6 hours. Or 300 mg diluted in 100 ml 5% dextrose solution or other compatible I.V. solution by I.V. infusion over 15 to 20 minutes q 6 hours. To increase dose, give 300 mg doses more frequently to maximum daily dose of 2,400 mg.

SIDE EFFECTS
Blood: *agranulocytosis*, neutropenia, *thrombocytopenia, aplastic anemia.*
CNS: mental confusion, dizziness, headaches, depression.
CV: bradycardia.
GI: mild and transient diarrhea, perforation of chronic peptic ulcers after abrupt cessation of drug, phytobezoars in the elderly.
GU: interstitial nephritis, *transient elevations in BUN and serum creatinine,* reduced sperm count.
Hepatic: jaundice.
Skin: acne-like rash, urticaria, *exfoliative dermatitis.*
Other: hypersensitivity, muscle pain, mild gynecomastia after use longer than 1 month (but no change in endocrine function).

INTERACTIONS
Antacids: interfere with absorption of

---

cimetidine. Separate cimetidine and antacids by at least 1 hour if possible.

NURSING CONSIDERATIONS
• I.M. route of administration may be painful.
• I.V. solutions compatible for dilution with cimetidine: 0.9% sodium chloride solution, 5% and 10% dextrose (and combinations of these) solutions, lactated Ringer's solution, and 5% sodium bicarbonate injection. Do not dilute with sterile water for injection.
• Hemodialysis reduces blood levels of cimetidine. Schedule cimetidine dose at end of hemodialysis treatment.
• Up to 10 g overdosage has been reported without untoward effects.
• Effectiveness in treatment of gastric ulcers not as great as in duodenal ulcer. Cimetidine may prove useful but is still unapproved in pancreatic insufficiency, short-bowel syndrome, psoriasis, prevention and treatment of GI bleeding, relief of symptoms and acid sensitivity in reflux esophagitis, and prevention of gastric inactivation of oral enzyme preparations by gastric acid and pepsin.
• Taking tablets with meals will ensure a more consistent therapeutic effect.
• Large parenteral doses should be avoided in asthmatics.
• Blue dye in Tagamet tablets may produce a false-positive Hemoccult test for blood in gastric juice. This can be avoided by administering the tablet at least 15 minutes before obtaining gastric juice by aspiration.
• Elderly patients more susceptible to cimetidine-induced mental confusion. Dose should be decreased in elderly and in patients with hepatic or renal insufficiency.
• I.V. cimetidine often used in critically ill patients prophylactically to prevent GI bleeding.
• Also effective in the treatment of gastric ulcers.
• Cimetidine is being used investigationally to treat chronic hives.
• When administering cimetidine I.V.

in 100 ml of diluent solution, do not infuse so rapidly that circulatory overload is produced. Some authorities recommend that the drug be infused over at least 30 minutes, to minimize the risk of adverse cardiac effects.
• Available in liquid form (300 mg/ 5 ml).
• Tablets available in two strengths: 200 mg (SKF T12) and 300 mg (SKF T13). Both tablets are pale green. Identify tablet when obtaining a drug history.

dexpanthenol
Ilopan♦, Intrapan, Motilyn♦♦, Tonestat

INDICATIONS & DOSAGE
Postoperative abdominal distention (resulting from flatus retention)—
Adults and children: 250 to 500 mg I.M., repeat in 2 hours and again q 6 hours until distention is relieved. May require therapy for 48 to 72 hours or longer. Or, 500 mg infused slow I.V. drip in glucose or lactated Ringer's solution.
Treatment and postoperative prevention of paralytic ileus—
Adults and children: 500 mg I.M., repeat in 2 hours; then q 4 to 6 hours until distention is relieved. May require therapy for 48 to 72 hours or longer.

SIDE EFFECTS
Blood: prolonged bleeding time.
GI: excessive passage of flatus with increased doses or prolonged use, increased frequency of bowel movements, hyperperistalsis.

INTERACTIONS
None significant.

NURSING CONSIDERATIONS
• Contraindicated in hemophilia because bleeding time is prolonged.
• Don't administer full-strength solution I.V.; always dilute.

Unmarked trade names available in the United States only.
♦ Also available in Canada.   ♦ ♦ Available in Canada only.

• Dexpanthenol use shouldn't delay treatment of mechanical ileus if present.
• A smooth-muscle stimulant; used postoperatively against delayed resumption of intestinal motility. Also used as adjunctive treatment of peripheral neuritis and lupus erythematosus.
• Hypokalemia may cause a decreased response. If this occurs, potassium supplements should be started. Increased doses of dexpanthenol may be needed.
• May also be useful during laxative withdrawal after long-term use.
• Wait 12 hours after giving parasympathomimetics before starting dexpanthenol.

metoclopramide hydrochloride
Maxeran♦♦,Reglan♦

INDICATIONS & DOSAGE
Preventing or reducing nausea and vomiting induced by cisplatin—
Adults: 2 mg/kg I.V. q 2 hours for 5 doses, beginning 30 minutes prior to cisplatin administration.
To facilitate small-bowel intubation and to aid in radiologic examinations—
Adults: 10 mg (2 ml) I.V. as a single dose over 1 to 2 minutes.
Children 6 to 14 years: 2.5 to 5 mg (0.5 to 1 ml).
Children under 6 years: 0.1 mg/kg.
Delayed gastric emptying secondary to diabetic gastroparesis—
Adults: 10 mg P.O. 30 minutes before meals and at bedtime for 2 to 8 weeks, depending on response.

SIDE EFFECTS
CNS: restlessness, *drowsiness,* fatigue, *lassitude,* insomnia, headache, dizziness, extrapyramidal symptoms, tardive dyskinesia, dystonic reactions, sedation.
Endocrine: prolactin secretion, loss of libido.
GI: nausea, bowel disturbances.

INTERACTIONS
Anticholinergics, narcotic analgesics: antagonize effects of metoclopramide. Use together cautiously.

NURSING CONSIDERATIONS
• Contraindicated whenever stimulation of GI motility might be dangerous (hemorrhage, obstruction, perforation), and in pheochromocytoma and epilepsy.
• Should not be taken for longer than 12 weeks.
• Speeds gastric emptying by stimulating smooth muscle in upper GI tract.
• If I.V. injection is too rapid, a transient but intense feeling of anxiety and restlessness occurs, followed by drowsiness.
• Warn patient to avoid activities requiring alertness for 2 hours after taking each dose.
• Give oral form with meals.
• Also used to treat gastroesophageal reflux.
• Extrapyramidal symptoms occur more frequently in children and young adults.

sucralfate
Carafate, Sulcrate**

INDICATIONS & DOSAGE
Short-term (up to 8 weeks) treatment of duodenal ulcer—
Adults: 1 g P.O. q.i.d. 1 hour before meals and at bedtime.

SIDE EFFECTS
CNS: dizziness, sleepiness.
GI: *constipation,* nausea, gastric discomfort, diarrhea.

INTERACTIONS
Antacids: May decrease binding of drug to gastroduodenal mucosa, impairing effectiveness. Don't give within 30 minutes of each other.

Italicized side effects are common or life-threatening.
*Liquid form contains alcohol.   **May contain tartrazine.

NURSING CONSIDERATIONS
• No known contraindications.
• Symptomatic improvement doesn't preclude possibility of gastric cancer.
• Drug is minimally absorbed. Incidence of side effects is low.
• Tell patient for best results to take sucralfate on an empty stomach (1 hour before each meal and at bedtime).
• Pain and ulcer symptoms may subside within first few weeks of therapy. However, for complete healing, be sure patient continues on prescribed regimen.
• Monitor for severe, persistent constipation.
• Studies suggest that drug is as effective as cimetidine in healing duodenal ulcers.
• Drug has been used to treat gastric ulcers, but effectiveness of this use is still under investigation.
• Drug contains aluminum, but isn't classified as an antacid.

49

Corticosteroids

beclomethasone dipropionate
betamethasone
betamethasone acetate and
   betamethasone sodium
   phosphate
betamethasone disodium
   phosphate
betamethasone sodium
   phosphate
cortisone acetate
desoxycorticosterone acetate
desoxycorticosterone pivalate
dexamethasone
dexamethasone acetate
dexamethasone sodium
   phosphate
fludrocortisone acetate
hydrocortisone
hydrocortisone acetate
hydrocortisone sodium
   phosphate
hydrocortisone sodium
   succinate
hydrocortisone retention enema
methylprednisolone
methylprednisolone acetate
methylprednisolone sodium
   succinate
paramethasone acetate
prednisolone
prednisolone acetate
prednisolone sodium phosphate
prednisolone tebutate
prednisone
triamcinolone
triamcinolone acetonide
triamcinolone diacetate
triamcinolone hexacetonide

MECHANISM OF ACTION
• Glucocorticoids (beclomethasone,

betamethasone, cortisone, dexamethasone, hydrocortisone, methylprednisolone, paramethasone, prednisolone, prednisone, and triamcinolone) influence protein metabolism by increasing protein catabolism, decreasing use of amino acids for protein synthesis, and converting amino acids to glucose. Conversion of amino acids to glucose results in accelerated protein breakdown, and muscle weakness and wasting. Interference with wound healing, suppression of the immune response, temporary growth arrest, and osteoporosis may also be related to protein catabolism.

Glucocorticoids influence fat metabolism by inducing lipogenesis, which decreases adipose tissue formation. In high doses they cause fat redistribution—fat loss from the extremities and fat accumulation in the neck, back, and cheeks.

These drugs influence carbohydrate metabolism by converting amino acids to glucose and decreasing peripheral utilization of glucose. This raises blood glucose levels, which triggers pancreatic release of insulin. Prolonged treatment in patients with controlled diabetes may cause resistance to exogenous insulin and necessitate adjustment of insulin levels.

By interfering with histamine synthesis, glucocorticoids influence the blood and blood-forming elements. They also block fibroblast formation, collagen deposition, capillary proliferation, increased capillary permeability in response to tissue trauma, microvascular dilation, plasma exudation, migration of polymorphonuclear leukocytes into inflamed areas, and phagocytosis. Glucocorticoids stabilize cell membranes and inhibit release of proteolytic enzymes, preventing normal inflammatory response. They also have an antilymphocytic action in the treatment of some neoplasms.

Glucocorticoids also potentiate vasoconstriction of norepinephrine in treatment of shock; inhibit release of pituitary ACTH, leading to adrenocortical suppression; and lower blood calcium levels by antagonizing vitamin D effects on calcium absorption from the bowel and by decreasing calcium reabsorption from bone in multiple myeloma.

• Mineralocorticoids (desoxycorticosterone and fludrocortisone) increase sodium reabsorption, and potassium and hydrogen secretion at the nephron's distal convoluted tubule. They also increase water retention, resulting in increased plasma volume and elevated blood pressure.

COMBINATION PRODUCTS
DECADRON WITH XYLOCAINE: dexamethasone phosphate 4 mg and lidocaine hydrochloride 10 mg/ml.

beclomethasone dipropionate
Beclovent♦ Vanceril♦

INDICATIONS & DOSAGE
Steroid-dependent asthma—
Adults: 2 to 4 inhalations t.i.d. or q.i.d. Maximum 20 inhalations daily.
Children 6 to 12 years: 1 to 2 inhalations t.i.d. or q.i.d. Maximum 10 inhalations daily.

SIDE EFFECTS
EENT: hoarseness, fungal infections of mouth and throat.
GI: dry mouth.

INTERACTIONS
None significant.

NURSING CONSIDERATIONS
• Contraindicated in status asthmaticus. Not for asthma controlled by bronchodilators or other noncorticosteroids, or for nonasthmatic bronchial diseases.
• Oral therapy should be tapered slowly. Acute adrenal insufficiency and death have occurred in asthmatics who changed abruptly from oral corticosteroids to beclomethasone.
• During times of stress (trauma, surgery, infection) systemic corticosteroids may be needed to prevent adrenal insufficiency in previously steroid-dependent patients.
• Instruct patient to carry a card indicating his need for supplemental systemic glucocorticoids during stress.
• Patient requiring bronchodilator should use it several minutes before beclomethasone.
• Don't store near heat or open flame.
• Glucocorticoid with potent antiinflammatory action.
• Oral fungal infections can be prevented by following inhalations with glass of water.

betamethasone
Betnelan♦♦, Celestone♦*

betamethasone acetate and betamethasone sodium phosphate
Celestone Soluspan♦

betamethasone disodium phosphate
Betnesol♦♦

betamethasone sodium phosphate
Celestone Phosphate

INDICATIONS & DOSAGE
Severe inflammation or immunosuppression—

Adults: 0.6 to 7.2 mg P.O. daily; or 0.5 to 9 mg (sodium phosphate) I.M., I.V., or into joint or soft tissue daily; or 1.5 to 12 mg (sodium phosphate-acetate suspension) into joint or soft tissue q 1 to 2 weeks, p.r.n.

Prevention of Neonatal Respiratory Distress Syndrome (R.D.S.)—

Adults (pregnant female): 12 mg I.M. Celestone Soluspan 36 to 48 hours before premature delivery. Repeated in 24 hours.

SIDE EFFECTS
Most side effects of corticosteroids are dose- or duration-dependent.

CNS: *euphoria, insomnia,* psychotic behavior, pseudotumor cerebri.

CV: *congestive heart failure,* hypertension, edema.

EENT: cataracts, glaucoma.

GI: *peptic ulcer,* gastrointestinal irritation, increased appetite.

Metabolic: *possible hypokalemia, hyperglycemia and carbohydrate intolerance,* growth suppression in children.

Skin: delayed wound healing, acne, various skin eruptions.

Other: muscle weakness, pancreatitis, hirsutism, susceptibility to infections. Acute adrenal insufficiency may follow increased stress (infection, surgery, trauma) or abrupt withdrawal after long-term therapy.

Withdrawal symptoms: rebound inflammation, fatigue, weakness, arthralgia, fever, dizziness, lethargy, depression, fainting, orthostatic hypotension, dyspnea, anorexia, hypoglycemia. *Sudden withdrawal may be fatal.*

INTERACTIONS
Barbiturates, phenytoin, rifampin: decreased corticosteroid effect. Corticosteroid dose may need to be increased. *Indomethacin, aspirin:* increased risk of GI distress and bleeding. Give together cautiously.

NURSING CONSIDERATIONS
• Contraindicated in systemic fungal infections. Use cautiously in patients with GI ulceration or renal disease, hypertension, osteoporosis, varicella, vaccinia, exanthema, diabetes mellitus, Cushing's syndrome, thromboembolic disorders, seizures, myasthenia gravis, congestive heart failure, tuberculosis, ocular herpes simplex, hypoalbuminemia, emotional instability, or psychotic tendencies.

• Don't use for alternate-day therapy.

• Adrenal suppression may last up to 1 year after drug is stopped. Gradually reduce drug dosage after long-term therapy. Tell patient not to stop drug abruptly or without doctor's consent.

• Always titrate to lowest effective dose.

• To prevent muscle atrophy, give by deep I.M. injection.

• Monitor blood and urine sugars, along with serum potassium, regularly.

• Teach patients about the effects and side effects of the medication. Warn patients who are on long-term therapy about cushingoid symptoms.

• Observe for signs of infection, especially after steroid withdrawal. Tell patients to report slow healing.

• Instruct patient to carry a card indicating his need for supplemental glucocorticoids during stress.

• Give with milk or food to reduce gastric irritation.

• Glucocorticoid with little mineralocorticoid effect.

• Watch for additional potassium depletion from diuretics and amphotericin B.

• Immunizations may show decreased antibody response.

• Obtain baseline weight before starting therapy, and weigh patient daily; report any sudden weight gain to doctor.

• Check for glycosuria in patients using glucose oxidase reagent sticks instead of tablets.

Italicized side effects are common or life-threatening.
*Liquid form contains alcohol.   **May contain tartrazine.

cortisone acetate
Cortistan, Cortone Acetate♦

INDICATIONS & DOSAGE
Adrenal insufficiency, allergy, inflammation—
Adults: 25 to 300 mg P.O. or I.M. daily or on alternate days. Doses highly individualized, depending on severity of disease.

SIDE EFFECTS
Most side effects of corticosteroids are dose- or duration-dependent.
CNS: *euphoria, insomnia,* psychotic behavior, pseudotumor cerebri.
CV: *congestive heart failure,* hypertension, edema.
EENT: cataracts, glaucoma.
GI: *peptic ulcer,* gastrointestinal irritation, increased appetite.
Metabolic: *possible hypokalemia, hyperglycemia and carbohydrate intolerance,* growth suppression in children.
Skin: delayed wound healing, acne, various skin eruptions.
Local: atrophy at I.M. injection sites.
Other: muscle weakness, pancreatitis, hirsutism, susceptibility to infections. Acute adrenal insufficiency may follow increased stress (infection, surgery, trauma) or abrupt withdrawal after long-term therapy.
Withdrawal symptoms: rebound inflammation, fatigue, weakness, arthralgia, fever, dizziness, lethargy, depression, fainting, orthostatic hypotension, dyspnea, anorexia, hypoglycemia. *Sudden withdrawal may be fatal.*

INTERACTIONS
Barbiturates, phenytoin, rifampin: decreased corticosteroid effect. Corticosteroid dose may need to be increased.
Indomethacin, aspirin: increased risk of GI distress and bleeding. Give together cautiously.

NURSING CONSIDERATIONS
• Contraindicated in systemic fungal infections. Use cautiously in patients with GI ulceration or renal disease, hypertension, osteoporosis, varicella, vaccinia, exanthema, diabetes mellitus, Cushing's syndrome, thromboembolic disorders, seizures, myasthenia gravis, congestive heart failure, tuberculosis, ocular herpes simplex, hypoalbuminemia, emotional instability, or psychotic tendencies.
• Gradually reduce drug dosage after long-term therapy. Tell patient not to discontinue drug abruptly or without doctor's consent.
• Always titrate to lowest effective dose.
• Patient may need salt-restricted diet and potassium supplement.
• I.M. route causes slow onset of action. Don't use in acute conditions where rapid effect required. May use on a b.i.d. schedule matching diurnal variation.
• Glucocorticoid with potent mineralocorticoid effect; report sudden weight gain or edema to doctor.
• Observe for signs of infection, especially after steroid withdrawal. Tell patients to report slow healing.
• Drug of choice for replacement therapy in adrenal insufficiency.
• Monitor serum electrolytes and blood and urine sugars.
• Warn patients on long-term therapy about cushingoid symptoms.
• Give with milk or food to reduce gastric irritation.
• Instruct patient to carry a card indicating his need for supplemental glucocorticoids during stress.
• Not for I.V. use.
• Watch for additional potassium depletion from diuretics and amphotericin B.
• Immunizations may show decreased antibody response.

desoxycorticosterone acetate
Doca Acetate, Percorten Acetate

desoxycorticosterone pivalate
Percorten Pivalate

INDICATIONS & DOSAGE
Adrenal insufficiency (partial replacement), salt-losing adrenogenital syndrome—
Adults: 2 to 5 mg (acetate) I.M. daily; or 25 to 100 mg (pivalate) I.M. q 4 weeks. Or implant 1 pellet for each 0.5 mg of the daily injected maintenance dose. Pellets last for 8 to 12 months.

SIDE EFFECTS
CV: *sodium and water retention,* hypertension, cardiac hypertrophy, edema.
Metabolic: *hypokalemia.*

INTERACTIONS
None significant.

NURSING CONSIDERATIONS
• Contraindicated in hypertension, congestive heart failure, cardiac disease. Use cautiously in Addison's disease. Patients may have exaggerated side effects.
• Has no anti-inflammatory effect.
• Most potent mineralocorticoid. Has little glucocorticoid effect.
• Use with glucocorticoid for full treatment of adrenal insufficiency.
• Report significant weight gain, edema, hypertension, or cardiac symptoms to doctor. Drug may have to be stopped.
• Injection is sesame oil solution. Withdraw dose with 19G needle, but give with 23G needle. Inject in upper, outer quadrant of buttocks. Not for I.V. use.
• Monitor sodium and potassium levels, fluid intake. Patient may need salt-restricted diet, potassium supplement.
• Watch for additional potassium depletion from diuretics and amphotericin B.

dexamethasone
Decadron♦, Dexasone♦♦, Dexone, Hexadrol, SK-Dexamethasone

dexamethasone acetate
Decadron-LA, Decameth-LA, Dexacen-LA, Dexasone-LA, Dalalone

dexamethasone sodium phosphate
Decadron Phosphate, Decaject, Decameth, Dexacen-4, Dexasone, Dexone, Dezone, Hexadrol Phosphate♦, Savacort-D

INDICATIONS & DOSAGE
Cerebral edema—
Adults: initially, 10 mg (phosphate) I.V., then 4 to 6 mg I.M. q 6 hours for 2 to 4 days, then taper over 5 to 7 days.
Children: 0.2 mg/kg P.O. daily in divided doses.
Inflammatory conditions, allergic reactions, neoplasias—
Adults: 0.25 to 4 mg P.O. b.i.d., t.i.d., or q.i.d.; or 4 to 16 mg (acetate) I.M. into joint or soft tissue q 1 to 3 weeks; or 0.8 to 1.6 mg (acetate) into lesions q 1 to 3 weeks.
Shock—
Adults: 1 to 6 mg/kg (phosphate) I.V. single dose; or 40 mg I.V. q 2 to 6 hours, p.r.n.
Dexamethasone suppression test—
0.5 mg P.O. q 6 hours for 48 hours.

SIDE EFFECTS
Most side effects of corticosteroids are dose- or duration-dependent.
CNS: *euphoria, insomnia,* psychotic behavior, pseudotumor cerebri.
CV: *congestive heart failure,* hypertension, edema.
EENT: cataracts, glaucoma.
GI: *peptic ulcer,* gastrointestinal irritation, increased appetite.

Metabolic: *possible hypokalemia, hyperglycemia and carbohydrate intolerance,* growth suppression in children.
Skin: delayed wound healing, acne, various skin eruptions.
Local: atrophy at I.M. injection sites.
Other: muscle weakness, pancreatitis, hirsutism, susceptibility to infections. Acute adrenal insufficiency may follow increased stress (infection, surgery, trauma) or abrupt withdrawal after long-term therapy.
Withdrawal symptoms: rebound inflammation, fatigue, weakness, arthralgia, fever, dizziness, lethargy, depression, fainting, orthostatic hypotension, dyspnea, anorexia, hypoglycemia. *Sudden withdrawal may be fatal.*

INTERACTIONS
Barbiturates, phenytoin, rifampin: decreased corticosteroid effect. Corticosteroid dose may need to be increased.
Indomethacin, aspirin: increased risk of GI distress and bleeding. Give together cautiously.

NURSING CONSIDERATIONS
• Contraindicated in systemic fungal infections and for alternate-day therapy. Use cautiously in patients with GI ulceration or renal disease, hypertension, osteoporosis, varicella, vaccinia, exanthema, diabetes mellitus, Cushing's syndrome, thromboembolic disorders, seizures, myasthenia gravis, metastatic cancer, congestive heart failure, tuberculosis, ocular herpes simplex, hypoalbuminemia, emotional instability or psychotic tendencies, and in children.
• Gradually reduce drug dosage after long-term therapy. Tell patient not to discontinue drug abruptly or without doctor's consent.
• Always titrate to lowest effective dose.
• Monitor patient's weight, blood pressure, serum electrolytes.
• Instruct patient to carry a card indicating his need for supplemental systemic glucocorticoids during stress, especially as dose is decreased.
• Teach patient signs of early adrenal insufficiency: fatigue, muscular weakness, joint pain, fever, anorexia, nausea, dyspnea, dizziness, fainting.
• May mask or exacerbate infections.
• Watch for depression or psychotic episodes, especially in high-dose therapy.
• Inspect patient's skin for petechiae. Warn patient about easy bruising.
• Patients with diabetes may need increased insulin; monitor urine for sugar.
• Monitor growth in infants and children on long-term therapy.
• Give I.M. injection deep into gluteal muscle. Avoid subcutaneous injection, as atrophy and sterile abscesses may occur.
• Give P.O. dose with food when possible.
• Warn patients on long-term therapy about cushingoid symptoms.
• Watch for additional potassium depletion from diuretics and amphotericin B.
• Immunizations may show decreased antibody response.
• Follow your hospital's guidelines when performing dexamethasone suppression test.
• Not used for alternate-day therapy.

---

fludrocortisone acetate
Florinef♦

INDICATIONS & DOSAGE
Adrenal insufficiency (partial replacement), salt-losing adrenogenital syndrome—
Adults: 0.1 to 0.2 mg P.O. daily.

SIDE EFFECTS
CV: *sodium and water retention,* hypertension, cardiac hypertrophy, edema.
Metabolic: hypokalemia.

INTERACTIONS
None significant.

NURSING CONSIDERATIONS
• Contraindicated in hypertension, congestive heart failure, cardiac disease. Use cautiously in Addison's disease.
• Monitor patient's blood pressure and serum electrolytes. Weigh patient daily; report sudden weight gain to doctor.
• Warn patient that mild peripheral edema is common.
• Unless contraindicated, give salt-restricted diet rich in potassium and protein. Potassium supplement may be needed.
• Has potent mineralocorticoid effects. Little glucocorticoid effect with usual doses.
• Used with cortisone or hydrocortisone in adrenal insufficiency.
• Watch for additional potassium depletion from diuretics and amphotericin B.

hydrocortisone
Cortef♦, Hydrocortone♦

hydrocortisone acetate
Hydrocortone Acetate, Cortef Acetate

hydrocortisone retention enema
Cortenema, Rectoid

hydrocortisone sodium phosphate
Hydrocortone Phosphate

hydrocortisone sodium succinate
A-HydroCort, S-Cortilean♦♦, Solu-Cortef♦, Solu-Ject♦♦

INDICATIONS & DOSAGE
Severe inflammation, adrenal insufficiency—
Adults: 5 to 30 mg P.O. b.i.d., t.i.d., or q.i.d. (as much as 80 mg P.O. q.i.d. may be given in acute situations); or initially, 100 to 250 mg (succinate) I.M. or I.V., then 50 to 100 mg I.M., as indicated; or 15 to 240 mg (phosphate) I.M. or I.V. q 12 hours; or 5 to 75 mg (acetate) into joints and soft tissue. Dose varies with size of joint. Often local anesthetics are injected with dose.
Shock—
Adults: 500 mg to 2 g (succinate) q 2 to 6 hours.
Children: 0.16 to 1 mg/kg (phosphate or succinate) I.M. or I.V. b.i.d. or t.i.d.
Adjunctive treatment of ulcerative colitis and proctitis—
Adults: 1 enema (100 mg) nightly for 21 days.

SIDE EFFECTS
Most side effects of corticosteroids are dose- or duration-dependent.
CNS: *euphoria, insomnia,* psychotic behavior, pseudotumor cerebri.

CV: *congestive heart failure,* hypertension, edema.
EENT: cataracts, glaucoma.
GI: *peptic ulcer,* gastrointestinal irritation, increased appetite.
Metabolic: *possible hypokalemia, hyperglycemia and carbohydrate intolerance,* growth suppression in children.
Skin: delayed wound healing, acne, various skin eruptions.
Other: muscle weakness, pancreatitis, hirsutism, susceptibility to infections. Acute adrenal insufficiency may occur with increased stress (infection, surgery, trauma) or abrupt withdrawal after long-term therapy.
Withdrawal symptoms: rebound inflammation, fatigue, weakness, arthralgia, fever, dizziness, lethargy, depression, fainting, orthostatic hypotension, dyspnea, anorexia, hypoglycemia. *Sudden withdrawal may be fatal.*

INTERACTIONS

Barbiturates, phenytoin, rifampin: decreased corticosteroid effect. Corticosteroid dose may need to be increased.
Indomethacin, aspirin: increased risk of GI distress and bleeding. Give together cautiously.

NURSING CONSIDERATIONS

• Contraindicated in systemic fungal infections. Use cautiously in patients with GI ulceration or renal disease, hypertension, osteoporosis, varicella, vaccinia, exanthema, diabetes mellitus, Cushing's syndrome, thromboembolic disorders, seizures, myasthenia gravis, metastatic cancer, congestive heart failure, tuberculosis, ocular herpes simplex, hypoalbuminemia, emotional instability or psychotic tendencies, and in children.
• Gradually reduce drug dosage after long-term therapy. Tell patient not to discontinue drug abruptly or without doctor's consent.
• Always titrate to lowest effective dose.

• Glucocorticoid and mineralocorticoid effect.
• Monitor patient's weight, blood pressure, serum electrolytes.
• May mask or exacerbate infections.
• Stress (fever, trauma, surgery, emotional problems) may increase adrenal insufficiency. Dose may have to be increased.
• Instruct patient to carry a card identifying his need for supplemental systemic glucocorticoids during stress.
• Teach patient signs of early adrenal insufficiency: fatigue, muscular weakness, joint pain, fever, anorexia, nausea, dyspnea, dizziness, fainting.
• Watch for depression or psychotic episodes, especially in high-dose therapy.
• Inspect patient's skin for petechiae. Warn patient about easy bruising.
• Patients with diabetes may need increased insulin; monitor urine for sugar.
• Monitor growth in infants and children on long-term therapy.
• Give I.M. injection deep into gluteal muscle. Avoid subcutaneous injection as atrophy and sterile abscesses may occur.
• Unless contraindicated, give salt-restricted diet rich in potassium and protein. Potassium supplement may be needed. Watch for additional potassium depletion from diuretics and amphotericin B.
• Give P.O. dose with food when possible.
• Warn patients on long-term therapy about cushingoid symptoms.
• Acetate form not for I.V. use.
• Enema may produce same systemic effects as other forms of hydrocortisone. If enema therapy must exceed 21 days, discontinue gradually by reducing administration to every other night for 2 or 3 weeks.
• Immunizations may show decreased antibody response.
• Do not confuse Solu-Cortef with Solu-Medrol.

Unmarked trade names available in the United States only.
♦ Also available in Canada.   ♦ ♦ Available in Canada only.

• Injectable forms not for alternate-day therapy.

methylprednisolone
Medrol♦**

methylprednisolone acetate
Depo-Medrol♦, D-Med, Medralone, Pre-Dep, Rep-Pred

methylprednisolone sodium succinate
A-Methapred, Solu-Medrol♦

INDICATIONS & DOSAGE
Severe inflammation or immunosuppression—
Adults: 2 to 60 mg P.O. in four divided doses; or 40 to 80 mg (acetate) daily, I.M. or 10 to 250 mg (succinate) I.M. or I.V. q 4 hours; or 4 to 30 mg (acetate) into joints and soft tissue, p.r.n.
Children: 117 mcg to 1.66 mg/kg (succinate) I.V. in three or four divided doses.
Shock—100 to 250 mg (succinate) I.V. at 2- to 6-hour intervals.

SIDE EFFECTS
Most side effects of corticosteroids are dose- or duration-dependent.
CNS: *euphoria, insomnia,* psychotic behavior, pseudotumor cerebri.
CV: *congestive heart failure,* hypertension, edema.
EENT: cataracts, glaucoma.
GI: *peptic ulcer,* gastrointestinal irritation, increased appetite.
Metabolic: *possible hypokalemia, hyperglycemia and carbohydrate intolerance,* growth suppression in children.
Skin: delayed wound healing, acne, various skin eruptions.
Other: muscle weakness, pancreatitis, hirsutism, susceptibility to infections. Acute adrenal insufficiency may occur with increased stress (infection, surgery, trauma) or abrupt withdrawal after long-term therapy.
Withdrawal symptoms: rebound inflammation, fatigue, weakness, arthralgia, fever, dizziness, lethargy, depression, fainting, orthostatic hypotension, dyspnea, anorexia, hypoglycemia. *Sudden withdrawal may be fatal.*

INTERACTIONS
Barbiturates, phenytoin, rifampin: decreased corticosteroid effect. Corticosteroid dose may need to be increased.
Indomethacin, aspirin: increased risk of GI distress and bleeding. Give together cautiously.

NURSING CONSIDERATIONS
• Contraindicated in systemic fungal infections. Use cautiously in patients with GI ulceration or renal disease, hypertension, osteoporosis, varicella, vaccinia, exanthema, diabetes mellitus, Cushing's syndrome, thromboembolic disorders, seizures, myasthenia gravis, metastatic cancer, congestive heart failure, tuberculosis, ocular herpes simplex, hypoalbuminemia, emotional instability, or psychotic tendencies.
• Gradually reduce drug dosage after long-term therapy. Tell patient not to discontinue drug abruptly or without doctor's consent.
• Always titrate to lowest effective dose.
• Glucocorticoid with little mineralocorticoid effect.
• Discard reconstituted solutions after 48 hours.
• Don't use acetate salt when immediate onset of action needed.
• Dermal atrophy may occur with large doses of acetate salt. Use multiple small injections into lesions.
• Monitor weight, blood pressure, serum electrolytes, sleep patterns. Euphoria may initially interfere with sleep, but patient generally adjusts to the medication after 1 to 3 weeks.
• May mask or exacerbate infections.
• Instruct patient to carry a card identifying his need for supplemental systemic glucocorticoids during stress.
• Teach patient signs of early adrenal

Italicized side effects are common or life-threatening.
*Liquid form contains alcohol.   **May contain tartrazine.

insufficiency: fatigue, muscular weakness, joint pain, fever, anorexia, nausea, dyspnea, dizziness, fainting.
• Watch for depression or psychotic episodes, especially in high-dose therapy.
• Patients with diabetes may need increased insulin; monitor urine for sugar.
• Give I.M. injection deep into gluteal muscle. Avoid subcutaneous injection as atrophy and sterile abscesses may occur.
• Unless contraindicated, give salt-restricted diet rich in potassium and protein. Potassium supplement may be needed. Watch for additional potassium depletion from diuretics and amphotericin B.
• Give P.O. dose with food when possible.
• Give I.V. dose slowly over 1 minute; in shock, give massive I.V. doses over 3 to 15 minutes to prevent cardiac arrhythmias and circulatory collapse.
• Warn patients on long-term therapy about cushingoid symptoms.
• Acetate form not for I.V. use.
• Do not confuse Solu-Medrol with Solu-Cortef.
• Immunizations may show decreased antibody response.
• May be used for alternate-day therapy.

paramethasone acetate
Haldrone

INDICATIONS & DOSAGE
Inflammatory conditions—
Adults: 0.5 to 6 mg P.O. t.i.d. or q.i.d.
Children: 58 to 800 mcg/kg daily divided t.i.d. or q.i.d.

SIDE EFFECTS
Most side effects of corticosteroids are dose- or duration-dependent.
CNS: *euphoria, insomnia,* psychotic behavior, pseudotumor cerebri.
CV: *congestive heart failure,* hypertension, edema.
EENT: cataracts, glaucoma.
GI: *peptic ulcer,* gastrointestinal irritation, increased appetite.
Metabolic: *possible hypokalemia, hyperglycemia and carbohydrate intolerance,* growth suppression in children.
Skin: delayed wound healing, acne, various skin eruptions.
Other: muscle weakness, pancreatitis, hirsutism, susceptibility to infections. Acute adrenal insufficiency may occur with increased stress (infection, surgery, trauma) or abrupt withdrawal after long-term therapy.
Withdrawal symptoms: rebound inflammation, fatigue, weakness, arthralgia, fever, dizziness, lethargy, depression, fainting, orthostatic hypotension, dyspnea, anorexia, hypoglycemia. *Sudden withdrawal may be fatal.*

INTERACTIONS
Barbiturates, phenytoin, rifampin: decreased corticosteroid effect. Corticosteroid dose may need to be increased. *Indomethacin, aspirin:* increased risk of GI distress and bleeding. Give together cautiously.

NURSING CONSIDERATIONS
• Contraindicated in systemic fungal infections and alternate-day therapy. Use cautiously in patients with GI ulceration or renal disease, hypertension, osteoporosis, varicella, vaccinia, exanthema, diabetes mellitus, Cushing's syndrome, thromboembolic disorders, seizures, myasthenia gravis, metastatic cancer, congestive heart failure, tuberculosis, ocular herpes simplex, hypoalbuminemia, emotional instability, or psychotic tendencies.
• Gradually reduce drug dosage after long-term therapy. Tell patient not to discontinue drug abruptly or without doctor's consent.
• Always titrate to lowest effective dose.

- Glucocorticoid with little mineralo-corticoid effect.
- Monitor patient's weight, blood pressure, serum electrolytes.
- May mask or exacerbate infections.
- Instruct patient to carry a card identifying his need for supplemental systemic glucocorticoids during stress.
- Teach patient signs of early adrenal insufficiency: fatigue, muscular weakness, joint pain, fever, anorexia, nausea, dyspnea, dizziness, fainting.
- Watch for depression or psychotic episodes, especially in high-dose therapy.
- Patients with diabetes may need increased insulin; monitor urine for sugar.
- Monitor growth in infants and children on long-term therapy.
- Unless contraindicated, give salt-restricted diet rich in potassium and protein. Potassium supplement may be needed. Watch for additional potassium depletion from diuretics and amphotericin B.
- Give P.O. dose with food when possible, especially if GI irritation occurs.
- Warn patients on long-term therapy about cushingoid symptoms.
- Immunizations may show decreased antibody response.

---

prednisolone
Cordrol, Delta-Cortef♦, Predoxine, Ropredlone, Ster 5, Sterane

prednisolone acetate
Fernisolone, Savacort

prednisolone sodium phosphate
Hydeltrasol, PSP-I.V.

prednisolone tebutate
Hydeltra-TBA, Metalone-TBA

INDICATIONS & DOSAGE
Severe inflammation or immunosuppression—

Adults: 2.5 to 15 mg P.O. b.i.d., t.i.d., or q.i.d.; 2 to 30 mg I.M. (acetate, phosphate), or I.V. (phosphate) q 12 hours; or 2 to 30 mg (phosphate) into joints, lesions, and soft tissue; or 4 to 40 mg (tebutate) into joints and lesions; or 0.25 to 1 ml (acetate-phosphate suspension) into joints weekly, p.r.n.

SIDE EFFECTS
Most side effects of corticosteroids are dose- or duration-dependent.
CNS: *euphoria, insomnia,* psychotic behavior, pseudotumor cerebri.
CV: *congestive heart failure,* hypertension, edema.
EENT: cataracts, glaucoma.
GI: *peptic ulcer,* gastrointestinal irritation, increased appetite.
Metabolic: *possible hypokalemia, hyperglycemia and carbohydrate intolerance,* growth suppression in children.
Skin: delayed wound healing, acne, various skin eruptions.
Other: muscle weakness, pancreatitis, hirsutism, susceptibility to infections. Acute adrenal insufficiency may occur with increased stress (infection, surgery, trauma) or abrupt withdrawal after long-term therapy.
Withdrawal symptoms: rebound inflammation, fatigue, weakness, arthralgia, fever, dizziness, lethargy, depression, fainting, orthostatic hypotension, dyspnea, anorexia, hypoglycemia. *Sudden withdrawal may be fatal.*

INTERACTIONS
Barbiturates, phenytoin, rifampin: decreased corticosteroid effect. Corticosteroid dose may need to be increased. *Indomethacin, aspirin:* increased risk of GI distress and bleeding. Give together cautiously.

NURSING CONSIDERATIONS
- Contraindicated in systemic fungal infections. Use cautiously in patients with GI ulceration or renal disease, hypertension, osteoporosis, varicella, vaccinia, exanthema, diabetes mellitus,

---

Italicized side effects are common or life-threatening.
*Liquid form contains alcohol. **May contain tartrazine.

Cushing's syndrome, thromboembolic disorders, seizures, myasthenia gravis, metastatic cancer, congestive heart failure, tuberculosis, ocular herpes simplex, hypoalbuminemia, emotional instability, or psychotic tendencies.
- Gradually reduce drug dosage after long-term therapy. Tell patient not to discontinue drug abruptly or without doctor's consent.
- Always titrate to lowest effective dose.
- Glucocorticoid with slight mineralo-corticoid action.
- Prednisolone salts (acetate, sodium phosphate, and tebutate) are used parenterally less often than other corticosteroids that have more potent anti-inflammatory action.
- May use for alternate-day therapy.
- Monitor patient's weight, blood pressure, serum electrolytes.
- May mask or exacerbate infections. Tell patient to report slow healing.
- Instruct patient to carry a card identifying his need for supplemental systemic glucocorticoids during stress.
- Teach patient signs of early adrenal insufficiency: fatigue, muscular weakness, joint pain, fever, anorexia, nausea, dyspnea, dizziness, fainting.
- Watch for depression or psychotic episodes, especially in high-dose therapy.
- Patients with diabetes may need increased insulin; monitor urine for sugar.
- Give I.M. injection deep into gluteal muscle. Avoid subcutaneous injection, as atrophy and sterile abscesses may occur.
- Unless contraindicated, give salt-restricted diet rich in potassium and protein. Potassium supplement may be needed. Watch for additional potassium depletion from diuretics and amphotericin B.
- Give P.O. dose with food when possible, to reduce GI irritation.
- Warn patients on long-term therapy about cushingoid symptoms.

- Acetate form not for I.V. use.
- Immunizations may show decreased antibody response.

prednisone
Colisone♦♦, Deltasone♦, Fernisone, Liquid Pred, Meticorten, Orasone, Prednicen-M, SK-Prednisone, Sterapred, Wojtab

INDICATIONS & DOSAGE
Severe inflammation or immunosuppression—
Adults: 2.5 to 15 mg P.O. b.i.d., t.i.d., or q.i.d. Maintenance dose given once daily or every other day.
Children: 0.14 to 2 mg/kg daily P.O. divided q.i.d.

SIDE EFFECTS
Most side effects of corticosteroids are dose- or duration-dependent.
CNS: *euphoria, insomnia,* psychotic behavior, pseudotumor cerebri.
CV: *congestive heart failure,* hypertension, edema.
EENT: cataracts, glaucoma.
GI: *peptic ulcer,* gastrointestinal irritation, increased appetite.
Metabolic: *possible hypokalemia, hyperglycemia and carbohydrate intolerance,* growth suppression in children.
Skin: delayed wound healing, acne, various skin eruptions.
Other: muscle weakness, pancreatitis, hirsutism, susceptibility to infections. Acute adrenal insufficiency may occur with increased stress (infection, surgery, trauma) or abrupt withdrawal after long-term therapy.
Withdrawal symptoms: rebound inflammation, fatigue, weakness, arthralgia, fever, dizziness, lethargy, depression, fainting, orthostatic hypotension, dyspnea, anorexia, hypoglycemia. *Sudden withdrawal may be fatal.*

INTERACTIONS
Barbiturates, phenytoin, rifampin: de-

---

creased corticosteroid effect. Corticosteroid dose may need to be increased. *Indomethacin, aspirin:* increased risk of GI distress and bleeding. Give together cautiously.

NURSING CONSIDERATIONS
• Contraindicated in systemic fungal infections. Use cautiously in patients with GI ulceration or renal disease, hypertension, osteoporosis, varicella, vaccinia, exanthema, diabetes mellitus, Cushing's syndrome, thromboembolic disorders, seizures, myasthenia gravis, metastatic cancer, congestive heart failure, tuberculosis, ocular herpes simplex, hypoalbuminemia, emotional instability, or psychotic tendencies.
• Gradually reduce drug dosage after long-term therapy. Tell patient not to discontinue drug abruptly or without doctor's consent.
• Always titrate to lowest effective dose.
• Monitor patient's blood pressure, sleep patterns, serum potassium levels.
• Weigh patient daily; report sudden weight gain to doctor.
• May mask or exacerbate infections. Tell patient to report slow healing.
• Instruct patient to carry a card identifying his need for supplemental systemic glucocorticoids during stress.
• Teach patient signs of early adrenal insufficiency: fatigue, muscular weakness, joint pain, fever, anorexia, nausea, dyspnea, dizziness, fainting.
• Watch for depression or psychotic episodes, especially in high-dose therapy.
• Patients with diabetes may need increased insulin; monitor urine for sugar.
• Monitor growth in infants and children on long-term therapy.
• Give salt-restricted diet rich in potassium and protein. Potassium supplement may be needed. Watch for additional potassium depletion from diuretics and amphotericin B.
• Unless contraindicated, give P.O.

dose with food when possible, to reduce GI irritation.
• May use for alternate-day therapy.
• Warn patients on long-term therapy about cushingoid symptoms.
• Immunizations may show decreased antibody response.
• Now available in a pleasant tasting, grape-flavored syrup (Liquid Pred).

triamcinolone
Aristocort♦, Kenacort♦**,
Spencort, Tricilone

triamcinolone acetonide
Kenalog♦

triamcinolone diacetate
Amcort, Aristocort Forte Parenteral,
Cenocort Forte, Cino-40, Tracilon,
Triam-Forte, Tristoject

triamcinolone hexacetonide
Aristospan♦

INDICATIONS & DOSAGE
Severe inflammation or immunosuppression—
Adults: 4 to 48 mg P.O. daily divided b.i.d., t.i.d., or q.i.d., or 40 mg I.M. (diacetate or acetonide) weekly; or 5 to 48 mg (diacetate or acetonide) into lesions; or 2 to 40 mg (diacetate or acetonide) into joints and soft tissue; or up to 0.5 mg (hexacetonide) per square inch of affected skin intralesional; or 2 to 20 mg (hexacetonide) intra-articular or intrasynovial into soft tissue or into joint or lesion. Often, a local anesthetic is injected into the joint with triamcinolone.

SIDE EFFECTS
Most side effects of corticosteroids are dose- or duration-dependent.
CNS: *euphoria, insomnia,* psychotic behavior, pseudotumor cerebri.
CV: *congestive heart failure,* hypertension, edema.
EENT: cataracts, glaucoma.

Italicized side effects are common or life-threatening.
*Liquid form contains alcohol.   **May contain tartrazine.

GI: *peptic ulcer*, gastrointestinal irritation, increased appetite.
Metabolic: *possible hypokalemia, hyperglycemia and carbohydrate intolerance,* growth suppression in children.
Skin: delayed wound healing, acne, various skin eruptions.
Other: muscle weakness, pancreatitis, hirsutism, susceptibility to infections. Acute adrenal insufficiency may occur with increased stress (infection, surgery, trauma) or abrupt withdrawal after long-term therapy.
Withdrawal symptoms: rebound inflammation, fatigue, weakness, arthralgia, fever, dizziness, lethargy, depression, fainting, orthostatic hypotension, dyspnea, anorexia, hypoglycemia. *Sudden withdrawal may be fatal.*

INTERACTIONS
Barbiturates, phenytoin, rifampin: decreased corticosteroid effect. Corticosteroid dose may need to be increased.
Indomethacin, aspirin: increased risk of GI distress and bleeding. Give together cautiously.

NURSING CONSIDERATIONS
• Contraindicated in systemic fungal infections. Use cautiously in patients with GI ulceration or renal disease, hypertension, osteoporosis, varicella, vaccinia, exanthema, diabetes mellitus, Cushing's syndrome, thromboembolic disorders, seizures, myasthenia gravis, metastatic cancer, congestive heart failure, tuberculosis, ocular herpes simplex, hypoalbuminemia, emotional instability, or psychotic tendencies.
• Gradually reduce drug dosage after long-term therapy. Tell patient not to discontinue drug abruptly or without doctor's consent.

• Always titrate to lowest effective dose.
• Monitor patient's weight, blood pressure, serum electrolytes.
• May mask or exacerbate infections. Tell patient to report slow healing.
• Instruct patient to carry a card identifying his need for supplemental systemic glucocorticoids during stress.
• Teach patient signs of early adrenal insufficiency: fatigue, muscular weakness, joint pain, fever, anorexia, nausea, dyspnea, dizziness, fainting.
• Watch for depression or psychotic episodes, especially in high-dose therapy.
• Patients with diabetes may need increased insulin; monitor urine for sugar.
• Give I.M. injection deep into gluteal muscle. Avoid subcutaneous injection, as atrophy and sterile abscesses may occur.
• Unless contraindicated, give salt-restricted diet rich in potassium and protein. Potassium supplement may be needed. Watch for additional potassium depletion from diuretics and amphotericin B.
• Give P.O. dose with food when possible, to reduce GI irritation.
• Glucocorticoid with very little mineralocorticoid effect.
• Discard unused diluted suspension within 7 days.
• Don't use diluents that contain preservatives. Flocculation may occur.
• Warn patients on long-term therapy about cushingoid symptoms.
• Immunizations may show decreased antibody response.
• Not for alternate-day therapy.
• No forms for I.V. use. Hexacetonide not for I.V. or I.M. use.

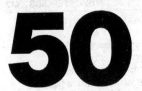

Androgens and anabolic steroids

danazol
ethylestrenol
fluoxymesterone
methyltestosterone
nandrolone decanoate
nandrolone phenpropionate
oxandrolone
oxymetholone
stanozolol
testosterone
testosterone cypionate
testosterone enanthate
testosterone propionate

MECHANISM OF ACTION

● Androgens are simply exogenous replacements that stimulate target tissues to develop normally in androgen-deficient males.

● Anabolic steroids stimulate cellular protein synthesis in debilitated patients. The resulting positive nitrogen balance promotes anabolism. Anabolic steroids also promote a sense of well-being in debilitated patients. This may encourage the patient to eat more and gain weight.

Anabolic steroids improve calcium balance and decrease bone resorption. They also enhance erythropoiesis by stimulating secretion of renal or extrarenal erythropoietin and by directly stimulating heme synthesis, an action potentiated by erythropoietin.

COMBINATION PRODUCTS

DELADUMONE INJECTION (oil)♦: testosterone enanthate 90 mg, estradiol valerate 4 mg, and chlorobutanol 0.5%.
DEPO-TESTADIOL (oil): testosterone cy-
pionate 50 mg, estradiol cypionate 2 mg, and chlorobutanol 0.5%.
DITATE: estradiol valerate 4 mg, and testosterone enanthate 90 mg.
DITATE-DS: estradiol valerate 8 mg, and testosterone enanthate 180 mg.
ESTRATEST H.S.: esterified estrogens 0.625 mg, and methyltestosterone 1.25 mg.
FORMATRIX: conjugated estrogens 1.25 mg, methyltestosterone 10 mg, and ascorbic acid 400 mg.
LACTOSTAT (oil)♦♦: testosterone enanthate benzilic acid hydrazone 300 mg, estradiol dienanthate 15 mg, and estradiol benzoate 6 mg.
MEDIATRIC: conjugated estrogens 0.25 mg, methyltestosterone 2.5 mg, methamphetamine HCl 1 mg, vitamin C 100 mg, thiamine 10 mg, vitamin B_{12} 2.5 mcg, ferrous sulfate 30 mg, vitamin B_2 5 mg, vitamin B_6 3 mg, and nicotinamide 50 mg.
PREMARIN WITH METHYLTESTOSTERONE♦: conjugated estrogens 0.625 mg and methyltestosterone 5 mg.
TESTOJECT-E.P. Testosterone enanthate 200 mg, testosterone propionate 25 mg, and Chlorobutanol 0.5%.

---

danazol
Cyclomen♦♦, Danocrine

INDICATIONS & DOSAGE
Endometriosis—
Women: 400 mg P.O. b.i.d. uninterrupted for 3 to 6 months; may continue for 9 months.
Fibrocystic breast disease—
Women: 100 to 400 mg P.O. daily in 2

Italicized side effects are common or life-threatening.
*Liquid form contains alcohol.   **May contain tartrazine.

divided doses uninterrupted for 2 to 6 months.

Prevention of hereditary angioedema—
Adults: 200 mg P.O. 2 to 3 times a day, continued until favorable response is achieved. Then dosage should be decreased by half at 1- to 3-month intervals.

SIDE EFFECTS

Androgenic: acne, edema, *weight gain, hirsutism,* hoarseness, clitoral enlargement, *decrease in breast size,* changes in libido, male-pattern baldness, *oiliness of skin or hair.*
CNS: dizziness, headache, sleep disorders, fatigue, tremor, irritability, excitation, lethargy, mental depression, chills, paresthesias.
CV: elevated blood pressure.
EENT: visual disturbances.
GI: gastric irritation, nausea, vomiting, diarrhea, constipation, change in appetite.
GU: hematuria.
Hepatic: jaundice.
Hypoestrogenic: flushing; sweating; vaginitis, including itching, dryness, burning, and vaginal bleeding; nervousness, emotional lability.
Other: muscle cramps or spasms.

INTERACTIONS
None significant.

NURSING CONSIDERATIONS
• Contraindicated in patients with undiagnosed abnormal genital bleeding; impaired renal, cardiac, or hepatic function. Use cautiously in patients with epilepsy or migraine headache.
• Use with diet high in calories and protein unless contraindicated.
• Monitor closely for signs of virilization. Some androgenic effects, such as deepening of voice, may not be reversible upon discontinuation of drug.
• Advise patient who is taking danazol for fibrocystic disease to examine breasts regularly. If breast nodule en-

larges during treatment, tell patient to call doctor immediately.
• Instruct patient to wear cotton underwear only.
• Washing after intercourse is recommended to decrease the risk of vaginitis.

ethylestrenol
Maxibolin♦*

INDICATIONS & DOSAGE
Promote weight gain and combat tissue depletion, refractory anemias, catabolic effects of corticosteroid therapy, osteoporosis, prolonged immobilization, and debilitated states—
Adults: 4 to 8 mg P.O. daily, reduced to minimum levels at first evidence of clinical response.
Children: 1 to 3 mg P.O. daily; highly individualized.
A single course of therapy in both adults and children should not exceed 6 weeks; may be reinstituted after 4-week interval.

SIDE EFFECTS
Androgenic: in females—*acne, edema, oily skin, weight gain, hirsutism, hoarseness,* clitoral enlargement, changes in libido. In males—prepubertal: premature epiphyseal closure, acne, priapism, growth of body and facial hair, phallic enlargement; postpubertal: testicular atrophy, oligospermia, decreased ejaculatory volume, impotence, gynecomastia, epididymitis.
CV: edema.
GI: gastroenteritis, nausea, vomiting, diarrhea, constipation, change in appetite.
GU: bladder irritability.
Hepatic: jaundice.
Hypoestrogenic: in females—flushing; sweating; vaginitis with itching, drying, burning, or bleeding; menstrual irregularities.
Other: hypercalcemia.

INTERACTIONS
None significant.

NURSING CONSIDERATIONS
• Contraindicated in patients with prostatic hypertrophy with obstruction; carcinoma of male breast; hypercalcemia; prostatic cancer; cardiac, hepatic, or renal decompensation; nephrosis; and in premature infants. Use cautiously in prepubertal males; patients with diabetes or coronary disease; patients taking ACTH, corticosteroids, or anticoagulants.
• Hypercalcemia symptoms may be difficult to distinguish from symptoms of condition being treated unless anticipated and thought of as a symptom cluster. Hypercalcemia is particularly likely to occur in patients with metastatic breast cancer and may indicate bone metastases.
• Tell females to report menstrual irregularities; therapy should be discontinued pending etiologic determination.
• Watch for signs of virilization; may be irreversible despite prompt discontinuation of therapy. Doctor must decide if benefits outweigh effects.
• Closely monitor boys under 7 years for precocious development of male sexual characteristics.
• In children: therapy should be preceded by X-ray of wrist bones to establish level of bone maturation. During treatment, bone maturation may proceed more rapidly than linear growth; dosage should be intermittent and X-rays taken periodically.
• Edema is generally controllable with salt restriction and/or diuretics. Monitor weight routinely.
• Watch for symptoms of jaundice. Dose adjustment may reverse condition. If liver function tests are abnormal, discontinue therapy.
• Observe patient on concomitant anticoagulant therapy for ecchymotic areas, petechiae, or abnormal bleeding. Monitor prothrombin time.
• Watch for symptoms of hypogly-

cemia in patients with diabetes. Dosage of antidiabetic drug may need adjustment.
• Use with diet high in calories and protein unless contraindicated.
• Anabolic steroids may alter many laboratory studies during therapy and for 2 to 3 weeks after therapy is stopped.
• Involve the patient, family members, and a dietitian in developing a dietary regimen suitable to the anorexic or debilitated patient.

---

fluoxymesterone
Android-F, Halotestin♦**,
Oratestin♦♦, Oratestryl

INDICATIONS & DOSAGE
Hypogonadism and impotence due to testicular deficiency—
Adults: 2 to 10 mg P.O. daily.
Palliation of breast cancer in women—
15 to 30 mg P.O. daily in divided doses. All dosages should be individualized and reduced to minimum when effect is noted.
Postpartum breast engorgement—
2.5 mg P.O. followed by 5 to 10 mg daily for 5 days.

SIDE EFFECTS
Androgenic: in females—*acne, edema, oily skin, weight gain, hirsutism, hoarseness,* clitoral enlargement, change in libido. In males—prepubertal: premature epiphyseal closure, acne, priapism, growth of body and facial hair, phallic enlargement; postpubertal: testicular atrophy, oligospermia, decreased ejaculatory volume, impotence, gynecomastia, epididymitis.
CV: edema.
GI: gastroenteritis, nausea, vomiting, constipation, change in appetite, diarrhea.
GU: bladder irritability.
Hepatic: jaundice.
Hypoestrogenic: in females—flushing; sweating; vaginitis with itching, drying,

---

Italicized side effects are common or life-threatening.
*Liquid form contains alcohol.   **May contain tartrazine.

burning, or bleeding; menstrual irregularities; emotional lability.
Other: hypercalcemia.

INTERACTIONS
None significant.

NURSING CONSIDERATIONS
• Contraindicated in patients with prostatic hypertrophy with obstruction; carcinoma of male breast; prostatic cancer; cardiac, hepatic, or renal decompensation; nephrosis; hypercalcemia; and in premature infants. Use cautiously in prepubertal males; patients with diabetes or coronary disease; and patients taking ACTH, corticosteroids, or anticoagulants.
• Hypercalcemia symptoms may be difficult to distinguish from symptoms associated with condition being treated unless anticipated and thought of as a symptom cluster. Hypercalcemia is particularly likely to occur in patients with metastatic breast cancer and may indicate bone metastases.
• Explain to patient on drug for palliation of breast cancer that virilization usually occurs at dosage used. Give emotional support. Tell patient to report androgenic effects immediately. Stopping drug will prevent further androgenic changes but will probably not reverse those already existing.
• When used in breast cancer, subjective effects may not be seen for about 1 month; objective symptoms not for 3 months.
• Tell females to report menstrual irregularities; therapy should be discontinued pending etiologic determination.
• Edema is generally controllable with salt restriction and/or diuretics. Monitor weight routinely.
• Watch for symptoms of jaundice. Dose adjustment may reverse condition. If liver function tests are abnormal, therapy should be discontinued.
• Observe patient on concomitant anticoagulant therapy for ecchymotic

areas, petechiae, or abnormal bleeding. Monitor prothrombin time.
• Watch for symptoms of hypoglycemia in patients with diabetes. Dosage of antidiabetic drug may need adjustment.
• Use with diet high in calories and protein unless contraindicated.

---

methyltestosterone
Android-5, Android-10, Metandren♦, Oreton-Methyl, Testred, Virilon

INDICATIONS & DOSAGE
Adults:
Breast engorgement of nonnursing mothers—80 mg P.O. daily, or 40 mg buccal daily for 3 to 5 days.
Breast cancer in women 1 to 5 years postmenopausal—200 mg P.O. daily; or 100 mg buccal daily.
Eunuchoidism and eunuchism, male climacteric symptoms—10 to 40 mg P.O. daily; or 5 to 20 mg buccal daily.
Postpubertal cryptorchidism—30 mg P.O. daily; or 15 mg buccal daily.

SIDE EFFECTS
Androgenic: in females—*acne, edema, oily skin, weight gain, hirsutism, hoarseness,* clitoral enlargement, changes in libido. In males—prepubertal: premature epiphyseal closure, acne, priapism, growth of body and facial hair, phallic enlargement; postpubertal: testicular atrophy, oligospermia, decreased ejaculatory volume, impotence, gynecomastia, epididymitis.
CV: edema.
GI: gastroenteritis, constipation, nausea, vomiting, diarrhea, change in appetite.
GU: bladder irritability.
Hepatic: jaundice.
Hypoestrogenic: in females—flushing; sweating; vaginitis with itching, drying, burning, or bleeding; menstrual irregularities.

Local: irritation of oral mucosa with buccal administration.
Other: hypercalcemia.

INTERACTIONS
None significant.

NURSING CONSIDERATIONS
• Contraindicated in women of child-bearing potential (possible masculinization of female infant); in elderly, asthenic males who may react adversely to androgen overstimulation; in hypercalcemia; cardiac, hepatic, or renal decompensation; prostatic or breast cancer in males; benign prostatic hypertrophy with obstruction; conditions aggravated by fluid retention; hypertension; and in premature infants. Use cautiously in myocardial infarction or coronary artery disease.
• Treatment of breast cancer usually restricted to patients 1 to 5 years postmenopausal.
• Edema is generally controllable with salt restriction and/or diuretics.
• Periodic serum cholesterol and calcium determinations, and cardiac and liver function tests recommended. Watch closely for jaundice.
• In metastatic breast cancer, hypercalcemia may indicate progression of bone metastases. Report signs of hypercalcemia.
• Therapeutic response in breast cancer is usually apparent within 3 months. Therapy should be stopped if signs of disease progression appear.
• Enhances hypoglycemia; teach patient signs of hypoglycemia, and instruct him to report immediately if they occur.
• Watch for ecchymoses, petechiae, and abnormal bleeding in patients receiving concomitant anticoagulants.
• Promptly report signs of virilization in females.
• Use with diet high in calories and protein unless contraindicated.
• Buccal tablets twice as potent as oral tablets. Tell patient to avoid eating,

drinking, chewing, or smoking while buccal tablet is in place, and that tablet is not to be swallowed. Tablet requires 30 to 60 minutes to dissolve. Instruct patient to change tablet absorption site with each dose to minimize risk of buccal irritation.
• Erroneously thought to enhance athletic ability.

nandrolone decanoate
Deca-Durabolin♦, Hybolin Decanoate

nandrolone phenpropionate
Anabolin, Anorolone, Durabolin♦, Nandrolin, Nandrobolic

INDICATIONS & DOSAGE
Severe debility or disease states, refractory anemias (decanoate)—
Adults: 100 to 200 mg I.M. weekly. Therapy should be intermittent.
Tissue-building (decanoate)—
Adults: 50 to 100 mg I.M. q 3 to 4 weeks.
Children 2 to 13 years: 25 to 50 mg I.M. q 3 to 4 weeks.
Severe debility or disease states (phenpropionate)—
Adults: 50 to 100 mg I.M. weekly.
Children 2 to 13 years: 12.5 to 25 mg I.M. q 2 to 4 weeks.
Children under 2 years: 12.5 mg I.M. q 2 to 4 weeks.
Therapy should be intermittent, based on therapeutic response.
Tissue building and/or erythropoietic effects (phenpropionate)—
Adults: 25 to 50 mg I.M. weekly.

SIDE EFFECTS
Androgenic: in females—*acne, edema, oily skin, weight gain, hirsutism, hoarseness,* clitoral enlargement, decreased or increased libido. In males—prepubertal: premature epiphyseal closure, acne, priapism, growth of body and facial hair, phallic enlargement; postpubertal: testicular atrophy,

---

Italicized side effects are common or life-threatening.
*Liquid form contains alcohol.   **May contain tartrazine.

oligospermia, decreased ejaculatory volume, impotence, gynecomastia, epididymitis.

CV: edema.

GI: gastroenteritis, nausea, vomiting, diarrhea, change in appetite.

GU: bladder irritability.

Hepatic: jaundice.

Hypoestrogenic: in females—flushing; sweating; vaginitis with itching, drying, burning, or bleeding; menstrual irregularities with large doses.

Local: pain at injection site, induration.

Other: hypercalcemia, hypercalciuria.

INTERACTIONS
None significant.

NURSING CONSIDERATIONS
• Contraindicated in patients with prostatic hypertrophy with obstruction; male breast and prostatic cancer; cardiac, hepatic, or renal decompensation; nephrosis; and in premature infants. Use cautiously in prepubertal males; patients with diabetes or coronary disease; patients taking ACTH, corticosteroids, or anticoagulants.

• Inject drug deep I.M., preferably into upper outer quadrant of gluteal muscle in adults.

• Monitor serum cholesterol in cardiac patients.

• Hypercalcemia is most likely to occur in patients with mammary carcinoma; these patients should have quantitative urinary and serum calcium level determinations.

• Tell females to report menstrual irregularities; therapy should be discontinued pending etiologic determination.

• Watch for signs of virilization; they may be irreversible despite prompt discontinuation of therapy.

• Closely observe boys under 7 years for precocious development of male sexual characteristics.

• In children, therapy should be preceded by X-ray of wrist bones to establish level of bone maturation. During treatment, bone maturation may pro-

ceed more rapidly than linear growth; dosage should be intermittent and X-rays taken periodically.

• Edema is generally controllable with salt restrictions and/or diuretics.

• Watch for symptoms of jaundice. Dose adjustment may reverse condition. If liver function tests are abnormal, therapy should be discontinued.

• Observe patients receiving concomitant anticoagulant therapy for ecchymotic areas, petechiae, or abnormal bleeding. Monitor prothrombin time.

• Watch for symptoms of hypoglycemia in patients with diabetes. Dosage of antidiabetic drug may need adjustment.

• Use with diet high in calories and protein unless contraindicated.

• Erroneously thought to enhance athletic ability.

• Considered an adjunctive therapy.

• Anabolic steroids may alter many laboratory studies during therapy and for 2 to 3 weeks after therapy is stopped.

---

oxandrolone
Anavar

INDICATIONS & DOSAGE
To combat catabolic effects of corticosteroid therapy, osteoporosis, prolonged immobilization and debilitated states—
Adults: 2.5 mg P.O. b.i.d., t.i.d., or q.i.d.; up to 20 mg daily for 2 to 4 weeks.

Children: 0.25 mg/kg daily P.O. for 2 to 4 weeks.

Continuous therapy should not exceed 3 months.

SIDE EFFECTS
Androgenic: in females—*acne, edema, oily skin, weight gain, hirsutism, hoarseness,* clitoral enlargement, decreased or increased libido. In males—prepubertal: premature epiphyseal closure, acne, priapism, growth of body and facial hair, phallic enlarge-

ment; postpubertal: testicular atrophy, oligospermia, decreased ejaculatory volume, impotence, gynecomastia, epididymitis.
CV: edema.
GI: gastroenteritis, nausea, vomiting, constipation or diarrhea, change in appetite.
GU: bladder irritability.
Hepatic: jaundice.
Hypoestrogenic: in females—flushing; sweating; vaginitis with itching, drying, burning, or bleeding; menstrual irregularities.
Other: hypercalcemia.

INTERACTIONS
None significant.

NURSING CONSIDERATIONS
• Contraindicated in patients with prostatic hypertrophy with obstruction; prostatic and male breast cancer; cardiac, hepatic, or renal decompensation; nephrosis; and in premature infants. Use cautiously in prepubertal males; patients with diabetes or coronary disease; patients taking ACTH, corticosteroids, or anticoagulants.
• Hypercalcemia symptoms may be difficult to distinguish from symptoms of condition being treated unless anticipated and thought of as a cluster. Hypercalcemia most likely to occur with metastatic breast cancer and may indicate bone metastases.
• Tell females to report menstrual irregularities; therapy should be discontinued pending etiologic determination.
• Watch for signs of virilization; may be irreversible despite prompt discontinuation of therapy. Doctor must decide if benefits outweigh effects.
• Boys under 7 years should be closely observed for precocious development of male sexual characteristics.
• In children, therapy should be preceded by X-ray of wrist bones to establish level of bone maturation. During treatment, bone maturation may proceed more rapidly than linear growth;

dosage should be intermittent and X-rays taken periodically.
• Edema is generally controllable with salt restriction and/or diuretics. Monitor weight routinely.
• Watch for symptoms of jaundice. Dose adjustment may reverse condition. Periodic liver function tests are recommended.
• Observe patient on concomitant anticoagulant therapy for ecchymotic areas, petechiae, or abnormal bleeding. Monitor prothrombin time.
• Watch for symptoms of hypoglycemia in patients with diabetes. Change of dosage of antidiabetic drug may be required.
• Use with diet high in calories and protein unless contraindicated.
• Erroneously thought to enhance athletic ability.
• Anabolic steroids may alter many laboratory studies during therapy and for 2 to 3 weeks after therapy is stopped.

---

oxymetholone
Anadrol-50, Anapolon 50♦♦

INDICATIONS & DOSAGE
Aplastic anemia—
Adults and children: 1 to 5 mg/kg P.O. daily. Dose highly individualized; response not immediate. Trial of 3 to 6 months required.
Osteoporosis, catabolic conditions—
Adults: 5 to 15 mg P.O. daily, or up to 30 mg P.O. daily.
Children over 6 years: up to 10 mg P.O. daily.
Children under 6 years: 1.25 mg P.O. daily or up to q.i.d. Continuous therapy should not exceed 30 days in children; 90 days in any patient.

SIDE EFFECTS
Androgenic: in females—*acne, edema, oily skin, weight gain, hirsutism, hoarseness,* clitoral enlargement, decreased or increased libido, male-

---

Italicized side effects are common or life-threatening.
*Liquid form contains alcohol.   **May contain tartrazine.

pattern hair loss. In males—prepubertal: premature epiphyseal closure, acne, priapism, growth of body and facial hair, phallic enlargement; postpubertal: testicular atrophy, oligospermia, decreased ejaculatory volume, impotence, gynecomastia, epididymitis.
CV: edema.
GI: gastroenteritis, nausea, vomiting, constipation, diarrhea, change in appetite.
GU: bladder irritability.
Hepatic: jaundice.
Hypoestrogenic: in females—flushing; sweating; vaginitis with itching, drying, burning, or bleeding; menstrual irregularities.
Other: hypercalcemia.

INTERACTIONS
None significant.

NURSING CONSIDERATIONS
• Contraindicated in patients with prostatic hypertrophy with obstruction; prostatic and male breast cancer; cardiac, hepatic, or renal decompensation; nephrosis; and in premature infants. Use cautiously in prepubertal males; patients with diabetes or coronary diseases; patients taking ACTH, corticosteroids, or anticoagulants.
• Hypercalcemia symptoms may be difficult to distinguish from symptoms of condition being treated unless anticipated and thought of as a cluster. Hypercalcemia most likely to occur in metastatic breast cancer and may indicate bone metastases.
• Supportive treatment of anemias (transfusions, correction of iron, folic acid, vitamin B_{12}, or pyridoxine deficiency). Give 3 to 6 months for response.
• Effects in osteoporosis usually seen in 4 to 6 weeks.
• Tell females to report menstrual irregularities; therapy should be discontinued pending etiologic determination.
• Watch for signs of virilization; may be irreversible despite prompt stopping

of therapy. Doctor must decide if benefits outweigh effects.
• Boys under 7 years should be closely observed for precocious development of male sexual characteristics.
• In children, therapy should be preceded by X-ray of wrist bones to establish level of bone maturation. During treatment, bone maturation may proceed more rapidly than linear growth; dosage should be intermittent and X-rays taken periodically. Epiphyseal development may continue 6 months after stopping therapy.
• Edema is generally controllable with salt restriction and/or diuretics. Monitor weight routinely.
• Watch for symptoms of jaundice. Dose adjustment may reverse condition; if liver function tests are abnormal, therapy should be discontinued.
• Observe patient on concomitant anticoagulant therapy for ecchymotic areas, petechiae, or abnormal bleeding. Monitor prothrombin time.
• Watch for symptoms of hypoglycemia in patients with diabetes. Change of dosage in antidiabetic drug may be required.
• Use with diet high in calories and protein unless contraindicated.
• Erroneously thought to enhance athletic ability.
• Anabolic steroids may alter many laboratory studies during therapy and for 2 to 3 weeks after therapy is stopped.
• Has also been used to prevent hereditary angioedema.

stanozolol
Winstrol♦

INDICATIONS & DOSAGE
To increase hemoglobin in some cases of aplastic anemia—
Adults: 2 mg P.O. t.i.d.
Children 6 to 12 years: up to 2 mg P.O. t.i.d.

Children under 6 years: 1 mg P.O.
b.i.d.
Therapy should be intermittent.
Prevention of hereditary angioedema—
Adults: 0.5 to 2 mg P.O. daily for 2
years.

SIDE EFFECTS
Androgenic: in females—*acne,
edema, oily skin, weight gain, hirsutism, hoarseness,* clitoral enlargement,
decreased or increased libido. In
males— prepubertal: premature epiphyseal closure, acne, priapism, growth
of body and facial hair, phallic enlargement; postpubertal: testicular atrophy,
oligospermia, decreased ejaculatory
volume, impotence, gynecomastia, epididymitis.
CV: edema.
GI: gastroenteritis, nausea, vomiting,
constipation, diarrhea, change in
appetite.
GU: bladder irritability.
Hypoestrogenic: in females—flushing,
sweating; vaginitis with itching, drying,
burning or bleeding; menstrual irregularities.
Other: hypercalcemia.

INTERACTIONS
None significant.

NURSING CONSIDERATIONS
• Contraindicated in patients with
prostatic hypertrophy with obstruction;
prostatic and male breast cancer; cardiac, hepatic, or renal decompensation;
nephrosis; and in premature infants.
Use cautiously in prepubertal males;
patients with diabetes or coronary disease; patients taking ACTH, corticosteroids, or anticoagulants.
• Hypercalcemia symptoms may be
difficult to distinguish from symptoms
of condition being treated unless anticipated and thought of as a cluster.
Hypercalcemia most likely to occur in
metastatic breast cancer and may indicate bone metastases.
• Tell females to report menstrual ir-

regularities; therapy should be discontinued pending etiologic determination.
• Smaller dose (2 mg b.i.d.) is used in
females to avoid virilization. Watch for
these side effects; may be irreversible
despite prompt stopping of therapy.
Doctor must decide if benefits outweigh effects.
• Boys under 7 years should be closely
observed for precocious development
of male sexual characteristics.
• In children, therapy should be preceded by X-ray of wrist bones to establish level of bone maturation. During
treatment, bone maturation may proceed more rapidly than linear growth;
dosage should be intermittent and X-
rays taken periodically.
• Edema is generally controllable with
salt restriction and/or diuretics. Monitor weight routinely.
• Watch for symptoms of jaundice.
Dose adjustment may reverse condition; check liver function tests regularly. If abnormal, therapy should be
discontinued.
• Observe patient on concomitant anticoagulant therapy for ecchymotic
areas, petechiae, or abnormal bleeding.
Monitor prothrombin time.
• Watch for symptoms of hypoglycemia in patients with diabetes. Change
of dosage of antidiabetic drug may be
required.
• Use with diet high in calories and
protein unless contraindicated.
• Administer before or with meals to
minimize GI distress.
• Monitor serum cholesterol in cardiac
patients.
• Erroneously thought to enhance athletic ability.
• Anabolic steroids may alter many
laboratory studies during therapy and
for 2 to 3 weeks after therapy is
stopped.

Italicized side effects are common or life-threatening.
*Liquid form contains alcohol.   **May contain tartrazine.

testosterone

Andronaq, Histerone, Malogen♦,
Oreton, Testoject

INDICATIONS & DOSAGE

Eunuchoidism, eunuchism, male climacteric symptoms—
Adults: 10 to 25 mg I.M. 2 to 5 times weekly; or 2 to 6 pellets (75 mg each) implanted subcutaneously q 3 to 6 months.
*Breast engorgement of nonnursing mothers—*25 to 50 mg I.M. daily for 3 to 4 days, starting at delivery.
*Breast cancer in women 1 to 5 years postmenopausal—*100 mg I.M. 3 times weekly as long as improvement maintained.

SIDE EFFECTS

Androgenic: in females—*acne, edema, oily skin, weight gain, hirsutism, hoarseness,* clitoral enlargement, decreased or increased libido. In males—prepubertal: premature epiphyseal closure, acne, priapism, growth of body and facial hair, phallic enlargement; postpubertal: testicular atrophy, oligospermia, decreased ejaculatory volume, impotence, gynecomastia, epididymitis.
CV: edema.
GI: gastroenteritis, nausea, vomiting, constipation, diarrhea, change in appetite.
GU: bladder irritability.
Hepatic: jaundice.
Hypoestrogenic: in females—flushing; sweating; vaginitis with itching, drying, burning, or bleeding; menstrual irregularities.
Local: pain at injection site, induration, irritation and sloughing with pellet implantation, edema.
Other: hypercalcemia.

INTERACTIONS

None significant.

NURSING CONSIDERATIONS

• Contraindicated in women of childbearing potential (possible masculinization of female infant); in elderly, asthenic males who may react adversely to androgen overstimulation; in hypercalcemia; cardiac, hepatic, or renal decompensation; prostatic or breast cancer in males; benign prostatic hypertrophy with obstruction; conditions aggravated by fluid retention; hypertension; and in premature infants. Use cautiously in patients with myocardial infarction or coronary artery disease, and in prepubertal males.
• Periodic liver function tests should be performed.
• In metastatic breast cancer, hypercalcemia usually indicates progression of bone metastases. Report signs of hypercalcemia.
• Therapeutic response in breast cancer is usually apparent within 3 months. Stop therapy if signs of disease progression appear.
• Enhances hypoglycemia; tell patient to report signs of hyperinsulinism.
• Instruct males to report priapism, reduced ejaculatory volume, and gynecomastia. Withdraw drug if these occur.
• Report signs of virilization in females; reevaluate treatment.
• Monitor prepubertal males by X-ray for rate of bone maturation.
• Edema is generally controllable with salt restriction and/or diuretics. Monitor weight routinely.
• Use with diet high in calories and protein unless contraindicated.
• Inject deep into upper outer quadrant of gluteal muscle.
• Watch for irritation and sloughing with pellet implantation.
• Watch for ecchymotic areas, petechiae, or abnormal bleeding in patients on concomitant anticoagulant therapy. Monitor prothrombin time.
• Implantation of pellets may take place in doctor's office in a minor surgical procedure with aseptic precautions observed.

Unmarked trade names available in the United States only.
♦ Also available in Canada.   ♦♦ Available in Canada only.

- Many laboratory studies may be altered during therapy and for 2 to 3 weeks after therapy is stopped.

testosterone cypionate
Andro-Cyp, Androgen-860, Depotest, Depo-Test, Depo-Testosterone♦, Duratest

testosterone enanthate
Andryl, Arderone, Delatestryl♦, Everone, Malogex♦♦, Span-Test, Testate, Testone LA, Testostroval-P.A.

testosterone propionate
Androlan, Androlin, Testex

INDICATIONS & DOSAGE
Eunuchism, eunuchoidism, deficiency after castration and male climacteric—
Adults: 200 to 400 mg (cypionate or enanthate) I.M. q 4 weeks.
Oligospermia—
Adults: 100 to 200 mg (cypionate or enanthate) I.M. q 4 to 6 weeks for development and maintenance of testicular function.
Eunuchism and eunuchoidism, male climacteric, impotence—
Adults: 10 to 25 mg (propionate) I.M. 2 to 4 times weekly.
Metastatic breast cancer in women—50 to 100 mg (propionate) I.M. 3 times weekly.

SIDE EFFECTS
Androgenic: in females—*acne, edema, oily skin, weight gain, hirsutism, hoarseness,* clitoral enlargement, changes in libido. In males—prepubertal: premature epiphyseal closure, acne, priapism, growth of body and facial hair, phallic enlargement; postpubertal: testicular atrophy, oligospermia, decreased ejaculatory volume, impotence, gynecomastia, epididymitis.
CV: edema.
GI: gastroenteritis, nausea, vomiting, constipation, diarrhea, change in appetite.
GU: bladder irritability.
Hepatic: jaundice.
Local: pain at injection site, induration, postinjection furunculosis.
Other: hypercalcemia.

INTERACTIONS
None significant.

NURSING CONSIDERATIONS
- Contraindicated in women of childbearing potential (possible masculinization of female infant); in patients with hypercalcemia; cardiac, hepatic, or renal decompensation; prostatic or breast cancer in males; benign prostatic hypertrophy with obstruction; conditions aggravated by fluid retention; hypertension; elderly, asthenic males who may react adversely to androgen overstimulation; and in premature infants. Use cautiously in patients with myocardial infarction or coronary artery disease, and in prepubertal males.
- Periodic liver function tests should be performed.
- In metastatic breast cancer, hypercalcemia usually indicates progression of bone metastases. Report signs of hypercalcemia.
- Response in breast cancer is usually apparent within 3 months. Stop therapy if signs of disease progression appear.
- Enhances hypoglycemia; teach signs of hypoglycemia, and instruct the patient to report immediately if they occur.
- Instruct males to report priapism, reduced ejaculatory volume, and gynecomastia. Withdraw drug.
- Watch for signs of ecchymoses, petechiae with concomitant anticoagulant therapy. Monitor prothrombin time.
- Inject deep into upper outer quadrant of gluteal muscle. Report soreness at site; possibility of postinjection furunculosis.
- Report signs of virilization in females; reevaluate treatment.

Italicized side effects are common or life-threatening.
*Liquid form contains alcohol.   **May contain tartrazine.

• Monitor prepubertal males by X-ray for rate of bone maturation.
• Edema is generally controllable with salt restriction and/or diuretics. Monitor weight routinely.
• Use with diet high in calories and protein unless contraindicated.
• Daily requirements best administered in divided doses.
• May alter many laboratory studies during therapy and for 2 to 3 weeks after therapy is stopped.

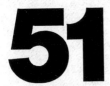

Oral contraceptives

estrogen with progestogen

MECHANISM OF ACTION
Oral contraceptives inhibit ovulation through a negative feedback mechanism directed at the hypothalamus. They may also prevent transport of the ovum through the fallopian tubes.
• Estrogen suppresses secretion of follicle-stimulating hormone, blocking follicular development and ovulation.
• Progestogen suppresses luteinizing hormone secretion so ovulation can't occur even if the follicle develops. Progestogen thickens cervical mucus, which interferes with sperm migration, and also causes endometrial changes that prevent implantation of the fertilized ovum.

estrogen with progestogen
Brevicon, Demulen♦, Enovid, Enovid-E, Loestrin 1/20, Loestrin 1.5/30♦, Lo/Ovral, Min-Ovral♦♦, Modicon, Norinyl 1 + 35, Norinyl 1 + 50♦, Norinyl 1 + 80♦, Norinyl 2 mg♦, Norlestrin♦, Ortho-Novum 1/50♦, Ortho-Novum 1/80♦, Ortho-Novum 2 mg♦, Ortho-Novum 10/11, Ovcon 35**, Ovcon 50**, Ovral, Ovulen♦

INDICATIONS & DOSAGE
Contraception—
Women: 1 tablet P.O. daily, beginning on day 5 of menstrual cycle (first day of menstrual flow is day 1). With 20- and 21-tablet packages, new dosing cycle begins 7 days after last tablet taken. With 28-tablet packages, dosage is 1 tablet daily without interruption; extra tablets are placebos or contain iron.
If only 1 or 2 doses are missed, dosage may continue on schedule. If 3 or more doses are missed, remaining tablets in monthly package must be discarded and another contraceptive method substituted. If next menstrual period doesn't begin on schedule, rule out pregnancy before starting new dosing cycle. If menstrual period begins, start new dosing cycle 7 days after last tablet was taken. If all doses have been taken on schedule and 1 menstrual period is missed, continue dosing cycle. If 2 consecutive menstrual periods are missed, pregnancy test is required before new dosing cycle is started.
Hypermenorrhea—
Women: use high-dose combinations only. Dose same as for contraception.
Endometriosis—
Women: Cyclic therapy: 1 tablet Ortho-Novum 10 mg P.O. daily for 20 days from day 5 to day 24 of menstrual cycle.
Suppressive therapy: Enovid 5 mg or 10 mg—1 tablet P.O. daily for 2 weeks starting on day 5 of menstrual cycle. Continue without interruption for 6 to 9 months, increasing dose by 5 to 10 mg q 2 weeks, up to 20 mg daily. Up to 40 mg daily may be needed if breakthrough bleeding occurs.

SIDE EFFECTS
CNS: *headache, dizziness,* depression, libido changes, lethargy, migraine.
CV: *thromboembolism,* hypertension, edema.

Italicized side effects are common or life-threatening.
*Liquid form contains alcohol.   **May contain tartrazine.

EENT: worsening of myopia or astigmatism, intolerance to contact lenses.
GI: *nausea,* vomiting, abdominal cramps, bloating, diarrhea, constipation, anorexia, changes in appetite, weight gain, *bowel ischemia,* pancreatitis.
GU: *breakthrough bleeding,* dysmenorrhea, amenorrhea, cervical erosion or abnormal secretions, enlargement of uterine fibromas, vaginal candidiasis.
Hepatic: gallbladder disease, cholestatic jaundice, liver tumors.
Metabolic: hyperglycemia, hypercalcemia, folic acid deficiency.
Skin: rash, acne, seborrhea, oily skin, erythema multiforme.
Other: *breast tenderness,* enlargement, secretion.
Adverse effects may be more serious, frequent, and rapid in onset with high-dose than with low-dose combinations.

INTERACTIONS

Ampicillin, tetracycline, barbiturates, anticonvulsants, rifampin: may diminish contraceptive effectiveness. Use supplemental form of contraception.

NURSING CONSIDERATIONS

• Contraindicated in thromboembolic disorders, cerebrovascular or coronary artery disease, myocardial infarction, known or suspected cancer of breasts or reproductive organs, benign or malignant liver tumors, undiagnosed abnormal vaginal bleeding, known or suspected pregnancy, lactation; and in adolescents with incomplete epiphyseal closure. Also contraindicated in women 35 years or older who smoke more than 15 cigarettes a day, and in all women over 40 years. Use cautiously in patients with systemic lupus erythematosus, hypertension, mental depression, migraine, epilepsy, asthma, diabetes mellitus, amenorrhea, scanty or irregular periods, fibrocystic breast disease, family history (mother, grandmother, sister) of breast or genital-tract cancer, renal or gallbladder disease. Report de-

velopment or worsening of these conditions to doctor. Prolonged therapy inadvisable in women who plan to become pregnant.
• If one menstrual period is missed and tablets have been taken on schedule, tell patient to continue taking them. If two consecutive menstrual periods are missed, tell patient to stop drug and to have pregnancy test. Progestogens may cause birth defects if taken early in pregnancy.
• Missed doses in midcycle greatly increase likelihood of pregnancy.
• Warn patient that headache, nausea, dizziness, breast tenderness, spotting, and breakthrough bleeding are common at first. These should diminish after 3 to 6 dosing cycles (months). However, breakthrough bleeding in patients taking high-dose estrogen-progestogen combinations for menstrual disorders may necessitate dosage adjustment.
• Warn patient to immediately report abdominal pain; numbness, stiffness, or pain in legs or buttocks; pressure or pain in chest; shortness of breath; severe headache; visual disturbances, such as blind spots, blurriness, or flashing lights; undiagnosed vaginal bleeding or discharge; two consecutive missed menstrual periods; lumps in the breast; swelling of hands or feet; severe pain in the abdomen (tumor rupture in the liver).
• Tell patient to take tablets at same time each day; nighttime dosing may reduce nausea and headaches.
• Stress importance of semiannual Pap smears and annual gynecologic examinations while taking estrogen-progestogen combinations.
• Warn the patient of signs and symptoms of gallbladder disease.
• Warn the patient of possible delay in achieving pregnancy when pill is discontinued.
• Teach the patient how to perform a breast self-examination.
• Advise the patient of increased risks

Unmarked trade names available in the United States only.
♦ Also available in Canada.   ♦ ♦ Available in Canada only.

associated with simultaneous use of cigarettes and oral contraceptives.

• Many laboratory tests are affected by oral contraceptives; some include: increase in serum bilirubin, alkaline phosphatase, SGOT, SGPT, and protein-bound iodine; decrease in glucose tolerance and urinary excretion of 17-hydroxycorticosteroids (17-OHCS).

• Estrogens and progestogens may alter glucose tolerance, thus changing requirements for antidiabetic drugs.

• Instruct patient to weigh herself at least twice a week and to report any sudden weight gain or edema to doctor.

• Many doctors recommend that women not become pregnant within 2 months after stopping the pill. Advise patient to check with her doctor about how soon pregnancy may be attempted after hormonal therapy is stopped.

• Advise patient not to take same drug for longer than 18 months without consulting doctor.

• Many doctors advise women on the pill for extended time (5 years or more) to stop drug and use other birth control methods in order to periodically reassess patient while off hormone therapy.

• The Centers for Disease Control (CDC) report that the use of oral contraceptives *may decrease* the incidence of ovarian and endometrial cancer. Also, oral contraceptives do not appear to increase a woman's chances of getting breast cancer. Reassure your patient and apprise her of these facts.

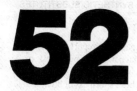

Estrogens

chlorotrianisene
dienestrol
diethylstilbestrol
diethylstilbestrol diphosphate
esterified estrogens
estradiol
estradiol cypionate
estradiol valerate
estrogenic substances,
    conjugated
estrone
ethinyl estradiol
quinestrol

MECHANISM OF ACTION
• Estrogens replace endogenous hormones to maintain normal hormonal balance.
• They suppress lactation by inhibiting prolactin secretion from the anterior pituitary.
• They antagonize the action of androgens that stimulate growth of tumor tissue.
• As oral contraceptives, estrogens suppress gonadotropin output from the anterior pituitary by a negative feedback effect. (Their mechanism of action is described in greater detail in Chapter 51.)

COMBINATION PRODUCTS
MENRIUM 5-2♦: chlordiazepoxide 5 mg and esterified estrogens 0.2 mg.
MENRIUM 5-4♦: chlordiazepoxide 5 mg and esterified estrogens 0.4 mg.
MENRIUM 10-4♦: chlordiazepoxide 10 mg, and esterified estrogens 0.4 mg.
MILPREM-200: conjugated estrogens 0.45 mg and meprobamate 200 mg.
MILPREM-400: conjugated estrogens 0.45 mg and meprobamate 400 mg.
PMB 200: conjugated estrogens 0.45 mg and meprobamate 200 mg.
PMB 400: conjugated estrogens 0.45 mg and meprobamate 400 mg.

See Chapter 51, ORAL CONTRACEPTIVES.

---

chlorotrianisene
Tace♦

INDICATIONS & DOSAGE
Men:
Prostatic cancer—12 to 25 mg P.O. daily.
Nonnursing mothers:
Postpartum breast engorgement—72 mg P.O. b.i.d. for 2 days; or 50 mg q 6 hours for 6 doses; or 12 mg q.i.d. for 7 days. Start dosing within 8 hours after delivery.
Women:
Menopausal symptoms—12 to 25 mg P.O. daily for 30 days or cyclic (3 weeks on, 1 week off).
Female hypogonadism—12 to 25 mg P.O. for 21 days, followed by 1 dose of progesterone 100 mg I.M. or 5 days of oral progestogen given concurrently with last 5 days of chlorotrianisene (i.e., medroxyprogesterone 5 to 10 mg).
Atrophic vaginitis—12 to 25 mg P.O. daily for 30 to 60 days.

SIDE EFFECTS
CNS: headache, dizziness, chorea, migraine, depression, libido changes.

CV: thrombophlebitis; *thromboembolism;* hypertension; edema; *increased risk of stroke, pulmonary embolism, and myocardial infarction.*
EENT: worsening of myopia or astigmatism, intolerance to contact lenses.
GI: *nausea,* vomiting, abdominal cramps, bloating, diarrhea, constipation, anorexia, increased appetite, excessive thirst, weight changes, pancreatitis.
GU: breakthrough bleeding, altered menstrual flow, dysmenorrhea, amenorrhea, cervical erosion or abnormal secretions, enlargement of uterine fibromas, vaginal candidiasis; *in males: gynecomastia, testicular atrophy, impotence.*
Hepatic: cholestatic jaundice.
Metabolic: hyperglycemia, hypercalcemia, folic acid deficiency.
Skin: melasma, urticaria, acne, seborrhea, oily skin, hirsutism or loss of hair.
Other: leg cramps, purpura, breast changes (tenderness, enlargement, secretion).

INTERACTIONS
None significant.

NURSING CONSIDERATIONS
• Contraindicated in thrombophlebitis or thromboembolic disorders; cancer of breast, reproductive organs, or genitals; undiagnosed abnormal genital bleeding. Use cautiously in patients with hypertension, asthma, mental depression, bone diseases, blood dyscrasias, gallbladder disease, migraine, seizures, diabetes mellitus, amenorrhea, heart failure, hepatic or renal dysfunction, and family history (mother, grandmother, sister) of breast or genital tract cancer. Development or worsening of these conditions may require discontinuation of the drug.
• FDA regulations require that female patients receive package insert explaining possible estrogen side effects before

first dose. Provide verbal explanation also.
• Warn patient to report immediately: abdominal pain; pain, numbness, or stiffness in legs or buttocks; pressure or pain in chest; shortness of breath; severe headaches; visual disturbances, such as blind spots, flashing lights, blurriness; vaginal bleeding or discharge; breast lumps; swelling of hands or feet; yellow skin and sclera; dark urine; and light-colored stools.
• Tell male patients on long-term therapy about possible gynecomastia and impotence, which will disappear when therapy is terminated.
• Not used for menstrual disorders because duration of action is very long.
• Pathologist should be advised of estrogen therapy when specimen is sent.
• Patients with diabetes should report positive urine tests so antidiabetic medication dose can be adjusted.
• Teach female patients how to perform routine breast self-examination.
• Explain to patient on cyclic therapy for postmenopausal symptoms that, although withdrawal bleeding may occur during week off drug, fertility has not been restored. Pregnancy is not possible since she has not ovulated.

dienestrol
Dienestrol Cream♦
Available in combination with sulfanilamide and aminacrine as AVC/Dienestrol, cream or suppositories

INDICATIONS & DOSAGE
Postmenopausal women:
Atrophic vaginitis and kraurosis vulvae—1 to 2 applicatorfuls of cream daily for 2 weeks, then half that dose for 2 more weeks; or 1 to 2 vaginal suppositories daily for 1 month, as directed.
Atrophic and senile vaginitis and kraurosis vulvae when complicated by infection—1 applicatorful AVC/Dienestrol

---

Italicized side effects are common or life-threatening.
♦Liquid form contains alcohol.　　**May contain tartrazine.

cream intravaginally daily or b.i.d. for 1 to 2 weeks, then every other day for 1 to 2 weeks.

SIDE EFFECTS
GU: vaginal discharge; with excessive use, uterine bleeding.
Local: increased discomfort, burning sensation. Systemic effects possible.
Other: breast tenderness.

INTERACTIONS
None significant.

NURSING CONSIDERATIONS
• Contraindicated in thrombophlebitis or thromboembolic disorders; cancer of breast, reproductive organs, or genitals; undiagnosed abnormal genital bleeding. Use cautiously in menstrual irregularities or endometriosis.
• Prolonged therapy with estrogen-containing products is contraindicated.
• FDA regulations require that female patients receive package insert explaining possible estrogen side effects before first dose. Provide verbal explanation also.
• Systemic reactions possible with normal intravaginal use. Monitor closely.
• Warn patient not to exceed the prescribed dose.
• Withdrawal bleeding may occur if estrogen is suddenly stopped.
• Teach patient how to insert suppositories or cream.

---

diethylstilbestrol
DES, Stibilium♦♦

diethylstilbestrol diphosphate
Honvol♦♦, Stilphostrol

INDICATIONS & DOSAGE
Women:
Atrophic vaginitis or kraurosis vulvae—0.1 to 1 mg as suppository daily for 10 to 14 days concurrently with oral ther-

apy; or up to 5 mg weekly as suppository.
Hypogonadism, castration, primary ovarian failure—0.2 to 0.5 mg P.O. daily.
Menopausal symptoms—0.1 to 2 mg P.O. daily in cycles of 3 weeks on and 1 week off.
Postcoital contraception ("morning-after pill")—25 mg P.O. b.i.d. for 5 days, starting within 72 hours after coitus.
Postpartum breast engorgement—5 mg P.O. daily or t.i.d. up to total dose of 30 mg.
Men:
Prostatic cancer—1 to 3 mg P.O. daily, initially; may be reduced to 1 mg P.O. daily, or 5 mg I.M. twice weekly initially, followed by up to 4 mg I.M. twice weekly. Or 50 to 200 mg (diphosphate) P.O. t.i.d.; or 0.25 to 1 g I.V. daily for 5 days, then once or twice weekly.
Men and postmenopausal women:
Breast cancer—15 mg P.O. daily.

SIDE EFFECTS
CNS: headache, dizziness, chorea, depression, lethargy.
CV: *thrombophlebitis; thromboembolism;* hypertension; edema; *increased risk of stroke, pulmonary embolism, and mycardial infarction.*
EENT: worsening of myopia or astigmatism, intolerance to contact lenses.
GI: *nausea,* vomiting, abdominal cramps, bloating, diarrhea, constipation, anorexia, increased appetite, excessive thirst, weight changes, pancreatitis.
GU: breakthrough bleeding, altered menstrual flow, dysmenorrhea, amenorrhea, cervical erosion, altered cervical secretions, enlargement of uterine fibromas, vaginal candidiasis, loss of libido; *in males:* gynecomastia, testicular atrophy, impotence.
Hepatic: cholestatic jaundice.
Metabolic: hyperglycemia, hypercalcemia, folic acid deficiency.
Skin: melasma, urticaria, acne, sebor-

---

rhea, oily skin, hirsutism or loss of hair.

Other: leg cramps, breast tenderness or enlargement.

INTERACTIONS
None significant.

NURSING CONSIDERATIONS
• Contraindicated in thrombophlebitis or thromboembolic disorders; undiagnosed abnormal genital bleeding. Use cautiously in patients with hypertension, asthma, mental depression, bone disease, migraine, seizures, blood dyscrasias, diabetes mellitus, gallbladder disease, amenorrhea, heart failure, hepatic or renal dysfunction, and family history (mother, grandmother, sister) of breast or genital tract cancer. Development or worsening of these conditions may require discontinuation of the drug.
• FDA regulations require that all female patients receive package insert explaining possible estrogen side effects before first dose. Provide verbal explanation also.
• Only the 25-mg tablet is approved by FDA as the "morning-after pill." To be effective, it must be taken within 72 hours after coitus.
• Warn patient to stop taking drug immediately if she becomes pregnant, since it can affect the fetus adversely.
• Warn patient to report immediately: abdominal pain; pain, numbness, or stiffness in legs or buttocks; pressure or pain in chest; shortness of breath; severe headache; visual disturbances, such as blind spots, flashing lights, or blurriness; vaginal bleeding or discharge; breast lumps; sudden weight gain; swelling of hands or feet; yellow sclera or skin; dark urine or light-colored stools.
• Pathologist should be advised of estrogen therapy when specimen is sent.
• Patients with diabetes should report positive urine tests so antidiabetic medication dose can be adjusted.

• High incidence of gross nonmalignant genital changes in offspring of women taking drug during pregnancy. Female offspring have higher than normal risk of developing cervical and vaginal adenocarcinoma. Male offspring may have higher than normal risk of developing testicular tumors.
• Increased number of cardiovascular deaths reported in men taking diethylstilbestrol tablet (5 mg daily) for prostatic cancer over long period of time. This effect not associated with 1 mg daily dose.
• Reassure male patients on estrogen therapy that such side effects as gynecomastia and impotence will disappear when therapy ends.
• Teach female patients how to perform routine breast self-examination.
• Explain to patient on cyclic therapy for postmenopausal symptoms that, although withdrawal bleeding may occur during week off drug, fertility has not been restored. Pregnancy is not possible since she has not ovulated.
• Use of estrogens associated with increased risk of endometrial cancer. Possible increased risk of breast cancer.

esterified estrogens
Amnestrogen, Climestrone♦♦, Estabs, Estratab, Menest, Menotrol♦♦, Ms-Med, Neo-Estrone♦♦

INDICATIONS & DOSAGE
Men:
Prostatic cancer—1.25 to 2.5 mg P.O. t.i.d.
Men and postmenopausal women:
Breast cancer—10 mg P.O. t.i.d. for 3 or more months.
Women:
Hypogonadism, castration, primary ovarian failure—2.5 mg daily to t.i.d. in cycles of 3 weeks on, 1 week off.
Menopausal symptoms—average 0.3 to 3.75 mg P.O. daily in cycles of 3 weeks on, 1 week off.

Italicized side effects are common or life-threatening.
♦Liquid form contains alcohol.   ♦♦May contain tartrazine.

SIDE EFFECTS
CNS: headache, dizziness, chorea, depression, libido changes, lethargy.
CV: thrombophlebitis; *thromboembolism;* hypertension; edema; *increased risk of stroke, pulmonary embolism, and myocardial infarction.*
EENT: worsening of myopia or astigmatism, intolerance to contact lenses.
GI: *nausea,* vomiting, abdominal cramps, bloating, diarrhea, constipation, anorexia, increased appetite, weight changes, pancreatitis.
GU: breakthrough bleeding, altered menstrual flow, dysmenorrhea, amenorrhea, cervical erosion, altered cervical secretions, enlargement of uterine fibromas, vaginal candidiasis; *in males:* gynecomastia, testicular atrophy, impotence.
Hepatic: cholestatic jaundice.
Metabolic: hyperglycemia, hypercalcemia, folic acid deficiency.
Skin: melasma, rash, acne, hirsutism or hair loss, seborrhea, oily skin.
Other: breast changes (tenderness, enlargement, secretion).

INTERACTIONS
None significant.

NURSING CONSIDERATIONS
● Contraindicated in thrombophlebitis or thromboembolic disorders; undiagnosed abnormal genital bleeding. Use cautiously in patients with history of hypertension, mental depression, gallbladder disease, migraine, seizures, diabetes mellitus, amenorrhea, or family history (mother, grandmother, sister) of breast or genital tract cancer. Development or worsening of these conditions may require discontinuation of the drug.
● FDA regulations require that female patients receive package insert explaining possible estrogen side effects before first dose. Provide verbal explanation also.
● Warn patient to report immediately: abdominal pain; pain, numbness, or stiffness in legs or buttocks; pressure or pain in chest; shortness of breath; severe headaches; visual disturbances, such as blind spots, flashing lights, or blurriness; vaginal bleeding or discharge; breast lumps; swelling of hands or feet; yellow skin or sclera; dark urine or light-colored stools.
● Pathologist should be advised of estrogen therapy when specimen is sent.
● Patients with diabetes should report positive urine tests so antidiabetic medication dose can be adjusted.
● Explain to patient on cyclic therapy for postmenopausal symptoms that, although she may experience withdrawal bleeding during week off drug, fertility has not been restored. Pregnancy cannot occur since she has not ovulated.
● Teach female patients how to perform routine breast self-examination.
● Reassure male patients on estrogen therapy that such side effects as gynecomastia and impotence will disappear when therapy ends.

estradiol
Estrace♦**

estradiol cypionate
Depo-Estradiol Cypionate, Depogen, Dura Estrin, E-Ionate P.A., Estro-Cyp, Estroject-L.A.

estradiol valerate
Delestrogen♦♦, Dioval♦, Duragen, Estate, Estradiol L.A., Estraval, Retestrin, Valergen

INDICATIONS & DOSAGE
Women:
Menopausal symptoms, hypogonadism, castration, primary ovarian failure—1 to 2 mg P.O. daily, in cycles of 21 days on and 7 days off, or cycles of 5 days on and 2 days off; or 0.2 to 1 mg I.M. weekly.
Kraurosis vulvae—1 to 1.5 mg I.M. once or more per week.
Menopausal symptoms—1 to 5 mg (cy-

pionate) I.M. q 3 to 4 weeks. Or 5 to 20 mg (valerate) I.M., repeated once after 2 to 3 weeks
Postpartum breast engorgement—10 to 25 mg (valerate) I.M. at end of first stage of labor.
Men:
Prostatic cancer—30 mg (valerate) I.M. q 1 to 2 weeks.

SIDE EFFECTS
CNS: headache, dizziness, chorea, depression, libido changes, lethargy.
CV: thrombophlebitis, *thromboembolism,* hypertension, edema.
EENT: worsening of myopia or astigmatism, intolerance to contact lenses.
GI: *nausea,* vomiting, abdominal cramps, bloating, diarrhea, constipation, anorexia, increased appetite, weight changes, pancreatitis.
GU: breakthrough bleeding, altered menstrual flow, dysmenorrhea, amenorrhea, cervical erosion, altered cervical secretions, enlargement of uterine fibromas, vaginal candidiasis; *in males:* gynecomastia, testicular atrophy, impotence.
Hepatic: cholestatic jaundice.
Metabolic: hyperglycemia, hypercalcemia, folic acid deficiency.
Skin: melasma, urticaria, acne, seborrhea, oily skin, hirsutism or hair loss.
Other: breast changes (tenderness, enlargement, secretion), leg cramps.

INTERACTIONS
None significant.

NURSING CONSIDERATIONS
• Contraindicated in thrombophlebitis or thromboembolic disorders; cancer of breast, reproductive organs; undiagnosed abnormal genital bleeding. Use cautiously in patients with hypertension, mental depression, bone diseases, blood dyscrasias, migraine, seizures, diabetes mellitus, amenorrhea, heart failure, hepatic or renal dysfunction, or family history (mother, grandmother, sister) of breast or genital tract cancer.

Development or worsening of these conditions may require discontinuation of the drug.
• FDA regulations require that female patients receive package insert explaining possible estrogen side effects before first dose. Provide verbal explanation also.
• Warn patient to report immediately: abdominal pain; pain, numbness, or stiffness in legs or buttocks; pressure or pain in chest; shortness of breath; severe headaches; visual disturbances, such as blind spots, flashing lights, or blurriness; vaginal bleeding or discharge; breast lumps; swelling of hands or feet; yellow skin or sclera; dark urine or light-colored stools.
• Risk of endometrial cancer is increased in postmenopausal women who take estrogens for more than 1 year.
• Patients with diabetes should report positive urine tests so antidiabetic medication dose can be adjusted.
• Pathologist should be advised of estrogen therapy when specimen is sent.
• Estradiol available as aqueous suspension or solution in peanut oil.
• Estradiol cypionate available as solution in cottonseed oil or vegetable oil.
• Estradiol valerate available as solution in castor oil, sesame oil, and vegetable oil. Check for allergy.
• Before injection, make sure drug is well dispersed in solution by rolling vial between palms. Inject deep I.M. into large muscle.
• Reassure male patient that possible side effects of gynecomastia and impotence disappear after termination of therapy.
• Teach female patients how to perform routine breast self-examination.
• Explain to patient on cyclic therapy for postmenopausal symptoms that, although withdrawal bleeding may occur during week off drug, fertility has not been reinstated. Pregnancy cannot occur since she has not ovulated.

Italicized side effects are common or life-threatening.
*Liquid form contains alcohol.   **May contain tartrazine.

estrogenic substances, conjugated

Premarin♦

INDICATIONS & DOSAGE
Women:

Abnormal uterine bleeding (hormonal imbalance)—25 mg I.V. or I.M. Repeat in 6 to 12 hours.

Breast cancer (at least 5 years after menopause)—10 mg P.O. t.i.d. for 3 months or more.

Castration, primary ovarian failure, and osteoporosis—1.25 mg P.O. daily in cycles of 3 weeks on, 1 week off.

Hypogonadism—2.5 mg P.O. b.i.d. or t.i.d. for 20 consecutive days each month.

Menopausal symptoms—0.3 to 1.25 mg P.O. daily in cycles of 3 weeks on, 1 week off.

Postpartum breast engorgement—3.75 mg P.O. q 4 hours for 5 doses or 1.25 mg q 4 hours for 5 days.

Men:

Prostatic cancer—1.25 to 2.5 mg P.O. t.i.d.

SIDE EFFECTS
CNS: headache, dizziness, chorea, depression, libido changes, lethargy.
CV: thrombophlebitis; *thromboembolism;* hypertension; edema; *increased risk of stroke, pulmonary embolism, and myocardial infarction.*
EENT: worsening of myopia or astigmatism, intolerance to contact lenses.
GI: *nausea,* vomiting, abdominal cramps, bloating, diarrhea, constipation, anorexia, increased appetite, weight changes, pancreatitis.
GU: breakthrough bleeding, altered menstrual flow, dysmenorrhea, amenorrhea, cervical erosion, altered cervical secretions, enlargement of uterine fibromas, vaginal candidiasis; *in males:* gynecomastia, testicular atrophy, impotence.
Hepatic: cholestatic jaundice.

Metabolic: hyperglycemia, hypercalcemia, folic acid deficiency.
Skin: melasma, urticaria, acne, seborrhea, oily skin, flushing (when given rapidly I.V.), hirsutism or loss of hair.
Other: breast changes (tenderness, enlargement, secretion), leg cramps.

INTERACTIONS
None significant.

NURSING CONSIDERATIONS
• Contraindicated in thrombophlebitis or thromboembolic disorders; undiagnosed abnormal genital bleeding. Use cautiously in hypertension, gallbladder disease, bone diseases, blood dyscrasias, migraine, seizures, diabetes mellitus, amenorrhea, heart failure, hepatic or renal dysfunction, or family history (mother, grandmother, sister) of breast or genital tract cancer. Development or worsening of these conditions may require discontinuation of the drug.
• FDA regulations require that female patients receive package insert explaining possible estrogen side effects before first dose. Provide verbal explanation also.
• Warn patient to report immediately: abdominal pain; pain, numbness, or stiffness in legs or buttocks; pressure or pain in chest; shortness of breath; severe headaches; visual disturbances, such as blind spots, flashing lights, or blurriness; vaginal bleeding or discharge; breast lumps; swelling of hands or feet; yellow skin or sclera; dark urine or light-colored stools.
• I.M. or I.V. use preferred for rapid treatment of dysfunctional uterine bleeding or reduction of surgical bleeding.
• Refrigerate before reconstituting. Agitate gently after adding diluent.
• Pathologist should be advised of estrogen therapy when specimen is sent.
• Patients with diabetes should report positive urine tests so antidiabetic medication dose can be adjusted.
• Use associated with increased risk of

Unmarked trade names available in the United States only.
♦ Also available in Canada.   ♦ ♦ Available in Canada only.

endometrial cancer. Possible increased risk of breast cancer.

• Teach female patients how to perform routine breast self-examination.

• Explain to patient on cyclic therapy for postmenopausal symptoms that, although withdrawal bleeding may occur during week off drug, fertility has not been restored. Pregnancy cannot occur since she has not ovulated.

• Reassure male patients that possible side effects of gynecomastia and impotence disappear after termination of therapy.

---

estrone
Foygen, Gravigen, Ogen♦, Theelin

INDICATIONS & DOSAGE
Women:
Atrophic vaginitis—0.2 mg intravaginal suppository daily or apply cream to vagina once nightly.
Hypogonadism, castration, ovarian failure—1.25 to 7.5 mg P.O. daily for 20 consecutive days each month; or 0.1 to 2 mg I.M. weekly.
Menopausal symptoms—0.625 to 5 mg P.O. daily in cycle of 3 weeks on, 1 week off; or 0.1 to 0.5 mg I.M. 2 to 3 times weekly.
Men:
Prostatic cancer—2 to 4 mg I.M. 2 to 3 times weekly.

SIDE EFFECTS
CNS: headache, dizziness, chorea, depression, libido changes, lethargy.
CV: thrombophlebitis, *thromboembolism*, hypertension, edema.
EENT: worsening of myopia or astigmatism, intolerance to contact lenses.
GI: *nausea*, vomiting, abdominal cramps, bloating, diarrhea, constipation, anorexia, increased appetite, weight changes, pancreatitis.
GU: breakthrough bleeding, altered menstrual flow, dysmenorrhea, amenorrhea, cervical erosion, altered cervical secretions, enlargement of uterine

fibromas, vaginal candidiasis; *in males:* gynecomastia, testicular atrophy, impotence.
Hepatic: cholestatic jaundice.
Metabolic: hyperglycemia, hypercalcemia, folic acid deficiency.
Skin: melasma, urticaria, acne, seborrhea, oily skin, hirsutism or hair loss.
Other: breast changes (tenderness, enlargement, secretion), leg cramps.

INTERACTIONS
None significant.

NURSING CONSIDERATIONS
• Contraindicated in thrombophlebitis or thromboembolic disorders; cancer of breast or reproductive organs; undiagnosed abnormal genital bleeding. Use cautiously in patients with hypertension, mental depression, migraine, seizures, diabetes mellitus, amenorrhea, hepatic or renal dysfunction, or family history (mother, grandmother, sister) of breast or genital tract cancer. Development or worsening of these conditions may require discontinuation of the drug.

• I.V. use contraindicated.

• FDA regulations require that female patients receive package insert explaining possible estrogen side effects before first dose. Provide verbal explanation also.

• Warn patient to report immediately: abdominal pain; pain, numbness, or stiffness in legs or buttocks; pressure or pain in chest; shortness of breath; severe headaches; visual disturbances, such as blind spots, flashing lights, or blurriness; vaginal bleeding or discharge; breast lumps; swelling of hands or feet.

• Oil preparation may become cloudy if chilled. Warm solution until clear before use. Also available in aqueous suspension.

• Pathologist should be advised of estrogen therapy when specimen is sent.

• Patients with diabetes should report

Italicized side effects are common or life-threatening.
*Liquid form contains alcohol.   **May contain tartrazine.

positive urine test so antidiabetic medication dose can be adjusted.
- Teach female patients how to perform routine breast self-examination.
- Use of estrogens associated with increased risk of endometrial cancer. Possible increased risk of breast cancer.
- Explain to patient on cyclic therapy for postmenopausal symptoms that, although withdrawal bleeding may occur during week off drug, fertility has not been restored. Pregnancy cannot occur since she has not ovulated.
- Reassure male patients that possible side effects of gynecomastia and impotence disappear after termination of therapy.

ethinyl estradiol
Estinyl♦**, Feminone

INDICATIONS & DOSAGE
Women:
Breast cancer (at least 5 years after menopause)—1 mg P.O. t.i.d.
Hypogonadism—0.05 mg daily to t.i.d. for 2 weeks a month, followed by 2 weeks progesterone therapy; continue for 3 to 6 monthly dosing cycles, followed by 2 months off.
Menopausal symptoms—0.02 to 0.05 mg P.O. daily for cycles of 3 weeks on, 1 week off.
Postpartum breast engorgement— 0.5 to 1 mg P.O. daily for 3 days, then taper over 7 days to 0.1 mg and discontinue.
Men:
Prostatic cancer—0.15 to 2 mg P.O. daily.

SIDE EFFECTS
CNS: headache, dizziness, chorea, depression, libido changes, lethargy.
CV: thrombophlebitis, *thromboembolism*, hypertension, edema.
EENT: worsening of myopia or astigmatism, intolerance to contact lenses.
GI: *nausea,* vomiting, abdominal cramps, bloating, diarrhea, constipation, anorexia, increased appetite, weight changes.
GU: breakthrough bleeding, altered menstrual flow, dysmenorrhea, amenorrhea, cervical erosion, altered cervical secretions, enlargement of uterine fibromas, vaginal candidiasis; *in males:* gynecomastia, testicular atrophy, impotence.
Hepatic: cholestatic jaundice.
Metabolic: hyperglycemia, hypercalcemia, folic acid deficiency.
Skin: melasma, urticaria, acne, seborrhea, oily skin, hirsutism or hair loss.
Other: breast changes (tenderness, enlargement, secretion), leg cramps.

INTERACTIONS
None significant.

NURSING CONSIDERATIONS
- Contraindicated in thrombophlebitis or thromboembolic disorders; undiagnosed abnormal genital bleeding. Use cautiously in patients with hypertension, mental depression, bone diseases, migraine, seizures, blood dyscrasias, diabetes mellitus, amenorrhea, heart failure, hepatic or renal dysfunction, or family history (mother, grandmother, sister) of breast or genital tract cancer. Development or worsening of these conditions may require discontinuation of the drug.
- FDA regulations require that female patients receive package insert explaining possible estrogen side effects before first dose. Provide verbal explanation also.
- Warn patient to report immediately: abdominal pain; pain, numbness, or stiffness in legs or buttocks; pressure or pain in chest; shortness of breath; severe headaches; visual disturbances, such as blind spots, flashing lights, or blurriness; vaginal bleeding or discharge; breast lumps; swelling of hands or feet; yellow skin or sclera; dark urine or light-colored stools.
- Pathologist should be advised of estrogen therapy when specimen is sent.

- Patients with diabetes should report positive urine test so antidiabetic medication dose can be adjusted.
- Teach female patients how to perform routine breast self-examination.
- Use of estrogens associated with increased risk of endometrial cancer. Possible increased risk of breast cancer.
- Explain to patient on cyclic therapy for postmenopausal symptoms that, although withdrawal bleeding may occur during week off drug, fertility has not been restored. Pregnancy cannot occur since she has not ovulated.
- Reassure male patients that possible side effects of gynecomastia and impotence disappear after termination of therapy.

quinestrol
Estrovis

INDICATIONS & DOSAGE
Women:
Moderate to severe vasomotor symptoms associated with menopause, and for atrophic vaginitis, kraurosis vulvae, female hypogonadism, female castration, and primary ovarian failure—100-mcg tablet once daily for 7 days, followed by 100 mcg weekly as maintenance dose beginning 2 weeks after start of treatment. Dosage may be increased to 200 mcg weekly.

SIDE EFFECTS
CNS: headache, dizziness, chorea, migraine, depression, libido changes.
CV: thrombophlebitis; *thromboembolism;* hypertension; edema; *increased risk of stroke, pulmonary embolism, and myocardial infarction.*
EENT: worsening of myopia or astigmatism, intolerance to contact lenses.
GI: *nausea,* vomiting, abdominal cramps, bloating, diarrhea, constipation, anorexia, increased appetite, excessive thirst, weight changes.
GU: breakthrough bleeding, altered menstrual flow, dysmenorrhea, amen-

orrhea, cervical erosion or abnormal secretions, enlargement of uterine fibromas, vaginal candidiasis.
Hepatic: cholestatic jaundice.
Metabolic: hyperglycemia, hypercalcemia, folic acid deficiency.
Skin: melasma, urticaria, acne, seborrhea, oily skin, hirsutism or loss of hair.
Other: leg cramps, purpura, breast changes (tenderness, enlargement, secretion).

INTERACTIONS
None significant.

NURSING CONSIDERATIONS
- Contraindicated in thrombophlebitis or thromboembolic disorders; cancer of breast or reproductive organs; undiagnosed abnormal genital bleeding. Use cautiously in patients with hypertension, mental depression, migraine, seizures, diabetes mellitus, amenorrhea, hepatic or renal dysfunction, or family history (mother, grandmother, sister) of breast or genital tract cancer. Development or worsening of these may require discontinuation of the drug.
- FDA regulations require that female patients receive package insert explaining possible estrogen side effects before first dose. Provide verbal explanation also.
- Warn patient to report immediately: abdominal pain; pain, numbness, or stiffness in legs or buttocks; pressure or pain in chest; shortness of breath; severe headaches; visual disturbances, such as blind spots, flashing lights, or blurriness; vaginal bleeding or discharge; breast lumps; swelling of hands or feet; yellw skin or sclera; dark urine or light-colored stools.
- Pathologist should be advised of estrogen therapy when specimen is sent.
- Patients with diabetes should report positive urine test so antidiabetic medication dose can be adjusted.
- Attempts to discontinue medication should be made at 3- to

6-month intervals.
• Similar in effectiveness to conjugated estrogens in treatment of postmenopausal symptoms. Biggest advantage is that quinestrol can be taken once a week.
• Use of estrogens associated with increased risk of endometrial cancer. Possible increased risk of breast cancer.
• Explain to patients on replacement therapy for postmenopausal symptoms that, although menstrual-like bleeding or spotting may occur, fertility has not been restored.
• Teach female patients how to perform breast self-examination.
• Reassure male patients that possible side effects of gynecomastia and impotence disappear after termination of therapy.

53

Progestogens

hydroxyprogesterone caproate
medroxyprogesterone acetate
norethindrone
norethindrone acetate
norgestrel
progesterone

MECHANISM OF ACTION
● Progestogens mimic the body's production of progesterone to reestablish a normal menstrual cycle in patients with amenorrhea.
● They promote glandular and vascular development of the endometrium by restoring progesterone levels.
● Progestogens suppress ovulation possibly by inhibiting pituitary gonadotropin secretion. They also form a thick cervical mucus that is relatively impermeable to sperm.

COMBINATION PRODUCTS
See Chapter 51, ORAL CONTRACEPTIVES.

---

hydroxyprogesterone caproate
Delalutin♦, Duralutin

INDICATIONS & DOSAGE
Women:
Menstrual disorders—125 to 375 mg I.M. q 4 weeks. Stop after 4 cycles.
Uterine cancer—1 to 5 g I.M. weekly.

SIDE EFFECTS
CNS: dizziness, migraine headache, lethargy, depression.

CV: hypertension, thrombophlebitis, *pulmonary embolism, edema.*
GI: nausea, vomiting, abdominal cramps.
GU: breakthrough bleeding, dysmenorrhea, amenorrhea; cervical erosion or abnormal secretions; uterine fibromas; vaginal candidiasis.
Hepatic: cholestatic jaundice.
Local: irritation and pain at injection site.
Metabolic: hyperglycemia.
Skin: melasma, rash.
Other: breast tenderness, enlargement, or secretion; decreased libido.

INTERACTIONS
None significant.

NURSING CONSIDERATIONS
● Contraindicated in thromboembolic disorders, breast cancer, undiagnosed abnormal vaginal bleeding, severe hepatic disease, missed abortion, or pregnancy. Use cautiously when diabetes mellitus, seizure disorder, migraine, cardiac or renal disease, asthma, or mental illness is present.
● FDA regulations require that, before receiving first dose, patients read package insert explaining possible progestogen side effects. Provide verbal explanation also. Patient should report any unusual symptoms immediately and should stop drug and call doctor if visual disturbances or migraine occurs.
● Don't use as test for pregnancy; drug may cause birth defects and masculinization of female fetus.
● Warn patient that edema and weight gain are likely.

Italicized side effects are common or life-threatening.
✶Liquid form contains alcohol.　　✶✶May contain tartrazine.

- Give oil solutions (sesame oil and castor oil) deep I.M. in gluteal muscle.
- Preliminary estrogen treatment is usually needed in menstrual disorders.
- Effect lasts 7 to 14 days.
- For I.M. use only.
- Teach patient how to perform a breast self-examination.

medroxyprogesterone acetate
Amen, Depo-Provera♦, Provera♦

INDICATIONS & DOSAGE
Women:
Abnormal uterine bleeding due to hormonal imbalance—5 to 10 mg P.O. daily for 5 to 10 days beginning on the 16th day of cycle. If patient has received estrogen—10 mg P.O. daily for 10 days beginning on 16th day of cycle.
Secondary amenorrhea—5 to 10 mg P.O. daily for 5 to 10 days.

SIDE EFFECTS
CNS: dizziness, migraine headache, lethargy, depression.
CV: hypertension, thrombophlebitis, *pulmonary embolism, edema.*
GI: nausea, vomiting, abdominal cramps.
GU: breakthrough bleeding, dysmenorrhea, amenorrhea; cervical erosion or abnormal secretions; uterine fibromas, vaginal candidiasis.
Hepatic: cholestatic jaundice.
Metabolic: hyperglycemia, decreased libido.
Skin: melasma, rash.
Other: breast tenderness, enlargement, or secretion.

INTERACTIONS
None significant.

NURSING CONSIDERATIONS
- Contraindicated in thromboembolic disorders, breast cancer, undiagnosed abnormal vaginal bleeding, pregnancy, missed abortion, hepatic dysfunction.

Use cautiously when diabetes mellitus, seizure disorder, migraine, cardiac or renal disease, asthma, or mental illness is present.
- FDA regulations require that, before receiving first dose, patients read package insert explaining possible progestogen side effects. Provide verbal explanation also. Patient should report any unusual symptoms immediately and should stop drug and call doctor if visual disturbances or migraine occurs.
- Don't use as test for pregnancy; drug may cause birth defects and masculinization of female fetus.
- Teach patient how to perform a breast self-examination.
- Has been used effectively to treat obstructive sleep apnea.

norethindrone
Norlutin, Nor-Q.D.

INDICATIONS & DOSAGE
Women:
Amenorrhea; abnormal uterine bleeding—5 to 20 mg P.O. daily on days 5 to 25 of menstrual cycle.
Endometriosis—10 mg P.O. daily for 14 days, then increase by 5 mg P.O. daily q 2 weeks up to 30 mg daily.

SIDE EFFECTS
CNS: dizziness, migraine headache, lethargy, depression.
CV: hypertension, thrombophlebitis, *pulmonary embolism, edema.*
GI: nausea, vomiting, abdominal cramps.
GU: breakthrough bleeding, dysmenorrhea, amenorrhea; cervical erosion or abnormal secretions; uterine fibromas; vaginal candidiasis.
Hepatic: cholestatic jaundice.
Metabolic: hyperglycemia, decreased libido.
Skin: melasma, rash.
Other: breast tenderness, enlargement, or secretion.

INTERACTIONS
None significant.

NURSING CONSIDERATIONS
• Contraindicated in thromboembolic disorders, breast cancer, undiagnosed abnormal vaginal bleeding, severe hepatic disease, missed abortion, or pregnancy. Use cautiously when diabetes mellitus, seizure disorder, migraine, cardiac or renal disease, asthma, or mental illness is present.
• Don't use as test for pregnancy; drug may cause birth defects and masculinization of female fetus.
• FDA regulations require that, before receiving first dose, patients read package insert explaining possible progestogen side effects. Provide verbal explanation also. Patient should report any unusual symptoms immediately and should stop drug and call doctor if visual disturbances or migraine occurs.
• Watch patient carefully for signs of edema.
• Preliminary estrogen treatment is usually needed in menstrual disorders.
• Teach the patient how to perform a breast self-examination.

norethindrone acetate
Norlutate♦

INDICATIONS & DOSAGE
Women:
Amenorrhea, abnormal uterine bleeding—2.5 to 10 mg P.O. daily on days 5 to 25 of menstrual cycle.
Endometriosis—5 mg P.O. daily for 14 days, then increase by 2.5 mg daily q 2 weeks up to 15 mg daily.

SIDE EFFECTS
CNS: dizziness, migraine headache, lethargy, depression.
CV: hypertension, thrombophlebitis, *pulmonary embolism, edema.*
GI: nausea, vomiting, abdominal cramps.
GU: breakthrough bleeding, dysmenor-

rhea, amenorrhea; cervical erosion or abnormal secretions; uterine fibromas; vaginal candidiasis.
Hepatic: cholestatic jaundice.
Metabolic: hyperglycemia, decreased libido.
Skin: melasma, rash.
Other: breast tenderness, enlargement, or secretion.

INTERACTIONS
None significant.

NURSING CONSIDERATIONS
• Contraindicated in thromboembolic disorders, breast cancer, undiagnosed abnormal vaginal bleeding, severe hepatic disease, missed abortion, or pregnancy. Use cautiously when diabetes mellitus, seizure disorder, migraine, cardiac or renal disease, asthma, or mental illness is present.
• FDA regulations require that, before receiving first dose, patients read package insert explaining possible progestogen side effects. Provide verbal explanation also. Patient should report any unusual symptoms immediately and should stop drug and call doctor if visual disturbances or migraine occurs.
• Don't use as test for pregnancy; drug may cause birth defects and masculinization of female fetus.
• Preliminary estrogen treatment is usually needed in menstrual disorders.
• Twice as potent as norethindrone.
• Teach patient how to perform a breast self-examination.

norgestrel
Ovrette**

INDICATIONS & DOSAGE
Women:
Contraception—1 tablet P.O. daily.

SIDE EFFECTS
CNS: cerebral thrombosis or hemorrhage, migraine headache, lethargy, depression.

Italicized side effects are common or life-threatening.
*Liquid form contains alcohol. **May contain tartrazine.

CV: hypertension, thrombophlebitis, *pulmonary embolism, edema*.
GI: nausea, vomiting, abdominal cramps, gallbladder disease.
GU: *breakthrough bleeding, change in menstrual flow*, dysmenorrhea, spotting, amenorrhea; cervical erosion, vaginal candidiasis.
Hepatic: cholestatic jaundice.
Skin: melasma, rash.
Other: breast tenderness, enlargement, or secretion.

INTERACTIONS
None significant.

NURSING CONSIDERATIONS
• Contraindicated in thromboembolic disorders, breast cancer, undiagnosed abnormal vaginal bleeding, severe hepatic disease, missed abortion, or pregnancy. Use cautiously when diabetes mellitus, seizure disorder, migraine, cardiac or renal disease, asthma, or mental illness is present.
• FDA regulations require that, before receiving first dose, patients read package insert explaining possible progestogen effects. Provide verbal explanation also. Patient should report any unusual symptoms immediately and should stop drug and call doctor if visual disturbances, migraine, or numbness or tingling in limbs occurs.
• Tell patient to take pill every day, even if menstruating. Pill should be taken at the same time every day.
• Progestogen-only oral contraceptive known as "minipill."
• Teach the patient how to perform a breast self-examination.
• Women using oral contraceptives should be advised of the increased risk of serious cardiovascular side effects associated with heavy cigarette smoking (15 or more cigarettes per day). These risks are quite marked in women over 35 years.
• Risk of pregnancy increases with each tablet missed. A patient who misses one tablet should take it as soon

as she remembers; she should then take the next tablet at the regular time. A patient who misses two tablets should take one as soon as she remembers and then take the next regular dose at the usual time; she should use a nonhormonal method of contraception in addition to norgestrel until 14 tablets have been taken. A patient who misses three or more tablets should discontinue the drug and use a nonhormonal method of contraception until after her menses. If her menstrual period does not occur within 45 days, pregnancy testing is necessary.
• Instruct the patient to report immediately excessive bleeding or bleeding between menstrual cycles.

progesterone
Profac-O, Progelan, Progestasert♦, Progestilin♦♦, Progestin

INDICATIONS & DOSAGE
Women:
Amenorrhea—5 to 10 mg I.M. daily for 6 to 8 days.
Dysfunctional uterine bleeding—5 to 10 mg I.M. daily for 6 doses.
Contraception (as an intrauterine device)—Progestasert system inserted into uterine cavity. Replace after 1 year.

SIDE EFFECTS
CNS: dizziness, migraine headache, lethargy, depression.
CV: hypertension, thrombophlebitis, *pulmonary embolism, edema*.
GI: nausea, vomiting, abdominal cramps.
GU: breakthrough bleeding, dysmenorrhea, amenorrhea; cervical erosion or abnormal secretions; uterine fibromas; vaginal candidiasis.
Hepatic: cholestatic jaundice.
Local: pain at injection site.
Metabolic: hyperglycemia, decreased libido.
Skin: melasma, rash.

Other: breast tenderness, enlargement, or secretion.

INTERACTIONS
None significant.

NURSING CONSIDERATIONS
• Contraindicated in thromboembolic disorders, breast cancer, undiagnosed abnormal vaginal bleeding, severe hepatic disease, or missed abortion. Use cautiously when diabetes mellitus, seizure disorder, migraine, cardiac or renal disease, asthma, or mental illness is present.
• FDA regulations require that, before receiving first dose, patients read package insert explaining possible progestogen side effects. Provide verbal explanation also. Patient should report any unusual symptoms immediately and should stop drug and call doctor if visual disturbances or migraine occurs.
• Give oil solutions (peanut oil or sesame oil) deep I.M.
• A progesterone-containing IUD (Progestasert) available that releases 65 mcg progesterone daily for 1 year.
• Instruct patient with Progestasert IUD how to check for proper IUD placement. Also, advise patient that she may experience cramps for several days after insertion and menstrual periods may be heavier. Patient should report excessively heavy menses and bleeding between menses to the doctor.
• Tell patient with Progestasert IUD that the progesterone supply is depleted in 1 year and the device must be changed. Pregnancy risk increases after 1 year if patient relies on progesterone-depleted device for contraception.
• Patients considering IUD contraception should be advised of side effects, including uterine perforation, increased risk of infection, pelvic inflammatory disease, ectopic pregnancy, abdominal cramping, increased menstrual flow, and expulsion of the device.
• Preliminary estrogen treatment is usually needed in menstrual disorders.
• Teach the patient how to perform a breast self-examination.

Italicized side effects are common or life-threatening.
*Liquid form contains alcohol.   **May contain tartrazine.

54

Gonadotropins

**chorionic gonadotropin, human
menotropins**

MECHANISM OF ACTION
- Human chorionic gonodotropin (HCG), when given on the day after the last dose of human menopausal gonadotropin (HMG or menotropins), serves as a substitute for luteinizing hormone (LH) to stimulate ovulation of an HMG-prepared follicle.
- HCG also promotes secretion of gonadal steroid hormones by stimulating production of androgen by the interstitial cells of the testes (Leydig's cells).
- Menotropins, when administered to women who have not had primary ovarian failure, mimics follicle-stimulating hormone (FSH) in inducing follicular growth, and LH in aiding follicular maturation.

COMBINATION PRODUCTS
None.

chorionic gonadotropin, human
Android HCG, A.P.L.♦, Chorex, Follutein, Glukor, Libigen, Pregnyl, Stemutrolin

INDICATIONS & DOSAGE
Anovulation and infertility—
Women: 10,000 units I.M. 1 day after last dose of menotropins.
Hypogonadism—
Men: 500 to 1,000 units I.M. 3 times weekly for 3 weeks, then twice weekly for 3 weeks; or 4,000 units I.M. 3 times weekly for 6 to 9 months, then 2,000 units 3 times weekly for 3 more months.
Nonobstructive cryptorchidism—
Boys 4 to 9 years: 5,000 units I.M. every other day for 4 doses.

SIDE EFFECTS
CNS: headache, fatigue, irritability, restlessness, depression.
GU: early puberty (growth of testes, penis, pubic and axillary hair; voice change; down on upper lip; growth of body hair).
Local: *pain at injection site.*
Other: gynecomastia, edema.

INTERACTIONS
None significant.

NURSING CONSIDERATIONS
- Contraindicated in pituitary hypertrophy or tumor, prostatic cancer, and early puberty (usual onset between 10 and 13 years of age). Use cautiously in epilepsy, migraine, asthma, cardiac or renal disease.
- Not for obesity control.
- When used with menotropins to induce ovulation, multiple births possible.
- In infertility, encourage daily intercourse from day before chorionic gonadotropin is given until ovulation occurs.
- Inspect genitalia of boys for signs of early puberty. Notify doctor, who may discontinue drug if early puberty occurs.

menotropins
Pergonal

INDICATIONS & DOSAGE

Anovulation—
Women: 75 international units (IU) each FSH and LH I.M. daily for 9 to 12 days, followed by 10,000 units chorionic gonadotropin I.M. 1 day after last dose of menotropins. Repeat for 1 to 3 menstrual cycles until ovulation occurs.

Infertility with ovulation—
Women: 75 IU each of FSH and LH I.M. daily for 9 to 12 days, followed by 10,000 units chorionic gonadotropin I.M. 1 day after last dose of menotropins. Repeat for 2 menstrual cycles and then increase to 150 IU each FSH and LH I.M. daily for 9 to 12 days, followed by 10,000 units chorionic gonadotropin I.M. 1 day after last dose of menotropins. Repeat for 2 menstrual cycles.

Infertility—
Men: 1 ampul I.M. 3 times weekly (given concomitantly with HCG 2,000 units twice weekly) for at least 4 months.
Menotropins are available in ampuls containing 75 IU each FSH and LH.

SIDE EFFECTS

Blood: hemoconcentration with fluid loss into abdomen.
GI: nausea, vomiting, diarrhea.
GU (women): *ovarian enlargement with pain and abdominal distention,* multiple births, ovarian hyperstimulation syndrome (sudden ovarian enlargement, ascites with or without pain, or pleural effusion).
GU (men): gynecomastia.
Other: fever.

INTERACTIONS
None significant.

NURSING CONSIDERATIONS

• Contraindicated in high urinary gonadotropin levels, thyroid or adrenal dysfunction, pituitary tumor, abnormal uterine bleeding, ovarian cysts or enlargement, and pregnancy.
• Tell patient that there is a possibility of multiple births.
• In infertility, encourage daily intercourse from day before chorionic gonadotropin is given until ovulation occurs.
• Reconstitute with 1 to 2 ml sterile saline injection. Use immediately.

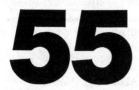

Antidiabetic agents and glucagon

acetohexamide
chlorpropamide
glucagon
insulins
tolazamide
tolbutamide

MECHANISM OF ACTION
• Glucagon raises blood glucose levels by promoting catalytic depolymerization of hepatic glycogen to glucose.
• Insulin increases glucose transport across muscle and fat-cell membranes to reduce blood glucose levels. It promotes conversion of glucose to its storage form, glycogen; triggers amino acid uptake and conversion to protein in muscle cells and inhibits protein degradation; stimulates triglyceride formation and inhibits release of free fatty acids from adipose tissue; and stimulates lipoprotein lipase activity, which converts circulating lipoproteins to fatty acids.
• Sulfonylureas stimulate insulin release from the pancreatic beta cells and reduce glucose output by the liver.

Chlorpropamide also exerts an antidiuretic effect in patients with pituitary-deficient diabetes insipidus.

COMBINATION PRODUCTS
MIXTARD INJECTION: 100 mg/ml isophane purified pork insulin suspension and purified pork insulin injection.

acetohexamide
Dimelor♦♦, Dymelor

INDICATIONS & DOSAGE
Stable, maturity-onset nonketotic diabetes mellitus uncontrolled by diet alone and previously untreated—
Adults: initially, 250 mg P.O. daily before breakfast; may increase dose q 5 to 7 days (by 250 to 500 mg) as needed to maximum 1.5 g daily, divided b.i.d. to t.i.d. before meals.
*To replace insulin therapy—*if insulin dose is less than 20 units daily, insulin may be stopped and oral therapy started with 250 mg P.O. daily, before breakfast, increased as above if needed. If insulin dose is 20 to 40 units daily, start oral therapy with 250 mg P.O. daily, before breakfast, while reducing insulin dose 25% to 30% daily or every other day, depending on response to oral therapy.

SIDE EFFECTS
Blood: *bone marrow aplasia.*
GI: nausea, heartburn, vomiting.
Metabolic: sodium loss, *hypoglycemia.*
Skin: rash, pruritus, facial flushing.
Other: hypersensitivity reactions.

INTERACTIONS
Alcohol, corticosteroids, dextrothyroxine, estrogens, glucagon, rifampin, thiazide diuretics, thyroxine: decreased hypoglycemic response. Monitor blood glucose.
Anabolic steroids, clofibrate, guanethidine, halofenate, MAO inhibitors, phenylbutazone, salicylates, sulfon-

---

amides, oral anticoagulants: increased hypoglycemic activity. Monitor blood glucose.
Beta blockers, clonidine: prolonged hypoglycemic effect and masked symptoms of hypoglycemia. Use together cautiously.

NURSING CONSIDERATIONS

• Contraindicated in treatment of juvenile, growth-onset, brittle, and severe diabetes; in diabetes mellitus adequately controlled by diet; and in maturity-onset diabetes complicated by ketosis, acidosis, diabetic coma, Raynaud's gangrene, renal or hepatic impairment, thyroid or other endocrine dysfunction. Use cautiously in patients with sulfonamide hypersensitivity.
• Instruct patient about nature of disease; importance of following therapeutic regimen and adhering to specific diet, weight reduction, exercise, personal hygiene, and avoiding infection; how and when to test for glycosuria and ketonuria; recognition of hypoglycemia and hyperglycemia.
• Be sure patient knows that the therapy relieves symptoms but doesn't cure the disease.
• Patient transferring from another oral sulfonylurea antidiabetic drug usually needs no transition period.
• Monitor patient transferring from insulin therapy to an oral antidiabetic for urine glucose and ketones at least t.i.d., before meals; emphasize the need for a double-voided specimen. Patient may require hospitalization during transition.
• During periods of increased stress, such as infection, fever, surgery, or trauma, patient may require insulin therapy. Monitor patient closely for hyperglycemia in these situations.
• Advise patient to avoid moderate to large intake of alcohol; disulfiram reaction possible.

chlorpropamide
Chloronase♦♦, Diabinese♦, Novopropamide♦♦, Stabinol♦♦

INDICATIONS & DOSAGE
Stable, maturity-onset nonketotic diabetes mellitus uncontrolled by diet alone and previously untreated—
Adults: 250 mg P.O. daily with breakfast or in divided doses if GI disturbances occur. First dosage increase may be made after 5 to 7 days due to extended duration of action, then dose may be increased q 3 to 5 days by 50 to 125 mg, if needed, to maximum 750 mg daily. Start with dose of 100 to 125 mg in older patients.
*To change from insulin to oral therapy—*If insulin dose less than 40 units daily, insulin may be stopped and oral therapy started as above. If insulin dose is 40 units or more daily, start oral therapy as above with insulin dose reduced 50%. Further insulin reductions should be made according to the patient's response.

SIDE EFFECTS
Blood: *bone marrow aplasia.*
GI: nausea, heartburn, vomiting, **GU:** tea-colored urine.
Metabolic: prolonged hypoglycemia, *dilutional hyponatremia.*
Skin: rash, pruritus, facial flushing.
Other: *hypersensitivity reactions.*

INTERACTIONS
Alcohol, corticosteroids, dextrothyroxine, glucagon, rifampin, thiazide diuretics: decreased hypoglycemic response. Monitor blood glucose.
Anabolic steroids, chloramphenicol, clofibrate, guanethidine, halofenate, MAO inhibitors, phenylbutazone, salicylates, sulfonamides, oral anticoagulants: increased hypoglycemic activity. Monitor blood glucose.
Beta blockers, clonidine: prolonged hypoglycemic effect and masked symp-

---

Italicized side effects are common or life-threatening.
∗Liquid form contains alcohol.   ∗∗May contain tartrazine.

toms of hypoglycemia. Use together cautiously.

NURSING CONSIDERATIONS
• Contraindicated in the treatment of juvenile, growth-onset, brittle, and severe diabetes.
• Contraindicated in diabetes mellitus adequately controlled by diet and in maturity-onset diabetes complicated by fever, ketosis, acidosis, diabetic coma, major surgery, severe trauma, Raynaud's gangrene, renal or hepatic impairment, thyroid or other endocrine dysfunction. Use cautiously in patients with sulfonamide hypersensitivity.
• Instruct patient about nature of the disease; importance of following therapeutic regimen and adhering to specific diet, weight reduction, exercise, personal hygiene, avoiding infection; how and when to test for glycosuria and ketonuria; and recognition of and intervention for hypoglycemia and hyperglycemia.
• Make sure patient understands that therapy relieves symptoms but does not cure the disease.
• Side effects, especially hypoglycemia, may be more frequent or severe than with some other sulfonylurea drugs (acetohexamide, tolazamide, and tolbutamide) because of its long duration of effect (36 hours).
• If hypoglycemia occurs, patient should be monitored closely for a minimum of 3 to 5 days.
• Patient transferring from another oral sulfonylurea antidiabetic drug usually needs no transition period.
• Patient may require hospitalization during transition from insulin therapy to an oral antidiabetic. Monitor patient for urine glucose and ketones at least t.i.d., before meals; emphasize the need for a double-voided specimen.
• Drug may accumulate in patients with renal insufficiency.
• Advise patient to avoid intake of alcohol. Chlorpropamide-alcohol flush (CPAF) is characterized by facial flush-

ing, lightheadedness, headache, and occasional breathlessness. Even very small amounts of alcohol can produce this reaction.
• Watch for signs of impending renal insufficiency, such as dysuria, anuria, and hematuria, and report them to the doctor immediately.

glucagon

INDICATIONS & DOSAGE
Coma of insulin-shock therapy—
Adults: 0.5 to 1 mg S.C., I.M., or I.V. 1 hour after coma develops; may repeat within 25 minutes, if necessary. In very deep coma, also give glucose 10% to 50% I.V. for faster response. When patient responds, give additional carbohydrate immediately.
Severe insulin-induced hypoglycemia during diabetic therapy—
Adults and children: 0.5 to 1 mg S.C., I.M., or I.V.; may repeat q 20 minutes for 2 doses, if necessary. If coma persists, give glucose 10% to 50% I.V.
Diagnostic aid for radiologic examination—
Adults: 0.25 to 2 mg I.V. or I.M. prior to initiation of radiologic procedure.

SIDE EFFECTS
GI: nausea, vomiting.
Other: hypersensitivity.

INTERACTIONS
Phenytoin: inhibited glucagon-induced insulin release. Use cautiously.

NURSING CONSIDERATIONS
• Use glucagon only under medical supervision.
• Hypoglycemic juvenile or unstable diabetics usually do not respond to glucagon. Give dextrose I.V. instead.
• It is vital to arouse the patient from coma as quickly as possible and to give additional carbohydrates orally to prevent secondary hypoglycemic reactions.

- For I.V. drip infusion, glucagon is compatible with dextrose solution, but forms a precipitate in chloride solutions.
- Instruct the patient and family in proper glucagon administration, recognition of hypoglycemia, and urgency of calling doctor immediately in emergencies.
- May be used as diagnostic aid in radiologic examination of the stomach, duodenum, small bowel, and colon when a hypotonic state is advantageous.
- May be stored for 3 months at 2° to 15° C. (35.6° to 59° F.) after reconstitution.

insulins

regular insulin
Actrapid, Beef Regular Iletin II (acid neutral CZI), Insulin-Toronto (beef or pork)♦♦, Pork Regular Iletin II, Velosulin

regular insulin concentrated
Regular (concentrated) Iletin

prompt insulin zinc suspension
Semilente Iletin, Semilente Insulin♦, Semitard

isophane insulin suspension (NPH)
Beef NPH Iletin II, Insulatard NPH, NPH Iletin, NPH Insulin♦♦, Pork NPH Iletin II, Protaphane NPH

insulin zinc suspension
Beef Lente Iletin, Beef Lente Iletin II, Lente Iletin, Lente Insulin♦, Pork Lente Iletin II, Lentard, Monotard

protamine zinc insulin suspension (PZI)
Beef Protamine Zinc Iletin II, Pork Protamine Zinc Iletin II, Protamine Zinc Iletin

extended insulin zinc suspension
Ultralente Iletin, Ultralente Insulin♦, Ultratard

INDICATIONS & DOSAGE
Diabetic ketoacidosis (use regular insulin only)—
Adults: 25 to 150 units I.V. immediately, then additional doses may be given q 1 hour based on blood sugar levels until patient is out of acidosis; then give S.C. q 6 hours thereafter. Alternative dosage schedule: 50 to 100 units I.V. and 50 to 100 units S.C. stat; additional doses may be given q 2 to 6 hours based on blood sugar levels; or 0.33 units/kg I.V. bolus, followed by 7 to 10 units/hour I.V. by continuous infusion. Continue infusion until blood sugar drops to 250 mg%, then start S.C. insulin q 6 hours.
Children: 0.5 to 1 unit/kg divided into 2 doses, 1 given I.V. and the other S.C., followed by 0.5 to 1 unit/kg I.V. q 1 to 2 hours; or 0.1 unit/kg I.V. bolus, then 0.1 unit/kg hourly continuous I.V. infusion until blood sugar drops to 250 mg%, then start S.C. insulin.
Preparation of infusion: add 100 units regular insulin and 1 g albumin to 100 ml 0.9% saline solution. Insulin concentration will be 1 unit/ml. (The albumin will adsorb to plastic, preventing loss of the insulin to plastic.)
Ketosis-prone and juvenile-onset diabetes mellitus, diabetes mellitus inadequately controlled by diet and oral hypoglycemics—
Adults and children: therapeutic regi-

Italicized side effects are common or life-threatening.
*Liquid form contains alcohol.   **May contain tartrazine.

men prescribed by doctor and adjusted according to patient's blood and urine glucose concentrations.

SIDE EFFECTS
Metabolic: *hypoglycemia, hyperglycemia (rebound, or Somogyi, effect).*
Skin: *urticaria.*
Local: *lipoatrophy, lipohypertrophy,* itching, swelling, redness, stinging, warmth at site of injection.
Other: *anaphylaxis.*

INTERACTIONS
Beta blockers: hyperglycemia or hypoglycemia may occur. Symptoms of hypoglycemia may be masked. Use together cautiously.
Alcohol, corticosteroids, dextrothyroxine, dobutamine, estrogens, glucagon, rifampin, thiazide diuretics, thyroxine: decreased insulin response. Monitor blood glucose.
Anabolic steroids, clofibrate, guanethidine, halofenate, MAO inhibitors, phenylbutazone, salicylates, sulfonamides, oral anticoagulants: increased insulin response. Monitor for blood glucose.

NURSING CONSIDERATIONS
• Use only regular insulin in patients with circulatory collapse, diabetic ketoacidosis, or hyperkalemia. Do not use regular insulin concentrated, I.V. Do not use intermediate or long-acting insulins for coma or other emergency requiring rapid drug action.
• During 1980, more purified forms of insulin became available. (These are called "new" insulin and are so labeled.) These new, highly purified forms may require dosage adjustment in patients previously stabilized on insulin. Patient should be made aware of this. Observe closely until dosage is established.
• Accuracy of measurement is very important, especially with regular insulin concentrated. Aids, such as magnifying sleeve, dose magnifier, or corn-

wall syringe, may help improve accuracy.
• With regular insulin concentrated, a deep secondary hypoglycemic reaction may occur 18 to 24 hours after injection.
• Dosage is always expressed in USP units.
• Regular, intermediate, and long-acting insulins may be mixed to meet the patient's needs. All insulins should be of the same concentration.
• Store insulin in cool area. Refrigeration desirable but not essential, except with regular insulin concentrated.
• Don't use insulin that has changed color.
• Check expiration date on vial before using contents.
• Administration route is subcutaneous because absorption rate and pain are less than with I.M. injections. Ketosis-prone juvenile-onset, severely ill, and newly diagnosed diabetics with very high blood sugar levels may require hospitalization and I.V. treatment with regular fast-acting insulin. Ketosis-resistant diabetics may be treated as outpatients with intermediate-acting insulin and instructions on how to alter dosage according to self-performed urine or blood glucose determinations. Some patients, primarily pregnant or brittle diabetics, may use a dextrometer to do fingerstick blood glucose tests at home.
• Press but do not rub site after injection. Rotate injection sites. Chart sites to avoid overuse of one area. However, unstable diabetics may achieve better control if injection site is rotated within same anatomic region.
• To mix insulin suspension, swirl vial gently or rotate between palms or between palm and thigh. Don't shake vigorously: this causes bubbling and air in syringe.
• Insulin requirements increase, sometimes drastically, in pregnant diabetics, then decline immediately postpartum.
• Be sure the patient knows that ther-

---

apy relieves symptoms but doesn't cure the disease.

• Tell patient about the nature of disease, the importance of following the therapeutic regimen and specific diet, weight reduction, exercise, personal hygiene, avoiding infection, and timing of injection and eating. Emphasize that meals must not be omitted. Teach that urine tests are essential guides to dosage and success of therapy; important to recognize hypoglycemic symptoms because insulin-induced hypoglycemia is hazardous and may cause brain damage if prolonged; most side effects are self-limiting and temporary.

• Advise patient to wear medical ID always; to carry ample insulin supply and syringes on trips; to have carbohydrates (lump of sugar or candy) on hand for emergency; to take note of time zone changes for dose schedule when traveling.

• Marijuana use may increase insulin requirements.

• Cigarette smoking decreases the amount of absorption of insulin administered subcutaneously. Advise patient not to smoke within 30 minutes after insulin injection.

• U-80 strength no longer certified by Food and Drug Administration. Instruct patient in use of U-100 strength.

• Some patients may develop insulin resistance and require large insulin doses to control symptoms of diabetes. U-500 insulin is available for such patients as Purified Pork Iletin Regular Insulin, U500. Although every pharmacy may not normally stock it, it is readily available. Patient should notify pharmacist several days before refill of prescription is needed. Nurse should give hospital pharmacy sufficient notice before needing to refill in-house prescription. Never store U-500 insulin in same area with other insulin preparations due to danger of severe overdose if given accidentally to other patients. U-500 insulin must be administered

with a U-100 syringe since no syringes are made for this drug.

tolazamide
Tolinase

INDICATIONS & DOSAGE
Stable, maturity-onset nonketotic diabetes mellitus uncontrolled by diet alone and previously untreated—
Adults: initially, 100 mg P.O. daily with breakfast if fasting blood sugar (FBS) under 200 mg%; or 250 mg if FBS is over 200 mg%. May adjust dose at weekly intervals by 100 to 250 mg. Maximum dose 500 mg b.i.d. before meals.
Elderly or debilitated patients: increase dose by 50 to 125 mg at weekly intervals.
*To change from insulin to oral therapy—*if insulin dose under 20 units daily, insulin may be stopped and oral therapy started at 100 mg P.O. daily with breakfast. If insulin dose is 20 to 40 units daily, insulin may be stopped and oral therapy started at 250 mg P.O. daily with breakfast. If insulin dose is over 40 units daily, decrease insulin dose 50% and start oral therapy at 250 mg P.O. daily with breakfast. Increase doses as above.

SIDE EFFECTS
Blood: *bone marrow aplasia.*
GI: nausea, vomiting.
Metabolic: hypoglycemia.
Skin: rash, urticaria, facial flushing.
Other: hypersensitivity reactions.

INTERACTIONS
Alcohol, corticosteroids, dextrothyroxine, estrogens, glucagon, rifampin, thiazide diuretics, thyroxine: decreased hypoglycemic response. Monitor blood glucose.
Anabolic steroids, clofibrate, guanethidine, halofenate, MAO inhibitors, phenylbutazone, salicylates, sulfonamides, oral anticoagulants: increased

---

Italicized side effects are common or life-threatening.
*Liquid form contains alcohol.   **May contain tartrazine.

hypoglycemic activity. Monitor blood glucose.

Beta blockers, clonidine: prolonged hypoglycemic effect and masked symptoms of hypoglycemia. Use together cautiously.

NURSING CONSIDERATIONS
• Contraindicated in juvenile, growth-onset, and severe diabetes mellitus; diabetes mellitus adequately controlled by diet or in maturity-onset diabetes mellitus complicated by fever, ketosis, acidosis, or coma; major surgery; severe trauma; Raynaud's gangrene; renal or hepatic impairment; thyroid or other endocrine dysfunction. Use cautiously in patients with sulfonamide hypersensitivity and in elderly, debilitated, or malnourished patients.
• Instruct patient about nature of disease; importance of following therapeutic regimen and specific diet, weight reduction, exercise, personal hygiene, avoiding infection; how and when to test for glycosuria and ketonuria; and recognition of hypoglycemia and hyperglycemia.
• Be sure patient knows that therapy relieves symptoms but doesn't cure disease.
• Patient transferring from another oral sulfonylurea antidiabetic drug usually needs no transition period.
• Patient transferring from insulin therapy to an oral hypoglycemic should test urine for glucose and ketones at least t.i.d., before meals; emphasize the need for a double-voided specimen. Hospitalization may be required during the transition.
• Advise patient to avoid moderate to large intake of alcohol; disulfiram reaction possible.

tolbutamide
Mobenol♦♦, Novobutamide♦♦, Oramide♦♦, Orinase♦, SK-Tolbutamide, Tolbutone♦♦

INDICATIONS & DOSAGE
Stable, maturity-onset nonketotic diabetes mellitus uncontrolled by diet alone and previously untreated—
Adults: initially, 1 to 2 g P.O. daily as single dose or divided b.i.d. to t.i.d. May adjust dose to maximum 3 g daily.
*To change from insulin to oral therapy—*if insulin dose is under 20 units daily, insulin may be stopped and oral therapy started at 1 to 2 g daily. If insulin dose is 20 to 40 units daily, insulin dose is reduced 30% to 50% and oral therapy started as above. If insulin dose is over 40 units daily, insulin dose is decreased 20% and oral therapy started as above. Further reductions in insulin dose are based on patient's response to oral therapy.

SIDE EFFECTS
Blood: *bone marrow aplasia.*
GI: nausea, heartburn.
Metabolic: hypoglycemia.
Skin: rash, pruritus, facial flushing.
Other: hypersensitivity reactions.

INTERACTIONS
Alcohol, corticosteroids, dextrothyroxine, estrogens, glucagon, rifampin, thiazide diuretics, thyroxine: decreased hypoglycemic response. Monitor blood glucose.
Anabolic steroids, chloramphenicol, clofibrate, guanethidine, halofenate, MAO inhibitors, phenylbutazone, salicylates, sulfonamides, oral anticoagulants: increased hypoglycemic activity. Monitor blood glucose.
Beta blockers, clonidine: prolonged hypoglycemic effect and masked symptoms of hypoglycemia. Use together cautiously.

NURSING CONSIDERATIONS

• Contraindicated in juvenile, growth-onset, brittle, and severe diabetes; diabetes mellitus adequately controlled by diet or in maturity-onset diabetes mellitus complicated by fever, ketosis, acidosis, or coma; major surgery; severe trauma; Raynaud's gangrene; renal or hepatic impairment; thyroid or other endocrine dysfunction; pregnancy. Use cautiously in patients with sulfonamide hypersensitivity.

• Instruct patient about nature of disease; importance of following therapeutic regimen and specific diet, weight reduction, exercise, personal hygiene, and avoiding infection; how and when to test for glycosuria and ketonuria; and recognition of hypoglycemia and hyperglycemia.

• Be sure patient knows that therapy relieves symptoms but doesn't cure disease.

• Patient transferring from another oral sulfonylurea antidiabetic drug usually needs no transition period.

• Patient transferring from insulin therapy to an oral hypoglycemic should test urine for glucose and ketones at least t.i.d., before meals; emphasize the need for a double-voided specimen. Hospitalization may be required during the transition.

• Advise patient to avoid moderate to large intake of alcohol: disulfiram reaction possible.

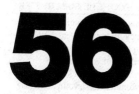

Thyroid hormones

levothyroxine sodium (T₄ or L-thyroxine sodium)
liothyronine sodium (T₃)
liotrix
thyroglobulin
thyroid USP (desiccated)
thyrotropin (thyroid-stimulating hormone or TSH)

MECHANISM OF ACTION

Thyroid hormones stimulate the metabolism of all body tissues by accelerating the rate of cellular oxidation. They enhance carbohydrate and protein biosynthesis by glyconeogenesis, which increases the mobilization and utilization of glycogen stores. They also affect lipid metabolism by decreasing cholesterol levels in the liver and blood.

• Thyrotropin stimulates the uptake of radioactive iodine in patients with thyroid carcinoma. It also promotes thyroid hormone production by the anterior pituitary.

COMBINATION PRODUCTS

EUTHROID-½: levothyroxine sodium 30 mcg and liothyronine sodium 7.5 mcg.
EUTHROID-1: levothyroxine sodium 60 mcg and liothyronine sodium 15 mcg.
EUTHROID-2: levothyroxine sodium 120 mcg and liothyronine sodium 30 mcg.
EUTHROID-3: levothyroxine sodium 180 mcg and liothyronine sodium 45 mcg.
THYROLAR-¼: levothyroxine sodium 12.5 mcg and liothyronine sodium 3.1 mcg.
THYROLAR-½♦: levothyroxine sodium 25 mcg and liothyronine sodium 6.25 mcg.
THYROLAR-1♦: levothyroxine sodium

50 mcg and liothyronine sodium 12.5 mcg.
THYROLAR-2♦: levothyroxine sodium 100 mcg and liothyronine sodium 25 mcg.
THYROLAR-3♦: levothyroxine sodium 150 mcg and liothyronine sodium 37.5 mcg.

---

levothyroxine sodium (T₄ or L-thyroxine sodium)
Eltroxin♦♦, Levoid, Levothroid, Noroxine, Synthroid♦**

INDICATIONS & DOSAGE

Cretinism in children younger than 1 year—initially, 0.025 to 0.05 mg P.O. daily, increased by 0.05 mg P.O. q 2 to 3 weeks to total daily dose 0.1 to 0.4 mg P.O.
Myxedema coma—
Adults: 0.2 to 0.5 mg I.V. If no response in 24 hours, additional 0.1 to 0.3 mg I.V. After condition stabilized, oral maintenance.
Thyroid hormone replacement—
Adults: initially, 0.025 to 0.1 mg P.O. daily, increased by 0.05 to 0.1 mg P.O. q 1 to 4 weeks until desired response. Maintenance dose 0.1 to 0.4 mg daily.
Children: initially, maximum 0.05 mg P.O. daily, gradually increased by 0.025 to 0.05 mg P.O. q 1 to 4 weeks until desired response.

SIDE EFFECTS

Side effects of thyroid hormones are extensions of their pharmacologic properties and reflect patient sensitivity to them.

Signs of overdosage:

CNS: *nervousness, insomnia, tremor.*

CV: *tachycardia, palpitations, arrhythmias, angina pectoris,* hypertension.

GI: change in appetite, nausea, diarrhea.

Other: headache, leg cramps, weight loss, sweating, heat intolerance, fever, menstrual irregularities.

INTERACTIONS

Cholestyramine: levothyroxine absorption impaired. Separate doses by 4 to 5 hours.

I.V. phenytoin: free thyroid released. Monitor for tachycardia.

NURSING CONSIDERATIONS

• Contraindicated in myocardial infarction, thyrotoxicosis (except with antithyroid drugs), or uncorrected adrenal insufficiency (thyroid hormones increase tissue demand for adrenocortical hormone and may cause acute adrenal crisis). Use with extreme caution in angina pectoris, hypertension, or other cardiovascular disorders; renal insufficiency; or ischemic states.

• Use carefully in myxedema; patients are unusually sensitive to thyroid hormone. Dose varies widely among patients; start at lowest and titrate in higher doses according to patient's symptoms and laboratory data until euthyroid state is reached.

• Rapid replacement in patients with arteriosclerosis may precipitate angina, coronary occlusion, or stroke. Use cautiously in such patients.

• In patients with coronary artery disease who must receive thyroid, observe carefully for possible coronary insufficiency if catecholamines must be given.

• Potentially dangerous; not indicated to relieve such vague symptoms as physical and mental sluggishness, irritability, depression, nervousness, ill-defined pains; to treat obesity in euthyroid persons; to treat metabolic insufficiency not associated with thyroid insufficiency; or to treat menstrual disorders or male infertility, unless associated with hypothyroidism.

• When changing from levothyroxine to liothyronine, stop levothyroxine and begin liothyronine. Increase in small increments after residual effects of levothyroxine have disappeared. When changing from liothyronine to levothyroxine, start levothyroxine several days before withdrawing liothyronine to avoid relapse.

• Different brands of levothyroxine may not be bioequivalent. Once the patient has been stabilized on one brand, warn him not to switch to another. Also advise him to avoid "generic" levothyroxine.

• Warn patient to tell doctor at once if chest pain (especially in elderly), palpitations, sweating, nervousness, or other signs of overdosage occur. Also notify doctor immediately if any signs of aggravated cardiovascular disease develop (chest pain, dyspnea, tachycardia).

• Tell patient to take thyroid hormones regularly, at the same time each day, to maintain constant hormone levels.

• Suggest morning dosage to prevent insomnia.

• Monitor pulse rate, blood pressure.

• Protect from moisture and light. Prepare I.V. dose immediately before injection.

• Thyroid hormones alter thyroid function test results. Monitor prothrombin time; patients taking these hormones usually require less anticoagulant. Alert patients to report unusual bleeding and bruising.

• Patients taking levothyroxine who need to have radioactive iodine uptake studies must discontinue drug 4 weeks before test.

Italicized side effects are common or life-threatening.
*Liquid form contains alcohol.   **May contain tartrazine.

liothyronine sodium (T₃)
Cytomel♦, Cytomine

INDICATIONS & DOSAGE
Cretinism—
Children 3 years and older: 50 to 100 mcg P.O. daily.
Children under 3 years: 5 mcg P.O. daily, increased by 5 mcg q 3 to 4 days until desired response occurs.
Myxedema—
Adults: initially 5 mcg daily, increased by 5 to 10 mcg q 1 or 2 weeks. Maintenance dose 50 to 100 mcg daily.
Nontoxic goiter—
Adults: initially, 5 mcg P.O. daily; may be increased by 12.5 to 25 mcg daily q 1 to 2 weeks. Usual maintenance dose 75 mcg daily.
Elderly: initially, 5 mcg P.O. daily, increased by 5-mcg increments at weekly intervals until desired response.
Children: initially, 5 mcg P.O. daily, increased by 5-mcg increments at weekly intervals until desired response.
Thyroid hormone replacement—
Adults: initially, 25 mcg P.O. daily, increased by 12.5 to 25 mcg q 1 to 2 weeks until satisfactory response. Usual maintenance dose 25 to 75 mcg daily.

SIDE EFFECTS
Side effects of thyroid hormones are extensions of their pharmacologic properties and reflect patient sensitivity to them.
CNS: hyperirritability, *nervousness, insomnia,* twitching, *tremors,* headache.
CV: increased cardiac output, *tachycardia,* cardiac arrhythmias, *angina pectoris,* increased blood pressure, *cardiac decompensation and collapse.*
GI: diarrhea, abdominal cramps, vomiting.
Other: weight loss, heat intolerance, hyperhidrosis, menstrual irregularities; in infants and children—accelerated rate of bone maturation.

INTERACTIONS
Cholestyramine: liothyronine absorption impaired. Separate doses by 4 to 5 hours.
I.V. phenytoin: free thyroid released. Monitor for tachycardia.

NURSING CONSIDERATIONS
• Contraindicated in myocardial infarction, thyrotoxicosis (except with antithyroid drugs), or uncorrected adrenal insufficiency (thyroid hormones increase tissue demand for adrenocortical hormone and may cause acute adrenal crisis). Use with extreme caution in angina pectoris, hypertension, or other cardiovascular disorders; renal insufficiency; or ischemic states.
• Rapid replacement in patients with arteriosclerosis may precipitate angina, coronary occlusion, or stroke. Use cautiously in such patients.
• In patients with coronary artery disease who must receive thyroid hormones, observe carefully for possible coronary insufficiency if catecholamines must be given.
• Use carefully in myxedema; patients are unusually sensitive to thyroid hormone.
• Potentially dangerous; not indicated to relieve vague symptoms, such as physical and mental sluggishness, irritability, depression, nervousness, and ill-defined aches and pains; to treat obesity in euthyroid persons; to treat metabolic insufficiency; or to treat menstrual disorders or male infertility, unless associated with hypothyroidism.
• When changing from levothyroxine to liothyronine, stop levothyroxine and begin liothyronine. Increase in small increments after residual effects of levothyroxine have disappeared. When changing from liothyronine to levothyroxine, start levothyroxine several days before withdrawing liothyronine to avoid relapse.
• Warn patient to tell doctor at once if chest pain (especially in elderly), palpitations, sweating, nervousness, or other

signs of overdosage occur. Also notify doctor immediately if any signs of aggravated cardiovascular disease develop (chest pain, dyspnea, tachycardia).
• Tell patient to take thyroid hormones regularly, at the same time each day, to maintain constant hormone levels.
• Suggest morning dosage to prevent insomnia.
• Monitor pulse rate, blood pressure.
• Thyroid hormones alter thyroid function tests. Monitor prothrombin time; patients taking these hormones may require less anticoagulant. Alert patients to report unusual bleeding and bruising.
• Patients taking liothyronine who need to have radioactive iodine uptake studies must discontinue drug 7 to 10 days before test.

---

liotrix
Euthroid**, Thyrolar◆

INDICATIONS & DOSAGE
Hypothyroidism—dosages must be individualized to approximate the deficit in the patient's thyroid secretion.
Adults and children: initially, 15 to 30 mg P.O. daily, increasing by 15 to 30 mg q 1 to 2 weeks to desired response; increments in children's dose q 2 weeks.
Elderly: initially, 15 to 30 mg. Usual adult dose doubled q 6 to 8 weeks to desired response.

SIDE EFFECTS
Side effects of thyroid hormones are extensions of their pharmacologic properties and reflect patient sensitivity to them.
CNS: hyperirritability, *nervousness, insomnia,* twitching, *tremors.*
CV: increased cardiac output, *tachycardia,* cardiac arrhythmia, *angina pectoris,* increased blood pressure, *cardiac decompensation and collapse.*
GI: diarrhea, abdominal cramps, vomiting.

Other: weight loss, menstrual irregularities, heat intolerance, hyperhidrosis; infants and children—accelerated rate of bone maturation.

INTERACTIONS
Cholestyramine: liotrix absorption impaired. Separate doses by 4 to 5 hours.
I.V. phenytoin: free thyroid released. Monitor for tachycardia.

NURSING CONSIDERATIONS
• Contraindicated in myocardial infarction, thyrotoxicosis (except with antithyroid drugs), or uncorrected adrenal insufficiency (thyroid hormones increase tissue demand for adrenocortical hormone and may cause acute adrenal crisis). Use with extreme caution in angina pectoris, hypertension, or other cardiovascular disorders; renal insufficiency; or ischemic states.
• Rapid replacement in patients with arteriosclerosis may precipitate angina, coronary occlusion, or stroke. Use cautiously in such patients.
• Use carefully in myxedema; patients are unusually sensitive to thyroid hormone.
• In patients with coronary artery disease who must receive thyroid hormones, observe carefully for possible coronary insufficiency if catecholamines must be given. Also observe carefully during surgery, since cardiac arrhythmias can be precipitated.
• Potentially dangerous; not indicated to relieve vague symptoms, such as physical and mental sluggishness, irritability, depression, nervousness, ill-defined pains; to treat obesity in euthyroid persons; to treat metabolic insufficiency not associated with thyroid insufficiency; or to treat menstrual disorders or male infertility, unless associated with hypothyroidism.
• Tell patient to take thyroid hormones regularly, at the same time each day, preferably before breakfast, to maintain constant hormone levels.
• Warn patient to tell doctor at once if

Italicized side effects are common or life-threatening.
*Liquid form contains alcohol.   **May contain tartrazine.

chest pain (especially in elderly), palpitations, sweating, nervousness, or other signs of overdosage occur. Also notify doctor immediately if any signs of aggravated cardiovascular disease develop (chest pain, dyspnea, tachycardia).
• The two commercially prepared liotrix drugs contain different amounts of each ingredient; do not change from one brand to the other without considering the differences in potency: Thyrolar-½ contains 25 mcg T₄ and 6.25 mcg T₃; Euthroid-½ contains 30 mcg T₄ and 7.5 mcg T₃.
• Monitor pulse rate, blood pressure.
• Protect from heat, light, moisture.
• Thyroid hormones alter thyroid function test results. Monitor prothrombin time; patients taking these hormones usually require less anticoagulant. Alert patients to report unusual bleeding and bruising.

thyroglobulin
Proloid♦

INDICATIONS & DOSAGE
Cretinism and juvenile hypo-thyroidism—
Children 1 year and older: dosage may approach adult dose (60 to 180 mg P.O. daily), depending on response.
Children 4 to 12 months: 60 to 80 mg P.O. daily.
Children 1 to 4 months: initially, 15 to 30 mg P.O. daily, increased at 2-week intervals. Usual maintenance dose 30 to 45 mg P.O. daily.
Hypothyroidism or myxedema—
Adults: initially, 15 to 30 mg P.O. daily, increased by 15 to 30 mg at 2-week intervals until desired response. Usual maintenance dose 60 to 180 mg P.O. daily, as a single dose.
Elderly: initially 7.5 to 15 mg P.O. daily; the dose is doubled at 6- to 8-week intervals until desired response is obtained.

SIDE EFFECTS
Side effects of thyroid hormones are extensions of their pharmacologic properties and reflect patient sensitivity to them.
CNS: hyperirritability, *nervousness, insomnia,* twitching, *tremors,* headache.
CV: increased cardiac output, *tachycardia,* cardiac arrhythmias, *angina pectoris,* increased blood pressure, *cardiac decompensation and collapse.*
GI: diarrhea, abdominal cramps, vomiting.
Other: weight loss, heat intolerance, hyperhidrosis, menstrual irregularities; in infants and children—accelerated rate of bone maturation.

INTERACTIONS
Cholestyramine: thyroglobulin absorption impaired. Separate doses by 4 to 5 hours.
I.V. phenytoin: free thyroid released. Monitor for tachycardia.

NURSING CONSIDERATIONS
• Contraindicated in myocardial infarction, thyrotoxicosis (except with antithyroid drugs), or uncorrected adrenal insufficiency (thyroid hormones increase tissue demand for adrenocortical hormone and may cause acute adrenal crisis). Use with extreme caution in angina pectoris, hypertension, or other cardiovascular disorders; renal insufficiency; or ischemic states.
• In patients with coronary artery disease who must receive thyroid hormones, observe carefully for possible coronary insufficiency if catecholamines must be given.
• Use carefully in myxedema; patients are unusually sensitive to thyroid hormone.
• Potentially dangerous; not indicated to relieve vague symptoms, such as physical and mental sluggishness, irritability, depression, nervousness, and ill-defined pains; to treat obesity in euthyroid persons; to treat metabolic insufficiency not associated with thyroid

insufficiency; or to treat menstrual disorders or male infertility, unless associated with hypothyroidism.
• Tell patient to take thyroid hormones regularly, at the same time each day, to maintain constant hormone levels.
• Warn patient to tell doctor at once if chest pain (especially in elderly), palpitations, sweating, nervousness, or other signs of overdosage occur. Also notify doctor immediately if any signs of aggravated cardiovascular disease develop (chest pain, dyspnea, tachycardia).
• Suggest morning dosage to prevent insomnia.
• Monitor pulse rate, blood pressure.
• Thyroid hormones alter thyroid function test results. Monitor prothrombin time; patients taking these hormones usually require less anticoagulant. Alert patients to report unusual bleeding and bruising.

thyroid USP (desiccated)
S-P-T, Thyrar, Thyro-Teric

INDICATIONS & DOSAGE
Adult hypothyroidism—
Adults: initially, 60 mg P.O. daily, increased by 60 mg q 30 days until desired response. Usual maintenance dose 60 to 180 mg P.O. daily, as a single dose.
Elderly: 7.5 to 15 mg P.O. daily; dose is doubled at 6- to 8-week intervals.
Adult myxedema—
Adults: 16 mg P.O. daily. May double dose q 2 weeks to maximum 120 mg.
Cretinism and juvenile hypothyroidism—
Children 1 year and older: dosage may approach adult dose (60 to 180 mg) daily, depending on response.
Children 4 to 12 months: 30 to 60 mg P.O. daily.
Children 1 to 4 months: initially, 15 to 30 mg P.O. daily, increased at 2-week intervals. Usual maintenance dose 30 to 45 mg P.O. daily.

SIDE EFFECTS
Side effects of thyroid hormones are extensions of their pharmacologic properties and reflect patient sensitivity to them.
CNS: *hyperirritability, nervousness, insomnia,* twitching, tremors, headache.
CV: increased cardiac output, *tachycardia,* cardiac arrhythmias, *angina pectoris,* increased blood pressure, *cardiac decompensation and collapse.*
GI: diarrhea, abdominal cramps, vomiting.
Other: weight loss, heat intolerance, hyperhidrosis, menstrual irregularities; in infants and children—accelerated rate of bone maturation.

INTERACTIONS
Cholestyramine: thyroid absorption impaired. Separate doses by 4 to 5 hours.
I.V. phenytoin: free thyroid released. Monitor for tachycardia.

NURSING CONSIDERATIONS
• Contraindicated in myocardial infarction, thyrotoxicosis (except with antithyroid drugs), or uncorrected adrenal insufficiency (thyroid hormones increase tissue demand for adrenocortical hormone and may cause acute adrenal crisis). Use with extreme caution in angina pectoris, hypertension, or other cardiovascular disorders; renal insufficiency; or ischemic states.
• Use carefully in myxedema; patients are unusually sensitive to thyroid hormone.
• In patients with coronary artery disease who must receive thyroid hormones, observe carefully for possible coronary insufficiency if catecholamines must be given.
• Potentially dangerous; not indicated to relieve vague symptoms, such as physical and mental sluggishness, irritability, depression, nervousness, ill-defined pains; to treat obesity in euthyroid persons; to treat metabolic insufficiency not associated with thyroid insufficiency; or to treat menstrual disor-

ders or male infertility, unless associated with hypothyroidism.

• Tell patient to take thyroid hormones regularly, at the same time each day, to maintain constant hormone levels.

• Warn patient to tell doctor at once if chest pain (especially in elderly), palpitations, sweating, nervousness, or other signs of overdosage occur. Also notify doctor immediately if any signs of aggravated cardiovascular disease develop (chest pain, dyspnea, tachycardia).

• Suggest morning dosage to prevent insomnia.

• Monitor pulse rate and blood pressure.

• In children, sleeping pulse rate and basal morning temperature are guides to treatment.

• Thyroid hormones alter thyroid function test results. Monitor prothrombin time; patients taking these hormones usually require less anticoagulant. Alert patients to report unusual bleeding and bruising.

thyrotropin
Thytropar♦

INDICATIONS & DOSAGE

Diagnosis of thyroid cancer remnant with ^{131}I *after surgery*—10 international units I.M. or S.C. for 3 to 7 days.
Differential diagnosis of primary and secondary hypothyroidism—10 units I.M. or S.C. for 1 to 3 days.
In PBI or ^{131}I *uptake determinations for differential diagnosis of subclinical hypothyroidism or low thyroid reserve*—10 units I.M. or S.C.
Therapy for thyroid carcinoma (local or metastatic) with ^{131}I—10 units I.M. or S.C. for 3 to 8 days.
To determine thyroid status of patient receiving thyroid—10 units I.M. or S.C. for 1 to 3 days.

SIDE EFFECTS
CNS: headache.
CV: *tachycardia*, atrial fibrillation, *angina pectoris, congestive failure,* hypotension.
GI: nausea, vomiting.
Other: thyroid hyperplasia (large doses), fever, menstrual irregularities, allergic reactions (postinjection flare, urticaria, *anaphylaxis*).

INTERACTIONS
None significant.

NURSING CONSIDERATIONS
• Contraindicated in coronary thrombosis, untreated Addison's disease. Use cautiously in angina pectoris, heart failure, hypopituitarism, adrenocortical suppression.
• May cause thyroid hyperplasia.
• Diagnostic use: to identify subclinical hypothyroidism or low thyroid reserve, to evaluate need for thyroid therapy, to distinguish between primary and secondary hypothyroidism, and to detect thyroid remnants and metastases of thyroid carcinoma.
• Therapeutic use: management of certain types of thyroid carcinoma and resulting metastases, and in conjunction with radioactive ^{131}I to enhance uptake of ^{131}I by the thyroid.
• Three-day dosage schedule may be used in long-standing pituitary myxedema or with prolonged use of thyroid medication.

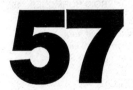

Thyroid hormone antagonists

iodine
radioactive iodine (sodium iodide) ^{131}I
methimazole
propylthiouracil (PTU)

MECHANISM OF ACTION
● Iodine inhibits thyroid hormone formation by blocking iodotyrosine and iodothyronine synthesis. It also limits iodide transport into the thyroid gland and blocks thyroid hormone release.
● Radioactive iodine limits thyroid hormone secretion by destroying thyroid tissue. The affinity of thyroid tissue for radioactive iodine facilitates uptake of the drug by cancerous thyroid tissue that has metastasized to other sites in the body.
● The thionamines inhibit oxidation of iodine in the thyroid gland, blocking iodine's ability to combine with tyrosine to form thyroxine. They may also prevent the coupling of monoiodotyrosine and diiodotyrosine to form thyroxine and triiodothyronine.

COMBINATION PRODUCTS
None.

---

iodine
Potassium Iodide Solution, USP;
Sodium Iodide, USP; Strong Iodine
Solution, USP (Lugol's Solution),
containing 5% iodine and 10%
potassium iodide

INDICATIONS & DOSAGE
Preparation for thyroidectomy—
Adults and children: Strong Iodine
Solution, USP, 0.1 to 0.3 ml t.i.d., or
Potassium Iodide Solution, USP,
5 drops in water t.i.d. after meals for
2 to 3 weeks before surgery.
Thyrotoxic crisis—
Adults and children: Strong Iodine
Solution, USP, 1 ml in water P.O. t.i.d.
after meals in refractory cases; Sodium
Iodide, USP, 250 to 500 mg (or up to 2
g) daily, slow I.V. infu-
sion with antithyroid drugs and pro-
pranolol.

SIDE EFFECTS
EENT: acute rhinitis, inflammation of
salivary glands, periorbital edema, conjunctivitis, hyperemia.
GI: burning, irritation, *nausea,* vomiting, *metallic taste.*
Skin: acneiform rash, mucous membrane ulceration.
Other: fever, frontal headache; with
I.V. use (sodium iodide): acute iodism,
shock, pulmonary edema.

INTERACTIONS
Lithium carbonate: hypothyroidism
may occur. Use with caution.

NURSING CONSIDERATIONS
● Contraindicated in tuberculosis, iodide hypersensitivity, hyperkalemia; after meals that contain excessive starch;
in laryngeal edema, swelling of salivary
glands.
● Generally use I.V. route only if patient is vomiting or cannot receive anything by mouth. Some prefer I.V. route
to prevent GI side effects, especially
during critical time at beginning of
treatment.

Italicized side effects are common or life-threatening.
*Liquid form contains alcohol. **May contain tartrazine.

• Dilute oral doses in water, milk, or fruit juice, and give after meals to prevent gastric irritation, to hydrate the patient, and to mask the very salty taste.
• Tell patient to ask the doctor about using iodized salt and eating shellfish during treatment. Iodine-rich foods may not be permitted.
• Warn the patient that sudden withdrawal may precipitate thyroid storm.
• Store in light-resistant container.
• Give iodides through straw to avoid tooth discoloration.
• Usually given with other antithyroid drugs.

---

radioactive iodine (sodium iodide) ^{131}I

INDICATIONS & DOSAGE

Hyperthyroidism—
Adults: usual dose is 4 to 10 millicuries P.O. Dose based on estimated weight of thyroid gland and thyroid uptake. Treatment may be repeated after 6 weeks, according to serum thyroxine levels.
Thyroid cancer—
Adults: 50 to 150 millicuries P.O. Dose based on estimated malignant thyroid tissue and metastatic tissue as determined by total body scan. Dose may be repeated according to clinical status.

SIDE EFFECTS

EENT: *feeling of fullness in neck,* metallic taste, "radiation mumps."
Endocrine: hypothyroidism, radiation thyroiditis.
GU: possible increased risk of birth defects in offspring after sufficient ^{131}I dose for thyroid ablation following cancer surgery.
Other: possible increased risk of developing leukemia later in life after sufficient ^{131}I dose for thyroid ablation following cancer surgery.

INTERACTIONS

Lithium carbonate: hypothyroidism may occur. Use with caution.

NURSING CONSIDERATIONS

• Contraindicated in pregnancy and lactation unless used to treat thyroid cancer.
• Stop all antithyroid medications, thyroid preparations, and iodine-containing preparations 1 week before ^{131}I dose. If medications are not stopped, patient may receive thyroid-stimulating hormone for 3 days before ^{131}I dose. When treating women of childbearing age, give dose during menstruation or within 7 days after menstruation.
• After therapy for hyperthyroidism, patient should not resume antithyroid drugs, but should continue propranolol or other drugs used to treat symptoms of hyperthyroidism until onset of full ^{131}I effect (usually 6 weeks).
• Monitor thyroid function with serum thyroxine levels.
• After dose for hyperthyroidism, patient's urine and saliva are slightly radioactive for 24 hours; vomitus is highly radioactive for 6 to 8 hours. Institute full radiation precautions during this time. Instruct patient to use appropriate disposal methods when coughing and expectorating.
• After dose for thyroid cancer, patient's urine, saliva, and perspiration remain radioactive for 3 days. Isolate patient and observe the following precautions: pregnant personnel should not take care of patient; disposable eating utensils and linens should be used; instruct patient to save all urine in lead containers for 24 to 48 hours so amount of radioactive material excreted can be determined. Patient should drink as much fluid as possible for 48 hours after drug administration to facilitate excretion. Limit contact with patient to 30 minutes per shift per person the first day. May increase time to 1 hour second day and longer on third day.

• If patient is discharged less than 7 days after ¹³¹I dose for thyroid cancer, warn him to avoid close, prolonged contact with small children (for example, holding children on lap), and instruct him not to sleep in same room with spouse for 7 days after treatment due to increased risk of thyroid cancer in persons exposed to ¹³¹I. Tell patient he may use same bathroom facilities as rest of family.

methimazole
Tapazole

INDICATIONS & DOSAGE
Hyperthyroidism—
Adults: 5 mg P.O. t.i.d. if mild; 10 to 15 mg P.O. t.i.d. if moderately severe; and 20 mg P.O. t.i.d. if severe. Continue until patient euthyroid, then start maintenance dose of 5 mg daily to t.i.d. Maximum dose 150 mg daily.
Children: 0.4 mg/kg daily divided q 8 hours. Continue until patient euthyroid, then start maintenance dose of 0.2 mg/kg daily divided q 8 hours.
Preparation for thyroidectomy—
Adults and children: same doses as for hyperthyroidism until patient is euthyroid; then iodine may be added for 10 days before surgery.
Thyrotoxic crisis—
Adults and children: same doses as for hyperthyroidism, with concomitant iodine therapy and propranolol.

SIDE EFFECTS
Blood: *agranulocytosis,* leukopenia, granulopenia, thrombocytopenia (appear to be dose-related).
CNS: headache, drowsiness, vertigo.
GI: diarrhea, nausea, vomiting (may be dose-related).
Hepatic: jaundice.
Skin: rash, urticaria, skin discoloration.
Other: arthralgia, myalgia, salivary gland enlargement, loss of taste, drug fever, lymphadenopathy.

INTERACTIONS
None significant.

NURSING CONSIDERATIONS
• Use cautiously in pregnancy. Pregnant women may require less drug as pregnancy progresses. Monitor thyroid function studies closely. Thyroid may be added to regimen. Drugs may be stopped during last few weeks of pregnancy.
• Watch for signs of hypothyroidism (mental depression; cold intolerance; hard, nonpitting edema). Dose may need to be adjusted.
• Monitor CBC periodically to detect impending leukopenia, thrombocytopenia, and agranulocytosis.
• Warn patient to report immediately: fever, sore throat, or mouth sores (possible signs of developing agranulocytosis). Agranulocytosis can develop too rapidly to be detected by periodic blood cell counts. Tell patient also to immediately report skin eruptions (sign of hypersensitivity).
• Drug should be stopped if severe rash or enlarged cervical lymph nodes develop.
• Tell patient to ask doctor about using iodized salt and eating shellfish during treatment.
• Warn patient against over-the-counter cough medicines; many contain iodine.
• Give with meals to reduce GI side effects.
• Store in light-resistant container.

propylthiouracil (PTU)
Propyl-Thyracil♦♦

INDICATIONS & DOSAGE
Hyperthyroidism—
Adults: 100 mg P.O. t.i.d.; up to 300 mg q 8 hours have been used in severe cases. Continue until patient euthyroid, then start maintenance dose of 100 mg daily to t.i.d.
Children over 10 years: 100 mg P.O.

Italicized side effects are common or life-threatening.
∗Liquid form contains alcohol.   ∗∗May contain tartrazine.

t.i.d. Continue until patient euthyroid, then start maintenance dose of 25 mg t.i.d. to 100 mg b.i.d.
Children 6 to 10 years: 50 to 150 mg P.O. divided doses q 8 hours.
Preparation for thyroidectomy—
Adults and children: same doses as for hyperthyroidism, then iodine may be added 10 days before surgery.
Thyrotoxic crisis—
Adults and children: same doses as for hyperthyroidism, with concomitant iodine therapy and propranolol.

SIDE EFFECTS
Blood: *agranulocytosis,* leukopenia, thrombocytopenia (appear to be dose-related).
CNS: headache, drowsiness, vertigo.
EENT: visual disturbances.
GI: diarrhea, *nausea, vomiting* (may be dose-related).
Hepatic: jaundice.
Skin: rash, urticaria, skin discoloration, pruritus.
Other: arthralgia, myalgia, salivary gland enlargement, loss of taste, drug fever, lymphadenopathy.

INTERACTIONS
None significant.

NURSING CONSIDERATIONS
• Use cautiously in pregnancy. Pregnant women may require less drug as pregnancy progresses. Monitor thyroid function studies closely. Thyroid may be added to regimen. Drugs may be stopped during last few weeks of pregnancy.
• Watch for signs of hypothyroidism (mental depression; cold intolerance; hard, nonpitting edema). Dose may need to be adjusted.
• Monitor CBC periodically to detect impending leukopenia, thrombocytopenia, and agranulocytosis.
• Warn patient to report immediately: fever, sore throat, or mouth sores (possible signs of developing agranulocytosis). Agranulocytosis can develop too rapidly to be detected by periodic blood cell counts. Tell patient to also report skin eruptions (sign of hypersensitivity) immediately.
• Drug should be stopped if severe rash or enlarged cervical lymph nodes develop.
• Tell patient to ask doctor about using iodized salt and eating shellfish during treatment.
• Warn patient against over-the-counter cough medicines; many contain iodine.
• Give with meals to reduce GI side effects.
• Store in light-resistant container.

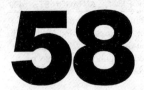

Pituitary hormones

corticotropin (ACTH)
cosyntropin
desmopressin acetate
lypressin
somatotropin (human growth
   hormone)
vasopressin (antidiuretic
   hormone)
vasopressin tannate

MECHANISM OF ACTION
• Corticotropin and cosyntropin, by replacing the body's own tropic hormone, stimulate the adrenal cortex to secrete its entire spectrum of hormones.
• Desmopressin, lypressin, and vasopressin increase the permeability of the renal tubular epithelium to adenosine monophosphate and water; the epithelium promotes reabsorption of water and produces a concentrated urine (antidiuretic hormone effect).
• Lypressin and vasopressin cause contraction of smooth muscle in the vascular bed (vasopressor effect). Vasopressin also causes contraction of smooth muscle in the gastrointestinal (GI) tract.
• Somatotropin stimulates linear growth in patients with pituitary growth deficiency by various mechanisms. These include facilitating intracellular transport of amino acids; increasing intestinal absorption and urinary excretion of calcium; increasing renal tubular reabsorption of phosphorus and decreasing that of calcium; promoting synthesis of collagen and chondroitin, which form cartilage; and inhibiting intracellular glucose metabolism.

COMBINATION PRODUCTS
None.

---

corticotropin (ACTH)
Acthar♦, Acton "X"♦♦, Cortigel-80, Cortrophin Gel, Cortrophin Zinc, Duracton♦♦, H.P. Acthar Gel

INDICATIONS & DOSAGE
Diagnostic test of adrenocortical function—
Adults: up to 80 units I.M. or S.C. in divided doses; or a single dose of repository form; or 10 to 25 units (aqueous form) in 500 ml dextrose 5% in water I.V. over 8 hours, between blood samplings.
Individual dosages generally vary with adrenal glands' sensitivity to stimulation as well as with specific disease. Infants and younger children require larger doses per kilogram than do older children and adults.
For therapeutic use—
Adults: 40 units S.C. or I.M. in 4 divided doses (aqueous); 40 units q 12 to 24 hours (gel or repository form).

SIDE EFFECTS
CNS: *convulsions, dizziness,* papilledema, headache, *euphoria, insomnia,* mood swings, personality changes, depression, psychosis.
EENT: cataracts, glaucoma.
GI: peptic ulcer with perforation and hemorrhage, pancreatitis, abdominal distention, ulcerative esophagitis, nausea, vomiting.
GU: menstrual irregularities.
Metabolic: *sodium and fluid retention,*

Italicized side effects are common or life-threatening.
♦Liquid form contains alcohol.   ♦♦May contain tartrazine.

calcium and potassium loss, hypokalemic alkalosis, negative nitrogen balance.

Skin: *impaired wound healing,* thin fragile skin, petechiae, ecchymoses, facial erythema, increased sweating, acne, hyperpigmentation, allergic skin reactions, hirsutism.

Other: muscle weakness, steroid myopathy, loss of muscle mass, osteoporosis, vertebral compression fractures, cushingoid state, suppression of growth in children, *activation of latent diabetes mellitus,* progressive increase in antibodies, and loss of ACTH stimulatory effect.

INTERACTIONS
None significant.

NURSING CONSIDERATIONS
• Contraindicated in scleroderma, osteoporosis, systemic fungal infections, ocular herpes simplex, recent surgery, peptic ulcer, congestive heart failure, hypertension, sensitivity to pork and pork products, concomitant smallpox vaccination, adrenocortical hyperfunction or primary insufficiency, or Cushing's syndrome. Use with caution in pregnant women or breast-feeding mothers and in women of childbearing age; patients being immunized; latent tuberculosis or tuberculin reactivity; hypothyroidism; cirrhosis; infection (use anti-infective therapy during and after ACTH treatment); acute gouty arthritis (limit ACTH treatment to a few days, and use conventional therapy during and for several days after ACTH treatment); emotional instability or psychotic tendencies; diabetes; abscess; pyogenic infections; renal insufficiency; myasthenia gravis.
• ACTH treatment should be preceded by verification of adrenal responsiveness and test for hypersensitivity and allergic reactions.
• ACTH should be adjunctive; not sole therapy. Oral agents are preferred for long-term therapy.

• Unusual stress may require additional use of rapidly acting corticosteroids. When possible, gradually reduce ACTH dosage to smallest effective dose to minimize induced adrenocortical insufficiency. Reinstitute therapy if stressful situation (trauma, surgery, severe illness) occurs shortly after stopping drug.
• Watch neonates of ACTH-treated mothers for signs of hypoadrenalism.
• Counteract edema by low-sodium, high-potassium intake; nitrogen loss by high-protein diet; and psychotic changes by reducing ACTH dosage or administering sedatives.
• ACTH may mask signs of chronic disease and decrease host resistance and ability to localize infection.
• Note and record weight changes, fluid exchange, and resting blood pressures until minimal effective dose is achieved.
• Refrigerate reconstituted solution and use within 24 hours.
• If administering gel, warm it to room temperature, draw into large needle, and give slowly deep I.M. with 21G or 22G needle. Warn patient that injection is painful.

cosyntropin
Cortrosyn♦, Synacthen Depot♦♦

INDICATIONS & DOSAGE
Diagnostic test of adrenocortical function—
Adults and children: 0.25 to 1 mg I.M. or I.V. (unless label prohibits I.V. administration) between blood samplings.
Children younger than 2 years: 0.125 mg I.M. or I.V.

SIDE EFFECTS
Skin: pruritus.
Other: flushing.

INTERACTIONS
None significant.

NURSING CONSIDERATIONS
- Use cautiously in hypersensitivity to natural corticotropin.
- Drug is synthetic duplication of the biologically active part of the ACTH molecule. It is less likely to produce sensitivity than natural ACTH from animal sources.

---

desmopressin acetate
DDAVP

INDICATIONS & DOSAGE
Nonnephrogenic diabetes insipidus, temporary polyuria and polydipsia associated with pituitary trauma—
Adults: 0.1 to 0.4 ml intranasally daily in 1 to 3 doses. Adjust morning and evening doses separately for adequate diurnal rhythm of water turnover.
Children 3 months to 12 years: 0.05 to 0.3 ml intranasally daily in 1 or 2 doses.

SIDE EFFECTS
CNS: headache.
CV: slight rise in blood pressure at high dosage.
EENT: nasal congestion, rhinitis.
GI: nausea.
GU: vulval pain.
Other: flushing.

INTERACTIONS
None significant.

NURSING CONSIDERATIONS
- Use with caution in patients with coronary artery insufficiency or hypertensive cardiovascular disease.
- Adjust fluid intake to reduce risk of water intoxication and sodium depletion, especially in very young or old patients.
- Titrate dosage to allow patient sufficient sleep.
- Give intranasally only.
- Overdose may cause oxytocic or vasopressor activity. Withhold drug until

effects subside. Furosemide may be used if fluid retention is excessive.
- Not effective in nephrogenic diabetes insipidus.
- Some patients may have difficulty measuring and inhaling drug into nostrils. Teach patient correct method of administration.

---

lypressin
Diapid

INDICATIONS & DOSAGE
Nonnephrogenic diabetes insipidus—
Adults and children: 1 or 2 sprays (approximately 2 USP posterior pituitary pressor units/spray) in either or both nostrils q.i.d. and an additional dose at bedtime, if needed, to prevent nocturia. If usual dosage is inadequate, increase frequency rather than number of sprays.

SIDE EFFECTS
CNS: headache, dizziness.
EENT: nasal congestion or ulceration, irritation, pruritus of nasal passages, rhinorrhea, conjunctivitis.
GI: heartburn due to drip of excess spray into pharynx, abdominal cramps, frequent bowel movements.
GU: possible transient fluid retention due to overdose.
Skin: hypersensitivity reaction.

INTERACTIONS
None significant.

NURSING CONSIDERATIONS
- Use with caution in patients with coronary artery disease.
- Particularly useful if diabetes insipidus is unresponsive to other therapy, or if antidiuretic hormones of animal origin cause adverse reactions.
- Nasal congestion, allergic rhinitis, or upper respiratory infections may diminish drug absorption and require larger dose or adjunctive therapy.
- Inadvertent inhalation of spray may

cause tightness in chest, coughing, and transient dyspnea.
• Test patients sensitive to antidiuretic hormone for sensitivity to lypressin.
• To administer a uniform, well-diffused spray, hold bottle upright with patient in vertical position holding head upright.
• Instruct the patient to carry the medication with him at all times because of its fairly short duration.

somatotropin (human growth hormone)
Asellacrin, Crescormon

INDICATIONS & DOSAGE
Growth failure due to pituitary growth hormone deficiency—
Children: 2 IU (1 ml) I.M. 3 times weekly, with a minimum of 48 hours between injections. Double dose if growth doesn't exceed 1″ in 6 months, or recheck diagnosis. Discontinue when epiphyses close, patient achieves satisfactory adult height, or patient fails to respond.

SIDE EFFECTS
GU: excess calcium in urine.
Metabolic: hyperglycemia.

INTERACTIONS
None significant.

NURSING CONSIDERATIONS
• Contraindicated in patients with closed epiphyses or intracranial lesions. Use with caution in patients with diabetes or family history of diabetes mellitus. Regular testing for glycosuria should be done.
• Subcutaneous administration not recommended.
• Should be used only by doctors experienced in treating patients with pituitary growth hormonal deficiency.
• Concurrent thyroid hormone or androgen therapy may accelerate epiphy-

seal closure and limit duration of somatotropin treatment.
• Monitor bone age progression annually.
• Store powder at or below room temperature.
• Reconstitute with 5 ml of bacteriostatic water per 10-IU vial. Refrigerate unused portion; discard after 1 month. Rotate injection sites.

vasopressin
Pitressin Synthetic◆

vasopressin tannate
Pitressin Tannate

INDICATIONS & DOSAGE
Nonnephrogenic, nonpsychogenic diabetes insipidus—
Adults: 5 to 10 units I.M. or S.C. b.i.d. to q.i.d., p.r.n.; or intranasally (spray or cotton balls) in individualized doses, based on response. For chronic therapy, inject 2.5 to 5 units Pitressin Tannate in oil suspension I.M. or S.C. every 2 to 3 days.
Children: 2.5 to 10 units I.M. or S.C. b.i.d. to q.i.d., p.r.n.; or intranasally (spray or cotton balls) in individualized doses. For chronic therapy, inject 1.25 to 2.5 units Pitressin Tannate in oil suspension I.M. or S.C. every 2 to 3 days.
Postoperative abdominal distention—
Adults: 5 units (aqueous) I.M. initially, then q 3 to 4 hours, increasing dose to 10 units, if needed. Reduce dose for children proportionately.
To expel gas before abdominal X-ray—
Adults: inject 10 units S.C. at 2 hours, then again at 30 minutes before X-ray. Enema before first dose may also help to eliminate gas.
Upper GI tract hemorrhage (intra-arterial)—
Adults: 0.2 to 0.4 units/minute. Do not use Tannate in oil suspension.

SIDE EFFECTS
CNS: tremor, dizziness, headache.

Unmarked trade names available in the United States only.
◆ Also available in Canada.   ◆◆ Available in Canada only.

CV: *angina in patients with vascular disease,* vasoconstriction. Large doses may cause hypertension, electrocardiographic changes. (With intraarterial infusion: *bradycardia, cardiac arrhythmias, pulmonary edema.*)
GI: abdominal cramps, nausea, vomiting, diarrhea, intestinal hyperactivity.
GU: uterine cramps, anuria.
Skin: circumoral pallor.
Other: water intoxication (drowsiness, listlessness, headache, confusion, weight gain), hypersensitivity reactions (urticaria, angioneurotic edema, bronchoconstriction, fever, rash, wheezing, dyspnea, *anaphylaxis),* sweating.

INTERACTIONS

Lithium, demeclocycline: reduced antidiuretic activity. Use together cautiously.
Chlorpropamide: increased antidiuretic response. Use together cautiously.

NURSING CONSIDERATIONS

• Contraindicated in chronic nephritis with nitrogen retention. Use cautiously in children, elderly persons, pregnant women, and patients with epilepsy, migraine, asthma, cardiovascular disease, or fluid overload.
• Never inject vasopressin tannate in oil I.V.
• Never inject during first stage of labor; may cause ruptured uterus.

• Monitor specific gravity of urine. Monitor intake and output to aid evaluation of drug effectiveness.
• Place tannate in oil in warm water for 10 to 15 minutes. Then shake thoroughly to make suspension uniform before withdrawing I.M. injection dose. Small brown particles must be seen in suspension. Use absolutely dry syringe to avoid dilution.
• Give with 1 to 2 glasses of water to reduce side effects and to improve therapeutic response.
• To prevent possible convulsions, coma, and death, observe patient closely for early signs of water intoxication.
• Overhydration more likely with long-acting tannate oil suspension than with aqueous vasopressin solution.
• Use minimum effective dose to reduce side effects.
• May be used for transient polyuria due to antidiuretic hormone deficiency related to neurosurgery or head injury.
• Synthetic desmopressin is sometimes preferred because of longer duration and less frequent side effects.
• Question the patient with abdominal distention about passage of flatus and stool.
• Monitor blood pressure of patient on vasopressin twice daily. Watch for excessively elevated blood pressure or lack of response to drug, which may be indicated by hypotension.

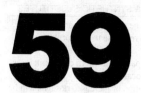

Parathyroid and parathyroid-like agents

calcifediol
calcitonin (Salmon)
calcitriol
dihydrotachysterol (AT-10)
etidronate disodium
parathyroid hormone (PTH)

MECHANISM OF ACTION
• Calcitonin and etidronate decrease osteoclastic activity by inhibiting osteocytic osteolysis. They also decrease mineral release and matrix or collagen breakdown in bone.
• Calcifediol, calcitriol and dihydrotachysterol stimulate calcium absorption from the GI tract and promote secretion of calcium from bone to blood, thereby raising serum calcium levels; they may also increase urinary excretion of inorganic phosphate.
• PTH enhances phosphate excretion by inhibiting renal tubular reabsorption of phosphate, mobilizing bone calcium and increasing GI absorption of calcium.

COMBINATION PRODUCTS
None.

calcifediol
Calderol

INDICATIONS & DOSAGE
Treatment and management of metabolic bone disease associated with chronic renal failure—
Adults: initially, 300 to 350 mcg P.O. weekly, given on a daily or alternate-day schedule. Dosage may be increased at 4-week intervals. Optimal dose must

be carefully determined for each patient.

SIDE EFFECTS
Vitamin D intoxication associated with hypercalcemia:
CNS: headache, somnolence.
EENT: conjunctivitis, photophobia, rhinorrhea.
GI: nausea, vomiting, constipation, metallic taste, dry mouth.
GU: polyuria.
Other: weakness, bone and muscle pain.

INTERACTIONS
Cholestyramine: may impair absorption of calcifediol. Monitor calcium levels.

NURSING CONSIDERATIONS
• Contraindicated in hypercalcemia or vitamin D toxicity. Withhold all preparations containing vitamin D in patients taking calcifediol. Use cautiously in patients on digitalis because hypercalcemia may precipitate cardiac arrhythmias.
• Monitor serum calcium; serum calcium times serum phosphate should not exceed 70. During titration, serum calcium levels should be determined at least weekly. If hypercalcemia occurs, calcifediol should be discontinued but resumed after serum calcium returns to normal.
• Patient should receive adequate daily intake of calcium—1,000 mg RDA.
• Advise patient to adhere to diet and calcium supplementation, and avoid nonprescription drugs.
• Most patients respond to doses be-

tween 50 and 100 mcg daily or between 100 and 200 mcg on alternate days.

calcitonin (Salmon)
Calcimar♦

INDICATIONS & DOSAGE
Paget's disease of bone (osteitis deformans)—
Adults: initially, 100 MRC units daily, S.C. or I.M. Maintenance: 50 to 100 units daily or every other day.
Hypercalcemia—
Adults: 100 to 400 MRC units I.M. once or twice daily.

SIDE EFFECTS
CNS: headaches.
GI: transient nausea with or without vomiting, diarrhea.
GU: transient diuresis.
Metabolic: hyperglycemia.
Local: inflammation at injection site, skin rashes.
Other: *facial flushing;* hypocalcemia; swelling, tingling, and tenderness of hands; unusual taste sensation; *anaphylaxis.*

INTERACTIONS
None significant.

NURSING CONSIDERATIONS
• Contraindicated in allergy to gelatin diluent used to prepare drug. Not recommended for breast-feeding mothers, or women who are or may become pregnant. Safe use in children not established.
• Periodic serum alkaline phosphatase and 24-hour urine hydroxyproline levels should be determined to evaluate drug effect.
• Skin test is usually done before beginning therapy.
• Systemic allergic reactions possible since hormone is protein. Keep epinephrine handy when administering.
• Patients with good initial clinical response to calcitonin who suffer relapse should be evaluated for antibody formation response to the hormone protein.
• Tell patient in whom calcitonin loses its hypocalcemic activity that further medication or increased dosages will be of no value.
• Teach patient aseptic method of preparing and administering injection, and stress the importance of rotating injection sites.
• Facial flushing and warmth occur in 20% to 30% of all patients within minutes of injection; usually last about 1 hour. Reassure patient that this is a transient effect.
• Observe patient for signs of hypocalcemic tetany during therapy (muscle twitching, tetanic spasms, and convulsions if hypocalcemia is severe).
• Monitor calcium levels closely. Watch for signs of hypercalcemic relapse: bone pain, renal calculi, polyuria, anorexia, nausea, vomiting, thirst, constipation, lethargy, bradycardia, muscle hypotonicity, pathologic fracture, psychosis, and coma.
• Periodic examinations of urine sediment advisable.
• Actually derived from the thyroid gland, not the parathyroid.
• Refrigerate solution.

calcitriol (1,25-dihydroxy-cholecalciferol)
Rocaltrol

INDICATIONS & DOSAGE
Management of hypocalcemia in patients undergoing chronic dialysis—
Adults: initially, 0.25 mcg daily. Dosage may be increased by 0.25 mcg daily at 2- to 4-week intervals. Maintenance: 0.25 mcg every other day up to 0.5 to 1.25 mcg daily.

SIDE EFFECTS
Vitamin D intoxication associated with hypercalcemia:

Italicized side effects are common or life-threatening.
*Liquid form contains alcohol.   **May contain tartrazine.

CNS: headache, somnolence.
EENT: conjunctivitis, photophobia, rhinorrhea.
GI: nausea, vomiting, constipation, metallic taste, dry mouth.
GU: polyuria.
Other: weakness, bone and muscle pain.

INTERACTIONS
None significant.

NURSING CONSIDERATIONS
• Contraindicated in hypercalcemia or vitamin D toxicity. Withhold all preparations containing vitamin D in patients taking calcitriol. Not recommended in breast-feeding mothers. Use cautiously in patients on digitalis; hypercalcemia may precipitate cardiac arrhythmias.
• Monitor serum calcium; serum calcium times serum phosphate should not exceed 70. During titration, determine serum levels twice weekly. If hypercalcemia occurs, discontinue, but resume after serum calcium level returns to normal. Patient should receive adequate daily intake of calcium—1,000 mg RDA.
• Protect from heat and light.
• Instruct patient to adhere to diet and calcium supplementation and to avoid unapproved nonprescription drugs.
• Patients should not use magnesium-containing antacids while taking this drug.
• Patients should report to doctor immediately any of the following symptoms: weakness, nausea, vomiting, dry mouth, constipation, muscle or bone pain, or metallic taste—early symptoms of vitamin D intoxication.
• Tell patient that although this drug is a vitamin, it must not be taken by anyone for whom it was not prescribed due to its potentially serious toxicities.
• Most potent form of vitamin D available.

dihydrotachysterol (AT-10)
Hytakerol♦

INDICATIONS & DOSAGE
Familial hypophosphatemia—
Adults and children: 0.5 to 2 mg P.O. daily. Maintenance: 0.3 to 1.5 mg daily.
Hypocalcemia associated with hypoparathyroidism and pseudohypoparathyroidism—
Adults: initially, 0.8 to 2.4 mg P.O. daily for several days. Maintenance: 0.2 to 2 mg daily, as required for normal serum calcium levels. Average dose 0.6 mg daily.
Children: initially, 1 to 5 mg for several days. Maintenance: 0.2 to 1 mg daily, as required for normal serum calcium levels.
Renal osteodystrophy in chronic uremia—
Adults: 0.1 to 0.6 mg P.O. daily.

SIDE EFFECTS
Vitamin D intoxication associated with hypercalcemia:
CNS: headache, somnolence.
EENT: conjunctivitis, photophobia, rhinorrhea.
GI: nausea, vomiting, constipation, metallic taste, dry mouth.
GU: polyuria.
Other: weakness, bone and muscle pain.

INTERACTIONS
None significant.

NURSING CONSIDERATIONS
• Contraindicated in hypercalcemia, hypocalcemia associated with renal insufficiency and hyperphosphatemia, renal stones, hypersensitivity to vitamin D, and in breast-feeding mothers.
• Monitor serum and urine calcium levels. Watch for signs of hypercalcemia.
• Adequate dietary calcium intake is necessary; usually supplemented with

10 to 15 g oral calcium lactate or gluconate daily.
• Report hypercalcemia reactions to doctor. Early signs of hypercalcemia include thirst, headache, vertigo, tinnitus, anorexia.
• 1 mg equal to 120,000 units ergocalciferol (vitamin D_2).
• Store in tightly closed, light-resistant containers. Don't refrigerate.

etidronate disodium
Didronel

INDICATIONS & DOSAGE
Symptomatic Paget's disease—
Adults: 5 mg/kg daily P.O. as a single dose 2 hours before a meal with water or juice. Patient should not eat for 2 hours after dose. May give up to 10 mg/kg daily in severe cases. Maximum dose 20 mg/kg daily.
Heterotopic ossification in spinal cord injuries—
Adults: 20 mg/kg daily for 2 weeks, then 10 mg/kg daily for 10 weeks. Total treatment period 12 weeks.
Heterotopic ossification after total hip replacement—
Adults: 20 mg/kg daily for 1 month prior to total hip replacement and for 3 months afterward.

SIDE EFFECTS
GI: (seen most frequently at 20 mg/kg daily) diarrhea, increased frequency of bowel movements, nausea.
Other: increased or recurrent bone pain at pagetic sites, pain at previously asymptomatic sites, increased risk of fracture, elevated serum phosphate.

INTERACTIONS
None significant.

NURSING CONSIDERATIONS
• Use cautiously in enterocolitis, impaired renal function.
• Therapy should not last more than 6 months. After 3 months, resume if

needed. Don't give longer than 3 months at doses above 10 mg/kg daily.
• Don't give drug with food, milk, or antacids; may reduce absorption.
• Monitor renal function before and during therapy.
• Monitor drug effect by serum alkaline phosphatase and urinary hydroxyproline excretion (both lowered if therapy effective).
• Tell patient that improvement may not occur for up to 3 months but may continue for months after drug is stopped. Stress importance of good nutrition, especially diet high in calcium and vitamin D.

parathyroid hormone (PTH)

INDICATIONS & DOSAGE
Acute hypoparathyroidism with tetany—
Adults: 20 to 40 units S.C., I.M., or I.V. q 12 hours.
Infants: (with transient congenital idiopathic true hypoparathyroidism) 25 to 50 units I.M. q 12 hours for 1 to 3 days.

SIDE EFFECTS
Allergic: *anaphylactic reactions* (parathyroid hormone is a foreign protein).
CNS: headache, vertigo.
GI: anorexia, nausea, vomiting, abdominal cramps, diarrhea.
Other: hypercalcemia (muscle weakness, bone and flank pain), lethargy, tinnitus, ataxia.

INTERACTIONS
None significant.

NURSING CONSIDERATIONS
• Contraindicated in hypercalcemia, hypercalciuria, and tetany unrelated to parathyroid failure; and by I.V. administration when serum calcium levels are above normal. Use cautiously in sarcoidosis, renal or cardiac disease, and in digitalized patients.

Italicized side effects are common or life-threatening.
*Liquid form contains alcohol.   **May contain tartrazine.

• Rarely used because calcium salts often effective alone.
• Subcutaneous injections may produce moderate inflammatory reaction.
• Therapy lasts only a few days; patients may soon become refractory to treatment due to parathyroid-initiated production of antihormone antibodies.
• If given I.V., skin-test for sensitivity. If positive, desensitize patient.
• Keep epinephrine injection handy when giving parathyroid hormone.
• Monitor serum calcium and serum phosphate levels, intake and output.
• Know and watch for signs of hypoparathyroidism and calcium deficiency. Test for Chvostek's and Trousseau's signs. Watch for drug-induced hypercalcemia.
• Use seizure precautions in patients with calcium deficiency: padded rails, soft light, no irritating noises until normal calcium level is restored.
• Do not dilute with saline solution, because a precipitate will form.
• Store ampuls at 2° to 8° C. (36° to 46° F.); do not freeze.

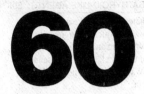

Diuretics

Thiazide diuretics
bendroflumethiazide
benzthiazide
chlorothiazide
cyclothiazide
hydrochlorothiazide
hydroflumethiazide
methyclothiazide
polythiazide
trichlormethiazide

Thiazide-like diuretics
chlorthalidone
metolazone
quinethazone

Loop diuretics
ethacrynate sodium
ethacrynic acid
furosemide

Carbonic anhydrase inhibitors
acetazolamide
acetazolamide sodium
dichlorphenamide
methazolamide

Miscellaneous diuretics
amiloride
mannitol
spironolactone
triamterene
urea

MECHANISM OF ACTION

● The thiazide and thiazide-like diuretics increase urinary excretion of sodium and water by inhibiting sodium reabsorption in the cortical diluting site of the ascending loop of Henle. They also increase urinary excretion of chloride, potassium, and—to a lesser extent—bicarbonate ions.

● Loop diuretics inhibit reabsorption of sodium and chloride at the proximal portion of the ascending loop of Henle, enhancing water excretion. These very potent diuretics can be effective in patients with markedly reduced glomerular filtration rates (in whom other diuretics usually fail).

● Carbonic anhydrase inhibitors, by enzymatic blocking, promote renal excretion of sodium, potassium, bicarbonate, and water. Bicarbonate-ion excretion makes the urine alkaline; blood bicarbonate levels are accordingly reduced, leading to metabolic acidosis. In this condition, the carbonic anhydrase inhibitors become less effective as diuretics. (Carbonic anhydrase inhibitors also decrease secretion of aqueous humor in the eye, thereby lowering intraocular pressure, but this mechanism is unrelated to their diuretic action.)

● Among miscellaneous diuretics, mannitol increases the osmotic pressure of glomerular filtrate, inhibiting tubular reabsorption of water and electrolytes.

Mercaptomerin works mainly in the ascending limb of the loop of Henle where the mercuric (Hg^{++}) ion interferes with renal tubular transport of chloride. During the ensuing diuresis, sodium, chloride, and water are excreted without profound potassium depletion. Diuresis is enhanced by acidifying agents.

Spironolactone antagonizes the hormone aldosterone in the distal tubule,

---

Italicized side effects are common or life-threatening.
*Liquid form contains alcohol.   **May contain tartrazine.

increasing excretion of sodium and water but sparing potassium.

Triamterene and amiloride depress sodium reabsorption and potassium secretion by direct action on the distal segment of the uriniferous tubule. This reduces potassium excretion.

Urea rapidly increases blood tonicity, which results in passage of fluid from the tissue (including the brain) to the blood.

COMBINATION PRODUCTS
ALDACTAZIDE♦: spironolactone 25 mg and hydrochlorothiazide 25 mg.
ALTEXIDE: spironolactone 25 mg and hydrochlorothiazide 25 mg.
DYAZIDE♦: triamterene 50 mg and hydrochlorothiazide 25 mg.
MODURETIC: amiloride hydrochloride 5 mg and hydrochlorthiazide 50 mg.

acetazolamide
Acetazolam♦♦, Diamox♦, Diamox Sequels♦, Hydrazol, Cetazol

acetazolamide sodium
Diamox Parenteral♦

INDICATIONS & DOSAGE
Narrow-angle glaucoma—
Adults: 250 mg q 4 hours; or 250 mg b.i.d. P.O., I.M., or I.V. for short-term therapy.
Edema, in congestive heart failure—
Adults: 250 to 375 mg P.O., I.M., or I.V. daily in a.m.
Children: 5 mg/kg daily in a.m.
Epilepsy—
Children: 8 to 30 mg/kg daily P.O., I.M., or I.V. in divided doses.
Open-angle glaucoma—
Adults: 250 mg daily to 1 g P.O., I.M., or I.V. divided q.i.d.

SIDE EFFECTS
Blood: *aplastic anemia,* hemolytic anemia, leukopenia.
CNS: drowsiness, paresthesias.
EENT: transient myopia.
GI: nausea, vomiting, anorexia.
GU: crystalluria, renal calculi.
Metabolic: *hyperchloremic acidosis,* hypokalemia, asymptomatic hyperuricemia.
Skin: rash.

INTERACTIONS
None significant.

NURSING CONSIDERATIONS
• Contraindicated in long-term therapy for chronic noncongestive narrow-angle glaucoma; also in depressed sodium or potassium serum levels, renal or hepatic disease or dysfunction, adrenal gland failure, and hyperchloremic acidosis. Use cautiously in respiratory acidosis, emphysema, chronic pulmonary disease, or patients receiving other diuretics.
• Monitor intake/output and electrolytes, especially serum potassium. When used in diuretic therapy, consult with doctor and dietitian to provide high-potassium diet.
• Weigh patient daily. Rapid weight loss may cause hypotension.
• Diuretic effect is decreased when acidosis occurs but can be reestablished by withdrawing drug for several days and then restarting, or by using intermittent administration schedules.
• Reconstitute 500-mg vial with at least 5 ml sterile water for injection. Use within 24 hours of reconstitution.
• I.M. injection painful because of alkalinity of solution. Direct I.V. administration preferred (100 to 500 mg/minute).
• Elderly patients are especially susceptible to excessive diuresis.
• Sustained-release form available.
• May cause false-positive urine protein tests by alkalinizing the urine.
• The drug's acidotic effects limit usefulness for daily treatment of edema.
• Used investigationally to prevent "mountain sickness."

amiloride hydrochloride
Midamor

INDICATIONS & DOSAGE
Hypertension; or edema associated with congestive heart failure, usually in patients who are also taking thiazide or other potassium-wasting diuretics—
Adults: Usual dosage is 5 mg P.O. daily. Dosage may be increased to 10 mg daily, if necessary. As much as 20 mg daily can be given.

SIDE EFFECTS
CNS: *headache,* weakness, dizziness.
CV: orthostatic hypotension.
GI: *nausea, anorexia, diarrhea, vomiting,* abdominal pain, constipation.
GU: *impotence.*
Metabolic: *hyperkalemia.*

INTERACTIONS
None significant.

NURSING CONSIDERATIONS
• Contraindicated with elevated serum potassium levels (greater than 5.5 mEq/liter). Don't administer to patients receiving other potassium-sparing diuretics, such as spironolactone and triamterene. Also contraindicated in anuria.
• Use cautiously in patients with renal impairment, because potassium retention is increased.
• Risk of hyperkalemia is greater when a potassium-wasting drug is not taken concurrently. When amiloride is taken this way, be sure to monitor daily potassium levels.
• Discontinue immediately if potassium level exceeds 6.5 mEq/liter.
• Warn patient to avoid excessive ingestion of potassium-rich foods or potassium-containing salt substitutes. Concomitant potassium supplement can lead to serious hyperkalemia.
• Administer amiloride with or after meals to prevent nausea.

bendroflumethiazide
Naturetin♦**

INDICATIONS & DOSAGE
Edema, hypertension—
Adults: 5 to 20 mg P.O. daily or b.i.d. in divided doses.
Children: initially, 0.1 to 0.4 mg/kg daily in 1 or 2 doses.
Maintenance: 0.05 to 0.1 mg/kg daily in 1 or 2 doses.

SIDE EFFECTS
Blood: *aplastic anemia, agranulocytosis,* leukopenia, thrombocytopenia.
CV: *volume depletion and dehydration,* orthostatic hypotension.
GI: anorexia, nausea, pancreatitis.
Hepatic: hepatic encephalopathy.
Metabolic: *hypokalemia, asymptomatic hyperuricemia, hyperglycemia and impairment of glucose tolerance,* fluid and electrolyte imbalances including dilutional hyponatremia and hypochloremia, metabolic alkalosis, hypercalcemia, gout.
Skin: dermatitis, photosensitivity, rash.
Other: hypersensitivity reactions, such as pneumonitis and vasculitis.

INTERACTIONS
Cholestyramine, colestipol: intestinal absorption of thiazides decreased. Keep doses as separate as possible.
Diazoxide: increased antihypertensive, hyperglycemic, hyperuricemic effects. Use together cautiously.

NURSING CONSIDERATIONS
• Contraindicated in anuria and in hypersensitivity to other thiazides or other sulfonamide-derived drugs. Use cautiously in severe renal disease and impaired hepatic function.
• Monitor intake/output, weight, and serum electrolytes regularly. Monitor serum creatinine and BUN levels regularly. Not effective if these levels are more than twice normal.
• Monitor serum potassium levels;

Italicized side effects are common or life-threatening.
*Liquid form contains alcohol.   **May contain tartrazine.

consult with doctor and dietitian to provide high-potassium diet. Watch for signs of hypokalemia (for example, muscle weakness, cramps). Patients on digitalis have an increased risk of digitalis toxicity due to potassium-depleting side effect of this diuretic. May use with potassium-sparing diuretic to prevent potassium loss.

• Foods rich in potassium include citrus fruits, bananas, tomatoes, dates, and apricots.

• Monitor blood sugar. Check insulin requirements in patients with diabetes. May treat severe hyperglycemia with oral antidiabetic agents.

• Monitor blood uric acid levels, especially in patients with a history of gout.

• Give in a.m. to prevent nocturia.

• Elderly patients are especially susceptible to excessive diuresis.

• In hypertension, therapeutic response may be delayed several days.

• Thiazides and thiazide-like diuretics should be discontinued before tests for parathyroid function are performed.

---

benzthiazide
Aquapres, Aquasec, Aquatag**, Diretic, Exna**, Hydrex, Lemazide, Marazide, Proaqua, Ridema, S-Aqua, Urazide

INDICATIONS & DOSAGE
Edema—
Adults: 50 to 200 mg P.O. daily or in divided doses.
Children: 1 to 4 mg/kg daily in 3 divided doses.
Hypertension—
Adults: 50 mg P.O. daily b.i.d., t.i.d., or q.i.d., adjusted to patient's response.

SIDE EFFECTS
Blood: *aplastic anemia, agranulocytosis,* leukopenia, thrombocytopenia.
CV: *volume depletion and dehydration,* orthostatic hypotension.
GI: anorexia, nausea, pancreatitis.

Hepatic: hepatic encephalopathy.
Metabolic: *hypokalemia, asymptomatic hyperuricemia, hyperglycemia and impairment of glucose tolerance,* fluid and electrolyte imbalances including dilutional hyponatremia and hypochloremia, metabolic alkalosis, hypercalcemia, gout.
Skin: dermatitis, photosensitivity, rash.
Other: hypersensitivity reactions, such as pneumonitis and vasculitis.

INTERACTIONS
Cholestyramine, colestipol: intestinal absorption of thiazides decreased. Keep doses as separate as possible.
Diazoxide: increased antihypertensive, hyperglycemic, hyperuricemic effects. Use together cautiously.

NURSING CONSIDERATIONS
• Contraindicated in anuria; hypersensitivity to other thiazides or other sulfonamide-derived drugs. Use cautiously in severe renal disease, impaired hepatic function.

• Monitor intake/output, weight, and serum electrolytes regularly. Monitor serum potassium levels; consult with doctor and dietitian to provide high-potassium diet. Watch for signs of hypokalemia (for example, muscle weakness, cramps). Patients on digitalis have an increased risk of digitalis toxicity due to the potassium-depleting side effect of this diuretic. May use with potassium-sparing diuretic to prevent potassium loss.

• Foods rich in potassium include citrus fruits, bananas, tomatoes, dates, and apricots.

• Monitor serum creatinine and BUN levels regularly. Not effective if these levels are more than twice normal.

• Monitor blood sugar. Check insulin requirements in patients with diabetes. May treat severe hyperglycemia with oral antidiabetic agents.

• Monitor blood uric acid levels, especially in patients with a history of gout.

• Give in a.m. to prevent nocturia.

Unmarked trade names available in the United States only.
♦ Also available in Canada.   ♦ ♦ Available in Canada only.

• Elderly patients are especially susceptible to excessive diuresis.
• In hypertension, therapeutic response may be delayed several days.
• Thiazides and thiazide-like diuretics should be discontinued before tests for parathyroid function are performed.

---

chlorothiazide
Diuril♦, Ro-Chlorozide,
SK-Chlorothiazide

INDICATIONS & DOSAGE
Diuresis—
Children over 6 months: 20 mg/kg
P.O. or I.V. daily in divided doses.
Children under 6 months: may require 30 mg/kg P.O. or I.V. daily in 2 divided doses.
Edema, hypertension—
Adults: 500 mg to 2 g P.O. or I.V. daily or in 2 divided doses.

SIDE EFFECTS
Blood: *aplastic anemia, agranulocytosis,* leukopenia, thrombocytopenia.
CV: *volume depletion and dehydration,* orthostatic hypotension.
GI: anorexia, nausea, pancreatitis.
Hepatic: hepatic encephalopathy.
Metabolic: *hypokalemia, asymptomatic hyperuricemia, hyperglycemia and impairment of glucose tolerance,* fluid and electrolyte imbalances including dilutional hyponatremia and hypochloremia, metabolic alkalosis, hypercalcemia, gout.
Skin: dermatitis, photosensitivity, rash.
Other: hypersensitivity reactions such as pneumonitis and vasculitis.

INTERACTIONS
Cholestyramine, colestipol: intestinal absorption of thiazides decreased. Keep doses as separate as possible.
Diazoxide: increased antihypertensive, hyperglycemic, hyperuricemic effects. Use together cautiously.

NURSING CONSIDERATIONS
• Contraindicated in anuria; hypersensitivity to other thiazides or other sulfonamide-derived drugs; impaired hepatic function; progressive hepatic disease. Use cautiously in severe renal disease.
• Monitor intake/output, weight, and serum electrolytes regularly.
• Monitor potassium levels; consult with doctor and dietitian to provide high-potassium diet. Watch for signs of hypokalemia (for example, muscle weakness, cramps). Patients on digitalis have an increased risk of digitalis toxicity due to the potassium-depleting effect of the diuretic. May use with potassium-sparing diuretic to prevent potassium loss.
• Foods rich in potassium include citrus fruits, tomatoes, bananas, dates, and apricots.
• Monitor blood sugar. Check insulin requirements in patients with diabetes. May treat severe hyperglycemia with oral antidiabetic agents.
• Monitor serum creatinine and BUN levels regularly. Not effective if these levels are more than twice normal.
• Monitor blood uric acid levels, especially in patients with a history of gout.
• Watch for decreased calcium excretion, progressive renal impairment.
• Only injectable thiazide. For I.V. use only—not I.M. or subcutaneous. Reconstitute with 18 ml of sterile water for injection/500 mg vial. May store reconstituted solutions at room temperature up to 24 hours. Compatible with intravenous dextrose or sodium chloride solutions.
• Avoid I.V. infiltration; can be very painful.
• Give in a.m. to prevent nocturia.
• In hypertension, therapeutic response may be delayed several days.
• Elderly patients are especially susceptible to excessive diuresis.
• A thiazide diuretic.
• The only thiazide available in liquid form.

Italicized side effects are common or life-threatening.
♦Liquid form contains alcohol.   ♦♦May contain tartrazine.

- Thiazides and thiazide-like diuretics should be stopped before tests for parathyroid function are performed.

chlorthalidone
Hygroton♦, Novothalidone♦♦, Uridon♦♦

INDICATIONS & DOSAGE
Edema, hypertension—
Adults: 25 to 100 mg P.O. daily, or 100 mg 3 times weekly or on alternate days.
Children: 2 mg/kg P.O. 3 times weekly.

SIDE EFFECTS
Blood: *aplastic anemia, agranulocytosis,* leukopenia, thrombocytopenia.
CV: *volume depletion and dehydration,* orthostatic hypotension.
GI: anorexia, nausea, pancreatitis.
GU: impotence.
Hepatic: hepatic encephalopathy.
Metabolic: *hypokalemia, asymptomatic hyperuricemia, hyperglycemia and impairment of glucose tolerance,* fluid and electrolyte imbalances including dilutional hyponatremia and hypochloremia, metabolic alkalosis, hypercalcemia, gout.
Skin: dermatitis, photosensitivity, rash.
Other: hypersensitivity reactions, such as pneumonitis and vasculitis.

INTERACTIONS
Cholestyramine, colestipol: intestinal absorption of thiazides decreased. Keep doses as separate as possible.
Diazoxide: increased antihypertensive, hyperglycemic, hyperuricemic effects. Use together cautiously.

NURSING CONSIDERATIONS
- Contraindicated in anuria; hypersensitivity to thiazides or other sulfonamide-derived drugs. Use cautiously in severe renal disease, progressive hepatic disease, impaired hepatic function.
- Monitor intake/output, weight, and serum electrolytes regularly.
- Monitor serum potassium levels; consult with doctor and dietitian to provide high-potassium diet. Watch for signs of hypokalemia (for example, muscle weakness, cramps). Patients on digitalis have an increased risk of digitalis toxicity due to the potassium-depleting effect on this diuretic. May use with potassium-sparing diuretic to prevent potassium loss.
- Foods rich in potassium include citrus fruits, tomatoes, bananas, dates, and apricots.
- Monitor serum creatinine and BUN levels regularly. Not effective if these levels are more than twice normal.
- Monitor blood uric acid levels, especially in patients with a history of gout.
- Monitor blood sugar. Check insulin requirements in patients with diabetes. May treat severe hyperglycemia with oral antidiabetic agents.
- In hypertension, therapeutic response may be delayed several days.
- Give in a.m. to prevent nocturia.
- Elderly patients are especially susceptible to excessive diuresis.
- Thiazides and thiazide-like diuretics should be stopped before tests for parathyroid function are performed.

cyclothiazide
Anhydron, Fluidil

INDICATIONS & DOSAGE
Edema—
Adults: 1 to 2 mg P.O. daily. May be used on alternate days as maintenance dose.
Children: 0.02 to 0.04 mg/kg P.O. daily.
Hypertension—
Adults: 2 mg P.O. daily; up to 2 mg b.i.d. or t.i.d.

SIDE EFFECTS
Blood: *aplastic anemia, agranulocytosis,* leukopenia, thrombocytopenia.
CV: *volume depletion and dehydration,* orthostatic hypotension.
GI: anorexia, nausea, pancreatitis.
Hepatic: hepatic encephalopathy.
Metabolic: *hypokalemia, asymptomatic hyperuricemia, hyperglycemia and impairment of glucose tolerance,* fluid and electrolyte imbalances including dilutional hyponatremia and hypochloremia, metabolic alkalosis, hypercalcemia, gout.
Skin: dermatitis, photosensitivity, rash.
Other: hypersensitivity reactions, such as pneumonitis and vasculitis.

INTERACTIONS
Cholestyramine, colestipol: intestinal absorption of thiazides decreased. Keep doses as separate as possible.
Diazoxide: increased antihypertensive, hyperglycemic, hyperuricemic effects. Use together cautiously.

NURSING CONSIDERATIONS
• Contraindicated in anuria; hypersensitivity to other thiazides or other sulfonamide-derived drugs. Use cautiously in severe renal disease, impaired hepatic function, progressive hepatic disease.
• Monitor intake/output, weight, and serum electrolytes regularly.
• Monitor serum potassium levels; consult with doctor and dietitian to provide high-potassium diet. Watch for signs of hypokalemia (for example, muscle weakness, cramps). Patients on digitalis have an increased risk of digitalis toxicity due to the potassium-depleting effect of this diuretic. May use with potassium-sparing diuretic to prevent potassium loss.
• Foods rich in potassium include citrus fruits, tomatoes, bananas, dates, and apricots.
• Monitor blood sugar. Check insulin requirements in patients with diabetes.

May treat severe hyperglycemia with oral antidiabetic agents.
• Monitor serum creatinine and BUN levels regularly. Not effective if these levels are more than twice normal.
• Monitor blood uric acid levels, especially in patients with a history of gout.
• In hypertension, therapeutic response may be delayed several days.
• Give in a.m. to prevent nocturia.
• Elderly patients are especially susceptible to excessive diuresis.
• Thiazides and thiazide-like diuretics should be stopped before tests for parathyroid function are performed.

dichlorphenamide
Daranide, Oratrol

INDICATIONS & DOSAGE
Adjunct in glaucoma—
Adults: initially, 100 to 200 mg P.O., followed by 100 mg q 12 hours until desired response obtained. Maintenance: 25 to 50 mg P.O. daily b.i.d. or t.i.d. Give miotics concomitantly.

SIDE EFFECTS
Blood: *aplastic anemia,* hemolytic anemia, leukopenia.
CNS: drowsiness, paresthesias.
EENT: transient myopia.
GI: nausea, vomiting, anorexia.
GU: crystalluria, renal calculi.
Metabolic: *hyperchloremic acidosis,* hypokalemia, asymptomatic hyperuricemia.
Skin: rash.

INTERACTIONS
None significant.

NURSING CONSIDERATIONS
• Contraindicated in hepatic insufficiency, renal failure, adrenocortical insufficiency, hyperchloremic acidosis, depressed sodium or potassium levels, severe pulmonary obstruction with inability to increase alveolar ventilation,

---

Italicized side effects are common or life-threatening.
*Liquid form contains alcohol.   **May contain tartrazine.

Addison's disease. Long-term use contraindicated in severe, absolute, or chronic noncongestive narrow-angle glaucoma. Use cautiously in respiratory acidosis, monitoring blood pH and blood gases.

• Monitor electrolytes, especially serum potassium in initial treatment. Usually no problem in long-term glaucoma therapy unless risk for hypokalemia from other causes; potassium supplements may be necessary.

• May cause false-positive results in urine protein tests.

• Anticipate that drug will be given every day for glaucoma but intermittently for edema.

• Evaluate patient with glaucoma for eye pain to make sure drug is effective in decreasing intraocular pressure.

---

ethacrynate sodium
Sodium Edecrin

ethacrynic acid
Edecrin♦

INDICATIONS & DOSAGE
Acute pulmonary edema—
Adults: 50 to 100 mg of ethacrynate sodium I.V. slowly over several minutes.
Edema—
Adults: 50 to 200 mg P.O. daily. Refractory cases may require up to 200 mg b.i.d.
Children: initial dose 25 mg P.O., cautiously, increased in 25-mg increments daily until desired effect is obtained.

SIDE EFFECTS
Blood: *agranulocytosis,* thrombocytopenia.
CV: *volume depletion and dehydration, orthostatic hypotension.*
EENT: transient deafness with too–rapid I.V. injection.
GI: abdominal discomfort and pain, diarrhea.
Metabolic: *hypokalemia; hypochlore-*

mic alkalosis; asymptomatic hyperuricemia; fluid and electrolyte imbalances including dilutional hyponatremia and hypochloremia, hypocalcemia, hypomagnesemia; hyperglycemia and impairment of glucose tolerance.
Skin: dermatitis.

INTERACTIONS
Aminoglycoside antibiotics: potentiated ototoxic side effects of both ethacrynic acid and aminoglycosides. Use together cautiously.

NURSING CONSIDERATIONS
• Contraindicated in patients with anuria and in infants. Use cautiously in electrolyte abnormalities. If electrolyte imbalance, azotemia, or oliguria develops, may require discontinuing drug.

• Monitor intake/output, weight, and serum electrolytes regularly.

• Monitor serum potassium levels; consult with doctor and dietitian to provide high-potassium diet. Watch for signs of hypokalemia (e.g., muscle weakness, cramps).

• Foods rich in potassium include citrus fruits, tomatoes, bananas, dates, and apricots.

• Patients also on digitalis have an increased risk of digitalis toxicity due to the potassium-depleting effect of this diuretic.

• I.V. injection painful; may cause thrombophlebitis. Don't give subcutaneously or I.M. Give slowly through tubing of running infusion over several minutes.

• Salt and potassium chloride supplement may be needed during therapy.

• Reconstitute vacuum vial with 50 ml of 5% dextrose injection or NaCl injection. Discard unused solution after 24 hours. Don't use cloudy or opalescent solutions.

• Elderly patients are especially susceptible to excessive diuresis.

• Give P.O. doses in a.m. to prevent nocturia.

Unmarked trade names available in the United States only.
♦ Also available in Canada.   ♦ ♦ Available in Canada only.

- Severe diarrhea may necessitate discontinuing drug.
- Monitor blood uric acid levels, especially in patients with history of gout.
- May potentiate effects of the anticoagulant warfarin; carefully monitor patients receiving both drugs.

furosemide

Lasix◆**, Novosemide◆◆, SK-Furosemide, Uritol◆◆

INDICATIONS & DOSAGE

Acute pulmonary edema—
Adults: 40 mg I.V. injected slowly; then 40 mg I.V. in 1 to 1½ hours if needed.
Edema—
Adults: 20 to 80 mg P.O. daily in a.m., second dose can be given in 6 to 8 hours; carefully titrated up to 600 mg daily if needed; or 20 to 40 mg I.M. or I.V. Increase by 20 mg q 2 hours until desired response is achieved. I.V. dose should be given slowly over 1 to 2 minutes.
Infants and children: 2 mg/kg daily; dose increased by 1 to 2 mg/kg in 6 to 8 hours if needed; carefully titrated up to 6 mg/kg daily if needed.
Hypertensive crisis, acute renal failure—
Adults: 100 to 200 mg I.V. over 1 to 2 minutes.
Chronic renal failure—
Adults: initially, 80 mg P.O. daily. Increase by 80 to 120 mg daily until desired response is achieved.

SIDE EFFECTS

Blood: *agranulocytosis,* thrombocytopenia.
CV: *volume depletion and dehydration, orthostatic hypotension.*
EENT: transient deafness with too rapid I.V. injection.
GI: abdominal discomfort and pain, diarrhea (with oral solution).
Metabolic: *hypokalemia; hypochlore-*mic alkalosis; asymptomatic hyperuricemia, fluid and electrolyte imbalances including dilutional hyponatremia and hypochloremia, hypocalcemia, hypomagnesemia; hyperglycemia and impairment of glucose tolerance.
Skin: dermatitis.

INTERACTIONS

Aminoglycoside antibiotics: potentiated ototoxicity. Use together cautiously.
Chloral hydrate: sweating, flushing with I.V. furosemide. Observe patient.
Clofibrate: enhanced furosemide effects. Use cautiously.
Indomethacin: inhibited diuretic response. Use cautiously.

NURSING CONSIDERATIONS

- Use cautiously in cardiogenic shock complicated by pulmonary edema, anuria, hepatic coma, or electrolyte imbalances. Drug is not routinely administered to women of childbearing age because its safety in pregnancy hasn't been established.
- Potent loop diuretic; can lead to profound water and electrolyte depletion. Monitor blood pressure and pulse rate during rapid diuresis.
- Sulfonamide-sensitive patients may have allergic reactions to furosemide.
- If oliguria or azotemia develops or increases, may require stopping drug.
- Monitor serum electrolytes, BUN, and CO_2 frequently.
- Monitor serum potassium levels. Watch for signs of hypokalemia (for example, muscle weakness, cramps). Patients also on digitalis have an increased risk of digitalis toxicity due to the potassium-depleting effect of this diuretic.
- Consult with doctor and dietitian to provide high-potassium diet.
- Foods rich in potassium include citrus fruits, tomatoes, bananas, dates, and apricots.
- Monitor blood sugar levels in patients with diabetes. May treat severe

hyperglycemia with oral antidiabetic agents.
- Monitor blood uric acid levels, especially in patients with a history of gout.
- Give I.V. doses over 1 to 2 minutes.
- Don't use parenteral route in infants and children unless oral dosage form is not practical.
- I.M. injection causes transient pain; moderate by using "Z" track to limit leakage into subcutaneous tissues.
- Give P.O. and I.M. preparations in a.m. to prevent nocturia. Give second doses in early afternoon.
- Elderly patients are especially susceptible to excessive diuresis, with potential for circulatory collapse and thromboembolic complications.
- Store tablets in light-resistant container to prevent discoloration (doesn't affect potency). Don't use discolored (yellow) injectable preparation. Oral furosemide solution should be stored in the refrigerator to ensure stability of the drug.
- Promotes calcium excretion. I.V. furosemide often used to treat hypercalcemia.
- Advise patients taking furosemide to stand slowly to prevent dizziness, and to limit alcohol intake and strenuous exercise in hot weather since these exacerbate orthostatic hypotension.
- Advise patients to report immediately ringing in ears, severe abdominal pain, or sore throat and fever; may indicate furosemide toxicity.
- Discourage patients receiving furosemide therapy at home from storing different types of medication in the same container. This increases the risk of drug errors, especially for patients taking both furosemide and digoxin, since the most popular strengths of these drugs pills are white tablets approximately equal in size.
- To prepare parenteral furosemide for I.V. infusion, mix drug with 5% dextrose in water, 0.9% sodium chloride solution, or lactated Ringer's solution.

Use prepared infusion solution within 24 hours.

hydrochlorothiazide
Chlorzide, Diuchlor-H♦♦, Diu-Scrip, Esidrix♦, Hydrid♦♦, HydroAquil♦♦, Hydro Diuril♦, Hydromal, Hydro-Z-50, Hydrozide♦♦, Hyperetic, Kenazide, Lexor, Neo-Codema♦♦, Novohydrazide♦♦, Oretic, Ro-Hydrazide, Urozide♦♦, Zide

INDICATIONS & DOSAGE
Edema—
Adults: initially, 25 to 100 mg P.O. daily or intermittently for maintenance to minimize electrolyte imbalance.
Children over 6 months: 2.2 mg/kg P.O. daily divided b.i.d.
Children under 6 months: up to 3.3 mg/kg P.O. daily divided b.i.d.
Hypertension—
Adults: 25 to 100 mg P.O. daily or divided dosage. Daily dosage increased or decreased according to blood pressure.

SIDE EFFECTS
Blood: *aplastic anemia, agranulocytosis,* leukopenia, thrombocytopenia.
CV: *volume depletion and dehydration,* orthostatic hypotension.
GI: anorexia, nausea, pancreatitis.
Hepatic: hepatic encephalopathy.
Metabolic: *hypokalemia, asymptomatic hyperuricemia, hyperglycemia and impairment of glucose tolerance,* fluid and electrolyte imbalances including dilutional hyponatremia and hypochloremia, metabolic alkalosis, hypercalcemia, gout.
Skin: dermatitis, photosensitivity, rash.
Other: hypersensitivity reactions, such as pneumonitis and vasculitis.

INTERACTIONS
Cholestyramine, colestipol: intestinal absorption of thiazides decreased. Keep doses as separate as possible.
Diazoxide: increased antihypertensive,

hyperglycemic, hyperuricemic effects.
Use together cautiously.

NURSING CONSIDERATIONS
• Contraindicated in anuria; hypersensitivity to other thiazides or other sulfonamide derivatives. Use cautiously in severe renal disease, impaired hepatic function, progressive hepatic disease.
• Monitor intake/output, weight, and serum electrolytes regularly.
• Monitor serum potassium levels; consult with doctor and dietitian to provide high-potassium diet. Watch for hypokalemia (for example, muscle weakness, cramps). Patients also on digitalis have an increased risk of digitalis toxicity due to the potassium-depleting effect of this diuretic. May use with potassium-sparing diuretic to prevent potassium loss.
• Foods rich in potassium include citrus fruits, tomatoes, bananas, dates, and apricots.
• Monitor serum creatinine and BUN levels regularly. Not effective if these levels are more than twice normal.
• Monitor blood uric acid levels, especially in patients with a history of gout.
• Check insulin requirements in patients with diabetes. May treat severe hyperglycemia with oral antidiabetic agents.
• In hypertension, therapeutic response may be delayed several days.
• Give in a.m. to prevent nocturia. Studies have shown that the drug is as effective when administered once daily as it is when given more frequently.
• Elderly patients are especially susceptible to excessive diuresis.
• Thiazides and thiazide-like diuretics should be stopped before tests for parathyroid function are performed.

hydroflumethiazide
Diucardin♦, Saluron

INDICATIONS & DOSAGE
Edema—
Adults: 25 mg to 200 mg P.O. daily in divided doses. Maintenance doses may be on intermittent or alternate-day schedule.
Children: 1 mg/kg P.O. daily.
Hypertension—
Adults: 50 to 100 mg P.O. daily or b.i.d.

SIDE EFFECTS
Blood: *aplastic anemia, agranulocytosis,* leukopenia, thrombocytopenia.
CV: *volume depletion and dehydration,* orthostatic hypotension.
GI: anorexia, nausea, pancreatitis.
Hepatic: hepatic encephalopathy.
Metabolic: *hypokalemia, asymptomatic hyperuricemia, hyperglycemia and impairment of glucose tolerance,* fluid and electrolyte imbalances including dilutional hyponatremia and hypochloremia, metabolic alkalosis, hypercalcemia, gout.
Skin: dermatitis, photosensitivity, rash.
Other: hypersensitivity reactions, such as pneumonitis and vasculitis.

INTERACTIONS
Cholestyramine, colestipol: intestinal absorption of thiazides decreased. Keep doses as separate as possible.
Diazoxide: increased antihypertensive, hyperglycemic, hyperuricemic effects. Use together cautiously.

NURSING CONSIDERATIONS
• Contraindicated in anuria; hypersensitivity to other thiazides or other sulfonamide-derived drugs. Use cautiously in severe renal disease, impaired hepatic function, progressive hepatic disease.
• Monitor intake/output, weight, and serum electrolytes regularly.
• Monitor serum potassium levels;

consult with doctor and dietitian to provide high-potassium diet. Food rich in potassium include citrus fruits, tomatoes, bananas, dates, and apricots. Watch for hypokalemia (for example, muscle weakness, cramps). May use with potassium-sparing diuretic to prevent potassium loss. Patients also on digitalis have an increased risk of digitalis toxicity due to the potassium-depleting effects of this diuretic.

• Monitor serum creatinine and BUN levels regularly. Not effective if these levels are more than twice normal.

• Monitor blood uric acid levels, especially in patients with history of gout.

• Check insulin requirements in patients with diabetes. May treat severe hyperglycemia with oral antidiabetic agents.

• Give in a.m. to prevent nocturia.

• In hypertension, therapeutic response may be delayed several days.

• Elderly patients are especially susceptible to excessive diuresis.

• Thiazides and thiazide-like diuretics should be stopped before tests for parathyroid function are performed.

mannitol
Osmitrol♦

INDICATIONS & DOSAGE
Adults and children over 12 years:
Test dose for marked oliguria or suspected inadequate renal function—200 mg/kg or 12.5 g as a 15% or 20% solution I.V. over 3 to 5 minutes. Response adequate if 30 to 50 ml urine/hour is excreted over 2 to 3 hours.
Treatment of oliguria—50 to 100 g I.V. as a 15% to 20% solution over 90 minutes to several hours.
Prevention of oliguria or acute renal failure—50 to 100 g I.V. of a concentrated (5% to 25%) solution. Exact concentration is determined by fluid requirements.

Edema—100 g as a 10% to 20% solution over 2- to 6-hour period.
To reduce intraocular pressure or intracranial pressure—1.5 to 2 g/kg as a 15% to 25% solution I.V. over 30 to 60 minutes.
To promote diuresis in drug intoxication—5% to 10% solution continuously up to 200 g I.V., while maintaining 100 to 500 ml urinary output/hour and a positive fluid balance.

SIDE EFFECTS
CNS: rebound increase in intracranial pressure 8 to 12 hours after diuresis, headache, confusion.
CV: *transient expansion of plasma volume during infusion causing circulatory overload and pulmonary edema,* tachycardia, angina-like chest pain.
EENT: blurred vision, rhinitis.
GI: thirst, nausea, vomiting.
GU: urinary retention.
Metabolic: *fluid and electrolyte imbalances, water intoxication, cellular dehydration.*

INTERACTIONS
None significant.

NURSING CONSIDERATIONS
• Contraindicated in anuria, severe pulmonary congestion, frank pulmonary edema, severe congestive heart disease, severe dehydration, metabolic edema, progressive renal disease or dysfunction, progressive heart failure during administration, active intracranial bleeding except during craniotomy.
• Monitor vital signs (including CVP) at least hourly; intake/output hourly (report increasing oliguria). Monitor daily: weight, renal function, fluid balance, serum and urine sodium and potassium levels.
• Solution often crystallizes, especially at low temperatures. To redissolve, warm bottle in hot water bath, shake vigorously. Cool to body temperature before giving. Concentrations greater than 15% have greater tendency to

crystallize. Do not use solution with undissolved crystals.

• Infusions should always be given I.V. via an in-line filter.

• Avoid infiltration; observe for inflammation, edema, potential necrosis.

• For maximum pressure reduction before surgery, give 1 to 1½ hours preoperatively.

• Can be used to measure glomerular filtration rate.

• Give frequent mouth care or fluids as permitted to relieve thirst.

• Urethral catheter is inserted in comatose or incontinent patients because therapy is based on strict evaluation of intake and output. In patients with urethral catheters, use an hourly urometer collection bag to facilitate accurate evaluation of output.

• An osmotic diuretic.

methazolamide
Neptazane

INDICATIONS & DOSAGE
Glaucoma (open-angle, or preoperatively in obstructive or narrow-angle)—
Adults: 50 to 100 mg b.i.d. or t.i.d.

SIDE EFFECTS
Blood: *aplastic anemia,* hemolytic anemia, leukopenia.
CNS: drowsiness, paresthesias.
EENT: transient myopia.
GI: nausea, vomiting, anorexia.
GU: crystalluria, renal calculi.
Metabolic: *hyperchloremic acidosis,* hypokalemia, asymptomatic hyperuricemia.
Skin: rash.

INTERACTIONS
None significant.

NURSING CONSIDERATIONS
• Contraindicated in severe or absolute glaucoma; for long-term use in chronic noncongestive narrow-angle glaucoma;

in patients with depressed sodium or potassium serum levels, renal or hepatic disease or dysfunction, adrenal gland dysfunction, and hyperchloremic acidosis. Use cautiously in respiratory acidosis, emphysema, chronic pulmonary disease.

• Monitor intake/output, weight, and serum electrolytes frequently.

• May cause false-positive urine protein tests by alkalinizing urine.

• A carbonic anhydrase inhibitor.

• Elderly patients are especially susceptible to excessive diuresis.

• Diuretic effect decreases in acidosis.

• Anticipate that drug will be given every day for glaucoma but intermittently for edema. Caution patient to comply with prescribed dosage and schedule to lessen risk of metabolic acidosis.

• Carefully evaluate the patient with glaucoma for eye pain to make sure drug is effective in decreasing intraocular pressure.

methyclothiazide
Aquatensen, Duretic♦♦, Enduron

INDICATIONS & DOSAGE
Edema, hypertension—
Adults: 2.5 to 10 mg P.O daily.

SIDE EFFECTS
Blood: *aplastic anemia, agranulocytosis,* leukopenia, thrombocytopenia.
CV: *volume depletion and dehydration,* orthostatic hypotension.
GI: anorexia, nausea, pancreatitis.
Hepatic: hepatic encephalopathy.
Metabolic: *hypokalemia, asymptomatic hyperuricemia, hyperglycemia and impairment of glucose tolerance,* fluid and electrolyte imbalances including dilutional hyponatremia and hypochloremia, metabolic alkalosis, hypercalcemia, gout.
Skin: dermatitis, photosensitivity, rash.
Other: hypersensitivity reactions, such as pneumonitis and vasculitis.

INTERACTIONS
Cholestyramine, colestipol: intestinal absorption of thiazides decreased. Keep doses as separate as possible.
Diazoxide: increased antihypertensive, hyperglycemic, hyperuricemic effects. Use together cautiously.

NURSING CONSIDERATIONS
• Contraindicated in renal decompensation; anuria; hypersensitivity to other thiazides or other sulfonamide-derived drugs. Use cautiously in potassium depletion, renal disease or dysfunction, impaired hepatic function, progressive hepatic disease.
• Monitor intake/output, weight, and serum electrolytes regularly.
• Monitor serum potassium levels; consult with doctor and dietitian to provide high-potassium diet. Foods rich in potassium include citrus fruits, tomatoes, bananas, dates, and apricots. Watch for hypokalemia (for example, muscle weakness, cramps). Patients also on digitalis have an increased risk of digitalis toxicity due to the potassium-depleting effect of this diuretic. May use with potassium-sparing diuretic to prevent potassium loss.
• Check insulin requirements in patients with diabetes. May treat severe hyperglycemia with oral antidiabetic agents.
• Monitor serum creatinine and BUN levels regularly. Not effective if these levels are more than twice normal.
• Monitor blood uric acid levels, especially in patients with a history of gout.
• In hypertension, therapeutic response may be delayed several days.
• Give in a.m. to prevent nocturia.
• Elderly patients are especially susceptible to excessive diuresis.
• Thiazides and thiazide-like diuretics should be stopped before tests for parathyroid function are performed.

metolazone
Diulo, Zaroxolyn♦**

INDICATIONS & DOSAGE
Edema (heart failure)—
Adults: 5 to 10 mg P.O. daily.
Edema (renal disease)—
Adults: 5 to 20 mg P.O. daily.
Hypertension—
Adults: 2.5 to 5 mg P.O. daily. Maintenance dose determined by patient's blood pressure.

SIDE EFFECTS
Blood: *aplastic anemia, agranulocytosis,* leukopenia, thrombocytopenia.
CV: *volume depletion and dehydration,* orthostatic hypotension.
GI: anorexia, nausea, pancreatitis.
Hepatic: hepatic encephalopathy.
Metabolic: *hypokalemia, asymptomatic hyperuricemia, hyperglycemia and impairment of glucose tolerance,* fluid and electrolyte imbalances including dilutional hyponatremia and hypochloremia, metabolic alkalosis, hypercalcemia, gout.
Skin: dermatitis, photosensitivity, rash.
Other: hypersensitivity reactions, such as pneumonitis and vasculitis.

INTERACTIONS
Cholestyramine, colestipol: intestinal absorption of thiazides decreased. Keep doses as separate as possible.
Diazoxide: increased antihypertensive, hyperglycemic, hyperuricemic effects. Use together cautiously.

NURSING CONSIDERATIONS
• Contraindicated in anuria; hepatic coma or precoma; hypersensitivity to thiazides or other sulfonamide-derived drugs. Use cautiously in hyperuricemia or gout and severely impaired renal function.
• Monitor intake/output, weight, and serum electrolytes regularly.
• Monitor serum potassium levels; consult with doctor and dietitian to pro-

vide high-potassium diet. Foods rich in potassium include citrus fruits, tomatoes, bananas, dates, and apricots. Watch for hypokalemia (for example, muscle weakness, cramps). Patients also on digitalis may have an increased risk of digitalis toxicity due to the potassium-depleting effect of this diuretic. May use with potassium-sparing diuretic to prevent potassium loss.

• Check insulin requirements in patients with diabetes. May treat severe hyperglycemia with oral antidiabetic agents.

• Monitor blood uric acid levels, especially in patients with a history of gout.

• In hypertension, therapeutic response may be delayed several days.

• Give in a.m. to prevent nocturia.

• Elderly patients are especially susceptible to excessive diuresis.

• A thiazide-related diuretic. However, unlike thiazide diuretics, metolazone is effective in patients with decreased renal function.

• Used as an adjunct in furosemide-resistant edema.

• Thiazides and thiazide-like diuretics should be stopped before tests for parathyroid function are performed.

polythiazide
Renese♦

INDICATIONS & DOSAGE
Hypertension—
Adults: 2 to 4 mg P.O. daily.
Edema (heart failure, renal failure)—
Adults: 1 to 4 mg P.O. daily.

SIDE EFFECTS
Blood: *aplastic anemia, agranulocytosis,* leukopenia, thrombocytopenia.
CV: *volume depletion and dehydration,* orthostatic hypotension.
GI: anorexia, nausea, pancreatitis.
Hepatic: hepatic encephalopathy.
Metabolic: *hypokalemia, asymptomatic hyperuricemia, hyperglycemia and*

impairment of glucose tolerance, fluid and electrolyte imbalances including dilutional hyponatremia and hypochloremia, metabolic alkalosis, hypercalcemia, gout.
Skin: dermatitis, photosensitivity, rash.
Other: hypersensitivity reactions, such as pneumonitis and vasculitis.

INTERACTIONS
Cholestyramine, colestipol: intestinal absorption of thiazides decreased. Keep doses as separate as possible.
Diazoxide: increased antihypertensive, hyperglycemic, hyperuricemic effects. Use together cautiously.

NURSING CONSIDERATIONS
• Contraindicated in anuria; hypersensitivity to other thiazides or other sulfonamide-derived drugs. Use cautiously in severe renal disease, impaired hepatic function, allergies.

• Monitor intake/output, weight, and serum electrolytes regularly.

• Monitor serum potassium levels; consult with doctor and dietitian to provide high-potassium diet. Foods rich in potassium include citrus fruits, tomatoes, bananas, dates, and apricots. Watch for hypokalemia (for example, muscle weakness, cramps). Patients also on digitalis may have an increased risk of digitalis toxicity due to the potassium-depleting effect of this diuretic. May use with potassium-sparing diuretic to prevent potassium loss.

• Monitor serum creatinine and BUN levels regularly. Not effective if these levels are more than twice normal.

• Monitor blood uric acid levels, especially in patients with a history of gout.

• Check insulin requirements in patients with diabetes. May treat severe hyperglycemia with oral antidiabetic agents.

• In hypertension, therapeutic response may be delayed several days.

• Give in a.m. to prevent nocturia.

• Elderly patients are especially susceptible to excessive diuresis.
• Thiazides and thiazide-like diuretics should be stopped before tests for parathyroid function are performed.

quinethazone
Aquamox♦♦, Hydromox

INDICATIONS & DOSAGE
Edema—
Adults: 50 to 100 mg P.O. daily or 50 mg P.O. b.i.d. Occasionally, up to 150 to 200 mg P.O. daily may be needed.

SIDE EFFECTS
Blood: *aplastic anemia, agranulocytosis,* leukopenia, thrombocytopenia.
CV: *volume depletion and dehydration,* orthostatic hypotension.
GI: anorexia, nausea, pancreatitis.
Hepatic: *hepatic encephalopathy.*
Metabolic: *hypokalemia, asymptomatic hyperuricemia, hyperglycemia and impairment of glucose tolerance,* fluid and electrolyte imbalances including dilutional hyponatremia and hypochloremia, metabolic alkalosis, hypercalcemia, gout.
Skin: dermatitis, photosensitivity, rash.
Other: hypersensitivity reactions, such as pneumonitis and vasculitis.

INTERACTIONS
Cholestyramine, colestipol: intestinal absorption of thiazides decreased. Keep doses as separate as possible.
Diazoxide: increased antihypertensive, hyperglycemic, hyperuricemic effects. Use together cautiously.

NURSING CONSIDERATIONS
• Contraindicated in anuria; hypersensitivity to quinethazones, thiazides, or other sulfonamide-derived drugs. Use cautiously in severe renal disease, impaired hepatic function, allergies.
• Monitor intake/output, weight, and serum electrolytes regularly.

• Monitor serum potassium levels; consult with doctor and dietitian to provide high-potassium diet. Foods rich in potassium include citrus fruits, tomatoes, bananas, dates, and apricots. Watch for hypokalemia (for example, muscle weakness, cramps). Patients also on digitalis have an increased risk of digitalis toxicity due to the potassium-depleting effect of this diuretic. May use with potassium-sparing diuretic to prevent potassium loss.
• Monitor serum creatinine and BUN levels regularly. Not effective if these levels are more than twice normal.
• Check insulin requirements in patients with diabetes. May treat severe hyperglycemia with oral antidiabetic agents.
• Monitor blood uric acid levels, especially in patients with a history of gout.
• In hypertension, therapeutic response may be delayed several days.
• Give in a.m. to prevent nocturia.
• Elderly patients are especially susceptible to excessive diuresis.
• Thiazides and thiazide-like diuretics should be stopped before tests for parathyroid function are performed.

spironolactone
Aldactone♦, Altex

INDICATIONS & DOSAGE
Edema—
Adults: 25 to 200 mg P.O. daily in divided doses.
Children: initially, 3.3 mg/kg P.O. daily in divided doses.
Hypertension—
Adults: 50 to 100 mg P.O. daily in divided doses.
Treatment of diuretic-induced hypokalemia—
Adults: 25 to 100 mg P.O. daily when oral potassium supplements are considered inappropriate.

Detection of primary hyper-aldosteronism—

Adults: 400 mg P.O. daily for 4 days (short test) or for 3 to 4 weeks (long test). If hypokalemia and hypertension are corrected, a presumptive diagnosis of primary hyperaldosteronism is made.

SIDE EFFECTS
CNS: headache.
GI: anorexia, nausea, diarrhea.
Metabolic: *hyperkalemia,* dehydration, hyponatremia, transient rise in BUN, acidosis.
Skin: urticaria.
Other: gynecomastia in males, breast soreness and menstrual disturbances in females.

INTERACTIONS
Aspirin: possible blocked spironolactone effect. Watch for diminished spironolactone response.

NURSING CONSIDERATIONS
• Contraindicated in anuria, acute or progressive renal insufficiency, hyperkalemia. Use cautiously in fluid or electrolyte imbalances, impaired renal function, and hepatic disease.
• A mild acidosis may occur during therapy. This may be dangerous in patients with hepatic cirrhosis.
• Monitor serum potassium levels, electrolytes, intake/output, weight, and blood pressure regularly.
• Potassium-sparing diuretic; useful as an adjunct to other diuretic therapy. Less potent diuretic than thiazide and loop types. Diuretic effect delayed 2 to 3 days when used alone.
• Maximum antihypertensive response may be delayed up to 2 weeks.
• Warn patient to avoid excessive ingestion of potassium-rich foods or potassium-containing salt substitutes. Concomitant potassium supplement can lead to serious hyperkalemia.
• Elderly patients are more susceptible to excessive diuresis.

• Protect drug from light.
• Breast cancer reported in some patients taking spironolactone, but cause-and-effect relationship not confirmed. Warn against taking drug indiscriminately.
• Give with meals to enhance absorption.

triamterene
Dyrenium♦

INDICATIONS & DOSAGE
Diuresis—
Adults: initially, 100 mg P.O. b.i.d. after meals. Total daily dosage should not exceed 300 mg.

SIDE EFFECTS
Blood: megaloblastic anemia related to low folic acid levels.
CNS: dizziness.
CV: hypotension.
EENT: sore throat.
GI: dry mouth, nausea, vomiting.
Metabolic: *hyperkalemia,* dehydration, hyponatremia, transient rise in BUN, acidosis.
Skin: photosensitivity, rash.
Other: *anaphylaxis,* muscle cramps.

INTERACTIONS
None significant.

NURSING CONSIDERATIONS
• Contraindicated in anuria, severe or progressive renal disease or dysfunction, severe hepatic disease, hyperkalemia. Use cautiously in impaired hepatic function, diabetes mellitus, pregnancy, or lactation.
• Watch for blood dyscrasias.
• Monitor BUN and serum potassium, electrolytes.
• A potassium-sparing diuretic, useful as an adjunct to other diuretic therapy. Less potent than thiazides and loop diuretics. Full diuretic effect delayed 2 to 3 days.
• Warn patients to avoid excessive

Italicized side effects are common or life-threatening.
∗Liquid form contains alcohol.   ∗∗May contain tartrazine.

ingestion of potassium-rich foods or potassium-containing salt substitutes. Concomitant potassium supplement can lead to serious hyperkalemia.
• Give medication after meals to prevent nausea.
• Should be withdrawn gradually to prevent excessive rebound potassium excretion.
• Concomitant use of spironolactone is not recommended.

trichlormethiazide
Diurese, Metahydrin**, Naqua, Rochlomethiazide, Trichlorex

INDICATIONS & DOSAGE
Edema—
Adults: 1 to 4 mg P.O. daily or in 2 divided doses.
Hypertension—
Adults: 2 to 4 mg P.O. daily.

SIDE EFFECTS
Blood: *aplastic anemia, agranulocytosis,* leukopenia, thrombocytopenia.
CV: *volume depletion and dehydration,* orthostatic hypotension.
GI: anorexia, nausea, pancreatitis.
Hepatic: hepatic encephalopathy.
Metabolic: *hypokalemia, asymptomatic hyperuricemia, hyperglycemia and impairment of glucose tolerance,* fluid and electrolyte imbalances including dilutional hyponatremia and hypochloremia, metabolic alkalosis, hypercalcemia, gout.
Skin: dermatitis, photosensitivity, rash.
Other: hypersensitivity reactions, such as pneumonitis and vasculitis.

INTERACTIONS
Cholestyramine, colestipol: intestinal absorption of thiazides decreased. Keep doses as separate as possible.
Diazoxide: increased antihypertensive, hyperglycemic, hyperuricemic effects. Use together cautiously.

NURSING CONSIDERATIONS
• Contraindicated in anuria; hypersensitivity to other thiazides or other sulfonamide-derived drugs. Use cautiously in severe renal disease, impaired hepatic function.
• Monitor intake/output, weight, and electrolytes regularly.
• Monitor serum potassium levels; consult with doctor and dietitian to provide high-potassium diet. Foods rich in potassium include citrus fruits, tomatoes, bananas, dates, and apricots. Watch for hypokalemia (for example, muscle weakness, cramps). Patients also on digitalis have an increased risk of digitalis toxicity due to the potassium-depleting effect of this diuretic. May use with potassium-sparing diuretic to prevent potassium loss.
• Monitor serum creatinine and BUN levels regularly. Not effective if these levels are more than twice normal.
• Check insulin requirements in patients with diabetes. May treat severe hyperglycemia with oral antidiabetic agents. Monitor blood sugar.
• Monitor blood uric acid levels, especially in patients with a history of gout.
• In hypertension, therapeutic response may be delayed several days.
• Give in a.m. to prevent nocturia.
• Elderly patients are especially susceptible to excessive diuresis.
• Thiazides and thiazide-like diuretics should be stopped before tests for fparathyroid function are performed.

urea (carbamide)
Ureaphil

INDICATIONS & DOSAGE
Intracranial or intraocular pressure—
Adults: 1 to 1.5 g/kg as a 30% solution by slow I.V. infusion over 1 to 2.5 hours.
Children over 2 years: 0.5 to 1.5 g/kg slow I.V. infusion.
Children under 2 years: as little as

Unmarked trade names available in the United States only.
♦ Also available in Canada. ♦♦ Available in Canada only.

0.1 g/kg slow I.V. infusion. Maximum 4 ml/minute.

Maximum adult daily dose 120 g. To prepare 135 ml 30% solution, mix contents of 40-g vial of urea with 105 ml dextrose 5% or 10% in water or 10% invert sugar in water. Each ml of 30% solution provides 300 mg urea.

SIDE EFFECTS
CNS: *headache*.
CV: tachycardia, volume expansion.
GI: *nausea, vomiting*.
Metabolic: sodium and potassium depletion.
Local: irritation or necrotic sloughing may occur with extravasation.

INTERACTIONS
None significant.

NURSING CONSIDERATIONS
• Contraindicated in severely impaired renal function, marked dehydration, frank hepatic failure, active intracranial bleeding. Use cautiously in pregnancy, lactation, cardiac disease, hepatic impairment, or sickle cell damage with CNS involvement.
• Avoid rapid I.V. infusion; may cause hemolysis or increased capillary bleeding. Avoid extravasation; may cause reactions ranging from mild irritation to necrosis.
• Don't administer through the same infusion as blood.
• Don't infuse into leg veins; may cause phlebitis or thrombosis, especially in the elderly.
• Watch for hyponatremia or hypokalemia (muscle weakness, lethargy); may indicate electrolyte depletion before serum levels are reduced.
• Maintain adequate hydration; monitor fluid and electrolyte balance.
• In renal disease, monitor BUN frequently.
• Indwelling urethral catheter should be used in comatose patients to assure bladder emptying. Use an hourly urometer collection bag to facilitate accurate evaluation of diuresis.
• If satisfactory diuresis does not occur in 6 to 12 hours, urea should be discontinued and renal function reevaluated.
• Use freshly reconstituted urea only for I.V. infusion; solution becomes ammonia upon oxidation when standing.
• Use within minutes of reconstitution.

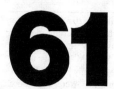

Electrolytes and replacement solutions

calcium chloride
calcium gluceptate
calcium gluconate
calcium lactate
dextrans (low molecular weight)
dextrans (high molecular weight)
hetastarch
magnesium sulfate
potassium acetate
potassium bicarbonate
potassium chloride
potassium gluconate
potassium phosphate
Ringer's injection
Ringer's injection, lactated
sodium chloride

MECHANISM OF ACTION
Electrolytes and replacement solutions replace and maintain specific anion or cation levels. Dextrans and hetastarch expand plasma volume and provide fluid replacement.

COMBINATION PRODUCTS
CALCIUM-SANDOZ FORTE♦♦: calcium lactate-gluconate 2.94 g, calcium carbonate 0.3 g, elemental sodium 275.8 mg; provides 500 mg elemental calcium.

DUO-K: 20 mEq potassium, 3.4 mEq chloride (from potassium gluconate and potassium chloride).

GRAMCAL♦♦: calcium lactate-gluconate 3,080 mg, calcium carbonate 1,500 mg, and potassium 390 mg; provides 1,000 mg of elemental calcium.

KAOCHLOR-EFF:20 mEq potassium, 20 mEq chloride (from potassium chloride, potassium citrate, potassium bicarbonate, and betaine hydrochloride).

KEFF: 20 mEq each potassium and chloride (potassium chloride, potassium carbonate, potassium bicarbonate, and betaine hydrochloride).

KLORVESS*: 20 mEq each potassium and chloride (from potassium chloride, potassium bicarbonate, and l-lysine monohydrochloride).

KOLYUM: 20 mEq potassium, 3.4 mEq chloride (from potassium gluconate and potassium chloride).

NEUTRA-PHOS: phosphorus 250 mg, sodium 164 mg, potassium 278 mg (from dibasic and monobasic sodium and potassium phosphate).

POTASSIUM-SANDOZ♦♦: potassium chloride 600 mg and potassium bicarbonate 400 mg (provides 12 mEq potassium and 8 mEq chloride).

POTASSIUM TRIPLEX: 45 mEq potassium (from potassium acetate, potassium bicarbonate, and potassium citrate) per 15 ml.

THERMOTABS: 450 mg sodium chloride, 30 mg potassium chloride, 18 mg calcium carbonate, and 200 mg dextrose.

TWIN-K: 20 mEq potassium (as potassium gluconate and potassium citrate).

TWIN-K-CL: 15 ml supplies 15 mEq of potassium ions as a combination of potassium gluconate, potassium citrate, and ammonium chloride.

calcium chloride

calcium gluceptate

calcium gluconate

calcium lactate

INDICATIONS & DOSAGE

Hypocalcemia, hypocalcemic tetany, hypocalcemia during exchange transfusions, cardiac resuscitation for inotropic effect when epinephrine has failed; magnesium intoxication; hypoparathyroidism—
Adults and children: initially 500 mg to 1 g elemental calcium I.V., with further dosage based on serum calcium determinations.

Dosage with calcium chloride (1 g [10 ml] yields 13.5 mEq Ca^{++}):
Magnesium intoxication—
Adults and children: initially 500 mg I.V., with further doses based on calcium and magnesium determination.
Cardiac arrest—0.5 to 1 g I.V., not to exceed 1 ml/minute; or 200 to 800 mg into the ventricular cavity.
Hypocalcemia—500 mg to 1 g I.V. at intervals of 1 to 3 days, determined by serum calcium levels.

Dosage with calcium gluconate (1 g [10 ml] yields 4.5 mEq Ca^{++}):
Hypocalcemia—
Adults: 500 mg to 1 g I.V., repeated q 1 to 3 days p.r.n. as determined by serum calcium levels. Further doses depend on serum calcium determination.
Children: 500 mg/kg I.V. daily. Rate of infusion should not exceed 0.5 ml/minute.

Dosage with calcium gluceptate (1.1 g [5 ml] yields 4.5 mEq Ca^{++}) and calcium salts (18 mg [1 ml] yields 0.898 mEq Ca^{++}):
Hypocalcemia—
Adults: initially 5 to 20 ml I.V., with further doses based on serum calcium determinations. If I.V. injection is impossible, 2 to 5 ml I.M. Average adult oral dose, 1 to 2 g daily P.O. in divided doses, t.i.d. or q.i.d. Average oral dose for children, 45 to 65 mg/kg P.O. daily, in divided doses, t.i.d. or q.i.d.
During exchange transfusions—
Adults and children: 0.5 ml I.V. after each 100 ml blood exchanged.

SIDE EFFECTS

CNS: from I.V. use, tingling sensations, sense of oppression or heat waves; with rapid I.V. injection, syncope.
CV: mild fall in blood pressure; with rapid I.V. injection, vasodilation, *bradycardia, cardiac arrhythmias, and cardiac arrest.*
GI: with oral ingestion, irritation, hemorrhage, *constipation;* with I.V. administration, chalky taste; with oral calcium chloride, gastrointestinal hemorrhage, nausea, vomiting, thirst, abdominal pain.
GU: hypercalcemia, polyuria, renal calculi.
Skin: local reaction if calcium salts given I.M.: burning, necrosis, sloughing of tissue, cellulitis, soft-tissue calcification.
Local: with S.C. injection, pain and irritation; *with I.V., venous irritation.*

INTERACTIONS

Cardiotonic glycosides: increased digitalis toxicity; administer calcium very cautiously (if at all) to digitalized patients.

NURSING CONSIDERATIONS

● Contraindicated in ventricular fibrillation, hypercalcemia, renal calculi. Use cautiously in patients with sarcoidosis and renal or cardiac disease, and in digitalized patients. Use calcium chloride cautiously in cor pulmonale,

---

Italicized side effects are common or life-threatening.
*Liquid form contains alcohol.   **May contain tartrazine.

respiratory acidosis, or respiratory failure.

• Monitor EKG when giving calcium I.V. Such injections should not exceed 0.7 to 1.5 mEq/minute. Stop if patient complains of discomfort. Following I.V. injection, patient should remain recumbent for a short while.

• I.M. injection should be given in the gluteal region in adults; lateral thigh in infants. I.M. route used only in emergencies when no I.V. route available.

• Monitor blood calcium levels frequently. Report abnormalities.

• Hypercalcemia may result after large doses in chronic renal failure.

• I.V. route generally recommended in children, but not by scalp vein (can cause tissue necrosis).

• Solutions should be warmed to body temperature before administration.

• Calcium chloride and calcium gluconate should be given I.V. only.

• Severe necrosis and sloughing of tissues follow extravasation. Calcium gluconate is less irritating to veins and tissues than calcium chloride.

• If gastrointestinal upset occurs, give oral calcium products 1 to 1½ hours after meals.

• Oxalic acid (found in rhubarb and spinach), phytic acid (in bran and whole cereals), and phosphorus (in milk and dairy products) may interfere with absorption of calcium.

• Crash carts usually contain both gluconate and chloride. Make sure doctor specifies form he wants administered.

dextrans
(low molecular weight dextrans)
Dextran 40, Gentran 40, LMVD,
Rheomacrodex♦

INDICATIONS & DOSAGE
Plasma volume expansion—Dosage of 10% solution by I.V. infusion depends on amount of fluid loss.
First 500 ml of Dextran 40 may be infused rapidly with central venous pres-

sure monitoring. Infuse remaining dose slowly. Total daily dose not to exceed 2 g/kg body weight. If therapy continued past 24 hours, do not exceed 1 g/kg daily. Continue for no longer than 5 days.
Reduction of blood sludging—500 ml of 10% solution by I.V. infusion.

SIDE EFFECTS
Blood: *decreased level of hemoglobin and hematocrit;* with higher doses, increased bleeding time.
GI: nausea, vomiting.
GU: tubular stasis and blocking, increased viscosity of urine.
Hepatic: increased SGPT and SGOT levels.
Skin: hypersensitivity reaction, urticaria.
Other: *anaphylaxis.*

INTERACTIONS
None significant.

NURSING CONSIDERATIONS
• Contraindicated in marked hemostatic defects; marked cardiac decompensation or pulmonary edema; renal disease with severe oliguria or anuria; or extreme dehydration. Use cautiously in active hemorrhage; may cause additional blood loss. Evaluate patient's hydration status before administration.

• Hazardous when given to patients with heart failure, especially if in saline solution. Use dextrose solution instead.

• Works as plasma expander via colloidal osmotic effect, thereby drawing fluid from interstitial to intravascular space. Provides plasma expansion slightly greater than volume infused. Watch for circulatory overload, rise in central venous pressure readings.

• Monitor urine flow rate during administration. If oliguria or anuria occurs or is not relieved by infusion, stop dextran and give osmotic diuretic.

• Hydration should be assessed before starting therapy; otherwise, use urine or serum osmolarity because urine spe-

cific gravity is affected by urine dextran concentration.
• Check hemoglobin and hematocrit; don't allow to fall below 30% by volume.
• Draw blood samples *before* starting infusion.
• Observe patient closely during early phase of infusion: most anaphylactoid reactions occur during this time.
• May interfere with analysis of blood grouping, crossmatching, bilirubin, blood glucose, and protein.
• Store at constant 25° C. (77° F.). May precipitate in storage, but can be heated to dissolve if necessary.

dextrans
(high molecular weight dextrans)
Dextran 70, Dextran 75♦, Gentran 75, Macrodex♦

INDICATIONS & DOSAGE
Plasma expander—
Adults: usual dose 30 g (500 ml of 6% solution) I.V. In emergency situations, may be administered at rate of 1.2 to 2.4 g (20 to 40 ml) per minute. In normovolemic or nearly normovolemic patients, rate of infusion should not exceed 240 mg (4 ml)/minute.
Total dose during first 24 hours not to exceed 1.2 g/kg; actual dose depends on amount of fluid loss and resultant hemoconcentration, and must be determined for each patient.

SIDE EFFECTS
Blood: *decreased level of hemoglobin and hematocrit;* with doses of 15 ml/kg body weight, prolonged bleeding time and significant suppression of platelet function.
GI: nausea, vomiting.
GU: increased specific gravity and viscosity of urine, tubular stasis and blocking.
Hepatic: increased SGPT and SGOT levels.

Skin: hypersensitivity reaction, urticaria.
Other: fever, arthralgia, nasal congestion, *anaphylaxis.*

INTERACTIONS
None significant.

NURSING CONSIDERATIONS
• Contraindicated in marked hemostatic defects; marked cardiac decompensation or pulmonary edema; renal disease with severe oliguria or anuria; and extreme dehydration. Use cautiously in active hemorrhage; may cause additional blood loss.
• Hazardous when given to patients with heart failure, especially if in saline solution. Use dextrose solution instead.
• Works as plasma expander via colloidal osmotic effect, thereby drawing fluid from interstitial to intravascular space. Provides plasma expansion slightly greater than volume infused. Watch for circulatory overload.
• Monitor urine flow rate during administration. If oliguria or anuria occurs or is not relieved by infusion, stop dextran and give osmotic diuretic.
• Hydration should be assessed before starting therapy; otherwise, use urine or serum osmolarity because urine specific gravity is affected by the urine dextran concentration.
• Check hemoglobin and hematocrit; don't allow to fall below 30% by volume.
• Draw blood samples *before* starting infusion.
• Observe patient closely during early phase of infusion: most anaphylactoid reactions occur during this time.
• May interfere with analysis of blood grouping, crossmatching, bilirubin, blood glucose, and protein.
• May precipitate in storage, but can be heated to dissolve if necessary.
• Dextran 70 and Dextran 75 can be used interchangeably. Both differ significantly from Dextran 40—do not interchange.

Italicized side effects are common or life-threatening.
*Liquid form contains alcohol.   **May contain tartrazine.

hetastarch
Hespan, Volex

INDICATIONS & DOSAGE
Plasma expander—
Adults: 500 to 1,000 ml I.V. dependent on amount of blood lost and resultant hemoconcentration. Total dosage usually not to exceed 1,500 ml/day. Up to 20 ml/kg hourly may be used in hemorrhagic shock.

SIDE EFFECTS
CNS: headaches.
CV: peripheral edema of lower extremities.
EENT: periorbital edema.
GI: nausea, vomiting.
Skin: urticaria.
Other: wheezing, mild fever.

INTERACTIONS
None significant.

NURSING CONSIDERATIONS
• Contraindicated in severe bleeding disorders or with severe congestive heart failure and renal failure with oliguria and anuria.
• To avoid circulatory overload, monitor patients with impaired renal function carefully.
• Discontinue if allergic or sensitivity reactions occur. If necessary, administer an antihistamine.
• Hetastarch is *not* a substitute for blood or plasma.
• Available in 500-ml I.V. infusion bottles.

magnesium sulfate

INDICATIONS & DOSAGE
Hypomagnesemia—
Adults: 1 g, or 8.12 mEq, of 50% solution (2 ml) I.M. q 6 hours for 4 doses, depending on serum magnesium level.
*Severe hypomagnesemia (serum magnesium 0.8 mEq/liter or less, with symp-*toms)—6 g, or 50 mEq, of 50% solution I.V. in 1 liter of solution over 4 hours. Subsequent doses depend on serum magnesium levels.
Magnesium supplementation in hyperalimentation—
Adults: 8 to 24 mEq daily added to hyperalimentation solution.
Children over 6 years: 2 to 10 mEq daily added to hyperalimentation solution.
Each 2 ml of 50% solution contains 1 g, or 8.12 mEq, magnesium sulfate.
Acute treatment of preeclampsia and eclampsia—
Adults: loading dose: 2 to 4 g (4 to 8 ml of 50% solution) given by slow I.V. bolus (over 5 minutes). Maintenance: 1 to 2 g hourly as a constant infusion. Prepare by adding 8 ml of 50% solution to 230 ml dextrose 5% in water.

SIDE EFFECTS
CNS: toxicity: weak or absent deep-tendon reflexes, flaccid paralysis, hypothermia, drowsiness, respiratory depression or paralysis; hypocalcemia (perioral paresthesias, twitching carpopedal spasm, tetany, and seizures).
CV: slow, weak pulse; cardiac arrhythmias (hypocalcemia); hypotension.
Skin: flushing, sweating.

INTERACTIONS
None significant.

NURSING CONSIDERATIONS
• Contraindicated in impaired renal function, myocardial damage, heart block, and in actively progressing labor. Use parenteral magnesium with extreme caution in patients receiving digitalis preparations. Treating magnesium toxicity with calcium in such patients could cause serious alterations in cardiac conduction; heart block may result.
• I.V. bolus dose *must* be injected slowly in order to avoid respiratory or cardiac arrest.

Unmarked trade names available in the United States only.
♦ Also available in Canada.　　♦ ♦ Available in Canada only.

- If available, use a constant infusion pump when administering infusion.
- Maximum infusion rate 150 mg/minute. Rapid drip causes feeling of heat.
- Keep I.V. calcium available to reverse magnesium intoxication.
- Monitor vital signs every 15 minutes when giving I.V. for severe hypomagnesemia. Watch for respiratory depression and signs of heart block. Respirations should be more than 16/minute before dose is given.
- Monitor intake/output. Output should be 100 ml or more during 4-hour period before dose.
- Test knee jerk and patellar reflexes before each additional dose. If absent, give no more magnesium until reflexes return; otherwise, patient may develop temporary respiratory failure and need cardiopulmonary resuscitation or I.V. administration of calcium.
- Check magnesium levels after repeated doses.
- After giving to toxemic mothers within 24 hours before delivery, watch newborn for signs of magnesium toxicity, including neuromuscular and respiratory depression.

potassium acetate

INDICATIONS & DOSAGE
Potassium replacement—I.V. should be used for life-threatening hypokalemia or when oral replacement not feasible. Give no more than 20 mEq hourly in concentration of 40 mEq/liter or less. Total 24-hour dose should not exceed 150 mEq (3 mEq/kg in children). Potassium replacement should be done with EKG monitoring and frequent serum K+ determinations.
Prevention of hypokalemia—
Adults and children: 20 mEq P.O. daily, in divided doses b.i.d., t.i.d., or q.i.d.
Potassium depletion—
Adults and children: usual dose 40 to 100 mEq P.O. daily, in divided doses b.i.d., t.i.d., or q.i.d.

SIDE EFFECTS
Signs of hyperkalemia—
CNS: paresthesias of the extremities, listlessness, mental confusion, weakness or heaviness of legs, flaccid paralysis.
CV: *peripheral vascular collapse with fall in blood pressure, cardiac arrhythmias,* heart block, possible cardiac arrest, EKG changes (prolonged P-R intervals; wide QRS; ST segment depression; tall, tented T waves).
GI: nausea, vomiting, abdominal pain, diarrhea, bowel ulceration.
GU: oliguria.
Skin: cold skin, gray pallor.

INTERACTIONS
None significant.

NURSING CONSIDERATIONS
- Contraindicated in severe renal impairment with oliguria, anuria, azotemia, and untreated Addison's disease; acute dehydration, hyperkalemia, hyperkalemic form of familial periodic paralysis, and conditions associated with extensive tissue breakdown. Use cautiously in patients with cardiac disease, patients receiving potassium-sparing diuretics, and those with renal impairment.
- During therapy, monitor EKG, serum potassium level, renal function, BUN, serum creatinine, and intake/output. Never give potassium postoperatively until urine flow is established.
- Give slowly as diluted solution; potentially fatal hyperkalemia may result from too rapid infusion.
- Parenteral potassium given by infusion only; never I.V. push or I.M.
- Observe for pain and redness at infusion site. Large-bore needle reduces local irritation.
- Watch for signs of GI ulceration: obstruction, hemorrhage, pain, distention, severe vomiting, bleeding.

Italicized side effects are common or life-threatening.
*Liquid form contains alcohol.   **May contain tartrazine.

- Reconstitute potassium acetate powder with liquids; give after meals with a full glass of water or fruit juice to minimize GI irritation.
- To prevent serious hyperkalemia, potassium deficits must be replaced gradually.

potassium bicarbonate
K-Lyte, K-Lyte DS

INDICATIONS & DOSAGE
Hypokalemia— 25 mEq or 50 mEq tablet dissolved in water 1 to 4 times a day.

SIDE EFFECTS
CNS: paresthesias of the extremities, listlessness, mental confusion, weakness or heaviness of legs, flaccid paralysis.
CV: *cardiac arrhythmias,* EKG changes (prolonged P-R interval; wide QRS; ST segment depression; tall, tented T waves).
GI: *nausea, vomiting, abdominal pain,* diarrhea, ulcerations, hemorrhage, obstruction, perforation.

INTERACTIONS
None significant.

NURSING CONSIDERATIONS
- Contraindicated in severe renal impairment with oliguria, anuria, azotemia, and untreated Addison's disease; also in acute dehydration, hyperkalemia, hyperkalemic familial periodic paralysis, and conditions associated with extensive tissue breakdown. Use with caution in cardiac disease and patients receiving potassium-sparing diuretics.
- Monitor serum potassium level, BUN, serum creatinine, and intake/output.
- Never switch potassium products without a doctor's order.
- Dissolve potassium bicarbonate tablets in 6 to 8 ounces of cold water.

- Have patient take with meals and sip slowly over a 5- to 10-minute period.
- Potassium bicarbonate cannot be given instead of potassium chloride.
- Potassium bicarbonate does not correct hypochloremic alkalosis.
- Available in lime and orange flavors. Check for patient's flavor preference.

potassium chloride
K-Lor, K-Lyte/Cl, K-10♦, Kaochlor 10%*, Kaochlor S-F 10%*, Kaon-Cl, Kaon-Cl 20%*, Kato Powder, KayCiel♦*, Klor-10%*, Kloride* **, Klor-Con, Klorvess, Klotrix, K Tab, Micro K Extencaps, SK-Potassium Chloride, Slow K♦

INDICATIONS & DOSAGE
Hypokalemia—
40 to 100 mEq P.O. divided into 3 to 4 doses daily for treatment; 20 mEq for prevention. Further dose based on serum potassium determinations.
I.V. route when oral replacement not feasible or when hypokalemia life-threatening. Usual dose 20 mEq hourly in concentration of 40 mEq/liter or less. Total daily dose not to exceed 150 mEq (3 mEq/kg in children). Potassium replacement should be done only with EKG monitoring and frequent serum K^+ determinations.

SIDE EFFECTS
Signs of hyperkalemia:
CNS: paresthesias of the extremities, listlessness, mental confusion, weakness or heaviness of limbs, flaccid paralysis.
CV: *peripheral vascular collapse with fall in blood pressure, cardiac arrhythmias, heart block, possible cardiac arrest,* EKG changes (prolonged P-R interval; wide QRS; ST segment depression; tall, tented T waves).
GI: *nausea, vomiting, abdominal pain,* diarrhea, GI ulcerations (possible stenosis, hemorrhage, obstruction, perforation).

Unmarked trade names available in the United States only.
♦ Also available in Canada.   ♦♦ Available in Canada only.

GU: oliguria.
Skin: cold skin, gray pallor.

INTERACTIONS
None significant.

NURSING CONSIDERATIONS
• Contraindicated in severe renal impairment with oliguria, anuria, azotemia, and untreated Addison's disease; also in acute dehydration, hyperkalemia, hyperkalemic form of familial periodic paralysis, conditions associated with extensive tissue breakdown. Use with caution in cardiac disease, patients receiving potassium-sparing diuretics.
• Potassium should not be given during immediate postoperative period until urine flow is established.
• Parenteral potassium given by infusion only; never I.V. push or I.M.
• Give slowly as dilute solution; potentially fatal hyperkalemia may result from too rapid infusion.
• Give oral potassium supplements with extreme caution because its many forms deliver varying amounts of potassium. Never switch products without a doctor's order. Tell the doctor if patient tolerates one product better than another.
• Sugar-free liquid available (Kaochlor S-F 10%).
• Use a liquid preparation for potassium supplementation if tablet or capsule passage is likely to be delayed, such as in GI obstruction.
• Have patient sip liquid potassium slowly to minimize GI irritation.
• Give with or after meals with full glass of water or fruit juice to lessen GI distress.
• Make sure powders are completely dissolved before giving.
• Enteric-coated tablets not recommended due to potential GI bleeding and small-bowel ulcerations.
• Tablets in wax matrix sometimes lodge in esophagus and cause ulceration in cardiac patients who have esophageal compression due to en-

larged left atrium. In such patients and in those with esophageal stasis or obstruction, use liquid form.
• Often used orally with diuretics that cause potassium excretion. Potassium chloride most useful since diuretics waste chloride ion. Hypokalemic alkalosis treated best with potassium chloride.
• Monitor EKG, serum potassium levels, and other electrolytes during therapy.

---

potassium gluconate
Kaon Liquid*, Kaon Tablets♦,
Potassium Rougier♦♦

INDICATIONS & DOSAGE
Hypokalemia—40 to 100 mEq P.O. divided into 3 to 4 doses daily for treatment; 20 mEq daily for prevention. Further dose based on serum potassium determinations.

SIDE EFFECTS
CNS: paresthesias of the extremities, listlessness, mental confusion, weakness or heaviness of legs, flaccid paralysis.
CV: cardiac arrhythmias, EKG changes (prolonged P-R interval; wide QRS; ST segment depression; tall, tented T waves).
GI: *nausea, vomiting, abdominal pain,* diarrhea, GI ulcerations with oral products (especially enteric-coated tablets); ulcerations may be accompanied by stenosis, hemorrhage, obstruction, perforation.

INTERACTIONS
None significant.

NURSING CONSIDERATIONS
• Contraindicated in severe renal impairment with oliguria, anuria, azotemia, and untreated Addison's disease; also in acute dehydration, hyperkalemia, hyperkalemic form of familial periodic paralysis, and conditions associ-

---

Italicized side effects are common or life-threatening.
*Liquid form contains alcohol.   **May contain tartrazine.

ated with extensive tissue breakdown. Use with caution in patients with cardiac disease, and in those receiving potassium-sparing diuretics.
• Monitor serum potassium level, BUN, serum creatinine, and intake/output.
• Give oral potassium supplements with extreme caution because their many forms deliver varying amounts of potassium. Never switch products without doctor's order. If one product is tolerated better than another, tell doctor so brand and dosage can be changed.
• Have patient sip liquid potassium slowly to minimize GI irritation.
• Give with or after meals with full glass of water or fruit juice to lessen GI distress.
• Potassium gluconate does not correct hypokalemic hypochloremic alkalosis.
• Enteric-coated tablets not recommended due to potential for GI bleeding and small-bowel ulcerations.
• Monitor EKG, serum potassium, and other electrolytes during therapy.

potassium phosphate

INDICATIONS & DOSAGE
Hypokalemia—I.V. should be used when oral replacement not feasible or when hypokalemia life-threatening. Dosage up to 20 mEq hourly in concentration of 60 mEq/liter or less. Total daily dose not to exceed 150 mEq. Should be done only with EKG monitoring and frequent serum K$^+$ determinations.
Average P.O. dose: 40 to 100 mEq.
Hypophosphatemia—3 mM/ml is administered I.V. after diluting in a larger volume of fluid. Dosage is adjusted according to individual needs of patient.

SIDE EFFECTS
Signs of hyperkalemia—
CNS: paresthesias of the extremities, listlessness, mental confusion, weakness or heaviness of legs, flaccid paralysis; hypocalcemia—perioral paresthesias, twitching, carpopedal spasm, tetany, and seizures.
CV: *peripheral vascular collapse with fall in blood pressure, cardiac arrhythmias, heart block, possible cardiac arrest,* EKG changes (prolonged P-R interval; wide QRS; ST segment depression; tall, tented T waves).
GI: nausea, vomiting, abdominal pain, diarrhea.
GU: oliguria.
Skin: cold skin, gray pallor.
Other: soft-tissue calcification.

INTERACTIONS
None significant.

NURSING CONSIDERATIONS
• Contraindicated in severe renal impairment with oliguria, anuria, azotemia, and untreated Addison's disease; also in acute dehydration, hyperkalemia, hyperkalemic form of familial periodic paralysis, extensive tissue damage, and hypocalcemia. Use with caution in patients with cardiac disease, and in those receiving potassium-sparing diuretics.
• Never give potassium postoperatively until urine flow is established.
• Monitor EKG for indications of tissue potassium levels; plasma potassium and calcium levels as well as BUN and creatinine for renal function; inorganic phosphorus levels; intake/output.
• Give slowly as dilute solution; potentially fatal hyperkalemia may result from too rapid an infusion.
• Parenteral potassium given by infusion only; never I.V. push or I.M.
• Reconstitute powder in juice. Give after meals.

Ringer's injection

INDICATIONS & DOSAGE
Fluid and electrolyte replacement—
Adults and children: dose highly individualized, but generally 1.5 to 3 liters

---

(2% to 6% body weight) infused I.V. over 18 to 24 hours.

SIDE EFFECTS
CV: fluid overload.

INTERACTIONS
None significant.

NURSING CONSIDERATIONS
• Contraindicated in renal failure, except as emergency volume expander. Use cautiously in congestive heart failure, circulatory insufficiency, renal dysfunction, hypoproteinemia, or pulmonary edema.
• Ringer's injection contains sodium, 147 mEq/liter; potassium, 4 mEq/liter; calcium, 4.5 mEq/liter; and chloride, 155.5 mEq/liter. This electrolyte content is insufficient for treating severe electrolyte deficiencies, although it does provide electrolytes in levels approximately equal to those of the blood.
• May be given with dextrose infusion, other carbohydrates, or sodium lactate.

Ringer's injection, lactated
(Hartmann's solution, Ringer's lactate solution)

INDICATIONS & DOSAGE
Fluid and electrolyte replacement—
Adults and children: dose highly individualized, but generally 1.5 to 3 liters (2% to 6% body weight) infused I.V. over 18 to 24 hours.

SIDE EFFECTS
CV: fluid overload.

INTERACTIONS
None significant.

NURSING CONSIDERATIONS
• Contraindicated in renal failure, except as emergency volume expander. Use cautiously in congestive heart failure, circulatory insufficiency, renal dys-

function, hypoproteinemia, and pulmonary edema.
• Ringer's injection, lactated, contains sodium, 130 mEq/liter; potassium, 4 mEq/liter; calcium, 2.7 mEq/liter; chloride, 109.7 mEq/liter; and lactate, 27 mEq/liter.
• Approximates more closely the electrolyte concentration in blood plasma than Ringer's injection.
• May be given with dextrose infusion.

sodium chloride

INDICATIONS & DOSAGE
Highly individualized fluid and electrolyte replacement in hyponatremia due to electrolyte loss or in severe salt depletion—
400 ml of 3% or 5% solutions only with frequent electrolyte determination and only if given slow I.V.; *with 0.45% solution:* 3% to 8% of body weight, according to deficiencies, over 18 to 24 hours; *with 0.9% solution:* 2% to 6% of body weight, according to deficiencies, over 18 to 24 hours.
Management of "heat cramp" due to excessive perspiration—
Adults: 1 g P.O. with every glass of water.

SIDE EFFECTS
CV: aggravation of congestive heart failure; edema and pulmonary edema if too much given or given too rapidly.
Metabolic: hypernatremia and aggravation of existing acidosis with excessive infusion; serious electrolyte disturbance, loss of potassium.

INTERACTIONS
None significant.

NURSING CONSIDERATIONS
• Use with caution in congestive heart failure, circulatory insufficiency, renal dysfunction, hypoproteinemia.
• Infuse 3% and 5% solutions very slowly and with caution to avoid pul-

---

Italicized side effects are common or life-threatening.
*Liquid form contains alcohol. **May contain tartrazine.

monary edema. Use only for critical situations. Observe patient constantly.
• Concentrates available for addition to parenteral nutrient solutions. Don't confuse these small volumes of paren-

terals with sodium chloride injection isotonic 0.9%. *Read label carefully.*
• Monitor serum electrolytes during therapy.

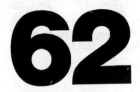

Potassium-removing resin

sodium polystyrene sulfonate

MECHANISM OF ACTION
The potassium-removing resin exchanges sodium ions for potassium ions in the intestine: 1 g of sodium polystyrene sulfonate is exchanged for 0.5 to 1 mEq of potassium. The resin is then eliminated. Much of the exchange capacity is used for cations other than potassium (calcium and magnesium) and possibly for fats and proteins.

COMBINATION PRODUCTS
None.

sodium polystyrene sulfonate
Kayexalate♦

INDICATIONS & DOSAGE
Hyperkalemia—
Adults: 15 g daily to q.i.d. in water or sorbitol (3 to 4 ml/g of resin).
Children: 1 g of resin for each mEq of potassium to be removed.
Oral administration preferred since drug should remain in intestine for at least 6 hours; otherwise, consider nasogastric administration.
Nasogastric administration: mix dose with appropriate medium: aqueous suspension or diet appropriate for renal failure; instill in plastic tube.
Rectal administration:
Adults: 30 to 50 g/100 ml of sorbitol q 6 hours as warm emulsion deep into sigmoid colon (20 cm). In persistent vomiting or paralytic ileus, high retention enema of sodium polystyrene sulfonate (30 g) suspended in 200 ml of 10% methylcellulose, 10% dextrose, or 25% sorbitol solution.

SIDE EFFECTS
GI: *constipation,* fecal impaction (in elderly), anorexia, gastric irritation, nausea, vomiting, *diarrhea (with sorbitol emulsions).*
Other: *hypokalemia,* hypocalcemia, hypomagnesemia, sodium retention.

INTERACTIONS
Antacids and laxatives (nonabsorbable cation-donating type, including magnesium hydroxide): systemic alkalosis, reduced potassium exchange capability. Don't use together.

NURSING CONSIDERATIONS
• Use with caution in elderly patients and those on digitalis therapy, with severe congestive heart failure, severe hypertension, and marked edema.
• Treatment may result in potassium deficiency. Monitor serum potassium at least once daily. Usually stopped when potassium level is reduced to 4 or 5 mEq/liter. Watch for other signs of hypokalemia: irritability, confusion, cardiac arrhythmias, EKG changes, severe muscle weakness and sometimes paralysis, and digitalis toxicity in digitalized patients.
• Monitor for symptoms of other electrolyte deficiencies (magnesium, calcium) since drug is nonselective. Monitor serum calcium determination in patients receiving sodium polystyrene therapy for more than 3 days. Supplementary calcium may be needed.

Italicized side effects are common or life-threatening.
*Liquid form contains alcohol.   **May contain tartrazine.

• Watch for sodium overload. About ⅓ of resin's sodium is retained.

• Use only fresh suspensions. Stir just before use. Discard unused portions after 24 hours.

• Do not heat resin. This will impair effectiveness of drug. Mix resin only with water or sorbitol for P.O. administration. Above all, *never* mix with orange juice (high K⁺ content) to disguise taste.

• Chill oral suspension for greater palatability.

• If sorbitol is given, it may be mixed with resin suspension.

• Consider solid form. Resin cookie and candy recipes are available; perhaps pharmacist or dietitian can supply.

• Watch for constipation in oral or nasogastric administration. Use sorbitol (10 to 20 ml of 70% syrup every 2 hours as needed) to produce one or two watery stools daily.

• Mix polystyrene resin only with water and sorbitol for rectal use. Do not use other vehicles (that is, mineral oil) for rectal administration to prevent impactions. Ion exchange requires aqueous medium. Sorbitol content prevents impaction.

• Prevent fecal impaction in elderly by administering resin rectally. Give cleansing enema before rectal administration. Explain necessity of retaining enema to patient. Retention for 6 to 10 hours is ideal, but 30 to 60 minutes is acceptable.

• Prepare rectal dose at room temperature. Stir emulsion gently during administration.

• Use #28 French rubber tube for rectal dose; insert 20 cm into sigmoid colon. Tape tube in place. Alternatively, consider a Foley catheter with a 30-ml balloon inflated distal to anal sphincter to aid in retention. This is especially helpful for patients with poor sphincter control (for example, after cerebrovascular accident). Use gravity flow. Drain returns constantly through Y-tube connection. When giving rectally, place patient in knee-chest position or with hips on pillow for a while if back-leakage occurs.

• After rectal administration, flush tubing with 50 to 100 ml of nonsodium fluid to ensure delivery of all medication.

• If hyperkalemia is severe, more drastic modalities should be added; for example, dextrose 50% with regular insulin I.V. push. Do not depend solely on polystyrene resin to lower serum potassium levels in severe hyperkalemia.

63

Hematinics

ferrocholinate
ferrous fumarate
ferrous gluconate
ferrous sulfate
iron dextran

MECHANISM OF ACTION
After absorption into the blood, iron is immediately bound to transferrin. Transferrin carries iron to bone marrow, where it's used to synthesize hemoglobin. Some iron is also used to synthesize myoglobin or other nonhemoglobin heme units.

COMBINATION PRODUCTS
FERMALOX: ferrous sulfate 200 mg, and magnesium hydroxide and dried aluminum hydroxide gel 200 mg.
FEROCYL: iron (as fumarate) 50 mg and docusate sodium 100 mg.
FER-REGULES: iron (as fumarate) 150 mg and docusate sodium 100 mg.
FERRO-SEQUELS: iron (as fumarate) 50 mg and docusate sodium 100 mg.
SIMRON: iron (as gluconate) 10 mg and polysorbate 20, 400 mg.

ferrocholinate
Chel-Iron, Firon, Kelex

INDICATIONS & DOSAGE
Iron deficiency—
Adults: 333-mg tablet P.O. t.i.d.
Children: 6 mg/kg P.O. daily in divided doses t.i.d.
Prevention of iron deficiency—
Children: 1 mg/kg P.O. daily as single or divided dose.

SIDE EFFECTS
GI: *nausea,* vomiting, *constipation, black stools.*
Other: stained tooth enamel.

INTERACTIONS
Antacids, cholestyramine resin, pancreatic extracts, vitamin E: decreased iron absorption. Separate doses if possible.
Chloramphenicol: watch for delayed response to iron therapy.
Vitamin C: may increase iron absorption. Beneficial drug interaction.

NURSING CONSIDERATIONS
• Contraindicated in hemosiderosis, hemochromatosis, and hemolytic anemia. Usually contraindicated in peptic ulcer or ulcerative colitis. Use cautiously on long-term basis.
• GI upset related to dose. Between-meal dosing preferable, but can be given with some foods although absorption may be decreased. Enteric-coated products reduce GI upset but also reduce amount of iron absorbed.
• Iron is toxic; parents should be aware of iron poisoning in children.
• Dilute liquid preparations in juice (preferably orange juice) or water, but not in milk or antacids. Give tablets with orange juice to promote iron absorption.
• To avoid staining teeth, give liquid iron preparations with glass straw.
• Check for constipation; record color and amount of stool. Teach dietary measures for preventing constipation.
• Monitor hemoglobin and reticulocyte counts periodically during therapy.

Italicized side effects are common or life-threatening.
∗Liquid form contains alcohol.   ∗∗May contain tartrazine.

ferrous fumarate

Eldofe, F&B Caps, Farbegen, Feco-T, Feostat, Ferranol, Ferrofume♦♦, Fersamal♦♦, Fumasorb, Fumerin, Hematon♦♦, Hemocyte, Ircon, Laud-Iron, Maniron, Novofumar♦♦, Palafer♦♦, Palmiron, Span-FF, Toleron

INDICATIONS & DOSAGE

Iron deficiency states—
Adults: 200 mg P.O. daily t.i.d. or q.i.d.

SIDE EFFECTS

GI: *nausea,* vomiting, *constipation, black stools.*
Other: stained tooth enamel.

INTERACTIONS

Antacids, cholestyramine resin, pancreatic extracts, vitamin E: decreased iron absorption. Separate doses if possible.
Chloramphenicol: watch for delayed response to iron therapy.
Vitamin C: may increase iron absorption. Beneficial drug interaction.

NURSING CONSIDERATIONS

• Contraindicated in peptic ulcer, regional enteritis, ulcerative colitis, hemosiderosis, and hemochromatosis. Use cautiously on long-term basis and in patients with anemia.
• GI upset related to dose. Between-meal dosing preferable, but can be given with some foods although absorption may be decreased. Enteric-coated products reduce GI upset but also reduce amount of iron absorbed.
• Iron is toxic; parents should be aware of iron poisoning in children.
• Tablets may be given with juice or water, but not in milk or antacids. Give with orange juice to promote iron absorption.
• To avoid staining teeth, give liquid iron preparations with glass straw.
• Check for constipation; record color and amount of stool. Teach dietary measures for preventing constipation.
• Monitor hemoglobin and reticulocyte counts during therapy.
• Combination products—Simron, Ferro-Sequels, Ferocyl, Fer-Regules—contain stool softeners to help prevent constipation. Fermalox contains antacids to help relieve GI upset, if present; don't use this product unless absolutely necessary because of decreased iron absorption.

ferrous gluconate

Fergon♦*, Ferralet, Ferrous-G, Fertinic♦♦, Novoferrogluc♦♦

INDICATIONS & DOSAGE

Iron deficiency—
Adults: 200 to 600 mg P.O., t.i.d.
Children 6 to 12 years: 300 to 900 mg P.O. daily.
Children under 6 years: 100 to 300 mg P.O. daily.
1 tablet contains 320 mg ferrous gluconate (37 mg elemental iron).
5 ml of elixir contains 300 mg ferrous gluconate (35 mg elemental iron).

SIDE EFFECTS

GI: *nausea,* vomiting, *constipation, black stools.*
Other: elixir may stain teeth.

INTERACTIONS

Antacids, cholestyramine resin, pancreatic extracts, vitamin E: decreased iron absorption. Separate doses if possible.
Chloramphenicol: watch for delayed response to iron therapy.
Vitamin C: may increase iron absorption. Beneficial drug interaction.

NURSING CONSIDERATIONS

• Contraindicated in peptic ulcer, regional enteritis, ulcerative colitis, hemosiderosis, and hemochromatosis. Use cautiously on long-term basis and in patients with anemia.

Unmarked trade names available in the United States only.
♦ Also available in Canada.   ♦♦ Available in Canada only.

- GI upset related to dose. Between-meal dosing preferable, but can be given with some foods although absorption may be decreased. Enteric-coated products reduce GI upset but also reduce amount of iron absorbed.
- Iron is toxic; parents should be aware of iron poisoning in children.
- Dilute liquid preparations in juice (preferably orange juice) or water, but not in milk or antacids. Give tablets with orange juice to promote absorption.
- To avoid staining teeth, give liquid iron preparations with glass straw.
- Check for constipation; record color and amount of stool. Teach dietary measures for preventing constipation.
- Monitor hemoglobin and reticulocyte counts during therapy.

ferrous sulfate
Arne Modified Caps, Feosol*, Fer-In-Sol♦*, Fero-Grad♦♦, Fero-Gradumet, Ferolix, Ferospace, Ferralyn, Fesofor♦♦, Irospan, Mol-Iron*, Novo-ferrosulfa♦♦, Slow-Fe♦♦, Telefon

INDICATIONS & DOSAGE
Iron deficiency—
Adults: 750 mg to 1.5 g P.O. daily divided t.i.d.; or 225 to 525 mg P.O. sustained-release preparations once daily or q 12 hours.
Children 6 to 12 years: 600 mg P.O. daily in divided doses.
Prophylaxis for iron deficiency anemia—
Pregnant women: 300 to 600 mg P.O. daily in divided doses.
Premature or undernourished infants: 3 to 6 mg/kg P.O. daily in divided doses.

SIDE EFFECTS
GI: *nausea,* vomiting, *constipation, black stools.*
Other: elixir may stain teeth.

INTERACTIONS
Antacids, cholestyramine resin, pancreatic extracts, vitamin E: decreased iron absorption. Separate doses if possible.
Chloramphenicol: watch for delayed response to iron therapy.
Vitamin C: may increase iron absorption. Beneficial drug interaction.

NURSING CONSIDERATIONS
- Contraindicated in peptic ulcer, ulcerative colitis, regional enteritis, hemosiderosis and hemochromatosis. Use cautiously on long-term basis and in patients with anemia.
- GI upset related to dose. Between-meal dosing preferable, but can be given with some foods although absorption may be decreased. Enteric-coated products reduce GI upset but also reduce amount of iron absorbed.
- Iron is toxic; parents should be aware of iron poisoning in children.
- Dilute liquid preparations in juice or water, but not in milk or antacids. Dilute liquids in orange juice; give tablets with orange juice to promote iron absorption.
- To avoid staining teeth, give liquid iron preparations with glass straw.
- Check for constipation; record color and amount of stool. Teach dietary measures for preventing constipation.
- Monitor hemoglobin and reticulocyte counts during therapy.

iron dextran
Hematran, Hydextran, Imferon♦, K-FeRON

INDICATIONS & DOSAGE
Iron deficiency anemia—
Adults: I.M. or I.V. injections of iron are advisable only for patients for whom oral administration is impossible or ineffective. Test dose (0.5 ml) required before administration.
I.M. (by Z-track): inject 0.5 ml test dose. If no reactions, next daily dose

---

Italicized side effects are common or life-threatening.
♦Liquid form contains alcohol.   **May contain tartrazine.

should ordinarily not exceed 0.5 ml (25 mg) for infants under 5 kg; 1 ml (50 mg) for children under 9 kg; 2 ml (100 mg) for patients under 50 kg; 5 ml (250 mg) for patients over 50 kg.

I.V. push: inject 0.5 ml test dose. If no reactions, within 2 to 3 days the dosage may be raised to 2 ml daily I.V., 1 ml/ minute undiluted and infused slowly until total dose is achieved. No single dose should exceed 100 mg of iron.

I.V. infusion: dosages are expressed in terms of elemental iron. Dilute in 250 to 1,000 ml of normal saline solution; dextrose increases local vein irritation. Infuse test dose of 25 mg slowly over 5 minutes. If no reaction occurs in 5 minutes, infusion may be started. Infuse total dose slowly over approximately 6 to 12 hours. 1 ml iron dextran = 50 mg elemental iron.

SIDE EFFECTS
CNS: headache, transitory paresthesias, arthralgia, myalgia, dizziness, malaise, syncope.
CV: *hypotensive reaction, peripheral vascular flushing with overly rapid I.V. administration, tachycardia.*
GI: nausea, vomiting, metallic taste, transient loss of taste perception.
Local: *soreness and inflammation at injection site (I.M.); brown skin discoloration at injection site (I.M.); local phlebitis at injection site (I.V.).*
Skin: rash, urticaria.
Other: *anaphylaxis.*

INTERACTIONS
None significant.

NURSING CONSIDERATIONS
• Contraindicated in all anemias other than iron deficiency anemia. Use with extreme caution in patients with impaired hepatic function and rheumatoid arthritis.
• Monitor vital signs for drug reaction. Reactions are varied and severe, ranging from pain, inflammation, and myalgia to hypotension, shock, and death.
• Inject deeply into upper outer quadrant of buttock—never into arm or other exposed area—with a 2- to 3-inch, 19G or 20G needle. Use Z-track technique to avoid leakage into subcutaneous tissue and tattooing of skin.
• Hemoglobin concentration, hematocrit, and reticulocyte count should be determined periodically.
• Use I.V. in these situations: insufficient muscle mass for deep intramuscular injection; impaired absorption from muscle due to stasis or edema; possibility of uncontrolled intramuscular bleeding from trauma (as may occur in hemophilia); and when massive and prolonged parenteral therapy is indicated (as may be necessary in cases of chronic substantial blood loss).
• Upon completion of I.V. iron dextran infusion, flush the vein with 10 ml of 0.9% sodium chloride injection.
• Patient should rest 15 to 30 minutes after I.V. administration.
• Check hospital policy before administering I.V. In some hospitals, only doctor may administer iron I.V.
• Not removed by hemodialysis.

64

Anticoagulants and heparin antagonist

anisindione
dicumarol
heparin calcium
heparin sodium
phenindione
phenprocoumon
protamine sulfate
warfarin potassium
warfarin sodium

MECHANISM OF ACTION
• Heparin accelerates formation of an antithrombin III-thrombin complex. It inactivates thrombin and prevents conversion of fibrinogen to fibrin.
• The oral anticoagulants inhibit vitamin K–dependent activation of clotting factors II, VII, IX, and X, which are formed in the liver.
• Protamine sulfate, a strong base, forms a physiologically inert complex with heparin sodium, a strong acid.

COMBINATION PRODUCTS
None.

---

anisindione
Miradon

INDICATIONS & DOSAGE
Treatment of pulmonary emboli; prevention and treatment of deep vein thrombosis, myocardial infarction, rheumatic heart disease with heart valve damage, atrial arrhythmias—
Adults: 300 mg P.O. first day, 200 mg P.O. second day, 100 mg P.O. third day. Maintenance dose: 25 to 250 mg daily based on prothrombin times.

SIDE EFFECTS
Blood: *hemorrhage with excessive dosage, agranulocytosis,* leukopenia, leukocytosis, eosinophilia.
CNS: headache.
CV: myocarditis, tachycardia.
EENT: conjunctivitis, blurred vision, paralysis of ocular accommodation.
GI: diarrhea, sore mouth and throat.
GU: *nephropathy with renal tubular necrosis,* albuminuria.
Hepatic: jaundice.
Skin: *rash, severe exfoliative dermatitis.*
Other: *fever.*

INTERACTIONS
Allopurinol, chloramphenicol, danazol, clofibrate, diflunisal, dextrothyraxine, thyroid drugs, heparin, anabolic steroids, cimetidine, disulfiram, glucagon, inhalation anesthetics, metronidazole, quinidine, influenza vaccine, sulindac, sulfonamides: increased prothrombin time. Monitor patient carefully for bleeding. Consider anticoagulant dose reduction.
Ethacrynic acid, indomethacin, mefenamic acid, oxyphenbutazone, phenylbutazone, salicylates: increased prothrombin time; ulcerogenic effects. Don't use together.
Griseofulvin, haloperiodol, carbamazepine, paraldehyde, rifampin: decreased prothrombin time with reduced anticoagulant effect. Monitor patient carefully.
Glutethimide, chloral hydrate, sulfinpyrazone, triclofos sodium: increased or decreased prothrombin time. Avoid use if possible, or monitor patient carefully.

Italicized side effects are common or life-threatening.
*Liquid form contains alcohol.   **May contain tartrazine.

Barbiturates: inhibition of hypoprothrombinemic effect of anticoagulants. If barbiturates are withdrawn, reduce anticoagulant dose; inhibition may last weeks after barbiturate is withdrawn, but fatal hemorrhage can occur when inhibiting effect disappears.
Cholestyramine: decreased response when administered too close together. Administer 6 hours after oral anticoagulants.

NURSING CONSIDERATIONS

• Contraindicated in hemophilia, thrombocytopenic purpura, leukemia with pronounced bleeding tendency, open wounds or ulcers, impaired hepatic or renal function, severe hypertension, acute nephritis, subacute bacterial endocarditis. Use cautiously in pregnancy or lactation, during menses, during use of any drainage tube in any orifice, and in any patient in whom slight bleeding is dangerous. Use with extreme caution (if at all) in psychiatric patients, debilitated patients, or cachectic patients.
• Use caution when adding or stopping any drug for patient receiving anticoagulants. May change the clotting status and result in hemorrhage.
• Fever and skin rash signal severe complications.
• Give drug at same time daily. Stress importance of complying with recommended dosage and keeping follow-up appointments. Patient should carry a card that identifies him as a potential bleeder.
• Regularly inspect patient for bleeding gums, bruises on arms or legs, petechiae, nosebleeds, melena, tarry stools, hematuria, hematemesis. Tell patient and family to watch for these signs and notify doctor immediately.
• Warn patient to avoid over-the-counter products containing aspirin, other salicylates, or any drugs that may interact with anisindione.
• Because onset of action is delayed, heparin sodium is often given during

first few days of treatment. When heparin is being given simultaneously, don't draw blood for prothrombin time within 5 hours after I.V. heparin administration.
• Schedule doses according to prothrombin time (PT). Doctors usually try to maintain PT at 1.5 to 2 times normal. Numerical PT values depend on procedure and reagents used in individual laboratory.
• Tell patient to notify doctor if menses is heavier than usual. May require adjusting dose.
• Tell patient to use electric razor when shaving to avoid scratching skin, and to brush teeth with a soft toothbrush.
• Warn patient that alkaline urine may turn red-orange.
• Duration of action 1½ to 5 days.
• Light to moderate alcohol intake does not significantly affect prothrombin time.

dicumarol

INDICATIONS & DOSAGE

Treatment of pulmonary emboli; prevention and treatment of deep vein thrombosis, myocardial infarction, rheumatic heart disease with heart valve damage, atrial arrhythmias—
Adults: 200 to 300 mg P.O. on first day, 25 to 200 mg P.O. daily thereafter, based on prothrombin times.

SIDE EFFECTS

Blood: *hemorrhage with excessive dosage,* leukopenia, *agranulocytosis.*
GI: anorexia, nausea, vomiting, cramps, *diarrhea,* mouth ulcers.
GU: hematuria.
Skin: dermatitis, urticaria, alopecia, *rash.*
Other: *fever.*

INTERACTIONS

Allopurinol, chloramphenicol, danazol, clofibrate, diflunisal, dextrothyraxine, thyroid drugs, heparin, anabolic ste-

---

Unmarked trade names available in the United States only.
♦ Also available in Canada.   ♦ ♦ Available in Canada only.

roids, cimetidine, disulfiram, glucagon, inhalation anesthetics, metronidazole, quinidine, influenza vaccine, sulindac, sulfonamides: increased prothrombin time. Monitor patient carefully for bleeding. Consider anticoagulant dose reduction.

Ethacrynic acid, indomethacin, mefenamic acid, oxyphenbutazone, phenylbutazone, salicylates: increased prothrombin time; ulcerogenic effects. Don't use together.

Griseofulvin, haloperiodol, carbamazepine, paraldehyde, rifampin: decreased prothrombin time with reduced anticoagulant effect. Monitor patient carefully.

Glutethimide, chloral hydrate, sulfinpyrazone, triclofos sodium: increased or decreased prothrombin time. Avoid use if possible, or monitor patient carefully.

Barbiturates: inhibition of hypoprothrombinemic effect of anticoagulants. If barbiturates are withdrawn, reduce anticoagulant dose; inhibition may last weeks after barbiturate is withdrawn, but fatal hemorrhage can occur when inhibiting effect disappears.

Cholestyramine: decreased response when administered too close together. Administer 6 hours after oral anticoagulants.

NURSING CONSIDERATIONS

• Contraindicated in hemophilia, thrombocytopenic purpura, leukemia with pronounced bleeding tendency, open wounds or ulcers, impaired hepatic or renal function, severe hypertension, acute nephritis, subacute bacterial endocarditis. Use cautiously in pregnancy or lactation, during menses, during use of any drainage tube, and in any patient in whom slight bleeding is dangerous. Use with extreme caution (if at all) in psychiatric patients, debilitated patients, or cachectic patients.

• Use caution when adding or stopping any drug for patient receiving anticoagulants. May change the clotting status and result in hemorrhage.

• Fever and skin rash signal severe complications.

• Give drug at same time daily. Stress importance of complying with recommended dosage and keeping follow-up appointments. Patient should carry a card that identifies him as a potential bleeder.

• Regularly inspect patient for bleeding gums, bruises on arms or legs, petechiae, nosebleeds, melena, tarry stools, hematuria, hematemesis. Tell patient and family to watch for these signs and notify doctor immediately.

• Warn patient to avoid over-the-counter products containing aspirin, other salicylates, or drugs that may interact with dicumarol.

• Because onset of action is delayed, heparin sodium is often given during first few days of treatment. When heparin is being given simultaneously, don't draw blood for prothrombin time within 5 hours after I.V. heparin administration.

• Dose given depends on prothrombin time (PT). Doctors usually try to maintain PT at 1.5 to 2 times normal. PT values depend on procedure and reagents used in individual laboratory.

• Tell patient to notify doctor if menses is heavier than usual. May require adjusting dose.

• Tell patient to use electric razor when shaving to avoid scratching skin and to brush teeth with a soft toothbrush.

• May turn alkaline urine red-orange.

• Duration of action 2 to 6 days.

• Light to moderate alcohol intake does not significantly affect prothrombin times.

Italicized side effects are common or life-threatening.
∗Liquid form contains alcohol.   ∗∗May contain tartrazine.

heparin calcium
Calciparine

heparin sodium
Hepalean♦♦, Lipo-Hepin,
Liquaemin Sodium, Panheprin

INDICATIONS & DOSAGE
Treatment of deep vein thrombosis, myocardial infarction—
Adults: initially, 5,000 to 7,500 units I.V. push, then adjust dose according to PTT results and give dose I.V. q 4 hours (usually 4,000 to 5,000 units); or 5,000 to 7,500 units I.V. bolus, then 1,000 units/hour by I.V. infusion pump. Wait 8 hours following bolus dose, and adjust hourly rate according to PTT.
Treatment of pulmonary embolism—
Adults: initially, 7,500 to 10,000 units I.V. push, then adjust dose according to PTT results and give dose I.V. q 4 hours (usually 4,000 to 5,000 units); or 7,500 to 10,000 units I.V. bolus, then 1,000 units hourly by I.V. infusion pump. Wait 8 hours following bolus dose, and adjust hourly rate according to PTT.
Prophylaxis of embolism—
Adults: 5,000 units S.C. q 12 hours.
Open heart surgery—
Adults: (total body perfusion) 150 to 300 units/kg continuous I.V infusion.
Treatment of pulmonary emboli; prevention and treatment of deep vein thrombosis—
Children: initially, 50 units/kg I.V. drip. Maintenance dose 100 units/kg I.V. drip q 4 hours. Constant infusion: 20,000 units/m² daily. Dosages adjusted according to PTT.
Heparin dosing is highly individualized, depending upon disease state, age, renal and hepatic status.

SIDE EFFECTS
Blood: *hemorrhage with excessive dosage, overly prolonged clotting time, thrombocytopenia.*
Local: irritation, mild pain.

Other: hypersensitivity reactions including chills, fever, pruritus, rhinitis, burning of feet, conjunctivitis, lacrimation, arthralgia, urticaria.

INTERACTIONS
Salicylates: increased anticoagulant effect. Don't use together.
Anticoagulants, oral: additive anticoagulation. Monitor prothrombin time and partial thromboplastin time.

NURSING CONSIDERATIONS
• Conditionally contraindicated in active bleeding; blood dyscrasias; or bleeding tendencies such as hemophilia, thrombocytopenia, or hepatic disease with hypoprothrombinemia; suspected intracranial hemorrhage; suppurative thrombophlebitis; inaccessible ulcerative lesions (especially of GI tract); open ulcerative wounds; extensive denudation of skin; ascorbic acid deficiency and other conditions causing increased capillary permeability; during or after brain, eye, or spinal cord surgery; during continuous tube drainage of stomach or small intestine; in subacute bacterial endocarditis; shock; advanced renal disease; threatened abortion; severe hypertension. Although the use of heparin is clearly hazardous in these conditions, a decision to use it depends on the comparative risk in failure to treat the coexisting thromboembolic disorder.
• Use cautiously during menses; in mild hepatic or renal disease; alcoholism; in patients in occupations with the risk of physical injury; immediately postpartum; and in patients with history of allergies, asthma, or GI ulcers.
• Monitor platelet counts regularly. Thrombocytopenia caused by heparin may be associated with arterial thrombosis.
• Measure partial thromboplastin time (PTT) carefully and regularly. Anticoagulation present when PTT values are 1.5 to 2 times control values.
• Drug requirements are higher in

early phases of thrombogenic diseases and febrile states; lower when patient becomes stabilized.

• Regularly inspect patient for bleeding gums, bruises on arms or legs, petechiae, nosebleeds, melena, tarry stools, hematuria, hematemesis. Tell patient and family to watch for these signs and notify doctor immediately.

• Tell patient to avoid over-the-counter medications containing aspirin, other salicylates, or drugs that may interact with heparin.

• Heparin comes in various concentrations. Check order and vial carefully.

• Low-dose injections given sequentially between iliac crests in lower abdomen deep into subcutaneous fat. Inject drug slowly subcutaneously into fat pad. Leave needle in place for 10 seconds after injection; then withdraw needle. Alternate site every 12 hours—right for a.m., left for p.m.

• Don't massage after subcutaneous injection. Watch for signs of bleeding at injection site. Rotate sites and keep accurate record.

• Check constant I.V. infusions regularly, even when pumps are in good working order, to prevent overdosage or underdosage.

• I.M. administration not recommended.

• I.V. administration preferred because of long-term effect and irregular absorption when given subcutaneously. Whenever possible, administer I.V. heparin using infusion pump to provide maximum safety.

• Concentrated heparin solutions (greater than 100 units/ml) can irritate blood vessels.

• Place notice above patient's bed to inform I.V. team or lab personnel to apply pressure dressings after taking blood.

• Avoid excessive I.M. injections of other drugs to prevent or minimize hematomas. If possible, don't give I.M. injections at all.

• Elderly patients should usually start at lower doses.

• When intermittent I.V. therapy is utilized, always draw blood ½ hour before next scheduled dose to avoid falsely elevated PTT.

• Blood for PTT can be drawn any time after 8 hours of initiation of continuous I.V. heparin therapy. Never draw blood for PTT from the I.V. tubing of the heparin infusion, or from vein of infusion. Falsely elevated PTT will result. Always draw blood from opposite arm.

• Give on time; try not to skip a dose or "catch up" with an I.V. containing heparin. If I.V. is out, get it restarted as soon as possible, and reschedule bolus dose immediately.

• Never piggyback other drugs into an infusion line while heparin infusion is running. Many antibiotics and other drugs inactivate heparin. Never mix any drug with heparin in syringe when bolus therapy is used.

• Abrupt withdrawal may cause increased coagulability. Usually, heparin therapy is followed by oral anticoagulants for prophylaxis.

phenindione
Danilone♦♦, Eridione, Hedulin

INDICATIONS & DOSAGE
Treatment of pulmonary emboli; prevention and treatment of deep vein thrombosis, myocardial infarction, rheumatic heart disease with heart valve damage, atrial arrhythmias—
Adults: 300 mg P.O. first day; 200 mg P.O. second day. Maintenance dose: 50 to 150 mg daily, based on prothrombin times.

SIDE EFFECTS
Blood: *hemorrhage with excessive dosage, agranulocytosis,* leukopenia, leukocytosis, eosinophilia.
CNS: headache.
CV: myocarditis, tachycardia.

Italicized side effects are common or life-threatening.
∗Liquid form contains alcohol.　　∗∗May contain tartrazine.

EENT: conjunctivitis, blurred vision, paralysis of ocular accommodation.
GI: diarrhea, sore mouth and throat.
GU: *nephropathy with renal tubular necrosis,* albuminuria.
Hepatic: jaundice.
Skin: *rash, severe exfoliative dermatitis.*
Other: *fever.*

INTERACTIONS

Allopurinol, chloramphenicol, danazol, clofibrate, diflunisal, dextrothyraxine, thyroid drugs, heparin, anabolic steroids, cimetidine, disulfiram, glucagon, inhalation anesthetics, metronidazole, quinidine, influenza vaccine, sulindac, sulfonamides: increased prothrombin time. Monitor patient carefully for bleeding. Consider anticoagulant dose reduction.

Ethacrynic acid, indomethacin, mefenamic acid, oxyphenbutazone, phenylbutazone, salicylates: increased prothrombin time; ulcerogenic effects. Don't use together.

Griseofulvin, haloperiodol, carbamazepine, paraldehyde, rifampin: decreased prothrombin time with reduced anticoagulant effect. Monitor patient carefully.

Glutethimide, chloral hydrate, sulfinpyrazone, triclofos sodium: increased or decreased prothrombin time. Avoid use if possible, or monitor patient carefully.

Barbiturates: inhibition of hypoprothrombinemic effect of anticoagulants. If barbiturates are withdrawn, reduce anticoagulant dose; inhibition may last weeks after barbiturate is withdrawn, but fatal hemorrhage can occur when inhibiting effect disappears.

Cholestyramine: decreased response when administered too close together. Administer 6 hours after oral anticoagulants.

NURSING CONSIDERATIONS

• Contraindicated in hemophilia, thrombocytopenic purpura, leukemia with pronounced bleeding tendency, open wounds or ulcers, impaired hepatic or renal function, severe hypertension, acute nephritis, and subacute bacterial endocarditis. Use cautiously in pregnancy or lactation, during menses, during use of any drainage tube in any orifice, and in any patient in whom slight bleeding is dangerous. Use with extreme caution (if at all) in psychiatric patients, debilitated patients, or cachectic patients.

• Use caution when adding or stopping any drug. May cause alteration in clotting status and result in hemorrhage.

• Fever and skin rash signal severe complications.

• Give drug at same time daily. Stress importance of complying with recommended dosage and keeping follow-up appointments. Patient should carry a card that identifies him as a potential bleeder.

• Regularly inspect patient for bleeding gums, bruises on arms or legs, petechiae, nosebleeds, melena, tarry stools, hematuria, hematemesis. Tell patient and family to watch for these signs and notify doctor immediately.

• Warn patient to avoid over-the-counter products containing aspirin, salicylates, or other drugs that may interact with phenindione.

• Because onset of action is delayed, heparin sodium is often given during first few days of treatment. When heparin is being given simultaneously, don't draw blood for prothrombin time within 5 hours after I.V. heparin administration.

• Dose given depends on prothrombin time (PT). Doctors usually try to maintain PT at 1.5 to 2 times normal. Numerical PT values depend on procedure and reagents used in individual laboratory.

• Tell patient to notify doctor if menses is heavier than usual. May require adjusting dose.

• Tell patient to use electric razor when

shaving to avoid scratching skin and to brush teeth with a soft toothbrush.
• Warn patient that alkaline urine may turn red-orange.
• Duration of action is 2 to 4 days.
• Light to moderate alcohol intake does not significantly affect prothrombin time.

phenprocoumon
Liquamar

INDICATIONS & DOSAGE
Treatment of pulmonary emboli; prevention and treatment of deep vein thrombosis, myocardial infarction, rheumatic heart disease with heart valve damage, atrial arrhythmias—
Adults: initially, 24 mg P.O. Maintenance dose: 0.75 to 6 mg daily, based on prothrombin time.

SIDE EFFECTS
Blood: *hemorrhage with excessive dosage, agranulocytosis,* leukopenia.
GI: paralytic ileus and intestinal obstruction (both resulting from hemorrhage), nausea, vomiting, cramps, diarrhea, mouth ulcers.
GU: nephropathy, hematuria.
Skin: *rash,* alopecia, necrosis.
Other: *fever.*

INTERACTIONS
Allopurinol, chloramphenicol, danazol, clofibrate, diflunisal, dextrothyraxine, thyroid drugs, heparin, anabolic steroids, cimetidine, disulfiram, glucagon, inhalation anesthetics, metronidazole, quinidine, influenza vaccine, sulindac, sulfonamides: increased prothrombin time. Monitor patient carefully for bleeding. Consider anticoagulant dose reduction.
Ethacrynic acid, indomethacin, mefenamic acid, oxyphenbutazone, phenylbutazone, salicylates: increased prothrombin time; ulcerogenic effects. Don't use together.
Griseofulvin, haloperiodol, carbamaze-

pine, paraldehyde, rifampin: decreased prothrombin time with reduced anticoagulant effect. Monitor patient carefully.
Glutethimide, chloral hydrate, sulfinpyrazone, triclofos sodium: increased or decreased prothrombin time. Avoid use if possible, or monitor patient carefully.
Barbiturates: inhibition of hypoprothrombinemic effect of anticoagulants. If barbiturates are withdrawn, reduce anticoagulant dose; inhibition may last weeks after barbiturate is withdrawn, but fatal hemorrhage can occur when inhibiting effect disappears.
Cholestyramine: decreased response when administered too close together. Administer 6 hours after oral anticoagulants.

NURSING CONSIDERATIONS
• Contraindicated in hemophilia, thrombocytopenic purpura, leukemia with pronounced bleeding tendency, open wounds or ulcers, impaired hepatic or renal function, severe hypertension, acute nephritis, and subacute bacterial endocarditis. Use cautiously in pregnancy or lactation, during menses, during use of any drainage tube in any orifice, and in any patient in whom slight bleeding is dangerous. Use with extreme caution (if at all) in psychiatric, debilitated, or cachectic patients.
• Use caution when adding or stopping any drug for patient receiving anticoagulants. May change the clotting status and result in hemorrhage.
• Fever and skin rash signal severe complications.
• Give drug at same time daily. Stress importance of complying with recommended dosage and keeping follow-up appointments. Patient should carry a card that identifies him as a potential bleeder.
• Regularly inspect patient for bleeding gums, bruises on arms or legs, petechiae, nosebleeds, melena, tarry stools, hematuria, hematemesis. Tell patient

---

Italicized side effects are common or life-threatening.
∗Liquid form contains alcohol.   ∗∗May contain tartrazine.

and family to watch for these signs and notify doctor immediately.

• Warn patient to avoid over-the-counter products containing aspirin, other salicylates, or drugs that may interact with phenprocoumon.

• Because onset of action is delayed, heparin sodium is often given during first few days of treatment. When heparin is being given simultaneously, don't draw blood for protrombin time within 5 hours of I.V. heparin administration.

• Dose given depends on prothombin time (PT). Doctors usually try to maintain PT at 1.5 to 2 times normal. Numerical PT values depend on procedure and reagents used in individual laboratory.

• Tell patient to notify doctor if menses is heavier than usual. May require adjusting dose.

• Tell patient to use electric razor when shaving to avoid scratching skin and to brush teeth with a soft toothbrush.

• Warn patient that alkaline urine may turn orange-red.

• A coumarin derivative.

• Duration of action is 7 to 14 days.

• Light to moderate alcohol intake does not significantly affect prothrombin times.

---

protamine sulfate

INDICATIONS & DOSAGE

Heparin overdose—
Adults: dosage based on venous blood coagulation studies, generally 1 mg for each 78 to 95 units of heparin. Give diluted to 1% (10 mg/ml) slow I.V. injection over 1 to 3 minutes. Maximum 50 mg/10 minutes.

SIDE EFFECTS

CV: fall in blood pressure, bradycardia.
Other: transitory flushing, feeling of warmth, dyspnea.

INTERACTIONS

None significant.

NURSING CONSIDERATIONS

• Use cautiously after cardiac surgery.

• Doctor gives this drug. Should be given slowly to reduce side effects. Have equipment available to treat shock.

• Monitor patient continually. Check vital signs frequently.

• Watch for spontaneous bleeding (heparin "rebound"), especially in patients undergoing dialysis and those who have had cardiac surgery.

• Protamine sulfate may act as anticoagulant in very high doses.

• 1 mg of protamine neutralizes 78 to 95 units of heparin.

• Heparin antagonist.

---

warfarin potassium
Athrombin-K♦

warfarin sodium
Coumadin♦, Panwarfin, Warfilone Sodium♦♦, Warnerin Sodium♦♦

INDICATIONS & DOSAGE

Treatment of pulmonary emboli; prevention and treatment of deep vein thrombosis, myocardial infarction, rheumatic heart disease with heart valve damage, atrial arrhythmias—
Adults: 10 to 15 mg P.O. for 3 days, then dosage based on daily prothrombin times. Usual maintenance dose 2 to 10 mg P.O. daily. Alternate regimen: initially, 40 to 60 mg P.O. daily; then 2 to 10 mg daily based on PT determinations.
Warfarin sodium also available for I.V. use (50 mg/vial). Reconstitute with sterile water for injection. I.V. form rarely used and may be in periodic short supply.

SIDE EFFECTS

Blood: *hemorrhage with excessive dosage,* leukopenia.

GI: paralytic ileus, intestinal obstruction (both resulting from hemorrhage), diarrhea, vomiting, cramps, nausea.
GU: excessive uterine bleeding.
Skin: dermatitis, urticaria, *rash*, necrosis, alopecia.
Other: *fever*.

INTERACTIONS

Allopurinol, chloramphenicol, danazol, clofibrate, diflunisal, dextrothyraxine, thyroid drugs, heparin, anabolic steroids, cimetidine, disulfiram, glucagon, inhalation anesthetics, metronidazole, quinidine, influenza vaccine, sulindac, sulfonamides: increased prothrombin time. Monitor patient carefully for bleeding. Consider anticoagulant dose reduction.

Ethacrynic acid, indomethacin, mefenamic acid, oxyphenbutazone, phenylbutazone, salicylates: increased prothrombin time; ulcerogenic effects. Don't use together.

Griseofulvin, haloperiodol, carbamazepine, paraldehyde, rifampin: decreased prothrombin time with reduced anticoagulant effect. Monitor patient carefully.

Glutethimide, chloral hydrate, sulfinpyrazone, triclofos sodium: increased or decreased prothrombin time. Avoid use if possible, or monitor patient carefully.

Barbiturates: inhibition of hypoprothrombinemic effect of anticoagulants. If barbiturates are withdrawn, reduce anticoagulant dose; inhibition may last weeks after barbiturate is withdrawn, but fatal hemorrhage can occur when inhibiting effect disappears.

Cholestyramine: decreased response when administered too close together. Administer 6 hours after oral anticoagulants.

NURSING CONSIDERATIONS

• Contraindicated in bleeding or hemorrhagic tendencies resulting from open wounds, visceral cancer, GI ulcers, severe hepatic or renal disease, severe uncontrolled hypertension, subacute bacterial endocarditis, vitamin K deficiency; after recent operations in eye, brain, or spinal cord. Use cautiously in diverticulitis, colitis, mild or moderate hypertension, mild or moderate hepatic or renal disease, lactation; in presence of drainage tubes in any orifice; with regional or lumbar block anesthesia; or in any condition increasing risk of hemorrhage.

• Observe nursing infants of mothers on drug for unexpected bleeding.

• PT determinations essential for proper control. High incidence of bleeding when PT exceeds 2.5 times control values. Doctors usually try to maintain PT at 1.5 to 2 times normal.

• Give at same time daily. Stress importance of complying with recommended dosage and keeping follow-up appointments. Patient should carry a card that identifies him as a potential bleeder.

• Elderly patients and patients with renal or hepatic failure are especially sensitive to warfarin effect.

• Half-life of warfarin is 36 to 44 hours.

• Warfarin effect can be neutralized by vitamin K injections.

• Regularly inspect patient for bleeding gums, bruises on arms or legs, petechiae, nosebleeds, melena, tarry stools, hematuria, hematemesis. Tell patient and family to watch for these signs and notify doctor immediately.

• Warn patient to avoid over-the-counter products containing aspirin, other salicylates, or drugs that may interact with warfarin potassium or warfarin sodium.

• Food and enteral feedings that contain vitamin K may cause inadequate anticoagulation. Warn patient to read labels.

• Because onset of action is delayed, heparin sodium is often given during first few days of treatment. When heparin is being given simultaneously, don't draw blood for prothrombin time

---

within 5 hours of I.V. heparin administration.
• Fever and skin rash signal severe complications.
• Tell patient to notify doctor if menses is heavier than usual. May require adjusting dose.
• Tell patient to use electric razor when shaving to avoid scratching skin and to brush teeth with a soft toothbrush.
• Best oral anticoagulant when patient must receive antacids or phenytoin.
• Light to moderate alcohol intake does not significantly affect prothrombin time.
• Possibly effective in treatment of transient cerebral ischemic attacks.

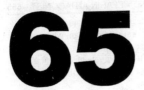

Hemostatics

absorbable gelatin sponge
aminocaproic acid
antihemophilic factor (AHF)
carbazochrome salicylate
Factor IX complex
microfibrillar collagen hemostat
negatol
oxidized cellulose
thrombin

MECHANISM OF ACTION
• Absorbable gelatin sponge and oxidized cellulose absorb and hold many times their weight in blood. Absorbable gelatin sponge also provides a framework for growth of granulation tissue.
• Aminocaproic acid inhibits plasminogen activator substances. To a lesser degree, it blocks antiplasmin activity by inhibiting fibrinolysis.
• Antihemophilic factor and Factor IX complex directly replace deficient clotting factors.
• Carbazochrome salicylate decreases capillary permeability.
• Microfibrillar collagen hemostat attracts and aggregates platelets.
• Negatol is an astringent and protein denaturant.
• Thrombin clots to form fibrin in the presence of fibrinogen.

COMBINATION PRODUCTS
None.

absorbable gelatin sponge
Gelfoam

INDICATIONS & DOSAGE
Adults:

Decubitus ulcers—place aseptically deep into ulcer. Don't disturb or remove; may add extra p.r.n.
To provide hemostasis in surgery (adjunct)—apply saturated with isotonic NaCl injection or thrombin solution. Hold in place for 10 to 15 seconds. When bleeding is controlled, allow material to remain in place.

SIDE EFFECTS
None reported.

INTERACTIONS
None significant.

NURSING CONSIDERATIONS
• Contraindicated in frank infection, as sole hemostatic agent in abnormal bleeding, or in postpartum bleeding or hemorrhage.
• Avoid overpacking when placed into body cavities or closed tissue spaces.
• Systemically absorbed within 4 to 6 weeks; no need to remove.

aminocaproic acid
Amicar♦

INDICATIONS & DOSAGE
Excessive bleeding resulting from hyperfibrinolysis—
Adults: initially, 5 g P.O. or slow I.V. infusion, followed by 1 to 1.25 g hourly until bleeding is controlled. Maximum dose 30 g daily.

SIDE EFFECTS
Blood: generalized thrombosis.
CNS: dizziness, malaise, headache.

Italicized side effects are common or life-threatening.
*Liquid form contains alcohol.   **May contain tartrazine.

CV: hypotension, bradycardia, arrhythmia (with rapid I.V. infusion).
EENT: tinnitus, nasal stuffiness, conjunctival suffusion.
GI: nausea, cramps, diarrhea.
Skin: rash.
Other: malaise.

INTERACTIONS
Oral contraceptives: increased probability of hypercoagulability. Use together cautiously.

NURSING CONSIDERATIONS
• Contraindicated in active intravascular clotting. Use cautiously in thrombophlebitis and cardiac, hepatic, or renal disease.
• Monitor coagulation studies, heart rhythm, and blood pressure. Notify doctor of any change immediately.
• Also used as antidote for streptokinase or urokinase toxicity; not beneficial in the treatment of thrombocytopenia.
• Dilute solution with sterile water for injection, normal saline injection, 5% dextrose in water, or Ringer's injection.

antihemophilic factor (AHF)
Antihemophilic Globulin (AHG),
Factorate, Hemofil, Humafac,
Koate, Profilate

INDICATIONS & DOSAGE
Hemophilia A (Factor VIII deficiency)—
Adults and children: 10 to 20 units/kg I.V. push or infusion q 8 to 24 hours. Maintenance doses may be less. Infusion rate usually 10 to 20 ml reconstituted solution per 3 minutes. Dosage varies with individual needs.

SIDE EFFECTS
CNS: headache, paresthesias, clouding or loss of consciousness.
CV: tachycardia, hypotension, possible intravascular hemolysis in patients with blood type A, B, or AB.

EENT: disturbed vision.
GI: nausea, vomiting.
Skin: erythema, urticaria.
Other: *chills, fever, backache, flushing,* constriction in chest; hypersensitivity.

INTERACTIONS
None significant.

NURSING CONSIDERATIONS
• Use cautiously in neonates, infants, and patients with hepatic disease because of susceptibility to hepatitis, which may be transmitted in antihemophilic factor.
• Have blood typed and crossmatched to treat possible hemorrhage.
• Monitor vital signs regularly. Take baseline pulse rate before I.V. administration. If pulse rate increases significantly, flow rate should be reduced or administration stopped.
• Monitor patient for allergic reactions.
• For I.V. use only. Use plastic syringe; drug may interact with glass syringe, causing binding of ground-glass surface.
• Refrigerate concentrate until ready to use, but not after reconstituted. Refrigeration after reconstitution may cause the active ingredient to precipitate. Before reconstituting, concentrate and diluent bottles should be warmed to room temperature. To mix drug, gently roll vial between your hands. Reconstituted solution unstable; use within 3 hours. Store away from heat. Don't shake or mix with other I.V. solutions.
• Monitor coagulation studies before and during therapy.

carbazochrome salicylate
Adrenosem Salicylate

INDICATIONS & DOSAGE
Surgery with excessive capillary bleeding or oozing—
Adults and children over 12 years: 10

mg I.M. preoperatively on night before surgery and with on-call medication, and 5 mg P.O. or I.M. postoperatively q 2 to 4 hours.
Children under 12 years: 5 mg I.M. preoperatively on night before surgery and with on-call medication, and 2.5 mg P.O. or I.M. postoperatively q 2 to 4 hours.

SIDE EFFECTS
Local: pain at I.M. injection site.

INTERACTIONS
None significant.

NURSING CONSIDERATIONS
• Contraindicated in hypersensitivity to salicylates.
• Obtain patient history of allergies, especially to salicylates.
• Has no effect on clotting time, prothrombin time, and vitamin K levels.

Factor IX complex
Konyne, Proplex, Profilnine

INDICATIONS & DOSAGE
Factor IX deficiency (hemophilia B or Christmas disease), anticoagulant overdosage—
Adults and children: units required equal 0.6 × body weight in kg × percentage of desired increase of Factor IX level, by slow I.V. infusion or I.V. push. Dosage is highly individualized, depending on degree of deficiency, level of Factor IX desired, weight of patient, and severity of bleeding.

SIDE EFFECTS
CNS: headache.
CV: : *thromboembolic reactions,* possible intravascular hemolysis in patients with blood types A, B, AB.
Other: *transient fever, chills, flushing, tingling,* hypersensitivity.

INTERACTIONS
None significant.

NURSING CONSIDERATIONS
• Contraindicated in hepatic disease, intravascular coagulation, or fibrinolysis. Use cautiously in neonates and infants because of susceptibility to hepatitis, which may be transmitted with Factor IX complex.
• Have blood typed and crossmatched to treat possible hemorrhage. If given to patients with blood types A, B, AB, intravascular hemolysis may occur.
• Observe patient for allergic reactions, and monitor vital signs regularly.
• Avoid rapid infusion. If tingling sensation, fever, chills, or headache develops during I.V. infusion, decrease flow rate and notify the doctor.
• Reconstitute with 20 ml sterile water for injection for each vial of lyophilized drug. Keep refrigerated until ready to use; warm to room temperature before reconstituting. Use within 3 hours of reconstitution. Unstable in solution. Don't shake, refrigerate, or mix reconstituted solution with other I.V. solutions. Store away from heat.

---

microfibrillar collagen hemostat
Avitene

INDICATIONS & DOSAGE
To provide hemostasis in surgery (adjunct)—
Adults and children: amount depends on severity of bleeding. Compress area with dry sponges. Apply drug directly to bleeding site for 1 to 5 minutes. Gently remove excess. Reapply if needed.

SIDE EFFECTS
Blood: hematoma.
Local: exacerbation of wound dehiscence, abscess formation, foreign body reaction, adhesion formation.
Other: enhanced infection in contaminated wounds, mediastinitis, hypersensitivity.

Italicized side effects are common or life-threatening.
*Liquid form contains alcohol.   **May contain tartrazine.

INTERACTIONS
None significant.

NURSING CONSIDERATIONS
• Contraindicated in closure of skin incisions; it may interfere with healing.
• Not for injection.
• Don't spill on nonbleeding surfaces.
• Don't dilute. Always apply dry.
• Adheres to wet gloves, instruments, or tissue surfaces. Handle and apply with smooth, dry forceps. Apply directly to source of bleeding.

negatol
Negatan

INDICATIONS & DOSAGE
Cervical bleeding—
Women: apply 1-inch gauze dipped in 1:10 dilution of drug; insert in cervical canal. If tolerated, may increase to full-strength solution. Remove pack after 24 hours; give 2-quart douche of dilute negatol or vinegar.
Oral ulcers—
Adults and children: apply to dried lesion with applicator, leave for 1 minute, then neutralize with large amounts of water.

SIDE EFFECTS
Local: *burning sensation.*
Skin: erythema, superficial desquamation when applied to skin.

INTERACTIONS
None significant.

NURSING CONSIDERATIONS
• Vaginal membrane turns grayish after vaginal use.
• When used in vagina, patient should wear a perineal pad to prevent soiling of clothing.
• When used for oral ulcers, may apply topical anesthetic first to prevent burning sensation.
• Always clean and dry area to be treated.

• Astringent, styptic, and protein denaturant; highly acidic.

oxidized cellulose
Oxycel♦, Surgicel

INDICATIONS & DOSAGE
To provide hemostasis in surgery (adjunct)—
Adults and children: apply with sterile technique, p.r.n. Remove after hemostasis, if possible, with dry sterile forceps. Leave in place if necessary.

SIDE EFFECTS
CNS: headache when used as packing for epistaxis, or after rhinologic procedures or application to surface wounds.
EENT: sneezing, epistaxis or stinging, burning when used as packing for rhinologic procedures; nasal membrane necrosis or septal perforation.
Local: encapsulation of fluid, foreign body reaction, burning or stinging after application to surface wounds.
Other: possible prolongation of drainage in cholecystectomies.

INTERACTIONS
None significant.

NURSING CONSIDERATIONS
• Contraindicated in controlling hemorrhage from large arteries; in nonhemorrhagic, serous, oozing surfaces; in implantation in bone defects.
• Don't pack or wad unless it will be removed after hemostasis. Don't apply too tightly when used as wrap sheet in vascular surgery. Apply loosely against bleeding surface.
• Always remove after hemostasis when used in laminectomies or near optic nerve chain.
• Don't autoclave this product.
• Use only amount needed to produce hemostasis. Remove excess before surgical closure.
• Use minimal amounts in urologic procedures.

- In large wounds, don't overlap skin edges.
- Use sterile technique to remove from open wounds after hemostasis. Don't remove without irrigating material first; otherwise, fresh bleeding may occur.
- Don't moisten. Hemostatic effect is greater when applied dry.
- Should not be used for permanent packing in fractures because it may result in cyst formation.

thrombin
Fibrindex, Thrombinar

INDICATIONS & DOSAGE
Bleeding from parenchymatous tissue, cancellous bone, dental sockets, nasal and laryngeal surgery, and in plastic surgery and skin-grafting procedures—
Adults: apply 100 units per ml of sterile isotonic NaCl solution or sterile distilled water to area where clotting needed (or may apply dry powder in bone surgery); in major bleeding, apply 1,000 to 2,000 units/ml sterile isotonic NaCl solution. Sponge blood from area before application, but avoid sponging area after application.
GI hemorrhage—
Adults: give 2 oz of milk, followed by 2 oz of milk containing 10,000 to 20,000 units thrombin. Repeat t.i.d. for 4 to 5 days or until bleeding is controlled.

SIDE EFFECTS
Systemic: hypersensitivity and fever.

INTERACTIONS
None significant.

NURSING CONSIDERATIONS
- Contraindicated in hypersensitivity to thrombin or bovine products.
- Obtain patient history of reactions to thrombin or bovine products.
- Observe patient for allergic reactions, and monitor vital signs regularly.
- Have blood typed and crossmatched to treat possible hemorrhage.
- Don't inject topical thrombin or allow it to enter large blood vessels. I.V. injection may cause death because of severe intravascular clotting.
- May be used with absorbable gelatin sponge but not with oxidized cellulose. Check sponge labeling before use.
- Neutralize stomach acids before oral use in GI hemorrhage.
- Keep refrigerated, preferably frozen, until ready to use. Unstable in solution. Use within 24 hours of reconstitution; discard after 48 hours. Store away from heat.
- Broken down by diluted acid, alkali, and salts of heavy metals.

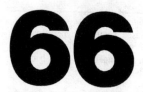

Blood derivatives

normal serum albumin
plasma protein fraction

MECHANISM OF ACTION
● Normal serum albumin 25% provides intravascular oncotic pressure in a 5:1 ratio, which causes a shift of fluid from interstitial spaces to the circulation and slightly increases plasma protein concentration.
● Normal serum albumin 5% and plasma protein fraction supply colloid to the blood and expand plasma volume.

COMBINATION PRODUCTS
None.

normal serum albumin 5%
Albuminar 5%, Albutein 5%, Buminate 5%, Plasbumin 5%

normal serum albumin 25%
Albuminar 25%, Albumisol 25%, Buminate 25%, Plasbumin 25%

INDICATIONS & DOSAGE
Shock—
Adults: initially, 500 ml (5% solution) by I.V. infusion, repeat q 30 minutes, p.r.n. Dose varies with patient's condition and response.
Children: 25% to 50% adult dose in nonemergency.
Hypoproteinemia—
Adults: 1,000 to 1,500 ml 5% solution by I.V. infusion daily, maximum rate 5 to 10 ml/minute; or 25 to 100 g 25% solution by I.V. infusion daily, maxi-

mum rate 3 ml/minute. Dose varies with patient's condition and response.
*Burns—*dosage varies according to extent of burn and patient's condition. Generally maintain plasma albumin at 2 to 3 g/100 ml.
Hyperbilirubinemia—
Infants: 1 g albumin (4 ml 25%)/kg before transfusion.

SIDE EFFECTS
CV: *vascular overload after rapid infusion,* hypotension, altered pulse rate.
GI: increased salivation, nausea, vomiting.
Skin: urticaria.
Other: chills, fever, altered respiration.

INTERACTIONS
None significant.

NURSING CONSIDERATIONS
● Contraindicated in severe anemia and heart failure. Use cautiously in low cardiac reserve, absence of albumin deficiency, and restricted salt intake.
● Do not give more than 250 g in 48 hours.
● Watch for hemorrhage or shock if used after surgery or injury.
● Monitor vital signs carefully.
● Watch for signs of vascular overload (heart failure or pulmonary edema).
● Patient should be properly hydrated before infusion of solution.
● Avoid rapid I.V. infusion. Specific rate is individualized according to patient's age, condition, diagnosis.
● Dilute with sterile water for injection, 0.9% NaCl solution, or 5% dextrose injection. Use solution

promptly; contains no preservatives. Discard unused solution.
- Don't use cloudy solutions or those containing sediment. Solution should be clear amber color.
- Freezing may cause bottle to break. Follow storage instructions on bottle.
- One volume of 25% albumin is equivalent to five volumes of 5% albumin in producing hemodilution and relative anemia.
- This product is very expensive, and random supply shortages occur often.
- Monitor intake and output, hemoglobin, hematocrit, and serum protein and electrolytes during therapy.

plasma protein fraction
Plasmanate, Plasmatein, Protenate

INDICATIONS & DOSAGE
Shock—
Adults: varies with patient's condition and response, but usual dose is 250 to 500 ml (12.5 to 25 g protein), usually not faster than 10 ml/minute.
Children: 22 to 33 ml/kg I.V. infused at rate of 5 to 10 ml/minute.
Hypoproteinemia—
Adults: 1,000 to 1,500 ml I.V. daily. Maximum infusion rate 8 ml/minute.

SIDE EFFECTS
CNS: headache.
CV: variable effects on blood pressure after rapid infusion or intra-arterial administration; *vascular overload after rapid infusion.*
GI: nausea, vomiting, hypersalivation.
Skin: erythema, urticaria.
Other: flushing, chills, fever, back pain, dyspnea.

INTERACTIONS
None significant.

NURSING CONSIDERATIONS
- Contraindicated in patients with severe anemia or heart failure, and in patients undergoing cardiac bypass. Use cautiously in hepatic or renal failure, low cardiac reserve, restricted salt intake.
- Monitor blood pressure. Infusion should be slowed or stopped if hypotension suddenly occurs.
- Vital signs should return to normal gradually; monitor hourly.
- Watch for signs of vascular overload (heart failure or pulmonary edema).
- Monitor intake and output. Watch for decreased urinary output.
- Check expiration date on container before using. Discard solutions in containers that have been opened for more than 4 hours. Solution contains no preservatives.
- Don't use solutions that are cloudy, contain sediment, or have been frozen.
- If patient is dehydrated, give additional fluids either P.O. or I.V.
- Do not give more than 250 g (5,000 ml 5%) in 48 hours.
- Contains 130 to 160 mEq sodium/liter.

Italicized side effects are common or life-threatening.
*Liquid form contains alcohol.   **May contain tartrazine.

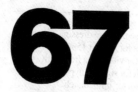

Thrombolytic enzymes

streptokinase
urokinase

MECHANISM OF ACTION
Both streptokinase and urokinase activate plasminogen and convert it to plasmin, which degrades fibrin clots, fibrinogen, and other plasma proteins.
• Streptokinase activates plasminogen in a two-step process. Plasminogen and streptokinase form a complex that exposes the plasminogen-activating site. Plasminogen is converted to plasmin by cleavage of the peptide bond.
• Urokinase activates plasminogen by directly cleaving peptide bonds at two different sites.

COMBINATION PRODUCTS
None.

streptokinase
Kabikinase, Streptase

INDICATIONS & DOSAGE
Arteriovenous cannula occlusion—
Adults: 250,000 IU in 2 ml I.V. solution by I.V. pump infusion into each occluded limb of the cannula over 25 to 35 minutes. Clamp off cannula for 2 hours. Then aspirate contents of cannula; flush with saline solution and reconnect.
Venous thrombosis, pulmonary embolism, and arterial thrombosis and embolism—
Adults: loading dose: 250,000 IU I.V. infusion over 30 minutes. Sustaining dose: 100,000 IU/hour I.V. infusion for 72 hours for deep vein thrombosis and

100,000 IU/hour over 24 to 72 hours by I.V. infusion pump for pulmonary embolism.
Lysis of coronary artery thrombi following acute myocardial infarction—
Adults: loading dose: 20,000 IU via coronary catheter, followed by a maintenance dose. Maintenance dose: 2,000 IU/minute for 60 minutes as an infusion.

SIDE EFFECTS
Blood: *bleeding, decreased hematocrit.*
CV: transient lowering or elevation of blood pressure.
EENT: periorbital edema.
Local: *phlebitis at injection site.*
Skin: urticaria.
Other: *hypersensitivity to drug, anaphylaxis,* musculoskeletal pain, minor breathing difficulty, bronchospasms, angioneurotic edema.

INTERACTIONS
Anticoagulants: concurrent use of anticoagulants with streptokinase is not recommended. Reversing the effects of oral anticoagulants must be considered before beginning therapy, and heparin must be stopped and its effect allowed to diminish.
Aspirin, indomethacin, phenylbutazone, drugs affecting platelet activity: increased risk of bleeding. Do not use together.

NURSING CONSIDERATIONS
• Contraindicated in ulcerative wounds, active internal bleeding, and recent cerebrovascular accident; recent trauma with possible internal injuries;

visceral or intracranial malignancy; ulcerative colitis; diverticulitis; severe hypertension; acute or chronic hepatic or renal insufficiency; uncontrolled hypocoagulation; chronic pulmonary disease with cavitation; subacute bacterial endocarditis or rheumatic valvular disease; recent cerebral embolism, thrombosis, or hemorrhage. Also contraindicated within 10 days after intra-arterial diagnostic procedure or any surgery, including liver or kidney biopsy, lumbar puncture, thoracentesis, paracentesis, or extensive or multiple cutdowns.

• Use cautiously when treating arterial emboli that originate from left side of heart because of danger of cerebral infarction.

• I.M. injections contraindicated during streptokinase therapy.

• Before initiating therapy, draw blood to determine PTT and PT. Rate of I.V. infusion depends on thrombin time and streptokinase resistance.

• If the patient has had either a recent streptococcal infection or recent treatment with streptokinase, a higher loading dose may be necessary.

• Preparation of I.V. solution: reconstitute each vial with 5 ml sodium chloride for injection. Further dilute to 45 ml. Don't shake; roll gently to mix. Use within 24 hours. Store at room temperature in powder form; refrigerate after reconstitution.

• Monitor patient for excessive bleeding; if evident, stop therapy. Pretreatment with heparin or drugs affecting platelets causes high risk of bleeding.

• Have typed and crossmatched packed red cells and whole blood available to treat possible hemorrhage.

• Keep aminocaproic acid available to treat bleeding. Corticosteroids are used to treat allergic reactions.

• Before using streptokinase to clear an occluded arteriovenous cannula, try flushing with heparinized saline solution.

• Bruising more likely during therapy; avoid unnecessary handling.

• Keep venipuncture sites to a minimum; use pressure dressing on puncture sites for at least 15 minutes.

• Monitor vital signs frequently.

• Watch for signs of hypersensitivity. Notify doctor immediately.

• Heparin by continuous infusion is usually started within an hour after stopping streptokinase. Use infusion pump to administer heparin.

• Should be used only by doctors with wide experience in thrombotic disease management where clinical and laboratory monitoring can be performed.

• In the treatment of acute myocardial infarction, streptokinase prevents primary or secondary thrombus formation in the microcirculation surrounding the necrotic area.

---

urokinase
Abbokinase, Breokinase, Win-Kinase

INDICATIONS & DOSAGE
Lysis of acute massive pulmonary emboli and lysis of pulmonary emboli accompanied by unstable hemodynamics—
Adults: for I.V. infusion only by constant infusion pump that will deliver a total volume of 195 ml.
Priming dose: 4,400 IU/kg hourly of urokinase-normal saline solution admixture given over 10 minutes.
Follow with 4,400 IU/kg hourly for 12 to 24 hours. Total volume should not exceed 200 ml.
Follow therapy with continuous I.V. infusion of heparin, then oral anticoagulants.

SIDE EFFECTS
Blood: *bleeding, decreased hematocrit.*
Local: *phlebitis at injection site.*
Other: hypersensitivity (not as frequent as streptokinase), musculoskeletal pain, bronchospasm, *anaphylaxis.*

Italicized side effects are common or life-threatening.
*Liquid form contains alcohol.   **May contain tartrazine.

INTERACTIONS

Anticoagulants: concurrent use of anti-coagulants with urokinase is not recommended. Reversing the effects of oral anticoagulants must be considered before beginning therapy, and heparin must be stopped and its effect allowed to diminish.

Aspirin, indomethacin, phenylbuta-zone, other drugs affecting platelet activity: increased risk of bleeding. Do not use together.

NURSING CONSIDERATIONS

• Contraindicated in ulcerative wounds, active internal bleeding, and cerebrovascular accident; recent trauma with possible internal injuries; visceral or intracranial malignancy; pregnancy and first 10 days postpartum; ulcerative colitis; diverticulitis; severe hypertension; acute or chronic hepatic or renal insufficiency; uncontrolled hypocoagulation; chronic pulmonary disease with cavitation; subacute bacterial endocarditis or rheumatic valvular disease; and recent cerebral embolism, thrombosis, or hemorrhage. Also contraindicated within 10 days after intra-arterial diagnostic procedure or any surgery, including liver or kidney biopsy, lumbar puncture, thoracentesis, paracentesis, or extensive or multiple cutdowns.

• I.M. injections are contraindicated during urokinase therapy.

• Preparation of I.V. solution: add 5.2 ml sterile water for injection to vial. Dilute further with 0.9% saline solution before infusion. Don't use bacteriostatic water for injection to reconstitute; it contains preservatives.

• Monitor patient for bleeding. Pretreatment with drugs affecting platelets places patient at high risk of bleeding.

• Have typed and crossmatched red cells and whole blood available to treat possible hemorrhage.

• Keep aminocaproic acid available to treat bleeding. Corticosteroids are used to treat allergic reactions.

• Watch for signs of hypersensitivity. Notify doctor immediately.

• Monitor vital signs.

• Keep venipuncture sites to a minimum; use pressure dressing on puncture sites for at least 15 minutes.

• Heparin by continuous infusion usually started within an hour after urokinase has been stopped. Use infusion pump to administer heparin.

• Bruising during therapy more likely; avoid unnecessary handling of patient.

• Should be used only by doctors with wide experience in thrombotic disease management where clinical and laboratory monitoring can be performed.

• Also used to clear intravenous catheters that are obstructed by clotted blood or fibrin deposits.

68

Alkylating agents

busulfan
carmustine (BCNU)
chlorambucil
cisplatin (cis-platinum)
cyclophosphamide
dacarbazine (DTIC)
lomustine (CCNU)
mechlorethamine hydrochloride
  (nitrogen mustard)
melphalan
pipobroman
streptozocin
thiotepa
uracil mustard

MECHANISM OF ACTION
Alkylating agents cross-link strands of
cellular DNA, causing an imbalance of
growth that leads to cell death.

COMBINATION PRODUCTS
None.

---

busulfan
Myleran♦

INDICATIONS & DOSAGE
*Chronic myelocytic (granulocytic) leu-
kemia—*
Adults: 4 to 6 mg P.O. daily up to
8 mg P.O. daily until WBC falls to
10,000/mm³; stop drug until WBC rises
to 50,000/mm³, then resume treatment
as before; or 4 to 8 mg P.O. daily until
WBC falls to 10,000 to 20,000/mm³,
then reduce daily dose as needed to
maintain WBC at this level (usually
2 mg daily).
Children: 0.06 to 0.12 mg/kg or 2.3 to
4.6 mg/m²/day P.O.; adjust dose to

maintain WBC at 20,000/mm³, but
never less than 10,000/mm³.

SIDE EFFECTS
Blood: WBC falling after about
10 days and continuing to fall for 2
weeks after stopping drug; *thrombocytopenia,* pancytopenia, anemia.
GI: nausea, vomiting, diarrhea, cheilosis, glossitis.
GU: amenorrhea, testicular atrophy,
impotence.
Metabolic: Addison-like wasting syndrome, profound hyperuricemia due to
increased cell lysis.
Skin: transient hyperpigmentation, anhidrosis.
Other: gynecomastia; alopecia; *irreversible pulmonary fibrosis, commonly
termed "busulfan lung."*

INTERACTIONS
None significant.

NURSING CONSIDERATIONS
• Use cautiously in patients recently
given other myelosuppressive drugs or
radiation treatment, and in those with
depressed neutrophil or platelet count.
• Watch for signs of infection (fever,
sore throat).
• Warn patient that pulmonary fibrosis
may be delayed for at least 4 to 6
months.
• Persistent cough, progressive dyspnea with alveolar exudate may result
from drug toxicity, not pneumonia.
• Monitor uric acid and CBC.
• Patient response usually begins
within 1 to 2 weeks (increased appetite,
sense of well-being, decreased total

Italicized side effects are common or life-threatening.
*Liquid form contains alcohol.   **May contain tartrazine.

leukocyte count, reduction in size of spleen).
• Can cause false-positive cytology in all body secretions.
• Anticoagulants should be used cautiously. Watch closely for signs of bleeding.
• Avoid all I.M. injections when platelets are low.

carmustine (BCNU)
BiCNU♦

INDICATIONS & DOSAGE
Brain, colon, and stomach cancer; Hodgkin's disease; non-Hodgkin's lymphomas; melanomas; multiple myeloma; and hepatoma—
Adults: 100 mg/m² I.V. by slow infusion daily for 2 days; repeat q 6 weeks if platelets are above 100,000/mm³ and WBC is above 4,000/mm³. Dose is reduced 50% when WBC less than 2,000/mm³ and platelets less than 25,000/mm³.
Alternate therapy: 200 mg/m² I.V. slow infusion as a single dose, repeated q 6 to 8 weeks; or 40 mg/m² I.V. slow infusion for 5 consecutive days, repeated q 6 weeks.

SIDE EFFECTS
Blood: *cumulative bone marrow depression, delayed 4 to 6 weeks, lasting 1 to 2 weeks; leukopenia; thrombocytopenia.*
GI: *nausea, which lasts 2 to 6 hours after giving (can be severe); vomiting.*
Hepatic: *hepatotoxicity.*
Metabolic: possible hyperuricemia in lymphoma patients when rapid cell lysis occurs.
Local: *intense pain at infusion site.*
Other: *pulmonary fibrosis.*

INTERACTIONS
None significant.

NURSING CONSIDERATIONS
• To reduce pain on infusion, dilute further or slow infusion rate.
• Warn patient to watch for signs of infection and bone marrow toxicity (fever, sore throat, anemia, fatigue, easy bruising, nose or gum bleeds, melena). Take temperature daily.
• Monitor uric acid, CBC.
• To reduce nausea, give antiemetic before administering.
• Don't mix with other drugs during administration.
• To reconstitute, dissolve 100 mg carmustine in 3 ml absolute alcohol. Dilute solution with 27 ml sterile water for injection. Resultant solution contains 3.3 mg carmustine/ml in 10% alcohol. Dilute in normal saline solution or dextrose 5% in water for I.V. infusion. Give at least 250 ml over 1 to 2 hours.
• May store reconstituted solution in refrigerator for 24 hours.
• If powder liquefies or appears oily, it is a sign of decomposition. Discard.
• Can cause false-positive cytology in all body secretions.
• To prevent hyperuricemia with resulting uric acid nephropathy, allopurinol may be used with adequate hydration. Screen urine for stones.
• Avoid contact with skin, as carmustine will cause a brown stain. If drug comes into contact with skin, wash off thoroughly.
• Anticoagulants should be used cautiously. Watch closely for signs of bleeding.
• Avoid all I.M. injections when platelets are low.

chlorambucil
Leukeran♦

INDICATIONS & DOSAGE
Chronic lymphocytic leukemia, lymphosarcoma, giant follicular lymphoma, Hodgkin's disease, ovarian carcinoma, mycosis fungoides—

Adults: 0.1 to 0.2 mg/kg P.O. daily for 3 to 6 weeks, then adjust for maintenance (usually 2 mg daily).
Children: 0.1 to 0.2 mg/kg daily or 4.5 mg/m^2/day P.O. as single dose or in divided doses.

SIDE EFFECTS
Blood: leukopenia, delayed up to 3 weeks, lasting up to 10 days after last dose; thrombocytopenia; anemia; myelosuppression (usually moderate, gradual, and rapidly reversible).
Metabolic: hyperuricemia.
Skin: *exfoliative dermatitis,* rashes.
Other: allergic febrile reactions.

INTERACTIONS
None significant.

NURSING CONSIDERATIONS
• Severe neutropenia reversible up to cumulative dose of 6.5 mg/kg in a single course.
• Monitor uric acid, CBC.
• To prevent hyperuricemia with resulting uric acid nephropathy, allopurinol may be used with adequate hydration. Screen urine for stones.
• Can cause false-positive cytology in all body secretions.
• Avoid all I.M. injections when platelets are low.
• Anticoagulants should be used cautiously. Watch closely for signs of bleeding.

cisplatin (cis-platinum)
Platinol

INDICATIONS & DOSAGE
Adjunctive therapy in metastatic testicular cancer—
Adults: 20 mg/m^2 I.V. daily for 5 days. Repeat every 3 weeks for 3 cycles or longer.
*Adjunctive therapy in metastatic ovarian cancer—*100 mg/m^2 I.V. Repeat every 4 weeks; or 50 mg/m^2 I.V. every 3 weeks with concurrent doxorubicin

HCl therapy. Give as I.V. infusion in 2 liters normal saline solution with 37.5 g mannitol over 6 to 8 hours.
Treatment of advanced bladder cancer—
Adults: 50 to 70 mg/m^2 I.V. once every 3 to 4 weeks. Patients who have received other antineoplastics or radiation therapy should receive 50 mg/m^2 every 4 weeks.
Note: Prehydration and mannitol diuresis may reduce renal toxicity and ototoxicity significantly.

SIDE EFFECTS
Blood: *reversible myelosuppression in 25% to 30% of patients, leukopenia, thrombocytopenia,* anemia; nadirs in circulating platelets and leukocytes on days 18 to 23, with recovery by day 39.
CNS: peripheral neuritis, loss of taste, seizures.
EENT: *tinnitus, hearing loss.*
GI: *nausea, vomiting, beginning 1 to 4 hours after dose and lasting 24 hours; diarrhea.*
GU: *more prolonged and severe renal toxicity with repeated courses of therapy.*
Other: *anaphylactoid reaction.*

INTERACTIONS
Aminoglycoside antibiotics: additive nephrotoxicity. Monitor renal function studies very carefully.

NURSING CONSIDERATIONS
• Use cautiously in preexisting renal impairment, myelosuppression, and hearing impairment.
• Hydrate patient with normal saline solution before giving drug. Maintain urine output of 100 ml/hour for 4 consecutive hours before therapy and for 24 hours after therapy.
• Don't use aluminum needles for reconstitution or administration of cisplatin; a black precipitate may form.
• Mannitol may be given as 12.5 g I.V. bolus before starting cisplatin infusion.

Italicized side effects are common or life-threatening.
*Liquid form contains alcohol.   **May contain tartrazine.

Follow by infusion of mannitol at rate up to 10 g/hour p.r.n. to maintain urine output during and 6 to 24 hours after cisplatin infusion.

• Do not repeat dose unless platelets are over 100,000/mm³, WBC is over 4,000/mm³, creatinine is under 1.5 mg%, or BUN is under 25 mg%.

• Monitor CBC, platelets, and renal function studies before initial and subsequent doses.

• Tell patient to report tinnitus immediately to prevent permanent hearing loss. Do audiometry prior to initial dose and subsequent courses.

• Nausea and vomiting may be severe and protracted (up to 24 hours). Antiemetics can be started 24 hours before therapy. Monitor intake and output. Continue I.V. hydration until patient can tolerate adequate oral intake.

• Reconstitute with sterile water for injection. Stable for 24 hours in normal saline solution at room temperature. Don't refrigerate.

• Given with bleomycin and vinblastine for testicular cancer and with doxorubicin HCl for ovarian cancer.

• Renal toxicity becomes more severe with repeated doses. Renal function must return to normal before next dose can be given.

• Avoid all I.M. injections when platelets are low.

• Metoclopramide has been used very effectively to treat and prevent nausea and vomiting.

• Anaphylactoid reaction usually responds to immediate treatment with epinephrine, corticosteroids, or antihistamines.

---

cyclophosphamide
Cytoxan♦**, Procytox♦♦, Neosar

INDICATIONS & DOSAGE
Breast, colon, head, neck, lung, ovarian, and prostatic cancer; Hodgkin's disease; chronic lymphocytic leukemia; chronic myelocytic leukemia; acute lymphoblastic leukemia; neuroblastoma; retinoblastoma; non-Hodgkin's lymphomas; multiple myeloma; mycosis fungoides; sarcomas—

Adults: 40 to 50 mg/kg P.O. or I.V. in single dose or in 2 to 5 daily doses, then adjust for maintenance; or 2 to 4 mg/kg P.O. daily for 10 days, then adjust for maintenance. Maintenance dose 1.5 to 3 mg/kg daily P.O.; or 10 to 15 mg/kg q 7 to 10 days I.V.; or 3 to 5 mg/kg twice weekly I.V.

Children: 2 to 8 mg/kg daily or 60 to 250 mg/m² daily P.O. or I.V. for 6 days (dose depends on susceptibility of neoplasm); divide oral dosages; give I.V. dosages once weekly. Maintenance dose 2 to 5 mg/kg or 50 to 150 mg/m² twice weekly P.O.

SIDE EFFECTS
Blood: *leukopenia,* nadir between days 8 to 15, recovery in 17 to 28 days; thrombocytopenia; anemia.

CV: *cardiotoxicity* (with very high doses and in combination with doxorubicin).

GI: anorexia; *nausea and vomiting beginning within 6 hours, lasting 4 hours;* stomatitis; mucositis.

GU: gonadal suppression (may be irreversible), *hemorrhagic cystitis,* bladder fibrosis, sterility, nephrotoxicity.

Metabolic: hyperuricemia; syndrome of inappropriate ADH secretion (with high doses).

Other: *reversible alopecia in 50% of patients, especially with high doses;* secondary malignancies, *pulmonary fibrosis (high doses).*

INTERACTIONS
Corticosteroids, chloramphenicol: reduced activity of cyclophosphamide. Use cautiously.
Succinylcholine: may cause apnea. Don't use together.

NURSING CONSIDERATIONS
• Use cautiously in severe leukopenia, thrombocytopenia, malignant cell infil-

---

tration of bone marrow, recent radiation therapy or chemotherapy, hepatic or renal disease.
- Advise both male and female patients to practice contraception while taking this drug and for 4 months after; drug is potentially teratogenic.
- Monitor uric acid, CBC, renal and hepatic functions.
- To reduce nausea, give antiemetic before administering.
- Push fluid (3 liters daily) to prevent hemorrhagic cystitis. Don't give drug at bedtime, since voiding is too infrequent to avoid cystitis. If hemorrhagic cystitis occurs, drug is stopped. Cystitis can occur months after therapy has been stopped.
- Reconstituted solution is stable 6 days refrigerated or 24 hours at room temperature.
- Can cause false-positive cytology in all body secretions.
- Avoid all I.M. injections when platelets are low.
- Can be given by direct I.V. push into a running I.V. line or by infusion in normal saline solution or dextrose 5% in water.
- To prevent hyperuricemia with resulting uric acid nephropathy, keep patient well hydrated.
- Warn patient that alopecia is likely to occur, but that it is reversible.
- Anticoagulants should be used cautiously. Watch closely for signs of bleeding.
- Monitor for cyclophosphamide toxicity if patient's corticosteroid therapy is discontinued.
- Has been used successfully to treat many nonmalignant conditions.

dacarbazine (DTIC)
DTIC-Dome♦

INDICATIONS & DOSAGE

Hodgkin's disease, metastatic malignant melanoma, neuroblastoma, sarcomas—

Adults: 2 to 4.5 mg/kg or 70 to 160 mg/m² I.V. daily for 10 days, then repeat q 4 weeks as tolerated; or 250 mg/m² I.V. daily for 5 days, repeated at 3-week intervals.

SIDE EFFECTS

Blood: *leukopenia and thrombocytopenia,* nadir between 3 and 4 weeks.
GI: *severe nausea and vomiting begin within 1 to 3 hours in 90% of patients, last 1 to 12 hours; anorexia.*
Local: severe pain if I.V. infiltrates or if solution is too concentrated; tissue damage.
Skin: phototoxicity.
Other: *flu-like syndrome* (fever, malaise, myalgia beginning 7 days after treatment stopped and possibly lasting 7 to 21 days), alopecia.

INTERACTIONS
None significant.

NURSING CONSIDERATIONS
- Use lower dose if renal function or bone marrow is impaired. Stop drug if WBC falls to 3,000/mm³ or platelets drop to 100,000/mm³.
- Take temperature daily. Observe for signs of infection.
- Monitor uric acid, CBC.
- Discard refrigerated solution after 72 hours, room temperature solution after 8 hours.
- Can cause false-positive cytology in all body secretions.
- Avoid all I.M. injections when platelets are low.
- Give I.V. infusion in 50 to 100 ml dextrose 5% in water over 30 minutes. May dilute further or slow infusion to decrease pain at infusion site. Make sure drug does not infiltrate.
- For Hodgkin's disease, usually given with bleomycin, vinblastine, doxorubicin.
- Advise patient to avoid sunlight and sunlamps for first 2 days after treatment.
- Anticoagulants should be used cau-

Italicized side effects are common or life-threatening.
∗Liquid form contains alcohol.   ∗∗May contain tartrazine.

tiously. Watch closely for signs of bleeding.
• Administering antiemetics before giving dacarbazine may help decrease nausea. Nausea and vomiting usually subside after several doses.

lomustine (CCNU)
CeeNU♦

INDICATIONS & DOSAGE
Brain, colon, lung, and renal cell cancer; Hodgkin's disease; lymphomas; melanomas; multiple myeloma—
Adults and children: 130 mg/m² P.O. as single dose q 6 weeks. Reduce dose according to bone marrow depression. Repeat doses should not be given until WBC is more than 4,000/mm³ and platelet count is more than 100,000/mm³.

SIDE EFFECTS
Blood: *leukopenia, delayed up to 6 weeks, lasting 1 to 2 weeks; thrombocytopenia, delayed up to 4 weeks, lasting 1 to 2 weeks.*
GI: *nausea and vomiting beginning within 4 to 5 hours, lasting 24 hours;* stomatitis.
Other: alopecia.

INTERACTIONS
None significant.

NURSING CONSIDERATIONS
• Give 2 to 4 hours after meals. To avoid nausea, give antiemetic before administering.
• May be useful in cancer involving CNS, since CSF level equals 30% to 50% of plasma level 1 hour after administration.
• Monitor blood counts weekly. Don't give more often than every 6 weeks; bone marrow toxicity is cumulative and delayed.
• Monitor uric acid, CBC.
• Can cause false-positive cytology in all body secretions.

• Avoid all I.M. injections when platelets are low.
• For Hodgkin's disease, usually given with mechlorethamine.
• Anticoagulants should be used cautiously. Watch closely for signs of bleeding.
• Advise patient that drug can cause alopecia but hair will grow back.

mechlorethamine hydrochloride (nitrogen mustard)
Mustargen♦

INDICATIONS & DOSAGE
Breast, lung, and ovarian cancer; Hodgkin's disease; non-Hodgkin's lymphomas; lymphosarcoma—
Adults: 0.4 mg/kg or 10 mg/m² I.V. as single or divided dose q 3 to 6 weeks. Give through running I.V. infusion. Dose reduced in prior radiation or chemotherapy to 0.2 to 0.4 mg/kg. Dose based on ideal or actual body weight, whichever is less.
Neoplastic effusions—
Adults: 10 to 20 mg intracavitarily.

SIDE EFFECTS
Blood: *nadir of leukopenia, thrombocytopenia, myelosuppression occuring by days 4 to 10, lasting 10 to 21 days;* mild anemia begins in 2 to 3 weeks, possibly lasting 7 weeks.
EENT: tinnitus, *metallic taste* (immediately after dose); deafness in high doses.
GI: *nausea, vomiting, and anorexia* begin within minutes, last 8 to 24 hours.
Metabolic: hyperuricemia.
Local: *thrombophlebitis, sloughing, severe irritation if drug extravasates or touches skin.*
Other: *alopecia,* may precipitate herpes zoster.

INTERACTIONS
None significant.

Unmarked trade names available in the United States only.
♦ Also available in Canada.   ♦♦ Available in Canada only.

NURSING CONSIDERATIONS

• Use cautiously in severe anemia, depressed neutrophil or platelet count, patients recently treated with radiation or chemotherapy.
• Avoid contact with skin or mucous membranes. Wear gloves when preparing solution to prevent accidental skin contact. If contact occurs, wash with copious amounts of water.
• Giving antiemetic before drug not always effective in reducing nausea.
• Be sure I.V. doesn't infiltrate. If drug extravasates, apply cold compresses and infiltrate the area with isotonic sodium thiosulfate.
• When given intracavitarily, turn patient from side to side every 15 minutes to 1 hour to distribute drug.
• Monitor uric acid, CBC.
• Severe herpes zoster may require stopping drug.
• Very unstable solution. Prepare immediately before infusion. Use within 15 minutes. Discard unused solution.
• To prevent hyperuricemia with resulting uric acid nephropathy, allopurinol may be given; keep patient well hydrated.
• Can cause false-positive cytology in all body secretions.
• Avoid all I.M. injections when platelets are low.
• One of the most effective drugs in treatment of Hodgkin's disease.
• Has been used topically in treatment of mycosis fungoides.
• Anticoagulants should be used cautiously. Watch closely for signs of bleeding.

melphalan
Alkeran♦

INDICATIONS & DOSAGE

Multiple myeloma, malignant melanoma, testicular seminoma, reticulum cell sarcoma, osteogenic sarcoma, breast cancer—
Adults: 6 mg P.O. daily for 2 to

3 weeks, then stop drug for up to 4 weeks or until WBC and platelets stop dropping and begin to rise again; resume with maintenance dose of 2 to 4 mg daily. Stop drug if WBC below 3,000/mm³ or platelets below 100,000/mm³. Alternate therapy: 0.15 mg/kg daily P.O. for 7 days, wait for WBC and platelets to recover, then resume with 0.05 mg/kg daily P.O.
Nonresectable advanced ovarian cancer—
Adults: 0.2 mg/kg daily, P.O. in divided doses, for 5 days. Repeat every 4 weeks, depending on bone marrow recovery.

SIDE EFFECTS

Blood: *thrombocytopenia, leukopenia, agranulocytosis.*
Other: *pneumonitis and pulmonary fibrosis.*

INTERACTIONS
None significant.

NURSING CONSIDERATIONS

• Not recommended in severe leukopenia, thrombocytopenia, or anemia; chronic lymphocytic leukemia; or suppurative inflammation.
• Monitor uric acid, CBC.
• Can cause false-positive cytology in all body secretions.
• Avoid all I.M. injections when platelets are low.
• May need dose reduction in renal impairment.
• Drug of choice in multiple myeloma.
• Anticoagulants should be used cautiously. Watch closely for signs of bleeding.
• Administer on empty stomach, because absorption is decreased by food.

pipobroman
Vercyte♦

INDICATIONS & DOSAGE
Polycythemia vera—

Italicized side effects are common or life-threatening.
✳Liquid form contains alcohol.　　✳✳May contain tartrazine.

Adults and children over 15 years:
1 mg/kg P.O. daily for 30 days; may increase to 1.5 to 3 mg/kg P.O. daily until hematocrit reduced to 50% to 55%, then 0.1 to 0.2 mg/kg daily maintenance.
Chronic myelocytic leukemia—
Adults and children over 15 years:
1.5 to 2.5 mg/kg P.O. daily until WBC drops to 10,000/mm³, then start maintenance 7 to 175 mg daily. Stop drug if WBC below 3,000/mm³ or platelets below 150,000/mm³.

SIDE EFFECTS
Blood: *anemia, leukopenia, and thrombocytopenia, delayed up to 4 weeks or longer.*
GI: nausea, vomiting, cramping, diarrhea, anorexia.
Skin: rash.

INTERACTIONS
None significant.

NURSING CONSIDERATIONS
• Use cautiously in bone marrow depression.
• Do WBC and platelet count until desired response or toxicity occurs (platelets less than 150,000/mm³ or WBC less than 3,000/mm³).
• Monitor CBC.
• Anticoagulants should be used cautiously. Watch closely for signs of bleeding.

streptozocin
Zanosar

INDICATIONS & DOSAGE
Treatment of metastatic islet cell carcinoma of the pancreas—
Adults and children: 500 mg/m² for 5 consecutive days every 6 weeks until maximum benefit or until toxicity is observed. Alternatively, 1,000 mg/m² at weekly intervals for the first 2 weeks. Don't exceed a single dose 1,500 mg/m².

SIDE EFFECTS
Blood: *aplastic anemia,* mild decreases in hematocrit values.
GI: *nausea, vomiting,* diarrhea.
Hepatic: elevated liver enzymes.
Metabolic: hyperglycemia and hypoglycemia.
Renal: *renal toxicity (evidenced by azotemia, glycosuria, and renal tubular acidosis),* mild proteinuria.

INTERACTIONS
Other potentially nephrotoxic drugs such as aminoglycosides: increased risk of renal toxicity. Use cautiously.

NURSING CONSIDERATIONS
• Use cautiously in patients with preexisting renal disease.
• Renal toxicity resulting from streptozocin therapy is dose-related and cumulative. Monitor renal function before and after each course of therapy. Urinalysis, BUN, creatinine, serum electrolytes and creatinine clearance should be obtained before, and at least weekly during, drug administration. Weekly monitoring should continue for 4 weeks after each course.
• Mild proteinuria is one of the first signs of renal toxicity. Make sure doctor is aware if and when this occurs. The dose of the drug may have to be reduced.
• Monitor CBC and liver function studies at least weekly.
• Reconstitute the streptozocin powder with 0.9% sodium chloride injection. This will produce a pale gold solution. After reconstitution, the drug must be used within 12 hours.
• The product contains no preservatives and is not intended as a multiple-dose vial.
• When preparing the solution, wear gloves to protect the skin from contact.
• Unopened and unreconstituted vials of streptozocin should be stored in the refrigerator.

thiotepa
Thiotepa♦

INDICATIONS & DOSAGE
Adults and children over 12 years:
*Breast, lung, and ovarian cancer;
Hodgkin's disease; lymphomas—*
0.2 mg/kg I.V. daily for 5 days; then
maintenance dose of 0.2 mg/kg I.V. q 1
to 3 weeks.
*Bladder tumor—*60 mg in 60 ml water
instilled in bladder once weekly for
4 weeks.
*Neoplastic effusions—*10 to 15 mg intracavitarily, p.r.n. Stop drug or decrease dosage if WBC below 4,000/
mm³ or if platelets below 150,000/
mm³.

SIDE EFFECTS
Blood: *leukopenia begins within
5 to 30 days; thrombocytopenia;
neutropenia.*
GU: amenorrhea, decreased spermatogenesis.
Metabolic: hyperuricemia.
Skin: hives, rash.
Local: intense pain at administration
site.
Other: headache, fever, tightness of
throat, dizziness.

INTERACTIONS
None significant.

NURSING CONSIDERATIONS
• Use cautiously in bone marrow
depression, chronic lymphocytic leukemia, renal or hepatic dysfunction.
• Do WBC, RBC counts weekly for at
least 3 weeks after last dose. Warn patient to report even mild infections.
• GU side effects reversible in 6 to
8 months.
• May require use of local anesthetic at
injection site if intense pain occurs.
• For bladder instillation: dehydrate
patient 8 to 10 hours before therapy. Instill drug into bladder by catheter; ask
patient to retain solution for 2 hours.

Volume may be reduced to 30 ml if discomfort is too great with 60 ml. Reposition patient every 15 minutes for maximum area contact.
• Toxicity delayed and prolonged because drug binds to tissues and stays in
body several hours.
• Monitor uric acid, CBC.
• Refrigerate dry powder; protect from
light.
• Use only sterile water for injection to
reconstitute. Refrigerated solution stable 5 days.
• To prevent hyperuricemia with resulting uric acid nephropathy, allopurinol may be given; keep patient well hydrated.
• Can cause false-positive cytology in
all body secretions.
• Avoid all I.M. injections when platelets are low.
• Can be given by all parenteral routes,
including direct injection into the tumor.
• Anticoagulants should be used cautiously. Watch closely for signs of
bleeding.
• Discuss possible amenorrhea with
female patients when drug therapy is
initiated.

uracil mustard

INDICATIONS & DOSAGE
*Chronic lymphocytic and myelocytic
leukemia; Hodgkin's disease; non-
Hodgkin's lymphomas of the histiocytic
and lymphocytic types; reticulum cell
sarcoma; lymphomas; mycosis fungoides; polycythemia vera; cancer of
ovaries, cervix, and lungs—*
Adults: 1 to 2 mg P.O. daily for
3 months or until desired response or
toxicity; maintenance 1 mg daily for
3 out of 4 weeks until optimum response or relapse; or 3 to 5 mg P.O. for
7 days not to exceed total dose 0.5 mg/
kg, then 1 mg daily until response, then
1 mg daily 3 out of 4 weeks.

SIDE EFFECTS

Blood: bone marrow depression, delayed 2 to 4 weeks; *thrombocytopenia; leukopenia;* anemia.

CNS: irritability, nervousness, mental cloudiness and depression.

GI: *nausea, vomiting, diarrhea, epigastric distress,* abdominal pain, anorexia.

Metabolic: hyperuricemia.

Skin: pruritus, dermatitis, hyperpigmentation, alopecia.

INTERACTIONS

None significant.

NURSING CONSIDERATIONS

● Not recommended in severe thrombocytopenia, aplastic anemia or leukopenia, acute leukemias.

● Give at bedtime to reduce nausea.

● Watch for signs of ecchymoses, easy bruising, petechiae.

● Monitor uric acid. Do regular platelet count. Do CBC 1 to 2 times weekly for 4 weeks; then 4 weeks after stopping drug.

● Don't give drug within 2 to 3 weeks after maximum bone marrow depression from past radiation or chemotherapy.

● To prevent hyperuricemia and resulting uric acid nephropathy, allopurinol can be given; keep patient hydrated.

● Can cause false-positive cytology in all body secretions.

● Avoid all I.M. injections when platelets are low.

● Anticoagulants should be used cautiously. Watch closely for signs of bleeding.

69

Antimetabolites

azathioprine
cytarabine
floxuridine
fluorouracil
hydroxyurea
mercaptopurine
methotrexate
methotrexate sodium
thioguanine

MECHANISM OF ACTION
All the antimetabolites interfere with DNA synthesis as follows:
• Azathioprine, mercaptopurine, and thioguanine inhibit purine synthesis.
• Cytarabine, floxuridine, and fluorouracil inhibit pyrimidine synthesis.
• Hydroxyurea inhibits ribonucleotide reductase.
• Methotrexate prevents reduction of folic acid to tetrahydrofolate by binding to dihydrofolate reductase.

COMBINATION PRODUCTS
None.

azathioprine
Imuran♦

INDICATIONS & DOSAGE
Immunosuppression in renal transplants—
Adults and children: initially, 3 to 5 mg/kg P.O. daily. Maintain at 1 to 2 mg/kg daily (dose varies considerably according to patient response).
Treatment of severe, refractory rheumatoid arthritis—
Adults: initially, 1 mg/kg taken as a single dose or as 2 doses. If patient response not satisfactory after 6 to 8 weeks, dosage may be increased by 0.5 mg/kg daily (up to a maximum of 2.5 mg/kg daily) at 4-week intervals.

SIDE EFFECTS
Blood: *leukopenia, bone marrow depression,* anemia, pancytopenia, thrombocytopenia.
GI: nausea, vomiting, anorexia, *pancreatitis,* ascites, steatorrhea, mouth ulceration, esophagitis.
Hepatic: hepatoxicity, jaundice.
Skin: rash.
Other: *immunosuppression (possibly profound),* arthralgia, muscle wasting, alopecia.

INTERACTIONS
Allopurinol: impaired inactivation of azathioprine. Decrease azathioprine dose to ¼ or ⅓ normal dose.

NURSING CONSIDERATIONS
• Use cautiously in hepatic or renal dysfunction.
• Watch for clay-colored stools, dark urine, pruritus, and yellow skin and sclera; and for increased alkaline phosphatase, bilirubin, SGOT, and SGPT.
• In renal homotransplants, start drug 1 to 5 days before surgery.
• Hemoglobin, WBC, platelet count should be done at least once a week; more often at beginning of treatment. Drug should be stopped immediately when WBC is less than 3,000/mm³ to prevent extension to irreversible bone marrow depression.
• This is a potent immunosuppressive. Warn patient to report even mild infec-

Italicized side effects are common or life-threatening.
*Liquid form contains alcohol.   **May contain tartrazine.

tions (coryza, fever, sore throat, malaise).

• Patient should avoid conception during therapy and up to 4 months after stopping therapy.

• Warn patient that some thinning of hair is possible.

• Avoid I.M. injections of any drugs in patients with severely depressed platelet counts (thrombocytopenia) to prevent bleeding.

• When used to treat refractory rheumatoid arthritis, inform patient that it may take up to 12 weeks to be effective.

cytarabine (ARA-C, cytosine arabinoside)
Cytosar-U♦

INDICATIONS & DOSAGE
Acute myelocytic and other acute leukemias—
Adults and children: 200 mg/m² daily by continuous I.V. infusion for 5 days; or 10 to 30 mg/m² intrathecally, up to 3 times weekly.

SIDE EFFECTS
Blood: WBC nadir 5 to 7 days after drug stopped; *leukopenia,* anemia, *thrombocytopenia,* reticulocytopenia; platelet nadir occurring on day 10; *megaloblastosis.*
GI: *nausea, vomiting,* diarrhea, dysphagia; reddened area at juncture of lips, followed by sore mouth, oral ulcers in 5 to 10 days; high dose given via rapid I.V. may cause projectile vomiting.
Hepatic: hepatotoxicity (usually mild and reversible).
Skin: rash.
Other: flu-like syndrome.

INTERACTIONS
None significant.

NURSING CONSIDERATIONS
• Use cautiously in inadequate bone marrow reserve. Use cautiously in renal or hepatic disease and after other chemotherapy or radiation therapy.

• Watch for signs of infection (leukoplakia, fever, sore throat).

• Excellent mouth care can help prevent oral side effects.

• Monitor intake/output carefully. Maintain high fluid intake and give allopurinol, if ordered, to avoid urate nephropathy in leukemia induction therapy.

• Check uric acid, CBC with platelets, and hepatic function.

• Use preservative-free normal saline or Elliot's B solution for intrathecal use.

• Optimum schedule is continuous infusion.

• To reduce nausea, give antiemetic before administering.

• Store dry powder in refrigerator; refrigerated, reconstituted solution stable 48 hours. Discard cloudy reconstituted solution.

• Avoid I.M. injections of any drugs in patients with severely depressed platelet count (thrombocytopenia) to prevent bleeding.

• Modify or discontinue therapy if polymorphonuclear granulocyte count is 1,000/mm³ or if platelet count is 50,000/mm³.

floxuridine
FUDR

INDICATIONS & DOSAGE
Brain, breast, head, neck, liver, gallbladder, and bile duct cancer—
Adults: 0.1 to 0.6 mg/kg daily by intra-arterial infusion (use pump for continuous, uniform rate); or 0.4 to 0.6 mg/kg daily into hepatic artery.

SIDE EFFECTS
Blood: *leukopenia, anemia,* thrombocytopenia.
CNS: cerebellar ataxia, vertigo, nystagmus, convulsions, depression, hemiplegia, hiccups, lethargy.

EENT: blurred vision.
GI: *stomatitis, cramps, nausea, vomiting, diarrhea, bleeding, enteritis.*
Skin: *erythema,* dermatitis, pruritus, rash.

INTERACTIONS
None significant.

NURSING CONSIDERATIONS
• Use cautiously in poor nutritional state, bone marrow depression, or serious infection. Use cautiously following high-dose pelvic irradiation or use of alkylating agent, and in impaired hepatic or renal function.
• Severe skin and GI side effects require stopping drug. Use of antacid eases but probably won't prevent GI distress.
• Excellent mouth care can help prevent oral side effects.
• Monitor intake/output, CBC, and renal and hepatic function.
• Discontinue if WBC falls below 3,500/mm³ or if platelet count below 100,000/mm³.
• Therapeutic effect may be delayed 1 to 6 weeks. Make sure patient is aware of time it may take for improvement to be noted.
• Reconstitute with sterile water for injection. Dilute further in 5% dextrose in water or normal saline solution for actual infusion.
• Always use infusion pump.
• Avoid I.M. injections of any drugs in patients with thrombocytopenia to prevent bleeding.
• Refrigerated solution stable no more than 2 weeks.
• Observe arterial perfused area. Check line for bleeding, blockage, displacement, or leakage.

fluorouracil (5-fluorouracil)
Adrucil, 5-FU

INDICATIONS & DOSAGE
Colon, rectal, breast, ovarian, cervical, bladder, liver, and pancreatic cancer—
Adults: 12.5 mg/kg I.V. daily for 3 to 5 days q 4 weeks; or 15 mg/kg weekly for 6 weeks. (Doses recommended based on lean body weight.) Maximum single recommended dose is 800 mg, although higher single doses (up to 1.5 g) have been used. The injectable form has been given orally but is not recommended.

SIDE EFFECTS
Blood: *leukopenia,* thrombocytopenia, anemia. WBC nadir 9 to 14 days after first dose; platelet nadir in 7 to 14 days.
GI: *stomatitis, GI ulcer may precede leukopenia, nausea, vomiting in 30% to 50% of patients; diarrhea.*
Skin: *dermatitis,* hyperpigmentation (especially in Blacks), nail changes, pigmented palmar creases.
Other: *reversible alopecia in 5% to 20% of patients, weakness, malaise.*

INTERACTIONS
None significant.

NURSING CONSIDERATIONS
• Use cautiously following major surgery; in poor nutritional state, serious infections, and bone marrow depression. Use cautiously following high-dose pelvic irradiation or use of alkylating agents, in impaired hepatic or renal function, or in widespread neoplastic infiltration of bone marrow.
• Watch for stomatitis or diarrhea (signs of toxicity). May use topical oral anesthetic to soothe lesions. Discontinue if diarrhea occurs.
• Give antiemetic before administering to reduce GI side effects.
• Do WBC and platelet counts daily. Drug should be stopped when WBC is

---

Italicized side effects are common or life-threatening.
*Liquid form contains alcohol.   **May contain tartrazine.

less than 3,500/mm³. Watch for ecchymoses, petechiae, easy bruising,
and anemia. Drug should be stopped if
platelet count is less than 100,000/
mm³.

• Skin and ocular side effects reversible when drug is stopped. Patient
should use highly protective sun blockers to avoid inflammatory erythematous dermatitis.

• Therapeutic concentrations don't
reach cerebrospinal fluid.

• Slowing infusion rate so it takes from
2 to 8 hours lessens toxicity but also
lessens efficacy compared with rapid
injection.

• Monitor intake/output, CBC, and
renal and hepatic functions.

• Do not refrigerate fluorouracil.

• Don't use cloudy solution. If crystals
form, redissolve by warming.

• Sometimes ordered as 5-FU. The
number 5 is part of the drug name and
should not be confused with dosage
units.

• Sometimes administered via hepatic
arterial infusion in treatment of hepatic
metastases.

• Warn patient that alopecia may occur
but is reversible.

• To prevent bleeding, avoid I.M. injections of any drugs in patients with
thrombocytopenia.

• Fluorouracil toxicity is delayed for 1
to 3 weeks.

hydroxyurea
Hydrea**

INDICATIONS & DOSAGE
*Melanoma; resistant chronic myelocytic
leukemia; recurrent, metastatic, or inoperable ovarian cancer—*
Adults: 80 mg/kg P.O. as single dose q
3 days; or 20 to 30 mg/kg P.O. daily.

SIDE EFFECTS
Blood: *leukopenia,* thrombocytopenia,
anemia, *megaloblastosis; dose-limiting*

*and dose-related bone marrow depres-
sion, with rapid recovery.*
CNS: drowsiness.
GI: *anorexia, nausea, vomiting, diar-
rhea,* stomatitis.
GU: increased BUN, serum creatinine.
Metabolic: hyperuricemia.
Skin: rash, pruritus.

INTERACTIONS
None significant.

NURSING CONSIDERATIONS
• Use cautiously following other chemotherapy or radiation therapy.

• Use with caution in renal dysfunction. Discontinue if WBC is less than
2,500/mm³ or if platelet count is less
than 100,000/mm³.

• If patient can't swallow capsule, he
may empty contents into water and take
immediately.

• Monitor intake/output; keep patient
hydrated.

• Routinely measure BUN, uric acid,
serum creatinine.

• Drug crosses blood-brain barrier.

• Auditory and visual hallucinations
and blood toxicity increase when decreased renal function exists.

• May exacerbate postirradiation
erythema.

• Avoid all I.M. injections when platelets are low.

mercaptopurine
Purinethol♦

INDICATIONS & DOSAGE
*Acute lymphoblastic leukemia (in chil-
dren), acute myeloblastic leukemia,
chronic myelocytic leukemia—*
Adults: 80 to 100 mg/m² P.O. daily as
a single dose up to 5 mg/kg daily.
Children: 70 mg/m² P.O. daily.
Usual maintenance for adults and children: 1.5 to 2.5 mg/kg daily.

SIDE EFFECTS
Blood: *decreased RBC; leukopenia,*

---

*thrombocytopenia, and anemia; all
may persist several days after drug is
stopped.*
GI: *nausea, vomiting, and anorexia in
25% of patients;* painful oral ulcers.
Hepatic: *jaundice, hepatic necrosis.*
Metabolic: hyperuricemia.

INTERACTIONS
Allopurinol: slowed inactivation of mercaptopurine. Decrease mercaptopurine
to ¼ or ⅓ normal dose.

NURSING CONSIDERATIONS
• Use cautiously following chemotherapy or radiation therapy, in depressed
neutrophil or platelet count, and in impaired hepatic or renal function.
• Observe for signs of bleeding and infection.
• Hepatic dysfunction reversible when
drug is stopped. Watch for jaundice,
clay-colored stools, frothy dark urine.
Drug should be stopped if hepatic tenderness occurs.
• Do weekly blood counts; watch for
precipitous fall.
• Monitor intake/output. Push fluids (3
liters daily).
• Sometimes ordered as 6-mercaptopu-
rine or 6-MP. The number 6 is part of
drug name and does not signify number
of dosage units.
• Warn patient that improvement may
take 2 to 4 weeks or longer.
• GI side effects less common in children than in adults.
• Avoid all I.M. injections when platelets are low.
• Monitor serum uric acid. If allopurinol is necessary, use very cautiously.

methotrexate

methotrexate sodium
Mexate

INDICATIONS & DOSAGE
*Trophoblastic tumors (choriocarci-
noma, hydatidiform mole)—*
Adults: 15 to 30 mg P.O. or I.M. daily
for 5 days. Repeat after 1 or more
weeks, according to response or toxicity.
*Acute lymphoblastic and lymphatic leu-
kemia—*
Adults and children: 3.3 mg/m² P.O.,
I.M., or I.V. daily for 4 to 6 weeks or
until remission occurs; then 20 to
30 mg/m² P.O. or I.M. twice weekly.
Meningeal leukemia—
Adults and children: 10 to 15 mg/m²
intrathecally q 2 to 5 days until cerebrospinal fluid is normal. Use only 20-,
50-, or 100-mg vials of powder with no
preservatives; dilute using 0.9% NaCl
injection *without* preservatives, Elliot's
B solution, or patient's own cerebrospi-
nal fluid. Use only new vials of drug
and diluent. Use immediately.
Burkitt's lymphoma (Stage I or
Stage II)—
Adults: 10 to 25 mg P.O. daily for 4 to
8 days with 1-week rest intervals.
Lymphosarcoma (Stage III)—
Adults: 0.625 to 2.5 mg/kg daily P.O.,
I.M., or I.V.
Mycosis fungoides—
Adults: 2.5 to 10 mg P.O. daily or
50 mg I.M. weekly; or 25 mg I.M.
twice weekly.
Psoriasis—
Adults: 10 to 25 mg P.O., I.M., or I.V.
as single weekly dose.
To detect idiosyncratic reactions, 5 to
10 mg test dose recommended 1 week
before methotrexate regimen.

SIDE EFFECTS
Blood: WBC and platelet nadir occurring on day 7; anemia, *leukopenia,
thrombocytopenia* (all dose-related).
CNS: *arachnoiditis within hours of intrathecal use;* subacute neurotoxicity
which may begin a few weeks later;
necrotizing demyelinating leukoen-
cephalopathy a few years later.
GI: *stomatitis; diarrhea leading to
hemorrhagic enteritis and intestinal
perforation; nausea; vomiting.*

Italicized side effects are common or life-threatening.
*Liquid form contains alcohol.   **May contain tartrazine.

GU: *tubular necrosis.*
Hepatic: hepatic dysfunction leading to cirrhosis or hepatic fibrosis.
Metabolic: hyperuricemia.
Skin: exposure to sun may aggravate psoriatic lesions, rash, photosensitivity.
Other: alopecia; *pulmonary interstitial infiltrates;* long-term use in children may cause osteoporosis.

INTERACTIONS

Alcohol: increased hepatotoxicity; warn patient not to drink alcoholic beverages.
Probenecid, phenylbutazone, salicylates, sulfonamides: increased methotrexate toxicity; don't use together if possible.

NURSING CONSIDERATIONS

• Use cautiously in impaired hepatic or renal function, bone marrow depression, aplasia, leukopenia, thrombocytopenia, anemia. Use cautiously in infection, peptic ulcer, ulcerative colitis, and in very young, old, or debilitated patients.
• Warn patient to avoid conception during and immediately after therapy because of possible abortion or congenital anomalies.
• GI side effects may require stopping drug.
• Rash, redness, or ulcerations in mouth or pulmonary side effects may signal serious complications.
• Monitor uric acid.
• Check thirst and urinary frequency.
• Monitor intake/output daily. Force fluids (2 to 3 liters daily).
• Alkalinize urine by giving NaHCO₃ tablets to prevent precipitation of drug, especially with high doses. Maintain urine pH at more than 6.5. Reduce dose if BUN 20 to 30 mg% or creatinine 1.2 to 2 mg%. Stop drug if BUN more than 30 mg% or creatinine more than 2 mg%.
• Watch for increases in SGOT, SGPT, alkaline phosphatase; may signal hepatic dysfunction.

• Watch for bleeding (especially GI) and infection.
• Warn patient to use highly protective sun screening agent when exposed to sunlight.
• Take temperature daily, and watch for cough, dyspnea, cyanosis; corticosteroids may help reduce pulmonary side effects.
• Leucovorin rescue is necessary with high dose protocols (greater than 100-mg doses): Leucovorin calcium (folinic acid) is given within 4 hours of administration of methotrexate and is usually continued 24 to 72 hours. Don't confuse with folic acid. This rescue technique is effective against systemic toxicity but does not interfere with the tumor cells' absorption of the methotrexate.
• Avoid all I.M. injections in patients with thrombocytopenia.
• Has been used investigationally to treat rheumatoid arthritis that is refractory to other therapy.

thioguanine
Lanvis♦♦

INDICATIONS & DOSAGE

Acute leukemia, chronic granulocytic leukemia—
Adults and children: initially, 2 mg/kg daily P.O. (usually calculated to nearest 20 mg); then increased gradually to 3 mg/kg daily if no toxic effects occur.

SIDE EFFECTS

Blood: *leukopenia,* anemia, *thrombocytopenia* (occurs slowly over 2 to 4 weeks).
GI: nausea, vomiting, stomatitis, diarrhea, anorexia.
Hepatic: hepatotoxicity, jaundice.
Metabolic: hyperuricemia.

INTERACTIONS
None significant.

NURSING CONSIDERATIONS
• Use cautiously in renal or hepatic dysfunction.
• Stop drug if hepatotoxicity or hepatic tenderness occurs. Watch for jaundice; may reverse if drug stopped promptly.
• Do CBC daily during induction, then weekly during maintenance therapy.
• Monitor serum uric acid.
• Sometimes ordered as 6-thioguanine. The number 6 is part of drug name and does not signify dosage units.
• Avoid all I.M. injections when platelets are low.

70

Antibiotic antineoplastic agents

bleomycin sulfate
dactinomycin (actinomycin D)
daunorubicin hydrochloride
doxorubicin hydrochloride
mithramycin
mitomycin
procarbazine hydrochloride

MECHANISM OF ACTION
• Bleomycin inhibits deoxyribonucleic acid (DNA) synthesis and causes scission of single- and double-stranded DNA.
• Dactinomycin, daunorubicin, doxorubicin, and mithramycin interfere with DNA-dependent ribonucleic acid (RNA) synthesis by intercalation.
• Mithramycin also inhibits osteocytic activity, blocking calcium and phosphorus resorption from bone.
• Mitomycin acts like an alkylating agent, cross-linking strands of DNA. This causes an imbalance of cell growth, leading to cell death.
• Procarbazine inhibits DNA, RNA, and protein synthesis.

COMBINATION PRODUCTS
None.

---

bleomycin sulfate
Blenoxane♦

INDICATIONS & DOSAGE
Dosage and indications may vary.
Check patient's protocol with doctor.
Cervical, esophageal, head, neck, and testicular cancer—
Adults: 10 to 20 units/m² I.V., I.M., or S.C. 1 or 2 times weekly to total 300 to 400 units.
Hodgkin's disease—
Adults:
10 to 20 units/m² I.V., I.M., or S.C. 1 or 2 times weekly. After 50% response, maintenance 1 unit I.M. or I.V. daily or 5 units I.M. or I.V. weekly.
Lymphomas—
Adults:
first 2 doses should be 5 units or less, and patient should be monitored for any allergic reaction. If no reaction occurs, then follow above dosing schedule.

SIDE EFFECTS
CNS: hyperesthesia of scalp and fingers, headache.
GI: *stomatitis, prolonged anorexia in 13% of patients, nausea, vomiting, diarrhea.*
Skin: *erythema, vesiculation, and hardening and discoloration of palmar and plantar skin in 8% of patients; desquamation of hands, feet, and pressure areas; hyperpigmentation; acne.*
Other: *reversible alopecia,* swelling of interphalangeal joints, *pulmonary fibrosis in 10% of patients, pulmonary side effects (fine rales, fever, dyspnea), leukocytosis and nonproductive cough, allergic reaction (fever up to 106° F. [41.1° C.] with chills up to 5 hours after injection; anaphylaxis in 1% to 6% of patients).*

INTERACTIONS
None significant.

NURSING CONSIDERATIONS
- Use cautiously in renal or pulmonary impairment.
- Drug concentrates in keratin of squamous epithelium. To prevent linear streaking, don't use adhesive dressings on skin.
- Allergic reactions may be delayed for several hours, especially in lymphoma.
- Monitor chest X-ray and listen to lungs.
- Pulmonary function tests should be performed to establish baseline. Drug should be stopped if pulmonary function test shows a marked decline.
- Pulmonary side effects common in patients over 70 years. Fatal pulmonary fibrosis occurs in 1% of patients, especially when cumulative dose exceeds 400 units.
- Advise patient that alopecia may occur, but that it is usually reversible.
- Refrigerated, reconstituted solution stable 4 weeks; at room temperature, stable 2 weeks. Solutions prepared in ampuls should be discarded if not used immediately.
- Bleomycin-induced fever is common and may be treated with antipyretics.

---

dactinomycin (actinomycin D)
Cosmegen◆

INDICATIONS & DOSAGE
Dosage and indications may vary. Check patient's protocol with doctor.
Melanomas, sarcomas, trophoblastic tumors in women, testicular cancer—
Adults: 500 mcg I.V. daily for 5 days; wait 2 to 4 weeks and repeat; or 2 mg I.V. single weekly dose for 3 weeks; wait for bone marrow recovery, then repeat in 3 to 4 weeks.
Wilms' tumor, rhabdomyosarcoma—
Children: 15 mcg/kg I.V. daily for 5 days. Maximum dose 500 mcg daily. Wait for marrow recovery.

SIDE EFFECTS
Blood: anemia, *leukopenia, thrombocytopenia, pancytopenia.*
GI: *anorexia, nausea, vomiting,* abdominal pain, diarrhea, *stomatitis.*
Skin: *erythema;* desquamation; *hyperpigmentation of skin, especially in previously irradiated areas; acne-like eruptions (reversible).*
Local: phlebitis, severe damage to soft tissue.
Other: reversible alopecia.

INTERACTIONS
None significant.

NURSING CONSIDERATIONS
- Contraindicated in renal, hepatic, or bone marrow impairment; viral infection; or during chickenpox or herpes zoster infection. Use cautiously in metastatic testicular tumors, in combination with chlorambucil and methotrexate therapy. Extreme bone marrow and GI toxicity can occur with this combined therapy.
- Stomatitis, diarrhea, leukopenia, thrombocytopenia may require stopping therapy.
- Give antiemetic before administering to reduce nausea.
- Monitor renal, hepatic functions.
- Monitor CBCs daily and platelet counts every third day.
- Observe for signs of bleeding.
- Warn patient that alopecia may occur but is usually reversible.
- Use only sterile water (without preservatives) as diluent for injection.
- Administer through a running I.V. infusion. Avoid infiltration.

---

daunorubicin hydrochloride
Cerubidine◆

INDICATIONS & DOSAGE
Dosage and indications may vary. Check patient's protocol with doctor.
Remission induction in acute nonlym-

---

phocytic leukemia (myelogenous, mono-cytic, erythroid) in adults—
As a single agent: 60 mg/m² daily I.V. on days 1, 2, and 3 q 3 to 4 weeks.
In combination: 45 mg/m² daily I.V. on days 1, 2, and 3 of the first course and on days 1 and 2 of subsequent courses with cytosine arabinoside infusions.
Note: Dose should be reduced if hepatic function is impaired.

SIDE EFFECTS
Blood: *bone marrow depression* (lowest blood counts 10 to 14 days after administration).
CV: *cardiomyopathy (dose-related), EKG changes, arrhythmias,* pericarditis, myocarditis.
GI: *nausea, vomiting, stomatitis, esophagitis,* anorexia, diarrhea.
Skin: rash.
Local: *severe cellulitis or tissue slough if drug extravasates.*
Other: *generalized alopecia,* fever, chills.

INTERACTIONS
Heparin: don't mix. May form a precipitate.

NURSING CONSIDERATIONS
• Use cautiously in myelosuppression, impaired cardiac function.
• Stop drug immediately in signs of congestive heart failure or cardiomyopathy. Prevent by limiting cumulative dose to 550 mg/m²; 450 mg/m² when patient has been receiving radiation therapy that encompasses the heart or any other cardiotoxic agent.
• Monitor EKG before treatment, monthly during therapy.
• Note if resting pulse rate is high (a sign of cardiac side effects).
• *Avoid extravasation;* inject into tubing of freely flowing I.V. *Never* give I.M. or subcutaneously.
• Monitor CBC and hepatic function.
• Warn patient urine may be red for

1 to 2 days and that it's a normal side effect, not hematuria.
• Advise patient that alopecia may occur, but that it's usually reversible.
• Don't use a scalp tourniquet or apply ice to prevent alopecia. May compromise effectiveness of drug.
• Nausea and vomiting may be very severe and last 24 to 48 hours.
• Refrigerated, reconstituted solution stable for at least 36 hours; 24 hours at room temperature. Optimally, use within 8 hours of preparation.
• Reddish color looks very similar to doxorubicin (Adriamycin). *Do not confuse the two drugs.*

doxorubicin hydrochloride
Adriamycin♦

INDICATIONS & DOSAGE
Dosage and indications may vary. Check patient's protocol with doctor.
Bladder, breast, cervical, head, neck, liver, lung, ovarian, prostatic, stomach, testicular, and thyroid cancer; Hodgkin's disease; acute lymphoblastic and myeloblastic leukemia; Wilms' tumor; neuroblastomas; lymphomas; sarcomas—
Adults: 60 to 75 mg/m² I.V. as single dose q 3 weeks; or 30 mg/m² I.V. in single daily dose, days 1 to 3 of 4-week cycle. Maximum cumulative dose 550 mg/m².

SIDE EFFECTS
Blood: *leukopenia, especially agranulocytosis, during days 10 to 15, with recovery by day 21; thrombocytopenia.*
CV: *cardiac depression, seen in such EKG changes as sinus tachycardia, T-wave flattening, ST segment depression, voltage reduction; arrhythmias in 11% of patients; cardiomyopathy (sometimes with pulmonary edema) with mortality of 30% to 75%.*
GI: *nausea, vomiting,* diarrhea, *stomatitis,* esophagitis.

GU: enhancement of cyclophospha-mide-induced bladder injury.
Skin: *hyperpigmentation of skin, especially in previously irradiated areas.*
Local: *severe cellulitis or tissue slough if drug extravasates.*
Other: hyperpigmentation of nails and dermal creases, *complete alopecia within 3 to 4 weeks;* hair may regrow 2 to 5 months after drug is stopped.

INTERACTIONS
None significant.

NURSING CONSIDERATIONS
• Use cautiously in myelosuppression, impaired cardiac function.
• Stop drug or slow rate of infusion if tachycardia develops.
• Stop drug immediately in signs of congestive heart failure. Prevent by limiting cumulative dose to 550 mg/m^2; 450 mg/m^2 when patient is also receiving cyclophosphamide.
• Monitor EKG before treatment, monthly during therapy.
• Note if resting pulse is high: a signal of cardiac side effects.
• *Avoid extravasation;* inject into tubing of freely flowing I.V. *Never* give I.M. or subcutaneously.
• Monitor CBC and hepatic function.
• Warn patient urine will be red for 1 to 2 days.
• Dose should be reduced in hepatic dysfunction.
• Warn patient that alopecia will occur. A scalp tourniquet or application of ice may decrease alopecia. However, *do not* use if treating leukemias or other neoplasms where tumor stem cells may be present in scalp.
• Refrigerated, reconstituted solution stable 48 hours; at room temperature, stable 24 hours.
• If cumulative dose exceeds 550 mg/m^2 body surface area, 30% of patients develop cardiac side effects, which begin 2 weeks to 6 months after stopping drug.
• Decrease dose if serum bilirubin is

increased: 50% dose when bilirubin is 1.2 to 3 mg/100 ml; 25% dose when bilirubin is greater than 3 mg/100 ml.
• Esophagitis very common in patients who have also received radiation therapy.
• Reddish color looks very similar to daunorubicin. *Do not confuse the two drugs.*

mithramycin
Mithracin

INDICATIONS & DOSAGE
Dosage and indications may vary. Check patient's protocol with doctor.
Hypercalcemia—
Adults: 25 mcg/kg I.V. daily for 1 to 4 days.
Testicular cancer—
Adults: 25 to 30 mcg/kg I.V. daily for up to 8 to 10 days (based on ideal body weight or actual weight, whichever is less).

SIDE EFFECTS
Blood: *thrombocytopenia; bleeding syndrome, from epistaxis to generalized hemorrhage; facial flushing.*
GI: *nausea, vomiting,* anorexia, diarrhea, stomatitis.
GU: proteinuria; increased BUN, serum creatinine.
Metabolic: *decreased serum calcium,* potassium, and phosphorus.
Skin: periorbital pallor, usually the day before toxic symptoms occur.
Local: extravasation causes irritation, cellulitis.

INTERACTIONS
None significant.

NURSING CONSIDERATIONS
• Contraindicated in thrombocytopenia and in coagulation and bleeding disorders. Use cautiously in renal, hepatic, or bone marrow impairment.
• Slow infusion reduces nausea that develops with I.V. push.

Italicized side effects are common or life-threatening.
∗Liquid form contains alcohol.　　∗∗May contain tartrazine.

- Monitor LDH, SGOT, SGPT, alkaline phosphatase, BUN, creatinine, potassium, calcium, phosphorus.
- Monitor platelet count and prothrombin time before and during therapy.
- Observe for signs of bleeding. Facial flushing early indicator of bleeding.
- Give antiemetic before administering to reduce nausea.
- Avoid extravasation. If I.V. infiltrates, stop immediately; use ice packs. Restart I.V.
- Avoid contact with skin or mucous membranes.
- Therapeutic effect in hypercalcemia may not be seen for 24 to 48 hours; may last 3 to 15 days.
- Precipitous drop in calcium possible. Monitor patient for tetany, carpopedal spasm, Chvostek's sign, muscle cramps; check serum calcium levels.
- Store lyophilized powder in refrigerator. Remains stable after reconstitution for 24 hours; 48 hours in refrigerator.

sation causes cellulitis, ulceration, sloughing.
Other: *reversible alopecia, purple coloration of nail beds.*

INTERACTIONS
None significant.

NURSING CONSIDERATIONS
- Use cautiously when platelet count is less than 75,000/mm³, WBC is less than 4,000/mm³; in coagulation or bleeding disorders, serious infections, impaired renal function.
- Continue CBC and blood studies at least 7 weeks after therapy is stopped. Observe for signs of bleeding.
- Advise patient that alopecia may occur, but that it's usually reversible.
- Reconstituted solution stable 1 week at room temperature, 2 weeks refrigerated.
- Has been administered topically by bladder instillation and has been given intraarterially through the hepatic artery.

mitomycin
Mutamycin♦

INDICATIONS & DOSAGE
Dosage and indications may vary. Check patient's protocol with doctor.
Breast, colon, head, neck, lung, pancreatic, and stomach cancer; malignant melanoma—
Adults: 2 mg/m² I.V. daily for 5 days. Stop drug for 2 days, then repeat dose for 5 more days; or 20 mg/m² as a single dose. Repeat cycle 6 to 8 weeks. Stop drug if WBC less than 4,000/mm³ or platelets less than 75,000/mm³.

SIDE EFFECTS
Blood: *thrombocytopenia, leukopenia (may be delayed up to 8 weeks and may be cumulative with successive doses).*
CNS: paresthesias.
GI: nausea, vomiting, anorexia, stomatitis.
Local: desquamation, induration, pruritus, *pain at site of injection.* Extrava-

procarbazine hydrochloride
Matulane, Natulan♦♦

INDICATIONS & DOSAGE
Dosage and indications may vary. Check patient's protocol with doctor.
Hodgkin's disease, lymphomas, brain and lung cancer—
Adults: 100 to 150 mg/m² P.O. for 10 days until WBC falls below 4,000/mm³ or platelets fall below 100,000/mm³. After bone marrow recovers, resume maintenance dose 50 to 100 mg P.O. daily.
Children: 50 mg P.O. daily for first week, then 100 mg/m² until response or toxicity occurs. Maintenance dose is 50 mg P.O. daily after bone marrow recovery.

SIDE EFFECTS
Blood: bleeding tendency, *thrombocytopenia, leukopenia,* anemia.

CNS: nervousness, depression, insomnia, nightmares, *hallucinations,* confusion.
EENT: retinal hemorrhage, nystagmus, photophobia.
GI: *nausea, vomiting, anorexia,* stomatitis, dry mouth, dysphagia, diarrhea, constipation.
Skin: dermatitis.
Other: reversible alopecia, pleural effusion.

INTERACTIONS
Alcohol: disulfiram (Antabuse)-like reaction. Warn patient not to drink alcohol.

NURSING CONSIDERATIONS
• Use cautiously in inadequate bone marrow reserve, leukopenia, thrombocytopenia, anemia, impaired hepatic or renal function.
• Observe for signs of bleeding.
• Warn patient not to drink alcoholic beverages while taking this drug.
• Procarbazine inhibits monoamine oxidase (MAO). Use cautiously with other MAO inhibitors, tricyclic antidepressants, phenothiazines, and foods with a large tyramine content.

71

Antineoplastics altering hormone balance

aminoglutethimide
dromostanolone propionate
estramustine phosphate sodium
megestrol acetate
mitotane
tamoxifen citrate
testolactone

MECHANISM OF ACTION
• Aminoglutethimide blocks conversion of cholesterol to delta-5-pregnenolone in the adrenal cortex, inhibiting the synthesis of glucocorticoids, mineralocorticoids, and other steroids.
• Dromostanolone, megestrol, and testolactone change the tumor's hormonal environment and alter the neoplastic process.
• Estramustine, a combination of estrogen and an alkylating agent, acts by its ability to bind selectively to a protein present in the human prostate. The exact mechanism is unknown.
• Mitotane selectively destroys adrenocortical tissue and hinders extra-adrenal metabolism of cortisol.
• Tamoxifen acts as an estrogen antagonist.

COMBINATION PRODUCTS
None.

---

aminoglutethimide
Cytadren

INDICATIONS & DOSAGE
Suppression of adrenal function in Cushing's syndrome and adrenal cancer; metastatic breast cancer—
Adults: 250 mg P.O. q.i.d. at 6-hour intervals. Dosage may be increased in increments of 250 mg daily every 1 to 2 weeks to a maximum total daily dose of 2 g.

SIDE EFFECTS
Blood: transient leukopenia, *severe pancytopenia.*
CNS: *drowsiness,* headache, dizziness.
CV: hypotension, tachycardia.
Endocrine: adrenal insufficiency, masculinization, hirsutism.
GI: *nausea, anorexia.*
Skin: *morbilliform skin rash,* pruritis, urticaria.
Other: fever, myalgia.

INTERACTIONS
None significant.

NURSING CONSIDERATIONS
• May cause adrenal hypofunction, especially under stressful conditions such as surgery, trauma, or acute illness. Patients may need hydrocortisone and mineralocorticoid supplements in these situations. Monitor patients carefully.
• Monitor blood pressure frequently. Advise patient to stand up slowly in order to minimize orthostatic hypotension.
• May cause a decrease in thyroid hormone production. Monitor thyroid function studies.
• Perform baseline hematologic studies and monitor CBC periodically.
• Warn patient that drug can cause drowsiness and dizziness. Advise him to avoid activities that require alertness and good psychomotor coordination

---

until response to drug has been determined.

• Tell patient to report if skin rash persists for more than 5 to 8 days.

Reassure patient that drowsiness, nausea, and loss of appetite will diminish within 2 weeks after start of aminoglutethimide therapy. However, if these symptoms persist, tell patient to notify doctor.

• Also used to produce a medical adrenalectomy in patients who have metastatic breast cancer.

dromostanolone propionate
Drolban

INDICATIONS & DOSAGE
Advanced, inoperable metastatic breast cancer, 1 to 5 years postmenopausal—
Women: 100 mg deep I.M. 3 times weekly.

SIDE EFFECTS
GU: clitoral enlargement.
Metabolic: hypercalcemia.
Skin: acne.
Other: *virilism (deepened voice, facial hair growth), which may be intense after long-term treatment;* edema, pain at injection site.

INTERACTIONS
None significant.

NURSING CONSIDERATIONS
• Contraindicated by any route other than I.M.; in male breast cancer; and in premenopausal women. Use cautiously in hepatic disease, cardiac decompensation, nephritis, nephrosis, and prostatic cancer.

• If severe hypercalcemia develops or disease accelerates, drug should be stopped.

• Therapeutic effect may be delayed 8 to 12 weeks. Reassure patient that results are not immediate.

• Do not store in refrigerator; drug precipitates at cold temperatures.

• Explain possible virilizing effects, skin and libido changes to female patients to prevent undue alarm.

• Dromostanolone is an androgen.

estramustine phosphate sodium
Emcyt

INDICATIONS & DOSAGE
Palliative treatment of metastatic or progressive cancer of the prostate—
Adults: 10 to 16 mg/kg P.O. in 3 to 4 divided doses. Usual dosage is 14 mg/kg daily. Therapy should continue for up to 3 months and, if successful, be maintained as long as the patient responds.

SIDE EFFECTS
Blood: leukopenia, thrombocytopenia.
CV: *myocardial infarction, cerebrovascular accident, edema, pulmonary emboli,* thrombophlebitis, congestive heart failure, hypertension.
GI: *nausea, vomiting,* diarrhea.
Skin: rash, pruritus.
Other: *painful gynecomastia and breast tenderness,* thinning of hair, hyperglycemia.

INTERACTIONS
None significant.

NURSING CONSIDERATIONS
• Contraindicated in patients hypersensitive to estradiol and nitrogen mustard. Also contraindicated in active thrombophlebitis or thromboembolic disorders, except in those cases where the actual tumor mass is the cause of the thromboembolic phenomenon.

• Use cautiously in patients with history of thrombophlebitis or thromboembolic disorders, cerebrovascular and coronary artery disease.

• Estramustine may exaggerate preexisting peripheral edema or congestive heart failure. Weight gain should be monitored regularly in these patients.

- Monitor blood pressure and glucose tolerance periodically throughout therapy.
- Because of the possibility of mutagenic effects, advise patient and spouse to use contraceptive measures if woman is of childbearing age.
- Estramustine is a combination of the estrogen estradiol and a nitrogen mustard. Shown to be effective in patients refractory to estrogen therapy alone.
- Patient may continue estramustine as long as he's responding favorably. Some patients have taken the drug for more than 3 years.
- Store capsules in refrigerator.

megestrol acetate
Megace♦**

INDICATIONS & DOSAGE
Breast cancer—
Women: 40 mg P.O. q.i.d.
Endometrial cancer—
Women: 40 to 320 mg P.O. daily in divided doses.

SIDE EFFECTS
None reported.

INTERACTIONS
None significant.

NURSING CONSIDERATIONS
- Use cautiously in patients with history of thrombophlebitis.
- Adequate trial is 2 months. Reassure patient that therapeutic response isn't immediate.

mitotane
Lysodren♦

INDICATIONS & DOSAGE
Inoperable adrenocortical cancer—
Adults: 9 to 10 g P.O. daily, divided t.i.d. to q.i.d. If severe side effects appear, reduce dose until maximum tolerated dose is achieved (varies from 2 to 16 g daily but is usually 8 to 10 g daily).

SIDE EFFECTS
CNS: *depression, somnolence, vertigo;* brain damage and dysfunction in long-term, high-dose therapy.
GI: *severe nausea, vomiting,* diarrhea, anorexia.
Metabolic: adrenal insufficiency.
Skin: dermatitis.

INTERACTIONS
None significant.

NURSING CONSIDERATIONS
- Use cautiously in hepatic disease.
- Drug should not be used in a patient with shock or trauma. Use of corticosteroids may avoid acute adrenocorticoid insufficiency.
- Assess and record behavioral and neurologic signs for baseline data daily throughout therapy.
- Give antiemetic before administering to reduce nausea.
- Dosage may be reduced if GI or skin side effects are severe.
- Obese patients may need higher dosage and may have longer-lasting side effects, since drug distributes mostly to body fat.
- Warn ambulatory patient of CNS side effects; advise him to avoid hazardous tasks requiring mental alertness or physical coordination.
- Monitor effectiveness by reduction in pain, weakness, anorexia.
- Adequate trial is at least 3 months, but therapy can continue if clinical benefits are observed.

tamoxifen citrate
Nolvadex♦

INDICATIONS & DOSAGE
Advanced premenopausal and postmenopausal breast cancer—
Women: 10 to 20 mg P.O. b.i.d.

SIDE EFFECTS
Blood: transient fall in WBC or platelets.
GI: nausea in 10% of patients, vomiting, anorexia.
GU: vaginal discharge and bleeding.
Skin: rash.
Other: temporary bone or tumor pain, hot flashes in 7% of patients. Brief exacerbation of pain from osseous metastases.

INTERACTIONS
None significant.

NURSING CONSIDERATIONS
• Use cautiously in preexisting leukopenia, thrombocytopenia.
• Use analgesic to relieve pain.
• Monitor WBC and platelet counts.
• Acts as an "antiestrogen." Best results in patients with positive estrogen receptors.
• Side effects are usually minor and are well tolerated.
• Reassure patient that acute exacerbation of bone pain during tamoxifen therapy usually indicates drug will produce good response.
• Short-term therapy induces ovulation in premenopausal women. *Mechanical* contraception recommended.
• Also used to treat breast cancer in males and advanced ovarian cancer in women.

---

testolactone
Teslac♦

INDICATIONS & DOSAGE
Advanced postmenopausal breast cancer—

Women: 100 mg deep I.M. 3 times weekly; or 250 mg P.O. q.i.d.

SIDE EFFECTS
Local: pain, inflammation at injection site.
Metabolic: hypercalcemia.

INTERACTIONS
None significant.

NURSING CONSIDERATIONS
• Contraindicated in male breast cancer and not recommended in premenopausal females.
• Adequate trial is 3 months. Reassure patient that therapeutic response isn't immediate.
• Monitor fluids and electrolytes, especially calcium levels.
• Immobilized patients are prone to hypercalcemia. Exercise may prevent it. Force fluids to aid calcium excretion.
• Shake vial vigorously before drawing up injection. Do not refrigerate.
• Use 1½" needle and inject into upper outer quadrant of gluteal region. Rotate injection sites.
• No advantage over testosterone, except less virilization.
• Higher than recommended doses do not increase incidence of remission.
• Testolactone is an androgen.

Italicized side effects are common or life-threatening.
*Liquid form contains alcohol.   **May contain tartrazine.

72

Vinca alkaloids, podophyllin derivatives, and asparaginase

asparaginase (L-asparaginase)
etoposide (VP-16)
vinblastine sulfate
vincristine sulfate
vindesine sulfate
teniposide (VM-26)

MECHANISM OF ACTION
● Asparaginase destroys the amino acid asparagine, which is needed for protein synthesis in acute lymphocytic leukemia. This leads to death of the leukemic cell.
● Podophyllin derivatives and vinca alkaloids all arrest mitosis in metaphase, blocking cell division.

COMBINATION PRODUCTS
None.

asparaginase (or L-asparaginase)
Elspar

INDICATIONS & DOSAGE
Acute lymphocytic leukemia (when used along with other drugs)—
Adults and children: 1,000 international units (IU)/kg I.V. daily for 10 days, injected over 30 minutes or by slow I.V. push; or 6,000 IU/m² I.M. at intervals specified in protocol.
Sole induction agent—200 IU/kg I.V. daily for 28 days.

SIDE EFFECTS
Blood: *hypofibrinogenemia* and depression of other clotting factors, thrombo-cytopenia, *leukopenia,* depression of serum albumin.
CNS: lethargy, somnolence.
GI: *vomiting (may last up to 24 hours), anorexia, nausea,* cramps, weight loss, pancreatitis.
GU: *azotemia,* renal failure, uric acid nephropathy, glycosuria, polyuria.
Hepatic: elevated SGOT, SGPT; *hepatotoxicity.*
Metabolic: elevated alkaline phosphatase and bilirubin (direct and indirect); increase or decrease in total lipids; *hyperglycemia; increased blood ammonia.*
Skin: *rash, urticaria.*
Other: *hemorrhagic pancreatitis, anaphylaxis (relatively common).*

INTERACTIONS
None significant.

NURSING CONSIDERATIONS
● Contraindicated in pancreatitis, previous hypersensitivity unless desensitized. Use cautiously in preexisting hepatic dysfunction.
● Should be administered in hospital setting with close supervision.
● Don't use as sole agent to induce remission unless combination therapy is inappropriate. Not recommended for maintenance therapy.
● Risk of hypersensitivity increases with repeated doses. Patient may be desensitized, but this doesn't rule out risk of allergic reactions. Routine administration of 2-unit I.V. test dose may identify high-risk patients.

• Intravenous administration of asparaginase with or immediately before vincristine or prednisone may increase toxicity reactions.

• Give I.V. injection over 30-minute period through a running infusion of sodium chloride injection or 5% dextrose injection.

• For I.M. injection, limit dose at single injection site to 2 ml.

• Due to vomiting, patient may need parenteral fluids for 24 hours or until oral fluids are tolerated.

• Monitor blood count and bone marrow levels. Bone marrow regeneration may take 5 to 6 weeks.

• Obtain frequent serum amylase determinations to check pancreatic status. If elevated, asparaginase should be discontinued.

• Watch for uric acid nephropathy. Prevent occurrence by increasing fluid intake. Allopurinol may be ordered.

• Watch for signs of bleeding, such as petechiae and melena.

• Monitor blood sugar and test urine for sugar before and during therapy. Watch for signs of hyperglycemia, such as glycosuria and polyuria.

• Reconstitute with 2 to 5 ml sterile water for injection or sodium chloride injection.

• Don't shake vial. May cause loss of potency. Don't use cloudy solutions.

• Refrigerate unopened dry powder. Reconstituted solution stable 6 hours at room temperature, 24 hours refrigerated.

• Keep epinephrine, diphenhydramine, and I.V. corticosteroids available for treatment of anaphylaxis.

etoposide (VP-16)

INDICATIONS & DOSAGE
Small cell carcinoma of the lung, acute nonlymphocytic leukemia, lymphosarcoma, Hodgkin's disease, testicular carcinoma—
Adults: 45 to 75 mg/m^2 daily I.V. for 3 to 5 days repeated q 3 to 5 weeks; or 200 to 250 mg/m^2 I.V. weekly; or 125 to 140 mg/m^2 daily I.V. 3 times a week q 5 weeks.

SIDE EFFECTS
Blood: *myelosuppression (dose-limiting), leukopenia,* thrombocytopenia.
CV: hypotension from rapid infusion.
GI: nausea and vomiting.
Local: infrequent phlebitis.
Other: occasional headache and fever, *reversible alopecia, anaphylaxis* (rare).

INTERACTIONS
None significant.

NURSING CONSIDERATIONS
• Intraperitoneal, intrapleural, and intrathecal administration of this drug is contraindicated.

• Give drug by slow I.V. infusion (over at least 30 minutes) to prevent severe hypotension.

• Patients receiving drug over less than 2 hours should be in the recumbent position.

• Blood pressure should be monitored before infusion and at 30-minute intervals during infusion. If systolic blood pressure falls below 90 mmHg, infusion should be stopped and doctor notified.

• Do *not* dilute in 5% dextrose in water due to physical incompatibility (precipitate will form).

• Drug must be diluted to a concentration of 1 mg/ml or less with normal saline solution before administration. Cloudy solutions should be discarded.

• Solutions containing 1 mg/ml stable for 30 minutes; 0.4 mg/ml stable 3 hours; 0.2 mg/ml stable 6 hours.

• Have diphenhydramine, hydrocortisone, epinephrine, and airway available in case of an anaphylactic reaction.

• Monitor CBC. Observe patient for signs of bone-marrow depression.

• An investigational drug.

---

vinblastine sulfate (VLB)
Velban, Velbe••

INDICATIONS & DOSAGE
Breast or testicular cancer, Hodgkin's and non-Hodgkin's lymphomas, choriocarcinoma, lymphosarcoma, neuroblastoma, mycosis fungoides, histiocytosis—
Adults and children: 0.1 mg/kg or 3.7 mg/m^2 I.V. weekly or q 2 weeks. May be increased to maximum dose (adults) of 0.5 mg/kg or 18.5 mg/m^2 I.V. weekly according to response. Dose should not be repeated if WBC less than 4,000/mm^3.

SIDE EFFECTS
Blood: *leukopenia* (nadir days 4 to 10 and lasts another 7 to 14 days), *thrombocytopenia.*
CNS: depression, *paresthesias, peripheral neuropathy and neuritis, numbness, loss of deep tendon reflexes, muscle pain and weakness.*
EENT: pharyngitis.
GI: *nausea, vomiting, stomatitis,* ulcer and bleeding, *constipation, ileus, anorexia, weight loss,* abdominal pain.
GU: oligospermia, aspermia, urinary retention.
Skin: dermatitis, vesiculation.
Local: *irritation, phlebitis,* cellulitis, necrosis if I.V. extravasates.
Other: reversible alopecia in 5% to 10% of patients; *pain in tumor site,* low fever.

INTERACTIONS
None significant.

NURSING CONSIDERATIONS
• Contraindicated in severe leukopenia, bacterial infection. Use cautiously in jaundice or hepatic dysfunction.
• Give antiemetic before administering to reduce nausea.
• Drug should be stopped if stomatitis occurs.
• Give laxatives as needed. May use stool softeners prophylactically.
• Don't repeat dose more frequently than every 7 days or severe leukopenia will develop.
• Less neurotoxic than vincristine.
• Should be injected directly into vein or tubing of running I.V. over 1 minute. May also be given in 50 ml dextrose in water or normal saline solution and infused over 15 minutes. If extravasation occurs, stop infusion. Apply ice packs on and off every 2 hours for 24 hours.
• Warn patient that alopecia may occur but is usually reversible.
• Adequate trial 12 weeks; reassure patient that therapeutic response isn't immediate.
• Reconstitute 10-mg vial with 10 ml of sodium chloride injection or sterile water. This yields 1 mg/ml.
• Refrigerate reconstituted solution. Discard after 30 days.
• Don't confuse vinblastine with vincristine or the investigational agent vindesine.

vincristine sulfate
Oncovin•

INDICATIONS & DOSAGE
Acute lymphoblastic and other leukemias, Hodgkin's disease, lymphosarcoma, reticulum cell sarcoma, neuroblastoma, rhabdomyosarcoma, Wilms' tumor, osteogenic and other sarcomas, lung and breast cancer—
Adults: 1 to 2 mg/m^2 I.V. weekly.
Children: 1.5 to 2 mg/m^2 I.V. weekly. Maximum single dose (adults and children) is 2 mg.

SIDE EFFECTS
Blood: rapidly reversible mild anemia and leukopenia.
CNS: *peripheral neuropathy,* sensory loss, *deep tendon reflex loss, paresthesias, wrist and foot drop,* ataxia, cranial nerve palsies (headache, *jaw pain,* hoarseness, vocal cord paralysis, visual

disturbances), *muscle weakness and cramps,* depression, agitation, insomnia; neurotoxicities may be permanent.
EENT: diplopia, optic and extraocular neuropathy, ptosis.
GI: *constipation, cramps,* ileus that mimics surgical abdomen, *nausea, vomiting,* anorexia, *stomatitis,* weight loss, dysphagia.
GU: urinary retention.
Local: *phlebitis,* cellulitis.
Other: *reversible alopecia (up to 71% of patients).*

INTERACTIONS
None significant.

NURSING CONSIDERATIONS
• Use cautiously in jaundice or hepatic dysfunction, neuromuscular disease, infection, or with other neurotoxic drugs.
• Because of neurotoxicity, don't give drug more than once a week. Children more resistant to neurotoxicity than adults.
• Should be given directly into vein or tubing of running I.V. slowly over 1 minute. May also be given in 50 ml dextrose in water or normal saline solution and infused over 15 minutes. If drug infiltrates, apply ice packs on and off every 2 hours for 24 hours.
• Check for depression of Achilles tendon reflex, numbness, tingling, foot or wrist drop, difficulty in walking, ataxia, slapping gait. Also check ability to walk on heels. Support patient when walking.
• Monitor bowel function. Give stool softener, laxative, or water before dosing. Constipation may be an early sign of neurotoxicity.
• Reconstitute with sodium chloride injection, normal saline solution, or sterile water.
• Refrigerate reconstituted solution. Discard after 14 days.
• Warn patient that alopecia may occur but is usually reversible.
• Be extremely careful about doses.

Don't confuse vincristine with vinblastine or the investigational agent vindesine.

---

vindesine
Eldesine, DAVA

INDICATIONS & DOSAGE
Acute lymphoblastic leukemia, breast cancer, malignant melanoma, lymphosarcoma, non–small-cell lung carcinoma—
Adults: 3 to 4 mg/m² I.V. q 7 to 14 days, or continuous I.V. infusion 1.2 to 1.5 mg/m² daily for 5 days every 3 weeks.

SIDE EFFECTS
Blood: *leukopenia, thrombocytopenia.*
CNS: *paresthesias, decreased deep tendon reflex, muscle weakness.*
GI: *constipation, abdominal cramping,* nausea, vomiting.
Local: *phlebitis,* necrosis on extravasation.
Other: *reversible alopecia,* jaw pain, fever with continuous infusions.

INTERACTIONS
None significant.

NURSING CONSIDERATIONS
• Do not give as a continuous infusion unless patient has a central I.V. line.
• To prevent paralytic ileus, encourage patient to force fluids, increase ambulation, and use stool softeners.
• Instruct patient to report any signs of neurotoxicity: numbness and tingling of extremities, jaw pain, constipation (may be early sign of neurotoxicity).
• Assess for depression of Achilles tendon reflex, foot or wrist drop, slapping gait (late signs of neurotoxicity).
• Neuropathy may be assessed by recording patient signatures before each course of therapy and observing for deterioration of handwriting.
• Monitor CBC.
• Avoid extravasation. Drug is a pain-

Italicized side effects are common or life-threatening.
*Liquid form contains alcohol.   **May contain tartrazine.

ful vesicant. Give 10 ml normal saline solution flush before drug to test vein patency, and 10 ml normal saline solution flush to remove any remaining drug from tubing after drug is given.
• When reconstituted with the 10 ml diluent provided or normal saline solution, the drug is stable for 2 weeks under refrigeration.
• Do not mix vindesine with other drugs; compatibility with other drugs has not yet been determined.
• An investigational drug.

teniposide (VM-26)

INDICATIONS & DOSAGE
Hodgkin's and non-Hodgkin's lymphomas, acute lymphocytic leukemia, bladder carcinoma—
Adults: 50 to 100 mg/m² I.V. once or twice weekly for 4 to 6 weeks, or 40 to 50 mg/m² daily I.V. for 5 days repeated every 3 to 4 weeks.

SIDE EFFECTS
Blood: *myelosuppression (dose-limiting), leukopenia,* some thrombocytopenia.
CV: hypotension from rapid infusion.
GI: nausea and vomiting.
Local: *phlebitis,* extravasation.

Other: alopecia (rare), *anaphylaxis* (rare).

INTERACTIONS
None significant.

NURSING CONSIDERATIONS
• May be diluted for infusion in either 5% dextrose in water or normal saline solution, but cloudy solutions should be discarded.
• Infuse over 45 to 90 minutes to prevent hypotension.
• Solutions containing 0.5 to 2 mg/ml are stable for 4 hours. Solutions containing 0.1 to 0.2 mg/ml are stable for 6 hours.
• Blood pressure should be monitored before infusion and at 30-minute intervals during infusion. If systolic blood pressure falls below 90 mmHg, infusion should be stopped and doctor notified.
• Have diphenhydramine, hydrocortisone, epinephrine, and airway available in case of an anaphylactic reaction.
• Monitor CBC. Observe patient for signs of bone marrow depression.
• Avoid extravasation.
• Drug may be given by local bladder instillation as a treatment for bladder cancer.
• An investigational drug.

73

Ophthalmic anti-infectives

bacitracin
benzalkonium chloride
boric acid
chloramphenicol
chlortetracycline hydrochloride
erythromycin
gentamicin sulfate
idoxuridine (IDU)
natamycin
polymyxin B sulfate
silver nitrate 1%
sulfacetamide sodium
tetracycline hydrochloride
tobramycin
trifluridine
vidarabine

MECHANISM OF ACTION

- Bacitracin, chloramphenicol, erythromycin, gentamicin, polymyxin B, the tetracyclines, and tobramycin inhibit protein synthesis in susceptible microorganisms.
- Benzalkonium chloride increases corneal permeability, enabling greater penetration of the drug.
- Boric acid's mechanism of action is unknown.
- Idoxuridine, trifluridine, and vidarabine interfere with DNA synthesis.
- Natamycin increases fungal cell-membrane permeability.
- Silver nitrate causes protein denaturation, which prevents gonorrheal ophthalmia neonatorum.
- Sulfacetamide prevents uptake of para-aminobenzoic acid, a metabolite of bacterial folic-acid synthesis.

COMBINATION PRODUCTS

BLEPHAMIDE LIQUIFILM SUSPENSION: sodium sulfacetamide 10%, prednisolone acetate 0.2%, and phenylephrine hydrochloride 0.12%.
BLEPHAMIDE S.O.P. OPHTHALMIC OINTMENT: sodium sulfacetamide 10% and prednisolone acetate 0.2%.
BPN OPHTHALMIC OINTMENT: bacitracin 500 units, polymyxin B sulfate 5,000 units, and neomycin sulfate 5 mg/g.
CETAPRED OINTMENT♦: sodium sulfacetamide 10% and prednisolone acetate 0.25%.
CHLOROMYCETIN HYDROCORTISONE OPHTHALMIC♦: chloramphenicol 1.25% and hydrocortisone acetate 2.5%.
CHLOROMYXIN OPHTHALMIC♦: chloramphenicol 10 mg and polymyxin B sulfate 5,000 units.
CHLOROPTIC-P S.O.P.: chloramphenicol 1% and prednisolone alcohol 0.5%.
CORTISPORIN OPHTHALMIC OINTMENT♦: polymyxin B sulfate 5,000 units, bacitracin zinc 400 units, neomycin sulfate 0.5%, and hydrocortisone 1%.
CORTISPORIN OPHTHALMIC SUSPENSION♦: polymyxin B sulfate 10,000 units, neomycin sulfate 0.5%, and hydrocortisone 1%.
ISOPTO CETAPRED SUSPENSION♦: sulfacetamide 10% and prednisolone acetate 0.25%.
MAXITROL OPHTHALMIC OINTMENT/SUSPENSION♦: dexamethasone 0.1%, neomycin sulfate 3.5 mg, and polymyxin B sulfate 6,000 units.
METIMYD OPHTHALMIC OINTMENT/SUSPENSION: sodium sulfacetamide 10% and prednisolone acetate 0.5%.

Italicized side effects are common or life-threatening.
*Liquid form contains alcohol. **May contain tartrazine.

MYCITRACIN OPHTHALMIC: polymyxin B sulfate 5,000 units, neomycin sulfate 5 mg, and bacitracin 500 units.

NEO-CORTEF OPHTHALMIC♦: hydrocortisone 0.5% or 1.5% and neomycin sulfate 0.5%.

NEODECADRON OPHTHALMIC OINTMENT: dexamethasone phosphate 0.5% and neomycin sulfate 0.5%.

NEODECADRON OPHTHALMIC SOLUTION♦: dexamethasone phosphate 1 mg and neomycin sulfate 0.5%.

NEO-DELTA CORTEF SUSPENSION: prednisolone acetate 0.25% and neomycin sulfate 0.5%.

NEO-MEDROL OINTMENT: methylprednisolone 0.1% and neomycin sulfate 0.5%.

NEOSPORIN OPHTHALMIC OINTMENT♦: polymyxin B sulfate 5,000 units, neomycin sulfate 5 mg, and bacitracin zinc 100 units/g.

NEOSPORIN OPHTHALMIC SOLUTION♦: polymyxin B sulfate 5,000 units, neomycin sulfate 2.5 mg, and gramicidin 0.025 mg.

NEOTAL OPHTHALMIC OINTMENT: polymyxin B sulfate 5,000 units, neomycin sulfate 5 mg, and bacitracin zinc 400 units.

OPHTHA P/S OPHTHALMIC DROPS: prednisolone acetate 0.5%, sodium sulfacetamide 10%, phenylephrine HCl 0.12%.

OPHTHOCORT OINTMENT: chloramphenicol 1.0%, polymyxin B sulfate 5,000 units, and hydrocortisone acetate 0.5%.

OPTIMYD SOLUTION: prednisolone phosphate 0.5% and sodium sulfacetamide 10%.

POLYSPORIN OPHTHALMIC OINTMENT: neomycin sulfate 5 mg, polymyxin B sulfate 10,000 units, and bacitracin zinc 500 units.

STATROL OPHTHALMIC OINTMENT: neomycin sulfate 5 mg and polymyxin B sulfate 6,000 units.

STATROL OPHTHALMIC SOLUTION: neomycin sulfate 5 mg and polymyxin B sulfate 16,250 units.

SULFAPRED OPHTHALMIC SUSPENSION: sodium sulfacetamide 10%, prednisolone acetate 0.25%, and phenylephrine HCl 0.125%.

VASOCIDIN OINTMENT: sodium sulfacetamide 10%, prednisolone acetate 0.2%, and phenylephrine HCl 0.125%.

VASOCIDIN SOLUTION♦: sodium sulfacetamide 10%, prednisolone phosphate 0.2%, and phenylephrine HCl 0.125%.

VASOSULF SOLUTION♦: sodium sulfacetamide 15% and phenylephrine HCl 0.125%

---

bacitracin
Baciguent Ophthalmic Ointment♦

INDICATIONS & DOSAGE
Ocular infections—
Adults and children: apply small amount into conjunctival sac several times a day or p.r.n. until favorable response is observed.

SIDE EFFECTS
Eye: slowed corneal wound healing, temporary visual haze.
Other: overgrowth of nonsusceptible organisms.

INTERACTIONS
Heavy metals (silver nitrate): inactivate bacitracin. Don't use together.

NURSING CONSIDERATIONS
• Use cautiously in patients with hereditary predisposition to antibiotic hypersensitivity.
• Warn patient to avoid sharing washcloths and towels with family members.
• Always wash hands before and after applying ointment.
• Cleanse eye area of excessive exudate before application.
• Tell patient to watch for signs of sensitivity, such as itching lids or constant burning. Patient who develops such signs should stop drug and notify doctor immediately.
• Show patient how to apply. Stress im-

portance of compliance with recommended therapy.
• Warn patient not to touch tip of tube to any part of eye or surrounding tissue.
• Solution not commercially available but may be prepared by pharmacy. May be stored up to 3 weeks in refrigerator.
• Bactericidal or bacteriostatic, depending on concentration and infection.
• Store in tightly closed, light-resistant container.
• Tell patient not to share eye medications with family members. If a family member develops the same symptoms, instruct him to contact the doctor.

benzalkonium chloride
Spensomide, Zephiran♦

INDICATIONS & DOSAGE
To increase transcorneal penetration of drugs—
Adults and children: 1:5,000 to 1:2,000 concentration used in some irrigating solutions for its antiseptic as well as its surface-active qualities.
To sterilize ophthalmic solutions: use 1:5,000 concentration.
An ingredient in germicidal cleaning solutions for contact lens.

SIDE EFFECTS
Eye: toxic to abraded cornea and to endothelial cells of cornea if introduced into anterior chamber.

INTERACTIONS
Fluorescein: destroys benzalkonium chloride antibacterial activity. May cause corneal staining. Don't use together.
Sulfonamides (ophthalmic): incompatible. Don't apply at same time.

NURSING CONSIDERATIONS
• Never prepare a straight benzalkonium chloride solution for use in eye.
• Warn patient to avoid sharing washcloths and towels with family members.

• Don't use concentrations greater than 1:5,000 in the eye; may be irritating.
• Tell patient to watch for signs of sensitivity, such as itching lids or constant burning. If he develops such signs, patient should stop drug and notify doctor immediately.
• Warn patient not to touch applicator to eye or surrounding tissue.
• Always wash hands before and after applying drug.
• Cleanse eye area of excessive exudate before application.
• Present in most commercially available combination topical eye preparations.
• Tell patient not to share eye medications with family members. If a family member develops the same symptoms, instruct him to contact the doctor.

boric acid
Blinx, Collyrium, Neo-Flo

INDICATIONS & DOSAGE
For irrigation following tonometry, gonioscopy, foreign body removal, or use of fluorescein; used to soothe and cleanse the eye; used in conjunction with contact lens—
Adults: irrigate eye with 2% solution or apply 5% or 10% ointment, p.r.n.

SIDE EFFECTS
Note: toxic if absorbed from abraded skin areas, granulating wounds, or ingestion.

INTERACTIONS
Polyvinyl alcohol (Liquifilm): may form insoluble complex. Check with pharmacy on contents in eye drugs and contact lens wetting solutions.

NURSING CONSIDERATIONS
• Contraindicated in eye abrasions.
• Don't apply to abraded cornea or skin.
• Always wash hands before and after instilling solution or ointment.

Italicized side effects are common or life-threatening.
*Liquid form contains alcohol.   **May contain tartrazine.

- Not for use with soft contact lenses.
- Weak bacteriostatic, fungistatic agent.
- Tell patient not to share eye medications with family members. If a family member develops the same symptoms, instruct him to contact the doctor.

chloramphenicol
Antibiopto, Chloromycetin Ophthalmic♦, Chloroptic Ophthalmic♦, Chloroptic S.O.P., Econochlor Ophthalmic, Fenicol♦♦, Isopto Fenicol♦♦, Nova-Phenicol♦♦, Ophthoclor Ophthalmic, Pentamycetin♦♦

INDICATIONS & DOSAGE
Surface bacterial infection involving conjunctiva or cornea—
Adults and children: instill 2 drops of solution in eye q 1 hour until condition improves, or instill q.i.d., depending on severity of infection. Apply small amount of ointment to lower conjunctival sac at bedtime as supplement to drops. May use ointment alone by applying a small amount of ointment to lower conjunctival sac q 3 to 6 hours or more frequently, if necessary. Continue until condition improves.

SIDE EFFECTS
Note: systemic adverse reactions have not been reported with short-term topical use.
Blood: *bone marrow hypoplasia with prolonged use, aplastic anemia.*
Eye: optic atrophy in children, stinging or burning of eye after instillation.
Other: overgrowth of nonsusceptible organisms; hypersensitivity, including itching and burning eye, dermatitis, angioedema.

INTERACTIONS
None significant.

NURSING CONSIDERATIONS
- Not for long-term use. Notify doctor if no improvement in 3 days.
- If patient has more than a superficial infection, systemic therapy should also be used.
- Apply light finger-pressure on lacrimal sac for 1 minute after drops are instilled.
- One of the safest topical ocular antibiotics, especially for endophthalmitis.
- Warn patient to avoid sharing washcloths and towels with family members.
- Always wash hands before and after applying ointment or solution.
- Cleanse eye area of excessive exudate before application.
- Tell patient to watch for signs of sensitivity, such as itching lids or constant burning. Patient who develops such signs should stop drug and notify doctor immediately.
- Show patient how to instill. Stress importance of compliance with recommended therapy.
- Warn patient not to touch tip of applicator to eye or surrounding tissue.
- If chloramphenicol drops are to be given q 1 hour, then tapered, follow order closely to ensure adequate anterior chamber levels.
- Store in tightly closed, light-resistant container.
- Tell patient not to share eye medications with family members. If a family member develops the same symptoms, instruct him to contact the doctor.

chlortetracycline hydrochloride
Aureomycin Ophthalmic

INDICATIONS & DOSAGE
Superficial ocular infection—
Adults and children: apply 1% ointment to eye q 2 hours or more, p.r.n.

SIDE EFFECTS
Eye: itching and burning.
Other: overgrowth of nonsusceptible

organisms with long-term use, dermatitis.

INTERACTIONS
None significant.

NURSING CONSIDERATIONS
• Contraindicated in tetracycline hypersensitivity.
• *Pseudomonas, Proteus,* and *Staphylococcus* resistant to drug. Used mainly for trachoma in conjunction with oral therapy. Trachoma treatment may continue 2 months or more. Trachoma may cause blindness if untreated or if treated improperly.
• Warn patient to avoid sharing washcloths and towels with family members.
• Always wash hands before and after applying ointment.
• Cleanse eye area of excessive exudate before application.
• Tell patient to watch for signs of sensitivity, such as itching lids or constant burning. Patient who develops such signs should stop drug and notify doctor immediately.
• Show patient how to instill. Stress importance of compliance with recommended therapy.
• Warn patient not to touch tip of tube to eye or surrounding tissue.
• Store in tightly closed, light-resistant container.
• Tell patient not to share eye medications with family members. If a family member develops the same symptoms, instruct him to contact the doctor.

---

erythromycin
Ilotycin Ophthalmic♦

INDICATIONS & DOSAGE
Acute and chronic conjunctivitis, other eye infections—
Adults and children: apply 0.5% ointment 1 or more times daily, depending upon severity of infection.

SIDE EFFECTS
Eye: slowed corneal wound healing.
Other: overgrowth of nonsusceptible organisms with long-term use; hypersensitivity, including itching and burning eye, urticaria, dermatitis, angioedema.

INTERACTIONS
None significant.

NURSING CONSIDERATIONS
• Bacteriostatic but may be bactericidal in high concentrations or against highly susceptible organisms.
• Has a limited antibacterial spectrum. Use only when sensitivity studies show it is effective against infecting organisms. Don't use in infections of unknown etiology.
• Warn patient to avoid sharing washcloths and towels with family members.
• Always wash hands before and after applying ointment.
• Cleanse eye area of excessive exudate before application.
• Tell patient to watch for signs of sensitivity, such as itching lids or constant burning. Patient who develops such signs should stop drug and notify doctor immediately.
• Show patient how to apply. Stress importance of compliance with recommended therapy.
• Warn patient not to touch tube to eye or surrounding tissue.
• Store at room temperature in tightly closed, light-resistant container.
• Tell patient not to share eye medications with family members. If a family member develops the same symptoms, instruct him to contact the doctor.

---

gentamicin sulfate
Garamycin Ophthalmic♦, Genoptic

INDICATIONS & DOSAGE
External ocular infections (conjunctivitis, keratoconjunctivitis, corneal ulcers, blepharitis, blepharoconjunctivitis,

---

Italicized side effects are common or life-threatening.
*Liquid form contains alcohol.   **May contain tartrazine.

*meibomianitis, and dacryocystitis) due
to susceptible organisms, especially*
Pseudomonas aeruginosa, Proteus,
Klebsiella pneumoniae, Escherichia
coli—
Adults and children: instill 1 to
2 drops in eye q 4 hours. In severe infections, may use up to 2 drops q
1 hour. Apply ointment to lower conjunctival sac b.i.d. to t.i.d.

SIDE EFFECTS
Note: systemic absorption from excessive use may cause systemic toxicities.
Eye: burning or stinging with
ointment, transient irritation from
solution.
Other: hypersensitivity, overgrowth of
nonsusceptible organisms with long-
term use.

INTERACTIONS
None significant.

NURSING CONSIDERATIONS
• Contraindicated in aminoglycoside
hypersensitivity. Use cautiously in impaired renal function.
• Have culture taken before giving
drug.
• Stress importance of following recommended therapy. *Pseudomonas* infections can cause complete vision loss
within 24 hours if infection is not controlled.
• Warn patient to avoid sharing washcloths and towels with family members.
• Always wash hands before and after
applying ointment or solution.
• Cleanse eye area of excessive exudate before application.
• Tell patient to watch for signs of sensitivity, such as itching lids or constant
burning. Patient who develops such
signs should stop drug and notify doctor immediately.
• Show patient how to instill.
• Apply light finger-pressure on lacrimal sac for 1 minute after drops are instilled.

• Warn patient not to touch tip of tube
or dropper to eye or surrounding tissue.
• Store away from heat.
• Tell patient not to share eye medications with family members. If a family
member develops the same symptoms,
instruct him to contact the doctor.

---

idoxuridine (IDU)
Dendrid, Herplex, Stoxil♦

INDICATIONS & DOSAGE
Herpes simplex keratitis—
Adults and children: instill 1 drop of
solution into conjunctival sac q 1 hour
during day and q 2 hours at night, or
apply ointment to conjunctival sac q 4
hours or 5 times daily, with last dose at
bedtime. A response should be seen in
7 days; if not, discontinue and begin alternate therapy. Therapy should not be
continued longer than 21 days.

SIDE EFFECTS
Eye: temporary visual haze; irritation,
pain, burning, or inflammation of eye;
mild edema of eyelid or cornea; photosensitivity; small punctate defects in
corneal epithelium; slowed corneal
wound healing with ointment.
Other: hypersensitivity.

INTERACTIONS
None significant.

NURSING CONSIDERATIONS
• Contraindicated in deep ulceration.
• Not for long-term use.
• Idoxuridine should not be mixed
with other medications.
• Don't use old solution; causes ocular
burning and has no antiviral activity.
• Warn patient to avoid sharing wash-
cloths and towels with family members.
• Always wash hands before and after
applying ointment or solution.
• Cleanse eye area of excessive exu-
date before application.
• Tell patient to watch for signs of sen-
sitivity, such as itching lids or constant

---

burning. Patient who develops such signs should stop drug and notify doctor immediately.

• Show patient how to apply. Stress importance of compliance with recommended therapy.

• Warn patient not to touch tip of tube or dropper to eye or surrounding tissue.

• Refrigerate idoxuridine 0.1% solution. Store in tightly closed, light-resistant container.

• Tell patient not to share eye medications with family members. If a family member develops the same symptoms, instruct him to contact the doctor.

• If sensitivity to light develops, patient should wear sunglasses.

natamycin
Natacyn

INDICATIONS & DOSAGE
Treatment of fungal keratitis—
Adults: initial dosage 1 drop instilled in conjunctival sac q 1 to 2 hours. After 3 to 4 days, reduce dosage to 1 drop 6 to 8 times daily.

SIDE EFFECTS
Eye: ocular edema, hyperemia.

INTERACTIONS
None significant.

NURSING CONSIDERATIONS
• Only antifungal available as ophthalmic preparation.

• Treatment of choice for fungal keratitis. May also be used to treat fungal blepharitis and conjunctivitis.

• Therapy should be continued for 14 to 21 days, or until active disease subsides.

• Reduce dosage gradually at 4- to 7-day intervals to assure that organism has been eliminated.

• If infection does not improve with 7 to 10 days of therapy, clinical and laboratory reevaluation is recommended.

• Apply light finger-pressure on lacrimal sac for 1 minute after drops are instilled.

• Warn patient to avoid sharing washcloths and towels with family members.

• Always wash hands before and after applying.

• Cleanse eye area of excessive exudate before application.

• Show patient how to apply. Stress importance of compliance with recommended therapy.

• Warn patient not to touch tip of dropper to eye or surrounding tissue.

• Tell patient not to share eye medications with family members. If a family member develops the same symptoms, instruct him to contact the doctor.

• Shake well before use. May be kept in refrigerator or at room temperature.

polymyxin B sulfate
Aerosporin♦

INDICATIONS & DOSAGE
Used alone or in combination with other agents for treating corneal ulcers resulting from Pseudomonas *infection or other gram-negative organism infections—*
Adults and children: instill 1 to 3 drops of 0.1% to 0.25% (10,000 to 25,000 units/ml) q 1 hour. Increase interval according to patient response; or up to 10,000 units subconjunctivally daily by doctor.

SIDE EFFECTS
Eye: eye irritation, conjunctivitis.
Other: overgrowth of nonsusceptible organisms, hypersensitivity (local burning, itching).

INTERACTIONS
None significant.

NURSING CONSIDERATIONS
• One of the most effective antibiotics against gram-negative organisms, especially *Pseudomonas*.

Italicized side effects are common or life-threatening.
∗Liquid form contains alcohol.   ∗∗May contain tartrazine.

- Often used in combination with neomycin sulfate.
- Warn patient to avoid sharing washcloths and towels with family members.
- Always wash hands before and after instilling solution.
- Cleanse eye area of excessive exudate before application.
- Tell patient to watch for signs of sensitivity, such as itching lids and lashes or constant burning. Patient who develops such signs should stop drug and notify doctor immediately.
- Show patient how to instill. Stress importance of compliance with recommended therapy.
- Apply light finger-pressure on lacrimal sac for 1 minute after drops are instilled.
- Warn patient not to touch tip of dropper to eye or surrounding tissue.
- Reconstitute carefully to ensure correct drug concentration in solution.
- Tell patient not to share eye medications with family members. If a family member develops the same symptoms, instruct him to contact the doctor.

---

silver nitrate 1%

INDICATIONS & DOSAGE
Prevention of gonorrheal ophthalmia neonatorum—
Neonates: cleanse lids thoroughly; instill 1 drop of 1% solution into each eye.

SIDE EFFECTS
Eye: periorbital edema, temporary staining of lids and surrounding tissue, conjunctivitis (with concentrations greater than 1%).

INTERACTIONS
Bacitracin: inactivates silver nitrate. Don't use together.

NURSING CONSIDERATIONS
- Legally required for neonates in most states.

- Don't use repeatedly.
- If 2% solution is accidentally used in eye, prompt irrigation with isotonic sodium chloride is advised to prevent eye irritation.
- May delay instillation slightly to allow neonate to bond with mother.
- Always wash hands before instilling solution.
- Store wax ampuls away from light and heat.
- Bacteriostatic, germicidal, and astringent.
- Handle solution carefully. May stain skin or utensils.
- Don't irrigate eyes after instillation.

---

sulfacetamide sodium 10%
Bleph-10 Liquifilm Ophthalmic♦, Cetamide Ophthalmic♦, Sodium Sulamyd 10% Ophthalmic, Sulf-10 Ophthalmic♦

sulfacetamide sodium 15%
Isopto Cetamide Ophthalmic♦, Sulfacel-15 Ophthalmic

sulfacetamide sodium 30%
Sodium Sulamyd 30% Ophthalmic♦

INDICATIONS & DOSAGE
Inclusion conjunctivitis, corneal ulcers, trachoma, prophylaxis to ocular infection—
Adults and children: instill 1 to 2 drops of 10% solution into lower conjunctival sac q 2 to 3 hours during day, less often at night; or instill 1 to 2 drops of 15% solution into lower conjunctival sac q 1 to 2 hours initially, increasing interval as condition responds; or instill 1 drop of 30% solution into lower conjunctival sac q 2 hours. Instill ½″ to 1″ of 10% ointment into conjunctival sac q.i.d. and at bedtime. May use ointment at night along with drops during the day.

SIDE EFFECTS
Eye: slowed corneal wound healing (ointment), *pain on instilling eye drop*.
Other: hypersensitivity (including itching or burning), overgrowth of nonsusceptible organisms, *Stevens-Johnson syndrome*.

INTERACTIONS
Local anesthetics (procaine, tetracaine),
p-aminobenzoic acid derivatives: decreased sulfacetamide sodium action. Wait ½ to 1 hour after instilling anesthetic or *p*-aminobenzoic acid derivative before instilling sulfacetamide.

NURSING CONSIDERATIONS
• Contraindicated in sulfonamide hypersensitivity.
• Often used with systemic tetracycline in treating trachoma and inclusion conjunctivitis.
• Replaced by antibiotics in treating major ocular infections; still used in minor ocular infections.
• Purulent exudate interferes with sulfacetamide action. Remove as much exudate as possible from lids before instilling sulfacetamide.
• Incompatible with silver preparations.
• Warn patient eye drop is painful.
• Warn patient to avoid sharing washcloths and towels with family members.
• Always wash hands before and after applying ointment or solution.
• Tell patient to watch for signs of sensitivity, such as itching lids or constant burning. Patient who develops such signs should stop drug and notify doctor immediately.
• Show patient how to instill. Stress importance of compliance with recommended therapy.
• Apply light finger-pressure on lacrimal sac for 1 minute after drops are instilled.
• Warn patient not to touch tip of tube or dropper to eye or surrounding tissue.

• Store in tightly closed, light-resistant container away from heat.
• Don't use discolored (dark brown) solution.
• Tell patient not to share eye medications with family members. If a family member develops the same symptoms, instruct him to contact the doctor.

---

tetracycline hydrochloride
Achromycin Ophthalmic◆

INDICATIONS & DOSAGE
Adults and children:
Superficial ocular infections and inclusion conjunctivitis— instill 1 to 2 drops in eye b.i.d., q.i.d., or more often, depending on severity of infection.
Trachoma—instill 2 drops in each eye b.i.d., t.i.d., or q.i.d. Continue for 1 to 2 months or longer, or use 1% ointment t.i.d. to q.i.d. for 30 days.

SIDE EFFECTS
Eye: itching.
Other: hypersensitivity (eye itching and dermatitis), overgrowth of nonsusceptible organisms with long-term use.

INTERACTIONS
None significant.

NURSING CONSIDERATIONS
• Tell patient or family that trachoma therapy should continue for 1 to 2 months or longer. Trachoma may cause blindness if left untreated or if not treated properly.
• Tell patient that gnats and flies are vectors of the trachoma organism. Warn patient with trachoma not to let them settle around eye area. Also explain that infection is spread by direct contact, so handwashing is essential to prevent spread.
• Apply light finger pressure on lacrimal sac for 1 minute after drops are instilled.
• Warn patient to avoid sharing washcloths and towels with family members.

Italicized side effects are common or life-threatening.
∗Liquid form contains alcohol.   ∗∗May contain tartrazine.

- Always wash hands before and after applying solution.
- Cleanse eye area of excessive exudate before application.
- Tell patient to watch for signs of sensitivity, such as itching lids or constant burning. Patient who develops such signs should stop drug and notify doctor immediately.
- Show patient how to instill. Stress importance of compliance with recommended therapy.
- Warn patient not to touch tip of dropper to eye or surrounding tissue.
- Store in tightly closed, light-resistant container.
- Tell patient not to share eye medications with family members. If a family member develops the same symptoms, instruct him to contact the doctor.

tobramycin
Tobrex

INDICATIONS & DOSAGE
Treatment of external ocular infections caused by susceptible bacteria—
Adults and children: In mild to moderate infections, instill 1 or 2 drops into the affected eye q 4 hours. In severe infections, instill 2 drops into the infected eye hourly.

SIDE EFFECTS
Eye: burning or stinging upon instillation.
Other: hypersensitivity.

INTERACTIONS
Tetracycline-containing eye preparations: incompatible with tyloxapol, an ingredient in Tobrex. Don't use together.

NURSING CONSIDERATIONS
- Prolonged use may result in overgrowth of nonsusceptible organisms, including fungi.
- Always wash hands before and after instilling solution.

- Warn patient to avoid sharing washcloths and towels with family members.
- Tell patient to watch for signs of sensitivity, such as itching lids or constant burning. Patient who develops such signs should discontinue drug and notify doctor immediately.
- Warn patient not to touch tip of dropper to eye or surrounding tissue.
- Show patient how to instill.
- Apply light finger-pressure on lacrimal sac for 1 minute after drops are instilled.

trifluridine
Viroptic Ophthalmic Solution 1%

INDICATIONS & DOSAGE
Primary keratoconjunctivitis and recurrent epithelial keratitis due to herpes simplex virus, types 1 and 2—
Adults 1 drop of solution q 2 hours while patient is awake, to a maximum of 9 drops daily, until re-epithelialization of the corneal ulcer occurs; then 1 drop q 4 hours (minimum 5 drops daily) for an additional 7 days.

SIDE EFFECTS
Eye: *stinging upon instillation,* edema of eyelids.

INTERACTIONS
None significant.

NURSING CONSIDERATIONS
- Should be prescribed only for those patients with clinical diagnosis of herpetic keratitis.
- Consider another form of therapy if improvement doesn't occur after 7 days' treatment or complete re-epithelialization after 14 days' treatment. Trifluridine shouldn't be used more than 21 days continuously due to potential ocular toxicity.
- Apply light finger-pressure on lacrimal sac for 1 minute after drops are instilled.
- Reassure patient that mild local irri-

tation of the conjunctiva and cornea that occurs when solution is instilled is usually temporary.
- Drug should be refrigerated.
- More effective drug than vidarabine with fewer side effects.
- Warn patient to avoid sharing washcloths and towels with family members.
- Wash hands before and after administration.
- Warn patient not to touch tip of dropper to eye or surrounding tissue.
- Tell patient not to share eye medications with family members. If a family member develops the same symptoms, instruct him to contact the doctor.

vidarabine
Vira-A Ophthalmic♦

INDICATIONS & DOSAGE
Acute keratoconjunctivitis, superficial keratitis, and recurrent epithelial keratitis resulting from herpes simplex types 1 and 2—
Adults and children: instill ½" ointment into lower conjunctival sac 5 times daily at 3-hour intervals.

SIDE EFFECTS
Eye: temporary visual burning, itching, mild irritation of eye, lacrimation, foreign body sensation, conjunctival injection, superficial punctate keratitis, eye pain, photosensitivity.
Other: hypersensitivity.

INTERACTIONS
None significant.

NURSING CONSIDERATIONS
- Not for long-term use.
- A relatively new alternative in treating herpes simplex ocular infections.
- Warn patient not to exceed recommended frequency or duration of dosage.
- Not effective against RNA virus or adenoviral ocular infections, or against bacterial, fungal, or chlamydial infections.
- Warn patient to avoid sharing washcloths and towels with family members.
- Always wash hands before and after applying ointment.
- Tell patient to watch for signs of sensitivity, such as itching lids or constant burning. Patient who develops such signs should stop drug and notify doctor immediately.
- Show patient how to instill.
- Warn patient not to touch tip of tube to eye or surrounding tissue.
- Store in tightly closed, light-resistant container.
- Tell patient not to share eye medications with family members. If a family member develops the same symptoms, instruct him to contact the doctor.
- Explain to patient that the ointment may produce a temporary visual haze.
- If sensitivity to light develops, patient should wear sunglasses.

Italicized side effects are common or life-threatening.
*Liquid form contains alcohol.   **May contain tartrazine.

74

Ophthalmic anti-inflammatory agents

dexamethasone
dexamethasone sodium phosphate
fluorometholone
hydrocortisone acetate
medrysone
prednisolone acetate
prednisolone sodium phosphate

MECHANISM OF ACTION
Corticosteroids decrease the infiltration of leukocytes at the site of inflammation.

COMBINATION PRODUCTS
Corticosteroids for ophthalmic use are commonly combined with antibiotics and sulfonamides. See Chapter 73, OPHTHALMIC ANTI-INFECTIVES.

dexamethasone
Maxidex Ophthalmic Suspension♦

dexamethasone sodium phosphate
Decadron Phosphate Ophthalmic♦, Maxidex Ophthalmic♦, Opto-Methasone♦♦

INDICATIONS & DOSAGE
Uveitis; iridocyclitis; inflammatory condition of eyelids, conjunctiva, cornea, anterior segment of globe; corneal injury from chemical or thermal burns, or penetration of foreign bodies; allergic conjunctivitis—
Adults and children: instill 1 to 2 drops into conjunctival sac. In severe disease, drops may be used hourly, tapering to discontinuation as condition improves. In mild conditions, drops may be used up to 4 to 6 times daily. Treatment may extend from a few days to several weeks.

SIDE EFFECTS
Eye: increased intraocular pressure, especially in elderly patients; thinning of cornea, interference with corneal wound healing, increased susceptibility to viral or fungal corneal infection, corneal ulceration; with excessive or long-term use, glaucoma exacerbations, cataracts, defects in visual acuity and visual field, optic nerve damage.
Other: systemic effects and adrenal suppression with excessive or long-term use.

INTERACTIONS
None significant.

NURSING CONSIDERATIONS
- Contraindicated in acute superficial herpes simplex (dendritic keratitis), vaccinia, varicella, or other fungal or viral diseases of cornea and conjunctiva; presence of active diabetes; ocular tuberculosis, or any acute, purulent, untreated infection of the eye. Use cautiously in corneal abrasions, since these may be infected (especially with herpes); patients with glaucoma (any form), due to possibility of increasing intraocular pressure (miotic medication drug regimen may need to be increased to compensate).
- Viral and fungal infections of the cornea may be exacerbated by the application of steroids.
- Warn patient to call doctor immedi-

Unmarked trade names available in the United States only.
♦ Also available in Canada. ♦♦ Available in Canada only.

ately and to stop drug if visual acuity changes or visual field diminishes.
● Not for long-term use.
● May use eye pad with ointment for increased effect.
● Show patient how to instill.
● Apply light finger-pressure on lacrimal sac for 1 minute following instillation.
● Watch for corneal ulceration; may require stopping drug.
● Dexamethasone has greater anti-inflammatory effect than dexamethasone sodium phosphate.
● Warn patient not to use leftover medication for a new eye infection; can cause serious problems.
● Tell patient never to share eye medications. If a family member develops similar symptoms, instruct him to contact the doctor.

---

fluorometholone
FML Liquifilm Ophthalmic◆

INDICATIONS & DOSAGE
Inflammatory and allergic conditions of cornea, conjunctiva, sclera, anterior uvea—
Adults and children: instill 1 to 2 drops q 1 hour for first 1 to 2 days, then b.i.d., t.i.d., or q.i.d.

SIDE EFFECTS
Eye: increased intraocular pressure, especially in elderly patients; thinning of cornea, interference with corneal wound healing, corneal ulceration, increased susceptibility to viral or fungal corneal infections; with excessive or long-term use, glaucoma exacerbations, cataracts, decreased visual acuity, diminished visual field; optic nerve damage.
Other: systemic effects and adrenal suppression in excessive or long-term use.

INTERACTIONS
None significant.

NURSING CONSIDERATIONS
● Contraindicated in vaccinia, varicella, acute superficial herpes simplex (dendritic keratitis), or other fungal or viral eye diseases; ocular tuberculosis; or any acute, purulent, untreated eye infection. Use cautiously in corneal abrasions since they are commonly contaminated (especially with herpes).
● Not for long-term use.
● Less likely to cause increased intraocular pressure with long-term use than other ophthalmic anti-inflammatory drugs (except medrysone).
● Store in tightly covered, light-resistant container.
● Warn patient to call doctor immediately and to stop drug if visual acuity decreases or visual field diminishes.
● Shake well before using.
● Show patient how to instill.
● Apply light finger-pressure on lacrimal sac for 1 minute following instillation.
● Warn patient not to use leftover medication for a new eye infection; can cause serious problems.
● Tell patient never to share eye medications. If a family member develops similar symptoms, instruct him to contact the doctor.

---

hydrocortisone acetate
Cortamed◆◆, Hydrocortone◆

INDICATIONS & DOSAGE
Uveitis, iridocyclitis, inflammatory condition of eyelids, conjunctiva, cornea, anterior segment of globe; to prevent corneal scarring in visual axis; corneal injury from chemical or thermal burns, or penetration of foreign bodies; allergic conjunctivitis—
Adults and children: instill 1 to 3 drops into conjunctival sac q 1 hour during the day and q 2 hours during the night in acute situations. May be decreased to 1 drop t.i.d. or q.i.d.; or instill ointment t.i.d. to q.i.d. initially. May decrease to daily or b.i.d.

Italicized side effects are common or life-threatening.
✳Liquid form contains alcohol.   ✳✳May contain tartrazine.

SIDE EFFECTS

Eye: increased intraocular pressure, especially in elderly patients; thinning of cornea, interference with corneal wound healing, increased susceptibility to viral or fungal corneal infection, corneal ulceration; with excessive or long-term use, glaucoma exacerbations, cataracts, visual acuity and visual field defects, optic nerve damage.

Other: systemic effects and adrenal suppression with excessive or long-term use.

INTERACTIONS

None significant.

NURSING CONSIDERATIONS

• Contraindicated in acute superficial herpes simplex (dendritic keratitis), vaccinia, varicella, or other fungal or viral diseases of cornea and conjunctiva; presence of active diabetes; ocular tuberculosis; or any acute, purulent, untreated eye infection. Use cautiously in corneal abrasions since they are commonly contaminated (especially with herpes).

• Viral and fungal infections of the cornea may be exacerbated by the application of steroids.

• Keep in mind possibility of increasing intraocular pressure.

• Warn patient to call doctor immediately and to stop drug if visual acuity changes or visual field diminishes.

• Not for long-term use.

• May use eye pad with ointment for increased effect.

• Show patient how to instill.

• Apply light finger-pressure on lacrimal sac for 1 minute following instillation.

• Watch for corneal ulceration; may require stopping drug.

• Warn patient not to use leftover medication for a new eye infection; can cause serious problems.

• Tell patient never to share eye medications. If a family member develops

similar symptoms, instruct him to contact the doctor.

---

medrysone
HMS Liquifilm Ophthalmic♦

INDICATIONS & DOSAGE

Allergic conjunctivitis, vernal conjunctivitis, episcleritis, ophthalmic epinephrine sensitivity reaction—

Adults and children: instill 1 drop in conjunctival sac b.i.d. to q.i.d. May use q hour during first 1 to 2 days if needed.

SIDE EFFECTS

Eye: thinning of cornea, interference with corneal wound healing, increased susceptibility to viral or fungal corneal infection, corneal ulceration; with excessive or long-term use, glaucoma exacerbations, cataracts, visual acuity and visual field defects, optic nerve damage.

Other: systemic effects and adrenal suppression with excessive or long-term use.

INTERACTIONS

None significant.

NURSING CONSIDERATIONS

• Contraindicated in vaccinia, varicella, acute superficial herpes simplex (dendritic keratitis), viral diseases of conjunctiva and cornea, ocular tuberculosis, fungal or viral eye diseases, iritis, uveitis, or any acute, purulent, untreated eye infection. Use cautiously in corneal abrasions since they are commonly contaminated (especially with herpes).

• Shake well before using. Don't freeze.

• Warn patient not to use leftover medication for a new eye infection; can cause serious problems.

• Tell patient never to share eye medications. If a family member develops

---

similar symptoms, instruct him to contact the doctor.

prednisolone acetate (suspensions)
Econopred Ophthalmic,
Econopred Plus Ophthalmic, Pred-
Forte♦, Pred Mild Ophthalmic♦,
Prednicon♦♦, Predulose
Ophthalmic

prednisolone sodium phosphate (solutions)
Ak-Pred, Hydeltrasol Ophthalmic,
Inflamase Forte♦, Inflamase
Ophthalmic♦, Metreton
Ophthalmic, Nova-Pred Forte♦♦

INDICATIONS & DOSAGE
*Inflammation of palpebral and bulbar
conjunctiva, cornea, and anterior segment of globe—*
Adults and children: instill 2 drops in
eye. In severe conditions, may be used
hourly, tapering to discontinuation as
inflammation subsides. In mild conditions, may be used up to 4 to 6 times
daily.

SIDE EFFECTS
Eye: increased intraocular pressure, especially in elderly patients; thinning of
cornea, interference with corneal
wound healing, increased susceptibility
to viral or fungal corneal infection, corneal ulceration; with excessive or long-
term use, glaucoma exacerbations, cataracts, visual acuity and visual field defects, optic nerve damage.
Other: systemic effects and adrenal
suppression with excessive or long-term
use.

INTERACTIONS
None significant.

NURSING CONSIDERATIONS
• Contraindicated in acute untreated
purulent ocular infections, acute superficial herpes simplex (dendritic keratitis), vaccinia, varicella, or other viral
or fungal eye diseases, ocular tuberculosis. Use cautiously in corneal abrasions since they are commonly contaminated (especially with herpes).
• Tell patient on long-term therapy to
have frequent tonometric examinations.
• Shake suspensions before using, and
store in tightly covered container.
• Show patient how to instill.
• Apply light finger-pressure on lacrimal sac for 1 minute following instillation.
• Don't stop therapy prematurely.
• Warn patient not to use leftover medication for a new eye infection; can
cause serious problems.
• Tell patient never to share eye medications. If a family member develops
similar symptoms, instruct him to contact the doctor.

Italicized side effects are common or life-threatening.
*Liquid form contains alcohol.   **May contain tartrazine.

75

Miotics

acetylcholine chloride
carbachol
demecarium bromide
echothiophate iodide
isoflurophate
physostigmine salicylate
pilocarpine hydrochloride
pilocarpine nitrate

MECHANISM OF ACTION

- Acetylcholine chloride, carbachol, and pilocarpine hydrochloride (cholinergic drugs) cause contraction of the sphincter muscles of the iris, resulting in miosis. They also produce ciliary spasm, deepening of the anterior chamber, and vasodilation of conjunctival vessels of the outflow tract.
- Demecarium bromide, echothiophate iodide, isoflurophate, and physostigmine salicylate (anticholinesterase drugs) inhibit the enzymatic destruction of acetylcholine by inactivating cholinesterase. This leaves acetylcholine free to act on the effector cells of the iridic sphincter and ciliary muscles, causing pupillary constriction and accommodation spasm.

COMBINATION PRODUCTS

E-CARPINE♦: epinephrine bitartrate 0.5% and pilocarpine hydrochloride 1%, 2%, 3%, 4%, or 6%.
E-PILO♦: epinephrine bitartrate 1% and pilocarpine hydrochloride 1%, 2%, 3%, 4%, or 6%.
ISOPTO P-ES: pilocarpine hydrochloride 2% and physostigmine salicylate 0.125%.
P_1E_1, P_2E_1, P_3E_1, P_4E_1, P_6E_1: epinephrine bitartrate 1% and pilocarpine hydrochloride 1%, 2%, 3%, 4%, or 6%.

acetylcholine chloride
Miochol♦

INDICATIONS & DOSAGE

Anterior segment surgery—
Adults and children: doctor instills 0.5 to 2 ml of 1% solution gently in anterior chamber of eye.

SIDE EFFECTS

None reported with 1% concentration. Iris atrophy possible with higher concentrations.

INTERACTIONS

None significant.

NURSING CONSIDERATIONS

- Shake vial gently until clear solution is obtained.
- Reconstitute immediately before using.
- Discard any unused solution.
- Complete miosis within seconds.
- Don't gas-sterilize vial. Ethylene oxide may produce formic acid.

carbachol (intraocular)
Miostat

carbachol (topical)
Carbacel, Isopto Carbachol♦

INDICATIONS & DOSAGE

Ocular surgery (to produce pupillary miosis)—

Unmarked trade names available in the United States only.
♦ Also available in Canada. ♦♦ Available in Canada only.

Adults: doctor should gently instill 0.5 ml into the anterior chamber for production of satisfactory miosis. It may be instilled before or after securing sutures.

Open-angle or narrow-angle glaucoma—

Adults: instill 1 drop into eye daily, b.i.d., t.i.d., or q.i.d. Ointment form also available with b.i.d. dosage.

SIDE EFFECTS
CNS: headache.
Eye: accommodative spasm, blurred vision, conjunctival vasodilation, eye and brow pain.
GI: abdominal cramps, diarrhea.
Other: sweating, flushing, asthma.

INTERACTIONS
None significant.

NURSING CONSIDERATIONS
• Contraindicated in acute iritis, corneal abrasion. Use cautiously in acute heart failure, bronchial asthma, peptic ulcer, hyperthyroidism, GI spasm, urinary tract obstruction, Parkinson's disease.
• Used in glaucoma, especially when patient is resistant or allergic to pilocarpine HCl or nitrate.
• Show patient how to instill. Warn him not to exceed recommended dosage.
• Apply light finger-pressure on lacrimal sac for 1 minute following instillation. This minimizes systemic absorption.
• For single-dose intraocular use only. Premixed; discard unused portions.
• Warn patient not to touch tip of dropper to eye or surrounding tissue.
• Tell glaucoma patient that long-term use may be necessary. Stress compliance. Tell him to remain under medical supervision for periodic tonometric readings.
• In case of toxicity, atropine should be given parenterally.

• Caution patient not to drive for 1 or 2 hours after administration.
• Reassure patient that blurred vision usually diminishes with prolonged use.

demecarium bromide
Humorsol

INDICATIONS & DOSAGE
Glaucoma, postiridectomy—
Adults: instill 1 drop 0.125% or 0.25% solution in eyes twice weekly up to b.i.d., depending on intraocular pressure.
Accommodative esotropia—
Children: instill 1 drop 0.125% solution in each eye daily for 2 to 3 weeks, taper to 1 drop q 2 days for 3 to 4 weeks, then 1 drop twice weekly. Therapy should be discontinued after 4 months if control of condition still requires q other day therapy or if patient shows no response.

SIDE EFFECTS
CNS: headache.
CV: hypotension, bradycardia.
Eye: iris cysts (reversible with discontinuation), lens opacity, ciliary or accommodative spasm, blurred vision, eye or brow pain, photosensitivity, eyelid twitching, congestive iritis, iridocyclitis, conjunctival and intraocular hyperemia, ocular pain, photophobia, acute attack of narrow-angle glaucoma.
GI: nausea, vomiting, abdominal pain, diarrhea, excessive salivation.
GU: frequent urination.
Skin: contact dermatitis.
Other: flushing, bronchial constriction.

INTERACTIONS
Systemic anticholinesterase for myasthenia gravis: additive effects. Monitor patient for signs of toxicity.
Echothiophate iodide: decreased duration of miosis if demecarium bromide is given first. Give echothiophate iodide first.

Organophosphorus insecticides: additive effects. Warn patient exposed to insecticides of this danger.

Pilocarpine: interferes with miosis. Do not use together.

Succinylcholine: respiratory or cardiovascular collapse. Don't use together.

NURSING CONSIDERATIONS

• Contraindicated in active uveal inflammation, narrow-angle glaucoma, secondary glaucoma resulting from iridocyclitis, ocular hypertension, vasomotor instability, bronchial asthma, spastic GI conditions, peptic ulcer, severe bradycardia, hypotension, recent myocardial infarction, epilepsy, parkinsonism, history of retinal detachment. Use cautiously in patients with myasthenia gravis receiving systemic anticholinesterase therapy; in patients exposed to organophosphorus insecticides.

• Dangerous drug capable of producing cumulative systemic side effects. Closely follow prescribed concentration and dosage schedule and monitor patient carefully.

• Atropine sulfate given subcutaneously or I.V., and pralidoxine chloride are antidotes of choice.

• Tell patient to stop drug and report immediately if excessive salivation, diaphoresis, urinary incontinence, diarrhea, or muscle weakness occurs.

• Instruct patient to use at bedtime since drug blurs vision.

• Warn patient not to exceed recommended dosage.

• Show patient how to instill. Warn him not to touch tip of dropper to eye or surrounding tissue.

• Apply light finger-pressure on lacrimal sac for 1 minute following instillation. This minimizes systemic absorption.

• Stop drug at least 2 weeks preoperatively.

• If solution contacts skin, wash promptly with large amount of water.

• Wash hands immediately before and after administering.

• Monitor patient for lenticular opacities every 6 months.

• Instruct patient that close and constant medical supervision is vital.

• Treat any extraocular pressure changes with rapid instillation of 1% to 2% epinephrine at 5-minute intervals.

• Antidote for atropine for glaucoma or preglaucoma patients, and used to control preoperative and postoperative intraocular pressure of glaucoma.

• Store in tightly closed container.

• An extremely potent, long-acting drug.

• Reassure patient that blurred vision usually diminishes with prolonged use.

echothiophate iodide
Echodide, Phospholine Iodide♦

INDICATIONS & DOSAGE

Open-angle glaucoma, conditions obstructing aqueous outflow, accommodative esotropia—

Adults and children: instill 1 drop 0.03% to 0.125% solution into conjunctival sac daily. Maximum 1 drop b.i.d. Use lowest possible dosage to continuously control intraocular pressure.

SIDE EFFECTS

CNS: fatigue, muscle weakness, paresthesias, headache.

CV: bradycardia, hypotension.

Eye: ciliary or accommodative spasm, ciliary or conjunctival injection, non-reversible cataract formation (time- and dose-related), reversible iris cysts, pupillary block, blurred or dimmed vision, eye or brow pain, lid twitching, hyperemia, photosensitivity, lens opacities, lacrimation, retinal detachment.

GI: diarrhea, nausea, vomiting, abdominal pain, intestinal cramps, salivation.

GU: frequent urination.

Other: flushing, sweating, bronchial constriction.

INTERACTIONS

Organophosphorus insecticides (parathion, malathion): may have an additive effect that could cause systemic effects. Warn patient exposed to insecticides of this danger.
Succinylcholine: respiratory and cardiovascular collapse. Don't use together.
Systemic anticholinesterase for myasthenia gravis: effects may be additive. Monitor patient for signs of toxicity.

NURSING CONSIDERATIONS

• Contraindicated in narrow-angle glaucoma, epilepsy, vasomotor instability, parkinsonism, iodide hypersensitivity, active uveal inflammation, ocular hypertension with intraocular inflammatory processes, bronchial asthma, spastic GI conditions, urinary tract obstruction, peptic ulcer, severe bradycardia or hypotension, vascular hypertension, myocardial infarction, history of retinal detachment. Use cautiously in patients routinely exposed to organophosphorus insecticides. May cause nausea, vomiting, and diarrhea, progressing to muscle weakness and respiratory difficulty. Use cautiously in patients with myasthenia gravis receiving anticholinesterase therapy.
• Toxicity is cumulative. Toxic systemic symptoms don't appear for weeks or months after initiating therapy.
• Reconstitute powder carefully to avoid contamination. Use only diluent provided. Discard refrigerated, reconstituted solution after 6 months; solution at room temperature after 1 month.
• Warn patient that transient browache or dimmed or blurred vision is common at first but usually disappears within 5 to 10 days.
• Instill at bedtime since drug causes transient blurred vision.
• Tell patient to remain under constant medical supervision. Warn him not to exceed recommended dosage.

• Report salivation, diarrhea, profuse sweating, urinary incontinence, or muscle weakness.
• Stop drug at least 2 weeks preoperatively if succinylcholine is to be used in surgery.
• Atropine sulfate (subcutaneous, I.M., or I.V.) is antidote of choice.
• A potent, long-acting, irreversible drug.
• Show patient how to instill. Warn him not to touch tip of dropper to eye or surrounding tissue.
• Apply light finger-pressure on lacrimal sac for 1 minute following instillation. This minimizes systemic absorption.
• Wash hands before and after administering medication.

isoflurophate
Floropryl

INDICATIONS & DOSAGE

Glaucoma—
Adults and children: instill ¼" strip 0.025% ointment in conjunctival sac q 8 to 72 hours.
Esotropia uncomplicated by amblyopia or anisometropia—
Adults and children: ¼" of ointment every night for 2 weeks.

SIDE EFFECTS

CNS: headache, muscle weakness.
Eye: moderate conjunctival hyperemia, eye pain, ciliary spasm causing discomfort, iris cysts, cataract formation, retinal detachment, paradoxical increase in intraocular pressure; precipitates attacks of acute narrow-angle glaucoma.
GI: diarrhea, salivation.
Other: sweating, bronchial constriction.

INTERACTIONS

Demecarium, physostigmine: competitive action. Decreased duration of miosis if isoflurophate given second. Give isoflurophate first.

Italicized side effects are common or life-threatening.
*Liquid form contains alcohol.   **May contain tartrazine.

Pilocarpine: interferes with miosis. Use cautiously for ciliary spasm.
Succinylcholine: respiratory or cardiovascular collapse. Don't use together.
Systemic anticholinesterase for myasthenia gravis: additive effects. Monitor patient for signs of toxicity.

NURSING CONSIDERATIONS

• Contraindicated in hypersensitivity to organophosphorus compounds, peanut oil, and polyethylene mineral oil; in patients with uveal inflammation, narrow-angle glaucoma, ocular hypertension, bronchial asthma, peptic ulcer, severe bradycardia, hypotension, recent MI, epilepsy, parkinsonism, or history of retinal detachment. Use cautiously in patients exposed to organophosphous insecticides; patients with myasthenia gravis receiving concurrent anticholinesterase drugs.

• Tell patient with glaucoma to use at bedtime if possible because of blurred vision and ciliary spasm.

• Show patient how to instill. Warn him not to touch tip of tube to eye, surrounding tissues, or moist surface.

• Apply light finger-pressure on lacrimal sac for 1 minute following instillation. This minimizes systemic absorption.

• Warn patient that close, constant medical supervision is vital and that he should not exceed prescribed dosage.

• Treat paradoxical pressure changes with rapid instillation of 1% to 2% epinephrine at 5-minute intervals.

• Instruct patient to stop therapy at once and notify doctor if he experiences excessive salivation, diarrhea, sweating, or muscle weakness.

• Unstable and inactivated in the presence of water.

• Store in refrigerator tightly closed container.

• Rapidly absorbed through skin.

• Wash hands before and after administering medication.

physostigmine salicylate
Eserine Salicylate, Isopto Eserine

INDICATIONS & DOSAGE
Atropine mydriasis, acute narrow-angle glaucoma—
Adults and children: instill ¼" 0.25% ophthalmic ointment in conjunctival sac, or instill 1 to 2 drops 0.25% to 0.5% solution in conjunctival sac t.i.d. Repeat p.r.n. to obtain miosis.

SIDE EFFECTS
CNS: *headache.*
Eye: twitching of eyelids, conjunctival irritation, reversible depigmentation of lid skin in Blacks allergic to ointment, eye and brow pain, marked miosis, lacrimation, dimmed or blurred vision, follicular cysts.
Skin: allergic dermatitis.

INTERACTIONS
Isoflurophate: decreased miosis if isoflurophate given second. Give isoflurophate first.
Organophosphorus insecticides: additive effect. Warn patients exposed to insecticides of this danger.
Pilocarpine: prolonged miosis. May be used together therapeutically.
Succinylcholine: additive effect. Don't use together.

NURSING CONSIDERATIONS
• Contraindicated in inflammatory diseases of iris or ciliary body, asthma, diabetes mellitus, gangrene, cardiovascular disease, mechanical obstruction of intestinal or urogenital tract, vagotonia, secondary glaucoma. Use cautiously in bradycardia, epilepsy, parkinsonism, and in patients exposed to organophosphorus insecticides.

• Glaucoma therapy is long term. Stress patient compliance. Warn not to exceed dosage.

• Lid twitching, temporarily blurred vision, and difficulty in seeing in the dark are common side effects.

• Irritating to eye. Watch for signs of conjunctivitis or allergic reactions.
• Show patient how to instill. Warn him not to touch dropper or tip of tube to eye or surrounding tissue.
• Apply light finger-pressure on lacrimal sac for 1 minute following instillation. This minimizes systemic absorption.
• Discard discolored (rusty or pink) solution or ointment. Aqueous solutions oxidize on exposure to light or air.
• Used in ocular myasthenia gravis.
• May be used alternately with atropine as a miotic to break adhesions between the iris and lens.
• Wash hands before and after administering medication.

---

pilocarpine hydrochloride
Adsorbocarpine, Almocarpine, Isopto Carpine♦, Miocarpine♦♦, Nova-Carpine♦♦, Ocusert Pilo♦, Opto-Pilo♦♦, Pilocar, Pilocel, Pilomiotin

pilocarpine nitrate
P.V. Carpine Liquifilm♦

INDICATIONS & DOSAGE
Chronic open-angle glaucoma, before emergency surgery in acute narrow-angle glaucoma—
Adults and children: instill 1 to 2 drops in eye daily b.i.d., t.i.d., q.i.d., or as directed by doctor.

SIDE EFFECTS
Eye: suborbital headache, *myopia,* ciliary spasm, *blurred vision,* conjunctival irritation, lacrimation, changes in visual field, *brow pain.*
GI: nausea, vomiting, abdominal cramps, diarrhea, salivation.
Other: bronchiolar spasm, pulmonary edema, hypersensitivity.

INTERACTIONS
Carbachol: additive effect. Do not use together.
Phenylephrine HCl: decreased dilation by phenylephrine HCl. Don't use together.

NURSING CONSIDERATIONS
• Contraindicated in acute iritis, acute inflammatory disease of anterior segment of eye, secondary glaucoma. Use cautiously in bronchial asthma, hypertension.
• Warn patient that vision will be temporarily blurred.
• Transient browache and myopia are common at first; usually disappear in 10 to 14 days.
• Warn patient not to exceed recommended dosage.
• Show patient how to instill. Warn him not to touch dropper to eye or surrounding tissue.
• Apply light finger-pressure on lacrimal sac for 1 minute following instillation. This minimizes systemic absorption.
• Glaucoma therapy is necessarily prolonged. Stress compliance. Warn that glaucoma can cause blindness.
• Most widely used drug in initial treatment of chronic open-angle glaucoma.
• Also used to counteract effects of mydriatics and cycloplegics after surgery or ophthalmoscopic examination.
• May be used alternately with atropine to break adhesions between iris and lens.
• In acute narrow-angle glaucoma before surgery, may be used alone or with physostigmine or mannitol, urea, or glycerol.
• Wash hands before and after administration.

Italicized side effects are common or life-threatening.
∗Liquid form contains alcohol.   ∗∗May contain tartrazine.

76

Mydriatics

atropine sulfate
cyclopentolate hydrochloride
epinephrine bitartrate
epinephrine hydrochloride
epinephryl borate
homatropine hydrobromide
hydroxyamphetamine
    hydrobromide
phenylephrine hydrochloride
scopolamine hydrobromide
tropicamide

MECHANISM OF ACTION
● Anticholinergics block acetylcholine, leaving the pupil under the unopposed influence of its sympathetic or adrenergic nerve supply. This causes the pupil to dilate. Relaxation of the ciliary muscle allows the lens to flatten.
● Adrenergics dilate the pupil by contracting the dilator muscle of the pupil.

COMBINATION PRODUCTS
CYCLOMYDRIL: cyclopentolate hydrochloride 0.2% and phenylephrine hydrochloride 1%.

---

atropine sulfate
Atropisol, BufOpto Atropine, Isopto Atropine♦, Opto-Tropinal♦♦

INDICATIONS & DOSAGE
Acute iris inflammation (iritis)—
Adults: 1 to 2 drops of 1% solution or small amount of ointment 2 to 3 times daily, b.i.d., or t.i.d.
Children: instill 1 to 2 drops of 0.5% solution daily, b.i.d., or t.i.d.
Cycloplegic refraction—

Adults: instill 1 to 2 drops of 1% solution 1 hour before refracting.
Children: instill 1 to 2 drops of 0.5% solution to each eye b.i.d. for 1 to 3 days before eye examination and 1 hour before refraction, or instill small amount ointment daily or b.i.d. 2 to 3 days before examination.

SIDE EFFECTS
Eye: increased intraocular pressure, ocular congestion in long-term use, conjunctivitis, contact dermatitis, edema, *blurred vision,* eye dryness, *photophobia.*
Systemic: flushing, dry skin and mouth, fever, tachycardia, abdominal distention in infants, ataxia, irritability, confusion, somnolence.

INTERACTIONS
None significant.

NURSING CONSIDERATIONS
● Contraindicated in primary glaucoma (shallow anterior chamber or narrow-angle), increased intraocular pressure. Use cautiously in infants, children, elderly or debilitated patients.
● Warn patient vision will be temporarily blurred. Dark glasses ease discomfort of photophobia.
● Not for internal use. Treat drops and ointment as poison. Keep physostigmine available as antidote for poisoning. Signs of poisoning are disorientation and confusion.
● Don't touch dropper or tip of tube to eye or surrounding tissue.
● Watch for signs of glaucoma: increased intraocular pressure, ocular

---

Unmarked trade names available in the United States only.
♦ Also available in Canada.   ♦♦ Available in Canada only.

pain, headache, progressive blurring of vision.
- Most potent mydriatic and cycloplegic available; long duration of action.
- Systemic side effects most commonly occur in children and the elderly.
- Warn patient not to operate machinery or drive a car until the temporary visual impairment caused by this drug wears off.
- Warn patient not to exceed recommended dosage.
- Show patient how to instill. Wash hands before and after administration.
- Apply light finger-pressure on lacrimal sac for 1 minute following instillation. This minimizes systemic absorption.

cyclopentolate hydrochloride
Cyclogyl♦, Mydplegic♦♦, Nova-Cyclo♦♦, Opto-Pentolate♦♦

INDICATIONS & DOSAGE
Diagnostic procedures requiring mydriasis and cycloplegia—
Adults: instill 1 drop 1% solution in eye, followed by 1 more drop in 5 minutes. Use 2% solution in heavily pigmented irises.
Children: instill 1 drop of 0.5%, 1%, or 2% solution in each eye, followed in 5 minutes with 1 drop 0.5% or 1% solution, if necessary. Not recommended for children under 6 years.

SIDE EFFECTS
Eye: burning sensation on instillation, increased intraocular pressure, blurred vision, eye dryness, *photophobia*, ocular congestion, contact dermatitis, conjunctivitis.
Systemic: flushing, tachycardia, urinary retention, dry skin, fever, ataxia, irritability, confusion, somnolence, convulsions, hallucinations, seizures.

INTERACTIONS
None significant.

NURSING CONSIDERATIONS
- Contraindicated in narrow-angle glaucoma. Use cautiously in elderly patients.
- Close container after each use to avoid contamination.
- Wash hands before and after administration.
- Potent drug with mydriatic and cycloplegic effect; superior to homatropine hydrobromide and has shorter duration of action.
- Instruct patient to wear dark glasses to ease discomfort of photophobia.
- Warn patient drug will burn when instilled.
- Warn patient not to operate machinery or drive until the temporary visual impairment caused by this drug has worn off.
- Show patient how to instill.
- Apply light finger-pressure on lacrimal sac for 1 minute following instillation. This minimizes systemic absorption.

epinephrine bitartrate
Epitrate♦, Mytrate

epinephrine hydrochloride
Epifrin♦, Glaucon♦

epinephryl borate
Epinal♦,

INDICATIONS & DOSAGE
Adults and children:
*Intraocular injection—*0.1 to 0.2 ml of 0.01% or 0.1% epinephrine HCl by doctor.
*Open-angle glaucoma—*instill 1 to 2 drops of 1% or 2% bitartrate solution in eye with frequency determined by tonometric readings (once q 2 to 4 days up to q.i.d.), or instill 1 drop 0.5%, 1%, or 2% HCl solution (or 0.25%,

---

Italicized side effects are common or life-threatening.
♦Liquid form contains alcohol.   ♦♦May contain tartrazine.

0.5%, or 1% epinephryl borate solution) in eye b.i.d.
During surgery—1 or more drops of 0.1% epinephrine HCl up to 3 times.

SIDE EFFECTS
Eye: corneal or conjunctival pigmentation or corneal edema in long-term use; follicular hypertrophy; chemosis; conjunctivitis; iritis; hyperemic conjunctiva; maculopapular rash; severe stinging, burning, and tearing upon instillation; browache.
Systemic: palpitations, tachycardia.

INTERACTIONS
Cyclopropane or halogenated hydrocarbons: arrhythmias, tachycardia. Use together cautiously, if at all.
Tricyclic antidepressants, antihistamines (diphenhydramine, dexchlorpheniramine): potentiated cardiac effects of epinephrine. Use together cautiously.

NURSING CONSIDERATIONS
• Contraindicated in shallow anterior chamber or narrow-angle glaucoma.
• Use cautiously in diabetes mellitus, hypertension, Parkinson's disease, hyperthyroidism, aphakia (eye without lens), cardiac disease, or cerebral arteriosclerosis; in elderly patients or pregnant women.
• May stain soft contact lenses.
• Use with pilocarpine: additive effect in lowering intraocular pressure.
• Monitor blood pressure and other systemic effects.
• Protect from light and heat.
• Don't use darkened solution.
• Also used during surgery to control local bleeding, or injected into the anterior chamber to produce rapid mydriasis during cataract removal.
• Warn patient not to touch dropper to eye or surrounding tissue.
• Wash hands before and after administration.
• Show patient how to instill.
• Apply light finger-pressure on lacri-

mal sac for 1 minute following instillation. This minimizes systemic absorption.

homatropine hydrobromide
Homatrocel Ophthalmic, Isopto Homatropine♦

INDICATIONS & DOSAGE
Adults and children:
Cycloplegic refraction—instill 1 to 2 drops 2% or 5% solution in eye; repeat in 5 to 10 minutes.
Uveitis—instill 1 to 2 drops 2% or 5% solution in eye up to every 3 to 4 hours.

SIDE EFFECTS
Eye: eye irritation, *blurred vision, photophobia.*
Systemic: flushing, dry skin and mouth, fever, tachycardia, ataxia, irritability, confusion, somnolence.

INTERACTIONS
None significant.

NURSING CONSIDERATIONS
• Contraindicated in primary glaucoma (shallow anterior chamber or narrow-angle). Use cautiously in infants, elderly or debilitated patients, or patients with hypertension, cardiac disease, or increased intraocular pressure.
• Warn patient vision will be temporarily blurred after instillation. Tell him not to drive a car or operate machinery until this wears off. Dark glasses should be worn to decrease photophobia.
• Long-term frequent use may produce symptoms of atropine SO_4 poisoning, such as severe dryness of mouth, tachycardia.
• Not for internal use. Treat as poison. Keep physostigmine available as antidote for poisoning.
• Show patient how to instill.
• Apply light finger-pressure on lacrimal sac for 1 minute following instilla-

tion. This minimizes systemic absorption.
• Warn patient not to touch dropper tip to eye or surrounding tissue.
• Wash hands before and after administration.
• Similar to atropine SO₄ but weaker, with a shorter duration of action.

---

hydroxyamphetamine hydrobromide
Paredrine

INDICATIONS & DOSAGE
Diagnosis of Horner's syndrome—
Adults and children over 12 years: instill 1 to 2 drops 1% solution into conjunctival sac.

SIDE EFFECTS
Eye: increased intraocular pressure, blurred vision, *photophobia.*

INTERACTIONS
None significant.

NURSING CONSIDERATIONS
• Contraindicated in narrow-angle glaucoma. Use cautiously in hypertension, hyperthyroidism, diabetes mellitus, increased intraocular pressure.
• Instruct patient to wear dark glasses to ease discomfort of photophobia.
• May cause blurred vision. Warn patient not to drive car or operate machinery until this effect wears off.
• Store in tightly closed container. Do not use discolored solution.
• Wash hands before and after administration.
• If ingested, toxic symptoms include arrhythmias, headache, nausea, vomiting. Contact doctor immediately.

---

phenylephrine hydrochloride
Mydfrin, Neo-Synephrine♦

INDICATIONS & DOSAGE
Adults and children:
Mydriasis (without cycloplegia)—instill 1 drop 2.5% or 10% solution in eye before examination.
Posterior synechia (adhesion of iris)— instill 1 drop 10% solution in eye.
Do not use 10% concentration in infants; use cautiously in elderly patients.

SIDE EFFECTS
Eye: transient burning or stinging on instillation, blurred vision, reactive hyperemia, allergic conjunctivitis, iris floaters, narrow-angle glaucoma, rebound miosis, allergic conjunctivitis, dermatitis.
CNS: headache, browache.
CV: *hypertension,* tachycardia, palpitations, premature ventricular contractions.
Other: pallor, trembling, sweating.

INTERACTIONS
Guanethidine: increased mydriatic and pressor effects of phenylephrine HCl. Use together cautiously.
Levodopa (systemic): reduced mydriatic effect of phenylephrine HCl. Use together cautiously.
MAO inhibitors and beta blockers: may cause arrhythmias due to increased pressor effect. Use together cautiously.
Tricyclic antidepressants: potentiated cardiac effects of epinephrine. Use together cautiously.

NURSING CONSIDERATIONS
• Contraindicated in narrow-angle glaucoma, soft contact lens use. Use cautiously in marked hypertension, cardiac disorders, and in children of low body weight.
• Should be avoided in patients with idiopathic orthostatic hypotension.

Italicized side effects are common or life-threatening.
♦Liquid form contains alcohol.   ♦♦May contain tartrazine.

May produce high blood pressure response.

• Protect from light and heat.

• Warn patient not to exceed recommended dosage. Systemic effects can result. Monitor blood pressure and pulse rate.

• Warn patient not to touch dropper tip to eye or surrounding tissue.

• Potential for systemic side effects less severe with 2.5% solution. Side effects and toxicity much more likely with 10% solution.

• Show patient how to instill.

• Apply light finger-pressure on lacrimal sac for 1 minute following instillation. This minimizes systemic absorption.

• Wash hands before and after administration.

• May cause blurred vision. Warn patient not to drive car or operate machinery until this effect wears off.

scopolamine hydrobromide
Isopto Hyoscine

INDICATIONS & DOSAGE
Cycloplegic refraction—
Adults: instill 1 to 2 drops 0.5% to 1% solution in eye 1 hour before refraction.
Children: instill 1 drop 0.2% or 0.25% solution or ointment b.i.d. for 2 days before refraction.
Iritis—
Adults: 1 to 2 drops of 0.1% solution daily, b.i.d., or t.i.d.

SIDE EFFECTS
Eye: ocular congestion with prolonged use, conjunctivitis, *blurred vision,* eye dryness, increased intraocular pressure, *photophobia,* contact dermatitis.
Systemic: flushing, fever, dry skin and mouth, tachycardia, hallucinations, ataxia, irritability, confusion, delirium, somnolence, acute psychotic reactions.

INTERACTIONS
None significant.

NURSING CONSIDERATIONS
• Contraindicated in primary glaucoma (shallow anterior chamber or narrow-angle). Use cautiously in cardiac disease, increased intraocular pressure, and in patients over 40 years.

• Observe patient closely for systemic effects (disorientation, delirium).

• Warn patient vision will be temporarily blurred; tell him not to drive car or operate machinery until this effect wears off.

• Instruct patient to wear dark glasses to ease discomfort of photophobia.

• May be used when patient is sensitive to atropine. Faster acting and has shorter duration of action and fewer side effects.

• Show patient how to instill. Warn him not to touch dropper tip to eye or surrounding tissue. Wash hands before and after administration.

• Apply light finger-pressure on lacrimal sac for 1 minute following instillation. This minimizes systemic absorption.

tropicamide
Mydriacyl♦

INDICATIONS & DOSAGE
Adults and children:
*Cycloplegic refractions—*instill 1 to 2 drops of 1% solution in each eye; repeat in 5 minutes. Additional drop may be instilled in 20 to 30 minutes.
*Fundus examinations—*instill 1 to 2 drops 0.5% solution in each eye 15 to 20 minutes before examination.

SIDE EFFECTS
EENT: *transient stinging on instillation,* increased intraocular pressure (less than with other mydriatic agents because of shorter duration of action), *blurred vision, photophobia,* dry mouth and throat.

INTERACTIONS
None significant.

NURSING CONSIDERATIONS
• Contraindicated in narrow-angle and shallow anterior chamber glaucoma. Use cautiously in elderly.
• Shortest acting cycloplegic, but mydriatic effect greater than cycloplegic effect.
• Causes transient stinging; vision temporarily blurred. Warn patient not to drive car or operate machinery until this effect wears off.
• Instruct patient to wear dark glasses if photosensitivity occurs (lasts about 2 hours).
• Store at room temperature in tightly closed container.

Italicized side effects are common or life-threatening.
*Liquid form contains alcohol.   **May contain tartrazine.

77

Ophthalmic vasoconstrictors

**naphazoline hydrochloride
phenylephrine hydrochloride
tetrahydrozoline hydrochloride
zinc sulfate**

MECHANISM OF ACTION
• Naphazoline, phenylephrine, and tetrahydrozoline produce vasoconstriction by local adrenergic action on the blood vessels of the conjunctiva.
• Zinc sulfate produces astringent action on the conjunctiva.

COMBINATION PRODUCTS
ALBALON-A♦: naphazoline hydrochloride 0.05% and antazoline phosphate 0.5%.
BLEPHAMIDE♦: phenylephrine hydrochloride 0.12%, sulfacetamide sodium 10%, and prednisolone acetate 0.2%.
M-Z: phenylephrine hydrochloride 0.12%, zinc sulfate 0.25%, and piperocaine hydrochloride 0.75%.
NEOZIN OPHTH: phenylephrine hydrochloride 0.125% and zinc sulfate 0.25%.
PHENYLZIN DROPS: zinc sulfate 0.25% and phenylephrine hydrochloride 0.12%.
PREFRIN-A♦: phenylephrine hydrochloride 0.12%, pyrilamine maleate 0.1%, and antipyrine 0.1%.
PREFIN-Z: phenylephrine hydrochloride 0.12% and zinc sulfate 0.24%.
VASOCIDIN♦: phenylephrine hydrochloride 0.125%, sodium sulfacetamide 10%, and prednisolone sodium phosphate 0.2%.
VASOCON-A♦: naphazoline hydrochloride 0.05% and antazoline phosphate 0.5%.

ZINCFRIN♦: phenylephrine hydrochloride 0.12% and zinc sulfate 0.25%.

**naphazoline hydrochloride
0.012%, 0.1%, 0.02%**
Albalon Liquifilm Ophthalmic♦,
Clear Eyes, Naphcon, Naphcon
Forte Ophthalmic♦, Opto-Zoline♦♦,
Vasoclear, Vasocon Regular
Ophthalmic♦

INDICATIONS & DOSAGE
Ocular congestion, irritation, itching—
Adults: instill 1 to 2 drops in eye q 3 to 4 hours.

SIDE EFFECTS
Eye: transient stinging, pupillary dilation, increased intraocular pressure, irritation.

INTERACTIONS
MAO inhibitors: hypertensive crisis if naphazoline HCl is systemically absorbed. Use together cautiously.

NURSING CONSIDERATIONS
• Contraindicated in narrow-angle glaucoma, hypersensitivity to any ingredients. Use cautiously in patients with hyperthyroidism, cardiac disease, hypertension, and diabetes mellitus, and in elderly patients.
• Can produce marked sedation and coma if ingested by child.
• Advise patient that photophobia may follow pupil dilation if he is sensitive to drug. Tell patient to report this to the doctor if it occurs.
• Warn patient not to exceed recom-

Unmarked trade names available in the United States only.
♦ Also available in Canada.   ♦♦ Available in Canada only.

mended dosage. Rebound congestion and rhinitis may occur with frequent or prolonged use.
• Notify doctor if blurred vision, pain, or lid edema develops.
• Store in tightly closed container.
• Most effective and widely used ocular decongestant.
• Show patient how to instill. Do not touch tip of dropper to eye or surrounding tissues.

phenylephrine hydrochloride
Isopto Frin, Prefrin, Tear-Efrin

INDICATIONS & DOSAGE
Decongestant, minor eye irritations—
Adults and children: 2 drops of 0.12% or 0.25% in affected eye. May repeat in 3 to 4 hours, p.r.n.

SIDE EFFECTS
CNS: headache.
Eye: transient stinging, iris floaters, narrow-angle glaucoma, blurred vision, reactive hyperemia, browache.

INTERACTIONS
MAO inhibitors: may cause hypertensive crisis. Don't use together.

NURSING CONSIDERATIONS
• Contraindicated in narrow-angle glaucoma, in patients taking tricyclic antidepressants or MAO inhibitors, and in hypersensitivity to any ingredient.
• May exacerbate hypertension in hypertensive patients.
• Do not use butacaine drops as local anesthetic, since phenylephrine and butacaine are incompatible.
• Do not exceed prescribed dose.
• Monitor blood pressure and pulse rate; watch for overdosage.
• Do not use if solution is dark brown or contains precipitate.
• Keep container tightly sealed and away from light.

• Do not touch tip of dropper to eye or surrounding tissues.
• Show patient how to instill.
• Caution patient not to share eye medications with others.

tetrahydrozoline hydrochloride
Clear & Bright, Soothe, Tetrasine, Visine

INDICATIONS & DOSAGE
Ocular congestion, irritation, and allergic conditions—
Adults and children over 2 years: instill 1 to 2 drops in eye b.i.d. or t.i.d., or as directed by doctor.

SIDE EFFECTS
Eye: transient stinging, pupillary dilation, increased intraocular pressure, irritation, iris floaters in elderly.
Systemic: drowsiness, CNS depression, cardiac irregularities, headache, dizziness, tremors, insomnia.

INTERACTIONS
MAO inhibitors: hypertensive crisis if tetrahydrozoline HCl is systemically absorbed. Don't use together.

NURSING CONSIDERATIONS
• Contraindicated in patients receiving MAO inhibitors, and in those with hypersensitivity to any ingredients or narrow-angle glaucoma. Use cautiously in patients with hyperthyroidism, heart disease, hypertension, and diabetes mellitus, and in elderly patients.
• Do not exceed recommended dosage. Rebound congestion and rhinitis may occur with frequent or prolonged use.
• Warn patient to stop drug and notify doctor if relief is not obtained within 48 hours, or if redness or irritation persists or increases.
• Available without prescription.
• Available in 0.05% concentration; less effective than naphazoline hydrochloride 0.1%.

Italicized side effects are common or life-threatening.
*Liquid form contains alcohol.   **May contain tartrazine.

- Warn patient not to touch dropper tip to eye or surrounding tissues.
- Show patient how to instill.
- Caution patient not to share eye medications with others.

zinc sulfate
Bufopto Zinc Sulfate, Eye-Sed Ophthalmic, Op-Thal-Zin

INDICATIONS & DOSAGE
Ocular congestion, irritation—
Adults and children: solution 0.2%— instill 1 to 2 drops in eye b.i.d. or t.i.d.

SIDE EFFECTS
Eye: irritation.

INTERACTIONS
None significant.

NURSING CONSIDERATIONS
- Use cautiously in patients with a shallow anterior chamber, predisposition to narrow-angle glaucoma.
- A decongestant astringent.
- Store in tightly closed container.
- Warn patient not to touch dropper tip to eye or surrounding tissues.
- Show patient how to instill drops.
- Caution patient not to share eye medications with others.

78

Topical ophthalmic anesthetics

cocaine hydrochloride
proparacaine hydrochloride
tetracaine hydrochloride

MECHANISM OF ACTION
Topical ophthalmic anesthetics produce anesthesia by preventing initiation and transmission of impulses at the nerve-cell membrane.
• Cocaine hydrochloride also has an adrenergic action that produces mydriasis and constriction of conjunctival vessels.

COMBINATION PRODUCTS
None.

cocaine hydrochloride

INDICATIONS & DOSAGE
Diagnosis of Horner's syndrome, topical anesthesia for minor surgery or examinations—
Adults and children: instill 1 to 2 drops 4% solution in eye just before procedure or examination.

SIDE EFFECTS
Eye: *blurring,* corneal ulceration or scarring in excessive or long-term use. Varying effects on intraocular pressure.
Systemic: excitation; nervousness; rapid, shallow respirations; emesis; chills; fever; tachycardia; hypertension; euphoria; anxiety; delirium; convulsions; respiratory and circulatory failure.

INTERACTIONS
Epinephrine (topical): increased epinephrine effect. Use together cautiously.

NURSING CONSIDERATIONS
• Use cautiously and sparingly in patients with known allergies, cardiac disease, hyperthyroidism, or open lesions.
• Patient should be given short-acting barbiturate before administering to avoid CNS stimulation.
• Solutions not commercially available; must be prepared specially by pharmacist. Rarely used.
• Monitor heart rate after instillation; observe for systemic effects.
• Warn patient that vision will be blurred for several hours.
• Warn patient not to rub eye for at least 20 minutes after instillation.
• Protective eyepatch recommended following procedure.
• Solution should be pink. Return discolored solution to pharmacy.
• Doesn't require refrigeration.

proparacaine hydrochloride
Alcaine♦, Ophthaine♦, Ophthetic♦

INDICATIONS & DOSAGE
Anesthesia for tonometry, gonioscopy; suture removal from cornea, removal of corneal foreign bodies—
Adults and children: instill 1 to 2 drops 0.5% solution in eye just before procedure.
Anesthesia for cataract extraction, glaucoma surgery—
Adults and children: instill 1 drop 0.5% solution in eye every 5 to 10 minutes for 5 to 7 doses.

SIDE EFFECTS
Eye: occasional conjunctival redness, transient pain.
Other: hypersensitivity.

INTERACTIONS
None significant.

NURSING CONSIDERATIONS
• Use cautiously in patients with cardiac disease and hyperthyroidism.
• *Not* for long-term use; may delay wound healing.
• Warn patient not to rub or touch eye while cornea is anesthetized, since this may cause corneal abrasion and greater discomfort when anesthesia wears off.
• Protective eyepatch recommended following procedure.
• Warn patient corneal pain is relieved only temporarily in abrasion.
• Systemic reactions unlikely when used in recommended doses.
• Topical ophthalmic anesthetic of choice in diagnostic and minor surgical procedures.
• Don't use discolored solution.
• Store in tightly closed container.
• Ophthaine brand packaged in bottle that looks similar in size and shape to Hemoccult. When taking bottle from shelf, check label carefully.

tetracaine hydrochloride
Anacel, Pontocaine♦

INDICATIONS & DOSAGE
Anesthesia for tonometry, gonioscopy; removal of corneal foreign bodies, su-ture removal from cornea; other diagnostic and minor surgical procedures—
Adults and children: instill 1 to 2 drops 0.5% solution in eye just before procedure.

SIDE EFFECTS
Eye: transient stinging in eye 30 seconds after initial instillation, epithelial damage in excessive or long-term use.
Other: sensitization in repeated use (allergic skin rash, urticaria).

INTERACTIONS
Sulfonamides: interference with sulfonamide antibacterial activity. Wait ½ hour after anesthesia before instilling sulfonamide.

NURSING CONSIDERATIONS
• Systemic absorption unlikely in recommended doses.
• Avoid repeated use.
• Does not dilate the pupil, paralyze accommodation, or increase intraocular pressure.
• Protective eyepatch recommended following procedure.
• Don't use discolored solution. Keep container tightly closed.

79

Artificial tears

artificial tears
eye irrigation solutions

MECHANISM OF ACTION
- Artificial tears augment insufficient tear production.
- External irrigation solutions clean the eye.

COMBINATION PRODUCTS
None.

artificial tears

Adsorbotear♦, Hypotears, Isopto Alkaline, Isopto Plain, Isopto Tears♦, Lacril♦, Lacrisert, Liquifilm Forte, Liquifilm Tears, Lyteers, Methulose, Neotears, Tearisol, Tears Naturale♦, Tears Plus, Ultra Tears, Visculose

INDICATIONS & DOSAGE
Insufficient tear production—
Adults and children: instill 1 to 2 drops in eye t.i.d., q.i.d., or p.r.n.
Moderate to severe dry eye syndromes, including keratoconjunctivitis sicca—
Adults: insert 1 Lacrisert rod daily into inferior cul-de-sac. Some patients may require twice daily use.

SIDE EFFECTS
Eye: discomfort; burning, pain on instillation; blurred vision (especially with Lacrisert); crust formation on eyelids and eyelashes in products with high viscosity, such as Adsorbotear, Isopto Tears, and Tearisol.

INTERACTIONS
Borate external irrigation solutions: may form gummy deposits on the lid when used with artificial tear products containing polyvinyl alcohol (Liquifilm Forte, Liquifilm Tears). Keep patient's eyelids clean.

NURSING CONSIDERATIONS
- Contraindicated in hypersensitivity to active product or preservatives.
- Show patient how to instill.
- Warn patient not to touch tip of container to eye, surrounding tissue, or other surface, to avoid contamination of solution.
- Instruct patient that product should be used by one person only.
- Lacrisert rod should be inserted with special applicator that is included in the package. Familiarize patient with illustrated instructions that are also included.

eye irrigation solutions

Blinx, Collyrium Eye Lotion♦, Dacriose, EyeStream, I-Lite Eye Drops, Lauro, Lavoptik Medicinal Eye Wash, Murine Eye Drops, Neo-Flow, Sterile Normal Saline (0.9%)

INDICATIONS & DOSAGE
Eye irrigation—
Adults and children: flush eye with 1 to 2 drops t.i.d., q.i.d., or p.r.n.

SIDE EFFECTS
None reported.

Italicized side effects are common or life-threatening.
✱Liquid form contains alcohol.   ✱✱May contain tartrazine.

INTERACTIONS
Products containing polyvinyl alcohol: may form gel and gummy deposits on the eye. Keep eyelids clean.

NURSING CONSIDERATIONS
• Contraindicated in hypersensitivity to active ingredient or preservatives.
• Don't touch tip of container to eye, surrounding tissue, or other surface, to avoid contamination.
• Check date of expiration to make sure solution is potent.
• Store in tightly closed, light-resistant container.
• Show patient how to instill.
• Should be used by one person only.
• When irrigating, have patient turn his head to side and irrigate from inner to outer canthus. Have tissues handy.

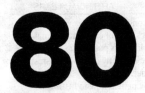

Miscellaneous ophthalmics

alpha-chymotrypsin
dipivefrin
fluorescein sodium
glycerin, anhydrous
isosorbide
sodium chloride, hypertonic
timolol maleate

MECHANISM OF ACTION
• Alpha-chymotrypsin dissolves filaments or zonules holding the lens.
• Dipivefrin is a prodrug of epinephrine (in the eye, dipivefrin is converted to epinephrine). The liberated epinephrine appears to decrease aqueous production and increase aqueous outflow.
• Fluorescein produces an intense green fluorescence in alkaline solution (pH 5.0 or less) or a bright yellow if viewed under cobalt blue illumination.
• Glycerin and sodium chloride remove excess fluid from the cornea.
• Isosorbide acts as an osmotic agent by promoting redistribution of water and thereby producing diuresis.
• Timolol, classified as a beta blocker, reduces aqueous formation and possibly increases aqueous outflow. It has little or no effect on pupil size.

COMBINATION PRODUCTS
FLURESS: sodium fluorescein 0.25% and benoxinate HCl 0.4%.

Adults over 20 years: 1 to 2 ml instilled into posterior chamber under the iris, by doctor.

SIDE EFFECTS
Eye: transient increase in intraocular pressure (dose-related), moderate uveitis, corneal edema and striation.

INTERACTIONS
Alcohol, surgical detergent: inactivated alpha-chymotrypsin. Rinse off all alcohol or detergents from surgical instruments and syringe with saline solution.

NURSING CONSIDERATIONS
• Contraindicated in high vitreous pressure with gaping incisional wound; congenital cataract.
• Solutions very unstable. Use only freshly reconstituted solution. Don't use if it is cloudy or has precipitated. Discard unused portions, including diluent, except for Zonulyn. Retains potency 1 week at room temperature, or for 1 month when refrigerated.
• Remove drug by irrigating with intraocular balanced saline solution.
• Don't autoclave powder or reconstituted solution; excess heat will inactivate the enzyme.
• Delayed healing of incision has been reported but not confirmed.

alpha-chymotrypsin
Alpha Chymar, Alpha Chymolean♦♦, Catarase♦, Zolyse♦

INDICATIONS & DOSAGE
Zonulysis in cataract surgery—

dipivefrin
Propine

INDICATIONS & DOSAGE
To reduce intraocular pressure in chronic open-angle glaucoma—

Italicized side effects are common or life-threatening.
*Liquid form contains alcohol. **May contain tartrazine.

Adults: for initial glaucoma therapy, 1 drop in eye q 12 hours.

SIDE EFFECTS
Eye: burning, stinging.
CV: tachycardia, hypertension.

INTERACTIONS
None significant.

NURSING CONSIDERATIONS
• Contraindicated in narrow-angle glaucoma.
• Use cautiously in patients with aphakia.
• Dipivefrin is a prodrug of epinephrine: converted to epinephrine when it enters the eye.
• May have fewer side effects than conventional epinephrine therapy.
• Often used concomitantly with other antiglaucoma drugs.
• Available as a 0.1% solution in 5-, 10-, and 15-ml dropper bottles.
• Teach patient how to instill.
• Wash hands before and after administration.
• Don't touch dropper to eye or surrounding tissue.

fluorescein sodium
Fluorescite, Fluor-I-Strip, Fluor-I-Strip-A.T.♦, Ful-Glo Strips♦, Funduscein Injections

INDICATIONS & DOSAGE
Diagnostic in corneal abrasions and foreign bodies; fitting hard contact lenses; lacrimal patency; fundus photography; applanation tonometry—
Topical: Solution: instill 1 drop of 2% solution followed by irrigation, or moisten strip with sterile water. Touch conjunctiva or fornix with moistened tip. Flush eye with irrigating solution. Patient should blink several times after application.
Indicated in retinal angiography—
Adults: 5 ml of 10% solution (500 mg) or 3 ml of 25% solution (750 mg) in-

jected rapidly into antecubital vein, by doctor.
Children: 0.077 ml of 10% solution (7.7 mg/kg body weight) or 0.044 ml of 25% solution (11 mg/kg body weight) injected rapidly into antecubital vein, by doctor.

SIDE EFFECTS
Topical use:
Eye: stinging, burning.
Intravenous use:
CNS: headache persisting for 24 to 36 hours.
GI: nausea, vomiting.
GU: bright yellow urine (persists for 24 to 36 hours).
Skin: yellow skin discoloration (fades in 6 to 12 hours).
Local: extravasation at injection site, thrombophlebitis.
Other: hypersensitivity, including urticaria and *anaphylaxis.*

INTERACTIONS
None significant.

NURSING CONSIDERATIONS
• Use with caution in patients with history of allergy or bronchial asthma.
• Use topical anesthetic before instilling to partially relieve burning and irritation.
• Always use aseptic technique. Easily contaminated by *Pseudomonas.*
• Yellow skin discoloration may persist 6 to 12 hours.
• Warn patient urine will be bright yellow after I.V. injection.
• Routine urinalysis will be abnormal within 1 hour after I.V. injection.
• A water-soluble dye.
• Don't freeze; store below 80° F. (26.7° C.).
• Defects appear green under normal light, or bright yellow under cobalt blue illumination. Foreign bodies are surrounded by a green ring. Similar lesions of the conjunctiva are delineated in orange-yellow.
• Always keep an emergency tray with

antihistamine, epinephrine, and oxygen available when giving parenterally.

glycerin, anhydrous
Ophthalgan

INDICATIONS & DOSAGE
Corneal edema before ophthalmoscopy or gonioscopy in acute glaucoma and bullous keratitis—
Adults and children: instill 1 to 2 drops glycerin, anhydrous after instilling a local anesthetic.

SIDE EFFECTS
Eye: pain if instilled without topical anesthetic.

INTERACTIONS
None significant.

NURSING CONSIDERATIONS
• Use topical tetracaine HCl or proparacaine HCl before instilling to prevent discomfort.
• Don't touch tip of dropper to eye, surrounding tissues, or tear-film; glycerin will absorb moisture.
• Used to temporarily restore corneal transparency when cornea is too edematous to permit diagnosis.
• Store in tightly closed container.

isosorbide
Ismotic

INDICATIONS & DOSAGE
Short-term reduction of intraocular pressure due to glaucoma—
Adults: Initially, 1.5 g/kg P.O. Usual dosage range is 1 to 3 g/kg.

SIDE EFFECTS
CNS: Vertigo, light-headedness, lethargy.
GI: gastric discomfort, diarrhea, anorexia.
Metabolic: hypernatremia, hyperosmolality.

INTERACTIONS
None significant.

NURSING CONSIDERATIONS
• Contraindicated in anuria due to severe renal disease, severe dehydration, frank or impending acute pulmonary edema, and hemorrhagic glaucoma.
• Repetitive doses should be used cautiously in patients with diseases associated with salt retention, such as congestive heart failure.
• Pour over cracked ice, and tell patient to sip the medication. This procedure improves palatability.
• Especially useful when a rapid reduction in intraocular pressure is desired.

sodium chloride, hypertonic
Adsorbonac Ophthalmic Solution, Hypersal Ophthalmic Solution, Methylcellulose Ophthalmic Solution, Muro Ointment, Murocoll, Sodium Chloride Ointment 5%

INDICATIONS & DOSAGE
Corneal edema (postoperative) after cataract extraction or corneal transplantation; also in trauma or bullous keratopathy—
Adults and children: instill 1 to 2 drops q 3 to 4 hours, or apply ointment at bedtime.

SIDE EFFECTS
Eye: slight stinging.
Other: hypersensitivity.

INTERACTIONS
None significant.

NURSING CONSIDERATIONS
• An osmotic agent used to reduce corneal edema when repeated instillation is indicated.
• May use few drops of sterile irrigation solution inside bottle cap to prevent caking on dropper bottle tip.

Italicized side effects are common or life-threatening.
*Liquid form contains alcohol.   **May contain tartrazine.

- Store in tightly closed container.
- Don't touch tip of dropper or tube to eye or surrounding tissue.
- Show patient how to instill.

timolol maleate
Timoptic Solution

INDICATIONS & DOSAGE
Chronic open-angle glaucoma, secondary glaucoma, aphakic glaucoma, ocular hypertension—
Adults: initially, instill 1 drop 0.25% solution in each eye b.i.d.; reduce to 1 drop daily for maintenance. If patient doesn't respond, instill 1 drop 0.5% solution in each eye b.i.d. If intraocular pressure is controlled, dosage may be reduced to 1 drop in each eye daily.

SIDE EFFECTS
CNS: headache, depression, fatigue.
CV: slight reduction in resting heart rate.
Eye: minor irritation. Long-term use may decrease corneal sensitivity.
GI: anorexia.
Other: apnea in infants, *evidence of beta blockade and systemic absorption (hypotension, bradycardia, syncope, exacerbation of asthma, and congestive heart failure).*

INTERACTIONS
Propranolol HCl, metoprolol tartrate, other oral beta-adrenergic blocking agents: increased ocular and systemic effect. Use together cautiously.
MAO inhibitors, other adrenergic-augmenting psychotropic drugs: hazardous increased effect. Use together cautiously.

NURSING CONSIDERATIONS
- Use cautiously in bronchial asthma, sinus bradycardia, second- and third-degree heart block, cardiogenic shock, right ventricular failure resulting from pulmonary hypertension, congestive heart failure, severe cardiac disease, and in infants with congenital glaucoma.
- Warn patient not to touch dropper to eye or surrounding tissue.
- Beta-adrenergic blocking agent in ophthalmic solution.
- Can be used safely in patients with glaucoma who wear conventional (PMMA) hard contact lenses.
- Show patient how to instill. Teach patient to lightly press lacrimal sac with finger after drug administration to decrease chance of systemic absorption.
- A systemic form of timolol is currently being investigated (trade name, Blocadren). May reduce the mortality associated with myocardial infarction.

81

Otics

acetic acid
benzocaine
boric acid
carbamide peroxide
chloramphenicol
colistin B sulfate
dexamethasone sodium
   phosphate
hydrocortisone
hydrocortisone acetate
methylprednisolone disodium
   phosphate
neomycin sulfate
oxytetracycline hydrochloride
polymyxin B sulfate
triethanolamine polypeptide
   oleate-condensate

MECHANISM OF ACTION
• Anti-infectives (acetic acid, boric acid, chloramphenicol, colistin B, neomycin, oxytetracycline, and polymyxin B) inhibit or destroy bacteria present in the ear canal.
• Corticosteroids (dexamethasone, hydrocortisone, and methylprednisolone) control inflammation, edema, and pruritus.
• The local anesthetic benzocaine produces analgesic effects.
• Ceruminolytics (carbamide peroxide and triethanolamine) emulsify and disperse accumulated cerumen.

COMBINATION PRODUCTS
ADRENOMYXIN♦♦: Each ml contains neomycin SO$_4$ 5 mg, polymyxin B SO$_4$ 10,000 units, and hydrocortisone 10 mg.
COLY-MYCIN S OTIC: Each ml contains neomycin SO$_4$ 5 mg, colistin SO$_4$ 3 mg, hydrocortisone acetate 10 mg, and thonzonium bromide 0.5%.
CORTISPORIN OTIC♦: Each ml contains neomycin SO$_4$ 5 mg, polymyxin B SO$_4$ 10,000 units, and hydrocortisone 1%.
LIDOSPORIN OTIC♦: Each ml contains polymyxin B SO$_4$ 10,000 units and lidocaine HCl 50 mg.
NEO-CORT-DOME OTIC: Each ml contains neomycin SO$_4$ 5 mg, acetic acid 2%, and hydrocortisone 1%.
NEOCORTEF♦♦: Each ml contains neomycin SO$_4$ 5 mg and hydrocortisone acetate 5 mg.
NEODECADRON♦♦: Each ml contains neomycin SO$_4$ 3.5 mg and dexamethasone phosphate 1 mg.
NEO-HYDRO: Neomycin sulfate 5 mg; polymixin B sulfate 2,000 I.V.; hydrocortisone O.1%; antipyrine 5%; dibucaine HCl 0.25%.
NEOMEDROL♦♦: Each ml contains neomycin SO$_4$ 5 mg and methylprednisolone acetate 2.5 mg.
NEOSPORIN♦♦: Each ml contains polymyxin B SO$_4$ 5,000 units, neomycin SO$_4$ 2.5 mg, and gramicidin 0.025 mg.
OTIZOL HC♦♦: Each ml contains neomycin SO$_4$ 0.5%, hydrocortisone 1%, and lidocaine HCl 3%.
OTOBIONE OTIC: Each ml contains neomycin SO$_4$ 5 mg, polymyxin B SO$_4$ 10,000 units, and hydrocortisone 1%.
PENTAMYCETIN HC♦♦: Each ml contains chloramphenicol 2 mg and hydrocortisone acetate 10 mg.
POLYSPORIN♦♦: Each ml contains polymyxin B SO$_4$ 10,000 units and gramicidin 0.25 mg.
PYOCIDIN-OTIC: Each ml contains po-

Italicized side effects are common or life-threatening.
∗Liquid form contains alcohol.   ∗∗May contain tartrazine.

lymyxin B sulfate 10,000 units and hydrocortisone 0.5%.
SOFRACORT♦♦: Each ml contains framycetin sulfate 5 mg, gramicidin 50 mcg, and dexamethasone 0.5 mg.
VOSOL HC♦: Each ml contains acetic acid 2% and hydrocortisone 1%.

acetic acid
Domeboro Otic♦, VoSol Otic♦

INDICATIONS & DOSAGE
External ear canal infection—
Adults and children: 4 to 6 drops into ear canal t.i.d. or q.i.d., or insert saturated wick for first 24 hours, then continue with instillations.
Prophylaxis of swimmer's ear—
Adults and children: 2 drops in each ear b.i.d.

SIDE EFFECTS
Ear: irritation or itching.
Skin: urticaria.
Other: overgrowth of nonsusceptible organisms.

INTERACTIONS
None significant.

NURSING CONSIDERATIONS
• Use cautiously in perforated eardrum.
• Has anti-infective, anti-inflammatory, and antipruritic effects.
• *Pseudomonas aeruginosa* particularly sensitive to drug.
• Reculture persistent drainage.

benzocaine
Americaine-Otic, Auralgan♦, Eardro, Myringacaine, Tympagesic

INDICATIONS & DOSAGE
Cerumen removal—
Adults and children: fill ear canal t.i.d. for 2 days.
Pain from otitis media—
Adults and children: fill ear canal

with solution and plug with cotton. May repeat q 1 to 2 hours, p.r.n.

SIDE EFFECTS
Ear: irritation or itching.
Skin: urticaria.
Other: edema.

INTERACTIONS
None significant.

NURSING CONSIDERATIONS
• Contraindicated in perforated eardrum.
• Local anesthetic effect only.
• Use with antibiotic to treat underlying cause of pain, because use alone may mask more serious condition.
• Tell patient to call doctor if pain lasts longer than 48 hours.
• Avoid touching ear with dropper. Do not rinse dropper.
• Irrigate ear gently to remove impacted cerumen.
• Keep container tightly closed and away from moisture.

boric acid
Ear-Dry, Swim-Ear, Swim 'n Clear

INDICATIONS & DOSAGE
External ear canal infection—
Adults and children: fill ear canal with solution and plug with cotton. Repeat t.i.d. or q.i.d.

SIDE EFFECTS
Ear: irritation or itching.
Skin: urticaria.
Other: overgrowth of nonsusceptible organisms.

INTERACTIONS
None significant.

NURSING CONSIDERATIONS
• Contraindicated in perforated eardrum or excoriated membranes in ear.
• Watch for signs of superinfection (continual pain, inflammation, fever).

- Weak bacteriostatic action; also fungistatic agent.
- If cotton plug used, always moisten with medication.
- Avoid touching ear with dropper.

carbamide peroxide
Benadyne Ear, Debrox♦

INDICATIONS & DOSAGE
Impacted cerumen—
Adults and children: 5 to 10 drops into ear canal b.i.d. for 3 to 4 days.

SIDE EFFECTS
None reported.

INTERACTIONS
None significant.

NURSING CONSIDERATIONS
- Contraindicated in perforated eardrum.
- Tell patient to call doctor if redness, pain, or swelling persists.
- Irrigation of ear may be necessary to aid in removal of cerumen.
- Tip of dropper should not touch ear or ear canal.

chloramphenicol
Chloromycetin Otic♦,
Sopamycetin♦♦

INDICATIONS & DOSAGE
External ear canal infection—
Adults and children: 2 to 3 drops into ear canal t.i.d. or q.i.d.

SIDE EFFECTS
Ear: itching or burning.
Local: pruritus, burning, urticaria, vesicular or maculopapular dermatitis.
Systemic: *sore throat, angioedema.*
Other: overgrowth of nonsusceptible organisms.

INTERACTIONS
None significant.

NURSING CONSIDERATIONS
- Avoid prolonged use.
- Obtain history of use and reaction to drug.
- Watch for signs of superinfection (continued pain, inflammation, fever).
- Reculture persistent drainage.
- Watch for signs of sore throat (early sign of toxicity).
- Avoid touching ear with dropper.

colistin B sulfate
available only in combination with neomycin and hydrocortisone (Coly-Mycin-S-Otic♦)

INDICATIONS & DOSAGE
External ear canal infection and otitis media—
Adults and children: 3 to 5 drops into ear canal t.i.d. or q.i.d.

SIDE EFFECTS
Ear: *ototoxicity* in patient with a perforated eardrum and in patient undergoing tympanoplasty; irritation, itching.
Other: overgrowth of nonsusceptible organisms.

INTERACTIONS
None significant.

NURSING CONSIDERATIONS
- Watch for signs of superinfection (continued pain, inflammation, fever).
- Reculture persistent drainage.
- Observe for signs of hearing loss.
- Avoid prolonged use.
- Shake well before using.
- Avoid touching ear with dropper.

dexamethasone sodium phosphate
Decadron♦

INDICATIONS & DOSAGE
Inflammation of external ear canal—
Adults and children: 1 to 2 drops into ear canal t.i.d. or q.i.d.

Italicized side effects are common or life-threatening.
♦Liquid form contains alcohol.   ♦♦May contain tartrazine.

SIDE EFFECTS
Systemic: adrenal suppression with long-term use.
Other: masking or exacerbation of underlying infection.

INTERACTIONS
None significant.

NURSING CONSIDERATIONS
• Contraindicated in perforated eardrum, fungal infections, herpes or other viral infections.
• Use with antibiotic to treat inflammation caused by infection.
• Use alone in allergic otitis externa.
• Anti-inflammatory agent.
• Avoid touching ear with dropper.

hydrocortisone

hydrocortisone acetate
Cortamed♦♦, Otall

INDICATIONS & DOSAGE
Inflammation of external ear canal—
Adults and children: 3 to 5 drops into ear canal t.i.d. or q.i.d.
Available in 0.25%, 0.5%, and 1% concentrations.

SIDE EFFECTS
Systemic: adrenal suppression with long-term use.
Other: may mask or exacerbate underlying infection.

INTERACTIONS
None reported.

NURSING CONSIDERATIONS
• Contraindicated in perforated eardrum, fungal infections, herpes or other viral infections.
• Use with antibiotic to treat inflammation caused by infection.
• Use alone in allergic otitis externa.
• Avoid touching ear with dropper.

methylprednisolone disodium phosphate
Medrol♦♦

INDICATIONS & DOSAGE
Inflammation of external ear canal—
Adults and children: 2 to 3 drops into ear canal t.i.d. or q.i.d.

SIDE EFFECTS
Systemic: adrenal suppression with long-term use.
Other: may mask or exacerbate underlying infection.

INTERACTIONS
None significant.

NURSING CONSIDERATIONS
• Contraindicated in perforated eardrum, fungal infection, herpes or other viral infections.
• Use with antibiotic to treat inflammation caused by infection.
• Use alone to treat seborrheic, contact, or uninfected eczematoid dermatitis.
• Avoid touching ear with dropper.

neomycin sulfate
Otobiotic

INDICATIONS & DOSAGE
External ear canal infection—
Adults and children: 2 to 5 drops into ear canal t.i.d. or q.i.d.

SIDE EFFECTS
Ear: ototoxicity (in patients undergoing tympanoplasty).
Local: burning, erythema, vesicular dermatitis, urticaria.
Other: overgrowth of nonsusceptible organisms.

INTERACTIONS
None significant.

NURSING CONSIDERATIONS
- Contraindicated in perforated eardrum.
- Obtain history of use and reaction to neomycin.
- Observe for signs of hearing loss.
- Watch for signs of superinfection (continued pain, inflammation, fever).
- Reculture persistent drainage.
- Best used in combination with other antibiotics.
- Avoid touching ear with dropper.

---

oxytetracycline hydrochloride
available only in combination with polymyxin B sulfate (Terramycin with Polymyxin B) or polymyxin B sulfate and hydrocortisone (Terra-Cortril♦♦)

INDICATIONS & DOSAGE
External ear canal infection—
Adults and children: instill ½″of ointment into external ear canal t.i.d. or q.i.d.

SIDE EFFECTS
Ear: irritation, itching, urticaria.
Other: overgrowth of nonsusceptible organisms.

INTERACTIONS
None significant.

NURSING CONSIDERATIONS
- Obtain history of reaction to tetracyclines.
- Watch for signs of superinfection (continued pain, inflammation, fever).
- Reculture persistent drainage.

---

polymyxin B sulfate

INDICATIONS & DOSAGE
Acute and chronic otitis externa, otitis media if tympanic membrane perforated; otomycosis—
Adults and children: 3 to 4 drops t.i.d. or q.i.d.

SIDE EFFECTS
Ear: irritation, itching, urticaria.
Other: overgrowth of nonsusceptible organisms.

INTERACTIONS
None significant.

NURSING CONSIDERATIONS
- Watch for signs of superinfection (continued pain, inflammation, fever).
- Reculture persistent drainage.
- Best used in combination with other antibiotics.
- Keep container tightly closed and away from moisture.
- Avoid touching ear with dropper.
- The combination drug containing polymyxin B, Cortisporin, is available as either a solution or a suspension. The solution is preferred when a clear otoscopic view is required. However, the solution causes more stinging than the suspension.

---

triethanolamine polypeptide oleate-condensate
Cerumenex♦

INDICATIONS & DOSAGE
Impacted cerumen—
Adults and children: fill ear canal with solution and insert cotton plug. After 15 to 30 minutes, flush ear with warm water.

SIDE EFFECTS
Ear: erythema, pruritus.
Skin: severe eczema.

INTERACTIONS
None significant.

NURSING CONSIDERATIONS
- Contraindicated in perforated eardrum, otitis media, and allergies. Do

---

Italicized side effects are common or life-threatening.
*Liquid form contains alcohol.   **May contain tartrazine.

patch test by placing 1 drop of drug on inner forearm; cover with small bandage. Read in 24 hours. If any reaction (redness, swelling) occurs, don't use drug.
• Tell patient not to use drops more often than prescribed. Flush ear gently with warm water, using soft rubber bulb ear syringe, within 30 minutes after instillation.
• Moisten cotton plug with medication before insertion.
• Keep container tightly closed and away from moisture.
• Avoid touching ear with dropper.

82

Oral and nasal agents

beclomethasone dipropionate
benzocaine
carbamide peroxide
cocaine hydrochloride
dexamethasone sodium
  phosphate
ephedrine sulfate
epinephrine hydrochloride
flunisolide
lidocaine hydrochloride
naphazoline hydrochloride
oxymetazoline hydrochloride
phenylephrine hydrochloride
piperocaine hydrochloride
tetrahydrozoline hydrochloride
triamcinolone acetonide
xylometazoline hydrochloride

MECHANISM OF ACTION
• Carbamide peroxide serves as a
source of hydrogen peroxide to produce
nascent oxygen, which aids in cleaning
and debriding.
• Corticosteroids reduce inflammation
and help heal oral ulcers and lesions by
interfering with the protein synthesis of
various enzymes. The mechanism of
beclomethasone and flunisolide in the
treatment of asthma is unknown.
• Local anesthetics block nerve conduction through sensory nerve fibers.
• Sympathomimetic agents produce local vasoconstriction of dilated arterioles to reduce blood flow and nasal
congestion.

COMBINATION PRODUCTS
CHLOROHIST NASAL SPRAY: phenylephrine hydrochloride 0.25%, metha-
pyriline hydrochloride 0.15%, and benzalkonium chloride 0.02%.

4-WAY NASAL SPRAY: phenylephrine
hydrochloride 0.5%, naphazoline hydrochloride 0.05%, and pyrilamine
maleate 0.2%.
NAZOTOC NASAL SPRAY: phenylephrine hydrochloride 0.5%, pyrilamine
maleate 0.15%, and 0.04% cetalko-
nium chloride.
NEO-VADRIN NASAL DECONGESTANT
DROPS: phenylephrine hydrochloride
0.15% and phenylpropanolamine hydrochloride 0.4%, with chlorobutanol
0.15% and benzalkonium chloride
0.005%.
NTZ NASAL DROPS: phenylephrine hydrochloride 0.5% and thenyldiamine
hydrochloride 0.1%, with benzalkonium chloride 1:5,000.

---

beclomethasone dipropionate
Beconase Nasal Inhaler,
Vancenase Nasal Inhaler

INDICATIONS & DOSAGE
*Relief of symptoms of seasonal or peren-
nial rhinitis*—
**Adults and children 12 years or
older:** Usual dosage is one spray
(42 mcg) in each nostril 2 to 4 times
daily (total dosage 168 to 336 mcg
daily). Most patients require one spray
in each nostril t.i.d. (252 mcg daily).
Not recommended for children under
age 12.

SIDE EFFECTS
CNS: headache.
EENT: *mild transient nasal burning*

Italicized side effects are common or life-threatening.
∗Liquid form contains alcohol.   ∗∗May contain tartrazine.

and stinging, nasal congestion, sneezing, epistaxis, watery eyes.
GI: nausea and vomiting.
Other: development of local fungal infections.

INTERACTIONS
None reported

NURSING CONSIDERATIONS
• Use cautiously, if at all, in patients with active or quiescent respiratory tract tubercular infections, or in untreated fungal, bacterial, or systemic viral or ocular herpes simplex infections.
• Use cautiously in patients who have recently had nasal septal ulcers or nasal surgery or trauma.
• Recommended dosages will not suppress hypothalamic-pituitary-adrenal (HPA) function. Warn patient not to exceed this dosage.
• Indicated when conventional treatment (antihistamines, decongestants) fails.
• Beclomethasone is not effective for active exacerbations. Nasal decongestants or oral antihistamines may be needed instead.
• Advise patients to use drug regularly, as prescribed; its effectiveness depends on regular use.
• Explain that the therapeutic effects of this corticosteroid, unlike those of decongestants, are not immediate. Most patients achieve benefit within a few days, but some may need 2 to 3 weeks for maximum benefit.
• If symptoms don't improve within 3 weeks or if nasal irritation persists, patient should stop drug and notify doctor.

benzocaine
Colrex, Orabase with Benzocaine, Oracin, Ora-Jel, Spec-T Anesthetic, Trocaine, Tyzomint

INDICATIONS & DOSAGE
Pain from toothache, cold sore, canker sore, oral irritation, minor sore throat—
Adults and children: apply syrup or jelly to affected area, or suck lozenges.

SIDE EFFECTS
Skin: hypersensitivity.
Other: possible tolerance.

INTERACTIONS
None significant.

NURSING CONSIDERATIONS
• Contraindicated in infants under 1 year. Use cautiously in children under 6 years and in severe oral trauma or sepsis.
• Not intended for use in the presence of infection.
• Obtain history of reactions to local anesthetics.
• Watch for allergic reactions, such as reddening or swelling. If condition persists, drug should be stopped and doctor notified.
• Show patient how to apply.

carbamide peroxide
Cank-aid, Clear Drops, Gly-Oxide, Proxigel

INDICATIONS & DOSAGE
Canker sores, herpetic and other lesions, gingivitis, denture irritation, traumatic or surgical wounds—
Adults and children over 3 years: apply, undiluted, to oral mucosa q.i.d. or p.r.n., leave for several minutes, then expectorate. Don't rinse out mouth.

SIDE EFFECTS
None reported.

INTERACTIONS
None significant.

NURSING CONSIDERATIONS
• Use only as adjunct to regular professional care.
• Don't dilute. Gently massage affected area with medication. Show patient how to apply. Tell him not to drink or rinse his mouth for 5 minutes after use.
• Warn patient that drug foams in mouth when mixed with saliva.
• Use after meals and at bedtime for best results.
• If severe or persistent inflammation continues, patient should notify doctor or dentist.
• Provides chemomechanical cleansing, debriding action, and has nonselective microbial activity.
• An oxygenating agent.
• Store in cool place.
• Only one person should use dropper bottle or tube.

cocaine hydrochloride
Controlled Substance Schedule II

INDICATIONS & DOSAGE
Adults and children:
Acute rhinosinusitis—use 1% solution with nasal pack.
Diagnostic nasal examination— apply 4% solution to nasal mucosa.
Local anesthesia of nose or throat—apply 5% to 10% solution to oral and nasal mucosa.

SIDE EFFECTS
CNS: nervousness, excitation, vasomotor collapse.

INTERACTIONS
None significant.

NURSING CONSIDERATIONS
• Store under lock and key with other controlled drugs.
• Patient should be given a short-

acting barbiturate before giving cocaine HCl to prevent excess CNS stimulation or vasomotor collapse.
• Nasal surgery performed with cocaine HCl anesthetic may cause a delayed capillary hemorrhage resulting from capillary dilation. Watch for postoperative nasal bleeding when effect of cocaine wears off.
• Obtain history of reactions to local anesthetics.

dexamethasone sodium phosphate
Decadron Phosphate♦, Decadron Phosphate Respihaler, Turbinaire

INDICATIONS & DOSAGE
Allergic or inflammatory conditions, nasal polyps—
Adults: 2 sprays in each nostril b.i.d. or t.i.d. Maximum 12 sprays daily.
Children 6 to 12 years: 1 or 2 sprays in each nostril b.i.d. Maximum 8 sprays daily.
Each spray delivers 0.1 mg dexamethasone sodium phosphate equal to 0.084 mg dexamethasone.

SIDE EFFECTS
EENT: nasal irritation, dryness, rebound nasal congestion.
Other: hypersensitivity, systemic side effects with prolonged use (pituitary-adrenal suppression, sodium retention, congestive heart failure, hypertension, hypokalemia, headaches, convulsions, peptic ulcer, ecchymoses, petechiae, masking of secondary infection).

INTERACTIONS
None significant.

NURSING CONSIDERATIONS
• Contraindicated in cutaneous tuberculosis, fungal and herpetic lesions. Use cautiously in diabetes mellitus, peptic ulcer, tuberculosis, as systemic absorption can activate disease.

• Mothers should not breast-feed, as systemic absorption can occur.
• Control underlying bacterial infection with anti-infectives.
• Irritation or sensitivity may require stopping drug.
• Don't break, incinerate, or store in extreme heat; contents under pressure.
• Gradually reduce dose as nasal condition improves.
• Fluid retention can occur as a result of systemic absorption.
• Show patient how to apply. Only one person should use nasal spray.
• Hypertension and hypokalemia can occur with systemic absorption. Monitor blood pressure, serum potassium frequently.
• Should not be used for prolonged periods.

ephedrine sulfate
Ephedsol-1%, Isofedrol, Nasdro

INDICATIONS & DOSAGE
Nasal congestion—
Adults and children: apply 3 to 4 drops 0.5% to 3% solution to nasal mucosa. Use no more frequently than q 4 hours.

SIDE EFFECTS
CNS: nervousness, excitation.
CV: *tachycardia.*
EENT: rebound nasal congestion with long-term or excessive use.
Local: mucosal irritation.

INTERACTIONS
MAO inhibitors: hypertensive crisis if ephedrine is absorbed. Don't use together.

NURSING CONSIDERATIONS
• Use cautiously in hyperthyroidism, coronary artery disease, hypertension, or diabetes mellitus, as systemic absorption can occur.
• Tell patient not to exceed recommended dose. Use only when needed.

• Show patient how to apply. Only one person should use dropper bottle or nasal spray.

epinephrine hydrochloride
Adrenalin Chloride

INDICATIONS & DOSAGE
Nasal congestion, local superficial bleeding—
Adults and children: apply 0.1% solution to oral or nasal mucosa.

SIDE EFFECTS
CNS: nervousness, excitation.
CV: *tachycardia.*
EENT: rebound nasal congestion, slight sting upon application.

INTERACTIONS
None significant.

NURSING CONSIDERATIONS
• Use cautiously in hyperthyroidism, coronary artery disease, hypertension, or diabetes mellitus, as systemic absorption can occur.
• Tell patient not to exceed recommended dose. Use only when needed.
• Show patient how to apply. Only one person should use dropper bottle or nasal spray.

flunisolide
Nasalide Nasal Solution

INDICATIONS & DOSAGE
Relief of symptoms of seasonal or perennial rhinitis—
Adults: Starting dose is 2 sprays (50 mcg) in each nostril b.i.d. Total daily dose is 200 mcg. If necessary, dose may be increased to 2 sprays in each nostril t.i.d. Maximum total daily dosage is 8 sprays in each nostril (400 mcg daily).
Children 6 to 14 years: Starting dose is 1 spray (25 mcg) in each nostril t.i.d. or 2 sprays (50 mcg) in each nostril

b.i.d. Total daily dose is 150 to 200 mcg. Maximum total daily dose is 4 sprays in each nostril (200 mcg daily).
Not recommended for children under age 6.

SIDE EFFECTS
CNS: headache.
EENT: *mild, transient nasal burning and stinging,* nasal congestion, sneezing, epistaxis, watery eyes.
GI: nausea, vomiting.
Other: development of local fungal infections.

INTERACTIONS
None reported

NURSING CONSIDERATIONS
• Use cautiously, if at all, in patients with active or quiescent respiratory tract tubercular infections or in untreated fungal, bacterial, or systemic viral, or ocular herpes simplex infections.
• Use cautiously in patients who have recently had nasal septal ulcers or nasal surgery or trauma.
• Recommended dosages will not suppress hypothalamic-pituitary-adrenal (HPA) function. Warn patient not to exceed this dosage.
• Indicated when conventional treatment (antihistamines, decongestants) fails.
• Flunisolide is not effective for acute exacerbations. Nasal decongestants or oral antihistamines may be needed instead.
• Advise patient to use drug regularly, as prescribed; its effectiveness depends on regular use.
• Explain that the therapeutic effects of this corticosteroid, unlike those of decongestants, are not immediate. Most patients achieve benefit within a few days, but some may need 2 to 3 weeks for maximum benefit.
• Patients with dryness and crusting of the nasal mucosa may prefer the liquid

spray of flunisolide to the aerosolized powder of beclomethasone.
• If symptoms don't improve within 3 weeks or if nasal irritation persists, patient should stop drug and notify doctor.

lidocaine hydrochloride
Xylocaine♦, Xylocaine Viscous♦

INDICATIONS & DOSAGE
Local anesthesia, pain from dental extractions, stomatitis—
Adults and children: apply 2% to 5% solution, ointment, or 15 ml of Xylocaine Viscous q 3 to 4 hours to oral or nasal mucosa.

SIDE EFFECTS
EENT: interference with pharyngeal stage of swallowing.
Other: hypersensitivity (CNS symptoms are excitatory or depressant; CV symptoms are depressant); systemic absorption when used repeatedly.

INTERACTIONS
None significant.

NURSING CONSIDERATIONS
• Use cautiously in cardiac disease, hyperthyroidism, or severe oral or nasal trauma or sepsis, as systemic absorption can occur.
• Chronic, prolonged use for oropharynx anesthesia can lead to systemic absorption and toxicity.
• Instruct patient how to use. Xylocaine Viscous should be swished around in mouth and can be swallowed. Warn patient to eat or drink cautiously within 60 minutes after oral application, to avoid food aspiration.
• Obtain history of reactions to local anesthetics.
• Taste can be improved by adding a drop of oil of peppermint.

---

naphazoline hydrochloride
Privine♦

INDICATIONS & DOSAGE
Nasal congestion—
Adults: apply 2 drops or sprays of 0.05% to 0.1% solution to nasal mucosa q 3 to 4 hours.
Children 6 to 12 years: 1 to 2 drops or sprays of 0.05% solution. Repeat q 3 to 6 hours, p.r.n. Use no longer than 3 to 5 days.

SIDE EFFECTS
EENT: rebound nasal congestion with excessive or long-term use, sneezing, stinging, dryness of mucosa.
Other: systemic side effects in children after excessive or long-term use; marked sedation.

INTERACTIONS
None significant.

NURSING CONSIDERATIONS
• Contraindicated in glaucoma. Use cautiously in hyperthyroidism, heart disease, hypertension, or diabetes mellitus, as systemic absorption can occur.
• Warn patient not to exceed recommended dosage.
• Tell patient to notify doctor if nasal congestion persists after 5 days.
• Show patient how to apply. Hold container upright. Only one person should use dropper bottle or nasal spray.
• Do not shake container.

oxymetazoline hydrochloride
Afrin, Duration, Nafrine♦♦, St. Joseph's Decongestant for Children

INDICATIONS & DOSAGE
Nasal congestion—
Adults and children over 6 years: apply 2 to 4 drops or sprays 0.05% solution to nasal mucosa b.i.d.

Children 2 to 6 years: apply 2 to 3 drops 0.025% solution to nasal mucosa b.i.d. Use no longer than 3 to 5 days. Dosage for younger children has not been established.

SIDE EFFECTS
CNS: headache, drowsiness, dizziness, insomnia.
CV: palpitations.
EENT: rebound nasal congestion or irritation with excessive or long-term use, dryness of nose and throat, increased nasal discharge, stinging, sneezing.
Other: systemic side effects in children with excessive or long-term use; possible sedation.

INTERACTIONS
None significant.

NURSING CONSIDERATIONS
• Use cautiously in hyperthyroidism, cardiac disease, hypertension, or diabetes mellitus, as systemic absorption can occur.
• Tell patient not to exceed recommended dose. Use only when needed.
• Show patient how to apply. Have patient bend head forward and sniff spray briskly. Only one person should use dropper bottle or nasal spray.

phenylephrine hydrochloride
Alconefrin, Coricidin Nasal Mist, Coryzine, Ephrine, Neo-Synephrine♦♦, Sinarest Nasal Spray, Sinophen Intranasal, SuperAnahist Nasal Spray, Vacon

INDICATIONS & DOSAGE
Nasal congestion—
Adults: 2 to 3 drops or sprays 0.25% to 1% solution; apply jelly or spray to nasal mucosa.
Children 6 to 12 years: apply 2 to 3 drops or sprays of 0.25% solution.

Children under 6 years: apply 2 to 3 drops or sprays 0.125% solution. Drops, spray, or jelly can be given q 4 hours, p.r.n.

SIDE EFFECTS
CNS: headache, tremors, dizziness, nervousness.
CV: *palpitations, tachycardia,* premature ventricular contractions, hypertension, pallor.
EENT: transient burning, stinging; dryness of nasal mucosa; rebound nasal congestion may occur with continued use.
GI: nausea.

INTERACTIONS
None significant.

NURSING CONSIDERATIONS
• Contraindicated in narrow-angle glaucoma. Use cautiously in hyperthyroidism, hypertension, diabetes mellitus, or ischemic cardiac disease, as systemic absorption may occur.
• Tell patient not to exceed recommended dose. Use only when needed.
• Show patient how to apply: keep head erect to minimize swallowing of medication. Only one person should use dropper bottle or nasal spray.

piperocaine hydrochloride
Metycaine HCl

INDICATIONS & DOSAGE
Anesthetic in dental procedures—
Adults and children: apply 5% to 10% solution as a spray or 1% to 2% solution by infiltration to oral or nasal mucosa.
Local anesthetic in rhinolaryngologic examinations—
Adults and children: apply 2% solution as a spray to oral or nasal mucosa.

SIDE EFFECTS
EENT: interference with pharyngeal stage of swallowing.
Other: hypersensitivity.

INTERACTIONS
None significant.

NURSING CONSIDERATIONS
• Use cautiously in cardiac disease, hyperthyroidism, severe trauma, or sepsis of oral or nasal mucosa, as systemic absorption can occur.
• Obtain history of reaction to topical anesthetics.
• Warn patient not to eat or drink for 60 minutes after oral application, to prevent possible food aspiration.

tetrahydrozoline hydrochloride
Tyzine HCl, Tyzine Pediatric

INDICATIONS & DOSAGE
Nasal congestion—
Adults and children over 6 years: apply 2 to 4 drops 0.1% solution or spray to nasal mucosa q 4 to 6 hours, p.r.n.
Children 2 to 6 years: apply 2 to 3 drops 0.05% solution to nasal mucosa q 4 to 6 hours, p.r.n.

SIDE EFFECTS
EENT: transient burning, stinging; sneezing, rebound nasal congestion in excessive or long-term use.

INTERACTIONS
None significant.

NURSING CONSIDERATIONS
• Contraindicated in glaucoma. Use cautiously in hyperthyroidism, hypertension, diabetes mellitus.
• Don't use 0.1% solution in children under 6 years.
• Tell patient not to exceed recommended dose. Use only as needed.
• Show patient how to apply. Only one

Italicized side effects are common or life-threatening.
∗Liquid form contains alcohol.   ∗∗May contain tartrazine.

person should use dropper or nasal spray.

triamcinolone acetonide
Kenalog in Orabase

INDICATIONS & DOSAGE
Stomatitis; erosive lichen planus; traumatic oral lesions, including sore denture spots—
Adults and children: press ¼″ of 0.1% emollient dental paste onto affected area until thin film develops. Repeat b.i.d. or t.i.d. Don't rub in or protection of film will be lost.

SIDE EFFECTS
Systemic: with prolonged use, adrenal insufficiency, altered glucose metabolism, peptic ulcer activation.

INTERACTIONS
None significant.

NURSING CONSIDERATIONS
• Contraindicated in oral herpetic or viral lesions. Use cautiously in diabetes mellitus, peptic ulcer, or tuberculosis, as systemic absorption can occur.
• Apply after meals and at bedtime for best results.

xylometazoline hydrochloride
4-Way Long Acting, Neo-Synephrine II, Otrivin♦, Sine-Off Nasal Spray, Sinex-L.A.

INDICATIONS & DOSAGE
Nasal congestion—
Adults and children over 12 years: apply 2 to 3 drops or 2 sprays of 0.1% solution to nasal mucosa q 8 to 10 hours.
Children under 12 years: apply 2 to 3 drops or 1 spray of 0.05% solution to nasal mucosa q 8 to 10 hours.

SIDE EFFECTS
EENT: rebound nasal congestion or irritation with excessive or long-term use; transient burning, stinging; dryness or ulceration of nasal mucosa; sneezing.

INTERACTIONS
None significant.

NURSING CONSIDERATIONS
• Contraindicated in narrow-angle glaucoma. Use cautiously in hyperthyroidism, cardiac disease, hypertension, diabetes mellitus, and advanced arteriosclerosis, as systemic absorption can occur.
• Tell patient not to exceed recommended dose.
• Show patient how to apply. Only one person should use dropper bottle or nasal spray.

83

Local anti-infectives

acyclovir
amphotericin B
bacitracin
carbol-fuchsin solution
chloramphenicol
chlortetracycline hydrochloride
clotrimazole
erythromycin
gentamicin sulfate
gentian violet (methylrosaniline chloride)
haloprogin
iodochlorhydroxyquin
mafenide acetate
meclocycline sulfosalicylate
miconazole nitrate 2%
neomycin sulfate
nitrofurazone
nystatin
silver sulfadiazine
tetracycline hydrochloride
tolnaftate
undecylenic acid (zinc undecylenate)

MECHANISM OF ACTION

• Acyclovir inhibits herpes virus DNA synthesis by interfering with the action of viral DNA polymerase.
• Amphotericin B and nystatin act mainly by altering the permeability of the cell membrane; the other antifungals act primarily by removing diseased tissue (softening and dissolving the horny layer of the epidermis).
• Bacitracin acts by inhibiting cell-wall synthesis; the other antibiotics act primarily by disrupting protein synthesis of bacterial ribosomes.

COMBINATION PRODUCTS

AUREOCORT OINTMENT♦♦: triamcinolone acetonide 0.1% and chlortetracycline HCl 3%/15-g tube.
BACIMYCIN OINTMENT: zinc bacitracin 500 units and neomycin sulfate 5 mg/g.
BACIMIN OINTMENT: polymyxin B sulfate 5,000 units, neomycin sulfate 5 mg, and bacitracin 400 units/g.
BIOTRES OINTMENT: polymyxin B sulfate 10,000 units and zinc bacitracin 500 units/g.
CORDRAN-N CREAM, OINTMENT: flurandrenolide 0.05% and neomycin sulfate 0.5%.
CORTISPORIN CREAM: hydrocortisone acetate 0.5%, neomycin sulfate 0.5%, gramicidin 0.25 mg, and polymyxin B sulfate 10,000/g.
CORTISPORIN OINTMENT♦: hydrocortisone 1%, neomycin sulfate 0.5%, bacitracin zinc 400 units and polymyxin B sulfate 5,000 units/g.
MYCITRACIN OINTMENT: polymyxin B sulfate 5,000 units, bacitracin 500 units, and neomycin sulfate 5 mg/g.
MYCOLOG CREAM, OINTMENT: triamcinolone acetonide 0.1%, gramidicin 0.25 mg, nystatin 100,000 units, and neomycin sulfate 0.25%.
NEO-CORTEF CREAM: hydrocortisone acetate 1% and 2.5%, and neomycin sulfate 0.5%.
NEO-CORTEF LOTION: hydrocortisone acetate 1% and neomycin sulfate 0.5%.
NEO-CORTEF OINTMENT♦: hydrocortisone acetate 0.5% and neomycin sulfate 0.5%.
NEODECADRON CREAM: dexametha-

Italicized side effects are common or life-threatening.
*Liquid form contains alcohol. **May contain tartrazine.

sone phosphate 0.1% and neomycin sulfate 0.5%.

NEO-DELTA-CORTEF OINTMENT: prednisolone acetate 0.5% and neomycin sulfate 0.5%.

NEO-POLYCON OINTMENT: polymyxin B sulfate 5,000 units, neomycin sulfate 5 mg, and zinc bacitracin 400 units/g.

POLYSPORIN CREAM♦♦: polymyxin B sulfate 10,000 units and gramicidin 0.25 mg/g.

POLYSPORIN OINTMENT♦: polymyxin B sulfate 10,000 units and zinc bacitracin 500 units/g.

SOFRAMYCIN OINTMENT♦♦: framycetin sulfate 15 mg, gramidicin 50 mcg, and anhydrous lanolin 10%/g.

SPECTROCIN OINTMENT: neomycin sulfate 3.6 mg and gramidicin 0.25 mg/g.

STERISPRAY♦♦: neomycin sulfate 500 mg, polymyxin B sulfate 165,000 units, and zinc bacitracin 10,000 units/110-g container.

TERRAMYCIN WITH POLYMYXIN B SULFATE OINTMENT♦, POWDER: oxytetracycline HCl 30 mg and polymyxin B sulfate 10,000 units/g.

TRICILONE NNG CREAM: triamcinolone acetonide 0.1%, nystatin 100,000 units, neomycin sulfate 0.25%, and gramicidin 0.25 mg/g.

VALISONE-G CREAM♦♦, OINTMENT♦♦: bethamethasone valerate NF 1.22 mg and gentamicin sulfate 1.67 mg/g.

Antifungal combinations

CORTIN CREAM: iodochlorhydroxyquin 3% and hydrocortisone 0.5% or 1%.

DRENIFORM CREAM♦♦: iodochlorhydroxyquin 3% and flurandrenolide 0.0125%/20-g tube.

HYSONE OINTMENT: iodochlorhydroxyquin 3% and hydrocortisone 1%.

IODOCORT CREAM♦: iodochlorhydroxyquin 3% and hydrocortisone 1%.

KOMED LOTION: sodium thiosulfate 8%, salicylic acid 2%, and isopropyl alcohol 25%/g.

LOCACORTEN-VIOFORM CREAM♦♦, OINTMENT♦♦: iodochlorhydroxy-

quin 3% and flumethasone pivalate 0.02%/g.

MYCOLOG CREAM, OINTMENT: gramicidin 0.25 mg, neomycin sulfate 0.25%, triamcinolone acetonide 0.1%, and nystatin 100,000 units/g.

NEO-POLYCIN HC OINTMENT♦♦: neomycin sulfate 3.5 mg, polymyxin B sulfate 5,000 units, zinc bacitracin 400 units, and hydrocortisone acetate 10 mg/g.

NEOSPORIN CREAM♦♦: polymyxin B sulfate 10,000 units, neomycin sulfate 5 mg, and gramicidin 0.25 mg/g.

NEOSPORIN OINTMENT♦: polymyxin B sulfate 5,000 units, zinc bacitracin 400 units, and neomycin sulfate 5 mg/g.

NEOSPORIN-G CREAM: polymyxin B sulfate 10,000 units, neomycin sulfate 5 mg, and gramicidin 0.25 mg/g.

NEO-SYNALAR CREAM♦: fluocinolone acetonide 0.025% and neomycin sulfate 0.5%.

NYSTAFORM OINTMENT♦: nystatin 100,000 units/g and iodochlorhydroxyquin 1%.

NYSTAFORM-HC CREME♦♦, LOTION♦♦, OINTMENT♦: nystatin 100,000 units per g, iodochlorhydroxyquin 3% and hydrocortisone alcohol, 5% or 1%.

P.B.N. OINTMENT: polymyxin B sulfate 5,000 units, neomycin sulfate 5 mg, and bacitracin 400 units/g.

RACET CREAM: iodochlorhydroxyquin 3% and hydrocortisone 0.5%.

TINVER LOTION♦: sodium thiosulfate 25%, salicylic acid 1%, and isopropyl alcohol 10%.

VIOFORM-HYDROCORTISONE CREAM♦, LOTION, OINTMENT♦: iodochlorhydroxyquin 3% and hydrocortisone 1%.

VIOFORM-HYDROCORTISONE MILD CREAM♦, OINTMENT♦: iodochlorhydroxyquin 3% and hydrocortisone 0.5%.

WHITFIELD'S OINTMENT: benzoic acid 12% and salicylic acid 6%.

Unmarked trade names available in the United States only.
♦ Also available in Canada.   ♦♦ Available in Canada only.

acyclovir
Zovirax

INDICATIONS & DOSAGE
Initial herpes genitalis; limited, non–life-threatening mucocutaneous herpes simplex virus infections in immunocompromised patients—
Adults and children: Apply sufficient quantity to adequately cover all lesions every 3 hours 6 times a day for 7 days.

SIDE EFFECTS
Skin: transient burning and stinging, rash, pruritus.

INTERACTIONS
None reported.

NURSING CONSIDERATIONS
• For cutaneous use only. Don't apply to the eye.
• Although the dose size for each application will vary depending upon the total lesion area, use approximately a ½" ribbon of ointment on each 4 sq in of surface area.
• Ointment must thoroughly cover all lesions.
• Apply with a finger cot or rubber glove to prevent autoinoculation of other body sites and transmission of infection to other persons.
• Therapy should be initiated as early as possible following onset of signs and symptoms of herpes.
• Most studies show that acyclovir is not effective when used to treat *recurrent* genital herpes.
• The intravenous dosage form, used for the treatment of life-threatening systemic herpes infections, will soon be available.

amphotericin B
Fungizone Cream, Lotion, Ointment
(3% amphotericin B)

INDICATIONS & DOSAGE
Cutaneous or mucocutaneous candidal infections—
Adults and children: apply liberally b.i.d., t.i.d., or q.i.d. for 1 to 3 weeks; up to several months for interdigital lesions, paronychias, and onychomycosis (where relapses are frequent).

SIDE EFFECTS
Skin: possible drying, contact sensitivity, erythema, burning, pruritus.

INTERACTIONS
None significant.

NURSING CONSIDERATIONS
• Cream or lotion preferred for such areas as folds of groin, armpit, and neck creases.
• Cream discolors skin slightly when rubbed in; lotion or ointment doesn't. Lotion may stain nail lesions.
• Watch for and report signs of local irritation.
• Avoid occlusive dressings and ointments.
• Store at room temperature; avoid freezing.
• Well tolerated, even by infants, for long periods.
• A fungistatic agent.
• Tell patient to continue using medication for full time prescribed even though condition has improved.

bacitracin
Baciguent♦, Bacitin♦♦

INDICATIONS & DOSAGE
Topical infections, impetigo, abrasions, cuts, minor wounds, seborrheic dermatitis, acne, contact dermatitis—
Adults and children: apply thin film

---

b.i.d. or t.i.d. or more often, depending on severity of condition.

SIDE EFFECTS
Skin: rashes and other allergic reactions; itching, burning, swelling of lips or face.
Other: *possible systemic side effects when used over large areas for prolonged periods: potentially nephrotoxic and ototoxic;* tightness in chest, hypotension.

INTERACTIONS
None significant.

NURSING CONSIDERATIONS
• Contraindicated for application in the external ear canal if the eardrum is perforated.
• If used on burns that cover more than 20% of body surface, and especially if patient suffers impaired renal function, apply only once daily.
• If no improvement or if condition worsens, stop using and notify doctor.
• Prolonged use may result in overgrowth of nonsusceptible organisms.
• Avoid excess application.
• A bacteriostatic agent.

carbol-fuchsin solution
Carfusin, Castaderm, Castellani's Paint

INDICATIONS & DOSAGE
Tinea, dermatophytosis, skin infections—
Adults and children: apply liberally 1 or 2 times daily.

SIDE EFFECTS
Blood: possibility of bone marrow hypoplasia with use over long periods or at frequent intervals.
Skin: *contact dermatitis.*

INTERACTIONS
None significant.

NURSING CONSIDERATIONS
• Do not use on large areas or on eroded skin.
• Do not continue use after 1 week if no improvement shown; consult doctor. Toxicities develop in long-term use.
• Poisonous; warn against swallowing.
• Clean and dry skin thoroughly before applying.
• A fungicidal and bactericidal agent.
• Instruct patient to continue using for full treatment period prescribed, even if condition has improved.
• Will stain clothing.

chloramphenicol
Chloromycetin♦
(1% chloramphenicol)

INDICATIONS & DOSAGE
Superficial skin infections caused by susceptible bacteria—
Adults and children: after thorough cleansing, apply t.i.d. or q.i.d.

SIDE EFFECTS
Skin: possible contact sensitivity; itching, burning, urticaria, angioneurotic edema in patients hypersensitive to any of the components.

INTERACTIONS
None significant.

NURSING CONSIDERATIONS
• If no improvement or if condition worsens, stop using and report to doctor.
• Prolonged use may result in overgrowth of nonsusceptible organisms.
• For all but very superficial infections, topical use of this drug should be supplemented by appropriate systemic medication.
• A bacteriostatic agent.
• Discontinue if signs of hypersensitivity develop.
• Tell patient to continue using for full treatment period prescribed, even if condition has improved.

chlortetracycline hydrochloride
Aureomycin 3%◆

INDICATIONS & DOSAGE
Superficial infections of the skin caused by susceptible bacteria—
Adults and children: rub into affected area b.i.d. or t.i.d.

SIDE EFFECTS
Skin: *rashes, dermatitis.*

INTERACTIONS
None significant.

NURSING CONSIDERATIONS
• Prolonged use may result in overgrowth of nonsusceptible organisms.
• If no improvement or if condition worsens, stop using and report to doctor.
• A bacteriostatic agent.

clotrimazole
Canesten◆◆, Gyne-Lotrimin, Lotrimin (1% clotrimazole)

INDICATIONS & DOSAGE
Superficial fungal infections (tinea pedis, tinea cruris, tinea versicolor, candidiasis, and tinea corporis)—
Adults and children: apply thinly and massage into affected and surrounding area, morning and evening, 1 to 8 weeks.
Candidal vulvovaginitis—
Adults: insert 1 applicatorful or 1 tablet intravaginally daily for 7 to 14 days at bedtime. Alternatively, insert 2 tablets once daily for 3 consecutive days.

SIDE EFFECTS
GU: *with vaginal use: mild vaginal burning, irritation.*
Skin: blistering, *erythema*, edema, pruritus, burning, stinging, peeling, urticaria, skin fissures, general irritation.

INTERACTIONS
None significant.

NURSING CONSIDERATIONS
• Not for ophthalmic use.
• Watch for and report irritation or sensitivity. Discontinue use.
• Improvement usually within a week; if none in 4 weeks, diagnosis should be reviewed.
• Shortened dosage schedule with tablets may be used when compliance is a problem.
• A fungicidal agent.
• Do not use occlusive dressings.

erythromycin
A/T/S, Eryderm, Staticin ◆

INDICATIONS & DOSAGE
Superficial skin infections due to susceptible organisms—
Adults and children: clean affected area; apply t.i.d. or q.i.d.

SIDE EFFECTS
Skin: sensitivity reactions.

INTERACTIONS
None significant.

NURSING CONSIDERATIONS
• Prolonged use may result in overgrowth of nonsusceptible organisms.
• If no improvement or if condition worsens, stop using and tell doctor.
• Usually a bacteriostatic agent, but in high concentrations or against highly susceptible organisms, may be bactericidal.

gentamicin sulfate
Garamycin◆

INDICATIONS & DOSAGE
Primary and secondary bacterial infections, superficial burns, skin ulcers, infected insect bites and stings, infected

---

Italicized side effects are common or life-threatening.
*Liquid form contains alcohol.   **May contain tartrazine.

lacerations and abrasions, wounds from minor surgery—
Adults and children over 1 year: rub in small amount gently t.i.d. or q.i.d., with or without gauze dressing.

SIDE EFFECTS
Skin: small percentage of minor skin irritation; possible photosensitivity.

INTERACTIONS
None significant.

NURSING CONSIDERATIONS
• If no improvement or if condition worsens, stop using and report to doctor.
• Avoid use on large skin lesions or over a wide area because of possible systemic toxic effects.
• Prolonged use may result in overgrowth of nonsusceptible organisms.
• May clear bacterial infections that have not responded to other antibacterial agents.
• Useful for treating patients who are sensitive to neomycin.
• Useful for infected skin cysts, preceded by incision and draining.
• Store in cool place.
• A bactericidal agent.
• Remove crusts before application of gentamicin in impetigo contagiosa.

gentian violet (methylrosaniline chloride)
Bismuth Violet Solution (1% and 2%), Crystal Violet

INDICATIONS & DOSAGE
Superficial infections of skin; lesions, except ulcerative lesions of face, particularly Candida albicans—
Adults and children: apply with swab b.i.d. or t.i.d. Keep affected area clean, dry, and exposed to air to prevent spread of infection.

SIDE EFFECTS
Skin: *permanent discoloration if ap-*

plied to granulation tissue; irritation or ulceration of mucous membranes.

INTERACTIONS
None significant.

NURSING CONSIDERATIONS
• Do not use on ulcerative lesions of the face.
• Apply carefully to avoid undue staining. Will stain skin and clothing.
• Fungistatic.
• When used in infant with oral candidiasis, turn infant face down after application to minimize amount swallowed.
• Do not use occlusive dressings.

haloprogin
Halotex♦

INDICATIONS & DOSAGE
Superficial fungal infections (tinea pedis, tinea cruris, tinea corporis, tinea manuum, and tinea versicolor)—
Adults and children: apply liberally b.i.d. for 2 to 3 weeks.

SIDE EFFECTS
Skin: burning sensation, irritation, vesicle formation, increased maceration, *pruritus or exacerbation of preexisting lesions.*

INTERACTIONS
None significant.

NURSING CONSIDERATIONS
• Diagnosis should be reconsidered if no improvement in 4 weeks.
• Fungistatic and fungicidal.
• Tell patient to continue using for full treatment period prescribed, even if condition has improved.

iodochlorhydroxyquin

Gentleline, Quinoform, Torofor, Vioform

INDICATIONS & DOSAGE

Inflamed skin conditions, including eczema, athlete's foot, other fungal infections; cutaneous or mucocutaneous mycotic infections caused by Candida species (Monilia)—

Adults and children: apply a thin layer b.i.d., t.i.d., q.i.d., or as directed. Continue for 1 week after clinical cure.

SIDE EFFECTS

Skin: *possible burning, itching, acneiform eruptions.*

INTERACTIONS

Systemic corticosteroids: possible increased absorption. Use together cautiously.

NURSING CONSIDERATIONS

• Contraindicated in hypersensitivity to iodine or iodine-containing preparations. Contraindicated in tuberculosis, vaccinia, and varicella.
• Note all side effects and precautions of each component in the combination antifungals.
• Presence in urine may cause false-positive result for phenylketonuria (PKU) or inaccurate thyroid function tests. Discontinue at least 1 month before thyroid function tests.
• Drug will stain fabric and hair.

mafenide acetate

Sulfamylon♦

INDICATIONS & DOSAGE

Adjunctive treatment of second- and third-degree burns—

Adults and children: apply 1/16″ daily or b.i.d. to cleansed, debrided wounds.

SIDE EFFECTS

Blood: eosinophilia.

Skin: pain, *burning sensation*, rash, itching, swelling, hives, blisters, erythema, facial edema.
Other: *metabolic acidosis.*

INTERACTIONS

None significant.

NURSING CONSIDERATIONS

• Use with caution in acute renal failure and in known hypersensitivity to mafenide.
• Closely monitor acid-base balance, especially in the presence of pulmonary and renal dysfunction.
• If acidosis occurs, discontinue use for 24 to 48 hours.
• Causes pain at application site. Check for pain and burning; if they occur, notify doctor. Severe and prolonged pain may indicate allergy. If other allergic reactions occur, treatment may have to be temporarily discontinued.
• Cleanse area before applying. Mafenide washes off with water.
• Accidental ingestion may cause diarrhea.
• Keep burn areas medicated at all times.
• Bathe patient daily, if possible.
• Safety of use during pregnancy has not yet been established.
• For burns, using reverse isolation technique with sterile gloves and instruments to apply cream prevents further wound contamination.
• Bacteriostatic against several gram-negative and gram-positive organisms.

meclocycline sulfosalicylate

Meclan

INDICATIONS & DOSAGE

Treatment of acne vulgaris—

Adults and adolescents: apply to affected area b.i.d. morning and evening.

Italicized side effects are common or life-threatening.
✦Liquid form contains alcohol.   ✦✦May contain tartrazine.

Less frequent application may be used depending on patient's response.

SIDE EFFECTS
Skin: *stinging and burning on application*, skin irritation, slight yellowing of treated skin (especially in patients with light complexions). Treated skin areas fluoresce under ultraviolet light.

INTERACTIONS
None significant.

NURSING CONSIDERATIONS
• Beneficial response will usually be seen within 2 weeks of start of treatment.
• If condition doesn't improve or worsens, medication should be discontinued and therapy reevaluated.
• Prolonged use may result in overgrowth of nonsusceptible organisms.
• Patient may continue use of cosmetics.
• Yellow-skin staining is generally worse when excessive amounts are applied.
• To minimize fluorescence under black lights in discotheques, medication should be removed from the skin by washing and reapplied at bedtime.

miconazole nitrate 2%
Monistat-Derm Cream and Lotion,
Monistat 7 Vaginal Suppository,
Monistat 7 Vaginal Cream

INDICATIONS & DOSAGE
Tinea pedis, tinea cruris, tinea corporis, cutaneous candidiasis (moniliasis), infections from common dermatophytes—
Adults and children: apply sparingly b.i.d. for 2 to 4 weeks.
Vulvovaginal candidiasis—
Adults: insert 1 full applicator or suppository intravaginally for 7 days at bedtime.

SIDE EFFECTS
Skin: isolated reports of irritation, burning, maceration.

INTERACTIONS
None significant.

NURSING CONSIDERATIONS
• For external use only. Keep out of eyes.
• Discontinue if sensitivity or chemical irritation occurs.
• Fungistatic.
• Tell patient to continue using for full treatment period prescribed, even if condition has improved.
• Do not use occlusive dressings.
• When using intravaginal forms, tell patient to insert high into the vagina with applicator provided.

neomycin sulfate
Mycifradin♦♦, Myciguent♦,
Neocin♦♦

INDICATIONS & DOSAGE
Topical bacterial infections, burns, wounds, skin grafts, following surgical procedure, lesions, pruritus, trophic ulcerations, edema—
Adults and children: rub in small quantity gently b.i.d., t.i.d., or as directed.

SIDE EFFECTS
Skin: *rashes*, contact dermatitis, urticaria.
Other: *possible nephrotoxicity, ototoxicity, and neuromuscular blockade; possible systemic absorption when used on extensive areas of the body.*

INTERACTIONS
None significant.

NURSING CONSIDERATIONS
• If no improvement or if condition worsens, stop using and report to doctor.
• If used on more than 20% of the

body surface and on patient with impaired renal function, apply only once daily.
• Prolonged use may result in overgrowth of nonsusceptible organisms.
• In those combination products that contain corticosteroids, use of occlusive dressings increases corticosteroid absorption and the likelihood of systemic effects.
• Particularly well absorbed on denuded or abraded areas.
• A bactericidal agent.
• Watch for signs of hypersensitivity and contact dermatitis.
• Evaluate patient for signs of ototoxicity.

---

nitrofurazone
Furacin♦, Furazyme

INDICATIONS & DOSAGE
Adjunctive treatment of second- and third-degree burns (especially when resistance to other antibiotics and sulfonamides occurs); skin grafting—
Adults and children: apply directly to lesion daily or every few days, depending on severity of burn.

SIDE EFFECTS
GU: possible renal toxicity.
Skin: *erythema, pruritus,* burning, edema, severe reactions (vesiculation, denudation, ulceration).

INTERACTIONS
None significant.

NURSING CONSIDERATIONS
• Use cautiously in patients with known or suspected renal impairment. Monitor BUN regularly.
• If irritation, sensitization, or infection occurs, discontinue use.
• When using wet dressing, protect skin around wound with zinc oxide.
• Cleanse wound as indicated by doctor at each dressing change.
• Remove adherent dressings by flushing with solution of nitrofurazone and sterile water or sterile normal saline solution.
• Solution should be stored in tight, light-resistant containers (brown bottles). Avoid exposure of solution at all times to direct light, prolonged heat, and alkaline materials.
• Drug may discolor in light but is still usable because it retains its potency.
• Discard cloudy solutions if warming to 55° to 60° C. (131° to 140° F.) does not restore clarity.
• Use reverse isolation and/or sterile application technique to prevent further wound contamination.

---

nystatin
Mycostatin♦, Nadostine♦♦, Nilstat

INDICATIONS & DOSAGE
Infant eczema, pruritus ani and vulvae, superficial bacterial infections, localized forms of candidiasis—
Adults and children: apply and rub into area b.i.d. for 2 weeks.

SIDE EFFECTS
Skin: occasional contact dermatitis from preservatives present in some formulations.
Systemic: possible nephrotoxicity or ototoxicity with prolonged or frequent use.

INTERACTIONS
None significant.

NURSING CONSIDERATIONS
• Contraindicated in viral diseases of the skin (vaccinia and varicella), fungal lesions (except candidiasis), and markedly impaired circulation.
• Generally well tolerated by all age-groups, including debilitated infants.
• Preparation does not stain skin or mucous membranes.
• Cream recommended for intertriginous areas, powder for very moist areas, ointment for dry areas.

Italicized side effects are common or life-threatening.
*Liquid form contains alcohol.   **May contain tartrazine.

- Fungistatic and fungicidal.
- Tell patient to continue using for full treatment period prescribed, even if condition has improved.
- Do not use occlusive dressings.

silver sulfadiazine
Flamazine♦♦, Silvadene

INDICATIONS & DOSAGE
Prevention and treatment of wound infection for second- and third-degree burns—
Adults and children: apply ¹⁄₁₆″ thickness of ointment to cleansed and debrided burn wound, then apply daily or b.i.d.

SIDE EFFECTS
Blood: *neutropenia (in 3% to 5%).*
Skin: pain, burning, rashes, itching.
Other: fungal infections.

INTERACTIONS
Topical proteolytic enzymes: inactivity of enzymes when used together. Do not use together.

NURSING CONSIDERATIONS
- Contraindicated in premature and newborn infants during first month of life. (Drug may increase possibility of kernicterus.) Use with caution in hypersensitivity to sulfonamides.
- If hepatic or renal dysfunction occurs, consider discontinuing drug.
- Inspect patient's skin daily, and note any changes. Notify doctor if burning or excessive pain develops.
- Use only on affected areas. Keep medicated at all times.
- For patients with extensive burns, monitor serum sulfa concentrations and renal function, and check urine for sulfa crystals.
- Bathe patient daily, if possible.
- Discard darkened cream.
- Reverse isolation and/or sterile application technique recommended to prevent wound contamination.

tetracycline hydrochloride
Achromycin♦, Topicycline

INDICATIONS & DOSAGE
Superficial skin infections caused by susceptible bacteria, acne—
Adults and children: rub into cleansed affected area b.i.d. or t.i.d.
Acne—
Adults: apply Topicycline generously to affected areas b.i.d. until skin is thoroughly wet.

SIDE EFFECTS
Skin: dermatitis with Achromycin; with Topicycline, temporary stinging or burning on application, slight yellowing of treated skin, especially in patients with light complexions; severe dermatitis; treated skin areas fluoresce under ultraviolet light.

INTERACTIONS
None significant.

NURSING CONSIDERATIONS
- If no improvement or if condition worsens, stop using and notify doctor.
- Prolonged use may result in overgrowth of nonsusceptible organisms.
- Primarily a bacteriostatic agent.
- Patient may continue normal use of cosmetics.
- Store at room temperature, away from excessive heat.
- Medication to be used by one person only. Tell patient not to share with family members.
- Apply in morning and evening. Warn that drug should be used within 2 months.
- Explain that floating plug in bottle of Topicycline—an inert and harmless result of proper reconstitution of the preparation—shouldn't be removed.
- Serum levels of topical tetracycline HCl are much lower than those for orally administered drug, so systemic effects are unlikely.
- To control flow rate of solution, in-

crease or decrease pressure of the applicator against the skin.

tolnaftate
Aftate, Tinactin♦

INDICATIONS & DOSAGE
Superficial fungal infections of the skin, infections due to common pathogenic fungi, tinea pedis, tinea cruris, tinea corporis, tinea manuum, tinea versicolor—
Adults and children: ¼″ to ½″ ribbon of cream or 1 or 3 drops of lotion to cover area of one hand; same amount of cream or 2 to 3 drops of lotion to cover the toes and interdigital webs of one foot. Apply and massage gently into skin b.i.d. for 2 or 3 weeks, up to 6 weeks.

SIDE EFFECTS
None significant.

INTERACTIONS
None significant.

NURSING CONSIDERATIONS
• Discontinue if condition worsens. Check with doctor.
• Odorless, greaseless. Won't stain or discolor skin, hair, nails, or clothing.
• Only a small quantity of cream or lotion is needed; area should not be wet with solution when application is completed.

• Fungistatic and fungicidal.
• Commonly available product used to treat athlete's foot (tinea pedis).
• Tell patient to continue using for full treatment period prescribed, even if condition has improved.

undecylenic acid (zinc undecylenate)
Desenex, Ting, Unde-Jen

INDICATIONS & DOSAGE
Athlete's foot and ringworm of the body exclusive of nails and hairy areas—
Adults and children: clean thoroughly. Apply ointment liberally at night and powder during the day. Use regularly to prevent fungal infections.

SIDE EFFECTS
Skin: possible irritation in hypersensitive person.

INTERACTIONS
None significant.

NURSING CONSIDERATIONS
• Consult doctor before using on person with peripheral neuropathy and peripheral vascular diseases or diabetes.
• Tell patient to continue using for full treatment period prescribed, even if condition has improved.

84

Scabicides and pediculicides

benzyl benzoate lotion
copper oleate solution
　(with tetrahydronaphthalene)
crotamiton
gamma benzene hexachloride
　(or lindane)
malathion
pyrethrins
sulfa (6%) in petrolatum

MECHANISM OF ACTION
Gamma benzene hexachloride appears
to inhibit neuronal membrane function
in arthropods. Pyrethrins act as contact
poison that disrupt the parasite's nervous system, resulting in the paralysis
and death of the parasite. The mechanism of action of the other agents is unknown.

COMBINATION PRODUCTS
None.

benzyl benzoate lotion
Scabanca♦♦

INDICATIONS & DOSAGE
Parasitic infestation (scabies, Phthirus
pubis)—
Adults and children: first, scrub entire
body with soap and water. Then apply
the 25% lotion undiluted over entire
body, except the face, while still damp.
Be sure to apply around nails. Let dry.
Apply second coat on the most involved
areas. Bathe after 24 to 48 hours.
Adults require 30 ml. Children require
20 ml.
Pediculosis capitis—
Adults and children: apply to scalp
and leave on overnight; shampoo out in
morning. Repeat next night if necessary.

SIDE EFFECTS
Skin: *irritation, itching; contact dermatitis with repeated applications.*

INTERACTIONS
None significant.

NURSING CONSIDERATIONS
• Contraindicated when skin is raw or
inflamed. Notify doctor immediately if
skin irritation or hypersensitivity develops; tell patient to discontinue drug and
to wash it off skin.
• Do not apply to face, eyes, mucous
membranes, or urethral meatus. If accidental contact with eyes does occur,
flush with water and notify doctor.
• Instruct patient to change and sterilize (boil, launder, dry clean, or apply
very hot iron) all clothing and bed linen
after drug is washed off.
• Itching may continue for several
weeks; this does not indicate that therapy is ineffective. To prevent acaropho-
bia, reassure patient that itching will
cease.
• Tendency to overuse this drug. Estimate amount needed.
• Topical corticosteroids may be
needed if dermatitis develops from
scratching.
• Question other family members
about possible infestation.
• After application, use a fine comb
dipped in white vinegar on hair to remove nits.
• Instruct patient to reapply if washed

Unmarked trade names available in the United States only.
♦ Also available in Canada.　　♦ ♦ Available in Canada only.

off (hands, for example) during treatment time.

• Hospitalized patients should be placed in isolation with linen handling precautions until treatment is completed.

• Tendency for overuse of pediculicides. Estimate amount needed.

• Hospitalized patients should be placed in isolation with linen handling precautions until treatment is completed.

copper oleate solution (with tetrahydronaphthalene)
Cuprex

INDICATIONS & DOSAGE
Parasitic infestation (pediculoses capitis and pubis)—
Adults and children: first, scrub entire body with soap and water. Apply gently and sparingly 3 to 4 tablespoonfuls onto affected areas; after 15 minutes wash off with soap and water.

SIDE EFFECTS
Skin: *irritation with repeated use, or if used on raw or inflamed skin.*

INTERACTIONS
None significant.

NURSING CONSIDERATIONS
• Contraindicated when skin is raw or inflamed, or when there is a severe infection. Notify doctor immediately if skin irritation or hypersensitivity develops; tell patient to discontinue drug and to wash it off skin.
• Do not apply more than twice within 48 hours.
• Do not apply to face, eyes, mucous membranes, or urethral meatus. If accidental contact with eyes does occur, flush with water and notify doctor.
• Instruct patient to change and sterilize (boil, launder, dry clean, or apply very hot iron) all clothing and bed linen after application.
• After application, use a fine comb dipped in white vinegar on hair to remove nits.
• Question other family members about possible infestation.

crotamiton
Eurax♦

INDICATIONS & DOSAGE
*Parasitic infestation (scabies)—***Adults and children:** scrub entire body with soap and water. Then, apply a thin layer of cream over entire body, from chin down, with special attention to folds, creases, interdigital spaces, genital area. Apply second coat within 24 hours. Wait 48 hours, then wash off.
*General itching—*apply locally b.i.d. or t.i.d.

SIDE EFFECTS
Skin: *irritation with repeated use.*

INTERACTIONS
None significant.

NURSING CONSIDERATIONS
• Contraindicated when skin is raw or inflamed. Notify doctor immediately if skin irritation or hypersensitivity develops; tell patient to discontinue drug and to wash it off skin.
• Do not apply to face, eyes, mucous membranes, or urethral meatus. If accidental contact with eyes does occur, flush with water and notify doctor.
• Instruct patient to change and sterilize (boil, launder, dry clean, or apply very hot iron) all clothing and bed linen after drug is washed off.
• Topical corticosteroids may be needed if dermatitis develops from scratching.
• Tendency to overuse scabicides. Estimate amount needed.
• Question other family members about possible infestation.
• Instruct patient to reapply if washed

Italicized side effects are common or life-threatening.
*Liquid form contains alcohol. **May contain tartrazine.

off (hands, for example) during treatment time.

• Hospitalized patients should be placed in isolation with special linen handling precautions until treatment is completed.

---

gamma benzene hexachloride (or lindane)
GBH♦♦, Kwell, Kwellada♦♦, Scabine

INDICATIONS & DOSAGE
Parasitic infestation (scabies, pediculosis)—
Adults and children: scrub entire body with soap and water.
Cream or lotion—apply thin layer over entire skin surface (with special attention to folds, creases, interdigital spaces, genital area) for scabies, or to hairy areas for pediculosis. After 8 to 12 hours, wash off drug. If second application needed for scabies, wait 1 week before repeating. For pediculosis, may be repeated after 7 days but never more than twice in a week.
Shampoo—apply 30 to 60 ml onto affected area and work into lather for 4 to 5 minutes. Rinse thoroughly and rub with dry towel.

SIDE EFFECTS
Skin: *irritation with repeated use.*

INTERACTIONS
None significant.

NURSING CONSIDERATIONS
• Contraindicated when skin is raw or inflamed. Notify doctor immediately if skin irritation or hypersensitivity develops; tell patient to discontinue drug and to wash it off skin.
Use cautiously in infants and small children.
• Do not apply to open areas or acutely inflamed skin, or to face, eyes, mucous membranes, or urethral meatus. If accidental contact with eyes does occur, flush with water and notify doctor.

• Warn parents not to let infants or children suck their fingers after drug application.
• Discourage repeated use, which can lead to skin irritation and possible systemic toxicity.
• Warn patient itching may continue several weeks, especially in scabies.
• Topical corticosteroids may be needed if dermatitis develops from scratching.
• Instruct patient to change and sterilize (boil, launder, dry clean, or apply very hot iron) all clothing and bed linen after drug is washed off.
• After application, use a fine comb dipped in white vinegar on hair to remove nits.
• Gamma benzene hexachloride shampoo can be used to clean comb or brushes; wash them thoroughly afterward. Warn patient not to use gamma benzene hexachloride as routine shampoo.
• Question other family members about possible infestation.
• Tendency for overuse. Estimate amount needed.
• Instruct patient to reapply if washed off (hands, for example) during treatment time.
• Hospitalized patients should be placed in isolation with special linen handling precautions until treatment is completed.

---

malathion
Prioderm Lotion

INDICATIONS & DOSAGE
Treatment of head lice and their eggs—
Adults and children: Sprinkle lotion on the hair and rub gently until scalp is thoroughly moistened, then allow to dry. After 8 to 12 hours, shampoo, rinse, and use a fine-tooth comb to remove dead lice and eggs. If necessary, repeat application in 7 to 9 days.

SIDE EFFECTS
Skin: irritation of scalp, stinging.

INTERACTIONS
None reported.

NURSING CONSIDERATIONS
• Prioderm lotion is highly flammable. Warn patient to avoid open flames and hair dryers during treatment period. Hair should be allowed to dry naturally and uncovered.
• If accidentally splashed in the eye, flush immediately with water and notify doctor.
• Lotion contains 70% alcohol. May be irritating if pyodermal lesions exist on the scalp.
• Instruct patient to change and sterilize (boil, launder, dry clean, or apply very hot iron) all clothing and bed linen after drug is washed off.
• More than two treatments are generally not necessary. Other family members should be evaluated to determine if infested and, if so, receive treatment.

pyrethrins
A-200 Pyrinate, Barc, Pyrin-Aid, Pyrinyl, Rid, TISIT, Triple X

INDICATIONS & DOSAGE
Treatment of infestations of head, body, and pubic (crab) lice and their eggs—
Adults and Children: apply to hair, scalp, or other infested area until entirely wet. Allow to remain for 10 minutes, but no longer. Wash thoroughly with warm water and soap, or shampoo. Remove dead lice and eggs with fine-toothed comb. Treatment may be repeated, if necessary, but don't exceed 2 applications within 24 hours.

SIDE EFFECTS
Skin: *irritation with repeated use.*

INTERACTIONS
None significant.

NURSING CONSIDERATIONS
• Contraindicated when skin is raw or inflamed. Notify doctor immediately if skin irritation develops; tell patient to discontinue drug and to wash it off skin. Also contraindicated in patients allergic to ragweed. Use cautiously in infants and small children.
• Do not apply to open areas or acutely inflamed skin, or to face, eyes, mucous membranes, or urethral meatus. If accidental contact with eyes does occur, flush with water and notify doctor.
• Warn parents not to let infants or children suck their fingers after drug application.
• Discourage repeated use, which can lead to skin irritation and possible systemic toxicity.
• Topical corticosteroids may be needed if dermatitis develops from scratching.
• Instruct patient to change and sterilize (boil, launder, dry clean, or apply very hot iron) all clothing and bed linen after drug is washed off.
• Products containing pyrethrins are available without prescription. Some authorities believe pyrethrins and gamma benzene hexachloride (Kwell) are equally effective for lice infestation.

sulfa (6%) in petrolatum

INDICATIONS & DOSAGE
Parasitic infestation (scabies)—
Adults and children (preferred treatment for infants and pregnant women): after taking a soapy bath, patient should apply drug nightly for 2 to 3 nights consecutively. He should take soapy bath 24 hours after last application.

SIDE EFFECTS
Skin: *may produce dermatitis if applied continually for several days.*

INTERACTIONS
None significant.

Italicized side effects are common or life-threatening.
∗Liquid form contains alcohol.   ∗∗May contain tartrazine.

NURSING CONSIDERATIONS

• Instruct patient to change and sterilize (boil, launder, dry clean, or apply very hot iron) all clothing and bed linen after drug is washed off.

• Warn patient product has an odor, is messy, and stains clothing.

• Question other members of family about possible infestation.

• Tendency to overuse scabicides. Estimate amount needed.

• Hospitalized patients should be placed in isolation with special linen handling precautions until treatment is completed.

85

Topical corticosteroids

amcinonide
betamethasone
betamethasone benzoate
betamethasone dipropionate
betamethasone valerate
clocortolone pivalate
desonide
desoximetasone
dexamethasone
dexamethasone sodium
   phosphate
diflorasone diacetate
flumethasone pivalate
fluocinolone acetonide
fluocinonide
fluorometholone
flurandrenolide
halcinonide
hydrocortisone
hydrocortisone acetate
hydrocortisone valerate
methylprednisolone acetate
prednisolone
triamcinolone acetonide

MECHANISM OF ACTION
Exactly how these drugs work is unknown. Some investigators believe that corticosteroids attach to tissue receptors, decreasing membrane permeability and inhibiting release of toxins. They may also control the rate of protein synthesis. Their actions on the inflammatory process include inhibition of edema, fibrin deposition, capillary dilation, migration of leukocytes into the inflamed area, and phagocytic activity. They may also moderate later inflammatory developments such as capillary and fibroblast proliferation and deposition of collagen.

Corticosteroid-induced vasoconstriction decreases extravasation of blood, swelling, and itching. The drugs also act as antimitotics, reducing cell multiplication in psoriasis.

COMBINATION PRODUCTS
Corticosteroids for topical use are commonly combined with antibiotics, antifungals, and sulfonamides. (See also Chapter 14, SULFONAMIDES, and Chapter 70, ANTIBIOTIC ANTINEOPLASTIC AGENTS.)

---

amcinonide
Cyclocort♦

INDICATIONS & DOSAGE
Inflammation of corticosteroid-responsive dermatoses—
Adults and children: apply a light film to affected areas 2 or 3 times daily. Cream should be rubbed in gently and thoroughly until it disappears.

SIDE EFFECTS
Skin: burning, itching, irritation, dryness, folliculitis, hypopigmentation, striae, acneiform eruptions, perioral dermatitis, hypertrichosis, allergic contact dermatitis. *With occlusive dressings: secondary infection, maceration, atrophy, striae, miliaria.*

INTERACTIONS
None significant.

NURSING CONSIDERATIONS
• Use cautiously in viral diseases of skin, such as varicella, vaccinia, herpes

---

Italicized side effects are common or life-threatening.
∗Liquid form contains alcohol.　　∗∗May contain tartrazine.

simplex; fungal infections; skin tuberculosis; impaired circulation.
• Avoid application in or near eyes. Do not use on face, armpits, groin, or under breasts unless specifically ordered.
• Due to alcohol content of vehicle, gel preparations may cause mild, transient stinging without irritation if used on or near excoriated skin.
• Systemic absorption especially likely with occlusive dressings, prolonged treatment, or extensive body-surface treatment.
• Stop drug and notify doctor if patient develops signs of systemic absorption, skin irritation or ulceration, signs of hypersensitivity, infection. (If antifungals or antibiotics are being used with corticosteroids and infection does not respond immediately, corticosteroids should be stopped until infection is controlled.)
• Before applying, gently wash skin. To prevent damage to skin, rub in medication gently, leaving a thin coat. When treating hairy sites, part hair and apply directly to lesion. Apply lotions to scalp immediately after shampoo, while scalp is still damp.
• Occlusive dressing: apply cream heavily, then cover with a thin, pliable, nonflammable plastic film; seal to adjacent normal skin with hypoallergenic tape. Minimize adverse reactions by using occlusive dressing intermittently.
• For patient with eczematous dermatitis who may develop irritation with adhesive material, hold dressing in place with gauze, elastic bandages, stockings, or stockinette.
• Notify doctor and remove occlusive dressing if body temperature rises.
• Occlusive dressings are generally not used in presence of infections or with weeping or exudative lesions.
• Change dressings as ordered by doctor. Inspect skin for infection, striae, and atrophy. Discontinue drug and notify doctor if these occur.
• Treatment should be continued for a few days after clearing of lesions to prevent recurrence.
• Instruct patient to report signs of drug sensitivity.

---

betamethasone
Celestone♦

INDICATIONS & DOSAGE
Inflammation of corticosteroid-responsive dermatoses—
Adults and children: clean area; apply cream sparingly b.i.d. or t.i.d. Massage gently until it disappears. Apply thick layer with occlusive dressing to manage deep-seated dermatoses, such as neurodermatitis.

SIDE EFFECTS
Skin: burning, itching, irritation, dryness, folliculitis, hypopigmentation, acneiform eruptions, hypertrichosis, allergic contact dermatitis. *With occlusive dressings: secondary infection, maceration, skin atrophy, striae, miliaria.*

INTERACTIONS
None significant.

NURSING CONSIDERATIONS
• Use cautiously in viral diseases of skin, such as vaccinia, varicella, herpes simplex; fungal infections; skin tuberculosis; impaired circulation.
• Avoid application in or near eyes.
• Systemic absorption especially likely with occlusive dressings, prolonged treatment, or extensive body-surface treatment.
• Stop drug and notify doctor if patient develops signs of systemic absorption, skin irritation or ulceration, hypersensitivity, infection. (If antifungals or antibacterials are being used with corticosteroids and infection does not respond immediately, corticosteroids should be stopped until infection is controlled.)
• Before applying, gently wash skin. To prevent damage to skin, rub medication in gently, leaving a thin coat.

• Occlusive dressing: apply cream heavily, then cover with a thin, pliable, nonflammable plastic film; seal to adjacent normal skin with hypoallergenic tape. Minimize adverse reactions by using occlusive dressing intermittently.

• For patient with eczematous dermatitis who may develop irritation with adhesive material, hold dressing in place with gauze, elastic bandages, stockings, or stockinette.

• Notify doctor and remove occlusive dressing if body temperature rises.

• Occlusive dressings are generally not used in presence of infection or with weeping or exudative lesions.

• Change dressing as ordered by doctor. Inspect skin for infection, striae, and atrophy. Discontinue drug and notify doctor if these occur.

• Treatment should be continued for a few days after clearing of lesions to prevent recurrence.

• Instruct patient to report signs of drug sensitivity.

betamethasone benzoate
Beben♦, Benisone, Uticort

INDICATIONS & DOSAGE
Inflammation of corticosteroid-responsive dermatoses—
Adults and children: clean area; apply cream, lotion, or gel sparingly daily to q.i.d.

SIDE EFFECTS
Skin: burning, itching, irritation, dryness, folliculitis, hypopigmentation, striae, acneiform eruptions, perioral dermatitis, hypertrichosis, allergic contact dermatitis. *With occlusive dressings: secondary infection, maceration, atrophy, striae, miliaria.*

INTERACTIONS
None significant.

NURSING CONSIDERATIONS
• Use cautiously in viral diseases of skin, such as varicella, vaccinia, herpes simplex; fungal infections; skin tuberculosis; impaired circulation.

• Avoid application in or near eyes.

• Due to alcohol content of vehicle, gel preparations may cause mild, transient stinging without irritation if used on or near excoriated skin.

• Systemic absorption especially likely with occlusive dressings, prolonged treatment, or extensive body-surface treatment.

• Stop drug and notify doctor if patient develops signs of systemic absorption, skin irritation or ulceration, signs of hypersensitivity, infection. (If antifungals or antibiotics are being used with corticosteroids and infection does not respond immediately, corticosteroids should be stopped until infection is controlled.)

• Before applying, gently wash skin. To prevent damage to skin, rub in medication gently, leaving a thin coat. When treating hairy sites, part hair and apply directly to lesion.

• Occlusive dressing: apply cream heavily, then cover with a thin, pliable, nonflammable plastic film; seal to adjacent normal skin with hypoallergenic tape. Minimize adverse reactions by using occlusive dressing intermittently.

• For patient with eczematous dermatitis who may develop irritation with adhesive material, hold dressing in place with gauze, elastic bandages, stockings, or stockinette.

• Notify doctor and remove occlusive dressing if body temperature rises.

• Occlusive dressings are generally not used in presence of infections or with weeping or exudative lesions.

• Change dressings as ordered by doctor. Inspect skin for infection, striae, and atrophy. Discontinue drug and notify doctor if these occur.

• Treatment should be continued for a few days after clearing of lesions to prevent recurrence.

• Instruct patient to report signs of drug sensitivity.

Italicized side effects are common or life-threatening.
*Liquid form contains alcohol.   **May contain tartrazine.

betamethasone dipropionate
Diprosone◆

INDICATIONS & DOSAGE
Inflammation of corticosteroid-responsive dermatoses—
Adults and children: clean area; apply cream, lotion, or ointment sparingly b.i.d.
Aerosol: Direct spray onto affected area from a distance of 6″ for only 3 seconds t.i.d.

SIDE EFFECTS
Skin: burning, itching, irritation, dryness, folliculitis, hypopigmentation, perioral dermatitis, allergic contact dermatitis, hypertrichosis, acneiform eruptions. *With occlusive dressings: maceration of skin, secondary infection, atrophy, striae, miliaria.*

INTERACTIONS
None significant.

NURSING CONSIDERATIONS
• Use cautiously in viral diseases of skin, such as varicella, vaccinia, herpes simplex; fungal infections; skin tuberculosis; impaired circulation.
• Avoid application in or near eyes.
• Systemic absorption especially likely with occlusive dressings, prolonged treatment, or extensive body-surface treatment.
• Stop drug and notify doctor if patient develops signs of systemic absorption, skin irritation or ulceration, hypersensitivity, infection. (If antifungals or antibiotics are being used with corticosteroids and infection does not respond immediately, corticosteroids should be stopped until infection is controlled.)
• Before applying, gently wash skin. To prevent damage to skin, rub in medication gently, leaving a thin coat. When treating hairy sites, part hair and apply directly to lesion.
• Aerosol preparation contains alcohol and may produce irritation or burning in open lesions. When using about the face, cover patient's eyes and warn against inhalation of spray. To avoid freezing tissues, do not spray longer than 3 seconds or closer than 6″.
• For patient with eczematous dermatitis who may develop irritation with adhesive material, hold dressing in place with gauze, elastic bandages, stockings, or stockinette.
• Occlusive dressings are generally not used in presence of infection or with weeping or exudative lesions.
• Change dressing as ordered by doctor. Inspect skin for infection, striae, and atrophy. Discontinue drug and notify doctor if these occur.
• Instruct patient to report signs of drug sensitivity.

betamethasone valerate
Betnovate◆◆, Betnovate 1/2◆◆, Celestoderm-V◆◆, Celestoderm-V/2◆◆, Valisone

INDICATIONS & DOSAGE
Inflammation of corticosteroid-responsive dermatoses—
Adults and children: clean area; apply cream, lotion, ointment, or aerosol sparingly daily to q.i.d.
Aerosol: shake can well. Direct spray onto affected area from a distance of 6″. Apply for only 3 seconds t.i.d. to q.i.d.
Betnovate 1/2 and Celestoderm V/2 contain less betamethasone.

SIDE EFFECTS
Skin: burning, itching, irritation, dryness, folliculitis, hypopigmentation, hypertrichosis, acneiform eruptions, perioral dermatitis, allergic contact dermatitis. *With occlusive dressings: maceration of skin, secondary infection, atrophy, striae, miliaria.*

INTERACTIONS
None significant.

Unmarked trade names available in the United States only.
◆ Also available in Canada.   ◆◆ Available in Canada only.

NURSING CONSIDERATIONS

• Use cautiously in viral diseases of skin, such as varicella, vaccinia, herpes simplex; fungal infections; skin tuberculosis; impaired circulation.
• Avoid application in or near eyes.
• Systemic absorption especially likely with occlusive dressings, prolonged treatment, or extensive body-surface treatment.
• Stop drug and notify doctor if patient develops signs of systemic absorption, skin irritation or ulceration, hypersensitivity, infection. (If antifungals or antibiotics are being used with corticosteroids and infection does not respond immediately, corticosteroids should be stopped until infection is controlled.)
• Before applying, gently wash skin. To prevent damage to skin, rub in medication gently, leaving a thin coat. When treating hairy sites, part hair and apply directly to lesions.
• Aerosol preparation contains alcohol and may produce irritation or burning in open lesions. When using about the face, cover patient's eyes and warn against inhalation of the spray. To avoid freezing tissues, do not spray longer than 3 seconds or closer than 6″.
• Occlusive dressing: apply cream or ointment heavily, then cover with a thin, pliable, nonflammable plastic film; seal to adjacent normal skin with hypoallergenic tape. Minimize adverse reactions by using occlusive dressing intermittently.
• For patient with eczematous dermatitis who may develop irritation with adhesive material, hold dressing in place with gauze, elastic bandages, stockings, or stockinette.
• Notify doctor and remove occlusive dressing if body temperature rises.
• Occlusive dressings are generally not used in presence of infection or with weeping or exudative lesions.
• Change dressing as ordered by doctor. Inspect skin for infection, striae, and atrophy. Discontinue drug and notify doctor if these occur.

• Treatment should be continued for a few days after clearing of lesions to prevent recurrence.
• Instruct patient to report signs of drug sensitivity.

clocortolone pivalate
Cloderm

INDICATIONS & DOSAGE

Inflammation of corticosteroid-responsive dermatoses, such as atopic dermatitis, contact dermatitis, seborrheic dermatitis—
Adults and children: apply cream sparingly to affected areas t.i.d. and rub in gently.

SIDE EFFECTS

Skin: burning, itching, irritation, dryness, folliculitis, hypopigmentation, striae, acneiform eruptions, perioral dermatitis, hypertrichosis, allergic contact dermatitis. *With occlusive dressings: secondary infection, maceration, atrophy, striae, miliaria.*

INTERACTIONS
None significant.

NURSING CONSIDERATIONS

• Use cautiously in viral diseases of skin, such as varicella, vaccinia, herpes simplex; fungal infections; skin tuberculosis; impaired circulation.
• Avoid application in or near eyes.
• Systemic absorption especially likely with occlusive dressings, prolonged treatment, or extensive body-surface treatment.
• Stop drug and notify doctor if patient develops signs of systemic absorption or hypersensitivity, skin irritation or ulceration, or infection. (If antifungals or antibiotics are being used with corticosteroids and infection does not respond immediately, corticosteroids should be stopped until infection is controlled.)
• Before applying, gently wash skin. To prevent damage to skin, rub in medi-

---

Italicized side effects are common or life-threatening.
*Liquid form contains alcohol.   **May contain tartrazine.

cation gently, leaving a thin coat. When treating hairy sites, part hair and apply direct to lesion.

• Occlusive dressing: apply cream heavily, then cover with a thin, pliable, nonflammable plastic film; seal to adjacent normal skin with hypoallergenic tape. Minimize adverse reactions by using occlusive dressing intermittently.

• For patient with eczematous dermatitis who may develop irritation with adhesive material, hold dressing in place with gauze, elastic bandages, or stockings.

• Notify doctor and remove occlusive dressing if body temperature rises.

• Occlusive dressings are generally not used in presence of infections or with weeping or exudative lesions.

• Change dressings as ordered by doctor. Inspect skin for infection, striae, and atrophy. Discontinue drug and notify doctor if these occur.

• Treatment should be continued for a few days after clearing of lesions to prevent recurrence.

• Instruct patient to report signs of drug sensitivity.

desonide
Tridesilon♦

INDICATIONS & DOSAGE
Adjunctive therapy for inflammation in acute and chronic corticosteroid-responsive dermatoses—
Adults and children: clean area; apply cream, lotion, or gel sparingly b.i.d. to t.i.d.

SIDE EFFECTS
Skin: burning, itching, irritation, dryness, folliculitis, hypopigmentation, perioral dermatitis, allergic contact dermatitis, hypertrichosis, acneiform eruptions. *With occlusive dressings: maceration of skin, secondary infection, atrophy, striae, miliaria.*

INTERACTIONS
None significant.

NURSING CONSIDERATIONS
• Use cautiously in viral diseases of skin, such as varicella, vaccinia, herpes simplex; fungal infections; skin tuberculosis; impaired circulation.

• Avoid application in or near eyes.

• Systemic absorption especially likely with occlusive dressings, prolonged treatment, or extensive body-surface treatment.

• Stop drug and notify doctor if patient develops signs of systemic absorption, skin irritation or ulceration, hypersensitivity, infection. (If antifungals or antibiotics are being used with corticosteroids and infection does not respond immediately, corticosteroids should be stopped until infection is controlled.)

• Before applying, gently wash skin. To prevent damage to skin, rub in medication gently, leaving a thin coat. When treating hairy sites, part hair and apply directly to lesion.

• Occlusive dressing: apply cream or ointment heavily, then cover with a thin, pliable, nonflammable plastic film; seal to adjacent normal skin with hypoallergenic tape. Minimize adverse reactions by using occlusive dressing intermittently.

• For patient with eczematous dermatitis who may develop irritation with adhesive material, hold dressing in place with gauze, elastic bandages, stockings, or stockinette.

• Notify doctor and remove occlusive dressing if body temperature rises.

• Occlusive dressings are generally not used in presence of infection or with weeping or exudative lesions.

• Change dressing as ordered by doctor. Inspect skin for infection, striae, and atrophy. Discontinue drug and notify doctor if these occur.

• Treatment should be continued for a few days after clearing of lesions to prevent recurrence.

• Instruct patient to report signs of drug sensitivity.

desoximetasone
Topicort♦

INDICATIONS & DOSAGE
Inflammation of corticosteroid-responsive dermatoses—
Adults and children: clean area; apply cream sparingly b.i.d.

SIDE EFFECTS
Skin: burning, itching, irritation, dryness, folliculitis, hypopigmentation, hypertrichosis, acneiform eruptions, perioral dermatitis, allergic contact dermatitis. *With occlusive dressings: maceration of skin, secondary infection, atrophy, striae, miliaria.*

INTERACTIONS
None significant.

NURSING CONSIDERATIONS
• Use cautiously in viral diseases of skin, such as varicella, vaccinia, herpes simplex; fungal infections; skin tuberculosis; impaired circulation.
• Avoid application in or near eyes.
• Systemic absorption especially likely with occlusive dressings, prolonged treatment, or extensive body-surface treatment.
• Stop drug and notify doctor if patient develops signs of systemic absorption, skin irritation or ulceration, hypersensitivity, infection. (If antifungals or antibiotics are being used with corticosteroids and infection does not respond immediately, corticosteroids should be stopped until infection is controlled.)
• Before applying, gently wash skin. To prevent damage to skin, rub in medication gently, leaving a thin coat. When treating hairy sites, part hair and apply directly to lesions.
• Occlusive dressing: apply cream heavily, then cover with a thin, pliable, nonflammable plastic film; seal to adja-

cent normal skin with hypoallergenic tape. To minimize adverse reactions, use occlusive dressing intermittently.
• For patient with eczematous dermatitis who may develop irritation with adhesive material, hold dressing in place with gauze, elastic bandages, stockings, or stockinette.
• Notify doctor and remove occlusive dressing if body temperature rises.
• Occlusive dressings are generally not used in presence of infection or with weeping or exudative lesions.
• Change dressing as ordered by doctor. Inspect skin for infection, striae, and atrophy. Discontinue drug and notify doctor if these occur.
• Treatment should be continued for a few days after clearing of lesions to prevent recurrence.
• Instruct patient to report signs of drug sensitivity.

dexamethasone
Aeroseb-Dex, Decaderm, Decaspray, Hexadrol♦

INDICATIONS & DOSAGE
Inflammation of corticosteroid-responsive dermatoses—
Adults and children: clean area; apply cream, gel, or aerosol sparingly b.i.d. to q.i.d.
Aerosol use on scalp: shake can well and apply to dry scalp after shampooing. Hold can upright. Slide applicator tube under hair so that it touches scalp. Spray while moving tube to all affected areas, keeping tube under hair and in contact with scalp throughout spraying, which should take about 2 seconds. Inadequately covered areas may be spot sprayed. Slide applicator tube through hair to touch scalp, press and immediately release spray button. Don't massage medication into scalp or spray forehead or eyes.

SIDE EFFECTS
Skin: burning, itching, irritation, dry-

ness, folliculitis, hypopigmentation, hypertrichosis, acneiform eruptions, perioral dermatitis, allergic contact dermatitis. *With occlusive dressings: maceration of skin, secondary infection, atrophy, striae, miliaria.*

INTERACTIONS
None significant.

NURSING CONSIDERATIONS
• Use cautiously in viral diseases of skin, such as varicella, vaccinia, herpes simplex; fungal infections; skin tuberculosis; impaired circulation.
• Avoid application in or near eyes.
• Systemic absorption especially likely with occlusive dressings, prolonged treatment, or extensive body-surface treatment.
• Stop drug and notify doctor if patient develops signs of systemic absorption, skin irritation or ulceration, signs of hypersensitivity, infection. (If antifungals or antibiotics are being used with corticosteroids and infection does not respond immediately, corticosteroids should be stopped until infection is controlled.)
• Before applying, gently wash skin. To prevent damage to skin, rub in medication gently, leaving a thin coat. When treating hairy sites, part hair and apply directly to lesions.
• Occlusive dressing: apply cream heavily and cover with a thin, pliable, nonflammable plastic film; seal to adjacent normal skin with hypoallergenic tape. To minimize adverse reactions, use occlusive dressing intermittently.
• For patient with eczematous dermatitis who may develop irritation with adhesive material, hold dressing in place with gauze, elastic bandages, stockings, or stockinette.
• Notify doctor and remove occlusive dressing if body temperature rises.
• Change dressing as ordered by doctor. Inspect skin for infection, striae, and atrophy. Discontinue drug and notify doctor if these occur.

• Occlusive dressings are generally not used in presence of infection or with weeping or exudative lesions.
• Aerosol preparation contains alcohol and may produce irritation or burning in open lesions. When using about the face, cover patient's eyes and warn against inhalation of the spray. To avoid freezing tissues, do not spray longer than 3 seconds or closer than 6″.
• Treatment should be continued for a few days after clearing of lesions to prevent recurrence.
• Instruct patient to report signs of drug sensitivity.

---

dexamethasone sodium phosphate
Decadron Phosphate♦

INDICATIONS & DOSAGE
Inflammation of corticosteroid-responsive dermatoses—
Adults and children: clean area; apply cream sparingly b.i.d. to t.i.d.

SIDE EFFECTS
Skin: burning, itching, irritation, dryness, folliculitis, hypopigmentation, hypertrichosis, acneiform eruptions, perioral dermatitis, allergic contact dermatitis. *With occlusive dressings: maceration of skin, secondary infection, atrophy, striae, miliaria.*

INTERACTIONS
None significant.

NURSING CONSIDERATIONS
• Use cautiously in viral diseases of skin, such as varicella, vaccinia, herpes simplex; fungal infections; skin tuberculosis; impaired circulation.
• Avoid application in or near eyes.
• Systemic absorption especially likely with occlusive dressings, prolonged treatment, or extensive body-surface treatment.
• Stop drug and notify doctor if patient develops signs of systemic absorption,

---

skin irritation or ulceration, hypersensitivity, infection. (If antifungals or antibiotics are being used along with corticosteroids and infection does not respond immediately, corticosteroids should be stopped until infection is controlled.)

• Before applying, gently wash skin. To prevent damage to skin, rub in medication gently, leaving a thin coat. When treating hairy sites, part hair and apply directly to lesions.

• Occlusive dressing: apply cream heavily, then cover with a thin, pliable, nonflammable plastic film; seal to adjacent normal skin with hypoallergenic tape. To minimize adverse reactions, use occlusive dressing intermittently. Occlusive dressings are generally not used in presence of infection or with weeping or exudative lesions.

• For patient with eczematous dermatitis who may develop irritation with adhesive material, hold dressing in place with gauze, elastic bandages, stockings, or stockinette.

• Notify doctor and remove occlusive dressing if body temperature rises.

• Change dressing as ordered by doctor. Inspect skin for infection, striae, and atrophy. Discontinue drug and notify doctor if these occur.

• Treatment should be continued for a few days after clearing of lesions to prevent recurrence.

• Instruct patient to report signs of drug sensitivity.

---

diflorasone diacetate
Florone, Maxiflor

INDICATIONS & DOSAGE

Inflammation of corticosteroid-responsive dermatoses—

Adults and children: clean area; apply ointment daily to t.i.d.; apply cream b.i.d. to q.i.d. Apply sparingly in a thin film.

SIDE EFFECTS

Skin: burning, itching, irritation, dryness, folliculitis, hypopigmentation, perioral dermatitis, hypertrichosis, acneiform eruptions. *With occlusive dressings: maceration, secondary infection, atrophy, striae, miliaria.*

INTERACTIONS
None significant.

NURSING CONSIDERATIONS

• Use cautiously in viral diseases of skin, such as varicella, vaccinia, herpes simplex; fungal infections; skin tuberculosis; impaired circulation.

• Avoid application in or near eyes.

• Systemic absorption especially likely with occlusive dressings, prolonged treatment, or extensive body-surface treatment.

• Stop drug and notify doctor if patient develops signs of systemic absorption, skin irritation or ulceration, hypersensitivity, infection. (If antifungals or antibiotics are being used concomitantly, corticosteroids should be stopped until infection is controlled.)

• Before applying, gently wash skin. To prevent damage to skin, rub in medication gently, leaving a thin coat. When treating hairy sites, part hair and apply directly to lesion.

• Occlusive dressing: apply cream or ointment heavily, then cover with a thin, pliable, nonflammable plastic film; seal to adjacent normal skin with hypoallergenic tape. Minimize adverse reactions by using occlusive dressing intermittently. Occlusive dressings are generally not used in presence of infection or with weeping or exudative lesions.

• For patient with eczematous dermatitis who may develop irritation with adhesive material, hold dressing in place with gauze, elastic bandages, stockings, or stockinette.

• Notify doctor and remove occlusive dressing if body temperature rises.

• Change dressing as ordered by doc-

---

tor. Inspect skin for infection, striae, and atrophy. Discontinue drug and notify doctor if these occur.
• Instruct patient to report signs of drug sensitivity.
• Diflorasone is often effective with once-daily application.

flumethasone pivalate
Locacorten♦♦, Locorten

INDICATIONS & DOSAGE
Inflammation of corticosteroid-responsive dermatoses—
Adults and children: clean area; apply cream sparingly t.i.d. to q.i.d.

SIDE EFFECTS
Skin: burning, itching, irritation, dryness, folliculitis, hypopigmentation, hypertrichosis, acneiform eruptions, perioral dermatitis, allergic contact dermatitis. *With occlusive dressings: maceration of skin, secondary infection, atrophy, striae, miliaria.*

INTERACTIONS
None significant.

NURSING CONSIDERATIONS
• Use cautiously in viral diseases of skin, such as varicella, vaccinia, and herpes simplex; fungal infections; skin tuberculosis; and impaired circulation.
• Avoid application in or near eyes.
• Systemic absorption especially likely with occlusive dressings, prolonged treatment, or extensive body-surface treatment.
• Stop drug and notify doctor if patient develops signs of systemic absorption, skin irritation or ulceration, hypersensitivity, infection. (If antifungals or antibiotics are being used along with corticosteroids and infection does not respond immediately, corticosteroids should be stopped until infection is controlled.)
• Before applying, gently wash skin. To prevent damage to skin, rub in medi-

cation gently, leaving a thin coat. When treating hairy sites, part hair and apply directly to lesion.
• Occlusive dressing: apply cream or ointment heavily, then cover with a thin, pliable, nonflammable plastic film; seal to adjacent normal skin with hypoallergenic tape. To minimize adverse reactions, use occlusive dressing intermittently. Occlusive dressings are generally not used in presence of infection or with weeping or exudative lesions.
• For patient with eczematous dermatitis who may develop irritation with adhesive material, hold dressing in place with gauze, elastic bandages, stockings, or stockinette.
• Notify doctor and remove occlusive dressing if body temperature rises.
• Change dressing as ordered by doctor. Inspect skin for infection, striae, and atrophy. Discontinue drug and notify doctor if these occur.
• Treatment should be continued for a few days after clearing of lesions to prevent recurrence.
• Instruct patient to report signs of drug sensitivity.

fluocinolone acetonide
Fluonid, Synalar♦, Synalar-HP♦, Synamol♦, Synemol

INDICATIONS & DOSAGE
Inflammation of corticosteroid-responsive dermatoses—
Adults and children over 2 years: clean area; apply cream, ointment, or solution sparingly b.i.d. to q.i.d. Treat multiple or extensive lesions sequentially, applying to only small areas at any one time.

SIDE EFFECTS
Skin: burning, itching, irritation, dryness, folliculitis, hypopigmentation, hypertrichosis, acneiform eruptions, perioral dermatitis, allergic contact dermatitis. *With occlusive dressings: macera-*

Unmarked trade names available in the United States only.
♦ Also available in Canada.   ♦♦ Available in Canada only.

tion of skin, secondary infection, atrophy, striae, miliaria.

INTERACTIONS
None significant.

NURSING CONSIDERATIONS
• Use cautiously in viral diseases of skin, such as varicella, vaccinia, herpes simplex; fungal infections; skin tuberculosis; impaired circulation.
• Avoid application in or near eyes.
• Systemic absorption especially likely with occlusive dressings, prolonged treatment, or extensive body-surface treatment.
• Stop drug and notify doctor if patient develops signs of systemic absorption, skin irritation or ulceration, hypersensitivity, infection. (If antifungals or antibiotics are being used with corticosteroids and infection does not respond immediately, corticosteroids should be stopped until infection is controlled.)
• Before applying, gently wash skin. To prevent damage to skin, rub in medication gently, leaving a thin coat. When treating hairy sites, part hair and apply directly to lesion.
• Occlusive dressing: apply gently and sparingly to the lesion until cream disappears. Then reapply, leaving a thin coat. Cover with a thin, pliable, nonflammable plastic film; seal to adjacent normal skin with hypoallergenic tape. To minimize adverse reactions, use occlusive dressing intermittently. Occlusive dressings are generally not used in presence of infection or with weeping or exudative lesions.
• For patient with eczematous dermatitis who may develop irritation with adhesive material, hold dressing in place with gauze, elastic bandages, stockings, or stockinette.
• Notify doctor and remove occlusive dressing if body temperature rises.
• Change dressing as ordered by doctor. Inspect skin for infection, striae, and atrophy. Discontinue drug and notify doctor if these occur.

• Instruct patient to report signs of drug sensitivity.
• Fluonid solution on dry lesions may increase dryness, scaling, or itching; on denuded or fissured areas, may produce burning or stinging. If burning or stinging persists and dermatitis has not improved, solution should be discontinued.

fluocinonide
Lidemol♦♦, Lidex♦, Lidex-E, Topsyn♦

INDICATIONS & DOSAGE
Inflammation of corticosteroid-responsive dermatoses—
Adults and children: clean area; apply cream, ointment, or gel sparingly t.i.d. to q.i.d.

SIDE EFFECTS
Skin: burning, itching, irritation, dryness, folliculitis, hypopigmentation, hypertrichosis, acneiform eruptions, perioral dermatitis, allergic contact dermatitis. *With occlusive dressings: maceration of skin, secondary infection, atrophy, striae, miliaria.*

INTERACTIONS
None significant.

NURSING CONSIDERATIONS
• Use cautiously in viral diseases of skin, such as varicella, vaccinia, and herpes simplex; untreated purulent bacterial skin infections; fungal infections; skin tuberculosis; impaired circulation.
• Avoid application in or near eyes.
• Systemic absorption especially likely with occlusive dressings, prolonged treatment, or extensive body-surface treatment.
• Stop drug and notify doctor if patient develops signs of systemic absorption, skin irritation or ulceration, hypersensitivity, infection. (If antifungals or antibiotics are being used with corticosteroids and infection does not respond

---

Italicized side effects are common or life-threatening.
*Liquid form contains alcohol. **May contain tartrazine.

immediately, corticosteroids should be stopped until infection is controlled.)
• Before applying, gently wash skin. To prevent damage to skin, rub in medication gently, leaving a thin coat. When treating hairy sites, part hair and apply directly to lesion.
• Occlusive dressing: apply cream or ointment heavily, then cover with a thin, pliable, nonflammable plastic film; seal to adjacent normal skin with hypoallergenic tape. To minimize adverse reactions, use occlusive dressing intermittently. Occlusive dressings are generally not used in presence of infection or with weeping or exudative lesions.
• For patient with eczematous dermatitis who may develop irritation with adhesive material, hold dressing in place with gauze, elastic bandages, stockings, or stockinette.
• Notify doctor and remove occlusive dressing if body temperature rises.
• Change dressing as ordered by doctor. Inspect skin for infection, striae, and atrophy. Discontinue drug and notify doctor if these occur.
• Treatment should be continued for a few days after clearing of lesions to prevent recurrence.
• Instruct patient to report signs of drug sensitivity.

---

fluorometholone
Oxylone

INDICATIONS & DOSAGE
Inflammation of corticosteroid-responsive dermatoses—
Adults and children: clean area; apply cream sparingly daily to t.i.d.

SIDE EFFECTS
Skin: burning, itching, irritation, dryness, folliculitis, hypopigmentation, hypertrichosis, acneiform eruptions, perioral dermatitis, allergic contact dermatitis. *With occlusive dressings: macera-*
tion of skin, secondary infection, atrophy, striae, miliaria.

INTERACTIONS
None significant.

NURSING CONSIDERATIONS
• Use cautiously in viral diseases of skin, such as varicella, vaccinia, herpes simplex; fungal infections; skin tuberculosis; impaired circulation.
• Avoid application in or near eyes.
• Systemic absorption especially likely with occlusive dressings, prolonged treatment, or extensive body-surface treatment.
• Stop drug and notify doctor if patient develops signs of systemic absorption, skin irritation or ulceration, hypersensitivity, infection. (If antifungals or antibiotics are being used with corticosteroids and infection does not respond immediately, corticosteroids should be stopped until infection is controlled.)
• Before applying, gently wash skin. To prevent damage to skin, rub in medication gently, leaving a thin coat. When treating hairy sites, part hair and apply directly to lesion.
• Occlusive dressing: apply cream heavily, then cover with a thin, pliable, nonflammable plastic film; seal to adjacent normal skin with hypoallergenic tape. To minimize adverse reactions, use occlusive dressing intermittently. Occlusive dressings are generally not used in presence of infection or with weeping or exudative lesions.
• For patient with eczematous dermatitis who may develop irritation with adhesive material, hold dressing in place with gauze, elastic bandages, stockings, or stockinette.
• Notify doctor and remove occlusive dressing if body temperature rises.
• Change dressing as ordered by doctor. Inspect skin for infection, striae, and atrophy. Discontinue drug and notify doctor if these occur.
• Treatment should be continued for a

few days after clearing of lesions to prevent recurrence.
• Instruct patient to report signs of drug sensitivity.

flurandrenolide
Cordran, Cordran SP, Cordran Tape, Drenison♦♦, Drenison 1/4♦♦, Drenison Tape♦♦

INDICATIONS & DOSAGE
Inflammation of corticosteroid-responsive dermatoses—
Adults and children: clean area; apply cream, lotion, or ointment sparingly b.i.d. or t.i.d. Apply tape q 12 to 24 hours. Before applying tape, cleanse skin carefully, removing scales, crust, and dried exudates. Allow skin to dry for 1 hour before applying new tape. Shave or clip hair to allow good contact with skin and comfortable removal. If tape ends loosen prematurely, trim off and replace with fresh tape. Lowest incidence of adverse reactions if tape is replaced q 12 hours, but may be left in place for 24 hours if well tolerated and adheres satisfactorily.
Drenison 1/4: for maintenance therapy of widespread or chronic lesions.

SIDE EFFECTS
Skin: burning, itching, irritation, dryness, folliculitis, hypopigmentation, hypertrichosis, acneiform eruptions, allergic contact dermatitis. *With occlusive dressings: maceration of skin, secondary infection, atrophy, striae, miliaria.* With tape: purpura, stripping of epidermis, furunculosis.

INTERACTIONS
None significant.

NURSING CONSIDERATIONS
• Use cautiously in viral diseases of skin, such as varicella, vaccinia, herpes simplex; fungal infections; skin tuberculosis; impaired circulation.
• Tape not advised for exudative lesions or those in intertriginous areas.
• Avoid application in or near eyes.
• Systemic absorption especially likely with occlusive dressings, prolonged treatment, or extensive body-surface treatment.
• Stop drug and notify doctor if patient develops signs of systemic absorption, skin irritation or ulceration, hypersensitivity, infection. (If antifungals or antibiotics are being used with corticosteroids and infection does not respond immediately, corticosteroids should be stopped until infection is controlled.)
• Before applying, gently wash skin. To prevent damage to skin, rub in medication gently, leaving a thin coat. When treating hairy sites, part hair and apply directly to lesion.
• Occlusive dressing: apply cream heavily, then cover with a thin, pliable, nonflammable plastic film; seal to adjacent normal skin with hypoallergenic tape. To minimize adverse reactions, use occlusive dressing intermittently. Occlusive dressings are generally not used in presence of infection or with weeping or exudative lesions.
• For patient with eczematous dermatitis who may develop irritation with adhesive material, hold dressing in place with gauze, elastic bandages, stockings, or stockinette.
• Notify doctor and remove occlusive dressing if body temperature rises.
• Change dressing as ordered by doctor. Inspect skin for infection, striae, and atrophy. Discontinue drug and notify doctor if these occur.
• Treatment should be continued for a few days after clearing of lesions to prevent recurrence.
• Instruct patient to report signs of drug sensitivity.

---

halcinonide
Halciderm, Halog♦

INDICATIONS & DOSAGE
Inflammation of acute and chronic corticosteroid-responsive dermatoses—
Adults and children: clean area; apply cream, ointment, or solution sparingly b.i.d. to t.i.d.

SIDE EFFECTS
Skin: burning, itching, irritation, dryness, folliculitis, hypopigmentation, hypertrichosis, acneiform eruptions, allergic contact dermatitis. *With occlusive dressings: maceration of skin, secondary infection, atrophy, striae, miliaria.*

INTERACTIONS
None significant.

NURSING CONSIDERATIONS
• Use cautiously in viral diseases of skin, such as varicella, vaccinia, herpes simplex; fungal infections; skin tuberculosis; impaired circulation.
• Avoid application in or near eyes.
• Systemic absorption especially likely with occlusive dressings, prolonged treatment, or extensive body-surface treatment.
• Stop drug and notify doctor if patient develops signs of systemic absorption, skin irritation or ulceration, hypersensitivity, infection. (If antifungals or antibiotics are being used with corticosteroids and infection does not respond immediately, corticosteroids should be stopped until infection is controlled.)
• Before applying, gently wash skin. To prevent damage to skin, rub in medication gently, leaving a thin coat. When treating hairy sites, part hair and apply directly to lesion.
• Occlusive dressing with cream: gently rub small amount into lesion until it disappears. Reapply, leaving a thin coating on lesion, and cover with occlusive dressing. With ointment: apply to lesion and cover with occlusive dress-

ing. Cover with a thin, pliable, nonflammable plastic film; seal to adjacent normal skin with hypoallergenic tape. To minimize adverse reactions, use occlusive dressing intermittently; or with extensive lesions, occlude one part of the body at a time.
• Good results have been obtained by applying occlusive dressings in the evening and removing them in the morning (i.e., 12-hour occlusion). Medication should then be reapplied in the morning, without using the occlusive dressings during the day.
• For patient with eczematous dermatitis who may develop irritation with adhesive material, hold dressing in place with gauze, elastic bandages, stockings, or stockinette.
• Notify doctor and remove occlusive dressing if body temperature rises.
• Occlusive dressings are generally not used in presence of infection or with weeping or exudative lesions.
• Change dressing as ordered by doctor. Inspect skin for infection, striae, and atrophy. Discontinue drug and notify doctor if these occur.
• Treatment should be continued for a few days after clearing of lesions to prevent recurrence.
• Instruct patient to report signs of drug sensitivity.

hydrocortisone

Acticort, Aeroseb-HC♦,
Alphaderm, Caladryl
Hydrocortisone, Carmol-HC,
Cetacort, ClearAid, Cortaid, Cort-
Dome♦, Corticreme♦♦, Cortinal,
Cortizone 5, Cortril♦, Cotacort,
Cremesone, Delacort, Dermacort,
Dermolate, Durel-Cort, Ecosone,
HC Cream, HI-COR-2.5, Hycort,
Hycortole, Hydrocortex, Hydro-
Cortilean♦♦, Ivocort, Manticor♦♦,
Maso-Cort, Microcort♦, Penetrate,
Proctocort, Rectocort♦♦, Relecort,
Rhus Tox HC, Rocort, Ulcort,
Unicort

INDICATIONS & DOSAGE

*Inflammation of corticosteroid-respon-
sive dermatoses; adjunctive typical
management of seborrheic dermatitis of
scalp; may be safely used on face,
groin, armpits, and under breasts—*
Adults and children: clean area; apply
cream, lotion, ointment, or aerosol
sparingly daily to q.i.d.
Aerosol: shake can well. Direct spray
onto affected area from a distance of
6″. Apply for only 3 seconds (to avoid
freezing tissues). Apply to dry scalp after shampooing; no need to massage or
rub medication into scalp after spraying. Apply daily until acute phase is
controlled, then reduce dosage to 1 to 3
times a week as needed to maintain
control.

SIDE EFFECTS

Skin: burning, itching, irritation, dryness, folliculitis, hypopigmentation, hypertrichosis, acneiform eruptions, allergic contact dermatitis. *With occlusive
dressings: maceration of skin, secondary infection, atrophy, striae, miliaria.*

INTERACTIONS

None significant.

NURSING CONSIDERATIONS

• Use cautiously in viral diseases of

skin, such as varicella, vaccinia, herpes
simplex; fungal infections; skin tuberculosis; impaired circulation.
• Avoid application in or near eyes.
• Systemic absorption especially likely
with occlusive dressings, prolonged
treatment, or extensive body-surface
treatment.
• Stop drug and notify doctor if patient
develops signs of systemic absorption,
skin irritation or ulceration, hypersensitivity, infection. (If antifungals or antibiotics are being used with corticosteroids and infection does not respond
immediately, corticosteroids should be
stopped until infection is controlled.)
• Before applying, gently wash skin.
To prevent damage to skin, rub in medication gently, leaving a thin coat. When
treating hairy sites, part hair and apply
directly to lesion.
• Occlusive dressing: apply cream
heavily, then cover with a thin, pliable,
nonflammable plastic film; seal to adjacent normal skin with hypoallergenic
tape. To minimize adverse reactions,
use occlusive dressing intermittently.
Occlusive dressings are generally not
used in presence of infection or with
weeping or exudative lesions.
• For patient with eczematous dermatitis who may develop irritation with adhesive material, it may be helpful to
hold dressing in place with gauze, elastic bandages, stockings, or stockinette.
• Notify doctor and remove occlusive
dressing if body temperature rises.
• Aerosol preparation contains alcohol
and may produce irritation or burning
in open lesions. When using about the
face, cover patient's eyes and warn
against inhalation of the spray. To avoid
freezing tissues, do not spray longer
than 3 seconds or closer than 6″.
• Change dressing as ordered by doctor. Inspect skin for infection, striae,
and atrophy. Discontinue drug and notify doctor if these occur.
• Treatment should be continued for a
few days following clearing of lesions
to prevent recurrence.

Italicized side effects are common or life-threatening.
*Liquid form contains alcohol.   **May contain tartrazine.

- Instruct patient to report signs of drug sensitivity.
- The 0.5% strength is available without prescription.

hydrocortisone acetate
Cortifoam, Cortiprel, Cortef Acetate, Epifoam, Hydrocortisone Acetate, Hydrocortone Acetate, My-Cort Lotion

hydrocortisone valerate
Westcort Cream

INDICATIONS & DOSAGE
Inflammation of corticosteroid-responsive dermatoses—
Adults and children: clean area; apply lotion, cream, ointment, or foam (acetate) sparingly daily to q.i.d. Massage gently (valerate) 2 to 3 times daily p.r.n.

SIDE EFFECTS
Skin: burning, itching, irritation, dryness, folliculitis, hypopigmentation, hypertrichosis, acneiform eruptions, perioral dermatitis, allergic contact dermatitis. *With occlusive dressings: maceration of skin, secondary infection, atrophy, striae, miliaria.*

INTERACTIONS
None significant.

NURSING CONSIDERATIONS
- Use cautiously in viral diseases of skin, such as varicella, vaccinia, herpes simplex; fungal infections; skin tuberculosis; impaired circulation.
- Avoid application in or near eyes.
- Systemic absorption especially likely with occlusive dressings, prolonged treatment, or extensive body-surface treatment.
- Stop drug and notify doctor if patient develops signs of systemic absorption, skin irritation or ulceration, hypersensitivity, infection. (If antifungals or antibiotics are being used with corticosteroids and infection does not respond immediately, corticosteroids should be stopped until infection is controlled.)
- Before applying, gently wash skin. To prevent damage to skin, rub in medication gently, leaving a thin coat. When treating hairy sites, part hair and apply directly to lesion.
- Occlusive dressing: apply cream or ointment heavily, then cover with a thin, pliable, nonflammable plastic film; seal to adjacent normal skin with hypoallergenic tape. To minimize adverse reactions, use occlusive dressings intermittently. Occlusive dressings are generally not used in presence of infection or with weeping or exudative lesions.
- For patient with eczematous dermatitis who may develop irritation with adhesive material, hold dressing in place with gauze, elastic bandages, stockings, or stockinette.
- Notify doctor and remove occlusive dressing if body temperature rises.
- Lotions and foams are not used with occlusive dressings.
- Change dressing as ordered by doctor. Inspect skin for infection, striae, and atrophy. Discontinue drug and notify doctor if these occur.
- Treatment should be continued for a few days after clearing of lesions to prevent recurrence.
- Instruct patient to report signs of drug sensitivity.
- The 0.5% strength of hydrocortisone acetate is available without prescription.

methylprednisolone acetate
Medrol Acetate♦

INDICATIONS & DOSAGE
Inflammation of corticosteroid-responsive dermatoses—
Adults and children: clean area; apply ointment daily to t.i.d.

SIDE EFFECTS
Skin: burning, itching, irritation, dryness, folliculitis, hypopigmentation, hypertrichosis, acneiform eruptions, allergic contact dermatitis. *With occlusive dressings: maceration of skin, secondary infection, atrophy, striae, miliaria.*

INTERACTIONS
None significant.

NURSING CONSIDERATIONS
• Use cautiously in viral diseases of skin, such as varicella, vaccinia, herpes simplex; fungal infections; skin tuberculosis; impaired circulation.
• Avoid application in or near eyes.
• Systemic absorption especially likely with occlusive dressings, prolonged treatment, or extensive body-surface treatment.
• Stop drug and notify doctor if patient develops signs of systemic absorption, skin irritation or ulceration, hypersensitivity, infection. (If antifungals or antibiotics agents are being used with corticosteroids and infection does not respond immediately, corticosteroids should be stopped until infection is controlled.)
• Before applying, gently wash skin. To prevent damage to skin, rub in medication gently, leaving a thin coat. When treating hairy sites, part hair and apply directly to lesion.
• Occlusive dressing: apply ointment heavily, then cover with a thin, pliable, nonflammable plastic film; seal to adjacent normal skin with hypoallergenic tape. To minimize adverse effects, use occlusive dressing intermittently. Occlusive dressings are generally not used in presence of infection or with weeping or exudative lesions.
• For patient with eczematous dermatitis who may develop irritation with adhesive material, hold dressing in place with gauze, elastic bandages, stockings, or stockinette.
• Notify doctor and remove occdusive dressing if body temperature rises.

• Change dressing as ordered by doctor. Inspect skin for infection, striae, and atrophy. Discontinue drug and notify doctor if these occur.
• Treatment should be continued for a few days after clearing of lesions to prevent recurrence.
• Instruct patient to report signs of drug sensitivity.

---

prednisolone
Meti-Derm

INDICATIONS & DOSAGE
Inflammation of corticosteroid-responsive dermatoses—
Adults and children: clean area; apply cream t.i.d. or q.i.d.

SIDE EFFECTS
Skin: burning, itching, irritation, dryness, folliculitis, hypopigmentation, hypertrichosis, acneiform eruptions, perioral dermatitis, allergic contact dermatitis. *With occlusive dressings: maceration of skin, secondary infection, atrophy, striae, miliaria.*

INTERACTIONS
None significant.

NURSING CONSIDERATIONS
• Use cautiously in viral diseases of skin, such as varicella, vaccinia, herpes simplex; fungal infections; skin tuberculosis; impaired circulation.
• Avoid application in or near eyes.
• Systemic absorption especially likely with occlusive dressings, prolonged treatment, or extensive body-surface treatment.
• Stop drug and notify doctor if patient develops signs of systemic absorption, skin irritation or ulceration, hypersensitivity, infection. (If antifungals or antibiotics are being used with corticosteroids and infection does not respond immediately, corticosteroids should be stopped until infection is controlled.)
• Before applying, gently wash skin.

Italicized side effects are common or life-threatening.
*Liquid form contains alcohol.   **May contain tartrazine.

To prevent damage to skin, rub in medication gently, leaving a thin coat. When treating hairy sites, part hair and apply directly to lesions.

• Occlusive dressing: apply cream heavily and cover with a thin, pliable, nonflammable plastic film; seal to adjacent normal skin with hypoallergenic tape. To minimize adverse reactions, use occlusive dressing intermittently. Occlusive dressings are generally not used in presence of infection or with weeping or exudative lesions.

• For patient with eczematous dermatitis who may develop irritation with adhesive material, hold dressing in place with gauze, elastic bandages, stockings, or stockinette.

• Notify doctor and remove occlusive dressing if body temperature rises.

• Change dressing as ordered by doctor. Inspect skin for infection, striae, and atrophy. Discontinue drug and notify doctor if these occur.

• Treatment should be continued for a few days after clearing of lesions to prevent recurrence.

• Instruct patient to report signs of drug sensitivity.

---

triamcinolone acetonide
Aristocort♦, Aristocort A, Kenalog♦, Trymex

INDICATIONS & DOSAGE
Inflammation of corticosteroid-responsive dermatoses—
Adults and children: clean area; apply cream, ointment, lotion, foam, or aerosol sparingly b.i.d. to q.i.d. Aerosol: shake can well. Direct spray onto affected area from a distance of approximately 6″ and apply for only 3 seconds.

SIDE EFFECTS
Skin: burning, itching, irritation, dryness, folliculitis, hypopigmentation, hypertrichosis, acneiform eruptions, perioral dermatitis, allergic contact dermatitis. *With occlusive dressings: macera-tion of skin, secondary infection, atrophy, striae, miliaria.*

INTERACTIONS
None significant.

NURSING CONSIDERATIONS
• Use cautiously in viral diseases of skin, such as varicella, vaccinia, herpes simplex; fungal infections; skin tuberculosis; impaired circulation.

• Avoid application in or near eyes.

• Systemic absorption especially likely with occlusive dressings, prolonged treatment, or extensive body-surface treatment.

• Stop drug and notify doctor if patient develops signs of systemic absorption, skin irritation or ulceration, hypersensitivity, infection. (If antifungals or antibiotics are being used with corticosteroids and infection does not respond immediately, corticosteroids should be stopped until infection is controlled.)

• Before applying, gently wash skin. To prevent damage to skin, rub in medication gently, leaving a thin coat. When treating hairy sites, part hair and apply directly to lesion.

• Aerosol preparation contains alcohol and may produce irritation or burning in open lesions. When using about the face, cover patient's eyes and warn against inhalation of the spray. To avoid freezing tissues, do not spray longer than 3 seconds or closer than 6″.

• Occlusive dressing: apply cream or ointment heavily, then cover with a thin, pliable, nonflammable plastic film; seal to adjacent normal skin with hypoallergenic tape. To minimize adverse reactions, use occlusive dressing intermittently. Occlusive dressings are generally not used in presence of infection or with weeping or exudative lesions.

• For patient with eczematous dermatitis who may develop irritation with adhesive material, hold dressing in place with gauze, elastic bandages, or stockings, or stockinette.

• Notify doctor and remove occlusive dressing if body temperature rises.
• Change dressing as ordered by doctor. Inspect skin for infection, striae, and atrophy. Discontinue drug and notify doctor if these occur.

• Treatment should be continued for a few days after clearing of lesions to prevent recurrence.
• Instruct patient to report signs of drug sensitivity.

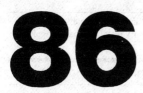

Antipruritics and topical anesthetics

benzocaine
camphor
dibucaine hydrochloride
dimethisoquin hydrochloride
diperodon monohydrate
dyclonine hydrochloride
ethyl chloride
lidocaine
lidocaine hydrochloride
menthol
phenol
pramoxine hydrochloride
tars
tetracaine
tetracaine hydrochloride

MECHANISM OF ACTION

• The general effect of all these drugs is to block conduction of impulses at the sensory nerve endings by interfering with the cell membrane's permeability to ions.
• Ethyl chloride produces local anesthesia by producing the sensation of cold.
• The specific mechanism of action of the other drugs is largely unknown. Menthol and phenol are general protoplasmic poisons.

COMBINATION PRODUCTS

BALNETAR♦: water-dispersible emollient tar 2.5% in lanolin fraction, mineral oil, and nonionic emulsifiers.
CARMOL HC: urea 10% and hydrocortisone acetate 1%.
CETACAINE LIQUID: benzocaine 14%, tetracaine HCl 2%, benzalkonium chloride 0.5%, butyl aminobenzoate 2%, and cetyl dimethyl ethyl ammonium bromide in a bland water-soluble base.

CETACAINE OINTMENT: benzocaine 14%, tetracaine HCl 2%, butyl aminobenzoate 2%, benzalkonium chloride 0.5%, and cetyl dimethyl ethyl ammonium bromide in a bland water-soluble base.
CHIGGER-TOX LIQUID: benzocaine 2.1% and benzyl benzoate in an isopropanol base.
COR-TAR-QUIN♦: coal tar solution USP 2%, diiodohydroxyquin 1% with hydrocortisone 0.25%, 0.5%, or 1% in an acid-mantle vehicle.
CUTAR BATH OIL EMULSION: coal tar solution 7.5% in liquid petrolatum isopropyl myristate, acetylated lanolin, lanolin alcohols extract, and water.
DERMA MEDICONE OINTMENT: benzocaine 2%, zinc oxide 13.7%, oxyquinoline sulfate 1.05%, ichthammol 1%, and menthol 0.48% in petrolatum and lanolin base.
DERMOPLAST SPRAY: benzocaine 20% and menthol 0.5%.
ESTAR GEL♦: coal tar 5% and alcohol 29%.
LAVATAR♦: tar distillate 33.3% in water-miscible emulsion base.
MEDICONE DRESSING (CREAM): benzocaine 0.5%, 8-hydroxyquinoline sulfate 0.05%, cod liver oil 12.5%, zinc oxide 12.5%, and menthol 0.18% with petrolatum, lanolin, talcum, and paraffin.
POLYTAR BATH: polytar 25% (juniper, pine, and coal tars, vegetable oil and solubilized crude coal tar) in water-miscible emulsion base.
PRAGMATAR OINTMENT♦: cetyl alcohol-coal tar distillate 4%, precipitated

---

Unmarked trade names available in the United States only.
♦ Also available in Canada. ♦♦ Available in Canada only.

sulfur 3%, and salicylic acid 3% in an
oil-in-water emulsion base.

SEBUTONE♦: tar (equivalent to 0.5%
coal tar) in surface-active soapless
cleansers and wetting agents, sulfur
2%, and salicylic acid 2%.

TAR DOAK LOTION♦: tar distillate 5%
and nonionic emulsifiers.

VANSEB-T♦: coal tar solution USP 5%
salicylic acid 1%, sulfur 2% in per-
fumed base.

ZETAR EMULSION♦: 30% colloidal
whole coal tar in polysorbates.

ZETAR SHAMPOO♦: whole coal tar 1%
and parachlorometaxylenol 0.5% in
foam shampoo base.

benzocaine
Americaine, Anbesol, Benzocol,
Col-Vi-Nol, Dermoplast, Hurricaine,
Rhulicream, Rhulihist, Solarcaine

INDICATIONS & DOSAGE
*Local anesthetic for pruritic
dermatoses, localized idiopathic pruritus, and sunburn—*
Adults and children: apply locally
2 or 3 times a day.
Hemorrhoids or rectal irritation—
Adults and children: apply ointment 2
or 3 times a day.

SIDE EFFECTS
Blood: methemoglobinemia (infants).
Local: sensitization, rash.

INTERACTIONS
None significant.

NURSING CONSIDERATIONS
• Contraindicated in hypersensitivity
to procaine or other para-aminobenzoic
acid (PABA) derivatives (often used in
topical sun-blocking agents).
• Discontinue if rash or irritation develops.
• Avoid contact with eyes.
• If spray preparation used, hold can 6″
to 12″ from affected area and spray liberally. Avoid inhalation.

• If using rectally, cleanse and thoroughly dry rectal area before applying.

camphor

INDICATIONS & DOSAGE
*Mild antipruritic and local anesthetic;
counterirritant for use in sprains and
rheumatic conditions—*
Adults and children: apply a 1% to
3% lotion or ointment of camphor, as
needed.

SIDE EFFECTS
Local: sensitization, rash.

INTERACTIONS
None significant.

NURSING CONSIDERATIONS
• Extremely toxic if taken orally.
• Avoid contact with eyes.
• Do not apply to broken skin or mu-
cous membranes.
• Discontinue use if rash develops.

dibucaine hydrochloride
D-Caine, Nupercainal Cream♦,
Nupercainal Ointment♦,
Nupercainal Suppositories

INDICATIONS & DOSAGE
*Abrasions, sunburn, minor burns, hem-
orrhoids, and other painful skin conditions—*
Adults and children: 0.5% to 1% lotion, cream, or ointment applied locally
several times a day.
Suppositories: insert rectally morning,
evening, and after every bowel movement.

SIDE EFFECTS
Local: sensitization, rash.

INTERACTIONS
None significant.

NURSING CONSIDERATIONS
- Avoid contact with eyes.
- Before applying cream or ointment rectally or inserting suppository, cleanse and thoroughly dry rectal area.
- Discontinue use if rash develops.
- Poisoning can occur if these preparations are swallowed. Keep out of reach of children

---

dimethisoquin hydrochloride
Quotane Cream♦♦, Quotane Ointment

INDICATIONS & DOSAGE
Surface pain and itching—
Adults and children: 0.5% ointment or lotion applied topically up to 4 times daily or as directed.

SIDE EFFECTS
Skin: *sensitization and contact dermatitis can develop but incidence is low.*

INTERACTIONS
None significant.

NURSING CONSIDERATIONS
- Useful in patients sensitive to ester- or amide-type agents.
- Don't apply to extensive areas.
- Avoid contact with eyes.
- Avoid prolonged use for patients with chronic conditions.
- Discontinue use if rash or irritation develops.

---

diperodon monohydrate
Diothane Ointment♦, Proctodon

INDICATIONS & DOSAGE
Pain caused by minor burns and cuts (cream); pain caused by anorectal disorders (ointment)—
Adults and children: apply 3 to 4 times a day.

SIDE EFFECTS
Skin: rash, irritation, and other allergic manifestations.

INTERACTIONS
None significant.

NURSING CONSIDERATIONS
- Before applying cream or ointment rectally, cleanse and thoroughly dry rectal area.
- Discontinue use if rash develops.

---

dyclonine hydrochloride
Dyclone

INDICATIONS & DOSAGE
To relieve surface pain and itching caused by minor burns or trauma, surgical wounds, pruritus ani or vulvae, insect bites, and pruritic dermatoses. Also, to anesthetize mucous membranes before endoscopic procedures—
Adults and children: 0.5% solution or 1% ointment applied 3 or 4 times daily.
Urethral dilation or cystourethroscopy—
Adults: 10 ml of 0.5% solution may be instilled into the urethra.

SIDE EFFECTS
Local: *irritation at site of application may occur.*

INTERACTIONS
None significant.

NURSING CONSIDERATIONS
- Avoid prolonged use in patients with chronic conditions.
- May be useful in patients hypersensitive to other local anesthetics because it is a ketone.
- Contraindicated in cystoscopic examinations following an intravenous pyelogram. Iodine-containing contrast material will cause precipitate to form with dyclonine.
- Can be combined with diphenhydramine elixir to provide an effective treatment for stomatitis.

Unmarked trade names available in the United States only.
♦ Also available in Canada.   ♦♦ Available in Canada only.

• Avoid accidental contact with drug; it produces temporary numbness.

ethyl chloride
Ethyl Chloride Spray

INDICATIONS & DOSAGE
For irritation—
Adults and children: hold container about 24″ from skin and spray rhythmically to cover area evenly once or twice. Application may be repeated.
As a local anesthetic in minor operative procedures; relieves pain caused by insect stings and burns, and irritation caused by myofascial and visceral pain syndromes—
Adults and children: dosage varies with different procedures. Use smallest dosage needed to produce desired effect. For local anesthesia, hold container about 12″ from area to produce a fine spray.
Infants: hold a cotton ball saturated with ethyl chloride to injection site, and make injection when site dries.

SIDE EFFECTS
Skin: sensitization; *frostbite and tissue necrosis may occur with prolonged spraying.*
Other: excessive cooling may increase pain and muscle spasms.

INTERACTIONS
None significant.

NURSING CONSIDERATIONS
• Do not apply to broken skin or mucous membranes.
• Protect skin adjacent to treated area with petrolatum to avoid tissue sloughing.
• Avoid use near eyes.
• Avoid inhalation when spraying.
• Highly flammable; do not use in areas where open flames or sparks are possible.
• Avoid accidental contact with drug; it produces temporary numbness.

lidocaine

lidocaine hydrochloride
Lida-Mantle Cream, Stanacaine, Xylocaine Jelly (2%), Xylocaine Ointment (2.5%)♦, Xylocaine Ointment (5%)♦, Xylocaine Solution (4%)♦, Xylocaine Viscous Solution (2%)

INDICATIONS & DOSAGE
Local anesthesia of skin or mucous membranes—
Adults and children: apply liberally.
In procedures involving the male or female urethra—
Adults: instill about 15 ml (male) or 3 to 5 ml (female) into urethra.
Pain, burning, or itching caused by burns, sunburn, or skin irritation—
Adults and children: apply liberally.

SIDE EFFECTS
Local: sensitization, rash.

INTERACTIONS
None significant.

NURSING CONSIDERATIONS
• Use with caution on severely traumatized mucosa or where sepsis is present or for anesthesia of oropharyngeal mucosa, since gag reflex may be suppressed by lidocaine and aspiration may occur.
• The 4% solution can be sprayed or poured onto abrasions to facilitate cleansing and removal of foreign substances (gravel, glass, etc.).
• Discontinue use if rash or irritation develops.
• Apply Xylocaine Ointment carefully to prevent contact with skin; it produces numbness.

menthol

INDICATIONS & DOSAGE
As an antipruritic—

Italicized side effects are common or life-threatening.
*Liquid form contains alcohol.   **May contain tartrazine.

Adults and children: apply 0.25% to 2% lotion or ointment, as needed. Often added with phenol to an ointment.

SIDE EFFECTS
None reported.

INTERACTIONS
None significant.

NURSING CONSIDERATIONS
• Relieves itching by substituting a cooling effect.
• Avoid contact with eyes.

phenol

INDICATIONS & DOSAGE
As an antipruritic—
Adults and children over 6 months: apply 0.5% to 2% preparations locally several times a day.

SIDE EFFECTS
None at recommended strengths.

INTERACTIONS
None significant.

NURSING CONSIDERATIONS
• Avoid accidental contact with normal skin. If contact occurs, remove phenol with alcohol or vegetable oil.
• Tissue necrosis possible with higher than usual concentration or extensive use.
• Avoid contact with eyes.
• Do not use under occlusive dressings, bandages, or diapers.

pramoxine hydrochloride
Proctofoam, Tronolane, Tronothane♦

INDICATIONS & DOSAGE
Pain and itching caused by dermatoses, minor burns, surgical wounds, insect bites, and hemorrhoids—

Adults and children: apply every 3 to 4 hours.

SIDE EFFECTS
Local: stinging or burning, sensitization.

INTERACTIONS
None significant.

NURSING CONSIDERATIONS
• Can be safely used in those allergic to other local anesthetics.
• May be applied with gauze or sprayed directly on skin. Avoid contact with eyes.
• Cleanse and thoroughly dry rectal area before applying ointment or cream, or inserting suppository.

tars

INDICATIONS & DOSAGE
As an antipruritic, antipsoriatic, antieczematic—
Adults and children: apply preparations 2 or 3 times daily.

SIDE EFFECTS
Skin: irritation, folliculitis, erythema, photosensitivity.

INTERACTIONS
None significant.

NURSING CONSIDERATIONS
• Use caution in applying tar preparations to patients with exacerbation of psoriasis. Excessive use may precipitate total body exfoliation.
• Never use under occlusive dressings.
• Avoid excessive exposure to sunlight. May produce photosensitization.
• Darkens color of blond hair when applied to scalp.
• May stain skin and clothing. Use mineral oil to remove from skin, especially if 1% to 5% crude coal tar is used.

---

tetracaine

tetracaine hydrochloride
Pontocaine♦

INDICATIONS & DOSAGE
For relief of pain in hemorrhoids, minor burns, ulcers, sunburn, and poison ivy—

Adults and children: apply 5% ointment or 1% cream—no more than 1 oz for adults or ¼ oz for children in 24 hours.

SIDE EFFECTS
Local: sensitization, rash.

INTERACTIONS
None significant.

NURSING CONSIDERATIONS
• Contraindicated in hypersensitivity to procaine or other para-aminobenzoic acid (PABA) derivatives (often used in topical sun-blocking agents).
• Before applying cream or ointment rectally, cleanse and thoroughly dry rectal area.
• Discontinue use if rash or irritation develops.

87

Astringents

acetic acid lotion
aluminum acetate
aluminum sulfate
hamamelis water
tannic acid

MECHANISM OF ACTION

Astringents precipitate protein, causing tissue to contract. The cement substance of the capillary endothelium is hardened so that transcapillary movement of plasma protein is inhibited. Local edema, inflammation, and exudation are thereby reduced.

Mucus or other secretions may also be reduced so that the affected area becomes drier.

COMBINATION PRODUCTS

ASTRINGENTS WITH ANESTHETICS, for example, Nupercainal Suppositories.
ASTRINGENTS WITH ANTIPRURITIC/ANTIHISTAMINE, for example, Caladryl, Ziradryl.
ASTRINGENTS WITH ANTIPRURITIC/ANTIHISTAMINE AND ANESTHETIC, for example, Rhulicream, Rhulihist, Rhulispray.
ASTRINGENTS WITH ANTISEPTICS, for example, Tucks Pads, Tanac, Lavoris.
ASTRINGENTS WITH ANTISEPTICS AND ANESTHETICS, for example, Rectal Medicone Suppositories and Unguent, Tanicaine Suppositories and Ointment, Wyanoid Ointment, Pazo Hemorrhoid Suppositories and Ointment.
ASTRINGENTS WITH DEODORANTS, for example, most antiperspirant/deodorants commonly available.

acetic acid lotion

(0.1% glacial acetic acid in alcohol)

INDICATIONS & DOSAGE

Superficial fungal or bacterial infection to toughen skin and prevent bedsores—
Adults and children: apply and work into area, p.r.n.

SIDE EFFECTS

Skin: burning and irritation of denuded skin and mucous membranes.

INTERACTIONS

Heavy metals: causes precipitation of the metal acetate.

NURSING CONSIDERATIONS

- Contraindicated under occlusive dressings.
- Never confuse acetic acid solutions with *glacial* acetic acid solutions. Glacial form is a concentrate.
- Keep away from eyes and mucous membranes.
- Always apply to freshly cleansed area, free of other medications.
- Especially good for treating topical infection due to *Pseudomonas aeruginosa*.

aluminum acetate

(modified Burow's solution)
Acid Mantle Creme and Lotion♦, Buro-sol, Burow's Emulsion, Burow's Lotion, Burow's Ointment

INDICATIONS & DOSAGE

Mild skin irritation from exposure to

Unmarked trade names available in the United States only.
♦ Also available in Canada. ♦♦ Available in Canada only.

soaps, detergents, chemicals, diaper rash, acne, scaly skin, eczema—
Adults and children: apply p.r.n.
Relieve inflammation of poison ivy, insect bites, athlete's foot—
Adults and children: apply as wet dressing, p.r.n.
Ulcerative skin conditions—
Adults and children: apply ointment, p.r.n.

SIDE EFFECTS
Skin: irritation; extension of inflammation possible.

INTERACTIONS
None significant.

NURSING CONSIDERATIONS
• Contraindicated under occlusive dressings.
• Keep away from eyes and mucous membranes.
• Always apply to freshly cleansed area, free of other medications.
• May be used in place of boric acid ointment.
• Powder must be diluted in water to prescribed concentration.
• Discontinue if irritation develops.
• Clear solution may be stored at room temperature for up to 7 days.

---

aluminum sulfate
Bluboro Powder, Domeboro Powder♦ and Tablets♦

INDICATIONS & DOSAGE
Skin inflammation, insect bites, poison ivy or other contact dermatoses, swelling, athlete's foot—
Adults and children: mix powder with 1 pint of lukewarm tap water and apply for 15 to 30 minutes every 4 to 8 hours; bandage loosely.

SIDE EFFECTS
Skin: irritation; extension of inflammation possible.

INTERACTIONS
None significant.

NURSING CONSIDERATIONS
• Contraindicated under occlusive dressings; use open wet dressings only.
• When solution is prepared, immediately decant clear portion. Discard precipitate. Use only clear solution, *not* precipitate, for soaks. Never strain or filter solutions. Decanted portion may be stored at room temperature for up to 7 days.
• In general, no more than a third of the body should be treated at any one time, since excessive wet dressings may cause chilling and hypothermia.
• Keep away from eyes and mucous membranes.
• Discontinue if irritation develops.

---

hamamelis water
(witch hazel)
Mediconet (wipes), Tucks (Cream, Ointment, Pads)

INDICATIONS & DOSAGE
Anal discomfort, itching, burning, minor external hemorrhoidal or outer vaginal discomfort, diaper rash—
Adults and children: apply t.i.d. or q.i.d.

SIDE EFFECTS
Skin: hypersensitivity.

INTERACTIONS
None significant.

NURSING CONSIDERATIONS
• Discontinue if irritation or itching does not improve.
• Use pads or wipes after toilet tissue to help prevent pruritus ani, vulvae.
• Cream can be used by breast-feeding mother for nipple care, but wash area clean before breast-feeding baby.
• Some products contain potential allergic sensitizers. Observe for allergic reactions.

---

tannic acid
Amertan Jelly, Dalidyne Lotion*, Tanac

INDICATIONS & DOSAGE
Denture irritation; teething irritation; trench mouth; gingivitis; throat irritation; herpes simplex; oral cavity lesions; adjunctive treatment of second- and third-degree thermal, chemical, or electrical burns—
Adults: apply with cotton applicator. As gargle or mouthwash, ½ teaspoon of solution in ½ glass of warm water, p.r.n.
Cold sores, throat irritation, oral cavity lesions, some second- and third-degree burns—
Children: apply with cotton applicator.

SIDE EFFECTS
Local: stinging.
Other: large amounts in burn treatment can cause hepatic damage.

INTERACTIONS
Organic salts of heavy metals: will precipitate tannate salt of heavy metal. Do not apply.

NURSING CONSIDERATIONS
• Incompatible with organic salts of heavy metals. Apply only to surfaces free of other medication.
• Produces a firm eschar on burned area that helps protect burned tissue from infection and loss of body fluids, and comforts patient.
• Apply only after proper debridement of burn.
• Prepare aqueous solutions freshly, as they are unstable.
• Light and air cause solution to darken, which reduces potency.
• Avoid extensive application and prolonged use on denuded tissue to decrease possibility of systemic toxicity from absorption.
• Slight stinging on application soon subsides.

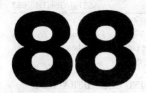

Antiseptics and disinfectants

alcohol, ethyl
alcohol, isopropyl
benzalkonium chloride
boric acid
chlorhexidine gluconate
formaldehyde
glutaraldehyde
hexachlorophene
hydrogen peroxide
iodine
merbromin
nitromersol
oxychlorosene calcium
oxychlorosene sodium
phenylmercuric nitrate
poloxamer iodine
potassium permanganate
povidone-iodine
silver protein, mild
sodium hypochlorite
thimerosal

MECHANISM OF ACTION
These drugs denature protein in micro-organisms, changing their chemical structure. They lower surface tension, increasing cell permeability and causing lysis of the cell's contents, and also interfere with cellular metabolic processes.

COMBINATION PRODUCTS
B.F.I. POWDER: bismuth-formici-iodide, zinc phenosulfonate, amol, potassium alum, bismuth subgallate, boric acid, menthol, eucalyptol, and thymol.
MERCRESIN: secondary-amyltricresols 0.1%, orthohydroxyphenylmercuric chloride 0.1%, acetone 10%, and alcohol 50%.

OBTUNDIA: camphor and metacresol in lanolin-petroleum base.
OBTUNDIA CALAMINE: camphor, metacresol, zinc oxide, and calamine.
S.T. 37: hexylresorcinol 0.1% in glycerin aqueous solution.
ZEASORB POWDER: parachlorometaxylenol 0.5%, aluminum dihydroxy allantoinate 0.2%, and microporous cellulose 45%.

---

alcohol, ethyl
Alcohol, Ethanol

INDICATIONS & DOSAGE
To disinfect skin, instruments, and ampuls—disinfect as needed.

SIDE EFFECTS
Skin: dryness, irritation.

INTERACTIONS
None significant.

NURSING CONSIDERATIONS
• Effective as fat solvent germicidal; ineffective against spore-forming organisms, tubercle bacilli, viruses.
• Alcohol used as 70% solution known commonly as "rubbing alcohol."
• Should be left on the skin for at least 2 minutes.
• Don't use on skin before insulin administration. May affect potency of insulin.
• Not recommended for treatment of an open wound.

Italicized side effects are common or life-threatening.
*Liquid form contains alcohol.   **May contain tartrazine.

alcohol, isopropyl

isopropyl alcohol 99%, isopropyl
rubbing alcohol 70%, isopropyl
aqueous alcohol 75%

INDICATIONS & DOSAGE
To disinfect skin, instruments, and ampuls— disinfect as needed.

SIDE EFFECTS
Skin: dryness, irritation.

INTERACTIONS
None significant.

NURSING CONSIDERATIONS
• Isopropyl alcohol is slightly more effective than ethyl alcohol as an antibacterial agent, but it also tends to cause more dryness.
• Should be left on the skin for at least 2 minutes.
• 75% solution for disinfection and storage of thermometers.
• Not effective against spore-forming organisms, tubercle bacilli, or viruses.
• Combined with formaldehyde, makes effective germicide.
• Not recommended for treatment of an open wound.

benzalkonium chloride

Benasept, Benzachlor-50♦♦, Benz-
All, Drapolex♦♦, Ionax Foam♦♦,
Ionax Scrub♦♦, Mercurochrome II,
Sabol♦♦, Spensomide, Zalkon,
Zalkonium Chloride, Zephiran

INDICATIONS & DOSAGE
Preoperative disinfection of unbroken skin—apply 1:750 to 1:1,000 tincture or spray.
Disinfection of mucous membranes and denuded skin—apply 1:10,000 to 1:5,000 aqueous solution.
Irrigation of vagina—instill 1:5,000 to 1:2,000 aqueous solution.

Irrigation of bladder or urethra—instill 1:20,000 to 1:5,000 aqueous solution.
Irrigation of deep infected wounds—instill 1:20,000 to 1:3,000 aqueous solution.
Preservation of metallic instruments, ampuls, thermometers, and rubber articles—wipe with or soak objects in 1:5,000 to 1:750 solution.
Disinfection of operating room equipment—wipe with 1:5,000 solution.

SIDE EFFECTS
Skin: hypersensitivity.

INTERACTIONS
Soaps: inactivate benzalkonium chloride. Remove soap traces with alcohol.

NURSING CONSIDERATIONS
• Germicidal for some nonspore-forming organisms and fungi. No effect on tubercle bacilli. Limited viricidal use.
• Used as preservative in ophthalmic solutions.
• Before applying to skin, remove all traces of soap with water and apply 70% alcohol.
• Don't store cotton, wool gauze, or sponges in solution. They absorb benzalkonium chloride and reduce the strength of the solution.
• Don't use with occlusive dressings or vaginal packs.
• Store in bottles with screw caps.
• Incompatible with iodine, silver nitrate, fluorescein, nitrates, peroxide, lanolin, potassium permanganate, aluminum, caramel, kaolin, pine oil, zinc sulfate, zinc oxide, and yellow oxide of mercury.
• To prevent rust of metallic instruments stored in benzalkonium chloride, add sodium nitrite to final solution. Change solution weekly.
• Available also as 17% concentrate (Zephiran). Even after dilution, this form of Zephiran should be used only on inanimate objects.

Unmarked trade names available in the United States only.
♦ Also available in Canada.   ♦♦ Available in Canada only.

boric acid
Bluboro, boric acid solution 5%,
Borofax♦, Ting

INDICATIONS & DOSAGE
Skin conditions (athlete's foot) as a compress, powder, or ointment (2% to 5%)—
Adults and children: apply as directed.
Vaginal candidiasis—
Adults: 600 mg powder intravaginally twice weekly for 3 weeks.

SIDE EFFECTS
Signs of systemic absorption:
CNS: delirium, convulsions, restlessness, headache.
CV: *circulatory collapse,* tachycardia.
GI: irritation, nausea, vomiting, diarrhea.
GU: renal damage.
Other: hypothermia.

INTERACTIONS
None significant.

NURSING CONSIDERATIONS
• Mild antiseptic and astringent.
• Not absorbed through intact skin, but, in high concentrations, may be absorbed through abraded skin or granulating wounds.
• Avoid long-term use.
• Ingestion of 5 g (infants) or 20 g (adults) may be fatal.

chlorhexidine gluconate
Hibiclens Liquid, Hibistat, Hibitane

INDICATIONS & DOSAGE
*Surgical hand scrub, hand wash, hand rinse, skin wound cleanser—*use p.r.n.

SIDE EFFECTS
EENT: irritating to eyes. Causes deafness if instilled into middle ear through perforated eardrum.

INTERACTIONS
None significant.

NURSING CONSIDERATIONS
• Bactericidal. Broad spectrum.
• Can be used many times a day without causing irritation or dryness.
• Low potential for producing skin reactions.
• Rinse skin thoroughly after use.
• Keep out of eyes and ears.
• Action is residual. Do not cleanse skin with alcohol after application.

formaldehyde
Formalin (37% solution of formaldehyde)

INDICATIONS & DOSAGE
*Cold sterilization of equipment—*disinfect as needed.
*Tissue preservative—*cover tissue.

SIDE EFFECTS
EENT: fumes cause eye, nose, and throat irritation.
Skin: irritation.
Other: pungent odor.

INTERACTIONS
None significant.

NURSING CONSIDERATIONS
• 0.5% solution germicidal against all forms of microorganisms, including spores, in 6 to 12 hours; 10% solution used to disinfect inanimate objects.
• Not affected by organic matter.
• Used with alcohol and sodium nitrite to disinfect instruments and articles that can't tolerate heat (cold sterilization).
• Avoid skin or mucous membrane contact with solutions greater than 0.5%.
• Always dilute 37% solution.

Italicized side effects are common or life-threatening.
*Liquid form contains alcohol.   **May contain tartrazine.

glutaraldehyde
Cidex♦

INDICATIONS & DOSAGE
Cold sterilization of surgical instruments—cover instruments with 2% solution.
Fumigate hospital and operating rooms—fog with aerosol.

SIDE EFFECTS
Skin: irritation.

INTERACTIONS
None significant.

NURSING CONSIDERATIONS
• Excellent disinfectant; broad spectrum of activity against gram-positive and gram-negative bacteria (vegetative and spores), viruses, and fungi.
• Use on inanimate objects only.
• Comes with activator that must be mixed before use to yield active acidic glutaraldehyde.
• Not affected by organic matter.
• Whenever possible, use commercially prepared 2% solution rather than diluting the 25% solution.

hexachlorophene
Germa-Medica "MG," pHisoHex♦, pHisoScrub, Sept-Soft, Septisol Soy-Dome Cleanser, WescoHEX

INDICATIONS & DOSAGE
Surgical scrub, bacteriostatic skin cleanser—use as directed in 0.25% to 3% concentrations.

SIDE EFFECTS
Note: systemic absorption can cause neurotoxic effects, including irritability, generalized clonic muscular contractions, decerebrate rigidity, convulsions, optic atrophy. (Systemic absorption has occurred only when used on premature infants, mucous membranes, and broken skin and burns.)

Skin: dermatitis, mild scaling, dryness (especially when combined with excessive scrubbing).

INTERACTIONS
None significant.

NURSING CONSIDERATIONS
• Use with caution in infants (especially premature infants) and burn patients. These patients tend to absorb hexachlorophene through the skin and may develop neurotoxic effects.
• Bacteriostatic agent. Spectrum of activity limited to gram-positive organisms, especially staphylococcus.
• Must be used preoperatively for at least 3 days for maximum effectiveness.
• After cleaning area, rinse thoroughly (especially the scrotum and perineum). Do not apply alcohol or organic solvents to cleansed area.

hydrogen peroxide
3% to 6% solution

INDICATIONS & DOSAGE
Cleansing wound—use 1.5% to 3% solution.
Mouth wash for necrotizing ulcerative gingivitis—gargle with 3% solution.
Cleansing douche—use 2% solution.

SIDE EFFECTS
EENT: excessive use as mouthwash causes "hairy tongue."

INTERACTIONS
None significant.

NURSING CONSIDERATIONS
• Germicidal, particularly against anaerobic organisms.
• Don't inject into closed body cavities or abscesses; generated gas can't escape.
• Dilute concentrate with 1 to 4 parts water.
• Useful to remove mucus from inner cannula of tracheostomy tube.

Unmarked trade names available in the United States only.
♦ Also available in Canada.   ♦♦ Available in Canada only.

- Store tightly capped in cool, dry place. Protect from light and heat.
- Do not shake bottle. This causes decomposition.

iodine

solution (2% iodine and 2.4% sodium and iodide in water)♦, tincture (2% iodine and 2.4% sodium iodide in diluted alcohol), Sepp Antiseptic Applicators (2% mild iodine tincture), strong iodine tincture (7% iodine and 5% potassium iodide in diluted alcohol)

INDICATIONS & DOSAGE

Preoperative disinfection of skin (small wounds and abraded areas)—apply p.r.n.

SIDE EFFECTS

Skin: irritation, redness, swelling (sign of hypersensitivity).

INTERACTIONS

None significant.

NURSING CONSIDERATIONS

- Microbicidal agent effective against bacteria, fungi, viruses, protozoa, and yeasts.
- If skin reaction develops, remove iodine residue from skin and stop use.
- To prevent skin irritation, do not cover areas treated with iodine.
- Aqueous solution less irritating.
- Sodium thiosulfate renders iodine colorless and is used to remove stains. It is also antidote of choice for accidental ingestion.

merbromin

Mercurochrome (2% aqueous solution)

INDICATIONS & DOSAGE

General antiseptic and first-aid prophylactic—

Adults and children: apply p.r.n. as 1% to 2% solution or tincture.

SIDE EFFECTS

Skin: sensitization.

INTERACTIONS

None significant.

NURSING CONSIDERATIONS

- Bacteriostatic.
- Don't use on large areas of abraded skin, because mercury may be absorbed and produce systemic toxicity.
- Least effective mercurial antiseptic. Its activity is decreased in presence of organic matter.
- Cleanse injury with soap and water before applying. Let dry.
- Stains may be removed with 2% permanganate solution, followed by 5% oxalic acid solution.
- Never heat solution.
- To prepare 1% solution, dilute with equal parts water.
- Note that a new product, Mercurochrome II, does *not* contain merbromin, but contains benzalkonium chloride.

nitromersol

Metaphen

INDICATIONS & DOSAGE

Disinfection of instruments—soak in 0.04% solution.
Disinfection of skin—apply 0.2% to 0.5% solution to area p.r.n.
Irrigation of mucous membranes (eye, urethra)—instill 0.01% to 0.02% solution as directed.
Skin antiseptic for abrasions—apply 0.2% solution to area.

SIDE EFFECTS

Skin: erythematous, papular, or vesicular eruptions indicate hypersensitivity; irritation.

Italicized side effects are common or life-threatening.
♦Liquid form contains alcohol.   ♦♦May contain tartrazine.

INTERACTIONS
None significant.

NURSING CONSIDERATIONS
• Contraindicated in hypersensitivity to mercury compounds.
• Do not use when aluminum may come in contact with skin.
• Incompatible with permanganates, strong acids, and heavy metal salts.
• Prepare as needed. Solutions tend to precipitate on standing.
• Remove rings when working with solution; the mercury component can damage the precious metals in jewelry.

oxychlorosene calcium
Clorpactin XCB

oxychlorosene sodium
Clorpactin WCS-90

INDICATIONS & DOSAGE
Topical antiseptic for local infections, preoperative skin cleanser (sodium salt)—apply as spray, soak, wet dressing, or irrigation as a 4% solution.
Ophthalmic and urologic irrigant (sodium salt)— 0.1% to 0.2% solution.
Local irrigation during surgery (calcium salt)—use 0.5% solution.

SIDE EFFECTS
Skin: local irritation.

INTERACTIONS
None significant.

NURSING CONSIDERATIONS
• Effective against bacteria, fungi, viruses, yeast, and spores.
• Powder reconstituted in saline solution.
• Refrigerate dry crystal until reconstitution.
• Oxychlorosene calcium has a special use as a local irrigating agent during surgery for neoplasms, to destroy loose viable neoplastic cells and thereby prevent iatrogenic metastasis. Oxychloro-

sene sodium is not used for this purpose.

phenylmercuric nitrate
Phe-Mer-Nite

INDICATIONS & DOSAGE
Preoperative disinfection—apply p.r.n. as a 0.1% to 0.2% solution.

SIDE EFFECTS
Skin: rash.

INTERACTIONS
None significant.

NURSING CONSIDERATIONS
• Contraindicated in hypersensitivity to mercury-containing compounds.
• Antiseptic and fungicidal.
• Frequent or prolonged use may cause mercury poisoning.
• Orange stain removed with soap and water.
• Commonly used as a preservative in ophthalmic solutions.

poloxamer iodine
Prepodyne

INDICATIONS & DOSAGE
Preoperative skin preparation and scrub, wound disinfection—use as directed.

SIDE EFFECTS
None reported.

INTERACTIONS
None significant.

NURSING CONSIDERATIONS
• Contraindicated in hypersensitivity to iodines.
• Prolonged germicidal action.
• Water-soluble solution releases iodine at predetermined rate, causing prolonged action.
• Relatively nonirritating to skin.

Unmarked trade names available in the United States only.
♦ Also available in Canada.   ♦ ♦ Available in Canada only.

potassium permanganate

INDICATIONS & DOSAGE
Topical antiseptic—apply 1:10,000 to 1:500 solution.
Vaginal douche—instill 1:5,000 to 1:1,000 solution as directed.

SIDE EFFECTS
Skin: solutions greater than 1:5,000 are irritating to skin.

INTERACTIONS
Iodine: precipitates iodine salt. Do not use together.

NURSING CONSIDERATIONS
• Antiseptic astringent with fungicidal properties.
• Germicidal effects reduced by organic matter.
• Stains caused by potassium permanganate removed with dilute acids (lemon juice, oxalic acid, or dilute hydrochloric acid).
• Never mix with charcoal or give charcoal as antidote. May explode.

povidone-iodine
ACU-dyne, Aerodine, Betadine♦, BPS, Bridine♦♦, Efodine, Final Step, Frepp, Frepp/Sepp, Isodine, Mallisol, Polydine, Proviodine♦♦, Sepp

INDICATIONS & DOSAGE
Many uses, including preoperative skin preparation and scrub, germicide for surface wounds, postoperative application to incisions, prophylactic application to urinary meatus of catheterized patients, miscellaneous disinfection—
Adults: apply p.r.n.

SIDE EFFECTS
Skin: local hypersensitivity reactions.

INTERACTIONS
None significant.

NURSING CONSIDERATIONS
• Use as a vaginal antiseptic should be discouraged during pregnancy.
• Germicidal activity of iodine without irritation to skin and mucous membranes.
• Thought to be superior to soap as a disinfectant; less effective than aqueous or alcoholic solutions of iodine.
• Treated areas may be bandaged or taped.
• Germicidal activity reduced if area cleansed with alcohol or other organic solvents after application of povidone-iodine.
• Prolonged, excessive use may lead to systemic absorption and toxicity.
• Betadine vaginal gel should not be used in patients hypersensitive to iodine.
• Don't combine with alcohol or hydrogen peroxide.

silver protein, mild
Argyrol S.S.♦, Silvol, Solargentum

INDICATIONS & DOSAGE
Topical application for inflammation of eye, nose, throat—
Adults and children: apply p.r.n. as a 5% to 25% solution.

SIDE EFFECTS
Skin: argyria in long-term use.

INTERACTIONS
None significant.

NURSING CONSIDERATIONS
• Store in amber glass bottles; protect from light.

Italicized side effects are common or life-threatening.
✳Liquid form contains alcohol.   ✳✳May contain tartrazine.

sodium hypochlorite
5% solution (instruments, swimming pools), 0.5% aqueous solution for wounds, Modified Dakin's solution

INDICATIONS & DOSAGE
Athlete's foot, wound irrigation, disinfection of walls and floors—apply as directed.

SIDE EFFECTS
Skin: irritation, bleeding.

INTERACTIONS
None significant.

NURSING CONSIDERATIONS
• Germicidal and weakly fungicidal.
• Interferes locally with thrombin formation, delaying blood clotting. Dissolves necrotic tissue.
• Unstable in solution. Make fresh solution and use immediately.
• Avoid contact with hair due to its bleaching properties.

thimerosal
Aeroaid Thimerosal, Merthiolate

INDICATIONS & DOSAGE
Preoperative disinfection of skin; antiseptic for open wounds—apply or instill to affected area daily, b.i.d., or t.i.d. as a 0.1% solution or tincture.

SIDE EFFECTS
Skin: erythematous, vesicular, papular eruptions (indicate hypersensitivity); irritation with tincture.

INTERACTIONS
None significant.

NURSING CONSIDERATIONS
• Contraindicated in hypersensitivity to mercury-containing compounds.
• Do not use when aluminum may come in contact with skin.
• Incompatible with permanganate, strong acids, and salts of heavy metals.
• Cleanse wound thoroughly before applying tincture.
• To prevent skin irritation, allow tincture to dry completely before applying dressing.
• Can be instilled into body cavities.
• Store in amber glass container.

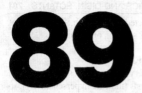

Emollients, demulcents, and protectants

aluminum paste
calamine
collodion
collodion, flexible
compound benzoin tincture
dexpanthenol
glycerin
hydrophilic lotion
hydrophilic ointment
hydrophilic petrolatum
hydrous wool fat lotion
hydrous wool fat and castor oil
liquid petrolatum
methyl salicylate
oatmeal
para-aminobenzoic acid
petrolatum
silicone
starch
talc
urea or carbamide
vitamins A and D ointment
zinc gelatin

MECHANISM OF ACTION
● Emollients soften dry skin by preventing evaporation of perspiration.

Methyl salicylate is a counterirritant that increases circulation to the area of application. This causes localized redness and warmth and helps reduce muscle soreness and stiffness.

● Demulcents have analgesic properties to soothe irritation and cool inflammation. Some (such as starch) absorb moisture when secretions are excessive, helping to dry skin.

● Protectants promote healing by reducing irritation and friction.

Talc and other dusting powders are not completely biologically inert and may cause irritation, granulomas, fibrosis, or adhesion.

Flexible collodion is collodion USP, a protectant to which castor oil has been added to improve pliability.

COMBINATION PRODUCTS
CALADRYL LOTION: diphenhydramine hydrochloride 1%, calamine, camphor, and alcohol 2%.
CALADRYL CREAM: diphenhydramine hydrochloride 1% with calamine.
GER-O-FOAM AEROSOL: methyl salicylate 30%, benzocaine 3%, in oil emulsion.
PANALGESIC: methyl salicylate 50%, aspirin 8%, menthol and camphor 4%, emollient oils 20%, alcohol 18%.

---

aluminum paste
(10% aluminum in zinc oxide ointment with liquid petrolatum)

INDICATIONS & DOSAGE
Emollient and protectant: colostomy area or other surgical sites—apply p.r.n.

SIDE EFFECTS
None.

INTERACTIONS
Topical enzymes: aluminum may inactivate preparations used to debride wounds. Don't use together.

NURSING CONSIDERATIONS
● Zinc oxide paste can be used as an alternative.
● Observe for inflammation or infec-

---

tion since protectants are occlusive layers that retain moisture, exclude air, and trap cutaneous bacteria.
- Skin should be cleaned daily or more often as needed.
- Emollients and protectants may be used alone, as vehicles for medications, or with other topical medications. Check with doctor.

calamine
liniment (15% calamine), lotion (8% calamine), ointment (17% calamine), Rhulihist (3% calamine), Rhulispray (1% calamine)

INDICATIONS & DOSAGE
Topical astringent and protectant: itching, poison ivy and poison oak, nonpoisonous insect bites, mild sunburn, minor skin irritations—apply p.r.n.

SIDE EFFECTS
Skin: transient light stinging, irritation, dry skin.

INTERACTIONS
None significant.

NURSING CONSIDERATIONS
- Contraindicated in hypersensitivity to any of the components.
- Watch for sensitivity reactions to calamine. Preparations containing antihistamines can cause sensitivity.
- Always shake well before use.
- Don't use cotton to apply; it will absorb the solute. Use gauze sponge.
- Do not apply to blistered, raw, or oozing areas of the skin.
- Toxic if taken internally.
- Observe for inflammation or infection since protectants are occlusive layers that retain moisture, exclude air, and trap skin bacteria.
- Skin should be cleaned daily or more often as needed.
- Emollients, demulcents, protectants may be used alone, as vehicles for med-

ications, or with other topical medications. Check with doctor.
- May irritate and dry skin.
- Keep away from eyes and mucous membranes.
- Keep container tightly closed so solvent won't evaporate.

collodion, USP
(5% pyroxylin in 1 part alcohol, 3 parts ether)

collodion, flexible
(5% pyroxylin in 1 part alcohol, 3 parts ether plus 20% camphor, 30% castor oil)

INDICATIONS & DOSAGE
Protectant; vehicle for other medicinal agents; and sealant for small wounds—apply to dry skin, p.r.n., or use flexible collodion when a flexible noncontracting film is desired.

SIDE EFFECTS
None.

INTERACTIONS
None significant.

NURSING CONSIDERATIONS
- Observe for inflammation or infection since protectants are occlusive layers that retain moisture, exclude air, and trap cutaneous bacteria.
- Skin should be cleaned daily or more often as needed.
- Protectants may be used alone, as vehicles for medications, or with other topical medications. Check with doctor.
- Camphor in flexible collodion is weakly antiseptic and antipruritic; may irritate and dry skin.
- Highly flammable; never use near flame.
- Keep container tightly closed so solvent won't evaporate.
- Toxic if taken internally.
- Avoid excessive inhalation of vapors.

Unmarked trade names available in the United States only.
♦ Also available in Canada.　　♦♦ Available in Canada only.

compound benzoin tincture
(10% benzoin in alcohol mixed with glycerin and water)
Benzoin Spray

INDICATIONS & DOSAGE
Demulcent and protectant: cutaneous ulcers, bedsores, cracked nipples, fissures of lips and anus—apply locally once daily or b.i.d.

SIDE EFFECTS
None.

INTERACTIONS
Skin: contact dermatitis.

NURSING CONSIDERATIONS
• Do not apply to acutely inflamed areas.
• Observe for inflammation or infection since protectants are occlusive layers that retain moisture, exclude air, and trap cutaneous bacteria.
• Skin should be cleaned daily or more often as needed.
• Protectants may be used alone, as vehicles for medications, or with other topical medications. Check with doctor.
• For demulcent and expectorant action in laryngitis or croup, use in boiling water and have patient inhale vapors.
• Spray is not intended for use as inhalant.
• Can be mixed with magnesium-aluminum hydroxide and applied on bedsores.

dexpanthenol
Panthoderm Cream♦
(dexpanthenol 2% in a water-miscible cream base), Panthoderm Lotion (dexpanthenol 2%, menthol 0.1%, and camphor 0.1%)

INDICATIONS & DOSAGE
Epithelial-bed stimulator in emollient base: itching, wounds, insect bites, poison ivy, poison oak, diaper rash, chafing, mild eczema, decubitus ulcers, dry lesions—apply topically, p.r.n.

SIDE EFFECTS
None.

INTERACTIONS
None significant.

NURSING CONSIDERATIONS
• Contraindicated in wounds of hemophilia patients.
• Before each new application *always* thoroughly cleanse affected area, removing all traces of previously applied medication. Observe for inflammation or infection.
• Dry lesions respond better than oozing lesions.
• May heal skin lesions in mild eczema and dermatoses.

glycerin
Corn Huskers Lotion (tragacanth 1 g, glycerin 30 ml, propylene glycol 10 ml)

INDICATIONS & DOSAGE
Emollient and lubricant: rectal tubes and catheters; dry skin, hands—apply p.r.n.

SIDE EFFECTS
None.

INTERACTIONS
None significant.

NURSING CONSIDERATIONS
• Applied undiluted to inflamed, dehydrated skin. Paradoxically, excessive use may dry the skin.
• Diluted with rose water, glycerin is useful for irritated or dry lips.

Italicized side effects are common or life-threatening.
*Liquid form contains alcohol.   **May contain tartrazine.

hydrophilic lotion
(white petrolatum 4.2 g, stearyl alcohol 4.2 g, methylparaben 0.004 g, propylparaben 0.002 g, sodium lauryl sulfate 0.167 g, propylene glycol 2 ml, perfume q.s., purified water)

INDICATIONS & DOSAGE
Protectant and emollient: dry skin, irritation—apply p.r.n.

SIDE EFFECTS
None.

INTERACTIONS
None significant.

NURSING CONSIDERATIONS
• Observe for inflammation or infection since protectants are occlusive layers that retain moisture, exclude air, and trap skin bacteria.
• Skin should be cleaned daily or more often as needed.
• Emollients and protectants may be used alone, as vehicles for medications, or with other topical medications. Check with doctor.

hydrophilic ointment
Cetaphil, Heb Cream Base, Multibase, Neobase, Unibase, Vanibase (methylparaben 0.025 g, propylparaben 0.015 g, stearyl alcohol 25 g, white petrolatum 25 g, propylene glycol 12 g, sodium lauryl sulfate 1 g, purified water)

INDICATIONS & DOSAGE
Protectant and emollient: dry skin, oozing lesions—apply p.r.n.

SIDE EFFECTS
None.

INTERACTIONS
None significant.

NURSING CONSIDERATIONS
• Easily removed with water.
• Use when little penetration of medicinal agent is desired.
• Observe for inflammation or infection since protectants are occlusive layers that retain moisture, exclude air, and trap skin bacteria.
• Skin should be cleaned daily or more often as needed.
• Emollients and protectants may be used alone, as vehicles for medications, or with other topical medications. Check with doctor.
• This nongreasy ointment is especially suited for application to hairy areas.

hydrophilic petrolatum
Aquaphor, Hydrosort, Plastibase Hydrophilic, Polysort (cholesterol 3 g, stearyl alcohol 3 g, white wax 8 g, white petrolatum 86 g)

INDICATIONS & DOSAGE
Protectant and emollient: dry skin, eczema, or psoriasis—mix with other medicinal ingredients as ordered, and apply p.r.n.

SIDE EFFECTS
None.

INTERACTIONS
None significant.

NURSING CONSIDERATIONS
• Not water-soluble; greasy.
• Observe for inflammation or infection since protectants are occlusive layers that retain moisture, exclude air, and trap skin bacteria.
• Skin should be cleaned daily or more often as needed.
• Emollients and protectants may be used alone, as vehicles for medications, or with other topical medications. Check with doctor.

Unmarked trade names available in the United States only.
♦ Also available in Canada.   ♦ ♦ Available in Canada only.

hydrous wool fat
Lanolin Lotion (stearic acid 2 g, triethanolamine 0.8 ml, light liquid petrolatum 10 ml, propylparaben 0.2 g, rose water)

hydrous wool fat and castor oil
(hydrous wool fat 25 g, castor oil 25 g, ceresin wax 5 g, polysorbate 60 5 g, white petrolatum)

INDICATIONS & DOSAGE
Protectant and emollient—apply hydrous wool fat p.r.n.
Protection against hydrocarbons, solvents, and cutting oils—apply hydrous wool fat and castor oil before exposure.

SIDE EFFECTS
Skin: allergic rash.

INTERACTIONS
None significant.

NURSING CONSIDERATIONS
• Contraindicated in hypersensitivity to lanolin.
• Don't confuse with anhydrous wool fat, which will dry skin if applied alone.
• Observe for inflammation or infection since protectants are occlusive layers that retain moisture, exclude air, and trap skin bacteria.
• Skin should be cleaned daily or more often as needed.
• Emollients and protectants may be used alone, as vehicles for medications, or with other topical medications. Check with doctor.

liquid petrolatum
Liquid Petrolatum, USP, Light Liquid Petrolatum, NF, Mineral Oil

INDICATIONS & DOSAGE
Protectant and emollient—apply locally, full strength, or diluted.

SIDE EFFECTS
None.

INTERACTIONS
None significant.

NURSING CONSIDERATIONS
• Occasionally used with other drugs.
• Available in two forms: light mineral oil and heavy mineral oil.
• Heavy mineral oil can be used internally as a laxative. Never use light mineral oil as a laxative. Mineral oil used as nose drops can cause lipid pneumonia.
• Observe for inflammation or infection since protectants are occlusive layers that retain moisture, exclude air, and trap skin bacteria.
• Skin should be cleaned daily or more often as needed.
• Emollients and protectants may be used alone, as vehicles for medications, or with other topical medications. Check with doctor.

methyl salicylate
Banalg, Baumodyne Gel and Ointment, Betula Oil, Gaultheria Oil, Sweet Birch Oil, Wintergreen Oil

INDICATIONS & DOSAGE
Counterirritant: minor pains of osteoarthritis, rheumatism, sprains, muscle and tendon soreness and tightness, lumbago, sciatica—
Adults: apply with gentle massage several times daily.
Not recommended for children.

SIDE EFFECTS
Skin: rash, irritation, burning, blistering.

INTERACTIONS
None significant.

NURSING CONSIDERATIONS
• Never apply directly, undiluted to skin.

Italicized side effects are common or life-threatening.
∗Liquid form contains alcohol.   ∗∗May contain tartrazine.

• Warning: as little as 4 ml ingested by children can cause fatal toxicity; in adults as little as 30 ml. Since GI absorption may be delayed, treat such ingestion with emetic lavage, then a saline cathartic. Continue lavage until no odor of methyl salicylate can be detected in the washings.

• Absorbed through skin; prolonged increased application can cause toxicity. Toxic effects include hyperpnea leading to respiratory alkalosis, nausea, vomiting, tinnitus, hyperpyrexia, and convulsions.

• Discontinue if rash or redness occurs. Consult doctor if pain or redness persists more than 10 days.

• Avoid getting near eyes, open wounds, mucous membranes.

• Do not use on sunburned membranes.

• Do not apply to broken or irritated skin.

• Do not wrap or bandage treated area.

• Store in tightly closed container.

---

oatmeal
Aveeno Colloidal, Aveeno Oilated Bath (with liquid petrolatum and hypoallergenic lanolin)

INDICATIONS & DOSAGE
Emollient and demulcent: local irritation—use as a lotion; 1 level tablespoon to a cup of warm water.
Skin irritation, pruritus, common dermatoses, sunburn, dry skin—
Adults: 1 packet in tub of warm water.
Children: 1 to 2 rounded tablespoons in 3″ to 4″ of bath water.
Infants: 2 or 3 level teaspoons, depending on size of bath.

SIDE EFFECTS
None.

INTERACTIONS
None significant.

NURSING CONSIDERATIONS
• Not to be ingested.
• Instruct patient to exercise caution to avoid slipping in tub.
• Avoid getting in eyes.

---

para-aminobenzoic acid
PABA♦, Pabagel♦, Pabanol♦, Pre-Sun♦, PreSun Gel, RV Paba Lipstick

INDICATIONS & DOSAGE
Topical protectant: sunburn protection, sun-sensitive skin, slow tanning—
Adults: apply evenly to dry skin; follow directions on various products for number and time of application, which vary from 2 to 6 hours; reapply after swimming.
Not recommended for children.

SIDE EFFECTS
Local: allergic reaction, irritation, sensitization.
Skin: photocontact dermatitis.

INTERACTIONS
None significant.

NURSING CONSIDERATIONS
• Contraindicated in hypersensitivity to any of the components and for persons with damaged or diseased skin.
• Discontinue if skin rash occurs.
• Encourage slow tanning and short exposure to sun.
• Avoid contact with eyes and lids.
• Avoid contact with open flame.
• May stain clothing.
• Observe for inflammation and infection since protectants produce an occlusive layer that retains perspiration, excludes air, and traps cutaneous bacteria, producing sites for anaerobic infections.

Unmarked trade names available in the United States only.
♦ Also available in Canada.   ♦♦ Available in Canada only.

petrolatum
Vaseline

INDICATIONS & DOSAGE
Topical protectant and emollient—use alone or with other drugs, as directed.

SIDE EFFECTS
None.

INTERACTIONS
None significant.

NURSING CONSIDERATIONS
• Stable, does not become rancid.
• Observe for inflammation or infection since protectants are occlusive layers that retain moisture, exclude air, and trap skin bacteria.
• Skin should be cleaned daily or more often as needed.
• Emollients and protectants may be used alone, as vehicles for medications, or with other topical medications. Check with doctor.

silicone
Silicone and Zinc Oxide Compound

INDICATIONS & DOSAGE
Topical protectant: dermatoses, diaper rash, decubitus ulcers—apply b.i.d. or t.i.d. in ointment.
Protection against water and corrosive chemicals—apply before exposure.

SIDE EFFECTS
None.

INTERACTIONS
None significant.

NURSING CONSIDERATIONS
• Protect eyes against spray.
• Very difficult to remove from skin; resistant to water and soap.
• Will not protect against oils or solvents.
• Observe for inflammation or infection since protectants are occlusive layers that retain moisture, exclude air, and trap cutaneous bacteria.
• Skin should be cleaned daily or more often as needed.
• Protectants may be used alone, as vehicles for medications, or with other topical medications. Check with doctor.

starch

INDICATIONS & DOSAGE
Demulcent: minor skin irritations, pruritus associated with common dermatoses—mix 2 cups of starch with 4 cups of water, add to tub of water, and soak affected area for 30 minutes.

SIDE EFFECTS
None.

INTERACTIONS
None significant.

NURSING CONSIDERATIONS
• Instruct patient to exercise caution to avoid slipping in tub.
• Use of cornstarch in intertriginous areas may promote or accelerate a yeast infection since yeast can feed on the sugar.

talc (magnesium silicate)

INDICATIONS & DOSAGE
Topical lubricant, protectant, drying agent, absorbent dusting powder: irritation, such as intertrigo prickly heat—sprinkle on affected areas p.r.n. for soothing and lubrication.

SIDE EFFECTS
None.

INTERACTIONS
None significant.

Italicized side effects are common or life-threatening.
∗Liquid form contains alcohol.   ∗∗May contain tartrazine.

NURSING CONSIDERATIONS
- Don't use on surgical gloves; causes granulation and adhesions in open wounds.
- Avoid dust entering eyes or inhalation of talc dust.
- Should not be used on open, weeping surfaces; it cakes and crusts.

urea or carbamide
Aquacare Dry Skin Cream and Lotion♦, Aquacare/HP Cream and Lotion♦, Aqua Lacten, Artra Ashy Skin Cream, Carmol Ten, Carmol Twenty, Gormel Cream, Nutraplus♦, Rea-Lo, Ultra-Mide, Uremol♦♦, Urtex♦♦

INDICATIONS & DOSAGE
Emollient: hard, dry skin on hands, elbows, or knees—
Adults: apply to affected area b.i.d. or t.i.d., particularly after exposure to sun or wind.
Not recommended for children.

SIDE EFFECTS
Skin: transient stinging when applied to irritated or fissured skin.

INTERACTIONS
None significant.

NURSING CONSIDERATIONS
- Contraindicated in viral skin diseases, or in impaired circulation. Use cautiously on face or broken skin.
- Wet skin before application. If irritation persists, discontinue.
- Avoid contact with eyes.
- Emollients produce an occlusive layer that retains perspiration, excludes air, and traps cutaneous bacteria, producing sites for anaerobic infections. Before each new application, *always* thoroughly cleanse affected area, removing all traces of previously applied medication. Observe for inflammation or infection.

vitamins A and D ointment
A&D, Balmex, Caldesene Medicated, Clocream, Comfortine, Desitin, Primaderm

INDICATIONS & DOSAGE
*Emollient, demulcent, and epithelial-bed stimulant: superficial burns, sunburn, abrasions, slow-healing lesions, chapped skin, diaper rash, skin care of infants or bedridden patients—*apply several times a day.

SIDE EFFECTS
Skin: irritation.

INTERACTIONS
None significant.

NURSING CONSIDERATIONS
- Discontinue if skin condition persists or irritation develops.
- Observe for inflammation or infection since emollients and demulcents are occlusive layers that retain moisture, exclude air, and trap cutaneous bacteria.
- Skin should be cleaned daily or more often as needed.
- Emollients and demulcents may be used alone, as vehicles for medications, or with other topical medications. Check with doctor.

zinc gelatin
Dome-Paste, Unna's Boot

INDICATIONS & DOSAGE
*Protectant: varicosities, lesions or injuries of lower legs or arms—*heat in hot bath till liquefied, clean skin, dust with talc, and apply gel with paint brush; make three layers, with gauze between each layer; retain 2 weeks. Dome-Paste, in 3″ and 4″ bandages, can be applied directly to arm or leg.

SIDE EFFECTS
None.

Unmarked trade names available in the United States only.
♦ Also available in Canada.   ♦♦ Available in Canada only.

INTERACTIONS
None significant.

NURSING CONSIDERATIONS
• Observe for inflammation and infection since protectants produce an occlusive layer that retains perspiration, excludes air, and traps cutaneous bacteria, producing sites for anaerobic infections. Before each new application *always* thoroughly cleanse affected area, removing all traces of previously applied medication.
• Zinc gelatin boot can be removed by unwinding outer bandage and soaking leg or arm in warm water until dressing floats off. Tell patient not to shower or take tub bath with zinc gelatin boot on leg.

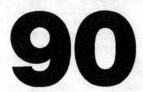

Keratolytics and caustics

cantharidin
dichloroacetic acid
podophyllum resin
resorcinol
resorcinol monoacetate
salicylic acid
silver nitrate
sulfur
sulfurated lime solution

MECHANISM OF ACTION
• Keratolytics soften keratin and loosen cornified epithelium, causing even viable cells to swell, soften, and dissolve.
• Caustics except podophyllum precipitate cell proteins, causing formation of a scab that eventually sloughs off.

Podophyllum inhibits cell division and other cellular processes, leading to the death of the cell.

COMBINATION PRODUCTS
ACNE-AID CREAM: sulfur 2.5%, resorcinol 1.25%, and parachlorometaxylenol 0.375% in a microporous cellulose base.
ACNE-DOME: colloidal sulfur 4% and resorcinol monoacetate 2% in an acid-mantle vehicle.
ACNOMEL CAKE♦: sulfur 4% and resorcinol 1% in a washable base.
ACNOMEL CREAM♦: sulfur 8%, resorcinol 2%, and alcohol 11% in a greaseless base.
BENSULFOID LOTION: fusion of finely divided sulfur (33% by weight) onto colloidal bentonite 6%, resorcinol 2%, zinc oxide 6%, thymol 0.5%, and alcohol 12% in a greaseless base.
CLEARASIL CREAM: benzoyl peroxide 10% and bentonite.

COMPOUND W WART REMOVER: salicylic acid 14%, acetic acid 11%, in castor oil, alcohol, ether, and collodion.
DUOFILM♦: salicylic acid 16.7% and lactic acid 16.7% in flexible collodion.
EXZIT: colloidal sulfur 4% and resorcinol monoacetate 2%.
FOSTEX CAKE♦: sulfur 2% and salicylic acid 2%.
FREEZONE CORN AND CALLUS REMOVER: salicylic acid 13.6%, zinc chloride 2.17%, in castor oil, and collodion, alcohol, and ether.
GETS-IT-LIQUID: salicylic acid, zinc chloride, and collodion in ether and alcohol.
REZAMID LOTION♦: sulfur 5%, resorcinol 2%, parachlorometaxylenol 0.5%, and alcohol 28.5% in a hydroalcoholic lotion base.
SULFORCIN BASE CREAM: sulfur 4% and resorcinol monoacetate 1.5%.

cantharidin
Cantharone

INDICATIONS & DOSAGE
Adults and children:
Molluscum contagiosum—coat each lesion. Repeat in a week on new or remaining lesions, this time covering with occlusive tape. Remove tape in 6 to 8 hours.
Palpebral warts—apply, leave lesion uncovered.
Plantar warts—pare away keratin, apply generously to affected area, allow to dry, apply protective padding, cover with nonporous tape for a week, then

---

debride. Repeat 3 times, if necessary, on large lesions.

Removal of ordinary and periungual warts and other benign epithelial growths—apply directly to lesion and cover completely. Allow to dry, then cover with nonporous adhesive tape. Remove tape in 24 hours (or less if extreme pain) and replace with loose bandage. Reapply, if necessary.

SIDE EFFECTS
Skin: annular warts, burning, tingling, extreme tenderness, inflammation.

INTERACTIONS
None significant.

NURSING CONSIDERATIONS
• If dropped on normal skin, remove immediately with acetone, alcohol, or tape remover. Scrub with warm, soapy water, and rinse well, as blistering of skin may result.
• If dropped on mucous membranes or in eyes, flush well with water to remove precipitated collodion, then continue to flush with water for 15 minutes.
• Treat only one or two lesions initially to test patient's sensitivity.
• Stop treatment if severe inflammation develops.
• If application causes burning, tenderness, or tingling, remove tape and soak area in cool water for 10 to 15 minutes; repeat, if necessary.
• If annular warts develop, assure patient that lesions are superficial; re-treat or substitute another procedure.
• Does not affect tissue layers below the epidermis and leaves no scar.
• Treatment should be supervised by a doctor.

dichloroacetic acid
Bichloracetic Acid

INDICATIONS & DOSAGE
All types of verrucae; calluses, corns; xanthelasma; ingrown toenails; cysts and benign erosion of the cervix; sebaceous adenoma; infectious granuloma; tattoo marks; epistaxis; spider nevi; tonsil tabs—
Adults: applied only by doctor at his discretion.

SIDE EFFECTS
Local: irritation, inflammation of normal skin.

INTERACTIONS
None significant.

NURSING CONSIDERATIONS
• Contraindicated for treatment of malignant or premalignant lesions.
• Protect adjacent areas with petrolatum, especially when using 50% solutions.
• Sodium bicarbonate is local antidote.
• Thoroughly dry area before application.
• Warn patient that when solution is applied, treated area will turn from white to red in about 4 hours.
• Peeling of skin usually is noticed in 4 days and is completed in a week.
• If acid comes in contact with normal skin, wipe off with cotton gauze and flush area with water.

podophyllum resin
Podoben

INDICATIONS & DOSAGE
Venereal warts and granuloma inguinale—
Adults: apply podophyllum resin preparation to the lesion, cover with waxed paper, and bandage. Leave covered for 8 to 12 hours, then wash lesion to remove medication. Repeat at weekly intervals.

SIDE EFFECTS
Blood: thrombocytopenia, leukopenia when systemically absorbed.
Local: irritation of normal skin.

Italicized side effects are common or life-threatening.
*Liquid form contains alcohol.   **May contain tartrazine.

Other: peripheral neuropathy when systemically absorbed.

INTERACTIONS
Other keratolytics: may cause extensive damage to the skin. Do not use together.

NURSING CONSIDERATIONS
• Use in pregnancy is controversial; may be harmful to fetus.
• Resin is irritating and cytotoxic, and should not be applied to normal skin. Petrolatum can be applied to adjacent areas to protect them during treatment.
• Should be applied only by a doctor because of toxicity.
• Do not use on extensive areas or for prolonged therapy; may be absorbed systemically.
• Warn patient that soreness from local irritation may develop 12 to 48 hours after treatment.

resorcinol

resorcinol monoacetate
Euresol, Resorcin

INDICATIONS & DOSAGE
Acute eczema, urticaria, and other inflammatory skin diseases (1% or 2% concentration in alcohol); acne or seborrhea (5% lotion or 10% soap liniment for scalp); chronic eczema, psoriasis (2% to 10% ointment); acne scarring (45% peeling paste)—
Adults and children: apply as directed.

SIDE EFFECTS
Skin: irritation, moderate erythema or scaling.
Other: darkening of light hair (resorcinol only).

INTERACTIONS
None significant.

NURSING CONSIDERATIONS
• Do not use preparations on or near eyes.
• If skin irritation persists, discontinue medication.
• Apply lotion with cotton ball to affected area.
• When applying the peeling paste, closely observe the patient and site of application until paste is removed.
• Use carefully with topical acne preparations because of local irritation.

salicylic acid
Calicylic, Keralyt♦, Salactic Liquifilm, Salonil

INDICATIONS & DOSAGE
Superficial fungal infections, acne, psoriasis, seborrheic dermatitis, other scaling dermatoses, hyperkeratosis, calluses, warts—
Adults and children: apply to affected area and place under occlusion at night.

SIDE EFFECTS
Skin: irritation, drying.
Other: salicylism with percutaneous absorption.

INTERACTIONS
Iodine, iron salts, and oxidizing substances: incompatible. Don't use together.

NURSING CONSIDERATIONS
• Use with caution in patients with diabetes or peripheral vascular disease. The skin inflammation that may result is difficult to treat. Limit use for children under 12 years. (Do not exceed 1 oz in 24 hours.)
• Avoid contact with eyes and mucous membranes.
• If excessive skin drying or irritation occurs, apply a bland cream or lotion.
• Rinse hands after application (unless they are being treated).
• Skin should be hydrated for at least 5

minutes before treatment and washed the morning after treatment.
- Most preparations are occlusive, which increases percutaneous absorption. Therefore, do not use on large surface areas for prolonged periods.
- Not for use on broken, inflamed, or ulcerated areas.
- Also has bacteristatic and fungistatic properties.

silver nitrate

INDICATIONS & DOSAGE
Cauterization of mucous membranes, fissures, aphthous lesions (5% to 10% solution); cauterization of granulomatous tissues and warts (solid form)—
Adults and children: applied only by doctor at his discretion.

SIDE EFFECTS
Local: *argyria (permanent silver discoloration of skin).*

INTERACTIONS
None significant.

NURSING CONSIDERATIONS
- May cause burns. Avoid accidental contact with skin and eyes. If accidental contact with skin occurs, flush with water for at least 15 minutes; accidental contact with eyes, call doctor at once.
- Not to be ingested; may cause altered respiration, coma, convulsions, paralysis, and even death. If ingested, call doctor at once. Give 1 tablespoon salt in warm water; repeat until emesis is clear. Or have patient drink milk or beaten egg whites mixed in warm water. Keep patient warm and lying down.
- Warn that silver nitrate stains skin and clothing.
- Silver nitrate pencils must be moistened with water before use.
- In low concentrations, as a wet dressing, is used as a local anti-infective in treatment of burn patients.

sulfur
Acne-Aid♦, Acnomead, Bensulfoid, Liquimat, Postacne♦, Transact, Xerac

INDICATIONS & DOSAGE
Acne, ringworm, psoriasis, seborrheic dermatitis, chigger infestation, scabies, favus, staphylococcal folliculitis—
Adults and children: apply preparation to affected areas b.i.d., t.i.d., or as directed.

SIDE EFFECTS
Local: excessive drying of skin, blackheads, contact dermatitis.

INTERACTIONS
None significant.

NURSING CONSIDERATIONS
- Prolonged use may cause severe contact dermatitis.
- When initiating therapy, use sparingly for patients with sensitive skin.
- Avoid contact with eyes. If accidental contact occurs, flush with water.
- Wash skin thoroughly before application. Tell patient that tingling sensation may be felt upon application.
- Skin is more reactive to drug in cold, dry climates, so decrease frequency of application. In hot, humid climates, increase frequency of application.
- Do not use on same area with topical acne preparation or preparations containing a peeling agent (for example, benzoyl peroxide); may cause severe irritation.
- Do not use on same area with any mercury-containing preparation; may cause a foul odor, irritate the skin, or stain skin black.
- Has antiseptic and parasiticide properties also.

---

sulfurated lime solution
Vlem-Dome, Vleminckx's solution

INDICATIONS & DOSAGE
Acne vulgaris, seborrhea—
Adults and children: dilute 1 packet in 1 pint hot water and apply as hot dressing for 15 to 20 minutes daily.
Generalized furunculosis—
Adults and children: add 30 to 60 ml solution to bath water.

SIDE EFFECTS
Local: may cause excessive drying of skin.

INTERACTIONS
None significant.

NURSING CONSIDERATIONS
• Discontinue use if excessive drying or skin irritation develops.
• Avoid contact with jewelry, metallic objects, or clothing.
• Avoid getting solution in eyes, nose, or mouth.
• Fumes are irritating and malodorous (rotten eggs). Ventilate adequately.
• Do not use in same area with topical acne preparations; may cause severe irritation.
• Do not use in same area with mercury-containing preparations; may cause a foul odor, irritate skin, or turn skin black.

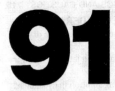

Miscellaneous dermatomucosal agents

ammoniated mercury
anthralin
benzoyl peroxide
collagenase
dextranomer
fluorouracil
hydroquinone
isotretinoin
methoxsalen
scarlet red
selenium sulfide
sutilains
tretinoin (vitamin A acid, retinoic
   acid)

MECHANISM OF ACTION

- Ammoniated mercury (Hg^{++}) inhibits sulfhydryl enzymes and combines with amino and other chemical groups.
- Anthralin acts as a local antieczematous and antipsoriatic irritant.
- Benzoyl peroxide has antimicrobial and keratolytic activity.
- Collagenase is an enzymatic debriding agent that digests undenatured collagen fibers in necrotic tissue and removes substrates for bacterial proliferation. It facilitates access to infected areas by antibiotics, antibodies, and leukocytes.
- Dextranomer is a synthetic polymer that aids in granulation.
- Fluorouracil acts as an antimetabolite. It interferes with DNA synthesis by inhibiting thymidylate synthetase.
- Hydroquinone inhibits tyrosinase, preventing the conversion of tyrosine to melanin.
- Methoxsalen is a potent photosensitizer of the skin that promotes melanin formation by facilitating the action of ultraviolet light. It does not promote pigmentation in the absence of light.
- Scarlet red stimulates proliferation of the basal layer of the skin.
- Selenium sulfide has irritant, antibacterial, and antifungal properties.
- Sutilains is a proteolytic enzyme that selectively digests necrotic tissue.
- Tretinoin (vitamin A acid) and isotretinoin are potent drying and peeling agents whose mechanisms of action are unknown.

COMBINATION PRODUCTS

EMERSAL: ammoniated mercury 5% and salicylic acid 2.5%.
LOROXIDE♦: benzoyl peroxide 5.5% and chlorhydroxyquinoline 0.25%.
LOROXIDE HC♦: benzoyl peroxide 5.5%, chlorhydroxyquinoline 0.25%, and hydrocortisone 0.5%.
SULFOXYL REGULAR: benzoyl peroxide 5% and sulfur 2%.
SULFOXYL STRONG: benzoyl peroxide 10% and sulfur 5%.
VANOXIDE♦: benzoyl peroxide 5% and chlorhydroxyquinoline 0.25%.
VANOXIDE-HC♦: benzoyl peroxide 5%, chlorhydroxyquinoline 0.25%, and hydrocortisone 0.5%.

---

ammoniated mercury

INDICATIONS & DOSAGE

Psoriasis, seborrheic dermatitis, impetigo contagiosa, tinea capitis, and favus—
Adults and children: apply to affected area b.i.d. or t.i.d.

Italicized side effects are common or life-threatening.
*Liquid form contains alcohol.   **May contain tartrazine.

SIDE EFFECTS
Systemic: acrodynia, mercury poisoning.

INTERACTIONS
None significant.

NURSING CONSIDERATIONS
• Don't apply to large areas of body or use for extended periods of time. Mercury poisoning could result. Signs of mercury poisoning include cloudy urine; headache; dizziness; irritation, soreness, or swelling of gums; nausea; skin rash.
• Don't apply to highly inflamed skin, sunburn, or open wounds.
• Has no odor. Doesn't stain.
• Don't use in same area with topical preparations containing sulfur; may cause foul odor or skin irritation or may stain skin black.

---

anthralin
Anthra-Derm

INDICATIONS & DOSAGE
Psoriasis, chronic dermatitis—
Adults and children: apply thinly daily or b.i.d. Concentrations range from 0.1% to 1%; start with lowest and increase, if necessary.

SIDE EFFECTS
GU: possible renal toxicity.
Skin: erythema on healthy skin.

INTERACTIONS
None significant.

NURSING CONSIDERATIONS
• Contraindicated in renal damage. Should not be used on acute or inflammatory eruptions.
• Partial excretion in urine may cause renal irritation, casts, and albuminuria. Check urine weekly.
• Discontinue if allergic reaction, pustular folliculitis, or renal irritation occurs.

• Don't get in eyes. May cause conjunctivitis, keratitis, corneal opacity.
• Wear plastic gloves to apply anthralin; wash hands thoroughly after using.
• May cause a temporary yellow-brown discoloration to hair, skin, and alkaline urine. May stain clothing.
• Avoid applying medication to normal skin by coating the area surrounding the lesion with petrolatum.

---

benzoyl peroxide
Benoxyl♦, Benzac, Benzagel♦, Clear by Design, Desquam-X♦♦, Dry and Clear, Oxy-5, Oxy-10, OxyCover, Panoxyl♦, Persadox, Persadox HP, Persa-Gel, Xerac BP

INDICATIONS & DOSAGE
Adjunctive treatment of acne—
Adults and children: apply once daily or b.i.d.

SIDE EFFECTS
Skin: transient stinging on application, feeling of warmth, painful irritation.

INTERACTIONS
Tretinoin: reduced effectiveness of benzoyl peroxide. Do not use together.

NURSING CONSIDERATIONS
• Contraindicated in sensitivity to any of the ingredients.
• Don't use on eyelids, mucous membranes, denuded or highly inflamed skin.
• Dryness, redness, peeling should occur 3 to 4 days after starting treatment. If these common reactions cause considerable discomfort, discontinue temporarily until they subside.
• If painful irritation develops, discontinue use.
• Cleanser (4%) may cause bleaching of hair or colored fabric.

---

collagenase
Biozyme-C, Santyl

INDICATIONS & DOSAGE
Debridement of dermal ulcers and severely burned areas—
Adults and children: apply ointment (250 units/g) to lesion daily or every other day.

SIDE EFFECTS
Skin: slight erythema of surrounding area, especially if ointment is not confined to lesion.
Other: hypersensitivity reactions.

INTERACTIONS
Detergents; hexachlorophene; antiseptics (especially those containing heavy metal ions, such as mercury or silver); iodine; soaks or acidic solutions containing metal ions, such as aluminum acetate (Burow's solution): decreased enzymatic activity. Do not use together.

NURSING CONSIDERATIONS
• Use with caution in debilitated patients, since debriding enzymes may increase risk of bacteremia; watch for signs of systemic infection.
• Before application, cleanse lesion with gauze saturated in normal saline, neutral buffer solution, or hydrogen peroxide; use topical antibacterial agent (such as neomycin-bacitracin-polymyxin B) if infection is present. Apply to lesion in powder form before using collagenase. If infection persists, discontinue collagenase until infection is healed. Confine collagenase ointment to area of lesion (Lassar's paste may protect surrounding skin). Apply ointment in thin layers to assure contact with necrotic tissue and complete wound coverage; apply collagenase ointment with tongue depressor on deep wounds; with gauze on shallow wounds. Remove any debris that comes off easily. Remove excess ointment, and cover wound with sterile gauze pad.

• Discontinue when sufficient debridement has occurred.
• Observe wound to monitor progress of therapy. Appearance of granulation may indicate effectiveness. Notify doctor if inflammation or color of drainage indicates any spread of infection.
• Watch for symptoms of protein sensitization (long-term therapy).
• If enzymatic action must be stopped for any reason, apply Burow's solution.
• Avoid getting ointment in eyes. If this occurs, flush with water at once.
• Protect drug from heat.

dextranomer
Debrisan

INDICATIONS & DOSAGE
To clean secreting wounds, such as venous stasis and decubitus ulcers, infected surgical wounds, and burns—
Adults and children: apply to affected area daily, b.i.d., or more often, p.r.n. Apply to ⅛″ or ¼″ thickness, and cover with sterile gauze pad.

SIDE EFFECTS
Skin: temporary pain.

INTERACTIONS
Ointment bases, such as Vaseline: negates action of dextranomer. Don't mix together.

NURSING CONSIDERATIONS
• Before application, cleanse wound with sterile water, saline solution, or other appropriate solution. Do not dry.
• Pack cratered wounds with beads, allowing room for expansion of beads. Cover with dressing to hold beads in place.
• When saturated, medication turns gray-yellow and should be removed.
• To remove, irrigate with sterile water, saline solution, or other cleansing solution.
• Dextranomer beads are not effective in cleaning nonsecreting wounds. When

the wound has healed to the point where it is no longer exuding, treatment should be discontinued.
• Dextranomer beads are hydrophilic; each gram of beads can absorb 4 ml of exudate.
• Keep drug away from moisture; store in tightly closed container.
• Avoid contact with eyes.
• Be careful not to spill beads onto floor, as the resultant slipperiness can be a safety hazard.

fluorouracil
Efudex♦, Fluoroplex♦

INDICATIONS & DOSAGE
Multiple actinic or solar keratoses; superficial basal cell carcinoma—
Adults and children: apply cream (5%) or solution (2% or 5%) b.i.d.

SIDE EFFECTS
Skin: erythema, pain, burning, scaling, pruritus, hyperpigmentation, dermatitis, soreness, suppuration, swelling.

INTERACTIONS
None significant.

NURSING CONSIDERATIONS
• Wash hands immediately after handling medication.
• Avoid use with occlusive dressings.
• Patient should avoid prolonged exposure to sunlight or ultraviolet light.
• Apply with caution near eyes, nose, and mouth.
• Warn patient that treated area may be unsightly during therapy and for several weeks after therapy is stopped. Complete healing may not occur until 1 or 2 months after treatment is stopped.
• Ingestion and systemic absorption may cause leukopenia, thrombocytopenia, stomatitis, diarrhea, or GI ulceration, bleeding, and hemorrhage.
• Topical application to large ulcerated areas may cause systemic toxicity.

• For basal cell carcinoma, use 5% strength.

hydroquinone
Artra Skin Tone Cream, Derma-Blanch, Eldopaque♦, Eldopaque-Forte♦ Eldoquin♦, Eldoquin Forte♦, Esoterica Medicated Cream, Golden Peacock, HQC Kit, Melanex, Quinnone

INDICATIONS & DOSAGE
Bleaching of blemished skin, lentigo, chloasma, freckles, old-age spots, and other skin conditions due to increased melanin—
Adults and children 12 years and over: apply 2% to 4% concentration daily or b.i.d.

SIDE EFFECTS
Skin: mild irritation, sensitization, rash.

INTERACTIONS
None significant.

NURSING CONSIDERATIONS
• Contraindicated in patients with prickly heat, sunburn, irritated skin; or as depilatory.
• Don't use near eyes.
• If rash or irritation develops, discontinue therapy.
• Sensitivity can be tested by applying a small amount of low-concentration medication on skin before treatment is started. Allergic reactions should appear within 24 hours.
• Doesn't cause permanent depigmentation.
• Advise patient to use opaque sunscreen when outdoors since sun can darken lesions faster than hydroquinone can lighten them.

isotretinoin
Accutane

INDICATIONS & DOSAGE
Severe cystic acne unresponsive to conventional therapy—
Adults and adolescents: 1 to 2 mg/kg daily P.O. given in 2 divided doses and continued for 15 to 20 weeks.

SIDE EFFECTS
Blood: anemia, elevated platelet count.
CNS: headache, fatigue.
EENT: *conjunctivitis*
GI: nonspecific gastrointestinal symptoms.
Hepatic: elevated SGOT, SPGT, alkaline phosphatase.
Skin: *cheilosis (lip inflammation), rash, dry skin,* peeling of palms and toes, skin infection, photosensitivity.
Other: *hypertriglyceridemia, musculoskeletal pain,* thinning of hair.

INTERACTIONS
Vitamin A and vitamin supplements containing vitamin A: increase in isotretinoin's toxic effects. Don't use together.

NURSING CONSIDERATIONS
• Contraindicated in patients hypersensitive to parabens, since parabens are used as a preservative in the medication.
• Isotretinoin shouldn't be used in women of childbearing age unless contraception is used during treatment and for 1 month posttreatment.
• Perform blood lipid studies before therapy begins and then at regular intervals until response to drug is established, usually about 4 weeks.
• If a second course of therapy is needed, it shouldn't be started until at least 8 weeks after the completion of the first course because patients may continue to improve after discontinuing the drug.
• Most adverse reactions appear to be dose related, with most occurring at doses greater than 1 mg/kg daily. They are generally reversible when therapy is discontinued.

methoxsalen
Oxsoralen♦

INDICATIONS & DOSAGE
Protect against sunburn, enhance pigmentation, and induce repigmentation in vitiligo—
Adults and children over 12 years: for small, well-defined lesions, apply topically weekly or less often and expose to ultraviolet A light gradually, as directed.

SIDE EFFECTS
CNS: nervousness, insomnia, mental depression.
GI: discomfort, nausea, diarrhea.
Hepatic: hepatic toxicity.
Skin: edema, erythema, painful blistering, burning, peeling, *photosensitivity.*

INTERACTIONS
Photosensitizing agents: do not use together.

NURSING CONSIDERATIONS
• Contraindicated in hepatic insufficiency, porphyria, acute systemic lupus erythematosus, and hydromorphic, polymorphic light eruptions. Use with caution in familial history of sunlight allergy, GI diseases, chronic infection.
• Regulate therapy carefully. Overdosage or overexposure to light can cause serious burning or blistering.
• Topical treatment should be directly supervised by a doctor.
• When applied topically to face or hands, patient should protect area from light (except during treatment exposure) for 24 hours after therapy.
• Protect eyes and lips during light exposure treatments.
• Monthly liver function tests should

be done on patients with vitiligo (especially at beginning of therapy).
• Significant changes require 6 to 9 months of therapy.

scarlet red
Decubitex Ointment
(also contains peruvian balsam, zinc oxide, starch, castor oil, petrolatum, xantham gum, sodium propionate, methylparaben, propylparaben, propylene glycol, and water)

INDICATIONS & DOSAGE
Aid in management of decubitus ulcers—
Adults and children: pour a small amount of 3% hydrogen peroxide or normal saline solution on the affected area. Cleanse thoroughly and apply ointment. Cover with dry sterile gauze.

SIDE EFFECTS
Systemic: gastroenteritis.

INTERACTIONS
None significant.

NURSING CONSIDERATIONS
• Change dressing twice daily, especially where seeping and secretions are present.
• Ointment should be in contact with newly forming tissue for maximum therapeutic results. Wound should be allowed to "breathe" by being loosely covered.
• Using excess ointment or covering the wound completely will retard wound healing.
• Use ointment until healing is complete.
• In advanced decubitus ulcers, use normal saline solution rather than hydrogen peroxide.

selenium sulfide
Exsel♦, Iosel 250, Selsun♦, Sul-Blue

INDICATIONS & DOSAGE
Dandruff, seborrheic scalp dermatitis—
Adults and children: massage 1 to 2 teaspoonfuls into clean, wet scalp. Leave on for 2 to 3 minutes. Rinse thoroughly, and repeat application. Apply twice weekly for 2 weeks, then once a week for 2 weeks, or as often as needed to maintain control.

SIDE EFFECTS
Skin: oily or dry scalp and hair, hair discoloration, hair loss, sensitivity reactions.

INTERACTIONS
None significant.

NURSING CONSIDERATIONS
• Contraindicated in sulfur hypersensitivity.
• Use with caution around areas of acute inflammation or exudation to avoid increased absorption.
• If sensitivity reactions occur, discontinue use.
• Reduce or prevent hair discoloration by thorough rinsing after treatment.
• Avoid contact with eyes.
• Highly toxic if ingested.
• Wash hands carefully after handling.
• Protect from heat.

sutilains
Travase♦

INDICATIONS & DOSAGE
Debridement of second- and third-degree burns, adjunctive debridement of decubitus ulcers, pyogenic wounds, or ulcers resulting from peripheral vascular disease—
Adults and children: apply thinly to area extending ¼″ to ½″ beyond area to be debrided. Cover with loose wet dressing t.i.d. or q.i.d.

SIDE EFFECTS
CNS: local paresthesias.
Skin: mild pain, bleeding, transient dermatitis.

INTERACTIONS
Detergents, anti-infectives (such as benzalkonium chloride, hexachlorophene, iodine, and nitrofurazone), and compounds containing metallic ions (such as silver nitrate and thimerosal): adversely affected enzymatic activity. Do not use together.

NURSING CONSIDERATIONS
• Contraindicated in wounds involving major body cavities or containing exposed nerves or nerve tissue, fungating neoplastic ulcers, wounds in women of childbearing age, persons having limited cardiac or pulmonary reserves.
• Use cautiously near eyes. If accidental contact occurs, flush eyes repeatedly with large amounts of normal saline solution or sterile water.
• Before application, cleanse and irrigate affected area with normal saline solution or sterile water to remove antiseptic or heavy metal antibacterial agents.
• May give mild analgesic to reduce painful reactions, but discontinue if pain is severe; also discontinue if bleeding or dermatitis occurs.
• For best response, keep affected area moist.
• In concomitant use of topical antimicrobial agent, apply sutilains first.
• Store at 35.6° to 50° F. (2° to 10° C.). Keep in refrigerator.

tretinoin (vitamin A acid, retinoic acid)

INDICATIONS & DOSAGE
Acne vulgaris (especially grades I, II, and III)—

Adults and children: cleanse affected area and lightly apply solution once daily at bedtime.

SIDE EFFECTS
Skin: *feeling of warmth, slight stinging, local erythema, peeling at site,* chapping and swelling, blistering and crusting, temporary hyperpigmentation or hypopigmentation.

INTERACTIONS
None significant.

NURSING CONSIDERATIONS
• Contraindicated in hypersensitivity to any tretinoin component. Use with caution in eczema.
• If severe local irritation develops, discontinue temporarily and readjust dosage when application is resumed.
• Some redness and scaling are normal reactions.
• Beneficial effects should be seen within 6 weeks of treatment.
• When treatment is stopped, relapses generally occur within 3 to 6 weeks.
• Patient should wash face with a mild soap no more than two or three times a day. Warn against using strong or medicated cosmetics, soaps, or other skin cleansers.
• Exposure to sunlight or ultraviolet rays should be minimal during treatment. If patient is sunburned, delay therapy until sunburn subsides.
• Avoid contact with eyes, mouth, and mucous membranes.
• Warn patient not to use topical products containing alcohol, astringents, spices, and lime. These may interfere with action of tretinoin.
• Warn patient to wait until skin is completely dry before applying tretinoin.

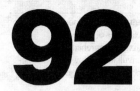

Local anesthetics

bupivacaine hydrochloride
chloroprocaine hydrochloride
dibucaine hydrochloride
etidocaine hydrochloride
lidocaine hydrochloride
mepivacaine hydrochloride
piperocaine hydrochloride
prilocaine hydrochloride
procaine hydrochloride
tetracaine hydrochloride

MECHANISM OF ACTION
Local anesthetics block depolarization by interfering with sodium-potassium exchange across the nerve-cell membrane, preventing generation and conduction of the nerve impulse.

When local anesthetics are combined with epinephrine, anesthesia is prolonged because the rate of absorption decreases. Vasoconstriction also helps control local bleeding.

COMBINATION PRODUCTS
None, although epinephrine is added to some solutions to prolong effect.

---

bupivacaine hydrochloride
Marcaine♦, Sensorcaine

INDICATIONS & DOSAGE
Available with or without epinephrine. Dosages given are for drug *without* epinephrine.
Epidural:

Sol.	Vol. (ml)	Dose (mg)
0.75%	10 to 20	75 to 150
0.50%	10 to 20	50 to 100
0.25%	10 to 20	25 to 50

Caudal:

Sol.	Vol. (ml)	Dose (mg)
0.50%	15 to 30	75 to 150
0.25%	15 to 30	37.5 to 75

Peripheral nerve block:

Sol.	Vol. (ml)	Dose (mg)
0.50%	5 to 80	25 to 400 (max.)

May repeat dose q 3 hours. Dose and interval may be increased with epinephrine. Maximum 400 mg daily.

SIDE EFFECTS
Skin: dermatologic reactions.
Other: edema, status asthmaticus, or *anaphylaxis* and anaphylactoid reactions.
Side effects of local anesthetics generally result from high blood levels of the drug. Examples of these are:
CNS: anxiety, apprehension, nervousness, convulsions followed by drowsiness, unconsciousness, and *respiratory arrest*.
CV: myocardial depression, *arrhythmias, cardiac arrest*.
EENT: blurred vision.
GI: nausea, vomiting.

INTERACTIONS
Chloroform, halothane, cyclopropane, trichloroethylene, and related drugs: cardiac arrhythmias may occur when used with bupivacaine *with* epinephrine. Use with extreme caution.
MAO inhibitors, tricyclic antidepressants: severe, sustained hypertension may occur when used with bupivacaine *with* epinephrine. Use with extreme caution.

Unmarked trade names available in the United States only.
♦ Also available in Canada. ♦ ♦ Available in Canada only.

NURSING CONSIDERATIONS
• Contraindicated in children under 12 years and for spinal, paracervical block, or topical anesthesia. Use cautiously in debilitated, elderly, or acutely ill patients; and in patients with severe hepatic disease or drug allergies.
• Use solutions with epinephrine cautiously in cardiovascular disorders and in body areas with limited blood supply (ears, nose, fingers, toes).
• Keep resuscitative equipment and drugs available.
• Don't use solution with preservatives for caudal or epidural block.
• Onset in 4 to 17 minutes; duration 3 to 6 hours.
• Causes less fetal depression than other local anesthetics.
• Discard partially used vials without preservatives.

---

chloroprocaine hydrochloride
Nesacaine (for infiltration and regional anesthesia), Nesacaine-CE (for caudal and epidural anesthesia)

INDICATIONS & DOSAGE
Available only without epinephrine.
Infiltration and nerve block:

Sol.	Vol. (ml)	Dose (mg)
1%	3 to 20	30 to 200
2%	2 to 40	20 to 400

Caudal and epidural:

Sol.	Vol. (ml)	Dose (mg)
2% to 3%	15 to 25	300 to 750

May repeat with smaller doses q 40 to 50 minutes. Dose and interval may be increased with epinephrine. Maximum adult dose 800 mg, or 1 g when mixed with epinephrine.

SIDE EFFECTS
Skin: dermatologic reactions.
Other: edema, status asthmaticus, or *anaphylaxis* and anaphylactoid reactions.
Side effects of local anesthetics generally result from high blood levels of the drug. Examples of these are:
CNS: anxiety, apprehension, nervousness, convulsions followed by drowsiness, unconsciousness, and *respiratory arrest.*
CV: myocardial depression, *arrhythmias, cardiac arrest.*
EENT: blurred vision.
GI: nausea, vomiting.

INTERACTIONS
None significant.

NURSING CONSIDERATIONS
• Contraindicated in hypersensitivity to procaine, tetracaine, or other para-aminobenzoic acid derivatives, and for spinal or topical anesthesia. Epidural and caudal contraindicated in CNS disease. Use cautiously in debilitated, elderly, or acutely ill patients; children; and in patients with drug allergies, paracervical block, or cardiovascular disease.
• A 3-ml test dose should be injected at least 10 minutes before giving total dose to check for intravascular or subarachnoid injection. Motor paralysis and extensive sensory anesthesia indicate subarachnoid injection.
• Repeat the test dose if patient is moved in a way that might displace the epidural catheter.
• At least 5 minutes should elapse after each test before proceeding further.
• Don't use solution with preservatives for caudal or epidural block.
• Don't use discolored solution.
• Keep resuscitative equipment and drugs available.
• Duration 30 to 60 minutes.
• Discard partially used vials without preservatives.

---

dibucaine hydrochloride
Nupercaine

INDICATIONS & DOSAGE
Available only without epinephrine.

Spinal anesthesia:
Perineum and lower limbs

Sol.	Vol. (ml)	Dose (mg)
0.5%	0.5 to 1	2.5 to 5

Lower abdomen

Sol.	Vol. (ml)	Dose (mg)
0.5%	1 to 1.5	5 to 7.5

Upper abdomen

Sol.	Vol. (ml)	Dose (mg)
0.5%	2	10

Spinal anesthesia:
Lower extremities as high as pelvis

Sol.	Vol. (ml)	Dose (mg)
1:1,500	6	4

Lower abdomen

Sol.	Vol. (ml)	Dose (mg)
1:1,500	10 to 15	6.67 to 10

Upper abdomen

Sol.	Vol. (ml)	Dose (mg)
1:1,500	15 to 18	10 to 12

SIDE EFFECTS
Skin: dermatologic reactions.
Other: edema, status asthmaticus, or *anaphylaxis* and anaphylactoid reactions.
Side effects of local anesthetics generally result from high blood levels of the drug. Examples of these are:
CNS: anxiety, apprehension, nervousness, convulsions followed by drowsiness, unconsciousness, and *respiratory arrest*.
CV: myocardial depression, *arrhythmias, cardiac arrest*.
EENT: blurred vision.
GI: nausea, vomiting.

INTERACTIONS
None significant.

NURSING CONSIDERATIONS
• Contraindicated in cerebrospinal disease, septicemia, pernicious anemia with spinal cord symptoms, arthritis, pyogenic skin infection in puncture area. Use cautiously in hysteria, chronic backache, headache of long duration, migraine, shock, hypotension, leaking spinal fluid, cardiac decompensation, pleural effusions, increased abdominal pressure, possibility of hemorrhage.
• Low spinal solution contraindicated in cesarean section or in presence of blood when doing lumbar puncture. Use low spinal solutions cautiously in patients with cardiac or neurologic disease or back problems and in uncooperative or hysterical patients.
• Use solutions with epinephrine cautiously in cardiovascular disorders and in body areas with limited blood supply (ears, nose, fingers, toes).
• Keep resuscitative equipment and drugs available.
• Don't use for nerve block or infiltration.
• Don't use discolored solution.
• Used primarily for spinal block and as topical anesthetic.
• Onset in 10 to 15 minutes; duration 6 hours.
• Discard partially used vials without preservatives.

etidocaine hydrochloride
Duranest

INDICATIONS & DOSAGE
Available with or without epinephrine. Doses cited are for drug *with* epinephrine.
Dose and interval may be decreased without epinephrine.

Infiltration:

Sol.	Vol. (ml)	Dose (mg)
0.5%	1 to 80	5 to 400

Peripheral nerve block:

Sol.	Vol. (ml)	Dose (mg)
0.5%	5 to 80	25 to 400
1%	5 to 40	50 to 400

Central neural block:
Lower limbs, cesarean section, lumbar peridural

Sol.	Vol. (ml)	Dose (mg)
1%	10 to 30	100 to 300
1.5%	10 to 20	150 to 300

Vaginal

Sol.	Vol. (ml)	Dose (mg)
0.5%	10 to 30	50 to 150
1%	5 to 20	50 to 200

Caudal:

Sol.	Vol. (ml)	Dose (mg)
0.5%	10 to 30	50 to 150
1%	10 to 30	100 to 300

SIDE EFFECTS
Skin: dermatologic reactions.
Other: edema, status asthmaticus, or *anaphylaxis* and anaphylactoid reactions.
Side effects of local anesthetics generally result from high blood levels of the drug. Examples of these are:
CNS: anxiety, apprehension, nervousness, convulsions followed by drowsiness, unconsciousness, and *respiratory arrest*.
CV: myocardial depression, *arrhythmias, cardiac arrest*.
EENT: blurred vision.
GI: nausea, vomiting.

INTERACTIONS
Chloroform, halothane, cyclopropane, trichloroethylene, and related drugs: cardiac arrhythmias may occur when used with etidocaine *with* epinephrine. Use with extreme caution.
MAO inhibitors, tricyclic antidepressants, phenothiazines: severe, sustained hypertension or hypotension may occur when used with etidocaine solution *with* epinephrine. Use with extreme caution.

NURSING CONSIDERATIONS
• Contraindicated in inflammation or infection in puncture region, children under 14 years, septicemia, severe hypertension, spinal deformities, neurologic disorders, and spinal block. Use cautiously in debilitated, elderly, or acutely ill patients; severe shock; heart block; epidural block in obstetrics; general drug allergies; hepatic and renal disease.
• Use solutions with epinephrine cautiously in cardiovascular disease and in body areas with limited blood supply (ears, nose, fingers, toes).
• Don't use solution with preservatives for caudal or epidural block.
• Keep resuscitative equipment and drugs available.
• Onset in 2 to 8 minutes; duration 3 to 6 hours.

---

lidocaine hydrochloride
Ardecaine, Canocaine, Dilocaine, Dolicaine, L-Caine, Nervocaine, Norocaine, Rocaine, Ultracaine, Xylocaine Hydrochloride♦

INDICATIONS & DOSAGE
Available with or without epinephrine. Doses cited are for drug *without* epinephrine except where indicated.
Caudal *(obstetrics)* **or epidural** *(thoracic):*

Sol.	Vol. (ml)	Dose (mg)
1%	20 to 30	200 to 300

Caudal *(surgery):*

Sol.	Vol. (ml)	Dose (mg)
1.5%	15 to 20	225 to 300

Epidural *(lumbar anesthesia):*

Sol.	Vol. (ml)	Dose (mg)
1.5%	15 to 20	225 to 300
2%	10 to 15	200 to 300

Maximum dose 200 to 300 mg/hour.
For anesthesia other than spinal—maximum single adult dose 4.5 mg/kg or 300 mg.
With epinephrine for anesthesia other than spinal—maximum single adult dose 7 mg/kg or 500 mg. Don't repeat dose more often than q 2 hours.
Spinal surgical anesthesia:

Sol.	Vol. (ml)	Dose (mg)
5% with 7.5% dextrose	1.5 to 2	75 to 100

Dose and interval may be increased with epinephrine.

SIDE EFFECTS
Skin: dermatologic reactions.
Other: edema, status asthmaticus, or *anaphylaxis* and anaphylactoid

---

reactions.

Side effects of local anesthetics generally result from high blood levels of the drug. Examples of these are:

CNS: anxiety, apprehension, nervousness, convulsions followed by drowsiness, unconsciousness, and *respiratory arrest*.

CV: myocardial depression, *arrhythmias, cardiac arrest*.

EENT: blurred vision.

GI: nausea, vomiting.

INTERACTIONS

Chloroform, halothane, cyclopropane, trichloroethylene, and related drugs: cardiac arrhythmias may occur when used with lidocaine *with* epinephrine. Use with extreme caution.

MAO inhibitors, tricyclic antidepressants: severe, sustained hypertension may occur when used with lidocaine *with* epinephrine. Use with extreme caution.

NURSING CONSIDERATIONS

• Contraindicated in inflammation or infection in puncture region, septicemia, severe hypertension, spinal deformities, neurologic disorders. Use cautiously in debilitated, elderly, or acutely ill patients; in severe shock; heart block; in obstetrics; general drug allergies; and paracervical block.

• Use solutions with epinephrine cautiously in cardiovascular disorders and in body areas with limited blood supply (ears, nose, fingers, toes).

• Keep resuscitative equipment and drugs available.

• A 2- to 5-ml test dose should be injected at least 5 minutes before giving total dose to check for intravascular or subarachnoid injection. Motor paralysis and extensive sensory anesthesia indicate subarachnoid injection.

• Solutions containing preservatives should not be used for spinal, epidural, or caudal block.

• Discard partially used vials without preservatives.

LOCAL ANESTHETICS **727**

mepivacaine hydrochloride
Carbocaine♦, Cavacaine, Isocaine

INDICATIONS & DOSAGE

Available with or without levonordefrin (vasoconstrictor). Doses cited are for drug *without* levonordefrin.

Nerve block:

Sol.	Vol. (ml)	Dose (mg)
1%	5 to 20	50 to 200
2%	5 to 20	100 to 400

Transvaginal block or infiltration (*maximum dose*):

Sol.	Vol. (ml)	Dose (mg)
1%	40	400

Paracervical block (*obstetrics*):

Sol.	Vol. (ml)	Dose (mg)
1%	10	100

Give on each side (200 mg total) per 90-minute period.

Caudal and epidural:

Sol.	Vol. (ml)	Dose (mg)
1%	15 to 30	150 to 300
1.5%	10 to 25	150 to 375
2%	10 to 20	200 to 400

Therapeutic block (*pain management*):

Sol.	Vol. (ml)	Dose (mg)
1%	1 to 5	10 to 50
2%	1 to 5	20 to 100

Adults: maximum single dose 7 mg/kg up to 550 mg. Don't repeat more often than q 90 minutes. Maximum total dose 1,000 mg daily.

Children: maximum dose 5 to 6 mg/kg. In children under 3 years or weighing less than 14 kg, use 0.5% or 1.5% solution only. Dose and interval may be increased with levonordefrin.

SIDE EFFECTS

Skin: dermatologic reactions.

Other: edema, status asthmaticus, or *anaphylaxis* and anaphylactoid reactions.

Side effects of local anesthetics generally result from high blood levels of the drug. Examples of these are:

CNS: anxiety, apprehension, nervousness, convulsions followed by drowsi-

ness, unconsciousness, and *respiratory arrest*.
CV: myocardial depression, *arrhythmias, cardiac arrest*.
EENT: blurred vision.
GI: nausea, vomiting.

INTERACTIONS
Chloroform, halothane, cyclopropane, trichloroethylene, and related drugs: cardiac arrhythmias may occur when used with mepivacaine *with* levonordefrin. Use with extreme caution.
MAO inhibitors, tricyclic antidepressants: severe, sustained hypertension may occur when used with mepivacaine *with* levonordefrin. Use with extreme caution.

NURSING CONSIDERATIONS
• Contraindicated in sensitivity to methylparaben, in heart block, or for spinal anesthesia. Use cautiously in debilitated, elderly, or acutely ill patients, or for paracervical block.
• Use solutions with levonordefrin cautiously in cardiovascular disease and in body areas with limited blood supply (nose, ears).
• Monitor fetal heart rate when paracervical block used in delivery.
• Keep resuscitative equipment and drugs available.
• Don't use solutions with preservatives for caudal or epidural block.
• Onset in 15 minutes; duration 3 hours.
• Discard partially used vials without preservatives.

---

piperocaine hydrochloride
Metycaine

INDICATIONS & DOSAGE
Caudal block *(obstetrics in women with normal-sized pelvic canals):*

Sol.	Vol. (ml)	Dose (mg)
1.5%	30	450

May give additional 20 ml doses

(300 mg) q 30 to 40 minutes, p.r.n.
Infiltration *(maximum dose):*

Sol.	Vol. (ml)	Dose (mg)
0.5%	200	1,000
1%	80	800

For dental infiltration, use a 1% to 2% solution.
For peripheral or sympathetic nerve block, use 0.5% to 2% solution.

SIDE EFFECTS
Skin: dermatologic reactions.
Other: edema, status asthmaticus, *anaphylaxis* and anaphylactoid reactions.
Side effects of local anesthetics generally result from high blood levels of the drug. Examples of these are:
CNS: anxiety, apprehension, nervousness, convulsions followed by drowsiness, unconsciousness, and *respiratory arrest*.
CV: myocardial depression, *arrhythmias, cardiac arrest*.
EENT: blurred vision.
GI: nausea, vomiting.

INTERACTIONS
None significant.

NURSING CONSIDERATIONS
• Contraindicated in hypersensitivity to procaine, tetracaine, or other para-aminobenzoic acid derivatives, CNS diseases, spinal deformities, infection at injection site, extreme obesity, profound anemia, or spinal block, in highly nervous women.
• Don't use solutions with preservatives for caudal block.
• Keep resuscitative equipment and drugs available.
• Effect peaks in 20 to 30 minutes, then decreases over next 10 minutes.
• Dilute 2% solutions to 0.5% or 1% with NaCl injection or Ringer's injection. Don't use sterile water for injection.
• An 8-ml dose of anesthetic solution should be injected a few minutes before giving total dose to check for subarach-

---

Italicized side effects are common or life-threatening.
*Liquid form contains alcohol.   **May contain tartrazine.

noid injection. Motor paralysis and extensive sensory anesthesia indicate subarachnoid injection.
• Discard partially used vials without preservatives.

prilocaine hydrochloride
Citanest♦, Propitocaine

INDICATIONS & DOSAGE
Infiltration:

Sol.	Vol. (ml)	Dose (mg)
1% to 2%	20 to 30	200 to 600

Peripheral nerve block (intercostal or paravertebral):

Sol.	Vol. (ml)	Dose (mg)
1% to 2%	3 to 5	30 to 100

Peripheral nerve block (sciatic [femoral or brachial plexus] or caudal nerve block [surgery]):

Sol.	Vol. (ml)	Dose (mg)
2%	20 to 30	400 to 600
3%	15 to 20	450 to 600

Caudal nerve block (obstetrics):

Sol.	Vol. (ml)	Dose (mg)
1%	20 to 30	200 to 300

Epidural:

Sol.	Vol. (ml)	Dose (mg)
1%	20 to 30	200 to 300
2%	20 to 30	400 to 600
3%	15 to 20	450 to 600

Maximum single adult dose 8 mg/kg up to 600 mg. In continuous caudal or epidural anesthesia, don't give maximum dose more often than q 2 hours.

SIDE EFFECTS
Skin: dermatologic reactions.
Other: edema, status asthmaticus, or *anaphylaxis* and anaphylactoid reactions.
With 4% solution: swelling and paresthesia of lips and mouth.
At maximum dose: methemoglobinemia.
Side effects of local anesthetics generally result from high blood levels of the drug. Examples of these are:
CNS: anxiety, apprehension, nervousness, convulsions followed by drowsiness, unconsciousness, and *respiratory arrest*.
CV: myocardial depression, *arrhythmias, cardiac arrest*.
EENT: blurred vision.
GI: nausea, vomiting.

INTERACTIONS
None significant.

NURSING CONSIDERATIONS
• Contraindicated in methemoglobinemia, severe shock, heart block, infection at injection site, or for spinal block. Use cautiously in debilitated, elderly, or acutely ill patients; children under 10 years; and in general drug sensitivities.
• Epidural and caudal contraindicated in CNS disease, spinal deformities, septicemia, severe hypertension, and in children.
• Keep resuscitative equipment and drugs available.
• Duration 1 to 3 hours.
• Don't use solutions with preservatives for caudal or epidural block.
• Discard partially used vials without preservatives.
• A 5-ml test dose should be injected at least 5 minutes before giving total dose to check for intravascular or subarachnoid injection. Motor paralysis and extensive sensory anesthesia indicate subarachnoid injection.

procaine hydrochloride
Novocain♦, Unicaine

INDICATIONS & DOSAGE
Spinal anesthesia—before using, dilute 10% solution with 0.9% NaCl injection, sterile distilled water, or cerebrospinal fluid.
For hyperbaric technique, use dextrose solution.
Perineum: use 0.5 ml 10% solution and 0.5 ml diluent injected at fourth lumbar interspace.
Perineum and lower extremities: use

1 ml 10% solution and 1 ml diluent injected at third or fourth lumbar interspace.
Up to costal margin: use 2 ml 10% solution and 1 ml diluent injected at second, third, or fourth lumbar interspace.
Epidural block:

Sol.	Vol. (ml)	Dose (mg)
1.5%	25	375

Peripheral nerve block:

Sol.	Vol. (ml)	Dose (mg)
1%	50	250
2%	25	500

Infiltration: use 250 to 600 mg 0.25% to 0.5% solution. Maximum initial dose 1 g. Dose and interval may be increased with epinephrine.

SIDE EFFECTS
Skin: dermatologic reactions.
Other: edema, status asthmaticus, or *anaphylaxis* and anaphylactoid reactions.
Side effects of local anesthetics generally result from high blood levels of the drug. Examples of these are:
CNS: anxiety, apprehension, nervousness, convulsions followed by drowsiness, unconsciousness, and *respiratory arrest*.
CV: myocardial depression, *arrhythmias, cardiac arrest*.
EENT: blurred vision.
GI: nausea, vomiting.

INTERACTIONS
Echothiophate iodide: reduced hydrolysis of procaine. Use together cautiously.

NURSING CONSIDERATIONS
• Contraindicated in traumatized urethra and in hypersensitivity to chloroprocaine, tetracaine, or other para-aminobenzoic acid derivatives. Use cautiously in hyperexcitable patients, and in patients with CNS diseases, infection at puncture site, shock, profound anemia, cachexia, sepsis, hypertension, hypotension, GI hemorrhage, bowel perforation or strangulation, peritonitis, cardiac decompensation,

massive pleural effusions, and increased intra-abdominal pressure.
• Contraindications to obstetric use: pelvic disproportion, placenta previa, abruptio placentae, floating fetal head, intrauterine manipulation.
• Keep resuscitative equipment and drugs available.
• A 1- to 5-ml test dose should be given 5 to 15 minutes before total epidural dose. Motor paralysis and extensive sensory anesthesia indicate subarachnoid injection.
• Use solution without preservatives for epidural block.
• Onset in 2 to 5 minutes; duration 60 minutes.
• Discard partially used vials without preservatives.

---

tetracaine hydrochloride
Pontocaine♦

INDICATIONS & DOSAGE
Low spinal (saddle block) in vaginal delivery: give 2 to 5 mg as hyperbaric solution (in 10% dextrose). Maximum dose 15 mg.
Perineum and lower extremities: give 5 to 10 mg.
Prolonged spinal anesthesia (2 to 3 hours): dilute 1% solution with equal volume of cerebrospinal fluid, or dissolve 5 mg powdered drug in 1 ml cerebrospinal fluid immediately before giving. Give 1 ml/5 seconds.
Up to costal margin: give 15 to 20 mg.

SIDE EFFECTS
Skin: dermatologic reactions.
Other: edema, status asthmaticus, or *anaphylaxis* and anaphylactoid reactions.
Side effects of local anesthetics generally result from high blood levels of the drug. Examples of these are:
CNS: anxiety, apprehension, nervousness, convulsions followed by drowsiness, unconsciousness, and *respiratory arrest*.

CV: myocardial depression, *arrhythmias, cardiac arrest.*
EENT: blurred vision.
GI: nausea, vomiting.

INTERACTIONS
None significant.

NURSING CONSIDERATIONS
• Contraindicated in infection at injection site, serious CNS diseases, and in hypersensitivity to procaine, chloroprocaine, tetracaine, or other para-aminobenzoic acid derivatives. Use cautiously in shock, profound anemia, cachexia, hypertension, hypotension, peritonitis, cardiac decompensation, massive pleural effusion, increased intracranial pressure, infection, and in highly nervous patients.
• Saddle block contraindicated in cephalopelvic disproportion, placenta previa, abruptio placentae, intrauterine manipulation, floating fetal head.
• Don't use cloudy, discolored, or crystallized solutions.
• Keep resuscitative equipment and drugs available.
• 10 times as strong as procaine HCl.
• Onset in 15 minutes; duration up to 3 hours.
• When cerebrospinal fluid is added to powdered drug or drug solution during spinal anesthesia, solution may be cloudy.
• Protect from light; store in refrigerator.

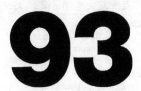

General anesthetics

fentanyl citrate with droperidol
ketamine hydrochloride
methohexital sodium
thiamylal sodium
thiopental sodium

MECHANISM OF ACTION
• Barbiturate anesthetics (methohexital, thiamylal, and thiopental) act by depressing the CNS. They inhibit the firing rate of neurons within the ascending reticular-activating system.
• Ketamine appears to interrupt association pathways in the brain, causing dissociative anesthesia, a feeling of dissociation from the environment.
• Fentanyl with droperidol acts as a CNS depressant to produce a general calming effect, reduced motor activity, and analgesia.

COMBINATION PRODUCTS
None.

fentanyl citrate with droperidol
Controlled Substance Schedule II
Innovar (Each ml contains [in a 1:50 ratio] fentanyl 0.05 mg as a citrate and droperidol 2.5 mg.)

INDICATIONS & DOSAGE
Doses vary depending on application, use of other agents, and patient's age, body weight, and physical status.
Anesthesia—
Adults:
*Premedication—*0.5 to 2 ml I.M. 45 to 60 minutes before surgery.
*Adjunct to general anesthesia—*Induction: 1 ml/20 to 25 lb body weight by slow I.V. to produce neuroleptanalgesia.
Maintenance: not indicated as sole agent for maintenance of surgical anesthesia. Used in combination with other measures. To prevent excessive accumulation of the relatively long-acting droperidol component, fentanyl alone should be used in increments of 0.025 to 0.05 mg (0.5 to 1 ml) for maintenance of analgesia. However, during prolonged surgery, additional 0.5- to 1-ml amounts of Innovar may be given with caution.
*Diagnostic procedures—*0.5 to 2 ml I.M. 45 to 60 minutes before procedure. In prolonged procedure, give 0.5 to 1 ml I.V. with caution and without a general anesthetic.
*Adjunct in regional anesthesia—*1 to 2 ml I.M. or slow I.V.
Children:
Premedication—0.25 ml/20 lb body weight I.M. 45 to 60 minutes before surgery.
*Adjunct to general anesthesia—*0.5 ml/20 lb body weight (total combined dose for induction and maintenance). Following induction with Innovar, fentanyl alone in a dose of ¼ to ⅓ of adult dose should be used to avoid accumulation of droperidol. However, during prolonged surgery, additional amounts of Innovar may be administered with caution. Safety of use in children under 2 years has not been established.

Italicized side effects are common or life-threatening.
∗Liquid form contains alcohol.　　　∗∗May contain tartrazine.

SIDE EFFECTS
CNS: emergence delirium and hallucinations, postoperative drowsiness.
CV: vasodilation, *hypotension,* decreased pulmonary arterial pressure, bradycardia, or tachycardia.
EENT: blurred vision, *laryngospasms.*
GI: *nausea, vomiting.*
Respiratory: *respiratory depression, apnea,* or *arrest.*
Other: drug dependence, muscle rigidity, chills, *shivering,* twitching, diaphoresis.

INTERACTIONS
CNS depressants (such as barbiturates, tranquilizers, narcotics, and general anesthetics): additive or potentiating effect. Dosage should be reduced.
MAO inhibitors: severe and unpredictable potentiation of Innovar. Do not use together or within 2 weeks of MAO inhibitor therapy.

NURSING CONSIDERATIONS
• Contraindicated in intolerance to either component. Use with caution in patients with head injuries and increased intracranial pressure, chronic obstructive pulmonary disease, hepatic and renal dysfunction, bradyarrhythmias, and in elderly or debilitated patients.
• Hypotension is a common side effect. However, if blood pressure drops, also consider hypovolemia as a possible cause. Use appropriate parenteral fluids to help restore blood pressure.
• Vital signs should be monitored frequently.
• Monitor pulmonary artery pressure.
• Be aware that respiratory depression, muscular rigidity of respiratory muscles, and respiratory arrest can occur. Have narcotic antagonist and CPR equipment on hand.
• Maintain airway.
• Postoperative EEG pattern may return to normal slowly.
• Postoperatively, if narcotic analgesics are required, use initially in reduced doses, as low as ¼ to ⅓ those usually recommended.
• When Innovar is given for anesthesia induction, fentanyl (Sublimaze) should be used for maintenance analgesia during procedure.
• Premedication with Innovar has sometimes been associated with patient agitation and refusal of surgery. Administration of diazepam may relieve this.

ketamine hydrochloride
Ketaject, Ketalar♦

INDICATIONS & DOSAGE
Induce anesthesia for procedures, especially short-term diagnostic or surgical, not requiring skeletal muscle relaxation; before giving other general anesthetics or to supplement low-potency agents, such as nitrous oxide—
Adults and children: 1 to 4.5 mg/kg I.V., administered over 60 seconds; or 6.5 to 13 mg/kg I.M. To maintain anesthesia, repeat in increments of half to full initial dose.

SIDE EFFECTS
CNS: *tonic and clonic movements resembling convulsions, respiratory depression, apnea when administered too rapidly.*
CV: *increased blood pressure and pulse rate,* hypotension, bradycardia.
EENT: diplopia, nystagmus, slight increase in intraocular pressure, *laryngospasms, salivation.*
GI: mild anorexia, nausea, vomiting.
Skin: transient erythema, measles-like rash.
Other: *dream-like states, hallucinations, confusion, excitement,* irrational behavior, psychic abnormalities.

INTERACTIONS
Thyroid hormones: may elevate blood pressure and cause tachycardia. Give cautiously.

NURSING CONSIDERATIONS

• Contraindicated in patients with history of cerebrovascular accident; patients who would be endangered by a significant rise in blood pressure; and those with severe hypertension; severe cardiac decompensation; surgery of the pharynx, larynx, or bronchial tree, unless used with muscle relaxants. Use with caution in chronic alcoholism, alcohol-intoxicated patients, patients with cerebrospinal fluid pressure elevated before anesthesia.
• Discourage giving anything orally at least 6 hours before elective surgery.
• Because of rapid induction, patient should be physically supported during administration.
• Do not inject barbiturates and ketamine HCl from same syringe, as they are chemically incompatible.
• Monitor vital signs before, during, and after anesthesia.
• Check cardiac function in patients with hypertension or cardiac depression.
• Maintain airway.
• Resuscitation equipment should be available and ready for use.
• Start supportive respiration if respiratory depression occurs. Use mechanical support if possible rather than administering analeptics.
• Keep verbal, tactile, and visual stimulation at a minimum during recovery phase to reduce incidence of emergent reactions.
• Hallucinations and excitement can occur on emergence from anesthesia; they can be abated by administering diazepam.
• A potent hallucinogen that can readily produce dissociative anesthesia (patient feels detached from environment). Dissociative effect and hallucinatory side effects have made this a popular drug of abuse among young people.

methohexital sodium
Controlled Substance Schedule IV
Brevital Sodium, Brietal Sodium••

INDICATIONS & DOSAGE

General anesthetic for short-term procedures (oral surgery, gynecologic and genitourinary examinations); reduction of fractures; before electroconvulsive therapy; for prolonged anesthesia when used with gaseous anesthetics—
Adults and children: 5 to 12 ml 1% solution (50 to 120 mg) I.V. at 1 ml/ 5 seconds. Dose required for induction may vary from 50 to 120 mg or more; average about 70 mg. Induction dose provides anesthesia for 5 to 7 minutes. Maintenance—intermittent injection: 2 to 4 ml 1% solution (20 to 40 mg) q 4 to 7 minutes; continuous I.V. drip: administer 0.2% solution (1 drop/second).

SIDE EFFECTS

CNS: *muscular twitching*, headache, emergence delirium.
CV: *temporary hypotension, tachycardia,* circulatory depression, *peripheral vascular collapse.*
GI: excessive salivation, *nausea, vomiting.*
Skin: tissue necrosis with extravasation.
Local: pain at injection site, injury to nerves adjacent to injection site.
Respiratory: *laryngospasm, bronchospasm, respiratory depression, apnea.*
Other: hiccups, coughing, acute allergic reactions, *twitching.* Extended use may cause cumulative effect.

INTERACTIONS
None significant.

NURSING CONSIDERATIONS
• Contraindicated in severe hepatic dysfunction, hypersensitivity to barbiturates, or porphyria; in shock or impending shock; and in patients for whom general anesthetics would be

---

Italicized side effects are common or life-threatening.
∗Liquid form contains alcohol.   ∗∗May contain tartrazine.

hazardous. Use with caution in debilitated patients, in patients with asthma, respiratory obstruction, severe hypertension or hypotension, myocardial disease, congestive heart failure, severe anemia, or extreme obesity.
• Maintain pulmonary ventilation.
• Avoid extravascular or intra-arterial injections.
• Monitor vital signs before, during, and after anesthesia.
• Have resuscitative equipment and drugs ready.
• Reduce postoperative nausea by having patient fast before administration.
• Incompatible with silicone; avoid contact with rubber stoppers or parts of syringes that have been treated with silicone.
• Incompatible with lactated Ringer's solution.
• Do not mix with acid solutions such as atropine sulfate.
• Solvents recommended are 5% glucose solution or isotonic (0.9%) sodium chloride solution instead of distilled water.
• Rate of flow must be individualized for each patient.
• Solutions may be stored and used as long as they remain clear and colorless. Solutions cannot be heated for sterilization.
• Has potential for abuse.

thiamylal sodium
Controlled Substance Schedule III
Surital♦

INDICATIONS & DOSAGE
General anesthetic for short-term procedures; anesthetic before administering other general anesthetics (dosage individualized to patient's response)—
Adults: 3 to 6 ml 2.5% solution I.V. at 1 ml/5 seconds. Additional intermittent injections of 0.5 to 1 ml. Maximum dose 1 g (40 ml 2.5% solution).
Rectal administration before diagnostic procedures—

Children: 800 mg to 1 g 5% solution/ 22.5 kg body weight.
Supplemental anesthetic—
Adults: 0.2% or 0.3% solution continuous I.V. drip. Recovery occurs within 20 to 30 minutes after last injection.

SIDE EFFECTS
CNS: excitement, headache, emergence delirium.
CV: hypotension, *circulatory depression*, thrombophlebitis, *hypoxia*.
GI: nausea, vomiting, excessive salivation.
Skin: rash, urticaria, tissue necrosis with extravasation.
Respiratory: *laryngospasm, bronchospasm, respiratory depression, apnea*.
Local: pain at injection site, injury to nerves adjacent to injection site.
Other: hiccups. Extended use can cause cumulative effects.

INTERACTIONS
None significant.

NURSING CONSIDERATIONS
• Contraindicated in hepatic dysfunction or disease, traumatic or impending shock, porphyria, hypersensitivity to barbiturates, and in those for whom general anesthetics would be hazardous. Use with caution in respiratory disease or obstruction, obesity, marked disturbance of arterial tension, heart failure, anemia, status asthmaticus, endocrine or renal dysfunction, and in debilitated patients.
• Maintain airway.
• Have resuscitative equipment and drugs ready.
• Monitor vital signs before, during, and after anesthesia.
• Avoid extravascular or intra-arterial injection.
• Incompatible with lactated Ringer's solution or solutions containing bacteriostatic or buffer agents, which tend to cause precipitation.
• Don't inject air into solution; may cause cloudiness.

- Sterile water is the preferred solvent for injections. For drip maintenance use 5% glucose or isotonic sodium chloride solution to avoid extreme hypotonicity.
- Solutions of atropine sulfate, d-tubocurarine, or succinylcholine may be given concurrently but should not be mixed together.
- Do not heat solutions for sterilization. Solutions should be stored in refrigerator and used within 6 days. If kept at room temperature, use within 24 hours.
- Has potential for abuse.

thiopental sodium
Controlled Substance Schedule III
Pentothal Sodium♦
(injection and rectal suspension)

INDICATIONS & DOSAGE
Induce anesthesia before administering other anesthetics—210 to 280 mg (3 to 4 ml/kg) usually required for average adult (70 kg).
General anesthetic for short-term procedures—
Adults: 2 to 3 ml 2.5% solution (50 to 75 mg) administered I.V. only at intervals of 20 to 40 seconds, depending on reaction. Dose may be repeated with caution, if necessary.
Convulsive states following anesthesia—75 to 125 mg (3 to 5 ml of 2.5% solution) immediately.
Psychiatric disorders (narcoanalysis, narcosynthesis)—100 mg/minute (4 ml/minute 2.5% solution) until confusion occurs and before sleep. Maximum dose 50 ml/minute.
Basal anesthesia by rectal administration—
Adults and children: administer up to 1 g/22.5 kg (50 lb) body weight, or 0.5 ml 10% solution/kg body weight. Maximum 1 to 1.5 g (children weighing 34 kg or more) and 3 to 4 g (adults weighing 91 kg or more).
Note: Thiopental is rarely administered rectally for basal sedation or anesthesia because of variable absorption from the rectum.

SIDE EFFECTS
CNS: *prolonged somnolence*, retrograde amnesia.
CV: *myocardial depression, arrhythmias.*
Skin: tissue necrosis with extravasation.
Respiratory: *respiratory depression (momentary apnea following each injection is typical)*, bronchospasm, laryngospasm.
Local: pain at injection site.
Other: sneezing, coughing, *shivering*.

INTERACTIONS
None significant.

NURSING CONSIDERATIONS
- Contraindicated in absence of suitable veins for intravenous administration, hypersensitivity to barbiturates, status asthmaticus, porphyria, respiratory depression or obstruction, decompensated cardiac disease, severe anemia, hepatic cirrhosis, shock, renal dysfunction, increased intracranial pressure, myxedema.
- Give test dose (1 to 3 ml 2.5% solution) to assess reaction to drug.
- When used as general anesthetic, give atropine sulfate as premedication to diminish laryngeal reflexes and to prevent laryngeal spasm.
- Have resuscitative equipment and oxygen ready. Maintain airway.
- Avoid extravasation.
- Monitor vital signs before, during, and after anesthesia.
- Solutions of atropine sulfate, d-tubocurarine, or succinylcholine may be given concurrently.
- Do not heat solutions for sterilization. Solutions should be stored in refrigerator and used within 6 days. If kept at room temperature, use within 24 hours.
- Has potential for abuse.

Italicized side effects are common or life-threatening.
*Liquid form contains alcohol.   **May contain tartrazine.

Vitamins and minerals

vitamin A
  oleovitamin A
vitamin B complex
  cyanocobalamin (B_{12})
  cyanocobalamin,
    hydroxocobalamin (B_{12a})
  folic acid (B_9)
  leucovorin calcium
  niacin (B_3)
  niacinamide
  pyridoxine hydrochloride (B_6)
  riboflavin (B_2)
  thiamine hydrochloride (B_1)
vitamin C
  ascorbic acid
vitamin D
  cholecalciferol (D_3)
  ergocalciferol (D_2)
vitamin E
vitamin K analogs
  menadione/menadiol sodium
    diphosphate (K_3)
  phytonadione (K_1)
multivitamins
sodium fluoride
trace elements
  chromium
  copper
  iodine
  manganese
  zinc
  zinc sulfate

MECHANISM OF ACTION

• Vitamins act as coenzymes or coenzyme precursors to catalyze protein, fat, and carbohydrate metabolism, and to facilitate energy-producing and anabolic reactions.
• Trace elements may act in metalloenzyme units (a metalloenzyme contains a metal atom in its structure). They participate in synthesis and stabilization of proteins and nucleic acids in subcellular and membrane transport systems.
• Sodium fluoride's mechanism is unknown; however, the compound may catalyze bone remineralization.

COMBINATION PRODUCTS

Vitamin A and D combinations
B vitamin combinations
B complex vitamins
B complex with vitamin C
Multivitamins
Multivitamins with B_{12}
Calcium and vitamin products
Fluoride with vitamins
B complex vitamins with iron
Miscellaneous vitamins and minerals
Geriatric supplements with multivitamins and minerals
Multivitamins and minerals with hormones

oleovitamin A
Acon, Afaxin♦♦, Alphalin, Aquasol A♦, Natola

INDICATIONS & DOSAGE
Severe vitamin A deficiency with xerophthalmia—
Adults and children over 8 years: 500,000 IU P.O. daily for 3 days, then 50,000 IU P.O. daily for 14 days, then maintenance with 10,000 to 20,000 IU P.O. daily for 2 months, followed by adequate dietary nutrition and RDA vitamin A supplements.
Severe vitamin A deficiency—

Unmarked trade names available in the United States only.
♦ Also available in Canada.   ♦♦ Available in Canada only.

Adults and children over 8 years:
100,000 IU P.O. or I.M. daily for
3 days, then 50,000 IU P.O. or I.M.
daily for 14 days, then maintenance
with 10,000 to 20,000 IU P.O. daily for
2 months, followed by adequate dietary
nutrition and RDA vitamin A supplements.

Children 1 to 8 years: 17,500 to
35,000 IU I.M. daily for 10 days.

Infants under 1 year: 7,500 to 15,000
IU I.M. daily for 10 days.

Maintenance only—

Children 4 to 8 years: 15,000 IU I.M.
daily for 2 months, then adequate dietary nutrition and RDA vitamin A supplements.

Children under 4 years: 10,000 IU
I.M. daily for 2 months, then adequate
dietary nutrition and RDA vitamin A
supplements.

SIDE EFFECTS
Side effects are usually seen only with
toxicity (hypervitaminosis A).

Blood: hypoplastic anemia, leukopenia.

CNS: irritability, headache, increased
intracranial pressure, fatigue, lethargy,
malaise.

EENT: miosis, papilledema, exophthalmos.

GI: anorexia, epigastric pain, diarrhea.

GU: hypomenorrhea.

Hepatic: jaundice, hepatomegaly.

Skin: alopecia; drying, cracking, scaling of skin; pruritus; lip fissures; massive desquamation; increased pigmentation; night sweating

Other: skeletal—slow growth, decalcification of bone, fractures, hyperostosis, painful periostitis, premature closure of epiphyses, migratory arthralgia,
cortical thickening over the radius and
tibia, bulging fontanelles; splenomegaly.

INTERACTIONS
Mineral oil, cholestyramine resin: reduced GI absorption of fat-soluble vitamins. If needed, give mineral oil at
bedtime.

NURSING CONSIDERATIONS
• Oral administration contraindicated
in presence of malabsorption syndrome;
if malabsorption is due to inadequate
bile secretion, oral route may be used
with concurrent administration of bile
salts (dehydrocholic acid). Also contraindicated in hypervitaminosis A. Intravenous administration contraindicated
except for special water-miscible forms
intended for infusion with large parenteral volumes. Intravenous push of vitamin A of any type is also contraindicated (anaphylaxis or anaphylactoid reactions and death have resulted).
• Caution: Evaluate intake from fortified foods, dietary supplements, selfadministered drugs, and prescription
drug sources.
• In pregnant women, avoid doses exceeding 6,000 IU daily.
• To avoid toxicity, discourage patient
self-administration of megavitamin
doses without specific indications. Also
stress that the patient should not share
prescribed vitamins with family or others. If family member feels vitamin
therapy may be of value, have him contact his doctor.
• Watch for side effects if dosage is
high.
• Acute toxicity has resulted from single doses of 25,000 IU/kg of body
weight; 350,000 IU in infants and over
2,000,000 IU in adults have also
proved acutely toxic.
• Chronic toxicity in infants (3 to
6 months) has resulted from doses of
18,500 IU daily for 1 to 3 months. In
adults, chronic toxicity has resulted
from doses of 50,000 IU daily for over
18 months; 500,000 IU daily for
2 months, and 1,000,000 IU daily for
3 days.
• Monitor patient closely during vitamin A therapy for skin disorders
since high dosages may induce chronic
toxicity.

Italicized side effects are common or life-threatening.
*Liquid form contains alcohol.   **May contain tartrazine.

- Liquid preparations available if nasogastric administration is necessary.
- Record eating and bowel habits. Report abnormalities to doctor.
- Adequate vitamin A absorption requires suitable protein intake, bile (give supplemental salts if necessary), concurrent RDA doses of vitamin E, and zinc (multivitamins usually supply zinc, but supplements may be necessary in long-term hyperalimentation).
- Absorption is fastest and most complete with water-miscible preparations, intermediate with emulsions, and slowest with oil suspensions.
- In severe hepatic dysfunction, diabetes, and hypothyroidism, use vitamin A rather than carotenes for vitamin therapy because the vitamin itself is more easily absorbed and the diseases adversely affect conversion of carotenes into vitamin A. If carotenes are prescribed, dosage should be doubled.
- Protect from light.

cyanocobalamin (vitamin B₁₂)

Anacobin◆◆, Bedoce, Bedoz◆◆, Berubigen, Betalin-12, Bio-12◆◆, Crystimin, Cyanabin◆◆, Cyanocobalamin, Cyano-Gel, DBH-B₁₂, Dodex, Kaybovite, Pernavite, Poyamin, Redisol, Rubesol, Rubion◆◆, Rubramin◆, Ruvite, Sigamine, Vibedoz, Vi-Twel

cyanocobalamin, hydroxocobalamin (vitamin B₁₂ₐ)

Alpha Redisol, Alpha-Ruvite, Codroxomin, Droxomin, Neo-Betalin 12, Rubesol-LA

INDICATIONS & DOSAGE

Vitamin B₁₂ deficiency due to inadequate diet, subtotal gastrectomy, or any other condition, disorder, or disease except malabsorption related to pernicious anemia or other gastrointestinal disease—

Adults: 25 mcg P.O. daily as dietary supplement, or 30 to 100 mcg S.C. or I.M. daily for 5 to 10 days, depending on severity of deficiency. Maintenance dose: 100 to 200 mcg I.M. once monthly. For subsequent prophylaxis, advise adequate nutrition and daily RDA vitamin B₁₂ supplements.
Children: 1 mcg P.O. daily as dietary supplement, or 1 to 30 mcg S.C. or I.M. daily for 5 to 10 days, depending on severity of deficiency. Maintenance: at least 60 mcg/month I.M. or S.C. For subsequent prophylaxis, advise adequate nutrition and daily RDA vitamin B₁₂ supplements.
Pernicious anemia or vitamin B₁₂ malabsorption—
Adults: initially, 100 to 1,000 mcg I.M. daily for 2 weeks, then 100 to 1,000 mcg I.M. once monthly for life. If neurologic complications are present, follow initial therapy with 100 to 1,000 mcg I.M. once every 2 weeks before starting monthly regimen.
Children: 1,000 to 5,000 mcg I.M. or S.C. given over 2 or more weeks in 100-mcg increments; then 60 mcg I.M. or S.C. monthly for life.
Methylmalonic aciduria—
Neonates: 1,000 mcg I.M. daily for 11 days with a protein-restricted diet.
Diagnostic test for vitamin B₁₂ deficiency without concealing folate deficiency in patients with megaloblastic anemias—
Adults and children: 1 mcg I.M. daily for 10 days with diet low in vitamin B₁₂ and folate. Reticulocytosis between days 3 and 10 confirms diagnosis of vitamin B₁₂ deficiency.
Schilling test flushing dose—
Adults and children: 1,000 mcg I.M. in a single dose.

SIDE EFFECTS
CV: peripheral vascular thrombosis.
GI: transient diarrhea.

Skin: itching, transitory exanthema, urticaria.
Local: pain, burning at S.C. or I.M. injection sites.
Other: *anaphylaxis,* anaphylactoid reactions.

INTERACTIONS
Neomycin, colchicine, para-aminosalicylic acid and salts, chloramphenicol: malabsorption of vitamin B_{12}. Don't use together.

NURSING CONSIDERATIONS
• Parenteral administration contraindicated in hypersensitivity to vitamin B_{12} or cobalt. Alternate use of large oral doses of vitamin B_{12} is controversial and should not be considered routine; combined with intrinsic factor increases risk of hypersensitive reactions and should be avoided. Therapeutic dose contraindicated before proper diagnosis; vitamin B_{12} therapy may mask folate deficiency.
• I.V. administration may cause anaphylactic reactions. Use cautiously and only if other routes are ruled out.
• Use cautiously in anemic patients with coexisting cardiac, pulmonary, or hypertensive disease; in patients with early Leber's disease; in patients with severe vitamin B_{12}–dependent deficiencies, especially those receiving cardiotonic glycosides (monitor closely the first 2 to 3 days for hypokalemia, fluid overload, pulmonary edema, congestive heart failure, and hypertension); and in patients with gouty conditions (monitor serum uric acid levels for hyperuricemia).
• Don't mix parenteral liquids in same syringe with other medication.
• Protect from light.
• Infection, tumors, or renal, hepatic, and other debilitating diseases may reduce therapeutic response.
• Deficiencies more common in strict vegetarians and their breast-fed infants.
• Stress need for patients with pernicious anemia to return for monthly injections. Although total body stores may last 3 to 6 years, anemia will recur if not treated monthly.
• May cause false-positive intrinsic factor antibody test.
• Hydroxocobalamin is approved for I.M. use only. Only advantage of hydroxocobalamin over vitamin B_{12} is longer duration.
• 50% to 98% of injected dose may appear in urine within 48 hours. Major portion is excreted within first 8 hours.
• Closely monitor serum potassium levels for first 48 hours. Give potassium if necessary.
• Physically incompatible with dextrose solutions, alkaline or strongly acidic solutions, oxidizing and reducing agents, and many other drugs.

folic acid (vitamin B_9)
Folvite♦, Novofolacid♦♦

INDICATIONS & DOSAGE
Megaloblastic or macrocytic anemia secondary to folic acid or other nutritional deficiency, hepatic disease, alcoholism, intestinal obstruction, excessive hemolysis—
Pregnant and lactating women: 0.8 mg P.O., S.C., or I.M. daily.
Adults and children over 4 years: 1 mg P.O., S.C., or I.M. daily for 4 to 5 days. After anemia secondary to folic acid deficiency is corrected, proper diet and RDA supplements are necessary to prevent recurrence.
Children under 4 years: up to 0.3 mg P.O., S.C., or I.M. daily.
Prevention of megaloblastic anemia of pregnancy and fetal damage—
Women: 1 mg P.O., S.C., or I.M. daily throughout pregnancy.
Nutritional supplement—
Adults: 0.1 mg P.O., S.C., or I.M. daily.
Children: 0.05 mg P.O. daily.
Treatment of tropical sprue—
Adults: 3 to 15 mg P.O. daily.

Italicized side effects are common or life-threatening.
*Liquid form contains alcohol.   **May contain tartrazine.

Test of megaloblastic anemia patients to detect folic acid deficiency without masking pernicious anemia—
Adults and children: 0.1 to 0.2 mg P.O. or I.M. for 10 days while maintaining a diet low in folate and vitamin B_{12}.
(Reticulosis, reversion to normoblastic hematopoiesis, and return to normal hemoglobin indicate folic acid deficiency.)

SIDE EFFECTS
Skin: allergic reactions (rash, pruritus, erythema).
Other: *allergic bronchospasms,* general malaise.

INTERACTIONS
Chloramphenicol: antagonism of folic acid. Monitor for decreased folic acid effect. Use together cautiously.

NURSING CONSIDERATIONS
• Contraindicated in normocytic, refractory, or aplastic anemias; as sole agent in treatment of pernicious anemia (since it may mask neurologic effects); in treatment of methotrexate, pyrimethamine, or trimethoprim overdose; and in undiagnosed anemia (since it may mask pernicious anemia).
• Patients with small-bowel resections and intestinal malabsorption may require parenteral administration routes.
• Don't mix with other medications in same syringe for I.M. injections.
• Protect from light.
• May use concurrent folic acid and vitamin B_{12} therapy if supported by diagnosis.
• Proper nutrition is necessary to prevent recurrence of anemia.
• Peak folate activity occurs in the blood in 30 to 60 minutes.
• Hematologic response to folic acid in patients receiving chloramphenicol concurrently with folic acid should be carefully monitored.

leucovorin calcium (citrovorum factor or folinic acid)
Calcium Folinate

INDICATIONS & DOSAGE
Overdose of folic acid antagonist—
Adults and children: P.O., I.M., or I.V. dose equivalent to the weight of the antagonist given.
Leucovorin rescue after high methotrexate dose in treatment of malignancy—
Adults and children: dose at doctor's discretion within 6 to 36 hours of last dose of methotrexate.
Toxic effects of methotrexate used to treat severe psoriasis—
Adults and children: 4 to 8 mg I.M. 2 hours after methotrexate dose.
Hematologic toxicity due to pyrimethamine therapy—
Adults and children: 5 mg P.O. or I.M. daily.
Hematologic toxicity due to trimethoprim therapy—
Adults and children: 400 mcg to 5 mg P.O. or I.M. daily.
Megaloblastic anemia due to congenital enzyme deficiency—
Adults and children: 3 to 6 mg I.M. daily, then 1 mg P.O. daily for life.
Folate-deficient megaloblastic anemias—
Adults and children: up to 1 mg of leucovorin I.M daily. Duration of treatment depends on hematologic response.

SIDE EFFECTS
Skin: allergic reactions (rash, pruritus, erythema).
Other: *allergic bronchospasms.*

INTERACTIONS
None significant.

NURSING CONSIDERATIONS
• Contraindicated in treatment of undiagnosed anemia, since it may mask pernicious anemia. Use cautiously in pernicious anemia; a hemolytic remission

may occur while neurologic manifestations remain progressive.

- Do not confuse leucovorin (folinic acid) with folic acid.
- Follow leucovorin rescue schedule and protocol closely to maximize therapeutic response. Generally, leucovorin should not be administered simultaneously with systemic methotrexate.
- Treat overdosage of folic acid antagonists; administer within 1 hour if possible; usually ineffective after 4-hour delay.
- Protect from light and heat, especially reconstituted parenteral preparations.
- Since allergic reactions have been reported with folic acid, the possibility of allergic reactions to leucovorin should be considered.

---

niacin
(vitamin B₃, nicotinic acid)

niacinamide (nicotinamide)
Diacin**, Lipo-Nicin, Niac, Nico400, Nicobid, Nicolar**, Nico-Span, Ni-Span, Vasotherm

INDICATIONS & DOSAGE
Pellagra—
Adults: 10 to 20 mg P.O., S.C., I.M., or I.V. infusion daily, depending on severity of niacin deficiency. Maximum daily dose recommended, 500 mg; should be divided into 10 doses, 50 mg each.
Children: up to 300 mg P.O. or 100 mg I.V. infusion daily, depending on severity of niacin deficiency. After symptoms subside, advise adequate nutrition and RDA supplements to prevent recurrence.
Hyperlipoproteinemia types III, IV, and V, and as secondary agent in type II—
Adults: up to 1 g 3 or 4 times a day.
Peripheral vascular disease and circulatory disorders—
Adults: 250 to 800 mg P.O. daily in divided doses.

SIDE EFFECTS
Most side effects are dose-dependent.
CNS: dizziness, transient headache.
CV: *excessive peripheral vasodilation (especially niacin).*
GI: *nausea, vomiting, diarrhea,* possible activation of peptic ulcer, epigastric or substernal pain.
Hepatic: hepatic dysfunction.
Metabolic: hyperglycemia, hyperuricemia.
Skin: *flushing,* pruritus, dryness.

INTERACTIONS
Antihypertensive drugs of the sympathetic blocking type: may have an additive vasodilating effect and cause postural hypotension. Use together cautiously. Warn patient about postural hypotension.

NURSING CONSIDERATIONS
- Contraindicated in hepatic dysfunction, active peptic ulcer disease, severe hypotension, arterial hemorrhage. Use with caution in patients with gallbladder disease, diabetes mellitus, gout.
- Monitor hepatic function and blood glucose early in therapy.
- Give with meals to minimize GI side effects.
- Aspirin may reduce the flushing response to niacin.
- Timed-release niacin or niacinamide may avoid excessive flushing effects with large doses. Give slow I.V. Explain harmlessness of flushing syndrome to ease patient's mind.
- Stress that medication used to treat hyperlipoproteinemia or to dilate peripheral vessels is not "just a vitamin." Explain importance of adhering to therapeutic regimen.

Italicized side effects are common or life-threatening.
*Liquid form contains alcohol.   **May contain tartrazine.

pyridoxine hydrochloride (vitamin B₆)
Bee six, Hexa-Betalin♦, Hexacrest

INDICATIONS & DOSAGE
Dietary vitamin B₆ deficiency—
Adults: 10 to 20 mg P.O., I.M., or I.V. daily for 3 weeks, then 2 to 5 mg daily as a supplement to a proper diet.
Children: 100 mg P.O., I.M., or I.V. to correct deficiency, then an adequate diet with supplementary RDA doses to prevent recurrence.
Seizures related to vitamin B₆ deficiency or dependency—
Adults and children: 100 mg I.M. or I.V. in single dose.
Vitamin B₆-responsive anemias or dependency syndrome (inborn errors of metabolism)—
Adults: up to 600 mg P.O., I.M., or I.V. daily until symptoms subside, then 50 mg daily for life.
Children: 100 mg I.M. or I.V., then 2 to 10 mg I.M. or 10 to 100 mg P.O. daily.
Prevention of vitamin B₆ deficiency during isoniazid therapy—
Adults: 25 to 50 mg P.O. daily.
Children: at least 0.5 to 1.5 mg daily.
Infants: at least 0.1 to 0.5 mg daily.
If neurologic symptoms develop in pediatric patients, increase dosage as necessary.
Treatment of vitamin B₆ deficiency secondary to isoniazid—
Adults: 100 mg P.O. daily for 3 weeks, then 50 mg daily.
Children: titrate dosages.

SIDE EFFECTS
CNS: drowsiness, paresthesias.

INTERACTIONS
None significant.

NURSING CONSIDERATIONS
• Contraindicated in hypersensitivity to parenteral pyridoxine and in doses larger than 5 mg for patients also receiving levodopa. Caution patient to check dosage, especially in multivitamins.
• Protect from light. Do not use injection solution if it contains a precipitate. Slight darkening is acceptable.
• Excessive protein intake increases daily pyridoxine requirements.
• If sodium bicarbonate is required to control acidosis in isoniazid toxicity, do not mix in same syringe with pyridoxine.
• If prescribed for maintenance therapy to prevent deficiency recurrence, stress importance of compliance and of good nutrition. Explain that pyridoxine in combination therapy with isoniazid has a specific therapeutic purpose and is not "just a vitamin." Emphasize need for adhering to therapeutic regimen.
• Patients receiving levodopa alone (not with carbidopa) shouldn't take pyridoxine.

riboflavin (vitamin B₂)

INDICATIONS & DOSAGE
Riboflavin deficiency or adjunct to thiamine treatment for polyneuritis or cheilosis secondary to pellagra—
Adults and children over 12 years: 5 to 50 mg P.O., S.C., I.M., or I.V. daily, depending on severity.
Children under 12 years: 2 to 10 mg P.O., S.C., I.M., or I.V. daily, depending on severity.
For maintenance, increase nutritional intake and supplement with vitamin B complex.

SIDE EFFECTS
GU: high doses make urine bright yellow.

INTERACTIONS
None significant.

NURSING CONSIDERATIONS
• Protect from light.

• Stress proper nutritional habits to prevent recurrence of deficiency.
• Riboflavin deficiency usually accompanies other vitamin B complex deficiencies and may require multivitamin therapy.

thiamine hydrochloride (vitamin B₁)

Apatate Drops, Betaline S*, Betaxin♦♦, Megamin♦♦, Thia

INDICATIONS & DOSAGE

Beriberi—
Adults: 10 to 500 mg, depending on severity, I.M. t.i.d. for 2 weeks, followed by dietary correction and multivitamin supplement containing 5 to 10 mg daily thiamine for 1 month.
Children: 10 to 50 mg, depending on severity, I.M. daily for several weeks with adequate dietary intake.
Anemia secondary to thiamine deficiency; polyneuritis secondary to alcoholism, pregnancy, or pellagra—
Adults: 100 mg P.O. daily.
Children: 10 to 50 mg P.O. daily in divided doses.
Wernicke's encephalopathy—
Adults: up to 500 mg to 1 g I.V. for crisis therapy, followed by 100 mg b.i.d. for maintenance.
"Wet beriberi," with myocardial failure—
Adults and children: 100 to 500 mg I.V. for emergency treatment.

SIDE EFFECTS

CNS: restlessness.
CV: *hypotension after rapid I.V. injection,* angioneurotic edema, cyanosis.
EENT: tightness of throat (allergic reaction).
GI: nausea, hemorrhage, diarrhea.
Skin: feeling of warmth, pruritus, urticaria, sweating.
Other: *anaphylactic reactions,* weakness, pulmonary edema.

INTERACTIONS
None significant.

NURSING CONSIDERATIONS
• Contraindicated in hypersensitivity to thiamine products. I.V. push contraindicated, except when treating life-threatening myocardial failure in "wet beriberi." Use with caution in I.V. administration of large doses (to prevent anaphylactic reactions); skin-test patients with history of hypersensitivity before therapy. Have epinephrine on hand to treat anaphylaxis should it occur after a large parenteral dose.
• Use parenteral administration only when P.O. route is not feasible.
• Clinically significant deficiency can occur in approximately 3 weeks of totally thiamine-free diet. Thiamine deficiency usually requires concurrent treatment for multiple deficiencies.
• Doses larger than 30 mg t.i.d. may not be fully utilized. After tissue saturation with thiamine, it is excreted in urine as pyrimidine.
• If beriberi occurs in a breast-fed infant, both mother and child should be treated with thiamine.
• Unstable in alkaline solutions; should not be used with materials that yield alkaline solutions.

ascorbic acid (vitamin C)

Adenex♦♦, Ascorbicap, Ascorbineed, Ascoril♦♦, Best-C, Cecon, Cemill, Cenolate, Cetane, Cevalin, Cevi-Bid, Ce-Vi-Sol♦*, Cevita, C-Long, C-Syrup-500, Megascorb♦♦, Redoxon♦♦, Saro-C, Solucap C, Vitacee, Viterra C

INDICATIONS & DOSAGE
Frank and subclinical scurvy—
Adults: 100 mg to 2 g, depending on severity, P.O., S.C., I.M., or I.V. daily, then at least 50 mg daily for maintenance.
Children: 100 to 200 mg, depending on severity, P.O., S.C., I.M., or I.V.

Italicized side effects are common or life-threatening.
*Liquid form contains alcohol.   **May contain tartrazine.

daily, then at least 35 mg daily for maintenance.

Infants: 50 to 100 mg P.O., I.M., I.V., or S.C. daily.

Extensive burns, delayed fracture or wound healing, postoperative wound healing, severe febrile or chronic disease states—

Adults: 200 to 500 mg S.C., I.M., or I.V. daily.

Children: 100 to 200 mg P.O., S.C., I.M., or I.V. daily.

Prevention of vitamin C deficiency in those with poor nutritional habits or increased requirements—

Adults: at least 45 to 50 mg P.O., S.C., I.M., or I.V. daily.

Pregnant or lactating women: at least 60 mg P.O., S.C., I.M., or I.V. daily.

Children: at least 40 mg P.O., S.C., I.M., or I.V. daily.

Infants: at least 35 mg P.O., S.C., I.M., or I.V. daily.

Potentiation of methenamine in urine acidification—

Adults: 4 to 12 g daily in divided doses.

Before gastrectomy—

Adults: 1 g daily for 4 to 7 days.

SIDE EFFECTS
CNS: faintness or dizziness with fast I.V. administration.
GI: diarrhea, epigastric burning.
GU: acid urine, oxaluria, renal calculi.
Skin: discomfort at injection site.

INTERACTIONS
None significant.

NURSING CONSIDERATIONS
• Use cautiously in G-6-PD deficiency to avoid possibility of hemolytic anemia.
• Avoid rapid I.V. administration.
• Protect solution from light.
• Discourage self-administration for colds; harmful side effects are possible.
• I.V. form used investigationally as adjunct to treat some forms of cancer.

vitamin D
(cholecalciferol: vitamin D$_3$; ergocalciferol: vitamin D$_2$)

Calciferol, Deltalin, Drisdol♦, Radiostol♦♦, Radiostol Forte♦♦

INDICATIONS & DOSAGE
Rickets and other vitamin D deficiency diseases—

Adults: 12,000 IU P.O. or I.M. daily initially, increased as indicated by response up to 500,000 IU daily in most cases and up to 800,000 IU daily for vitamin D–resistant rickets.

Children: 1,500 to 5,000 IU P.O. or I.M. daily for 2 to 4 weeks, repeated after 2 weeks, if necessary. Alternatively, a single dose of 600,000 IU. Monitor serum calcium daily to guide dosage. After correction of deficiency, maintenance includes adequate dietary nutrition and RDA supplements.

Hypoparathyroidism—

Adults and children: 50,000 to 200,000 IU P.O. or I.M. daily, with 4-g calcium supplement.

SIDE EFFECTS
Side effects listed are usually seen in vitamin D toxicity only.
CNS: headache, dizziness, ataxia, weakness, somnolence, decreased libido, overt psychosis, convulsions.
CV: calcifications of soft tissues, including the heart.
EENT: dry mouth, metallic taste, rhinorrhea, conjunctivitis (calcific), photophobia, tinnitus.
GI: anorexia, nausea, constipation, diarrhea.
GU: polyuria, albuminuria, hypercalciuria, nocturia, impaired renal function, renal calculi.
Metabolic: hypercalcemia, hyperphosphatemia.
Skin: pruritus.
Other: bone and muscle pain, bone demineralization, weight loss.

INTERACTIONS
Mineral oil, cholestyramine resin: inhibited GI absorption of oral vitamin D. Space doses. Use together cautiously.

NURSING CONSIDERATIONS
• Contraindicated in hypercalcemia, hypervitaminosis A, renal osteodystrophy with hyperphosphatemia.
• If I.V. route is necessary, use only water-miscible solutions intended for dilution in large-volume parenterals. Use cautiously in cardiac patients, especially if they are receiving cardiotonic glycosides.
• Monitor eating and bowel habits; dry mouth, nausea, vomiting, metallic taste, and constipation can be early signs of toxicity.
• Patients with hyperphosphatemia require dietary phosphate restrictions and binding agents to avoid metastatic calcifications and renal calculi.
• Dosage range between therapeutic and toxic effects is narrow. When high therapeutic doses are used, frequent serum and urine calcium, potassium, and urea determinations should be made.
• Malabsorption due to inadequate bile or hepatic dysfunction may require addition of exogenous bile salts to oral vitamin D.
• I.M. injection of vitamin D dispersed in oil is preferable in patients who are unable to absorb oral vitamin D.
• Protect solution from light.
• This vitamin is fat soluble. Warn patient of the dangers of increasing dosage without consulting the doctor. Also, discourage sharing of this drug: it is not "just a vitamin" and can have serious toxic effects.
• Patients taking vitamin D should restrict their intake of magnesium-containing antacids.

vitamin E
Aquasol E◆*, D-Alpha-E**, Daltose◆◆, Eprolin, Epsilan-M, Hy-E-Plex, Kell-E, Lethopherol, Maxi-E, Pertropin, Solucap E, Tocopher-Caps, Tokols, Viterra E

INDICATIONS & DOSAGE
Vitamin E deficiency in premature infants and in patients with impaired fat absorption—
Adults: 60 to 75 IU, depending on severity, P.O. or I.M. daily. Maximum 300 IU daily.
Children: 1 mg equivalent/0.6 g of dietary unsaturated fat P.O. or I.M. daily.

SIDE EFFECTS
None reported.

INTERACTIONS
Mineral oil, cholestyramine resin: inhibited GI absorption of oral vitamin E. Space doses. Use together cautiously.

NURSING CONSIDERATIONS
• Water-miscible forms more completely absorbed in GI tract than other forms.
• Adequate bile is essential for absorption.
• Requirements increase with rise in dietary polyunsaturated acids.
• May protect other vitamins against oxidation.
• Used for a variety of disorders with mixed successes and failures. Dosages not established.
• Megadoses can cause thrombophlebitis.
• This vitamin is fat soluble. Discourage patient from self-medication with megadoses, as they can cause undesirable side effects.

menadione/menadiol sodium diphosphate (vitamin K₃)
Kappadione, Synkavite♦♦, Synkayvite

INDICATIONS & DOSAGE
Hypoprothrombinemia secondary to vitamin K malabsorption or drug therapy, or when oral administration is desired and bile secretion is inadequate—
Adults: 2 to 10 mg menadione P.O. or 5 to 15 mg menadiol sodium diphosphate P.O. or parenterally, titrated to patient's requirements.

SIDE EFFECTS
CNS: headache, kernicterus.
GI: nausea, vomiting.
Skin: allergic rash, pruritus, urticaria.
Local: pain, hematoma at injection site.

INTERACTIONS
Mineral oil, cholestyramine resin: inhibited GI absorption of oral vitamin K. Space doses. Use together cautiously.

NURSING CONSIDERATIONS
• Contraindicated in treatment of oral anticoagulant overdose; in treatment of hereditary hypoprothrombinemia (because vitamin K₃ can paradoxically worsen it); in patients with hepatocellular disease, unless it is caused by biliary obstruction; or in treatment of heparin-induced bleeding. Use cautiously during last weeks of pregnancy to avoid toxic reactions in newborns and in G-6-PD deficiency to avoid hemolysis. In severe bleeding, do not delay other measures, such as giving fresh frozen plasma or whole blood. Use large doses cautiously in severe hepatic disease.
• Failure to respond to vitamin K₃ may indicate coagulation defects.
• Excessive use of vitamin K₃ may temporarily defeat oral anticoagulant therapy. Higher doses of oral anticoag-

ulant or interim use of heparin may be required.
• Protect parenteral products from light.
• When I.V. route must be used, rate shouldn't exceed 1 mg/minute.
• Effects of I.V. injections more rapid but shorter lived than S.C. or I.M. injections.
• Monitor prothrombin time to determine dosage effectiveness.
• Observe for signs of side effects and report them to doctor.
• Use caution in handling bulk menadione powder. It is irritating to the skin and the respiratory tract.
• Leafy vegetables are high in vitamin K content and may alter warfarin needs.
• This vitamin is fat soluble.

phytonadione (vitamin K₁)
AquaMephyton♦, Konakion♦, Mephyton

INDICATIONS & DOSAGE
Hypoprothrombinemia secondary to vitamin K malabsorption, drug therapy, or excess vitamin A—
Adults: 2 to 25 mg, depending on severity, P.O. or parenterally, repeated and increased up to 50 mg, if necessary.
Children: 5 to 10 mg P.O. or parenterally.
Infants: 2 mg P.O. or parenterally. I.V. injection rate for children and infants should not exceed 3 mg/m²/minute or a total of 5 mg.
Hypoprothrombinemia secondary to effect of oral anticoagulants—
Adults: 2.5 to 10 mg P.O., S.C., or I.M., based on prothrombin time, repeated, if necessary, 12 to 48 hours after oral dose or 6 to 8 hours after parenteral dose. In emergency, give 10 to 50 mg slow I.V., rate not to exceed 1 mg/minute, repeated q 4 hours, as needed.
Prevention of hemorrhagic disease in neonates—

Neonates: 0.5 to 1 mg S.C. or I.M. immediately after birth, repeated in 6 to 8 hours, if needed, especially if mother received oral anticoagulants or long-term anticonvulsant therapy during pregnancy.

Differentiation between hepatocellular disease or biliary obstruction as source of hypoprothrombinemia—
Adults and children: 10 mg I.M. or S.C.

Prevention of hypoprothrombinemia related to vitamin K deficiency in long-term parenteral nutrition—
Adults: 5 to 10 mg S.C. or I.M. weekly.
Children: 2 to 5 mg S.C. or I.M. weekly.

Prevention of hypoprothrombinemia in infants receiving less than 0.1 mg/liter vitamin K in breast milk or milk substitutes—
Infants: 1 mg S.C. or I.M. monthly.

SIDE EFFECTS
CNS: dizziness, convulsive movement.
CV: transient hypotension after I.V. administration, rapid and weak pulse, cardiac irregularities.
GI: nausea, vomiting.
Skin: sweating, flushing, erythema.
Local: pain, swelling, and hematoma at injection site.
Other: bronchospasms, dyspnea, cramp-like pain, *anaphylaxis and anaphylactoid reactions, usually after rapid I.V. administration.*

INTERACTIONS
Mineral oil, cholestyramine resin: inhibited GI absorption of oral vitamin K. Use together cautiously.

NURSING CONSIDERATIONS
• Contraindicated in hereditary hypoprothrombinemia; bleeding secondary to heparin therapy or overdose; hepatocellular disease, unless it is caused by biliary obstruction (vitamin K can paradoxically worsen the hypoprothrombinemia). Oral administration contra-

indicated if bile secretion is inadequate, unless supplemented with bile salts. Use cautiously, if at all, during last weeks of pregnancy to avoid toxic reactions in newborns; in G-6-PD deficiency to avoid hemolysis. Use large doses cautiously in severe hepatic disease.
• Failure to respond to vitamin K may indicate coagulation defects.
• In severe bleeding, don't delay other measures such as fresh frozen plasma or whole blood.
• Protect parenteral products from light. Wrap infusion container with aluminum foil.
• Effects of I.V. injections more rapid but shorter lived than S.C. or I.M. injections.
• Monitor prothrombin time to determine dosage effectiveness.
• Observe for signs of side effects and report them to the doctor.
• Phytonadione therapy for hemorrhagic disease in infants causes fewer adverse reactions than do other vitamin K analogs.
• Check brand name labels for administration route restrictions.
• Administer I.V. by slow infusion (over 2 to 3 hours). Mix in normal saline solution, dextrose 5% in water, or dextrose 5% in normal saline solution. Observe patient closely for signs of flushing, weakness, tachycardia, and hypotension; may progress to shock.
• Leafy vegetables are high in vitamin K content and may alter warfarin needs.
• This vitamin is fat soluble.

---

multivitamins
Available by many brand names. Contain vitamins A, B complex, C, D, and E in varying amounts.

INDICATIONS & DOSAGE
Prevention of vitamin deficiencies in patients with inadequate diets or increased daily requirements; treatment of multi-

---

plevitamin deficiencies and prevention of recurrence; additions to parenteral nutrition solutions to meet patient's normal or increased requirements—
Adults and children: dosage depends on nature and severity of deficiencies and composition of multivitamin preparation.

SIDE EFFECTS
None reported.

INTERACTIONS
Refer to each component of the multivitamin combination.

NURSING CONSIDERATIONS
• A single discovered vitamin deficiency usually coexists with others. After initial deficiencies are corrected, stress need for adequate nutrition and multivitamin supplements, if appropriate.
• Tell patient about possible interactions of vitamins in combinations and what precautions to take to avoid problems.
• Stress need to follow doctor's orders regarding daily dosages and follow-up therapy.
• Avoid excessive use of large-volume parenteral solutions of multivitamin supplements containing fat-soluble vitamins to prevent hypervitaminosis. I.V. solutions of water-soluble multivitamins may be used more freely.
• Chewable flavored multivitamins available for children. Prevent use of these drugs as candy.
• Liquid preparations may contain varying percentages of alcohol. Check label; alert patient to content.
• Warn against overdosing. Encourage patient to eat a well-balanced diet. Stress hazards of self-administered megadoses of vitamins. These medications are drugs, not just harmless vitamins. Explain possible side effects.
• Multivitamin preparations with ordinary doses of each component are usually nontoxic.

• Megavitamin combinations may promote significant accumulation of fat-soluble vitamins, with resultant toxicity.
• Multivitamins containing therapeutic doses of folic acid may mask pernicious anemia. Unless prescribed otherwise by doctor, patient should avoid folic acid in undiagnosed but suspected pernicious anemia.
• Other side effects depend on specific components and concentrations in each multivitamin preparation.
• Store vitamins in a cool place in light-resistant containers to limit loss of potency.

sodium fluoride
Fluor-A-Day ♦♦, Fluoritabs, Flura-Drops, Karidium♦, Luride Lozi-Tabs, Pediaflor

INDICATIONS & DOSAGE
Aid in the prevention of dental caries—
Oral—
Children over 3 years: 1 mg daily.
Children 3 years and under: 0.5 mg daily.
Topical—
Adults and children over 12 years: 10 ml. Use once daily after thoroughly brushing teeth and rinsing mouth. Rinse around and between teeth for 1 minute, then spit out.
Children 6 to 12 years: 5 ml.

SIDE EFFECTS
CNS: headaches, weakness.
GI: gastric distress.
Skin: hypersensitivity reactions such as atopic dermatitis, eczema, and urticaria.

INTERACTIONS
None significant.

NURSING CONSIDERATIONS
• Contraindicated when fluoride intake from drinking water exceeds 0.7 parts/

Unmarked trade names available in the United States only.
♦ Also available in Canada.   ♦ ♦ Available in Canada only.

million, and in patients on sodium-restricted diets.
- Chronic toxicity (fluorosis) may result from prolonged use of higher than recommended doses.
- Advise patient to notify dentist if tooth mottling occurs.
- Tablets may be dissolved in mouth, chewed, or swallowed whole.
- Drops may be administered orally undiluted or mixed with fluids or food.
- Topical forms (rinses and gels) should not be swallowed. Most effective when used immediately after brushing teeth.
- Tell patient to dilute drops or rinses in plastic containers rather than glass.
- Used investigationally in the treatment of osteoporosis.

trace elements
chromium, copper, iodine (as iodide), manganese, zinc

INDICATIONS & DOSAGE
Prevention of individual trace element deficiencies in patients receiving long-term hyperalimentation—
Chromium—
Adults: 10 to 15 mcg I.V. daily.
Children: 0.14 to 0.20 mcg/kg I.V. daily.
Copper—
Adults: 0.5 to 1.5 mg I.V. daily.
Children: 0.05 to 0.2 mg/kg I.V. daily.
Iodine—
Adults: 1 mcg/kg I.V. daily.
Manganese—
Adults: 1 to 3 mg I.V. daily.
Zinc—
Adults: 2 to 4 mg I.V. daily.
Children: 0.05 mg/kg I.V. daily.

SIDE EFFECTS
None reported.

INTERACTIONS
None significant at recommended dosages.

NURSING CONSIDERATIONS
- Check trace element serum levels of patients who have received total parenteral nutrition for 2 months or longer. Give supplement if ordered. Call doctor's attention to low serum levels of these elements.
- Normal serum levels are 0.07 to 0.15 mg/ml copper; 0.05 to 0.15 mg/100 ml zinc; 4 to 20 mcg/100 ml manganese.
- Solutions of trace elements are compounded by pharmacy for addition to total parenteral nutrition solutions according to various formulas. One common trace element solution is Shil's solution, which contains copper 1 mg/ml, iodide 0.06 mg/ml, manganese 0.4 mg/ml, and zinc 2 mg/ml.
- Trace element solutions are now also commercially available.

zinc sulfate
Orazinc

INDICATIONS & DOSAGE
Treatment of zinc deficiency or adjunct to treatment of disorders related to low serum zinc levels, including oral and decubitus leg ulcers, acne, granuloma of the ear, rheumatoid arthritis, idiopathic hypogeusia, anosmia; also, as adjunct to vitamin A therapy when patient fails to respond to vitamin A alone and in acrodermatitis enteropathica—
Adults: 200 to 220 mg P.O. t.i.d. (equivalent to 135 to 150 mg elemental zinc daily, 9 times the adult RDA of 15 mg daily).
Children: dosages not established. RDA is 0.3 mg/kg daily.

SIDE EFFECTS
GI: distress and irritation, nausea, vomiting with high doses.

INTERACTIONS
None significant.

Italicized side effects are common or life-threatening.
*Liquid form contains alcohol.   **May contain tartrazine.

NURSING CONSIDERATIONS

- Beneficial only if patient is zinc-deficient.
- Normal serum levels may not reliably show absence of zinc deficiency.
- Results may not appear for 6 to 8 weeks in zinc-depleted patients.
- Decreasing dosage to 100 mg b.i.d. may ease nausea or other GI side effects; zinc is thought to irritate gastric mucosa.
- Brown bread and dairy products may hinder zinc absorption.

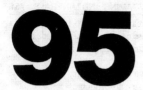

Calorics

amino acid solution
corn oil
dextrose (D-glucose)
essential crystalline amino acid solution
fat emulsions
fructose (levulose)
invert sugar
medium-chain triglycerides

MECHANISM OF ACTION
• Amino acids are used for protein synthesis of the viscera and skeletal muscle in the protein-depleted patient.
• I.V. carbohydrates minimize glyconeogenesis and promote anabolism in patients who can't receive sufficient oral caloric intake. I.V. solutions of dextrose, fructose, and invert sugar supply the energy equivalent of 3.4 kcal/g.
• I.V. fat emulsions provide neutral triglycerides, predominantly unsaturated fatty acids.

COMBINATION PRODUCTS
DEXTROSE 2½%, 5%, 10% and sodium chloride 0.45%.
DEXTROSE 2½%, 5%, 10% and sodium chloride 0.9%.
DEXTROSE 3⅓% and sodium chloride 0.3%.
DEXTROSE 5% and sodium chloride 0.11%, 0.2%, 0.33%.
POTASSIUM CHLORIDE 10 mEq, 20 mEq, 27 mEq, 30 mEq, 40 mEq, in 5% dextrose in water.
POTASSIUM CHLORIDE 10 mEq, 20 mEq, 30 mEq, 40 mEq in 5% dextrose, and 0.2% sodium chloride.
POTASSIUM CHLORIDE 10 mEq, 20 mEq, 30 mEq, 40 mEq in 5% dextrose, and 0.45% sodium chloride.
DEXTROSE 5% WITH ELECTROLYTE #75:50 g/L dextrose, 40 mEq/L Na^+, 35 mEq/L K^+, 40 mEq/L Cl^-, 15 mEq/L phosphate, and 20 mEq/L lactate.
ISOLYTE M WITH 5% DEXTROSE: 50 g/L dextrose, 40 mEq/L Na^+, 35 mEq/L K^+, 40 mEq/L Cl^-, 15 mEq/L phosphate, and 20 mEq/L acetate.
ISOLYTE G WITH 5% DEXTROSE: 50 g/L dextrose, 63 mEq/L Na^+, 17 mEq/L K^+, and 150 mEq/L Cl^-.
IONOSOL G IN 10%DEXTROSE: 100 g/L dextrose, 63 mEq/L Na^+, 17 mEq/L K^+, and 151 mEq/L Cl^-.
ISOLYTE G WITH 10% DEXTROSE: 100 g/L dextrose, 63 mEq/L Na^+, 17 mEq/L K^+, and 150 mEq/L Cl^-.
DEXTROSE 2.5% IN HALF-STRENGTH RINGER'S: 25 g/L dextrose, 74 mEq/L Na^+, 2 mEq/L K^+, 2 mEq/L Ca^{++}, and 78 mEq/L Cl^-.
DEXTROSE 5% IN RINGER'S: 50g/L dextrose, 147 mEq/L Na^+, 4 mEq/L K^+, 4 mEq/L Ca^{++}, and mEq/L 155 Cl^-.
DEXTROSE 2½% IN HALF-STRENGTH LACTATED RINGER'S: 25 g/L dextrose, 65 mEq/L Na^+, 2 mEq/L K^+, 1 mEq/L Ca^{++}, 54 mEq/L Cl^-, and 14 mEq/L lactate.
DEXTROSE 2½% IN LACTATED RINGER'S: 25 g/L dextrose, 130 mEq/L Na^+, 4 mEq/L K^+, 3 mEq/L Ca^{++}, 109 mEq/L Cl^-, and 28 mEq/L lactate.
DEXTROSE 5% IN LACTATED RINGER'S: 50 g/L dextrose, 130 mEq/L Na^+, 4 mEq/L K^+, 3 mEq/L Ca^{++}, 109 mEq/L Cl^-, and 28 mEq/L lactate.

Italicized side effects are common or life-threatening.
*Liquid form contains alcohol.   **May contain tartrazine.

DEXTROSE 10% IN LACTATED RINGER'S: 100 g/L dextrose, 130 mEq/L Na^+, 4 mEq/L K +, 3 mEq/L Ca^{++}, 109 mEq/L Cl^-, and 28 mEq/L lactate.

DEXTROSE 5% IN ACETATED RINGER'S: 50 g/L dextrose, 130 mEq/L Na^+, 4 mEq/L K^+, 3 mEq/L Ca^{++}, 109 mEq/L Cl^-, and 28 mEq/L acetate.

DEXTROSE 5% WITH ELECTROLYTE #48: 50 g/L dextrose, 25 mEq/L Na^+, 20 mEq/L K^+, 3 mEq/L Mg^{++}, 22 mEq/L Cl^-, 3 mEq/L phosphate, and 23 mEq/L lactate.

IONOSOL MB IN 5% DEXTROSE: 50 g/L dextrose, 25 mEq/L Na^+, 20 mEq/L K^+, 3 mEq/L Mg^{++}, 22 mEq/L Cl^-, 3 mEq/L phosphate, and 23 mEq/L lactate.

ELECTROLYTE #2 WITH 5% DEXTROSE: 50 g/L dextrose, 55 mEq/L Na^+, 23 mEq/L K^+, 5 mEq/L Mg^{++}, 45 mEq/L Cl^-, 12 mEq/L phosphate, and 25 mEq/L lactate.

IONOSOL B IN 5% DEXTROSE: 50 g/L dextrose, 57 mEq/L Na^+, 25 mEq/L K^+, 5 mEq/L Mg^{++}, 49 mEq/L Cl^-, 13 mEq/L phosphate, and 25 mEq/L lactate.

POLYONIC M-56 IN 5% DEXTROSE: 50 g/L dextrose, 40 mEq/L dextrose, 40 mEq/L Na^+, 13 mEq/L K^+, 3 mEq/L Mg^{++}, 40 mEq/L Cl^-, and 16 mEq/L acetate.

PLASMA-LYTE 56 IN 5% DEXTROSE: 50 g/L dextrose, 40 mEq/L Na^+, 13 mEq/L K^+, 3 mEq/L Mg^{++}, 40 mEq/L Cl^-, and 16 mEq/L acetate.

ISOLYTE P WITH 5% DEXTROSE: 50 g/L dextrose, 25 mEq/L Na^+, 20 mEq/L K^+, 3 mEq/L Mg^{++}, 22 mEq/L Cl^-, 3 mEq/L phosphate, and 23 mEq/L acetate.

ISOLYTE S WITH 5% DEXTROSE: 50 g/L dextrose, 140 mEq/L Na^+, 5 mEq/L K^+, 3 mEq/L Mg^{++}, 98 mEq/L Cl^-, and 27 mEq/L acetate.

PLASMA-LYTE 148 IN DEXTROSE: 50 g/L dextrose, 140 mEq/L Na^+, 5 mEq/L K^+, 3 mEq/L Mg^{++}, 98 mEq/L Cl^-, and 27 mEq/L acetate.

POLYONIC R-148 IN 5% DEXTROSE: 50 g/L dextrose, 140 mEq/L Na^+, 5 mEq/L K^+, 3 mEq/L mg^{++}, 98 mEq/L Cl^-, and 27 mEq/L acetate.

ISOLYTE R WITH 5% DEXTROSE: 50 g/L dextrose, 40 mEq/L Na^+, 16 mEq/L K^+, 5 mEq/L Ca^{++}, 3 mEq/L Mg^{++}, 40 mEq/L Cl^-, and 24 mEq/L acetate.

PLASMA-LYTE M IN 5% DEXTROSE: 50 g/L dextrose, 40 mEq/L Na^+, 16 mEq/L K^+, 5 mEq/L Ca^{++}, 3 mEq/L Mg^{++}, 40 mEq/L Cl^-, 12 mEq/L lactate, and 12 mEq/L acetate.

POLYSAL WITH 5% DEXTROSE: 50 g/L dextrose, 140 mEq/L Na^+, 10 mEq/L K^+, 5 mEq/L Ca^+, 3 mEq/L Mg^{++}, 103 mEq/L Cl^-, and 55 mEq/L acetate.

PLASMA-LYTE WITH 5% DEXTROSE: 50g/L dextrose, 140 mEq/L Na^+, 10 mEq/L K^+, 5 mEq/L Ca^{++}, 3 mEq/L Mg^{++}, 103 mEq/L Cl^-, 8 mEq/L lactate, and 47 mEq/L acetate.

ISONOSOL D-CM IN 5% DEXTROSE: 50 g/L dextrose, 138 mEq/L Na^+, 12 mEq/L K^+, 5 mEq/L Ca^{++}, 3 mEq/L Mg^{++}, 108 mEq/L Cl^-, and 50 mEq/L lactate.

ISOLYTE M WITH 5% FRUCTOSE: 50 g/L fructose, 40 mEq/L Na^+, 35 mEq/L K^+, 40 mEq/L Cl^-, 15 mEq/L phosphate, and 20 mEq/L acetate.

ISOLYTE P WITH 5% FRUCTOSE: 50 g/L fructose, 25 mEq/L Na^+, 26 mEq/L K^+, 3 mEq/L Mg^{++}, 23 mEq/L Cl^-, and 3 mEq/L phosphate, and 23 mEq/L acetate.

POLYONIC-M 900: 150 g/L fructose, 40 mEq/L Na^+, 13 mEq/L K^+, 3 mEq/L Mg^{++}, 40 mEq/L Cl^-, and 16 mEq/L acetate.

NORMOSOL-M 900♦: 150 g/L fructose, 40 mEq/L Na^+, 13 mEq/L K^+, 3 mEq/L Mg^{++}, 40 mEq/L Cl^-, and 16 mEq/L acetate.

IONOSOL G WITH 10% INVERT SUGAR: 100 g/L invert sugar, 60 mEq/L Na^+, 17 mEq/L K^+, and 147 mEq/L Cl^-.

5% TRAVERT WITH ELECTROLYTE #4: 50 g/L invert sugar, 30 mEq/L Na^+, 15 mEq/L K^+, 23 mEq/L Cl^-, 3 mEq/L phosphate, and 20 mEq/L lactate.

ELECTROLYTE #2 WITH 5% INVERT

SUGAR: 50 g/L invert sugar, 58 mEq/L Na^+, 25 mEq/L K^+, 6 mEq/L Mg^{++}, 51 mEq/L Cl^-, 13 mEq/L phosphate, and 25 mEq/L lactate.

5% TRAVERT WITH ELECTROLYTE #2: 50 g/L invert sugar, 56 mEq/L Na^+, 25 mEq/L K^+, 6 mEq/L Mg^{++}, 56 mEq/L Cl^-, 12.5 mEq/L phosphate, and 25 mEq/L lactate.

IONOSOL B WITH 10% INVERT SUGAR: 100 g/L invert sugar, 54 mEq/L Na^+, 25 mEq/L K^+, 5 mEq/L Mg^{++}, 49 mEq/L Cl^-, 13 mEq/L phosphate, and 22 mEq/L lactate.

10% TRAVERT WITH ELECTROLYTE #2: 100 g/L invert sugar, 56 mEq/L Na^+, 25 mEq/L K^+, 6 mEq/L Mg^{++}, 56 mEq/L Cl^-, 12.5 mEq/L phosphate, and 25 mEq/L lactate.

10% TRAVERT WITH ELECTROLYTE #1: 100 g/L invert sugar, 80 mEq/L Na^+, 36 mEq/L K^+, 5 mEq/L Ca^{++}, 3 mEq/L Mg^{++}, 64 mEq/L Cl^-, and 60 mEq/L lactate.

PLASMA-LYTE WITH 10% TRAVERT: 100 g/L invert sugar, 140 mEq/L Na^+, 10 mEq/L K^+, 5 mEq/L Ca^{++}, 3 mEq/L Mg^{++}, 103 mEq/L Cl^-, and 8 mEq/L lactate.

---

amino acid solution
(crystalline amino acid solution)
Aminosyn, FreAmine III ♦,
Travasol♦, Veinamine

INDICATIONS & DOSAGE
Total, supportive, or supplemental and protein-sparing parenteral nutrition when gastrointestinal system must rest during healing, or when patient can't, shouldn't, or won't eat at all or eat enough to maintain normal nutrition and metabolism—
Adults: 1 to 1.5 g/kg I.V. daily.
Children: 2 to 3 g/kg I.V. daily. Individualize dosage to metabolic and clinical response as determined by nitrogen balance and body weight corrected for fluid balance. Add electrolytes, vita-

mins, and nonprotein caloric solutions as needed.

SIDE EFFECTS
CNS: mental confusion, unconsciousness, headache, dizziness.
CV: hypervolemia related to congestive heart failure (in susceptible patients), *pulmonary edema,* exacerbation of hypertension (in predisposed patients).
GI: nausea, vomiting.
GU: glycosuria, osmotic diuresis.
Hepatic: fatty liver.
Metabolic: *rebound hypoglycemia* (when long-term infusions are abruptly stopped), *hyperglycemia,* metabolic acidosis, alkalosis, hypophosphatemia, *hyperosmolar syndrome, hyperosmolar-hyperglycemic-nonketotic syndrome,* hyperammonemia, *electrolyte imbalances,* and dehydration (if hyperosmolar solutions used).
Skin: chills, flushing, feeling of warmth.
Local: tissue sloughing at infusion site due to extravasation, *catheter sepsis, thrombophlebitis, thrombosis.*
Other: allergic reactions.

INTERACTIONS
None significant.

NURSING CONSIDERATIONS
• Contraindicated in patients with severe uncorrected electrolyte or acid-base imbalances, in hyperammonemia, and in decreased circulating blood volume. Use cautiously in renal insufficiency or failure, cardiac disease, and hepatic impairment. Long-term use for infants and children must be closely monitored.
• Monitor serum electrolytes, magnesium, glucose, BUN, renal and hepatic function. Check serum calcium levels frequently to avoid bone demineralization in children.
• If long-term therapy is needed, doctor may order trace element and vitamin supplements. Avoid overuse of fat-

---

soluble vitamins A and D—can cause toxic hypervitaminosis.

• Refrigerate solution until ½ hour before it will be infused.

• Don't mix medications, except electrolytes, vitamins, and trace elements with hyperalimentation solution without first consulting pharmacist.

• Control infusion rate carefully with infusion pump.

• If infusion rate falls behind, do not attempt to "catch up." Notify doctor.

• Check infusion site frequently for erythema, inflammation, irritation, tissue sloughing, necrosis, and phlebitis. Change I.V. sites routinely to prevent irritation and infection. I.V. catheter is usually introduced into subclavian vein.

• Watch closely for signs of fluid overload. Notify doctor promptly.

• Some crystalline amino acid solutions contain large amounts of acetates and lactates; use cautiously in patients with alkalosis or hepatic insufficiency.

• Most side effects are due to mixing amino acids with hypertonic dextrose solutions.

• Check fractional urines every 6 hours for glycosuria (if present, the doctor may order insulin coverage).

• Assess body temperature every 4 hours; elevation may indicate sepsis, infection.

• If patient has chills, fever, or other signs of sepsis, replace I.V. tubing and bottle and send them to the laboratory to be cultured.

corn oil
Lipomul♦

INDICATIONS & DOSAGE
As energy source—
Adults: 45 ml P.O. b.i.d. to q.i.d. after or between meals, alone or with proteins, milk, or other energy sources.
Children: 30 ml P.O. daily to q.i.d. after or between meals, alone or with proteins, milk, or other energy sources.

SIDE EFFECTS
GI: nausea, vomiting, diarrhea.

INTERACTIONS
Griseofulvin: increased GI absorption of griseofulvin. Space doses.

NURSING CONSIDERATIONS
• Contraindicated in gallbladder calculi or complete GI obstructions. Use cautiously in steatorrhea, partial GI obstruction, enterostomies, hepatic cirrhosis, portacaval shunts.
• To minimize nausea, diarrhea, and vomiting, give more frequent, smaller doses with meals or mixed with milk.

dextrose (D-glucose)

INDICATIONS & DOSAGE
Fluid replacement and caloric supplementation in patient who can't maintain adequate oral intake or who is restricted from doing so—
Adults and children: dosage depends on fluid and caloric requirements. Use peripheral I.V. infusion of 2.5%, 5%, or 10% solution, central I.V. infusion of 20% solution for minimal fluid needs. Use 50% solution to treat insulin-induced hypoglycemia. Solutions from 40% to 70% are used diluted in admixtures, normally with amino acid solutions, for total parenteral nutrition given through a central vein.

SIDE EFFECTS
CNS: mental confusion, unconsciousness in hyperosmolar syndrome.
CV: (with fluid overload) pulmonary edema, exacerbated hypertension, and congestive heart failure in susceptible patients. *Prolonged or concentrated infusions may cause phlebitis, sclerosis of vein, especially with peripheral route of administration.*
GU: glycosuria, osmotic diuresis.

Metabolic: (with rapid infusion of concentrated solution or prolonged infusion) hyperglycemia, hypervolemia, hyperosmolarity. Rapid termination of long-term infusions may cause hypoglycemia from rebound hyperinsulinemia.

Skin: sloughing and tissue necrosis, if extravasation occurs with concentrated solutions.

INTERACTIONS
None significant.

NURSING CONSIDERATIONS
• Contraindicated in hyperglycemia, diabetic coma, intracranial or intraspinal hemorrhage, delirium tremens. Use cautiously in cardiac or pulmonary disease, hypertension, renal insufficiency, urinary obstruction, or hypovolemia.
• Control infusion rate carefully. Maximal rate for dextrose infusion is 0.5 g/kg hourly. Use infusion pump when infusing dextrose with amino acids for total parenteral nutrition.
• Never infuse concentrated solutions rapidly; can cause hyperglycemia, fluid shift.
• Monitor serum glucose carefully. Prolonged therapy with 5% dextrose solution can cause depletion of pancreatic insulin production and secretion.
• Never stop abruptly. If necessary, have 10% dextrose solution available to treat hypoglycemia if rebound hyperinsulinemia occurs.
• Take care to prevent extravasation. Check injection site frequently to prevent irritation, tissue sloughing, necrosis, and phlebitis.
• Watch closely for signs of fluid overload, especially if fluid intake is restricted.
• Monitor intake/output and weight carefully, especially when renal function is impaired.
• Check vital signs frequently. Report side effects promptly.

• Don't give dextrose solutions without saline with blood transfusions; may cause clumping of red blood cells.

---

essential crystalline amino acid solution
Aminosyn-RF, Nephramine

INDICATIONS & DOSAGE
Management of potentially reversible renal decompensation—
Adults: 0.3 to 0.5 g/kg I.V., up to 26 g total daily (250 ml with 500 ml 70% dextrose injection), and infuse through central I.V. line at initial rate of 20 to 30 ml/hour, increased in steps of 10 ml/hour every 24 hours, to a maximum of 60 to 100 ml/hour. Individualize dose and infusion rate to tolerance for glucose, fluid, and nitrogen. Add electrolytes and vitamins as needed.
Children: up to 1 g/kg daily, individualized to patient's tolerance for glucose, fluid, and nitrogen. Add electrolytes, trace elements, and vitamins as needed.

SIDE EFFECTS
CNS: mental confusion, dizziness, unconsciousness, headache.
CV: hypervolemia related to congestive heart failure (in susceptible patients), *pulmonary edema,* exacerbation of hypertension (in predisposed patients).
GI: nausea, vomiting.
GU: glycosuria, osmotic diuresis.
Metabolic: *rebound hypoglycemia* (when long-term infusions are abruptly stopped), *hyperglycemia,* metabolic acidosis, alkalosis, hypophosphatemia, hyperosmolar syndrome, *hyperosmolar-hyperglycemic-nonketotic syndrome,* hyperammonemia, *electrolyte imbalances,* and dehydration (if hyperosmolar solutions used).
Skin: chills, flushing, feeling of warmth.
Local: tissue sloughing at infusion site due to extravasation, *catheter sepsis, thrombophlebitis.*
Other: allergic reactions.

Italicized side effects are common or life-threatening.
*Liquid form contains alcohol.   **May contain tartrazine.

INTERACTIONS
None significant.

NURSING CONSIDERATIONS
• Contraindicated in severe uncorrected electrolyte or acid-base imbalances, hyperammonemia, and decreased circulating blood volume.
• Monitor serum electrolytes, magnesium, glucose, BUN, renal and hepatic function. Check serum calcium levels frequently to avoid bone demineralization in children.
• In long-term therapy, doctor may order trace element and vitamin supplements. Avoid overuse of fat-soluble vitamins.
• Refrigerate solution until ½ hour before it will be infused.
• Don't mix medications, except electrolytes, vitamins, and trace elements with hyperalimentation solution without first consulting pharmacist.
• Control infusion rate carefully with infusion pump.
• If infusion rate falls behind, do not attempt to "catch up." Notify doctor.
• Check infusion site frequently for erythema, inflammation, irritation, tissue sloughing, necrosis, and phlebitis. Change I.V. sites routinely to prevent irritation. I.V. catheter is usually placed in subclavian vein.
• Watch closely for signs of fluid overload. Notify doctor promptly.
• Essential amino acid solution is used identically to other crystalline amino acid solutions, except that it contains only the essential amino acids. By controlling amino acid content, patients with impaired renal function have decreases in blood urea nitrogen level, minimized deterioration of serum potassium, magnesium, and phosphorus balances. May lead to earlier return of renal function in patients with potentially reversible acute renal failure and may decrease morbidity associated with acute renal failure.
• Most side effects due to mixing essential crystalline amino acid solution with hypertonic dextrose solutions.
• Check fractional urines every 6 hours for glycosuria (if present, the doctor may order insulin coverage).
• Assess body temperature every 4 hours; elevation may indicate sepsis, infection.
• If patient has chills, fever, or other signs of sepsis, replace I.V. tubing and bottle and send them to the laboratory to be cultured.

fat emulsions
Intralipid 10%♦, Intralipid 20%, Liposyn 10%, Liposyn 20%, Travamulsion 10%

INDICATIONS & DOSAGE
Intralipid:
Source of calories adjunctive to total parenteral nutrition—
Adults: 1 ml/minute I.V. for 15 to 30 minutes (10% emulsion); 0.5 ml/minute I.V. for 15 to 30 minutes (20% emulsion). If no adverse reactions, increase rate to deliver 500 ml over 4 to 8 hours. Total daily dose should not exceed 2.5 g/kg.
Children: 0.1 ml/minute for 10 to 15 minutes (10% emulsion), 0.05 ml/minute I.V. for 10 to 15 minutes (20% emulsion). If no adverse reactions, increase rate to deliver 1 g/kg over 4 hours. Daily dose should not exceed 4 g/kg. Equals 60% of daily caloric intake. Protein-carbohydrate hyperalimentation should supply remaining 40%.
Fatty acid deficiency—
Adults and children: 8% to 10% of total caloric intake I.V.
Liposyn:
Prevention of fatty acid deficiency—
Adults: 500 ml (10% emulsion) I.V. twice weekly. Infuse initially at a rate of 1 ml/minute for 30 minutes. Rate may be increased but should not exceed 500 ml over 4 to 6 hours.
Children: 5 to 10 ml/kg (10% emul-

sion) I.V. daily. Infuse initially at a rate of 0.1 ml/minute for 30 minutes. Rate may be increased but should not exceed 100 ml/hour.

SIDE EFFECTS
Early reactions of fat overload:
Blood: hyperlipemia, hypercoagulability, rarely thrombocytopenia in neonates.
CNS: headache, sleepiness, dizziness.
EENT: pressure over eyes.
GI: nausea, vomiting.
Skin: flushing, diaphoresis.
Local: irritation at infusion site.
Other: fever, dyspnea, chest and back pains, cyanosis, allergic reactions, deposition of I.V. fat.
Delayed reactions:
Blood: thrombocytopenia, leukopenia, leukocytosis.
CNS: focal seizures.
CV: *shock*.
Hepatic: transient increased liver function test, hepatomegaly.
Other: fever, splenomegaly, fat accumulation in lungs.

INTERACTIONS
None significant.

NURSING CONSIDERATIONS
• Contraindicated in hyperlipemia, lipid nephrosis, and acute pancreatitis accompanied by hyperlipemia. Use cautiously in severe hepatic disease, pulmonary disease, anemia, blood coagulation disorders, or patients with possible danger of fat embolism.
• Use very cautiously in premature infants, as they are very susceptible to I.V. fat overload. Carefully monitor triglycerides and free fatty acid levels in these infants.
• Never mix with electrolytes or other nutrient products or dilute manufactured fat emulsions. Infusion may be piggybacked into another I.V. line, but do not place additives in the fat emulsion bottle.
• Do not use an in-line filter when ad-

ministering this drug because the fat particles are larger than the 0.22-micron cellulose filter.
• Discard fat emulsion if it separates or becomes oily. Intralipid and Travamulsion may be refrigerated, although refrigeration is not essential. Liposyn needs no refrigeration.
• Avoid rapid infusion. Use an infusion pump to regulate rate.
• Check injection site daily. Report signs of inflammation or infection promptly.
• Watch closely for side effects, especially during first half hour of infusion.
• Monitor serum lipids closely when patient is receiving fat emulsion therapy. Lipemia must clear between dosing.
• Check platelet count frequently in neonates receiving fat emulsions I.V.
• Monitor hepatic function carefully in long-term use.
• Intralipid, Travamulsion, and Liposyn differ mainly by their fatty acid components.

fructose (levulose)

INDICATIONS & DOSAGE
Source of carbohydrate calories primarily when fluid replacement is also indicated and as a dextrose substitute for patients with diabetes—
Adults and children: dosage depends on caloric needs. I.V. infusion rate should not exceed 1 g/kg hourly. Single liter 10% solution yields 375 calories.

SIDE EFFECTS
CV: increased pulse rate, precipitation or exacerbation of congestive heart failure in susceptible patients, *pulmonary edema*.
Hepatic: hepatomegaly.
Metabolic: metabolic acidosis, hypervolemia.
Local: extravasation at infusion site

Italicized side effects are common or life-threatening.
*Liquid form contains alcohol.   **May contain tartrazine.

may cause sloughing of skin, thrombo-phlebitis.
Other: increased respiratory rate.

INTERACTIONS
None significant.

NURSING CONSIDERATIONS
• Contraindicated in hereditary fructose intolerance or in patients receiving therapy for hypoglycemia. Use cautiously in cardiac disease, hypertension, pulmonary disease, hypervolemia, renal insufficiency, or urinary tract obstructions.
• Control infusion rate carefully. Make sure rate does not exceed 1 g/kg hourly in infants.
• Change infusion sites regularly to avoid irritation with prolonged therapy. Take care to avoid extravasation.
• Watch closely for signs of fluid overload, pulmonary edema, or congestive heart failure.
• May be safely used in patients with diabetes.

---

invert sugar
Travert

INDICATIONS & DOSAGE
Nonelectrolyte fluid replacement and caloric supplementation solution—
Adults and children: dosage depends on patient's age, weight, clinical need. I.V. infusion rate should not exceed 1 g/kg hourly. Single liter 5% invert sugar yields 375 calories.

SIDE EFFECTS
CNS: mental confusion.
CV: increased pulse rate, precipitation or exacerbation of congestive heart failure in susceptible patients, *pulmonary edema,* hypertension.
GU: glycosuria, osmotic diuresis.
Metabolic: metabolic acidosis, hypervolemia, hyperglycemia, hypoglycemia.
Local: extravasation at infusion site

may cause sloughing of skin, thrombo-phlebitis.
Other: increased respiratory rate.

INTERACTIONS
None significant.

NURSING CONSIDERATIONS
• Contraindicated in hereditary fructose intolerance, hyperglycemia, diabetic coma, intracranial or intraspinal hemorrhage, or delirium tremens. Use cautiously in cardiac disease, hypertension, pulmonary disease, hypervolemia, renal insufficiency, or urinary tract obstructions.
• Control infusion rate carefully. Make sure rate does not exceed 1 g/kg hourly in infants.
• Change infusion sites regularly to avoid irritation with prolonged therapy. Take care to avoid extravasation.
• Watch closely for signs of fluid overload, pulmonary edema, or congestive heart failure. Monitor blood pressure frequently.
• May be safely used in patients with diabetes.
• Monitor serum glucose closely. Prolonged therapy can cause depletion of pancreatic insulin production and secretion.
• Don't stop abruptly. If necessary, have 10% dextrose available to prevent rebound hyperinsulinemia and subsequent hypoglycemia.
• Monitor intake/output and weight closely, especially if renal function is impaired.
• Check vital signs frequently. Tell doctor promptly if side effects develop.

---

medium-chain triglycerides
M.C.T. Oil♦

INDICATIONS & DOSAGE
Inadequate digestion or absorption of food fats—
Adults: 15 ml P.O. t.i.d. to q.i.d.

SIDE EFFECTS
CNS: reversible coma and precoma in susceptible patients.
GI: *nausea, vomiting, diarrhea.*

INTERACTIONS
None significant.

NURSING CONSIDERATIONS
• Contraindicated in advanced hepatic disease.
• To minimize GI side effects, give smaller doses more frequently with meals or mixed with fruit juice or salad dressing.
• More easily absorbed than long-chain fats; not dependent on bile salts for emulsification.
• Rapid metabolism provides quick energy.
• May be useful in obesity control and in lowering cholesterol levels. Also used in patients with short-bowel syndrome.

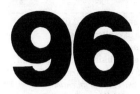

Immune serums

antirabies serum, equine
hepatitis B immune globulin, human
immune serum globulin
rabies immune globulin, human
Rh₀ (D) immune globulin, human
tetanus immune globulin, human
varicella-zoster immune globulin (VZIG)

MECHANISM OF ACTION
Immune serums contain preformed protective substances (antibodies) from the serum of human beings or animals, especially horses, that have been immunized by injection with the organisms or toxins of diseases. These antibodies, therefore, combat specific diseases.

COMBINATION PRODUCTS
None.

---

antirabies serum, equine

INDICATIONS & DOSAGE
Rabies exposure—
Adults and children: 40 to 55 units/kg at time of first dose of rabies vaccine. Use half dose to infiltrate wound area. Give remainder I.M. Don't give rabies vaccine and antirabies serum in same syringe or at same site.

SIDE EFFECTS
Local: pain at injection site.
Systemic: within 6 to 12 days serum sickness occurs in 15% to 25% of patients. Symptoms are skin eruptions, arthralgia, pruritus, lymphadenopathy, fever, headache, malaise, abdominal pain, *anaphylaxis.*

INTERACTIONS
None significant.

NURSING CONSIDERATIONS
• In hypersensitivity to equine serum, use rabies immune globulin, human, instead. If unavailable, desensitize before giving. Consult doctor or pharmacist.
• Do sensitivity test on all patients before giving. Dilute serum 1:100 or 1:1,000 with 0.9% sodium chloride for injection. Inject intradermally on inner forearm. Inject other arm with 0.1 ml of 0.9% sodium chloride for injection intradermally as control. Read within 20 minutes. Positive reaction: wheal 10 mm or more and erythematous flare 20 × 20 mm.
• Use only when rabies immune globulin, human, not available.
• Obtain history of animal bite, allergies (especially to equine serum and to eggs), and reaction to immunization.
• Epinephrine solution 1:1,000 should always be available when administering this drug.
• This immune serum provides immediate passive immunity (short-term).
• Do not confuse this drug with rabies vaccine, which is a suspension of attenuated or killed microorganisms used to confer long-term active immunity. These two drugs are often administered together prophylactically after exposure to known or suspected rabid animals.
• Ask patient when he received last tet-

anus immunization, since many doctors order a booster at this time.

hepatitis B immune globulin, human
H-BIG, HyperHep, Hep-B-Gammagee

INDICATIONS & DOSAGE
Hepatitis B exposure—
Adults and children: 0.06 ml/kg I.M. within 7 days after exposure. Repeat 28 days after exposure.

SIDE EFFECTS
Systemic: *anaphylaxis.*

INTERACTIONS
None significant.

NURSING CONSIDERATIONS
• Buttocks or deltoid areas preferred injection sites.
• Nurse should receive immunization if exposed to hepatitis B (for example, needle-stick, direct contact).
• Obtain history of allergies and reaction to immunization.

immune serum globulin
Gamastan, Gamimune, Gammar, Immuglobin

INDICATIONS & DOSAGE
Agammaglobulinemia or hypogammaglobulinemia—
Adults: 30 to 50 ml I.M. monthly.
Children: 20 to 40 ml I.M. monthly.
Hepatitis A exposure—
Adults and children: 0.02 to 0.04 ml/kg I.M. as soon as possible after exposure. Up to 0.1 ml/kg may be given after prolonged or intense exposure.
Serum hepatitis post-transfusion—
Adults and children: 10 ml I.M. within 1 week after transfusion and 10 ml I.M. 1 month later.
Measles exposure—

Adults and children: 0.02 ml/kg within 6 days after exposure.
Modification of measles—
Adults and children: 0.04 ml/kg I.M. within 6 days after exposure.
Measles vaccine complications—
Adults and children: 0.02 to 0.04 ml/kg I.M.
Poliomyelitis exposure—
Adults and children: 0.3 to 0.4 ml/kg I.M. within 7 days after exposure.
Chickenpox exposure—
Adults and children: 0.2 to 1.3 ml/kg I.M. as soon as exposed.
Rubella exposure in first trimester of pregnancy—
Women: 0.2 to 0.4 ml/kg I.M. as soon as exposed.

SIDE EFFECTS
Skin: urticaria.
Local: pain, erythema, muscle stiffness.
Systemic: angioedema, headache, malaise, fever, nephrotic syndrome, *anaphylaxis.*

INTERACTIONS
None significant.

NURSING CONSIDERATIONS
• Obtain history of allergies and reaction to immunization.
• Have drugs available for anaphylactic reaction.
• Divide dose of more than 10 ml, and inject into different sites, preferably buttocks. Do not inject more than 3 ml per injection site.
• Do not give for hepatitis A exposure if 6 weeks or more have elapsed since exposure or after onset of clinical illness.

rabies immune globulin, human
Hyperab, Imogam

INDICATIONS & DOSAGE
Rabies exposure—

Italicized side effects are common or life-threatening.
∗Liquid form contains alcohol.   ∗∗May contain tartrazine.

Adults and children: 20 IU/kg at time of first dose of rabies vaccine. Use half dose to infiltrate wound area. Give remainder I.M. Don't give rabies vaccine and rabies immune globulin in same syringe or at same site.

SIDE EFFECTS
Local: pain, redness, induration at injection site.
Other: slight fever, *anaphylaxis.*

INTERACTIONS
None significant.

NURSING CONSIDERATIONS
• Repeated doses contraindicated after rabies vaccine is started.
• Use only with rabies vaccine and immediate local treatment of wound. Give regardless of interval between exposure and initiation of therapy.
• Obtain history of animal bite, allergies, reaction to immunization.
• Corticosteroids decrease resistance to infection and decrease antibody response to vaccine. Stop corticosteroids after possible rabies exposure.
• This immune serum provides passive immunity.
• Do not confuse this drug with rabies vaccine, which is a suspension of attenuated or killed microorganisms used to confer active immunity. These two drugs are often given together prophylactically after exposure to known or suspected rabid animals.
• Ask the patient when he received his last tetanus immunization, since many doctors order a booster at this time.

Rh$_o$ (D) immune globulin, human
Gamulin Rh, HypRho-D, MICRhoGAM, RhoGam

INDICATIONS & DOSAGE
Rh exposure—
Women postabortion, postmiscarriage, ectopic pregnancy, or postpar-

tum: transfusion unit or blood bank determines fetal packed red blood cell volume entering woman's blood, then gives one vial I.M. if fetal packed RBC volume is less than 15 ml. More than one vial I.M. may be required if there is large fetomaternal hemorrhage. Must be given within 72 hours after delivery or miscarriage.
Transfusion accidents—
Adults and children: consult blood bank or transfusion unit at once. Must be given within 72 hours.
Postabortion or postmiscarriage to prevent Rh antibody formation—
Women: consult transfusion unit or blood bank. Ideally should be given within 3 hours, but may be given up to 72 hours after abortion or miscarriage.

SIDE EFFECTS
Local: discomfort at injection site.
Other: slight fever.

INTERACTIONS
None significant.

NURSING CONSIDERATIONS
• Contraindicated in Rh$_o$(D)-positive or D^u-positive patients and those previously immunized to Rh$_o$(D) blood factor.
• Immediately after delivery, send a sample of infant's cord blood to laboratory for type and crossmatch. Confirm mother is Rh$_o$ (D)-negative and D^u-negative. Infant must be Rh$_o$ (D)-positive or D^u-positive.
• Give only to postpartum mother.
• Obtain history of allergies and reaction to immunization.
• MICRhoGAM recommended for every woman undergoing abortion or miscarriage up to 12 weeks' gestation unless she is Rh$_o$ (D)-positive or D^u-positive, has Rh antibodies, or the father and/or fetus is Rh negative.
• Store at 36° to 46° F. (2° to 8° C.).
• This immune serum provides passive immunity to the woman exposed to

Rh$_o$-positive fetal blood during pregnancy. Prevents formation of maternal antibodies (active immunity), which would endanger future Rh$_o$-positive pregnancies.
• Explain to the patient how drug protects future Rh$_o$-positive infants.

tetanus immune globulin, human
Homo-Tet, Hu-Tet, Hyper-Tet

INDICATIONS & DOSAGE
Tetanus exposure—
Adults and children: 250 units I.M.
Tetanus treatment—
Adults and children: single doses of 3,000 to 6,000 units have been used. Optimal dosage schedules not established. Don't give at same site as toxoid.

SIDE EFFECTS
Local: pain, stiffness, erythema.
Other: slight fever, allergy, *anaphylaxis.*

INTERACTIONS
None significant.

NURSING CONSIDERATIONS
• Use tetanus immune globulin only if wound is over 24 hours old or patient has had less than two previous tetanus toxoid injections.
• Obtain history of injury, tetanus immunizations, last tetanus toxoid injection, allergies, and reaction to immunization.
• Thoroughly cleanse and remove all foreign matter from wound.
• This immune serum provides passive immunity. Antibodies remain at effective levels for 3 weeks or longer, which is several times the duration of antitoxin-induced antibodies. Protects the patient for the incubation period of most tetanus cases.
• Human globulin is not a substitute for tetanus toxoid, which should be

given at the same time to produce active immunization.
• Do not confuse this drug with tetanus toxoid.

varicella-zoster immune globulin (VZIG)

INDICATIONS & DOSAGE
Passive immunization of susceptible immunodeficient children after exposure to varicella (chicken pox or herpes zoster)—
Children to 10 kg: 125 units I.M.
Children 10.1 to 20 kg: 250 units I.M.
Children 20.1 to 30 kg: 375 units I.M.
Children 30.1 to 40 kg: 500 units I.M.
Children over 40 kg: 625 units I.M.

SIDE EFFECTS
Local: local discomfort at injection site, rash.
Systemic: gastrointestinal distress, malaise, headache, respiratory distress, *anaphylaxis.*

INTERACTIONS
None reported.

NURSING CONSIDERATIONS
• Contraindicated in patients with a history of severe reaction to human immune serum globulin or severe thrombocytopenia.
• VZIG is not recommended for non-immunosuppressed patients, including pregnant women.
• Not commercially distributed. Available only from 20 regional distribution centers throughout the United States. These centers will distribute to Canada and overseas. Call the Centers for Disease Control (404-329-3311) for the distribution center in your area.
• Should be administered only by deep I.M. injection. Never administer I.V.
• Store vial in refrigerator.

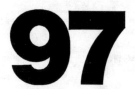

Vaccines and toxoids

BCG vaccine
cholera vaccine
diphtheria and tetanus toxoids,
   adsorbed
diphtheria and tetanus toxoids
   and pertussis vaccine (DPT)
diphtheria toxoid, adsorbed,
   pediatric
hepatitis B vaccine
influenza virus vaccine, trivalent
measles, mumps, and rubella
   virus vaccine, live
measles (rubeola) and rubella
   virus vaccine, live attenuated
measles (rubeola) virus vaccine,
   live attenuated
meningitis vaccines
mumps virus vaccine, live
plague vaccine
pneumococcal vaccine,
   polyvalent
poliovirus vaccine, live, oral,
   trivalent
rabies vaccine, human diploid
   cell (HDCV)
rubella and mumps virus
   vaccine, live
rubella virus vaccine, live
   attenuated (RA 27/3)
smallpox vaccine
tetanus toxoid
typhoid vaccine
yellow fever vaccine

MECHANISM OF ACTION
Vaccines and toxoids initiate formation
of specific antibodies by stimulating the
host's antigen-antibody mechanism,
providing active, acquired immunity.
(Active immunity can be induced by
exposure to an infectious disease or to
one of its antigens, or by vaccination.
The host has the ability to produce
these immune bodies even after the antigen is rendered harmless.)

COMBINATION PRODUCTS
None.

BCG vaccine

INDICATIONS & DOSAGE
*Tuberculosis exposure, cancer immuno-
therapy—*
Adults and children: 0.1 ml intrader-
mally.
Newborns: 0.05 ml intradermally.

SIDE EFFECTS
Local: lymphangitis, lymph node and
skin abscess, ulceration at site of injection (2 to 3 weeks after injection), lupus reaction.
Other: urticaria of trunk and limbs,
anaphylaxis.

INTERACTIONS
Isoniazid (INH): inhibited multiplication of BCG. Avoid using together.

NURSING CONSIDERATIONS
• Contraindicated in patients with
hypogammaglobulinemia, positive tuberculin reaction (when meant for use
as immunoprophylactic after exposure
to tuberculosis), immunosuppression,
fresh smallpox vaccination, and burns,
and in those receiving corticosteroid
therapy. Use cautiously in chronic skin
disease. Inject in area of healthy skin
only.

- Obtain history of allergies and reaction to immunization.
- Vaccine is of no value as immunoprophylactic in patients with positive tuberculin test.
- Keep epinephrine 1:1,000 available to treat anaphylaxis.
- Recommended injection site is over insertion of deltoid muscle.
- Do not shake vial following reconstitution.
- Expected lesion forms in 7 to 10 days.
- Live vaccine; destroy by autoclaving or formaldehyde solution before disposal.
- Patient should have tuberculin skin test 2 to 3 months after BCG vaccination to determine success of vaccine.
- Use of BCG has shown some value in treatment of various cancers, such as leukemia, some lung cancers, malignant melanoma, multiple myeloma, and some breast tumors. Currently, researchers are trying to find ways of augmenting the immune system's response to cancer. They hope to stimulate the body to destroy tumor cells.

cholera vaccine

INDICATIONS & DOSAGE
Primary immunization—
Adults and children over 10 years: 2 doses of 0.5 ml I.M. or 1 ml S.C., 1 week to 1 month before traveling in cholera area. Booster: 0.5 ml q 6 months as long as protection is needed.
Children 5 to 10 years: 0.3 ml I.M. or S.C.
Children 6 months to 4 years: 0.2 ml I.M. or S.C. Boosters of same dose should be given q 6 months as long as protection needed.

SIDE EFFECTS
Systemic: malaise, fever, flushing, urticaria, tachycardia, hypotension, headache, *anaphylaxis.*

Local: erythema, swelling, pain, induration.

INTERACTIONS
None significant.

NURSING CONSIDERATIONS
- Contraindicated in corticosteroid therapy or in immunosuppression. Defer in acute illness.
- Obtain history of allergies and reaction to immunization.
- Keep epinephrine 1:1,000 available.
- May be given intradermally, but I.M. and subcutaneous routes give higher levels of protection.

diphtheria and tetanus toxoids, adsorbed

INDICATIONS & DOSAGE
Primary immunization—
Adults and children 7 years and over: use adult strength; 0.5 ml I.M. 4 to 6 weeks apart for 2 doses and a third dose 1 year later. Booster: 0.5 ml I.M. q 10 years.
Children under 7 years: use pediatric strength; 0.5 ml I.M. 4 to 8 weeks apart for 2 doses and a third dose 6 to 12 months later. Booster: 0.5 ml when starting school.

SIDE EFFECTS
Systemic: chills, fever, malaise, *anaphylaxis.*
Local: stinging, edema, erythema, pain, induration.

INTERACTIONS
None significant.

NURSING CONSIDERATIONS
- Contraindicated in immunosuppression, radiation, or corticosteroid therapy. Defer in respiratory illness or polio outbreaks, or acute illness except in emergency. Use single antigen during polio risks. In children under 6 years, use only when diphtheria, tetanus, and

---

Italicized side effects are common or life-threatening.
*Liquid form contains alcohol.   **May contain tartrazine.

pertussis toxoid combination is contra-indicated because of pertussis component.
• Verify strength (pediatric or adult) of toxoid used.
• Don't use hot or cold compresses; may increase severity of local reaction.
• Obtain history of allergies and reaction to immunization.
• Keep epinephrine 1:1,000 available.
• Give in site not previously used for vaccines or toxoids.

diphtheria and tetanus toxoids and pertussis vaccine (DPT)
Tri-Immunol, Triple Antigen

INDICATIONS & DOSAGE
Primary immunization—
Children 6 weeks to 6 years: 0.5 ml I.M. 2 months apart for 3 doses and a fourth dose 1 year later. Booster: 0.5 ml I.M. when starting school. Not advised for adults or children over 6 years.

SIDE EFFECTS
Systemic: slight fever, chills, malaise, *convulsions, encephalopathy, anaphylaxis.*
Local: soreness, redness, expected nodule remaining several weeks.

INTERACTIONS
None significant.

NURSING CONSIDERATIONS
• Contraindicated in corticosteroid therapy or immunosuppression. Defer in acute illness.
• Stop immunization if CNS disorder occurs. Immunization may be continued with diphtheria and tetanus toxoids without pertussis component at doses of 0.05 to 0.1 ml.
• DPT injection may be given at same time as trivalent oral polio vaccine (TOPV).

• Obtain history of allergies and reaction to immunization.
• Keep epinephrine 1:1,000 available.
• Not to be used for active infection.
• Don't give subcutaneously.
• Shake before using. Refrigerate.

diphtheria toxoid, adsorbed, pediatric

INDICATIONS & DOSAGE
Diphtheria immunization—
Children under 6 years: 0.5 ml I.M. 6 to 8 weeks apart for 2 doses and a third dose 1 year later. Booster: 0.5 ml I.M. at 5- to 10-year intervals. Not advised for adults or for children over 6 years; instead, use adult strength of diphtheria toxoid (usually combined with tetanus toxoid).

SIDE EFFECTS
Systemic: fever, malaise, urticaria, tachycardia, flushing, pruritus, hypotension, aches and pains, *anaphylaxis.*
Local: erythema, pain, induration, expected nodule persistent for several weeks.

INTERACTIONS
None significant.

NURSING CONSIDERATIONS
• Contraindicated in immunosuppression, radiation or corticosteroid therapy, children under 12 months with cerebral damage. Defer in acute illness or polio outbreak, except in emergency.
• Don't use hot or cold compresses; may intensify local reaction.
• Obtain history of allergies and reaction to immunization.
• Keep epinephrine 1:1,000 available to treat anaphylaxis.
• Shake vial well before using. Store in refrigerator.

Unmarked trade names available in the United States only.
♦ Also available in Canada.   ♦ ♦ Available in Canada only.

hepatitis B vaccine
Hepatavax

INDICATIONS & DOSAGE
Immunization against infection caused by all known subtypes of hepatitis B virus. Recommended for immunization of selected populations who are considered to be at increased risk of contracting hepatitis B infection—
Adults and children over 10 years: initial dose 1 ml I.M. followed by another dose of 1 ml 1 month later. This is followed by a third dose of 1 ml 6 months after the first dose.
Children 3 months to 10 years: initial dose 0.5 ml I.M. followed by another dose of 0.5 ml 1 month later. This is followed by a third dose of 0.5 ml 6 months after the first dose.
Dialysis and immunocompromised patients: initial dose 2 ml I.M. followed by another dose of 2 ml 1 month later. This is followed by a third dose of 2 ml 6 months after the first dose. (The 2-ml doses should be divided into 2 1-ml doses and administered at different sites.)

SIDE EFFECTS
Local: discomfort at injection site, local inflammation.
Systemic: slight fever, transient malaise, headache, dizziness, nausea, vomiting.

INTERACTIONS
None reported.

NURSING CONSIDERATIONS
• Use cautiously in patients with any serious active infection, compromised cardiac or pulmonary status, and in those whom a febrile or systemic reaction could pose a serious risk.
• Although anaphylaxis has not been reported, epinephrine should always be available when administering this drug to counteract any possible reaction.
• Because the incubation period for hepatitis B is long, unrecognized hepatitis B infection may be present when the vaccine is given. The vaccine will not prevent hepatitis B in such patients.
• The recommended dosage regimen provides immunity for at least 5 years.
• The following are at increased risk of infection and should be considered for the vaccine: health-care personnel, selected patients and patient contacts, certain endemic populations (Alaskan Eskimos, Indo-Chinese and Haitian refugees), certain military personnel, morticians and embalmers, blood bank employees, sexually active homosexuals, prostitutes, prisoners, users of illicit injectable drugs.
• For I.M. use only.
• Thoroughly agitate vial just before administration to restore suspension.
• Store both opened and unopened vials in the refrigerator. Don't freeze.

influenza virus vaccine, trivalent types A & B (whole virus)
Fluax•, Fluzone-Connaught

influenza virus vaccine, trivalent types A & B (split virus)
Fluogen •

INDICATIONS & DOSAGE
Brazil, Bangkok, and Singapore influenza prophylaxis—
Adults and youths 13 years and older: 0.5 ml whole or split virus I.M. Only one dose is required.
Children 3 to 12 years: give 0.5 ml split virus I.M. Repeat dose in 4 weeks unless child received 1978 to 1982 vaccine.
Children 6 to 35 months: 0.25 ml split virus I.M. Repeat dose in 4 weeks unless child received 1978 to 1982 vaccine.
Recommendations are for 1983 only. Must check yearly for new recommendations.

Italicized side effects are common or life-threatening.
∗Liquid form contains alcohol.   ∗∗May contain tartrazine.

SIDE EFFECTS
Systemic: *fever, malaise, myalgia, Guillain-Barré syndrome, anaphylaxis.*
Local: erythema, induration. Side effects occur most often in children and in others not exposed to influenza viruses.

INTERACTIONS
None significant.

NURSING CONSIDERATIONS
• Contraindicated in egg allergy. Defer in acute respiratory or other active infection, or when there is risk of poliomyelitis infection.
• Obtain history of allergies, especially to eggs, and reaction to immunization.
• Give injections in deltoid or midlateral thigh.
• Keep epinephrine 1:1,000 available.
• Recommended for patients with chronic disease, metabolic disorders, and those over 65 years of age.
• Influenza vaccine available as whole virus and split virus preparations. Split virus vaccines cause somewhat fewer side effect than whole virus in children.
• Fever, malaise, and myalgia begin 6 to 12 hours after vaccination and persist 1 to 2 days.
• Allergic reactions, which occur immediately, are extremely rare.
• Paralysis associated with Guillain-Barré syndrome is uncommon, but patient should be made aware of risk as compared with risk of influenza and its complications.

measles, mumps, and rubella virus vaccine, live
M-M-R-II♦

INDICATIONS & DOSAGE
Immunization—
Children 12 months to puberty:
1 vial (1,000 units) S.C.

SIDE EFFECTS
Systemic: fever, rash, regional lymphadenopathy, urticaria, *anaphylaxis.*
Local: erythema.

INTERACTIONS
Immune serum globulin, whole blood, plasma: antibodies in serum may interfere with immune response. Don't use vaccine within 3 months of transfusion.

NURSING CONSIDERATIONS
• Contraindicated in immunosuppression; cancer; blood dyscrasias; corticosteroid or radiation therapy; gamma globulin disorders; fever; active, untreated tuberculosis. Use cautiously in hypersensitivity to neomycin, chickens, ducks, eggs, or feathers. Defer immunization in acute illness.
• Presence of maternal antibodies may prevent response in children under 12 months.
• Treat fever with antipyretics.
• Store in refrigerator; protect from light. Solution may be used if red, pink, or yellow, but must be clear.
• Use only diluent supplied. Discard 8 hours after reconstituting.
• Obtain history of allergies, especially to ducks, rabbits, antibiotics, and reaction to immunization.
• Inject in outer aspect of upper arm. Don't give I.V.
• Keep epinephrine 1:1,000 available.

measles (rubeola) and rubella virus vaccine, live attenuated
M-R-Vax-II

INDICATIONS & DOSAGE
Immunization—
Children 15 months to puberty:
1 vial (1,000 units) S.C.

SIDE EFFECTS
Systemic: fever, rash, lymphadenopathy, *anaphylaxis.*

INTERACTIONS

Immune serum globulin, whole blood, plasma: antibodies in serum may interfere with immune response. Don't use vaccine within 3 months of transfusion.
Tuberculin skin test: may temporarily decrease response to test. Defer skin testing.

NURSING CONSIDERATIONS

• Contraindicated in immunosuppression; cancer; blood dyscrasias; corticosteroid or radiation therapy; gamma globulin disorders; fever; active, untreated tuberculosis. Use cautiously in hypersensitivity to neomycin, chickens, ducks, eggs, or feathers, and when there is a history of febrile seizures or in cerebral injury. Defer immunization in acute illness.
• Do not give within 1 month of other live virus vaccines, except oral poliovirus vaccine.
• Store in refrigerator and protect from light. Solution may be used if red, pink, or yellow, but must be clear (with no precipitation).
• Use only diluent supplied. Discard 8 hours after reconstituting.
• Inject in outer aspect of upper arm. Don't inject I.V.

---

measles (rubeola) virus vaccine, live attenuated
Attenuvax♦

INDICATIONS & DOSAGE
Immunization—
Adults and children 15 months or over: 0.5 ml (1,000 units) S.C.

SIDE EFFECTS
Systemic: fever, rash, lymphadenopathy, *anaphylaxis,* febrile convulsions in susceptible children, anorexia, leukopenia.
Local: erythema, swelling, tenderness.

INTERACTIONS
Immune serum globulin, whole blood, plasma: antibodies in serum may interfere with immune response. Don't use vaccine within 3 months of transfusion.
Tuberculin skin test: may temporarily decrease response to test. Defer skin testing.

NURSING CONSIDERATIONS

• Contraindicated in immunosuppression; cancer; blood dyscrasias; corticosteroid or radiation therapy; gamma globulin disorders; active, untreated tuberculosis; fever. Use with caution in hypersensitivity to neomycin, chickens, eggs, or feathers. Defer in acute illness or after administration of blood or plasma.
• Warn patient to avoid pregnancy for 3 months after vaccination.
• Do not give I.V.
• Obtain history of allergies, especially to eggs, and reaction to immunization.
• Keep epinephrine 1:1,000 available.
• Store in refrigerator and protect from light. Solution may be used if red, pink, or yellow, but must be clear (with no precipitation).
• Use only diluent supplied. Discard 8 hours after reconstituting.
• May be given with oral poliovirus vaccine.

---

meningitis vaccines
Meningovax-A/C, Menomune-A, Menomune-C, Menomune-A/C, Menomune-A/C/Y/W-135

INDICATIONS & DOSAGE
Meningococcal meningitis prophylaxis—
Adults 18 years or older: 0.5 ml S.C. vaccine group A/C/Y/W-135 only.
Adults and children over 2 years: 0.5 ml S.C. Use vaccine group C or A, except in highly endemic areas; in these areas use A/C combination.
Children 3 months to 2 years: 0.5 ml S.C. Use vaccine group A.

SIDE EFFECTS

Systemic: headache, malaise, chills, fever, cramps, *anaphylaxis.*
Local: pain, erythema, induration.

INTERACTIONS

None significant.

NURSING CONSIDERATIONS

• Contraindicated in immunosuppression. Defer in acute illness.
• Tell patient to avoid pregnancy for 3 months after vaccination.
• Obtain history of allergies and reaction to immunization.
• Do not give I.V.
• Keep epinephrine 1:1,000 available.

mumps virus vaccine, live

Mumpsvax♦

INDICATIONS & DOSAGE

Immunization—
Adults and children over 12 months: 1 vial (5,000 units) S.C.

SIDE EFFECTS

Systemic: *slight fever,* rash, malaise, mild allergic reactions.

INTERACTIONS

Immune serum globulin, whole blood, plasma: antibodies in serum may interfere with immune response. Don't use vaccine within 3 months of transfusion.
Tuberculin skin test: may temporarily decrease response to test. Defer skin testing.

NURSING CONSIDERATIONS

• Contraindicated in immunosuppression; cancer; blood dyscrasias; corticosteroid or radiation therapy; gamma globulin disorders; active, untreated tuberculosis; pregnancy. Use cautiously in hypersensitivity to neomycin, chickens, ducks, eggs, or feathers. Defer in acute illness and for 3 months following transfusions or immune serum globulin.

• Keep epinephrine 1:1,000 available.
• Mumpsvax should not be given less than 1 month before or after immunization with other live virus vaccines, with the exception of Attenuvax, Meruvax, and/or monovalent or trivalent live, oral poliovirus vaccine, which may be administered simultaneously.
• The vaccine will not offer protection when given after exposure to natural mumps.
• Not recommended for infants younger than 12 months because retained maternal mumps antibodies may interfere with the immune response.
• Stress importance of avoiding pregnancy for 3 months after immunization. If necessary, provide contraceptive information.
• Treat fever with antipyretics.
• Don't give I.V.
• Store in refrigerator and protect from light. Solution may be used if red, pink, or yellow, but must be clear.
• Use only diluent supplied. Discard 8 hours after reconstituting.
• Obtain history of allergies, especially to antibiotics, and reaction to immunization.

plague vaccine

INDICATIONS & DOSAGE

Primary immunization and booster—
Adults and children over 10 years: 1 ml I.M. followed by 0.2 ml in 4 weeks, then 0.2 ml 6 months after the first dose. Booster: 0.1 to 0.2 ml q 6 months while in plague area.
Children 5 to 10 years: $^3/_5$ adult primary or booster dose.
Children 1 to 4 years: $^2/_5$ adult primary or booster dose.
Children under 1 year: $^1/_5$ adult primary or booster dose.

SIDE EFFECTS

Systemic: malaise, headache, slight fever, lymphadenopathy, *anaphylaxis.*
Local: swelling, *induration, erythema.*

Unmarked trade names available in the United States only.
♦ Also available in Canada. ♦ ♦ Available in Canada only.

INTERACTIONS
None significant.

NURSING CONSIDERATIONS
- Contraindicated in immunosuppression. Defer in respiratory infection.
- Deltoid area preferred injection site.
- Obtain history of allergies and reaction to immunization.
- Keep epinephrine 1:1,000 available.

---

pneumococcal vaccine, polyvalent
Pneumovax◆,Pnu-Imune

INDICATIONS & DOSAGE
Pneumococcal immunization—
Adults and children 2 years or over:
0.5 ml I.M. or S.C.
Not recommended for children under 2 years.

SIDE EFFECTS
Systemic: *slight fever, anaphylaxis.*
Local: severe local reaction can occur when revaccination takes place within 3 years.

INTERACTIONS
None significant.

NURSING CONSIDERATIONS
- Check immunization history carefully to avoid revaccination within 3 years.
- Inject in deltoid or midlateral thigh. Don't inject I.V.
- Keep refrigerated. Reconstitution or dilution not necessary.
- Treat fever with mild antipyretics.
- Protects against 14 pneumococcal types, which account for 80% of pneumococcal disease.
- Obtain history of allergies and reaction to immunization.
- Keep epinephrine 1:1,000 available.

poliovirus vaccine, live, oral, trivalent
Orimune

INDICATIONS & DOSAGE
Poliovirus immunization—
Adults and children over 6 weeks:
two drops or 0.5 ml P.O. in 5 ml of water or simple syrup, or on sugar cube. Repeat dose in 8 weeks. Give third dose at 18 months. Booster: two drops or 0.5 ml P.O.

SIDE EFFECTS
None reported.

INTERACTIONS
Immune serum globulin, whole blood, plasma: antibodies in serum may interfere with immune response. Don't use vaccine within 3 months of transfusion.

NURSING CONSIDERATIONS
- Contraindicated in immunosuppression, cancer, immunoglobulin abnormalities, and in radiation, antimetabolite, alkylating agent, or corticosteroid therapy. Defer in acute illness, vomiting, or diarrhea.
- Use with caution in siblings of child with known immunodeficiency syndrome.
- This vaccine not effective in modifying or preventing existing or incubating poliomyelitis.
- Check the parents' immunization history when they bring in child for vaccine; this is an excellent time for parents to receive booster immunizations.
- Keep frozen until used. Once thawed, if unopened, may store refrigerated up to 30 days. Opened vials may be refrigerated up to 7 days. Thaw before administration.
- Color change from pink to yellow has no effect on the efficiency of the vaccine. Yellow color results from vaccine being stored at low temperatures.

Italicized side effects are common or life-threatening.
*Liquid form contains alcohol.   **May contain tartrazine.

- Obtain history of allergies and reaction to immunization.
- Not for parenteral use.

rabies vaccine, human diploid cell (HDCV)
Wyvac

INDICATIONS & DOSAGE
Postexposure antirabies immunization—
Adults and children: 5 1-ml doses of HDCV I.M. (for example, in the deltoid region). Give first dose as soon as possible after exposure; give an additional dose on each of days 3, 7, 14, and 28 after first dose.
Preexposure prophylaxis immunization for persons in high-risk groups—
Adults and children: 3 1-ml injections administered I. M. Give first dose on day 0 (the first day of therapy), second dose on day 7, and third dose on either day 21 or 28.

SIDE EFFECTS
Systemic: headache, nausea, abdominal pain, muscle aches, dizziness.
Local: *pain, erythema, swelling or itching at injection site.*

INTERACTIONS
None significant.

NURSING CONSIDERATIONS
- Stop corticosteroids during immunization period.
- When postexposure immunization is indicated, pregnancy is not a contraindication.
- Persons with a history of hypersensitivity should be given rabies vaccine with caution. Persons allergic to duck embryo vaccine are less likely to be allergic to HDCV.
- Keep epinephrine 1:1,000 available.
- HDCV is the preferred rabies vaccine because of its presumed greater efficacy and because fewer adverse reactions are known to be associated with it.
- Although the intradermal route of administration for preexposure prophylaxis is being used in some centers, this route is not currently recommended.
- Contact state health department or Merieux Institute (1-800-327-8387) on vaccine availability.

rubella and mumps virus vaccine, live
Biavax-II

INDICATIONS & DOSAGE
Measles and mumps immunization—
Adults and children over 12 months: 1 vial (1,000 units) S.C.

SIDE EFFECTS
Systemic: fever, rash, thrombocytopenic purpura, urticaria, arthritis, arthralgia, polyneuritis, *anaphylaxis*.
Local: pain, erythema, induration, lymphadenopathy.

INTERACTIONS
Immune serum globulin, whole blood, plasma: antibodies in serum may interfere with immune response. Don't give vaccine within 3 months of transfusion.
Tuberculin skin test: may temporarily decrease response to test. Defer skin testing.

NURSING CONSIDERATIONS
- Contraindicated in immunosuppression; cancer; blood dyscrasias; corticosteroid or radiation therapy; gamma globulin disorders; active, untreated tuberculosis; fever; pregnancy. Use with caution in hypersensitivity to neomycin, chickens, ducks, eggs, or feathers. Defer in acute illness and after administration of immune serum globulin, blood, or plasma.
- Stress importance of avoiding pregnancy for 3 months after immunization. If necessary, provide contraceptive information.

Unmarked trade names available in the United States only.
♦ Also available in Canada.   ♦ ♦ Available in Canada only.

• Store in refrigerator and protect from light. Solution may be used if red, pink, or yellow, but must be clear.

• Use only diluent supplied. Discard 8 hours after reconstituting.

• Obtain history of allergies, especially to ducks, rabbits, and antibiotics, and reaction to immunization.

• Inject into outer aspect of upper arm. Don't inject I.V.

• Keep epinephrine 1:1,000 available.

rubella virus vaccine, live attenuated (RA 27/3)
Meruvax-II♦

INDICATIONS & DOSAGE
Measles immunization—
Adults and children 12 months or over: 1 vial (1,000 units) S.C.

SIDE EFFECTS
Systemic: fever, rash, thrombocytopenic purpura, urticaria, arthritis, arthralgia, polyneuritis, *anaphylaxis.*
Local: pain, erythema, induration, lymphadenopathy.

INTERACTIONS
Immune serum globulin, whole blood, plasma: antibodies in serum may interfere with immune response. Don't use vaccine within 3 months of transfusion.
Tuberculin skin test: may temporarily decrease response to test. Defer skin testing.

NURSING CONSIDERATIONS
• Contraindicated in immunosuppression; cancer; blood dyscrasias; corticosteroid or radiation therapy; gamma globulin disorders; active, untreated tuberculosis; fever. Use cautiously in hypersensitivity to neomycin, chickens, ducks, eggs, or feathers. Defer in acute illness and after administration of human immune serum globulin, blood, or plasma.

• Stress importance of avoiding pregnancy for 3 months after immunization.

If necessary, provide contraceptive information.

• Store in refrigerator and protect from light. Solution may be used if red, pink, or yellow, but must be clear.

• Use only diluent supplied. Discard 8 hours after reconstituting.

• Obtain history of allergies, especially to ducks and rabbits, and reaction to immunization.

• Inject into outer aspect of upper arm. Don't inject I.V.

• Keep epinephrine 1:1,000 available.

smallpox vaccine
Dryvax

INDICATIONS & DOSAGE
Immunization—
Adults: deposit drop of vaccine on cleansed site and make series of multiple pressures with sharp needle through drop. Use only for laboratory personnel working with virus.

SIDE EFFECTS
Systemic: encephalopathy, transverse myelitis, acute infection, polyneuritis, eczema vaccinatum, eye infection, rash, *anaphylaxis,* fever.
Local: necrosis, pustule (expected), infection.

INTERACTIONS
Immune serum globulin, whole blood, plasma: antibodies in serum may interfere with immune response. Don't use vaccine within 3 months of transfusion.
Methotrexate: may interfere with immune response. Don't use together.

NURSING CONSIDERATIONS
• Contraindicated in wounds or burns, skin disorders (for example, eczema), immunosuppression, antimetabolite and radiation therapy, and pregnancy. Also contraindicated in patients with active infections, and in those with leukemia, lymphomas, or other malignant neoplasms affecting the bone marrow

---

Italicized side effects are common or life-threatening.
*Liquid form contains alcohol.   **May contain tartrazine.

or lymphatic system. Weigh risks against benefits. Use cautiously in hypersensitivity to chickens, eggs, or feathers, or to neomycin or other antibiotic preservatives in this vaccine (polymyxin B, streptomycin, chlortetracycline).

• Don't expose site to direct sunlight for several days or to water for 2 hours. Don't cover site initially. In pustular stage, loose dressing may be applied. Warn patient against touching site: may spread lesion and cause secondary infection.

• Obtain history of allergies—especially to chickens or beef, and antibiotics—and reaction to immunization.

• Do not inject.

• Reconstituted solution may be stored for 3 months under refrigeration.

• A successful primary vaccination shows a typical jennerian vesicle. If none is observed, vaccination procedures should be checked and vaccination repeated with a different lot of vaccine until a successful result is obtained.

• After revaccination, two responses are possible. A "major reaction" is the formation of a vesicular or pustular lesion of an area of definite palpable induration, which indicates virus multiplication has most likely taken place and revaccination is successful. Any other reaction is regarded as "equivocal." When an equivocal reaction is observed, revaccination procedures should be checked and revaccination repeated with another lot of vaccine.

• Keep epinephrine 1:1,000 available.

tetanus toxoid, adsorbed
tetanus toxoid fluid

INDICATIONS & DOSAGE
Primary immunization—
Adults and children: 0.5 ml (adsorbed) I.M. 4 to 6 weeks apart for

2 doses, then third dose 1 year after the second.
Primary immunization—
Adults and children: 0.5 ml (fluid) I.M. or S.C. 4 to 8 weeks apart, for 3 doses, then fourth dose of 0.5 ml 6 to 12 months after third dose. Booster: 0.5 ml I.M. at 10-year intervals.

SIDE EFFECTS
Systemic: slight fever, chills, malaise, aches and pains, flushing, urticaria, pruritus, tachycardia, hypotension, *anaphylaxis*.
Local: erythema, induration, nodule.

INTERACTIONS
None significant.

NURSING CONSIDERATIONS
• Contraindicated in immunosuppression and immunoglobulin abnormalities. Defer in acute illness and polio outbreaks, except in emergencies.
• For prevention, not treatment, of tetanus infections.
• Determine date of last tetanus immunization.
• Don't use hot or cold compresses; may increase severity of local reaction.
• Obtain history of allergies and reaction to immunization.
• Keep epinephrine 1:1,000 available.
• Adsorbed form produces longer duration of immunity. Fluid form provides quicker booster effect in patients actively immunized previously.
• Do not confuse this drug with tetanus immune globulin, human.

typhoid vaccine

INDICATIONS & DOSAGE
Primary immunization—
Adults and children over 10 years: 0.5 ml S.C.; repeat in 4 weeks. Booster: same dose as primary immunization q 3 years.
Children 6 months to 10 years:

0.25 ml S.C.; repeat in 4 weeks.
Booster: same dose as primary immunization q 3 years.

SIDE EFFECTS
Systemic: *fever,* malaise, headache, nausea, *anaphylaxis.*
Local: swelling, pain, inflammation.

INTERACTIONS
None significant.

NURSING CONSIDERATIONS
• Contraindicated in corticosteroid therapy. Defer in acute illness.
• Treat fever with antipyretics.
• Do not give intradermally.
• Obtain history of allergies and reaction to immunization.
• Keep epinephrine 1:1,000 available.
• Store at 2° to 10° C. (35.6° to 50° F.).
• Shake thoroughly before withdrawal from vial.

---

yellow fever vaccine

INDICATIONS & DOSAGE
Primary vaccination—

Adults and children over 6 months:
0.5 ml S.C. Booster: repeat 0.5 ml S.C. q 10 years.

SIDE EFFECTS
Systemic: fever, malaise, *anaphylaxis.*

INTERACTIONS
None significant.

NURSING CONSIDERATIONS
• Contraindicated in gamma globulin deficiency, immunosuppression, cancer, corticosteroid or radiation therapy, allergies to chickens or eggs, and in pregnancy. Also contraindicated in infants under 6 months except in high-risk areas.
• Reconstitute with sodium chloride injection that contains no preservatives (preservatives decrease potency of vaccine).
• Must be kept frozen. Shake well before using. Use within 1 hour after reconstitution. Discard remainder.
• Obtain history of allergies, especially to eggs, and reaction to immunization.
• Don't give within 1 month of other live virus vaccines.
• Keep epinephrine 1:1,000 available.

Italicized side effects are common or life-threatening.
*Liquid form contains alcohol.   **May contain tartrazine.

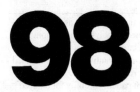

Antitoxins and antivenins

black widow spider antivenin
botulism antitoxin, bivalent
  equine
crotaline antivenin, polyvalent
diphtheria antitoxin, equine
Micrurus fulvius antivenin
tetanus antitoxin (TAT), equine

MECHANISM OF ACTION
• Antitoxins provide passive immunity. This type of immunity is acquired by inoculation with purified, concentrated antibodies that have been formed in the blood of horses immunized by specific toxins.
• Toxins and venoms are bound to and neutralized by the specific antitoxin or antivenin.

COMBINATION PRODUCTS
None.

---

black widow spider antivenin
Antivenin *(Latrodectus mactans)*◆

INDICATIONS & DOSAGE
Black widow spider bite—
Adults and children: 2.5 ml I.M. in deltoid. Second dose may be needed.

SIDE EFFECTS
Systemic: hypersensitivity, *anaphylaxis, neurotoxicity*.

INTERACTIONS
None significant.

NURSING CONSIDERATIONS
• If possible, hospitalize patient.

• Immobilize patient; splint bitten limb to prevent spread of venom.
• Test for sensitivity before giving.
• Epinephrine 1:1,000 should be available in case of adverse reaction.
• Venom is neurotoxic and may cause respiratory paralysis and convulsions. Watch patient carefully for 2 to 3 days.
• Obtain accurate patient history of allergies, especially to horses, and reaction to immunization.
• Earliest possible use of the antivenin is recommended for best results.
• Antivenin may also be given I.V. in severe cases (as when the patient is in shock). Drug is given in 10 to 50 ml of saline solution over a 15-minute period.

---

botulism antitoxin, bivalent equine

INDICATIONS & DOSAGE
Botulism—
Adults and children: 1 vial I.V. stat and q 4 hours, p.r.n., until patient's condition improves. Dilute antitoxin 1:10 in 5% or 10% dextrose in water or normal saline solution before giving. Give first 10 ml of dilution over 5 minutes; after 15 minutes, rate may be increased.

SIDE EFFECTS
Systemic: hypersensitivity, *anaphylaxis*, serum sickness (urticaria, pruritus, fever, malaise, arthralgia) may occur in 5 to 13 days.

INTERACTIONS
None significant.

NURSING CONSIDERATIONS
• Test for sensitivity before giving.
• Epinephrine 1:1,000 should be available in case of adverse reaction. Bivalent antitoxin contains antibodies against types A and B *Clostridium botulinum*. Antitoxins against all other types available only from Center for Disease Control in Atlanta, Georgia.
• Obtain accurate patient history of allergies, especially to horses, and reaction to immunization.
• Earliest possible use of antitoxin is recommended for best results.

crotaline antivenin, polyvalent

INDICATIONS & DOSAGE
Crotalid (rattlesnake) bites—
Adults and children: initially, 10 to 50 ml or more I.M. or S.C., depending on severity of bite and patient's response. If large amount of venom, 70 to 100 ml I.V. directly into superficial vein. Subsequent doses based on patient's response; may give 10 ml q ½ to 2 hours, p.r.n. If bite is in extremity, inject part of initial dose at various sites around limb above swelling; don't inject in finger or toe. The smaller the patient, the larger the initial dose.

SIDE EFFECTS
Systemic: hypersensitivity, *anaphylaxis.*

INTERACTIONS
Antihistamines: enhanced toxicity of crotaline venoms. Don't use together.

NURSING CONSIDERATIONS
• Test for sensitivity before giving.
• Immobilize patient immediately. Splint bite extremity.
• Epinephrine 1:1,000 should be available in case of adverse reaction.

• Type and crossmatch as soon as possible since hemolysis from venom prevents accurate crossmatching.
• Early use of antivenin recommended for best results.
• Watch patient carefully for delayed allergic reaction or relapse.
• Because children have less resistance and less body fluid to dilute venom, they may need twice the adult dose.
• Obtain accurate patient history of allergies, especially to horses, and reaction to immunization.
• Discard unused reconstituted drug.

diphtheria antitoxin, equine

INDICATIONS & DOSAGE
Diphtheria prevention—
Adults and children: 1,000 to 5,000 units I.M.
Diphtheria treatment—
Adults and children: 20,000 to 80,000 units or more slow I.V. Additional doses may be given in 24 hours. I.M. route may be used in mild cases.

SIDE EFFECTS
Systemic: hypersensitivity, *anaphylaxis,* serum sickness (urticaria, pruritus, fever, malaise, arthralgia) may occur in 7 to 12 days.

INTERACTIONS
None significant.

NURSING CONSIDERATIONS
• Test for sensitivity before giving.
• Epinephrine 1:1,000 should be available in case of adverse reaction.
• Obtain accurate patient history of allergies, especially to horses, and reaction to immunization.
• Therapy should be started immediately, without waiting for culture and sensitivity reports, if patient has clinical symptoms of diphtheria (sore throat, fever, tonsillar membrane).
• Refrigerate antitoxin at 2° to 10°C. (35.6° to 50° F.). May be warmed to

---

Italicized side effects are common or life-threatening.
*Liquid form contains alcohol.   **May contain tartrazine.

32.2° to 35° C. (90° to 95° F.), never higher.

Micrurus fulvius antivenin

INDICATIONS & DOSAGE
Eastern and Texas coral snake bite—
Adults and children: 3 to 5 vials slow I.V. through running I.V. of 0.9% normal saline solution. Give first 1 to 2 ml over 3 to 5 minutes, and watch for signs of allergic reaction. If no signs develop, continue injection. Up to 10 vials may be needed. Not effective for Sonoran or Arizona coral snake bites.

SIDE EFFECTS
Systemic: hypersensitivity, *anaphylaxis*.

INTERACTIONS
None significant.

NURSING CONSIDERATIONS
• Test for sensitivity before giving.
• Immobilize patient or splint bitten limb to prevent spread of venom.
• If possible, hospitalize patient.
• Early use of antivenin recommended for best results.
• Venom is neurotoxic and may cause respiratory paralysis. Watch patient carefully for 24 hours. Be ready to take supportive measures. Epinephrine 1:1,000 should be available in case of adverse reaction.
• Obtain accurate patient history of allergies, especially to horses, and reaction to immunization.

tetanus antitoxin (TAT), equine

INDICATIONS & DOSAGE
Tetanus prophylaxis—
Patients over 29.5 kg: 3,000 to 5,000 units I.M. or S.C.
Patients under 29.5 kg: 1,500 to 3,000 units I.M. or S.C.
Tetanus treatment—
All patients: 10,000 to 20,000 units injected into wound. Give additional 40,000 to 200,000 units I.V. Start tetanus toxoid at same time but at different site and with a different syringe.

SIDE EFFECTS
Local: pain, numbness, skin eruptions.
Systemic: joint pain, hypersensitivity, *anaphylaxis*.

INTERACTIONS
None significant.

NURSING CONSIDERATIONS
• Test for sensitivity before giving.
• Use only when tetanus immune globulin (human) not available.
• Obtain accurate patient history of allergies, especially to horses, and reaction to immunization. If respiratory difficulty develops, give 0.4 ml of 1:1,000 solution epinephrine HCl.
• Preventive dose should be given to those who have had two or fewer injections of tetanus toxoid and who have tetanus-prone injuries more than 24 hours old.

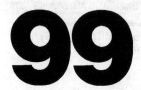

Acidifiers and alkalinizers

Acidifiers
ammonium chloride
dilute hydrochloric acid

Alkalinizers
sodium bicarbonate
sodium lactate
tromethamine

MECHANISM OF ACTION
• Acidifiers increase free hydrogen ion (H^+) concentration.
• Alkalinizers decrease free hydrogen ion concentration. Sodium bicarbonate restores the buffering capacity of the body. Sodium lactate is metabolized to sodium bicarbonate before it can produce a buffering effect. Tromethamine combines with hydrogen ions and associated acid anions; the resulting salts are excreted by the kidneys.

COMBINATION PRODUCTS
None.

---

ammonium chloride

INDICATIONS & DOSAGE
Metabolic alkalosis—
Adults and children: 4 mEq/kg slow I.V. or calculated by amount of chloride deficit. Infusion rate: 0.9 to 1.3 ml/minute 2.14% solution. Do not exceed 2 ml/minute. Hypodermoclysis has been used in infants and young children. One half calculated volume should be given, then patient should be reassessed.
As an acidifying agent—

Adults: 4 to 12 g P.O. daily in divided doses.
Children: 75 mg/kg daily P.O. in 4 divided doses.

SIDE EFFECTS
Side effects usually result from ammonia toxicity or too rapid I.V. administration.
CNS: headache, confusion, progressive drowsiness, excitement alternating with coma, hyperventilation, *calcium-deficient tetany, twitching, hyperreflexia, EEG abnormalities.*
CV: bradycardia.
GI: (with oral dose) *gastric irritation, nausea, vomiting,* thirst, anorexia, retching.
GU: glycosuria.
Metabolic: *acidosis, hyperchloremia, hypokalemia,* hyperglycemia.
Skin: rash, pallor.
Local: pain at injection site.
Other: irregular respirations with periods of apnea.

INTERACTIONS
Spironolactone: systemic acidosis. Use together cautiously.

NURSING CONSIDERATIONS
• Contraindicated in severe hepatic or renal dysfunction. Use cautiously in pulmonary insufficiency or cardiac edema and in infants.
• Give after meals to decrease GI side effects. Enteric-coated tablets may also minimize GI symptoms but are absorbed erratically.
• Pain of I.V. injection may be lessened by decreasing infusion rate.

Italicized side effects are common or life-threatening.
∗Liquid form contains alcohol. ∗∗May contain tartrazine.

- Determine CO_2 combining power and serum electrolytes before and during therapy to prevent acidosis.
- Monitor urine pH and output. Diuresis is normal for first 2 days.
- Dilute concentrated solutions (21.4%, 26.75%) to 2.14% before giving.
- Monitor rate and depth of respirations frequently.
- Hypodermoclysis should be into lateral aspect of thigh. Stop infusion immediately if pain occurs.

dilute hydrochloric acid

INDICATIONS & DOSAGE
Metabolic alkalosis— pharmacy prepares (0.1 normal HCl solution in sterile water) 100 mEq hydrogen and 100 mEq chloride/liter.

SIDE EFFECTS
None confirmed.

INTERACTIONS
None significant.

NURSING CONSIDERATIONS
- Not available commercially; prepared in pharmacy.
- Administer I.V. solution slowly through a central venous line.
- Monitor pH, blood gases, and electrolytes at 4- to 6-hour intervals.

sodium bicarbonate

INDICATIONS & DOSAGE
Cardiac arrest—
Adults and children: as a 7.5% or 8.4% solution, 1 to 3 mEq/kg I.V. initially; may repeat in 10 minutes. Further doses based on blood gases. If blood gases unavailable, use 0.5 mEq/kg q 10 minutes until spontaneous circulation returns.
Infants up to 2 years: 4.2% solution,

I.V. infusion. Rate not to exceed 8 mEq/kg daily.
Metabolic acidosis—
Adults and children: dose depends on blood CO_2 content, pH, and patient's clinical condition. Generally, 2 to 5 mEq/kg I.V. infused over 4- to 8-hour period.
Systemic or urinary alkalinization—
Adults: 325 mg to 2 g P.O. q.i.d.

SIDE EFFECTS
GI: gastric distention, belching, flatulence.
GU: renal calculi or crystals.
Metabolic: (with overdose) alkalosis, hypernatremia, hyperkalemia, hyperosmolarity.

INTERACTIONS
None significant.

NURSING CONSIDERATIONS
- No contraindications for use in life-threatening emergencies. Contraindicated in hypertension, in patients with tendency toward edema, in patients who are losing chlorides by vomiting or from continuous GI suction, in patients receiving diuretics known to produce hypochloremic alkalosis, and in patients on salt restriction or with renal disease.
- May be added to other I.V. fluids.
- Parenteral bicarbonate solutions will precipitate calcium salts. Do not mix in same infusion fluid. I.V. bolus injections should be given only through running I.V. lines free of calcium salts.
- Because sodium bicarbonate inactivates such catecholamines as norepinephrine and dopamine, do not mix with I.V. solutions of these agents.
- To avoid risk of alkalosis, determine blood pH, PaO_2, $PaCO_2$, and electrolytes. Keep doctor informed of laboratory results.
- Tell patient not to take with milk. May cause hypercalcemia, alkalosis, and possibly renal calculi.

sodium lactate

INDICATIONS & DOSAGE
Alkalinize urine—
Adults: 30 ml of a $\frac{1}{6}$ molar solution/kg of body weight given in divided doses over 24 hours.
Metabolic acidosis—
Adults: usually given as $\frac{1}{6}$ molar injection (167 mEq lactate/liter). Dosage depends on degree of bicarbonate deficit.

SIDE EFFECTS
Metabolic: (with overdose) alkalosis, hypernatremia, hyperosmolarity.

INTERACTIONS
None significant.

NURSING CONSIDERATIONS
• Contraindicated in severe hepatic disease, respiratory alkalosis, and acidosis associated with congenital heart disease with persistent cyanosis.
• Monitor serum electrolytes to avoid alkalosis.

tromethamine
Tham♦

INDICATIONS & DOSAGE
Metabolic acidosis (associated with cardiac bypass surgery or with cardiac arrest)—
Adults: dose depends on bicarbonate deficit. Calculate as follows: ml of 0.3 M tromethamine solution required = wt in kg × bicarbonate deficit (mEq/liter). Additional therapy based on serial determinations of existing bicarbonate deficit.
Children: calculate dose as above. Give slowly over 3 to 6 hours. Addi-

tional therapy based on degree of acidosis. Total 24-hour dose should not exceed 33 to 40 ml/kg.

SIDE EFFECTS
CNS: respiratory depression.
Metabolic: hypoglycemia, hyperkalemia (with decreased urinary output).
Local: venospasm; intravenous thrombosis; inflammation, necrosis, and sloughing if extravasation occurs.

INTERACTIONS
None significant.

NURSING CONSIDERATIONS
• Contraindicated in anuria, uremia, chronic respiratory acidosis, pregnancy (except acute, life-threatening situations). Use cautiously in renal disease or poor urinary output. Monitor EKG and serum K^+ in these patients.
• To prevent blood pH from rising above normal, adjust dose carefully.
• Give slowly through large needle (18G to 20G) into largest antecubital vein or by indwelling I.V. catheter.
• Before, during, and after therapy, make the following determinations: blood pH; carbon dioxide tension; bicarbonate, glucose, and electrolyte levels.
• Mechanical ventilation should be readily available. Use when giving drug to patient with associated respiratory acidosis.
• Except in life-threatening situations, do not use longer than 1 day.
• If extravasation occurs, infiltrate area with 1% procaine and hyaluronidase 150 units; may reduce vasospasm and dilute remaining drug in local area.
• Concentration of tromethamine should not exceed 0.3 M.

Italicized side effects are common or life-threatening.
*Liquid form contains alcohol.   **May contain tartrazine.

Uricosurics

probenecid
sulfinpyrazone

MECHANISM OF ACTION
Uricosurics block renal tubular reabsorption of uric acid, increasing excretion. They also inhibit active renal tubular secretion of many weak organic acids (for example, penicillins and cephalosporins).

COMBINATION PRODUCTS
COLBENEMID: probenecid 500 mg and colchicine 0.5 mg.
PROBEN-C: probenecid 500 mg and colchicine 0.5 mg.

---

probenecid
Benemid♦, Benn, Benuryl♦♦,
Probalan, Probenimead,
Robenecid, SK-Probenecid

INDICATIONS & DOSAGE
Adjunct to penicillin or cephalosporin therapy—
Adults and children over 50 kg: 500 mg P.O. q.i.d.
Children 2 to 14 years (under 50 kg): initially, 25 mg/kg P.O., then 40 mg/kg divided q.i.d.
Single-dose treatment of gonorrhea—
Adults: 3.5 g ampicillin P.O. with 1 g probenecid P.O. given together; or 1 g probenecid P.O. 30 minutes before dose of 4.8 million units of aqueous penicillin G procaine I.M., injected at 2 different sites.
Treatment of hyperuricemia of gout, gouty arthritis—
Adults: 250 mg P.O. b.i.d. for first

week, then 500 mg b.i.d., to maximum of 2 g daily. Maintenance: 500 mg daily for 6 months.

SIDE EFFECTS
Blood: *hemolytic anemia.*
CNS: headache, dizziness.
CV: hypotension.
GI: anorexia, nausea, vomiting, *gastric distress.*
GU: urinary frequency.
Skin: dermatitis, pruritus.
Other: flushing, sore gums, fever.

INTERACTIONS
Salicylates: inhibited uricosuric effect of probenecid, causing urate retention. Do not use together.

NURSING CONSIDERATIONS
• Contraindicated in blood dyscrasias; acute gout attack; penicillin therapy in presence of known renal impairment; gouty nephropathy; urinary tract stones or obstruction; azotemia, hyperuricemia secondary to cancer chemotherapy, radiation, or myeloproliferative neoplastic diseases. Use cautiously with peptic ulcer or renal impairment.
• Usually preferred over sulfinpyrazone because probenecid produces fewer, less severe GI and hematologic side effects.
• Contains no analgesic or anti-inflammatory agent, and is of no value during acute gout attacks. Don't initiate therapy until acute attack subsides.
• Suitable for long-term use; no cumulative effects or tolerance.
• Not effective with chronic renal in-

Unmarked trade names available in the United States only.
♦ Also available in Canada.　　　　♦ ♦ Available in Canada only.

sufficiency (glomerular filtration rate less than 30 ml/minute).

• Periodic BUN and renal function tests recommended in long-term therapy.

• May increase frequency, severity, and length of acute gout attacks during first 6 to 12 months of therapy. Prophylactic colchicine is given during first 3 to 6 months.

• Tell patient to avoid alcohol; it increases urate level.

• Patient should avoid all medications that contain aspirin. These may precipitate gout.

• Force fluids to maintain minimum daily output of 2 to 3 liters. Alkalinize urine with sodium bicarbonate or potassium citrate ordered by doctor. These measures will prevent hematuria, renal colic, urate stone development, and costovertebral pain.

• Give with milk, food, or antacids to minimize GI distress. Continued disturbances might indicate need to lower dose.

• Restrict foods high in purine: anchovies, liver, sardines, kidneys, sweetbreads, peas, lentils.

• Instruct patient and family that drug must be taken regularly as ordered or gout attacks may result. Tell him to visit doctor regularly so uric acid can be monitored and dosage can be adjusted if necessary. Lifelong therapy may be required in patients with hyperuricemia.

• May produce false-positive glucose tests with Benedict's solution or Clinitest, but not with glucose oxidase method (Clinistix, Diastix, Tes-Tape).

• Decreases urinary excretion of 17-ketosteroids, phenolsulfonphthalein (PSP), Bromsulphalein (BSP), aminohippuric acid, and iodine-related organic acids, interfering with laboratory procedures.

sulfinpyrazone
Anturan♦♦, Anturane

INDICATIONS & DOSAGE

Inhibition of platelet aggregation, increase of platelet survival time in treatment of thromboembolic disorders, angina, myocardial infarction, transient cerebral ischemic attacks, peripheral arterial atherosclerosis—
Adults: 200 mg P.O. q.i.d.
Maintenance therapy for common gout: reduction, prevention of joint changes and tophi formation—
Adults: 100 to 200 mg P.O. b.i.d. first week, then 200 to 400 mg P.O. b.i.d. Maximum 800 mg daily.

SIDE EFFECTS

GI: *nausea, dyspepsia,* epigastric pain, blood loss, reactivation of peptic ulcers.
Skin: rash.

INTERACTIONS

Probenecid: inhibited renal excretion of sulfinpyrazone. Use together with caution.
Salicylates: inhibited uricosuric effect of sulfinpyrazone. Do not use together.

NURSING CONSIDERATIONS

• Contraindicated in hypersensitivity to pyrazole derivatives (including oxyphenbutazone, phenylbutazone); active peptic ulcer; gouty nephropathy; urolithiasis or urinary obstruction; bone-marrow depression; azotemia; hyperuricemia secondary to cancer chemotherapy, radiation, or myeloproliferative neoplastic diseases; and during or within 2 weeks after gout attack. Use cautiously in diminished hepatic or renal function.

• Use in treating thromboembolic conditions is investigational and is most often directed at prevention of recurrent myocardial infarction.

• Recommended for patients unresponsive to probenecid. Suitable for long-

term use; no cumulative effects or tolerance.
• Contains no analgesic or anti-inflammatory agent, and is of no value during acute gout attacks.
• Periodic BUN, CBC, and renal function studies advised during long-term use.
• May increase frequency, severity, and length of acute gout attacks during first 6 to 12 months of therapy; prophylactic colchicine is given during first 3 to 6 months.
• Therapy, especially at start, may lead to renal colic and formation of uric acid stones. Until acid levels are normal (about 6 mg/100 ml), monitor intake and output closely.
• Force fluids to maintain minimum daily output of 2 to 3 liters. Alkalinize urine with sodium bicarbonate or other agent ordered by doctor.
• Give with milk, food, or antacids to minimize GI disturbances.

• Restrict foods high in purine: anchovies, liver, sardines, kidneys, sweetbreads, peas, lentils.
• Instruct patient and family that drug must be taken regularly as ordered or gout attacks may result. Tell him to visit doctor regularly so blood levels can be monitored and dosage adjusted if necessary.
• Lifelong therapy may be required in patients with hyperuricemia.
• Decreases urinary excretion of aminohippuric acid and phenolsulfonphthalein (PSP), interfering with laboratory procedures.
• Alkalinizing agents are used therapeutically to increase sulfinpyrazone activity, preventing urolithiasis.
• Warn patient not to take any aspirin-containing medications.
• Monitor patients taking oral hypoglycemic agents; these drugs' effects may be potentiated by sulfinpyrazone, causing hypoglycemia.

bromelains
chymotrypsin
fibrinolysin and
    desoxyribonuclease
hyaluronidase
papain
trypsin

MECHANISM OF ACTION

Enzymes reverse the decreased tissue permeability that develops with inflammation and edema. In this way, they restore flow of blood and other body fluids, and facilitate drainage and tissue repair.

They degrade protein of blood clots, necrotic tissue, and purulent exudate, which may block free flow of body fluids and impede resolution of inflammation and edema.

They digest protein matter, cleaning wounds by liquefaction and dissolution.

COMBINATION PRODUCTS

CHYMORAL ENTERIC-COATED TABLETS: 50,000 units enzymatic activity; trypsin and chymotrypsin in ratio of 6:1.

CHYMORAL-100: 100,000 units enzymatic activity; trypsin and chymotrypsin in ratio of 6:1.

GRANULEX AEROSOL: trypsin 0.1 mg, balsam Peru 72.5 mg, and castor oil 650 mg/0.82 ml.

ORENZYME BITABS ENTERIC-COATED TABLETS: 100,000 units trypsin and 8,000 units chymotrypsin.

ORENZYME ENTERIC-COATED TABLETS♦: 50,000 units trypsin and 4,000 units chymotrypsin.

bromelains
Ananase

INDICATIONS & DOSAGE

Adjunct to reduce inflammation and edema, ease pain, and speed tissue repair of traumatic injuries (contusions, sprains, strains, dislocations), cellulitis, furunculosis, ulcerations—
Adults: initially, 100,000 units P.O. q.i.d., then 50,000 units t.i.d. or q.i.d. for maintenance.

SIDE EFFECTS

Blood: bleeding tendencies.
GI: mild diarrhea, nausea, vomiting.
GU: menorrhagia, metrorrhagia.
Other: fever, hypersensitivity reactions (rash, urticaria).

INTERACTIONS

Alkaline solutions, antacids: dissolve enteric coating of tablet. Do not use within 1 hour of bromelains.

NURSING CONSIDERATIONS

• Contraindicated in hypersensitivity to pineapple or pineapple products. Use cautiously with anticoagulant therapy and in patients with blood-clotting abnormalities, including hemophilia; hepatic or renal disease; and systemic infection.

• Obtain history of allergies. Watch for hypersensitivity reactions and discontinue drug immediately if any occur.

• Destruction of enteric coating may decrease effectiveness. Tablets must be

---

Italicized side effects are common or life-threatening.
✱Liquid form contains alcohol.   ✱✱May contain tartrazine.

swallowed whole; do not crush or break.
- Observe wound to monitor progress of therapy. Appearance of granulation tissue may indicate effectiveness. Notify doctor if inflammation or color of drainage indicates spread of infection.
- Protect from heat.

chymotrypsin
Avazyme**

INDICATIONS & DOSAGE
Adjunct in general, rectal, oral, and dental surgery—
Adults: preoperatively, 2,500 units I.M.; then 2,500 units once or twice daily, as indicated.
Adjunct in treatment of respiratory conditions (asthma, bronchitis, rhinitis, sinusitis)—
Adults: 2,500 to 5,000 units I.M. once or twice weekly; more often if needed.
Children: ½ adult dose.
Chronic or recurrent inflammation (peptic ulcer, ulcerative colitis, phlebitis, thrombophlebitis, dermatologic conditions)—
Adults: 2,500 to 5,000 units I.M. once or twice weekly. Tablet containing 10,000 units may be given buccally q.i.d. alone or in conjunction with I.M. therapy.
Relief of episiotomy symptoms—
Adults: 5,000 units I.M. repeated twice at 12-hour intervals. Tablet containing 20 mg (20,000 units) may be given P.O. q.i.d.
Pelvic inflammatory diseases—
Adults: 2,500 units daily for 7 days; repeat course if needed.

SIDE EFFECTS
Blood: increased bleeding tendencies.
GI: nausea, vomiting, diarrhea with oral administration.
GU: hematuria, albuminuria, menorrhagia.
Local: pain, induration at injection site.
Other: chills, dizziness, fever, rapid

dissolution of animal-origin sutures, *hypersensitivity reactions (rash, urticaria, itching, anaphylaxis)*.

INTERACTIONS
Alkaline solutions, antacids: dissolve enteric coating of tablet. Do not use within 1 hour of oral administration of chymotrypsin.

NURSING CONSIDERATIONS
- Contraindicated in hypersensitivity to trypsin or to sesame oil (injectable form), septicemia, severe generalized or localized infection, and blood coagulation disorders such as hemophilia. Use with caution in severe hepatic or renal disease.
- Parenteral administration: Do not give I.V. Test for sensitivity before giving. Inject deep into gluteal muscle; rotate sites. Watch for hypersensitivity reactions, including changes in blood pressure and pulse rate. Watch for pain, induration at injection site. Stop if reaction occurs.
- Avoid getting in eyes. If drug does get into eyes, flood with water at once.
- Protect from heat.

fibrinolysin and desoxyribonuclease
Elase♦

INDICATIONS & DOSAGE
Debridement of inflammatory and infected lesions (surgical wounds, ulcerative lesions, second- and third-degree burns, circumcision, episiotomy, cervicitis, vaginitis, abscesses, fistulas, and sinus tracts)—
Intravaginally: 5 ml ointment may be inserted using applicator supplied, once daily for vaginitis or cervicitis.
Topical use: apply ointment 30 units fibrinolysin, 20,000 units desoxyribonuclease/30 g at intervals as long as enzyme action is desired.
Irrigating agent for infected wounds, empyema cavities, abscesses, otorhino-

---

laryngologic wounds, subcutaneous hematomas—dilution for irrigation depends on extent and severity of wound: 25 units fibrinolysin powder, 15,000 units desoxyribonuclease/30-ml vial.

SIDE EFFECTS
Local: hyperemia with high doses.

INTERACTIONS
None significant.

NURSING CONSIDERATIONS
• Contraindicated for parenteral use.
• Dense, dry eschar must be removed surgically before enzymatic debridement. Enzyme must be in constant contact with substrate. Accumulated necrotic debris must be removed periodically.
• Clean wound with water or peroxide and dry gently; cover with thin layer of Elase. Cover with nonadhering dressing.
• Change dressing at least once a day. Flush away necrotic debris and reapply ointment.
• Solution as wet dressing: Mix 1 vial of Elase powder with 10 to 50 ml saline solution; saturate strips of fine gauze with solution. Pack ulcerated area with Elase gauze. Allow gauze to dry in contact with ulcerated lesion for about 6 to 8 hours. Remove dried gauze and repeat 3 to 4 times daily.
• Solution as irrigating agent: Drain cavity and replace Elase every 6 to 10 hours to reduce amount of by-product accumulation and to minimize loss of enzyme activity. Although parenteral use is contraindicated, Elase is used as an irrigating agent in certain specific conditions.
• Prepare solution just before use. Discard after 24 hours.

hyaluronidase
Wydase♦

INDICATIONS & DOSAGE
Adjunct to increase absorption and dispersion of other injected drugs—
Adults and children: 150 units to injection medium containing other medication.
Hypodermoclysis—
Adults and children over 3 years: 150 units injected S.C. before clysis or injected into clysis tubing near needle for each 1,000 ml clysis solution.
Subcutaneous urography—
Adults and children: with patient prone, give 75 units S.C. over each scapula, followed by injection of contrast medium at same sites.

SIDE EFFECTS
Skin: rash, urticaria.
Local: irritation.

INTERACTIONS
Local anesthetics: increased potential for toxic local reaction. Use together cautiously.

NURSING CONSIDERATIONS
• Use with caution in patients with blood-clotting abnormalities, severe hepatic or renal disease.
• Do not inject into acutely inflamed or cancerous areas.
• In hypodermoclysis, adjust dose, rate of injection, and type of solution to patient response.
• Administration precautions: Skin-test for sensitivity. Avoid injecting into diseased areas (may spread infection). Observe injection site for local reactions.
• Avoid getting solution in eyes. If solution does get into eyes, flood with water at once.
• Protect from heat. Do not use cloudy or discolored solution.

Italicized side effects are common or life-threatening.
✳Liquid form contains alcohol.   ✳✳May contain tartrazine.

papain
Panafil, Papase♦

INDICATIONS & DOSAGE
Prevention of inflammation and edema in surgical procedures—
Adults and children: 10,000 to 20,000 units P.O. or buccally 1 to 2 hours before surgery, then 20,000 units q.i.d. for up to 5 days.
Treatment of inflammation and burns, enzymatic debridement, promotion of normal healing and deodorization of surface lesions, particularly in local infection, necrosis, fibrinous or purulent debris, sloughing—
Adults and children: apply ointment 10% directly to lesion 1 to 2 times daily. Cover with gauze.

SIDE EFFECTS
Blood: increased bleeding tendencies.
GI: nausea, vomiting, diarrhea with oral administration.
Local: tingling at site of buccal absorption, occasional itching or stinging with first application of ointment.
Other: fever, hypersensitivity reactions (rash, urticaria, pruritus).

INTERACTIONS
With topical use, detergents and antiseptics (benzalkonium chloride, hexachlorophene, iodine, hydrogen peroxide): decreased enzymatic activity. Do not use together.

NURSING CONSIDERATIONS
• Contraindicated in hypersensitivity to papaya fruit. Oral administration contraindicated in anticoagulant therapy; blood-clotting abnormalities, including hemophilia; and systemic infections. Use cautiously in severe hepatic or renal disease.
• Instruct patient on proper route to be used. Oral tablets may be swallowed with water or chewed.
• Before treatment, thoroughly cleanse and irrigate wound area with sterile normal saline solution or water to remove antiseptics, detergents, and heavy-metal antibacterials, which can decrease enzyme activity. Don't use hydrogen peroxide, as it inactivates topical papain. Moisten area for optimal enzymatic activity. Apply ointment in thin layers to assure contact with necrotic tissue. Cover with gauze.
• Irrigate lesion with mild cleansing solution (not hydrogen peroxide) at each redressing.
• Observe wound to monitor progress of therapy. Appearance of granulation tissue may indicate effectiveness. Notify doctor if inflammation or color of drainage indicates spread of infection.
• Avoid getting ointment in eyes. If it does get into eyes, flood with water at once.
• Protect drug from heat.

trypsin

INDICATIONS & DOSAGE
In general and oral surgical procedures to reduce inflammation, accelerate reabsorption of edema, facilitate restoration of local tissue circulation; to reduce inflammation and edema of bronchial mucosa; as adjunct in treatment of phlebothrombosis, thrombophlebitis, iritis, iridocyclitis, chorioretinitis, cutaneous ulcerative conditions—
Adults: 50,000 to 100,000 units P.O. q.i.d.; or 12,500 units I.M. daily or for severe conditions b.i.d. for 1 to 2 days, then 12,500 units daily.
Solution for wet dressings: 10,000 units in each ml normal saline solution or water for injection. Apply new dressings when dry.
Ointment: 5,000 units/g once daily or b.i.d.
Inhalation: 125,000 units dissolved in 3 ml saline solution or water inhaled at least once daily.

SIDE EFFECTS
Blood: increased bleeding tendencies.

Unmarked trade names available in the United States only.
♦ Also available in Canada.   ♦ ♦ Available in Canada only.

CNS: dizziness, fainting.
EENT: rhinorrhea, sneezing, with aerosol inhalation.
GI: nausea, vomiting, diarrhea, abdominal pain.
GU: albuminuria, hematuria.
Skin: rash, pruritus, urticaria.
Local: pain and induration, local irritation.
Other: febrile reactions, angioneurotic edema, rapid dissolution of sutures of animal origins, *anaphylaxis.*

INTERACTIONS
With topical use, detergents and antiseptics (benzalkonium chloride, hexachlorophene, iodine, hydrogen peroxide): decreased enzymatic activity. Do not use together.

NURSING CONSIDERATIONS
• Contraindicated in patients with history of allergic reactions to parenteral enzyme therapy. Use with extreme caution in severe hepatic or renal disease, abnormalities of blood-clotting mechanism.
• Test for possible hypersensitivity reactions before I.M. administration. Observe for 30 minutes after I.M. administration. Have epinephrine 1:1,000 available.
• Do not apply to actively bleeding areas, ocular lesions, or to ulcerated carcinomas.
• Do not give I.V.
• Enteric-coated tablets must be swallowed whole; do not crush or break.
• Give deep I.M. in gluteal muscle, alternating sites.
• Follow nasal inhalation with water or saline spray. Have patient take several swallows of water to remove large droplets from oropharynx.
• Store in tightly closed container. Protect from heat.

Italicized side effects are common or life-threatening.
*Liquid form contains alcohol.   **May contain tartrazine.

102

Oxytocics

carboprost tromethamine
dinoprost tromethamine
dinoprostone
ergonovine maleate
methylergonovine maleate
oxytocin, synthetic injection
oxytocin, synthetic nasal
sodium chloride 20% solution

MECHANISM OF ACTION
- Carboprost, dinoprost, and dinoprostone (prostaglandins) produce
strong, prompt contractions of uterine
smooth muscle, possibly mediated by
calcium and cyclic $3',5'$-adenosine
monophosphate. Endocrine levels also
influence contractions. These drugs
promote cervical dilation and softening, and exert uterine effects by direct
stimulation of the myometrium.
- Ergonovine and methylergonovine
(ergot alkaloids) increase motor activity of the uterus by direct stimulation.
A gravid uterus responds markedly
even to small doses.
- Oxytocin may act as a hormone in
potent and selective stimulation of uterine and mammary gland smooth muscle. It produces uterine contractions of
the same intensity, duration, and frequency as those in spontaneous labor.
Oxytocin may stimulate contractions of
uterine smooth muscle by increasing
the sodium permeability of uterine my-
ofibrils.
- Sodium chloride 20% solution may
damage decidual cells, causing release
of prostaglandins and leading to fetal
death and abortion.

COMBINATION PRODUCTS
None.

carboprost tromethamine
Prostin/M15

INDICATIONS & DOSAGE
*Abort pregnancy between 13th and 20th
weeks of gestation*—initially, 250 mcg
is administered deep I.M. Subsequent
doses of 250 mcg should be administered at intervals of 1½ to 3½ hours,
depending on uterine response. Increments in dosage may be increased to
500 mcg if contractility is inadequate
after several 250 mcg doses. Total dose
should not exceed 12 mg.

SIDE EFFECTS
GI: *vomiting, diarrhea.*
Other: *fever.*

INTERACTIONS
None significant.

NURSING CONSIDERATIONS
- Contraindicated in patients with pelvic inflammatory disease or active cardiac, pulmonary, renal, or hepatic disease. Use cautiously in patients with a
history of asthma; hypertension; cardiovascular, renal, or hepatic disease;
anemia; jaundice; diabetes; epilepsy;
previous uterine surgery.
- I.M. injection of this drug is techni-
cally less difficult and poses fewer potential risks than other prostaglandin
abortifacients.
- Carboprost can be used without concern that expulsion of vaginal supposi-

tories may occur in the presence of profuse vaginal bleeding.
- Live birth may result.
- Should be used only in a hospital setting by trained personnel.

dinoprost tromethamine
Prostin F$_2$ Alpha

INDICATIONS & DOSAGE
Abort second trimester pregnancy—
1 ml of amniotic fluid is withdrawn by transabdominal intra-amniotic catheter. If no blood is present in tap, 40 mg of dinoprost is injected directly into amniotic sac. Initially, 5 mg is given very slowly (1 mg/minute), and patient is watched for adverse reactions. Then, remainder is injected. If abortion not completed in 24 hours, another 10 to 40 mg may be given. Uterine activity may continue 10 to 30 minutes after drug is stopped.

SIDE EFFECTS
CNS: dizziness, fainting.
GI: *nausea, vomiting, diarrhea,* abdominal cramps, epigastric pain.
Other: bronchospasm, wheezing.

INTERACTIONS
Alcohol (I.V. infusions of 500 ml of 10% over 1 hour): inhibited uterine activity.
I.V. oxytocin: cervical perforation, especially in primigravida patients or in those with inadequately dilated cervices. Use with caution.

NURSING CONSIDERATIONS
- Contraindicated in patients with pelvic inflammatory disease. Use with caution in cardiovascular, renal, or hypertensive disease; asthma; glaucoma; epilepsy; previous uterine surgery.
- Observe and record character and amount of vaginal bleeding.
- Live birth may result.
- Other measures may be required if

dinoprost fails to terminate pregnancy completely. Utilization of hypertonic saline solution should be delayed until uterine contractions stop.
- Monitor vital signs. Report rapid fall in blood pressure or hypertonic uterine contractions.
- Instruct patient to remain in prone position.
- After abortion, observe patient frequently for cervical injuries.
- Store at 2° to 8° C. (35.6° to 46.4° F.). Discard 24 months after manufacture date.
- Should be used only in hospital setting by trained personnel.

dinoprostone
Prostin E$_2$♦

INDICATIONS & DOSAGE
*Abort second trimester pregnancy, evacuate uterus in cases of missed abortion, intrauterine fetal deaths up to 28 weeks of gestation, or benign hydatidiform mole—*insert 20 mg suppository high into posterior vaginal fornix. Repeat q 3 to 5 hours until abortion is complete.

SIDE EFFECTS
CNS: *headache.*
CV: hypotension (in large doses).
GI: *nausea, vomiting, diarrhea.*
GU: vaginal pain, vaginitis.
Other: *fever, shivering, chills.*

INTERACTIONS
None significant.

NURSING CONSIDERATIONS
- Contraindicated in patients with pelvic inflammatory disease or history of pelvic surgery, incisions, uterine fibroids, or cervical stenosis. Use with caution in asthma, epilepsy, anemia, diabetes, hyper- or hypotension, jaundice, or cardiovascular, renal, or hepatic disease.
- Live birth may result.

Italicized side effects are common or life-threatening.
*Liquid form contains alcohol.   **May contain tartrazine.

• Warm dinoprostone suppositories in their wrapping to room temperature.
• After insertion of suppository, patient should remain supine for 10 minutes.
• Store suppositories in freezer at temperature of $-20°$ C. $(-4°$ F.) or below.
• Should be administered only when critical-care facilities are readily available.
• Dinoprostone-induced fever is self-limiting and transient. Treat with water or alcohol sponging and increased fluid intake rather than with aspirin, which has not proved effective.
• Abortion should be complete within 30 hours.

---

ergonovine maleate
Ergotrate Maleate♦

INDICATIONS & DOSAGE
Prevent or treat postpartum and post-abortion hemorrhage due to uterine atony or subinvolution—0.2 mg I.M. q 2 to 4 hours, maximum 5 doses; or 0.2 mg I.V. (only for severe uterine bleeding or other life-threatening emergency) over 1 minute while blood pressure and uterine contractions are monitored. I.V. dose may be diluted to 5 ml with 0.9% sodium chloride injection. After initial I.M. or I.V. dose, may give 0.2 to 0.4 mg P.O. q 6 to 12 hours for 2 to 7 days. Decrease dose if severe uterine cramping occurs.

SIDE EFFECTS
CNS: dizziness, headache.
CV: hypertension, chest pain.
EENT: tinnitus.
GI: *nausea, vomiting*.
GU: uterine cramping.
Other: sweating, dyspnea, hypersensitivity.

INTERACTIONS
Regional anesthetics, dopamine, I.V. oxytocin: excessive vasoconstriction. Use together cautiously.

NURSING CONSIDERATIONS
• Contraindicated for induction or augmentation of labor, before delivery of placenta, in threatened spontaneous abortion, and in patients with allergy or sensitivity to ergot preparations. Use cautiously in hypertension, cardiac disease, venoatrial shunts, mitral valve stenosis, obliterative vascular disease, sepsis, and hepatic or renal impairment.
• Monitor blood pressure, pulse rate, and uterine response. Report sudden changes in vital signs, frequent periods of uterine relaxation, and/or character and amount of vaginal bleeding.
• Hypocalcemia may decrease patient response. If patient is not also taking digitalis, cautious administration of calcium gluconate I.V. may produce desired oxytocic action.
• Contractions begin 5 to 15 minutes after P.O. administration; immediately after I.V. injection. May continue 3 hours or more after P.O. or I.M. administration; 45 minutes after I.V. injection.
• Store in tightly closed, light-resistant container. Discard if discolored.
• Store I.V. solutions below 8° C. (46.4° F.). Daily stock may be kept at cool room temperature for 60 days.
• Keep patient warm.
• Have drug ready for immediate use if it is to be given postpartum.
• I.V. bolus doses of ergonovine are used to diagnose coronary artery spasm.

---

methylergonovine maleate
Methergine

INDICATIONS & DOSAGE
Prevent and treat postpartum hemorrhage due to uterine atony or subinvolution—0.2 mg I.M. q 2 to 5 hours for maximum of 5 doses; or I.V. (excessive uterine bleeding or other emergencies) over 1 minute while blood pressure and uterine contractions are monitored. I.V.

---

dose may be diluted to 5 ml with 0.9% sodium chloride injection. Following initial I.M. or I.V. dose, may give 0.2 to 0.4 mg P.O. q 6 to 12 hours for 2 to 7 days. Dose may be decreased if severe cramping occurs.

SIDE EFFECTS
CNS: dizziness, headache.
CV: hypertension, transient chest pain, dyspnea, palpitation.
EENT: tinnitus.
GI: *nausea, vomiting*.
Other: sweating, hypersensitivity.

INTERACTIONS
Regional anesthetics, dopamine, I.V. oxytocin: excessive vasoconstriction. Use together cautiously.

NURSING CONSIDERATIONS
• Contraindicated for induction of labor; before delivery of placenta; in patients with hypertension, toxemia, or sensitivity to ergot preparations; in threatened spontaneous abortion. Use with caution in sepsis, obliterative vascular disease, hepatic or renal disease, hypertension, cardiac disease, venoatrial shunts, mitral valve stenosis.
• Monitor and record blood pressure, pulse rate, uterine response; and report any sudden change in vital signs or frequent periods of uterine relaxation, and character and amount of vaginal bleeding.
• Contractions begin 5 to 15 minutes after P.O. administration; 2 to 5 minutes after I.M. injection; immediately following I.V. injection. May continue 3 hours or more after P.O. or I.M. administration; 45 minutes after I.V. injection.
• Store in tightly closed, light-resistant containers. Discard if discolored.
• Store I.V. solutions below 8° C. (46.4° F.). Daily stock may be kept at room temperature for 60 to 90 days.

oxytocin, synthetic injection
Oxytocin◆, Pitocin◆, Syntocinon◆, Uteracon

INDICATIONS & DOSAGE
Induction or stimulation of labor—initially, 1 ml (10 units) ampul in 1,000 ml of 5% dextrose injection or 0.9% sodium chloride solution I.V. infused at 1 to 2 milliunits/minute. Increase rate at 15- to 30-minute intervals until normal contraction pattern is established. Maximum 1 to 2 ml (20 milliunits)/minute. Decrease rate when labor is firmly established.
Reduction of postpartum bleeding after expulsion of placenta—10 to 40 units added to 1,000 ml of 5% dextrose in water or 0.9% sodium chloride solution infused at rate necessary to control bleeding.
Facilitate threatened abortion—10 to 40 units (1 to 4 ml) oxytocin added to 1,000 ml of 5% dextrose in water, normal saline solution, or other nonhydrating solution; infused at rate necessary to control uterine atony.

SIDE EFFECTS
Maternal
Blood: afibrinogenemia; may be related to increase in postpartum bleeding.
CNS: subarachnoid hemorrhage resulting from hypertension; *convulsions or coma resulting from water intoxication.*
CV: hypotension; increased heart rate, systemic venous return, and cardiac output; arrhythmia.
GI: nausea, vomiting.
Other: hypersensitivity, tetanic contractions, abruptio placentae, impaired uterine blood flow, and increased uterine motility.
Fetal
Blood: increased risk of hyperbilirubinemia.
CV: bradycardia, tachycardia, premature ventricular contractions.
Other: *anoxia, asphyxia*.

Italicized side effects are common or life-threatening.
✳Liquid form contains alcohol.   ✳✳May contain tartrazine.

INTERACTIONS

Cyclopropane anesthetics: less pronounced bradycardia; more severe hypotension than occurs with oxytocin alone. Use together cautiously.

Thiopental anesthetics: delayed induction reported. May require dosage adjustment.

Vasoconstrictors:
severe hypertension if oxytocin is given within 3 to 4 hours of vasoconstrictor in patient receiving caudal block anesthetic. Monitor patient closely.

NURSING CONSIDERATIONS

• Contraindicated in cases of cephalopelvic disproportion or where delivery requires conversion, as in transverse lie; fetal distress, when delivery isn't imminent; severe toxemia; and other obstetric emergencies. Use cautiously in history of cervical or uterine surgery, grand multiparity, uterine sepsis, traumatic delivery, or overdistended uterus, and in primipara over 35 years. Use with extreme caution during first and second stages of labor, since cervical laceration, uterine rupture, and maternal and fetal death are reported.

• Used to induce or reinforce labor only when pelvis is known to be adequate, when vaginal delivery is indicated, when fetal maturity is assured, and when fetal position is favorable. Should be used only in hospital where critical-care facilities and doctor are immediately available.

• Oxytocin should never be given simultaneously by more than one route.

• Incompatible with fibrinolysin, norepinephrine, prochlorperazine edisylate, protein hydrolysate, and warfarin sodium. Compatibility with other I.V. infusion fluids may be influenced by drug concentration, temperature, pH, and other factors. Rotate bottle gently to distribute drug in diluted solution.

• Monitor and record uterine contractions, heart rate, blood pressure, intrauterine pressure, fetal heart rate, and character and volume of blood loss.

• Store at temperature below 25° C. (77° F.), but do not freeze.

• Oxytocin may produce an antidiuretic effect; monitor fluid intake/output.

• If contractions occur less than 2 minutes apart and if contractions above 50 mmHg are recorded, or if contractions last 90 seconds or longer, stop infusion, turn patient on her side, and notify doctor.

• Oxygen administration may be necessary.

• Also used investigationally to evaluate fetal distress.

• Not recommended for I.M. use.

---

oxytocin, synthetic nasal

INDICATIONS & DOSAGE

To promote initial milk ejection; may be useful in relieving postpartum breast engorgement—one spray or three drops into one or both nostrils 2 or 3 minutes before breast-feeding or pumping breasts.

SIDE EFFECTS
None reported.

INTERACTIONS
None significant.

NURSING CONSIDERATIONS

• Instruct patient to clear nasal passages first. With patient's head in vertical position, hold squeeze bottle upright and eject solution into patient's nostril.

• Support patient's wish to breast-feed with quiet, nonstressful environment, and encouragement.

---

sodium chloride 20% solution

INDICATIONS & DOSAGE

To induce fetal death and abortion in second trimester of pregnancy (beyond

---

Unmarked trade names available in the United States only.
♦ Also available in Canada. ♦♦ Available in Canada only.

16th week of gestation)—after transabdominal tap of amniotic sac, at least 1 ml of fluid is withdrawn and examined. If no blood is found, 250 ml of amniotic fluid may be aspirated and 250 ml (maximum dose) of sodium chloride solution instilled over 20 to 30 minutes, while patient is observed for adverse reactions. Sodium chloride instillation may be repeated in 48 hours if membranes are still intact. I.V. infusion of oxytocin or intra-amniotic dinoprost tromethamine may be given to patients who fail to respond to second dose after oxytocic action of saline solution has ceased.

SIDE EFFECTS
Blood: mild, self-limiting disseminated intravascular coagulation; coagulation changes, including decreased platelet count, hematocrit, fibrinogen, and factors V and VIII; increased plasma volume, fibrin levels, and thrombin, PT, and PTT times. Occur within first 12 to 24 hours.
CV: *pulmonary embolism,* pneumonia.
GU: *cortical necrosis of kidneys,* cervical laceration and perforation, cervicovaginal fistula, and uterine rupture reported in primigravida patients receiving concomitant I.V. oxytocin before cervix is adequately dilated.
Local: infection at injection site.
Other: fever, flushing.

INTERACTIONS
Indomethacin: may prolong abortion if used within 4 to 6 hours after intra-amniotic instillation of sodium chloride solution. Defer indomethacin dose.
Oxytocin: intense uterine contractions and increased risk of uterine rupture or cervical laceration. Don't use together.

NURSING CONSIDERATIONS
• Contraindicated in blood disorders or in actively contracting or hypertonic uterus. Use with extreme caution in cardiac disease, hypertension, epilepsy, renal impairment, uterine incision, or pelvic adhesions, or in history of pelvic surgery.
• Should be done only by doctors trained in amniocentesis when critical-care facilities are immediately available.
• Monitor constantly for signs of accidental intravascular, endometrial, or intraperitoneal injection. Procedure usually painless. If patient complains of pain, burning, feeling of heat, thirst, severe headache, mental confusion, distress, tinnitus, numbness of fingertips, or anxiety, stop instillation at once. Inadvertent I.V. injection can cause hypernatremia, myometrial necrosis, with secondary vomiting, cerebral blood clots, cardiovascular collapse, and death.
• Patient should drink at least 2 liters of water on day of procedure to improve salt excretion.
• General anesthetics or sedatives should not be used during administration of hypertonic saline solution.

Italicized side effects are common or life-threatening.
*Liquid form contains alcohol.   **May contain tartrazine.

103

Spasmolytics

aminophylline
or theophylline
ethylenediamine
dyphylline
flavoxate hydrochloride
oxtriphylline
oxybutynin chloride
theophylline
theophylline sodium glycinate

MECHANISM OF ACTION

• Flavoxate has a direct spasmolytic effect on smooth muscles of the urinary tract. It also provides some local anesthesia and analgesia.

• Oxybutynin has both a direct spasmolytic effect and an atropine-like effect on urinary tract smooth muscles; it has little or no effect on smooth muscles of blood vessels. It increases urinary bladder capacity and provides some local anesthesia and mild analgesia.

• Of the xanthine derivatives, theophylline and its salts competitively inhibit phosphodiesterase, the enzyme that degrades cyclic adenosine monophosphate (AMP). This increases intracellular cyclic AMP, which in turn causes relaxation of the smooth muscle of the bronchial airways and pulmonary blood vessels. This action relieves bronchospasm and increases pulmonary vital capacity.

Dyphylline presumably has the same mechanism of action as theophylline, but this has not been proven.

COMBINATION PRODUCTS

THEOLAIR-PLUS LIQUID: 125 mg theophylline and 100 mg guaifenesin/15 ml.
THEOLAIR-PLUS TABLETS 125: 125 mg theophylline and 100 mg guaifenesin.
THEOLAIR-PLUS TABLETS 250: 250 mg theophylline and 200 mg guaifenesin.

aminophylline or theophylline ethylenediamine

Aminodur Dura-Tab, Aminophyllin, Corophyllin♦♦, Lixaminol*, Phyllocontin, Somophyllin, Somophyllin-DF

INDICATIONS & DOSAGE

For treatment of acute and chronic bronchial asthma, bronchospasm; also used for treatment of Cheyne-Stokes respiration—

Oral: **Adults:** 500 mg immediately; then 250 to 500 mg q 6 to 8 hours.
Children: 7.5 mg/kg immediately; then 3 to 6 mg/kg q 6 to 8 hours.
I.V.: inject very slowly, minimum time of 4 to 5 minutes; do not exceed 25 mg/minute infusion rate.
Loading dose: 5.6 mg/kg over 30 minutes.
Maintenance dose: **Adults:** 0.3 to 0.9 mg/kg hourly I.V. by continuous infusion.
Children less than 9 years: 1 mg/kg hourly.
I.M.: **Adults:** 500 mg. Painful. Not recommended.
Rectal: **Adults:** 500 mg suppository or by retention enema q 6 to 8 hours.

Unmarked trade names available in the United States only.
♦ Also available in Canada. ♦♦ Available in Canada only.

SIDE EFFECTS

CNS: *restlessness, dizziness,* headache, *insomnia,* light-headedness, *convulsions.*

CV: *palpitations, sinus tachycardia,* extrasystoles, flushing, marked hypotension, increase in respiratory rate.

GI: *nausea, vomiting, anorexia,* bitter aftertaste, dyspepsia, heavy feeling in stomach.

Skin: urticaria.

Local: *rectal suppositories may cause irritation.*

INTERACTIONS

Alkali-sensitive drugs: reduced activity. Do not add to I.V. fluids containing aminophylline.

Propranolol, nadolol, metoprolol, atenolol, timolol: antagonism. Propranolol and nadolol may cause bronchospasm in sensitive patients. Use together cautiously.

Troleandomycin, erythromycin, cimetidine, furosemide: decreased hepatic clearance of theophylline; elevated theophylline levels. Monitor for signs of toxicity.

Barbiturates: enhanced metabolism and decreased theophylline blood levels. Monitor for decreased aminophylline effect.

NURSING CONSIDERATIONS

• Contraindicated in hypersensitivity to xanthine compounds (caffeine, theobromine); preexisting cardiac arrhythmias, especially tachyarrhythmias. Use cautiously in young children; in elderly patients with congestive heart failure or other cardiac or circulatory impairment, cor pulmonale, hepatic disease; in patients with active peptic ulcer, since it may increase volume and acidity of gastric secretions; and in hyperthyroidism or diabetes mellitus.

• Individuals metabolize xanthines at different rates. Adjust dose by monitoring response, tolerance, pulmonary function, and theophylline blood levels;

therapeutic level = 10 to 20 mcg/ml; toxicity seen over 20 mcg/ml.

• Plasma clearance may be decreased in patients with congestive heart failure, hepatic dysfunction, or pulmonary edema. Smokers show accelerated clearance. Dose adjustments necessary.

• I.V. drug administration can cause burning; dilute with dextrose in water solution.

• Monitor vital signs; measure and record intake/output. Expected clinical effects include improvement in quality of pulse and respiration.

• Warn elderly patient of dizziness, common side effect at start of therapy.

• GI symptoms may be relieved by taking oral drug with full glass of water at meals, although food in stomach delays absorption. Enteric-coated tablets may also delay and impair absorption. No evidence that antacids reduce GI side effects.

• Suppositories slowly and erratically absorbed; retention enemas may be absorbed more rapidly. Rectally administered preparations can be given when patient cannot take drug orally. Schedule after evacuation, if possible; may be retained better if given before meal. Advise patient to remain recumbent 15 to 20 minutes after insertion.

• Question patient closely about other drugs used. Warn that over-the-counter remedies may contain ephedrine in combination with theophylline salts; excessive CNS stimulation may result. Tell him to check with doctor before taking *any* other medications.

• Before giving loading dose, check that patient has not had recent theophylline therapy.

• Supply instructions for home care and dosage schedule. Some patients may require round-the-clock dosage schedule.

• Warn patients with allergies that exposure to allergens may exacerbate bronchospasm.

Italicized side effects are common or life-threatening.
*Liquid form contains alcohol.   **May contain tartrazine.

dyphylline
Air-Tabs, Brophylline,
Coeurophylline♦♦, Dilin, Dilor,
Dyflex, Dylline, Emfabid, Lufyllin*,
Neothylline*, Protophylline♦♦

INDICATIONS & DOSAGE
For relief of acute and chronic bronchial asthma and reversible bronchospasm associated with chronic bronchitis and emphysema—
Adults: 200 to 800 mg P.O. q 6 hours; or 250 to 500 mg
I.M. injected slowly at 6-hour intervals.
Children over 6 years: 4 to 7 mg/kg P.O. daily, in divided doses.

SIDE EFFECTS
CNS: *restlessness, dizziness,* headache, insomnia, light-headedness, *convulsions.*
CV: *palpitations, sinus tachycardia,* extrasystoles, flushing, marked hypotension, increase in respiratory rate.
GI: *nausea, vomiting, anorexia,* bitter aftertaste, dyspepsia, heavy feeling in stomach.
Skin: urticaria.

INTERACTIONS
None significant.

NURSING CONSIDERATIONS
• Contraindicated in hypersensitivity to xanthine compounds (caffeine, theobromine); preexisting cardiac arrhythmias, especially tachycardias. Use cautiously in young children; in elderly patients with congestive heart failure, any impaired cardiac or circulatory function, cor pulmonale, renal or hepatic disease; in patients with peptic ulcer, hyperthyroidism, or diabetes mellitus.
• I.V. use not recommended.
• Dyphylline is metabolized faster than theophylline; dosage intervals may have to be decreased to ensure continual therapeutic effect. Higher daily doses may be needed.

• Dose should be decreased in renal insufficiency.
• Monitor vital signs; measure and record intake/output. Expected clinical effects include improvement in quality of pulse and respiration.
• Warn elderly patient of dizziness, a common side effect.
• Gastric irritation may be relieved by taking oral drug after meals; no evidence that antacids reduce this side effect. May produce less gastric discomfort than theophylline.
• Discard dyphylline ampul if precipitate is present. Protect from light.
• Question patient closely about other drugs used. Warn that over-the-counter remedies may contain ephedrine in combination with theophylline salts; excessive CNS stimulation may result. Tell him to check with doctor before taking *any* other medications.
• Supply instructions for home care and dosage schedule.

flavoxate hydrochloride
Urispas

INDICATIONS & DOSAGE
Symptomatic relief of dysuria, frequency, urgency, nocturia, incontinence, and suprapubic pain associated with urologic disorders—
Adults and children over 12 years: 100 to 200 mg P.O. q.i.d.

SIDE EFFECTS
CNS: *mental confusion* (especially in elderly), nervousness, dizziness, headache, drowsiness, difficulty with concentration.
CV: tachycardia, palpitations.
EENT: *dry mouth and throat, blurred vision,* disturbed eye accommodation.
GI: abdominal pain, constipation (with high doses), nausea, vomiting.
Skin: urticaria, dermatoses.
Other: fever.

Unmarked trade names available in the United States only.
♦ Also available in Canada.   ♦ ♦ Available in Canada only.

INTERACTIONS
None significant.

NURSING CONSIDERATIONS
• Contraindicated in pyloric or duodenal obstruction, obstructive intestinal lesions or ileus, achalasia, GI hemorrhage, obstructive uropathies of lower urinary tract. Use cautiously in patients suspected of having glaucoma.
• Check history for other drug use before giving drugs with anticholinergic side effects.
• Warn about possible drowsiness, mental confusion, and blurred vision.
• Tell the patient to report adverse effects or lack of response to drug.

oxtriphylline
Choledyl♦*, Theophylline Choline♦♦

INDICATIONS & DOSAGE
To relieve acute bronchial asthma and reversible bronchospasm associated with chronic bronchitis and emphysema—
Adults and children over 12 years: 200 mg P.O. q 6 hours.
Children 2 to 12 years: 4 mg/kg P.O. q 6 hours. Increase as needed to maintain therapeutic levels of theophylline (10 to 20 mcg/ml).

SIDE EFFECTS
CNS: *restlessness, dizziness,* headache, *insomnia,* light-headedness, *convulsions.*
CV: *palpitations, sinus tachycardia,* extrasystoles, flushing, marked hypotension, increase in respiratory rate.
GI: *nausea, vomiting, anorexia,* bitter aftertaste, dyspepsia, heavy feeling in stomach.
Skin: urticaria.

INTERACTIONS
Erythromycin, troleandomycin, furosemide, cimetidine: decreased hepatic clearance of theophylline; increased plasma level. Monitor for signs of toxicity.
Barbiturates: enhanced metabolism and decreased theophylline blood levels. Monitor for decreased effect.
Propranolol, nadolol, metoprolol, atenolol, timolol: antagonism. May cause bronchospasms in sensitive patients. Use together cautiously.

NURSING CONSIDERATIONS
• Contraindicated in hypersensitivity to xanthines (caffeine, theobromine); preexisting cardiac arrhythmias, especially tachyarrhythmias.
• Tell patient to report GI distress, palpitations, irritability, restlessness, nervousness, or insomnia; may indicate excessive CNS stimulation.
• Administer drug after meals and at bedtime.
• Store at 15° to 30° C. (59° to 86° F.). Protect elixir from light, tablets from moisture.
• Equivalent to 64% anhydrous theophylline.
• Monitor therapy carefully.
• Combination products that contain ephedrine not recommended; excessive CNS stimulation may result (nervousness, tremors, akathisia).

oxybutynin chloride
Ditropan

INDICATIONS & DOSAGE
Antispasmodic for neurogenic bladder—
Adults: 5 mg P.O. b.i.d. to t.i.d. to maximum of 5 mg q.i.d.
Children over 5 years: 5 mg P.O. b.i.d. to maximum of 5 mg t.i.d.

SIDE EFFECTS
CNS: *drowsiness,* dizziness, insomnia, *dry mouth,* flushing.
CV: *palpitations, tachycardia.*
EENT: *transient blurred vision,* mydriasis, cycloplegia.

Italicized side effects are common or life-threatening.
*Liquid form contains alcohol.   **May contain tartrazine.

GI: nausea, vomiting, *constipation*, bloated feeling.

GU: impotence, *urinary hesitance or retention*.

Skin: urticaria, severe allergic reactions in patients sensitive to anticholinergics.

Other: decreased sweating, fever, suppression of lactation.

INTERACTIONS
None significant.

NURSING CONSIDERATIONS
• Contraindicated in myasthenia gravis, GI obstruction, adynamic ileus, megacolon, severe or ulcerative colitis; in elderly or debilitated patients with intestinal atony; and in patients with obstructive uropathy. Use cautiously in elderly patients; in patients with autonomic neuropathy, reflux esophagitis, or hepatic or renal disease.
• May aggravate symptoms of hyperthyroidism, coronary artery disease, congestive heart failure, cardiac arrhythmias, tachycardia, hypertension, or prostatic hypertrophy.
• Therapy should be stopped periodically to determine whether patient can get along without it. Minimizes tendency toward tolerance.
• Rapid onset of action, peaks at 3 to 4 hours, lasts 6 to 10 hours.
• Neurogenic bladder should be confirmed by cystometry before oxybutynin is given. Evaluate patient response to therapy periodically by cystometry.
• Rule out partial intestinal obstruction in patients with diarrhea, especially those with colostomy or ileostomy, before giving oxybutynin.
• If urinary tract infection is present, patient should receive antibiotics concomitantly.
• Warn patient that drug may impair alertness or vision.
• Since oxybutynin suppresses sweating, its use during very hot weather may precipitate fever or heatstroke.

• Store in tightly closed containers at 59° to 86° F. (15° to 30° C.).

theophylline
Accurbron, Adophyllin, Aerolate*, Asthmophylline♦♦, Bronkodyl*, Bronkodyl S-R, Constant-T, Elixicon, Elixophyllin♦*, Labid, Lanophyllin*, Liquophylline, Norophylline, Optiphyllin, Oralphyllin, Physpan, Slo-bid Gyrocaps, Slo-Phyllin, Somophyllin♦, Theo-dur, Theo-Lix, Theo II, Theobid, Theocap, Theoclear, Theolair♦, Theolixir♦*, Theolline*, Theon*, Theophyl♦*, Theo-Span*, Theostat, Theotal, Theovent

theophylline sodium glycinate
Acet-Am♦♦, Panophylline Forte, Synophylate, Theocyne♦♦, Theo-tort

INDICATIONS & DOSAGE
Prophylaxis and symptomatic relief of bronchial asthma, bronchospasm of chronic bronchitis and emphysema—
Adults: 100 to 200 mg P.O. q 6 hours; or 250 to 500 mg rectally q 8 to 12 hours.
Children: 50 to 100 mg P.O. q 6 hours, not to exceed 10 to 12 mg/kg/24 hours, in divided doses q 8 to 12 hours.
Oral timed-release form given q 8 to 12 hours.
Symptomatic relief of bronchial asthma, pulmonary emphysema, and chronic bronchitis—
Adults: 330 to 660 mg (sodium glycinate) P.O. q 6 to 8 hours, after meals.
Children over 12 years: 220 to 330 mg (sodium glycinate) P.O. q 6 to 8 hours.
Children 6 to 12 years: 330 mg (sodium glycinate) P.O. q 6 to 8 hours.
Children 3 to 6 years: 110 to 165 mg (sodium glycinate) P.O. q 6 to 8 hours.

Unmarked trade names available in the United States only.
♦ Also available in Canada.   ♦♦ Available in Canada only.

Children 1 to 3 years: 55 to 110 mg (sodium glycinate) P.O. q 6 to 8 hours.

SIDE EFFECTS

CNS: *restlessness, dizziness,* headache, *insomnia,* light-headedness, *convulsions.*

CV: *palpitations, sinus tachycardia,* extrasystoles, flushing, marked hypotension, increase in respiratory rate.

GI: *nausea, vomiting, anorexia,* bitter aftertaste, dyspepsia, heavy feeling in stomach.

Skin: urticaria.

INTERACTIONS

Erythromycin, thiabendazole, troleandomycin, cimetidine, furosemide: decreased hepatic clearance of theophylline; increased plasma levels. Monitor for signs of toxicity.

Barbiturates: enhanced metabolism and decreased theophylline blood levels. Monitor for decreased effect.

Propranolol nadolol, metoprolol, atenolol, timolol: antagonism. May cause bronchospasms in sensitive patients. Use together cautiously.

NURSING CONSIDERATIONS

• Contraindicated in hypersensitivity to xanthine compounds (caffeine, theobromine); preexisting cardiac arrhythmias, especially tachyarrhythmias. Use cautiously in young children; in elderly patients with congestive heart failure or other circulatory impairment, cor pulmonale, renal or hepatic disease; and in patients with peptic ulcer, hyperthyroidism, or diabetes mellitus.

• Individuals metabolize xanthines at different rates; determine dose by monitoring response, tolerance, pulmonary function, and theophylline plasma levels: therapeutic level = 10 to 20 mcg/ml.

• Monitor vital signs; measure and record intake/output. Expected clinical effects include improvement in quality of pulse and respiration.

• Warn elderly patients of dizziness, a common side effect at start of therapy.

• GI symptoms may be relieved by taking oral drug with full glass of water after meals, although food in stomach delays absorption.

• Question patient closely about other drugs used. Warn that over-the-counter remedies may contain ephedrine in combination with theophylline salts; excessive CNS stimulation may result. Tell him to check with doctor before taking *any* other medications.

• Supply instructions for home care and dosage schedule.

• Daily dosage may need to be decreased in patients with congestive heart failure or hepatic disease, or in elderly patients, since metabolism and excretion may be decreased. Monitor carefully, using blood levels, observation, examination, and interview. Give drug around the clock, using sustained-release product at bedtime.

• Be careful not to confuse sustained-release dosage forms with standard-release dosage forms.

Italicized side effects are common or life-threatening.
∗Liquid form contains alcohol.   ∗∗May contain tartrazine.

104

Heavy metal antagonists

deferoxamine mesylate
dimercaprol
edetate calcium disodium
edetate disodium
D-penicillamine

MECHANISM OF ACTION
Heavy metal antagonists act as chelating agents to react with and neutralize calcium, cysteine, and heavy metals such as iron and copper. These substances bind more easily to heavy metal antagonists than to body tissues. The resulting complex (chelate) is stable, soluble, and easily excreted in urine.
• D-penicillamine's mechanism of action in rheumatoid arthritis is unknown but is probably due to inhibition of collagen formation.

COMBINATION PRODUCTS
None.

---

deferoxamine mesylate
Desferal♦

INDICATIONS & DOSAGE
Acute iron intoxication—
Adults and children: 1 g I.M. or I.V. followed by 500 mg I.M. or I.V. for two doses, q 4 hours; then 500 mg I.M. or I.V. q 4 to 12 hours. Infusion rate shouldn't exceed 15 mg/kg hourly.
Chronic iron overload and in patients requiring multiple transfusions—
Adults and children: 500 mg to 1 g I.M. daily and 2 g slow I.V. infusion in separate solution along with each unit of blood transfused. Maximum dose 6 g daily. I.V. infusion rate shouldn't exceed 15 mg/kg hourly.
S.C.: 1 to 2 g administered q 8 to 24 hours.

SIDE EFFECTS
Local: pain and induration at injection site. *After rapid I.V. administration: erythema, urticaria, hypotension.*
With long-term use: sensitivity reaction (cutaneous wheal formation, pruritus, rash, *anaphylaxis), diarrhea, leg cramps, fever, tachycardia, blurred vision, dysuria, abdominal discomfort.*

INTERACTIONS
None significant.

NURSING CONSIDERATIONS
• Contraindicated in severe renal disease or anuria. Use cautiously in impaired renal function.
• Monitor intake/output carefully.
• I.M. route preferred.
• Use I.V. only when patient has cardiovascular collapse or shock. For I.V. use, dissolve as for I.M. use; dilute in normal saline solution, 5% dextrose in water, or lactated Ringer's solution.
• If giving I.V., change to I.M. as soon as possible.
• For reconstitution, add 2 ml of sterile water for injection to each ampul. Make sure drug is completely dissolved. Reconstituted solution good for 1 week at room temperature. Protect from light.
• Warn patient urine may be red.
• Have epinephrine 1:1,000 readily available in case of allergic reaction.

---

dimercaprol
BAL in Oil♦

INDICATIONS & DOSAGE
Adults and children:
Severe arsenic or gold poisoning—
3 mg/kg deep I.M. q 4 hours for 2
days, then q.i.d. on 3rd day, then b.i.d.
for 10 days.
Mild arsenic or gold poisoning—
2.5 mg/kg deep I.M. q.i.d. for 2 days,
then b.i.d. on 3rd day, then once daily
for 10 days.
Mercury poisoning—5 mg/kg deep I.M.
initially, then 2.5 mg/kg daily or b.i.d.
for 10 days.
*Acute lead encephalopathy or lead level
more than 100 mcg/ml—* 4 mg/kg deep
I.M. injection, then q 4 hours with edetate calcium disodium (12.5 mg/kg
I.M.). Use separate sites. Maximum
dose 5 mg/kg per dose.

SIDE EFFECTS
CNS: pain or tightness in throat, chest,
or hands; headache; paresthesias; muscle pain or weakness.
CV: *transient increase in blood pressure, returns to normal in 2 hours;
tachycardia.*
EENT: blepharospasm, conjunctivitis,
lacrimation, rhinorrhea, excessive salivation.
GI: halitosis; nausea; vomiting; burning sensation in lips, mouth, and
throat.
GU: renal damage if alkaline urine not
maintained.
Metabolic: decreased iodine uptake.
Local: sterile abscess, pain at injection
site.
Other: fever (especially in children),
sweating, pain in teeth.

INTERACTIONS
^{131}I uptake thyroid tests: decreased;
don't schedule patient for this test during course of dimercaprol therapy.
Iron: formed toxic metal complex; concurrent therapy contraindicated.

NURSING CONSIDERATIONS
• Contraindicated in hepatic dysfunction (except postarsenical jaundice),
acute renal insufficiency.
• Don't use for iron, cadmium, or selenium toxicity. Complex formed is
highly toxic, even fatal.
• Ephedrine or antihistamine may prevent or relieve mild side effects.
• Ineffective in arsine gas poisoning.
• Solution with slight sediment usable.
• Keep urine alkaline to prevent renal damage. Oral NaHCO₃ may be
ordered.
• Don't give I.V.; give by deep I.M.
route only. The injection site can be
massaged after drug is given.
• Drug has an unpleasant, garlic-like
odor.
• Be careful when preparing and administering drug not to let drug come in
contact with skin, as it may cause a skin
reaction.

edetate calcium disodium
Calcium Disodium Versenate♦,
Calcium EDTA

INDICATIONS & DOSAGE
Lead poisoning—
Adults: 1 g/250 to 500 ml of 5% dextrose in water or 0.9% normal saline
solution I.V. over 1 to 2 hours daily or q
12 hours for 3 to 5 days; repeat after 2
days if indicated. Maximum dose
50 mg/kg daily.
Children: 35 mg/kg I.M. daily divided
q 8 to 12 hours. Maximum dose 50 mg/
kg daily.
*Acute lead encephalopathy or lead lev-
els above 100 mcg/ml—*
Adults and children: 12.5 mg/kg with
dimercaprol 4 mg/kg deep I.M. after
initial dose of dimercaprol 4 mg deep
I.M. Use separate sites. After first
dose, reduce to 3 mg/kg for 2 to 7 days.

SIDE EFFECTS
CNS: headache, paresthesias,
numbness.

Italicized side effects are common or life-threatening.
∗Liquid form contains alcohol.   ∗∗May contain tartrazine.

CV: cardiac arrhythmias, hypotension.
GI: anorexia, nausea, vomiting.
GU: *proteinuria, hematuria; nephrotoxicity with renal tubular necrosis leading to fatal nephrosis in excessive dose.*
Other: arthralgia, myalgia, hypercalcemia.
4 to 8 hours after infusion: sudden fever and chills, fatigue, excessive thirst, sneezing, nasal congestion.

INTERACTIONS
None significant.

NURSING CONSIDERATIONS
• Contraindicated in severe renal disease or anuria.
• I.V. use contraindicated in lead encephalopathy; may increase intracranial pressure. Use I.M. route instead.
• Force fluids to facilitate lead excretion in all patients except those with lead encephalopathy.
• Monitor intake/output, urinalysis, BUN, and EKGs.
• To avoid toxicity, use with dimercaprol.
• Procaine HCl may be added to I.M. solutions to minimize pain. Watch for local reactions.
• Avoid rapid I.V. infusions. I.M. route preferred.
• Do not confuse this drug with edetate disodium, which is used for the emergency treatment of hypercalcemia.

---

edetate disodium
Disodium EDTA, Disotate, Endrate, Sodium Versenate

INDICATIONS & DOSAGE
Hypercalcemic crisis—
Adults and children: 15 to 50 mg/kg slow I.V. infusion. Dilute in 500 ml of 5% dextrose in water or 0.9% normal saline solution. Give over 3 to 4 hours. Maximum adult dose 3 g/day; maximum children's dose 70 mg/kg daily.

SIDE EFFECTS
CNS: circumoral paresthesias, numbness, headache, malaise, fatigue, muscle pain or weakness.
CV: hypertension, thrombophlebitis.
GI: nausea, vomiting, diarrhea, anorexia, abdominal cramps.
GU: in excessive doses—nephrotoxicity with urgency, nocturia, dysuria, polyuria, proteinuria, renal insufficiency and failure, tubular necrosis.
Metabolic: *severe hypocalcemia,* decreased magnesium.
Local: pain at site of infusion, erythema, dermatitis.

INTERACTIONS
None significant.

NURSING CONSIDERATIONS
• Contraindicated in anuria, known or suspected hypocalcemia, or significant renal disease; active or healed tubercular lesions; history of seizures or intracranial lesions; generalized arteriosclerosis associated with aging. Use cautiously in limited cardiac reserve, incipient congestive heart failure, hypokalemia, diabetes.
• Avoid rapid I.V. infusion; profound hypocalcemia may occur.
• Monitor EKG and test renal function frequently.
• Obtain serum calcium levels after each dose.
• Keep I.V. calcium available.
• Keep patient in bed for 15 minutes after infusion to avoid postural hypotension.
• Don't use to treat lead toxicity; use edetate calcium disodium instead.
• Record I.V. site used, and try to avoid repeated use of the same site, as this increases likelihood of thrombophlebitis.
• Generalized systemic reactions may occur 4 to 8 hours after drug administration; these include fever, chills, back pain, emesis, muscle cramps, and urinary urgency. Report such reactions to doctor. Treatment is usually supportive.

Unmarked trade names available in the United States only.
♦ Also available in Canada.   ♦ ♦ Available in Canada only.

Symptoms generally subside within 12 hours.

• Do not confuse this drug with edetate calcium disodium, which is used to treat lead poisoning.

• Edetate disodium not currently drug of choice for treatment of hypercalcemia; other treatments are safer and more effective.

D-penicillamine
Cuprimine♦, Depen

INDICATIONS & DOSAGE
Wilson's disease—
Adults: 250 mg P.O. q.i.d. before meals. Adjust dose to achieve urinary copper excretion of 0.5 to 1 mg daily.
Children: 20 mg/kg daily P.O. divided q.i.d. before meals. Adjust dose to achieve urinary copper excretion of 0.5 to 1 mg daily.
Cystinuria—
Adults: 250 mg P.O. q.i.d. before meals. Adjust dose to achieve urinary cystine excretion of less than 100 mg daily when renal calculi present, or 100 to 200 mg daily when no calculi present. Maximum adult dose is 5 g daily.
Children: 30 mg/kg daily P.O. divided q.i.d. before meals. Adjust dose to achieve urinary cystine excretion of less than 100 mg daily when renal calculi present, or 100 to 200 mg daily when no calculi present.
Rheumatoid arthritis—
Adults: 250 mg P.O. daily initially, with increases of 250 mg q 2 to 3 months if necessary. Maximum dose 1 g daily.

SIDE EFFECTS
Blood: *leukopenia, eosinophilia, thrombocytopenia, monocytosis, granulocytopenia,* elevated sedimentation rate, lupus erythematosus-like syndrome.
EENT: tinnitus.
GU: *nephrotic syndrome, glomerulonephritis.*

Hepatic: hepatotoxicity.
Metabolic: *decreased pyridoxine (may cause optic neuritis),* decreased zinc and mercury.
Skin: friability, especially at pressure spots; wrinkling; erythema; urticaria; ecchymoses.
Other: reversible taste impairment, especially of salts and sweets; hair loss.
About ⅓ of patients develop allergic reactions (rash, pruritus, fever), arthralgia, lymphadenopathy, or pneumonitis. With long-term use, myasthenia gravis syndrome.

INTERACTIONS
Oral iron: decreased effectiveness of D-penicillamine. If used together, give at least 2 hours apart.

NURSING CONSIDERATIONS
• Contraindicated in pregnant women with cystinuria. Use cautiously in penicillin allergy; cross sensitivity may occur.
• Report to doctor if fever or other allergic reactions occur.
• Patient should receive pyridoxine daily.
• Handle patients carefully to avoid skin damage.
• Dose should be given on empty stomach to facilitate absorption of drug.
• Patient should drink large amounts of fluid, especially at night.
• Tell patient that therapeutic effect may be delayed up to 3 months.
• Monitor CBC, and renal and hepatic function regularly throughout therapy (every 2 weeks for the first 6 months, then monthly).
• Hold drug and notify doctor if WBC falls below 3,500/mm³ and/or platelet count falls below 100,000/mm³ (these are indications to stop drug). A progressive decline in platelet or WBC in three successive blood tests may necessitate temporary cessation of therapy, even if these counts are within normal limits.

Italicized side effects are common or life-threatening.
♦Liquid form contains alcohol.   ♦♦May contain tartrazine.

• Advise patient to report fever, sore throat, chills, bruising, increased bleeding time; may be early signs of granulocytopenia.

• Provide appropriate health teaching for patients with Wilson's disease and cystinuria.

105

Gold salts

aurothioglucose
gold sodium thiomalate

MECHANISM OF ACTION
The exact mechanism of action is unknown. Anti-inflammatory effects in the active stage of rheumatoid arthritis are probably due to inhibition of sulfhydryl systems, which alters cellular metabolism. Gold salts may also alter enzyme function and immune response, and suppress phagocytic activity.

COMBINATION PRODUCTS
None.

aurothioglucose
Solganal

gold sodium thiomalate
Myochrysine♦

INDICATIONS & DOSAGE
Rheumatoid arthritis—
Adults: initially, 10 mg (aurothioglucose) I.M., followed by 25 mg for second and third doses at weekly intervals. Then, 50 mg weekly until 1 g has been given. If improvement occurs without toxicity, continue 25 to 50 mg at 3- to 4-week intervals indefinitely as maintenance therapy.
Children 6 to 12 years: ¼ usual adult dose. Alternatively, 1 mg/kg I.M. once weekly for 20 weeks.
Rheumatoid arthritis—
Adults: initially, 10 mg (gold sodium thiomalate) I.M., followed by 25 mg in 1 week. Then, 50 mg weekly until 14 to 20 doses have been given. If improvement occurs without toxicity, continue 50 mg q 2 weeks for 4 doses; then, 50 mg q 3 weeks for 4 doses; then, 50 mg q month indefinitely as maintenance therapy. If relapse occurs during maintenance therapy, resume injections at weekly intervals.
Children: 1 mg/kg weekly I.M. for 20 weeks. If response is good, may be given q 3 to 4 weeks indefinitely.

SIDE EFFECTS
Adverse reactions to gold are considered severe and potentially life-threatening. Report any side effect to the doctor at once.
Blood: *thrombocytopenia* (with or without purpura), *aplastic anemia, agranulocytosis,* leukopenia, eosinophilia.
CNS: *dizziness,* syncope, sweating.
CV: bradycardia.
EENT: corneal gold deposition, corneal ulcers.
GI: *metallic taste, stomatitis,* difficulty swallowing, nausea, vomiting.
GU: *albuminuria, proteinuria, nephrotic syndrome,* nephritis, acute tubular necrosis.
Hepatic: hepatitis, jaundice.
Skin: *rash and dermatitis in 20% of patients. (If drug is not stopped, may lead to fatal exfoliative dermatitis.)*
Other: *anaphylaxis,* angioneurotic edema.

INTERACTIONS
None significant.

Italicized side effects are common or life-threatening.
*Liquid form contains alcohol.   **May contain tartrazine

NURSING CONSIDERATIONS

• Contraindicated in patients with severe uncontrollable diabetes, renal disease, hepatic dysfunction, marked hypertension, heart failure, systemic lupus erythematosus, Sjögren's syndrome, skin rash, and drug allergies or hypersensitivities. Use cautiously with other drugs that cause blood dyscrasias.

• Indicated only in active rheumatoid arthritis that has not responded adequately to salicylates, D-penicillamine, rest, and physical therapy.

• Should be administered only under constant supervision of a doctor who is thoroughly familiar with the drug's toxicities and benefits.

• Most side effects are readily reversible if drug is stopped immediately.

• Administer all gold salts I.M., preferably intragluteally. Color of drug is pale yellow; don't use if it darkens.

• Observe patient for 30 minutes after administration because of possible anaphylactic reaction.

• Inform patient that benefits of therapy may not appear for 6 to 8 weeks or longer.

• Gold therapy may alter liver function studies.

• Aurothioglucose is a suspension. Immerse vial in warm water and shake vigorously before injecting.

• When giving gold sodium thiomalate, advise patient to lie down and to remain recumbent for 10 to 20 minutes after injection.

• Complete blood counts including platelet estimation should be performed before every second injection for the duration of therapy.

• Dermatitis is the most common side effect of these drugs. Advise patient to report any skin rashes or problems immediately. Pruritus often precedes dermatitis and should be considered a warning of impending skin reactions. Any pruritic skin eruption while a patient is receiving gold therapy should be considered a reaction until proven otherwise. Therapy is stopped until reaction subsides.

• Stomatitis is the second most common side effect of gold therapy. Advise patient that stomatitis is often preceded by a metallic taste. This warning should be reported to the doctor immediately.

• Advise patient of the importance of close medical follow-up and the need for frequent blood and urine tests during therapy.

• Urine should be analyzed for protein and sediment changes before each injection.

• Platelet counts should be performed if patient develops purpura or ecchymoses.

• If side effects are mild, some rheumatologists may order resumption of gold therapy after 2 to 3 weeks' rest.

• Dimercaprol should be kept on hand to treat acute toxicity.

106

Diagnostic skin tests

coccidioidin
histoplasmin
mumps skin test antigen
tuberculin purified protein
  derivative
tuberculosis multiple-puncture
  tests

MECHANISM OF ACTION
Skin tests cause antigen-antibody reactions and nonspecific inflammatory reactions.

COMBINATION PRODUCTS
None.

coccidioidin

INDICATIONS & DOSAGE
Suspected coccidioidomycosis—
Adults and children: 0.1 ml intradermally into the volar surface of the forearm. Use tuberculin syringe with 26G or 27G ⅝" to ½" needle.

SIDE EFFECTS
Local: hypersensitivity (vesiculation, ulceration, necrosis).
Other: *anaphylaxis.*

INTERACTIONS
None significant.

NURSING CONSIDERATIONS
• Test is read at 24 and 48 hours. Reaction usually peaks at about 36 hours. Induration of 5 mm or more indicates a positive reaction (cell-mediated immune response). Erythema is not considered indicative of a delayed hypersensitivity reaction.
• Obtain history of allergies and reactions to skin tests.
• Obtain history of any recent residence or travel to endemic areas—southern California, Arizona, New Mexico, and western Texas.
• Keep epinephrine 1:1,000 available.
• Available as either a 1:100 or 1:10 dilution. The more dilute (1:100) is always tried first. The 1:10 dilution is never used as the initial test dose. If a patient is suspected of having coccidioidomycosis because of clinical manifestations or X-ray findings and the 1:100 dilution is negative, the 1:10 dilution may be applied.
• Reaction to this test may be depressed or suppressed for as long as 4 to 6 weeks in patients who have received concurrent or recent coccidioidomycosis or immunosuppressive agents
• Reaction may be depressed or suppressed in malnourished or immunosuppressed patients.

histoplasmin

INDICATIONS & DOSAGE
Suspected histoplasmosis—
Adults and children: 0.1 ml intradermally into the volar surface of the forearm. Use tuberculin syringe with 26G or 27G ⅝" to ½" needle.

SIDE EFFECTS
Local: urticaria, ulceration or necrosis in highly sensitive patients.

Italicized side effects are common or life-threatening.
*Liquid form contains alcohol.   **May contain tartrazine.

Other: shortness of breath, sweating, *anaphylaxis*.

INTERACTIONS
None significant.

NURSING CONSIDERATIONS
• Read test at 24 to 48 hours. Induration of 5 mm or more is positive response. In some instances, maximum reactions may not be present until the fourth day.
• Reaction may be depressed in malnourished or immunosuppressed patients.
• A positive reaction may indicate a past infection or a mild subacute, or chronic infection with histoplasmosis or such immunologically related organisms as coccidioidomycosis or blastomycosis.
• Obtain history of allergies and reactions to skin tests.
• Keep epinephrine 1:1,000 availabe.
• Cold packs or topical corticosteroids may relieve pain and itching if severe local reaction occurs.
• Serologic titers are often boosted by previous skin test. Wait 48 to 96 hours after skin test to obtain serologic sample.
• Tuberculin skin test is advisable concurrently with histoplasmin test.
• Obtain history of any residence or recent travel to endemic areas—central U.S. (Ohio Valley) and eastern U.S.
• Reactivity to this test may be depressed or suppressed for as long as 4 to 6 weeks in patients who have received concurrent or recent corticosteroids or immunosuppressive agents.

---

mumps skin test antigen

INDICATIONS & DOSAGE
Suspected mumps—
Adults and children: 0.1 ml intradermally into the volar surface of the forearm. Use tuberculin syringe with 26G or 27G ⅝" to ½" needle.

SIDE EFFECTS
Local: hypersensitivity (vesiculation, ulceration).
Other: *anaphylaxis*.

INTERACTIONS
None significant.

NURSING CONSIDERATIONS
• Test is read at 24-, 48-, and 72-hour intervals. A positive reaction (cell-mediated immune response) is 5 mm or more of induration. Erythema is not considered indicative of a delayed hypersensitivity reaction.
• Obtain history of allergies and reactions to skin tests. In patients hypersensitive to eggs, feathers, and chicken, a severe reaction may follow administration.
• Keep epinephrine 1:1,000 available.
• Store vials in refrigerator.
• Mumps skin test antigen is *not* used to assess exposure to mumps. This antigen is used in assessing T cell function and immunocompetence.
• Reactivity to this test may be depressed or suppressed for as long as 4 to 6 weeks in individuals who have received concurrent or recent immunization with certain virus vaccines (for example, measles or influenza), in those who are receiving corticosteroid or immunosuppressive agents, and in those who have had viral infections (rubeola, influenza, mumps, and probably others).
• Reaction may be depressed or suppressed in malnourished or immunosuppressed patients.

---

tuberculin purified protein derivative
Aplisol, Tubersol, PPD-Stablized Solution (Mantoux)

INDICATIONS & DOSAGE
Diagnosis of tuberculosis, evaluation of immunocompetence in patients with cancer, malnutrition—

Adults and children: 5 tuberculin units (0.1 ml) intradermally into volar surface of the forearm. Suspected sensitivity dose use 1 tuberculin unit. First strength equals 1 tuberculin unit/ 0.1 ml; intermediate strength, 5 tuberculin units/0.1 ml. Second strength equals 250 tuberculin units/0.1 ml. Use tuberculin syringe with 26G or 27G ⅝" to ½" needle.

SIDE EFFECTS
Local: pain, pruritus, vesiculation, ulceration, necrosis.
Other: *anaphylaxis.*

INTERACTIONS
None significant.

NURSING CONSIDERATIONS
• Contraindicated in known tuberculin-positive reactors; severe reactions may occur. Use cautiously with active tuberculosis.
• Read test in 48 to 72 hours. An induration of 10 mm or greater indicates a significant reaction (formerly called positive reaction). Significance of a reaction is determined not only by the size of the reaction but by circumstances. For example, a reaction of 5 mm or more may be considered significant in a close relative of a person with known tuberculosis. A reaction of 2 mm or more may also be considered significant in infants and children. The amount of induration at the site—not erythema—determines the significance of the reaction.
• Report all known cases of tuberculosis to the appropriate public health agency.
• Obtain history of allergies and reactions to skin tests.
• Reaction may be depressed in malnutrition, immunosuppression, or viral infections, or in patients who have received concurrent or recent corticosteroids or immunosuppressive agents (within 4 to 6 weeks).
• Antigen absorbed by plastic and glass. Use at once after drawing into plastic or glass syringe.
• Keep epinephrine 1:1,000 available.
• Subcutaneous injection invalidates test results. Bleb (6 to 10 mm in diameter) must form on skin upon intradermal injection.
• Cold packs or topical corticosteroids may relieve pain and itching of severe local reaction.
• Never give initial test with second test strength (250 tuberculin units). Use only when a patient has negative response to a 5–tuberculin unit PPD but has the clinical signs and symptoms of tuberculosis.
• Corticosteroids and other immunosuppressives may suppress skin test reaction.
• Significant response at the injection site in patients with cancer indicates immunocompetence (the patient's immune system can respond to a challenge). These patients have a better chance of responding to immunotherapy.

tuberculosis multiple-puncture tests
Tine Test (dried purified protein derivative [PPD], dried Old Tuberculin)
Mono-Vacc Test (liquid Old Tuberculin)
Aplitest (dried PPD)
Sclavo Test (dried PPD)
Sterneedle ([Heaf] liquid PPD)

INDICATIONS & DOSAGE
Screening for tuberculosis—
Adults and children: cleanse skin thoroughly with alcohol; make skin taut on volar surface of forearm and press points firmly into selected site. Hold device at injection site for about 3 seconds. This will assure stabilizing the dried tuberculin B in tissue lymph. All multiple-puncture tests are equivalent to 5 tuberculin units of PPD Mantoux.

SIDE EFFECTS
Local: hypersensitivity (vesiculation, ulceration, necrosis).
Other: *anaphylaxis.*

INTERACTIONS
None significant.

NURSING CONSIDERATIONS
• Contraindicated in known tuberculin-positive reactors.
• False-positive reaction can occur in sensitive patients.
• Reaction may be depressed in patients with malnutrition, immunosuppression, or miliary tuberculosis.
• Read test in 48 to 72 hours. Doubtful or positive reactions to any multiple-puncture test must be verified by the Mantoux test. The amount of induration—not erythema—at the site determines significance of the reaction.
• Induration of 1 to 2 mm is significant.
• Old Tuberculin Tine Test equals 5 tuberculin units purified protein derivative.
• Obtain history of allergies, especially to acacia (contained in the Tine Test as stabilizer), and reactions to skin tests.
• Keep epinephrine 1:1,000 available.
• Report all known cases of tuberculosis to appropriate public health agency.
• Corticosteroids and other immunosuppressive agents may suppress skin test reaction.
• Cold packs or topical corticosteroids may relieve pain and itching if severe local reaction occurs after test.

Uncategorized drugs

adenosine phosphate
allopurinol
alprostadil
amantadine hydrochloride
bromocriptine mesylate
clomiphene citrate
colchicine
cromolyn sodium
diazoxide, oral
dimethyl sulfoxide 50% (DMSO)
disulfiram
levodopa
levodopa-carbidopa
methoxsalen
pralidoxime chloride
ritodrine hydrochloride

MECHANISM OF ACTION

• Adenosine phosphate may correct biochemical imbalance or deficiency at the cellular level. Therapeutic effects may also result from the drug's vasodilation and ability to reduce tissue edema and inflammation.

• Allopurinol reduces uric-acid production by inhibiting the biochemical reactions preceding its formation.

• Amantadine increases dopamine release in animal brain, but its exact mechanism of action in humans is unknown.

• Bromocriptine inhibits secretion of prolactin. It acts as a dopamine-receptor antagonist by activating postsynaptic dopamine receptors.

• Clomiphene appears to stimulate release of pituitary gonadotropins, follicle-stimulating hormone, and luteinizing hormone. This results in maturation of the ovarian follicle, ovulation, and development of the corpus luteum.

• Colchicine inhibits migration of granulocytes to an area of inflammation. It decreases lactic acid production associated with phagocytosis and interrupts the cycle of urate crystal deposition and inflammatory response.

• Cromolyn inhibits the degranulation of sensitized mast cells that occurs after a patient's exposure to specific antigens. It also inhibits release of histamine and slow-reacting substance of anaphylaxis (SRS-A).

• Oral diazoxide inhibits the release of insulin from the pancreas and decreases peripheral utilization of glucose.

• Dimethyl sulfoxide acts nonspecifically as an anti-inflammatory agent. Its exact mechanism of action is unknown.

• Disulfiram blocks oxidation of alcohol at the acetaldehyde stage. Excess acetaldehyde produces a highly unpleasant reaction in the presence of even small amounts of alcohol.

• Levodopa and levodopa-carbidopa act as follows: levodopa is decarboxylated to dopamine, countering the depletion of striatal dopamine in extrapyramidal centers, which is thought to produce parkinsonism. Carbidopa inhibits the peripheral decarboxylation of levodopa without affecting levodopa's metabolism within the central nervous system. Therefore, more levodopa is available to be decarboxylated to dopamine in the brain.

• Methoxsalen may enhance melanogenesis, either directly or secondarily, to an inflammatory process.

• Pralidoxime reactivates cholinesterase that has been inactivated by organo-

---

Italicized side effects are common or life-threatening.
*Liquid form contains alcohol.   **May contain tartrazine.

phosphorus pesticides and related compounds. It permits degradation of accumulated acetylcholine and facilitates normal functioning of neuromuscular junctions.

• Ritodrine is a beta-receptor agonist that stimulates the beta$_2$-adrenergic receptors in uterine smooth muscle, inhibiting contractility.

COMBINATION PRODUCTS

COLBENEMID: probenecid 500 mg and colchicine 0.5 mg.
PROBENECID WITH COLCHICINE: probenecid 500 mg and colchicine 0.5 mg.

adenosine phosphate
Adenocrest, Adenyl, Cobalasine

INDICATIONS & DOSAGE

To relieve edema, pruritus, dermatitis, and erythema of varicose veins; symptomatic treatment of bursitis, tendinitis, intractable pruritus, and multiple sclerosis—
Adults: 20 to 100 mg I.M. (extended-release) daily for 3 or 4 days, reduced to same dosage every other day. Depending on patient response, reduce dose to 20 mg once or twice weekly; or 20 mg I.M. daily to t.i.d. (simple aqueous solution); or every hour for 5 doses for first 3 days, followed by 20 mg daily as needed; or 100 mg in aqueous solution injected as single dose daily for 3 days, followed by 100 mg on alternate days as needed.

SIDE EFFECTS

CNS: dizziness, headache.
CV: *palpitations, hypotension, dyspnea.*
GI: epigastric discomfort, nausea, diarrhea.
Skin: erythema, flushing.
Other: *anaphylaxis; local reaction at injection site; may increase symptoms of bursitis or tendinitis.*

INTERACTIONS
None significant.

NURSING CONSIDERATIONS

• Contraindicated in myocardial infarction and cerebral hemorrhage. Use cautiously in patients with history of allergy or asthma. Obtain accurate history of allergies before giving first dose.
• Anaphylactic reactions have occurred following use of gelatin I.M. solution. Discontinue if patient complains of dyspnea or tightness in chest.
• Don't give I.V.
• I.M. extended-release in gelatin vehicle: warm solution before using. Inject into gluteal muscle, using 22G to 20G 1″ to 1½″ needle.
• Assess patient for reduction of edema, inflammation.

allopurinol
Lopurin, Zyloprim♦

INDICATIONS & DOSAGE

Gout, primary or secondary to hyperuricemia; secondary to diseases such as acute or chronic leukemia, polycythemia vera, multiple myeloma, and psoriasis—
Dosage varies with severity of disease; can be given as single dose or divided, but doses larger than 300 mg should be divided.
Adults: mild gout, 200 to 300 mg P.O. daily; severe gout with large tophi, 400 to 600 mg P.O. daily. Same dose for maintenance in secondary hyperuricemia.
Hyperuricemia secondary to malignancies—
Children 6 to 10 years: 300 mg P.O. daily.
Children under 6 years: 150 mg P.O. daily.
Impaired renal function—
Adults: 200 mg P.O. daily if creatinine clearance is 10 to 20 ml/minute; 100 mg P.O. daily if creatinine is less than

10 ml/minute; 100 mg P.O. more than 24 hours apart if clearance is less than 3 ml/minute.

To prevent acute gouty attacks—
Adults: 100 mg P.O. daily; increase at weekly intervals by 100 mg without exceeding maximum dose (800 mg), until serum uric acid level falls to 6 mg/100 ml or less.

To prevent uric acid nephropathy during cancer chemotherapy—
Adults: 600 to 800 mg P.O. daily for 2 to 3 days, with high fluid intake.

SIDE EFFECTS

Blood: *agranulocytosis,* anemia, *aplastic anemia.*
CNS: drowsiness.
EENT: cataracts, retinopathy.
GI: nausea, vomiting, diarrhea, abdominal pain.
Hepatic: altered liver function studies, hepatitis.
Skin: *rash, usually maculopapular; exfoliative,* urticarial, and purpuric lesions; erythema multiforme; severe furunculosis of nose; ichthyosis, *toxic epidermal necrolysis.*

INTERACTIONS

Uricosuric agents: additive effect; may be used to therapeutic advantage.

NURSING CONSIDERATIONS

• Contraindicated in hypersensitivity, and in patients with idiopathic hemochromatosis or who have developed reactions to it. Use cautiously in patients with hepatic or renal disease.
• Obtain accurate patient history; note possible allergies with other drug use before first dose.
• Discontinue at first sign of rash, which may precede severe hypersensitivity reaction or any other adverse reaction. Tell patient to report all side effects immediately. Skin rash is more common in patients taking diuretics and in those with renal disorders.
• Monitor intake/output; daily urinary output of at least 2 liters and maintenance of neutral or slightly alkaline urine are desirable. Patient should be encouraged to drink plenty of fluids while taking this drug unless otherwise contraindicated.
• Periodically check CBC, hepatic and renal function, especially at start of therapy.
• Acute gouty attacks may occur in first 6 weeks of therapy; concurrent use of colchicine may be prescribed prophylactically.
• Minimize GI side effects by administering with meals or immediately after.
• Evaluate effectiveness, using serum uric acid levels. Goal is to lower serum level to 6 mg/100 ml, usually within 7 to 10 days; to gradually reduce size of tophi, with no new deposits within 6 months; and to relieve joint pain and increase mobility.
• Allopurinol may predispose patient to ampicillin-induced rash.
• Allopurinol may cause rash even weeks after discontinuation.
• Since drug may cause drowsiness, advise patient to refrain from driving car or performing tasks requiring mental alertness until CNS response to drug is known.

alprostadil
Prostin VR Pediatric

INDICATIONS & DOSAGE

Palliative therapy for temporary maintenance of patency of ductus arteriosus until surgery can be performed—
Infants: 0.1 mcg/kg/minute by I.V. infusion. When therapeutic response is achieved, reduce infusion rate to give lowest dosage that will maintain response. Maximum dosage is 0.4 mcg/kg/minute. Alternatively, administer through umbilical artery catheter placed at ductal opening.

Italicized side effects are common or life-threatening.
*Liquid form contains alcohol.   **May contain tartrazine.

SIDE EFFECTS
Blood: disseminated intravascular coagulation.
CNS: seizures.
CV: *flushing,* bradycardia, hypotension, tachycardia.
GI: diarrhea.
Other: *apnea, fever, sepsis.*

INTERACTIONS
None reported.

NURSING CONSIDERATIONS
• Contraindicated in neonatal respiratory distress syndrome.
• Because drug inhibits platelet aggregation, use cautiously in neonates with bleeding tendencies.
• Monitor arterial pressure by umbilical artery catheter, auscultation, or Doppler transducer. Slow rate of infusion if arterial pressure falls significantly.
• In infants with restricted pulmonary bloodflow, measure drug's effectiveness by monitoring blood oxygenation. In infants with restricted systemic bloodflow, measure drug's effectiveness by monitoring systemic blood pressure and blood pH.
• Drug must be diluted before being administered. Fresh solution must be prepared daily. Discard any solution more than 24 hours old.
• Apnea and bradycardia may reflect drug overdose. If the signs occur, stop infusion immediately.

---

amantadine hydrochloride
Symmetrel♦

INDICATIONS & DOSAGE
To treat drug-induced extrapyramidal reactions—
Adults: 100 mg P.O. b.i.d., up to 300 mg daily in divided doses. Patient may benefit from as much as 400 mg daily, but doses over 200 mg must be closely supervised.

To treat idiopathic parkinsonism, parkinsonian syndrome—
Adults: 100 mg P.O. b.i.d.; in patients who are seriously ill or receiving other antiparkinsonism drugs, 100 mg daily for at least 1 week, then 100 mg b.i.d., p.r.n.

SIDE EFFECTS
CNS: depression, fatigue, confusion, *dizziness,* psychosis, hallucinations, anxiety, irritability, *ataxia, insomnia,* weakness, headache.
CV: peripheral edema, *orthostatic hypotension,* congestive heart failure.
GI: anorexia, nausea, constipation, vomiting, dry mouth.
GU: urinary retention.
Skin: *livedo reticularis,* dermatitis.

INTERACTIONS
None significant.

NURSING CONSIDERATIONS
• Use cautiously in epilepsy or seizures, with congestive heart failure, renal impairment, peripheral edema, hepatic disease, eczematoid dermatitis, uncontrolled psychosis, or severe psychoneurosis.
• Don't stop abruptly, since this might precipitate a parkinsonian crisis; taper off gradually.
• Warn elderly patients about orthostatic hypotension. Suggest they change position slowly, dangle legs before getting up, and lie down if they feel faint or dizzy. Advise elderly males to sit down to urinate, especially at night.
• Last daily dose should be given as early as possible to avoid insomnia.
• Warn patient that drug may produce dizziness, blurred vision, impaired coordination; activities requiring mental alertness should be resumed gradually.
• Advise patient to report decrease in drug's effectiveness to doctor.

---

bromocriptine mesylate
Parlodel♦

INDICATIONS & DOSAGE
To treat amenorrhea and galactorrhea associated with hyperprolactinemia; treatment of female infertility—
2.5 mg P.O. b.i.d. or t.i.d. with meals for 14 days, but for no longer than 6 months.
Prevention of postpartum lactation—
2.5 mg P.O. b.i.d. with meals for 14 days. Treatment may be extended for up to 21 days, if necessary.
Treatment of Parkinson's disease—
1.25 mg P.O. b.i.d. with meals. Dosage may be increased every 14 to 28 days, up to 100 mg daily.

SIDE EFFECTS
CNS: *dizziness, headache,* fatigue, mania, delusions, nervousness, insomnia, depression.
CV: *hypotension,* syncope.
EENT: nasal congestion, tinnitus, blurred vision.
GI: *nausea,* vomiting, *abdominal cramps,* constipation, diarrhea.

INTERACTIONS
None significant.

NURSING CONSIDERATIONS
• Contraindicated in hypersensitivity to ergot derivatives.
• Patient should be examined carefully for pituitary tumor (Forbes-Albright syndrome). Use of Parlodel will not affect tumor size (cause tumor to regress) although it may alleviate amenorrhea or galactorrhea.
• May lead to early postpartum conception. Test for pregnancy every 4 weeks or whenever period is missed after menses are reinitiated.
• Advise patient to use contraceptive methods other than oral contraceptives during treatment.
• First-dose phenomenon occurs in 1% of patients. Sensitive patients may col-

lapse for 15 to 60 minutes but can usually tolerate subsequent treatment without ill effects.
• Incidence of adverse effects is high (68%); however, most are mild to moderate, and only 6% of patients discontinue drug for this reason. Nausea is the most common side effect.
• Recurrence rates when used to treat amenorrhea or galactorrhea associated with hyperprolactinemia are high (70% to 80%).
• Advise the patient that it may take 6 to 8 weeks or longer for menses to be reinstated and galactorrhea to be suppressed.
• Should be given with meals.
• Giving last daily dose at bedtime with a snack may help decrease nausea and dizziness.
• When used to treat Parkinson's disease, bromocriptine is usually given in addition to either levodopa alone or levidopa-carbidopa combination (Sinemet).
• Side effects are more frequent when drug is used for Parkinson's disease.

clomiphene citrate
Clomid♦

INDICATIONS & DOSAGE
*To induce ovulation—*50 to 100 mg P.O. daily for 5 days, starting any time; or 50 to 100 mg P.O. daily starting on day 5 of menstrual cycle (first day of menstrual flow is day 1). Repeat until conception occurs or until 3 courses of therapy are completed.

SIDE EFFECTS
CNS: headache, restlessness, insomnia, dizziness, light-headedness, depression, fatigue, tension.
CV: hypertension.
EENT: blurred vision, diplopia, scotoma, photophobia (signs of impending visual toxicity).
GI: nausea, vomiting, bloating, distention, increased appetite, weight gain.

Italicized side effects are common or life-threatening.
*Liquid form contains alcohol.   **May contain tartrazine.

GU: urinary frequency and polyuria; ovarian enlargement and cyst formation, which regress spontaneously when drug is stopped.
Metabolic: hyperglycemia.
Skin: urticaria, rash, dermatitis.
Other: *hot flashes*, reversible alopecia, *breast discomfort*.

INTERACTIONS
None significant.

NURSING CONSIDERATIONS
• Contraindicated in thrombophlebitis, thromboembolic disorders, or history of these conditions; cancer of breast or reproductive organs; undiagnosed abnormal genital bleeding; ovarian cyst; hepatic disease or dysfunction. Use cautiously in hypertension, mental depression, migraines, seizures, diabetes mellitus, or gonadotropin sensitivity. Report development or worsening of these conditions to doctor. May require stopping drug.
• Patient with visual disturbances should report symptoms to doctor immediately.
• Tell patient possibility of multiple births exists with this drug. Risk increases with higher doses.
• Teach patient to take basal body temperature and chart on graph to ascertain whether ovulation has occurred.
• Advise patient to stop drug and contact doctor immediately if abdominal symptoms or pain occurs because these indicate ovarian enlargement or ovarian cyst.
• Reassure patient that response (ovulation) generally occurs after the first course of therapy. If pregnancy does not occur, course of therapy may be repeated twice.
• Since drug may cause dizziness or visual disturbances, caution patient not to perform hazardous tasks until her response to the drug is known.
• Advise patient to stop drug and contact doctor immediately if she suspects she is pregnant (drug may have teratogenic effect).

colchicine
Colchicine, Colsalide, Novocolchine◆◆

INDICATIONS & DOSAGE
To prevent acute attacks of gout as prophylactic or maintenance therapy—
Adults: 0.5 or 0.6 mg P.O. daily; or 1 to 1.8 mg P.O. daily for more severe cases.
To prevent attacks of gout in patients undergoing surgery—
Adults: 0.5 to 0.6 mg P.O. t.i.d. 3 days before and 3 days after surgery.
To treat acute gout, acute gouty arthritis—
Adults: initially, 1 to 1.2 mg P.O., then 0.5 or 0.6 mg q hour, or 1 to 1.2 mg q 2 hours until pain is relieved or until nausea, vomiting, or diarrhea ensues. Or 2 mg I.V. followed by 2 mg I.V. in 12 hours if necessary. Total I.V. dose over 24 hours not to exceed 4 mg.
Note: Give I.V. by slow I.V. push over 2 to 5 minutes. Avoid extravasation. Don't dilute colchicine injection with 0.9% sodium chloride or 5% dextrose injection, or any other fluid that might change pH of colchicine solution. If lower concentration of colchicine injection needed, dilute with sterile water for injection. However, if diluted solution becomes turbid, don't inject.

SIDE EFFECTS
Blood: *aplastic anemia and agranulocytosis with prolonged use;* nonthrombocytopenic purpura.
CNS: peripheral neuritis.
GI: *nausea, vomiting, abdominal pain, diarrhea.*
Skin: urticaria, dermatitis.
Local: severe local irritation if extravasation occurs.
Other: alopecia.

Unmarked trade names available in the United States only.
◆ Also available in Canada.   ◆◆ Available in Canada only.

INTERACTIONS
None significant.

NURSING CONSIDERATIONS
• Use cautiously in hepatic dysfunction, cardiac disease, renal disease, GI disorders, and in aged or debilitated patients.
• Reduce dosage if weakness, anorexia, nausea, vomiting, or diarrhea appears. First sign of acute overdosage may be GI symptoms, followed by vascular damage, muscle weakness, ascending paralysis. Delirium and convulsions may occur without the patient losing consciousness.
• Do not administer I.M. or subcutaneously; severe local irritation occurs. Administer I.V. over 2 to 5 minutes.
• As maintenance therapy, give with meals to reduce GI effects. May be used with uricosuric agents.
• Baseline laboratory studies, including CBC, should precede therapy and be repeated periodically.
• Monitor fluid intake/output. Keep output at 2,000 ml daily.
• Store in tightly closed, light-resistant container.
• Change needle before making direct I.V. injection.

cromolyn sodium
Intal**, Intal P♦♦, Rynacrom♦♦

INDICATIONS & DOSAGE
Adjunct in treatment of severe perennial bronchial asthma—
Adults and children over 5 years: contents of 20-mg capsule inhaled q.i.d. at regular intervals.
Also available as an aqueous solution administered through a nebulizer.

SIDE EFFECTS
CNS: dizziness, headache.
EENT: *irritation of the throat and trachea, cough, bronchospasm following inhalation of dry powder; esophagitis;* nasal congestion; pharyngeal irritation; wheezing.
GI: nausea.
GU: dysuria, urinary frequency.
Skin: rash, urticaria.
Other: joint swelling and pain, lacrimation, swollen parotid gland, angioedema.

INTERACTIONS
None significant.

NURSING CONSIDERATIONS
• Contraindicated in acute asthma attacks and status asthmaticus.
• Capsule not to be swallowed; insert capsule into inhaler provided; follow manufacturer's directions.
• Watch for recurrence of asthmatic symptoms when dosage is decreased, especially when corticosteroids are also used.
• Use only when acute episode has been controlled, airway is cleared, and patient is able to inhale.
• Patient considered for cromolyn therapy should have pulmonary function tests to show significant bronchodilator-reversible component to his airway obstruction.
• Teach correct use of Spinhaler: insert capsule in device properly, exhale completely before placing mouthpiece between lips, then inhale deeply and rapidly with steady, even breath; remove inhaler from mouth, hold breath a few seconds, and exhale. Repeat until all powder has been inhaled.
• Store capsules at room temperature in a tightly closed container; protect from moisture and temperatures higher than 40° C. (104° F.).
• Instruct patient to avoid excessive handling of capsule.
• Esophagitis may be relieved by antacids or a glass of milk.
• Intranasal form for seasonal rhinitis is available in Canada.

Italicized side effects are common or life-threatening.
*Liquid form contains alcohol.   **May contain tartrazine.

diazoxide, oral
Proglycem

INDICATIONS & DOSAGE
Management of hypoglycemia due to a variety of conditions resulting in hyperinsulinism—
Adults and children: 3 to 8 mg/kg daily P.O., divided into 3 equal doses q 8 hours.
Infants and newborns: 8 to 15 mg/kg daily P.O., divided into 2 or 3 equal doses q 8 to 12 hours.

SIDE EFFECTS
Blood: *leukopenia, thrombocytopenia.*
CV: *cardiac arrhythmias.*
EENT: diplopia.
GI: nausea, vomiting.
Metabolic: sodium and fluid retention, ketoacidosis and hyperosmolar nonketotic coma, hyperuricemia.
Other: *severe hypertrichosis (hair growth) in 25% of adults and higher percentage of children.*

INTERACTIONS
Thiazide diuretics: may potentiate hyperglycemic, hyperuricemic, and hypotensive effects. Monitor appropriate laboratory values.

NURSING CONSIDERATIONS
• Contraindicated in thiazide hypersensitivity and functional hypoglycemia.
• Oral diazoxide does not significantly lower blood pressure in dosages used to treat hypoglycemia.
• A nondiuretic congener of thiazide diuretics.
• Most important use is in management of hypoglycemia due to hyperinsulinism in infants and children.
• Monitor urine regularly for glucose and ketones; report any abnormalities to doctor.
• If not effective after 2 or 3 weeks, drug should be stopped.
• Hair growth on arms and forehead is a common side effect that subsides when drug treatment is completed. Reassure patient.
• Available in capsules and oral suspension.

dimethyl sulfoxide 50% (DMSO)
Rimso-50, Rimso-100

INDICATIONS & DOSAGE
Symptomatic relief of interstitial cystitis—
Adults: instill 50 ml directly into bladder with catheter or syringe; allow to remain for 15 minutes. Repeat every 2 weeks until maximum symptomatic relief is obtained. Thereafter, intervals between therapy may be increased.

SIDE EFFECTS
Other: *garlic-like taste in mouth,* hypersensitivity.

INTERACTIONS
None significant.

NURSING CONSIDERATIONS
• Chronic use of DMSO has been associated with ophthalmic changes. Eyes should be examined periodically.
• After retention of Rimso-50 for 15 minutes, it's expelled by spontaneous voiding.
• Administration of oral analgesics or opium and belladonna suppositories before instillation can reduce bladder spasm in sensitive patients.
• Lidocaine jelly or similar local anesthetic should be applied to urethra before insertion of catheter to avoid spasm.
• Warn patient before administration that he may experience some discomfort as the drug is introduced into the bladder. Reassure patient that this generally subsides with repeated administration.
• Warn patient that he may experience a garlic-like taste several minutes after

---

Unmarked trade names available in the United States only.
♦ Also available in Canada.   ♦ ♦ Available in Canada only.

administration, which may persist for several hours.

• Not for I.M. or I.V. injection.

• Patients on DMSO therapy should have liver and kidney function studies and CBC every 6 months while receiving drug.

• Safety of DMSO in pregnancy has not been established. Use only if potential maternal benefits outweigh potential risks to fetus.

• Safety and effectiveness of DMSO in children not yet established.

• Used investigationally as a topical treatment for arthritis-inflamed joints.

disulfiram
Antabuse♦, Cronetal, Ro-Sulfiram

INDICATIONS & DOSAGE
Adjunct in management of chronic alcoholism—
Adults: maximum of 500 mg q morning for 1 to 2 weeks. Can be taken in evening if drowsiness occurs. Maintenance: 125 to 500 mg daily (average dose 250 mg) until permanent self-control is established. Treatment may continue for months or years.

SIDE EFFECTS
CNS: drowsiness, headache, fatigue, *delirium, depression,* neuritis.
EENT: optic neuritis.
GI: metallic or garlic-like aftertaste.
GU: impotence.
Skin: acneiform or allergic dermatitis.
Other: disulfiram reaction, which may include flushing, throbbing headache, dyspnea, nausea, copious vomiting, sweating, thirst, chest pain, palpitations, hyperventilation, hypotension, syncope, anxiety, weakness, blurred vision, confusion. *In severe reactions, respiratory depression, cardiovascular collapse, arrhythmias, myocardial infarction, acute congestive heart failure, convulsions, unconsciousness, and even death can occur.*

INTERACTIONS
Isoniazid (INH): ataxia or marked change in behavior. Avoid use.
Metronidazole: psychotic reaction. Do not use together.
Paraldehyde: toxic levels of the acetaldehyde. Do not use together.
Alcohol: disulfiram reaction.

NURSING CONSIDERATIONS
• Contraindicated in alcohol intoxication, psychoses, myocardial disease, coronary occlusion, or in patients receiving metronidazole, paraldehyde, alcohol, or alcohol-containing preparations. Use cautiously in diabetes mellitus, hypothyroidism, epilepsy, cerebral damage, nephritis, hepatic cirrhosis or insufficiency, abnormal EEG, multiple drug dependence.

• Used only under close medical and nursing supervision. Patient should clearly understand consequences of disulfiram therapy and give permission. Drug should be used only in patients who are cooperative, well motivated, and are receiving supportive psychiatric therapy.

• Complete physical examination and laboratory studies, including CBC, SMA-12, and transaminase, should precede therapy and be repeated regularly.

• If compliance is questionable, crush tablets and mix with juice or other liquid; observe patient.

• Warn patient to avoid all sources of alcohol: sauces, cough syrups. Even external application of liniments, shaving lotion, back-rub preparations may precipitate disulfiram reaction. Tell him that alcohol reaction may occur as long as 2 weeks after single dose of disulfiram; the longer patient remains on drug, the more sensitive he will become to alcohol.

• Patient should wear a bracelet or carry a card supplied by drug manufacturer identifying him as disulfiram user. Cards may be obtained from

---

Italicized side effects are common or life-threatening.
*Liquid form contains alcohol.   **May contain tartrazine.

Ayerst Laboratories, 685 Third Ave., New York, N.Y. 10017.

Note: Mild reactions may occur in sensitive patients with blood alcohol level of 5 to 10 mg/100 ml; symptoms are fully developed at 50 mg/100 ml; unconsciousness usually occurs at 125 to 150 mg/100 ml level. Reaction may last ½ hour to several hours, or as long as alcohol remains in blood.

• Caution patient's family that disulfiram should never be given to the patient without his knowledge; severe reaction or death could result if such a patient then ingested alcohol.

• Reassure patient that disulfiram-induced side effects, such as drowsiness, fatigue, impotence, headache, peripheral neuritis, and metallic- or garlic-like taste, subside after about 2 weeks of therapy.

levodopa
Dopar, Larodopa♦, Levopa, Parda, Rio-Dopa

INDICATIONS & DOSAGE
Treatment of idiopathic parkinsonism and parkinsonian syndrome resulting from encephalitis lethargica; carbon monoxide and chronic manganese intoxication; and cerebral arteriosclerosis—administered orally with food in dosages carefully adjusted to individual requirements, tolerance, response.
Adults: initially, 0.5 to 1 g P.O. daily, given b.i.d., t.i.d., or q.i.d. with food; increase by no more than 0.75 g daily q 3 to 7 days, until usual maximum of 8 g is reached. Larger dose requires close supervision.

SIDE EFFECTS
Blood: hemolytic anemia, leukopenia.
CNS: *choreiform, dystonic, dyskinetic movements; involuntary grimacing, head movements, myoclonic body jerks, ataxia, tremors, muscle twitching; bradykinetic episodes; psychiatric disturbances, memory loss, nervousness,* anxiety, disturbing dreams, euphoria, malaise, fatigue; severe depression, suicidal tendencies, dementia, delirium, hallucinations *(may necessitate reduction or withdrawal of drug)*.
CV: *orthostatic hypotension,* cardiac irregularities, flushing, hypertension, phlebitis.
EENT: blepharospasm, blurred vision, diplopia, mydriasis or miosis, widening of palpebral fissures, activation of latent Horner's syndrome, oculogyric crises, nasal discharge.
GI: *nausea, vomiting, anorexia;* weight loss may occur at start of therapy; constipation; flatulence; diarrhea; epigastric pain; hiccups; sialorrhea; dry mouth; bitter taste.
GU: urinary frequency, retention, incontinence; darkened urine; excessive and inappropriate sexual behavior; priapism.
Hepatic: hepatotoxicity.
Other: dark perspiration, hyperventilation.

INTERACTIONS
Anticholinergic drugs, tricyclic antidepressants, benzodiazepines, clonidine, papaverine, phenothiazines and other antipsychotics, phenytoin: watch for decreased levodopa effect.
Pyridoxine: reduced efficacy of levodopa. Examine vitamin preparations and nutritional supplements for content of vitamin B_6 (pyridoxine).
Antacids, propranolol: may increase levodopa effect. Use together cautiously.

NURSING CONSIDERATIONS
• Contraindicated in narrow-angle glaucoma, melanoma, or undiagnosed skin lesions. Use cautiously in cardiovascular, renal, hepatic, pulmonary disorders; in patients with peptic ulcer, psychiatric illness, myocardial infarction with residual arrhythmias; and in patients with bronchial asthma, emphysema, and endocrine disease.
• Carefully monitor patients also re-

ceiving antihypertensive medication, hypoglycemic agents. Stop MAO inhibitors at least 2 weeks before therapy is begun.
• Adjust dosage according to patient's response and tolerance. Observe and monitor vital signs, especially while adjusting dose. Report significant changes.
• Instruct patient to report adverse reactions and therapeutic effects.
• Warn patient of possible dizziness and orthostatic hypotension, especially at start of therapy. Patient should change position slowly and dangle legs before getting out of bed. Elastic stockings may control this side effect in some patients.
• Muscle twitching and blepharospasm (twitching of eyelids) may be an early sign of drug overdosage; report immediately.
• Patients on long-term use should be tested regularly for diabetes and acromegaly; repeat blood tests, liver and kidney function studies periodically.
• Advise patient and family that multivitamin preparations, fortified cereals, and certain over-the-counter medications may contain pyridoxine (vitamin B$_6$), which can reverse the effects of levodopa.
• If therapy is interrupted for long period, drug should be adjusted gradually to previous level.
• Therapeutic response usually occurs following each dose and disappears within 5 hours but varies considerably.
• Patient who must undergo surgery should continue levodopa as long as oral intake is permitted, generally 6 to 24 hours before surgery. Drug should be resumed as soon as patient is able to take oral medication.
• Protect from heat, light, moisture. If preparation darkens, it has lost potency and should be discarded.
• Coombs' test occasionally becomes positive during extended use. Expect uric acid elevations with colorimetric method but not with uricase method.

• Alkaline phosphatase, SGOT, SGPT, LDH, bilirubin, BUN, and PBI show transient elevations in patients receiving levodopa; WBC, hemoglobin, and hematocrit show occasional reduction.
• A doctor-supervised period of drug discontinuance (called a drug holiday) may re-establish the effectiveness of a lower dose regimen.
• Combination of levodopa-carbidopa usually reduces amount of levodopa needed by 75%, thereby reducing incidence of side effects.
• Pills may be crushed and mixed with applesauce or baby food fruits for patients who have difficulty swallowing pills.
• Warn patient and family not to increase drug dose without the doctor's orders (they may be tempted to do this as disease symptoms of parkinsonism progress). Daily dose should not exceed 8 g.

levodopa-carbidopa
(combination)
Sinemet♦

INDICATIONS & DOSAGE
Treatment of idiopathic Parkinson's disease, postencephalitic parkinsonism, and symptomatic parkinsonism; carbon monoxide and manganese intoxication—
Adults: 3 to 6 tablets of 25 mg carbidopa/250 mg levodopa daily given in divided doses. Do not exceed 8 tablets of 25 mg carbidopa/250 mg levodopa a day. Optimum daily dosage must be determined by careful titration for each patient.

SIDE EFFECTS
Blood: hemolytic anemia.
CNS: *choreiform, dystonic, dyskinetic movements; involuntary grimacing, head movements, myoclonic body jerks, ataxia,* tremors, muscle twitching; bradykinetic episodes; psychiatric disturbances, memory loss, nervousness,

---

Italicized side effects are common or life-threatening.
*Liquid form contains alcohol.   **May contain tartrazine.

anxiety, disturbing dreams, euphoria, malaise, fatigue; severe depression, suicidal tendencies, dementia, delirium, hallucinations (may necessitate reduction or withdrawal of drug).

CV: *orthostatic hypotension*, cardiac irregularities, flushing, hypertension, phlebitis.

EENT: blepharospasm, blurred vision, diplopia, mydriasis or miosis, widening of palpebral fissures, activation of latent Horner's syndrome, oculogyric crises, nasal discharge.

GI: nausea, vomiting, anorexia, weight loss may occur at start of therapy; constipation; flatulence; diarrhea; epigastric pain; hiccups; sialorrhea; dry mouth; bitter taste.

GU: urinary frequency, retention, incontinence; darkened urine; excessive and inappropriate sexual behavior; priapism.

Hepatic: hepatotoxicity.

Other: dark perspiration, hyperventilation.

INTERACTIONS

Papaverine, diazepam, clonidine, phenothiazines: may antagonize anti-Parkinson actions. Use together cautiously.

NURSING CONSIDERATIONS

• Contraindicated in narrow-angle glaucoma, melanoma, or undiagnosed skin lesions. Use cautiously in cardiovascular, renal, hepatic, pulmonary disorders; in history of peptic ulcer, psychiatric illness, myocardial infarction with residual arrhythmias; and in bronchial asthma, emphysema, and endocrine disease.

• Carefully monitor patients also receiving antihypertensive medication, hypoglycemic agents. Discontinue MAO inhibitors at least 2 weeks before therapy is begun.

• Dosage is adjusted according to patient's response and tolerance to drug. Therapeutic and adverse reactions occur more rapidly with levodopa-carbidopa than with levodopa alone. Observe and monitor vital signs, especially while dosage is being adjusted; report significant changes.

• Instruct patient to report adverse reactions and therapeutic effects.

• Warn patient of possible dizziness and orthostatic hypotension, especially at start of therapy. Patient should change position slowly and dangle legs before getting out of bed. Elastic stockings may control this side effect in some patients.

• Muscle twitching and blepharospasm (twitching of eyelids) may be an early sign of drug overdosage; report immediately.

• Patients on long-term therapy should be tested regularly for diabetes and acromegaly; blood tests, liver and kidney function studies should be repeated periodically.

• If patient is being treated with levodopa, discontinue at least 8 hours before starting levodopa-carbidopa.

• This combination drug usually reduces the amount of levodopa needed by 75%, thereby reducing the incidence of side effects.

• Pyridoxine (vitamin B_6) does not reverse the beneficial effects of Sinemet. Multivitamins can be taken without fear of losing control of symptoms.

• If therapy is interrupted temporarily, the usual daily dosage may be given as soon as patient resumes oral medication.

• Available as tablets with carbidopa-levodopa in a 1:10 ratio (Sinemet 10/100 and Sinemet 25/250); also in a 1:4 ratio (Sinemet 25/100).

• Sinemet 25/100 may reduce many side effects seen with 1:10 ratio strengths.

• Carbidopa (Lodosyn) as a single agent is available from Merck Sharp & Dohme on doctor's request.

• Warn the patient and his family not to increase dose without doctor's order.

---

methoxsalen
Oxsoralen♦

INDICATIONS & DOSAGE
To induce repigmentation in vitiligo—
Adults and children over 12 years: 20 mg P.O. daily, 2 to 4 hours before carefully timed exposure to ultraviolet light.

SIDE EFFECTS
CNS: nervousness, insomnia, depression.
GI: *discomfort, nausea, diarrhea.*
Skin: edema, erythema, painful blistering, burning, peeling.

INTERACTIONS
Photosensitizing agents: do not use together. May increase toxicity.

NURSING CONSIDERATIONS
• Contraindicated in hepatic insufficiency, porphyria, acute lupus erythematosus, hydromorphic and polymorphic light eruptions. Use with caution in familial history of sunlight allergy, GI diseases, or chronic infection.
• Regulate therapy carefully. Overdosage or overexposure to light can cause serious burning or blistering.
• Drug should be taken orally with meals or milk.
• During light exposure treatments, protect eyes and lips.
• Monthly liver function tests should be done on patients with vitiligo (especially at beginning of therapy).

pralidoxime chloride
Protopam♦

INDICATIONS & DOSAGE
Antidote for organophosphate poisoning—
Adults: I.V. infusion of 1 to 2 g in 100 ml of saline solution over 15 to 30 minutes. If pulmonary edema is present, give drug by slow I.V. push over 5 minutes. Repeat in 1 hour if muscle weakness persists. Additional doses may be given cautiously. I.M. or S.C. injection can be used if I.V. is not feasible; or 1 to 3 g P.O. q 5 hours.
Children: 20 to 40 mg/kg I.V.
To treat cholinergic crisis in myasthenia gravis—
Adults: 1 to 2 g I.V., followed by increments of 250 mg I.V. q 5 minutes.

SIDE EFFECTS
CNS: dizziness, headache, drowsiness, excitement, and manic behavior following recovery of consciousness.
CV: tachycardia.
EENT: blurred vision, diplopia, impaired accommodation, laryngospasm.
GI: nausea.
Other: muscular weakness, muscle rigidity, hyperventilation.

INTERACTIONS
None significant.

NURSING CONSIDERATIONS
• Contraindicated in poisoning with Sevin, a carbamate insecticide, since it increases drug's toxicity. Use with extreme caution in renal insufficiency or myasthenia gravis (overdosage may precipitate myasthenic crisis); also in patients with history of asthma or peptic ulcer.
• Use in hospitalized patients only; have respiratory and other supportive measures available. Obtain accurate medical history and chronology of poisoning if possible. Give as soon as possible after poisoning.
• I.V. preparation should be given slowly, as dilute solution.
• Initial measures should include removal of secretions, maintenance of patent airway, artificial ventilation if needed.
• Drug relieves paralysis of respiratory muscles but is less effective in relieving depression of respiratory center.
• Atropine along with pralidoxime should be given I.V., 2 to 4 mg, if cya-

---

Italicized side effects are common or life-threatening.
*Liquid form contains alcohol.   **May contain tartrazine.

nosis is not present. If cyanosis is present, atropine should be given I.M. Give atropine every 5 to 10 minutes until signs of atropine toxicity appear (flushing, tachycardia, dry mouth, blurred vision, excitement, delirium, hallucinations); maintain atropinization for at least 48 hours.

• Dilute with sterile water without preservatives.

• Not effective against poisoning due to phosphorus, inorganic phosphates, or organophosphates with no anticholinesterase activity.

• Difficult to distinguish between toxic effects produced by atropine or by organophosphate compounds and those resulting from pralidoxime. Observe patient for 48 to 72 hours if poison ingested. Delayed absorption may occur from lower bowel.

• Caution patients treated for organophosphate poisoning to avoid contact with insecticides for several weeks.

• Patients with myasthenia gravis treated for overdose of cholinergic drugs should be observed closely for signs of rapid weakening. These patients can pass quickly from a cholinergic crisis to a myasthenic crisis, and require more cholinergic drugs to treat the myasthenia. Keep edrophonium (Tensilon) available in such situations for establishing differential diagnosis.

ritodrine hydrochloride
Yutopar

INDICATIONS & DOSAGE
Management of preterm labor—
I.V. therapy: dilute 150 mg (3 ampuls) in 500 ml of fluid, yielding a final concentration of 0.3 mg/ml. Usual initial dose is 0.1 mg/minute, to be gradually increased according to the results by 0.05 mg/minute q 10 minutes until desired result obtained. Effective dosage range usually lies between 0.15 and 0.35 mg/minute.
Oral maintenance: 1 tablet (10 mg)

may be given approximately 30 minutes before termination of I.V. therapy. Usual dosage for first 24 hours of oral maintenance is 10 mg q 2 hours. Thereafter, usual dose is 10 to 20 mg q 4 to 6 hours. Total daily dose should not exceed 120 mg.

SIDE EFFECTS
Intravenous
CNS: nervousness, anxiety, headache.
CV: *dose-related alterations in blood pressure, palpitations, pulmonary edema, tachycardia,* EKG changes.
GI: nausea, vomiting.
Other: erythema.
Oral
CNS: tremors, nervousness.
CV: palpitations.
GI: nausea, vomiting.
Skin: rash.

INTERACTIONS
Corticosteroids: may produce pulmonary edema in mother. When these drugs are used concomitantly, monitor closely.
Beta blockers: may inhibit ritodrines' action. Avoid concurrent administration.

NURSING CONSIDERATIONS
• Contraindicated before 20th week of pregnancy and in the following conditions: antepartum hemorrhage, eclampsia, intrauterine fetal death, chorioamnionitis, maternal cardiac disease, pulmonary hypertension, maternal hyperthyroidism, uncontrolled maternal diabetes mellitus.

• Because cardiovascular responses are common and more pronounced during I.V. administration, cardiovascular effects—including maternal pulse rate and blood pressure, and fetal heart rate—should be closely monitored. A maternal tachycardia of over 140 or persistent respiratory rate of over 20/ minute may be a sign of impending pulmonary edema.

• Discontinue drug if pulmonary edema develops.
• Monitor amount of fluids administered intravenously, to prevent circulatory overload.

• Ritodrine decreases intensity and frequency of uterine contractions.
• Don't use ritodrine I.V. if solution is discolored or contains a precipitate.

Appendices and Index

FLOW-RATE CONVERTERS

Here's what a standard I.V. flow-rate converter might look like. Available from I.V. fluid manufacturers, these make flow-rate determinations fast and easy.

Note that the drop factor for this set is listed at the bottom of the chart (15 drops = 1 ml).

STANDARD I.V. SET CONVERSION CHART					
Drops per minute	Approximate volume infused in ml* per time interval				
	30 min	1 hr	2 hr	4 hr	8 hr
5	10	20	40	80	160
10	20	40	80	160	320
20	40	80	160	320	640
30	60	120	240	480	960
40	80	160	320	640	1,280
50	100	200	400	800	1,600
60	120	240	480	960	1,920
70	140	280	560	1,120	2,240
80	160	320	640	1,280	2,560
90	180	360	720	1,440	2,880
100	200	400	800	1,600	3,200
110	220	440	880	1,760	3,520
120	240	480	960	1,920	3,840
125	250	500	1,000	2,000	4,000
Approximately 15 drops = 1 ml					

*Actual flow rate may vary as much as ± 10% with the following factors: viscosity of solution; head pressure; rate of infusion; patient venous pressure; variation of drip orifice; patient position.

Note: Drip rates should be monitored periodically and control clamp adjustments made.

PEDIATRIC FLUID AND NUTRITIONAL REQUIREMENTS

Maintaining proper fluid and electrolyte levels in infants is critical. Why? Because an infant's body is 70% to 75% water, whereas an adult's is only 50% to 60%. Therefore, gastrointestinal upset in an infant may lead to severe dehydration and dangerous disturbance of acid-base and electrolyte balance. Also, administering I.V. fluids too fast can lead to dangerous fluid overload. To help guard against severe dehydration or fluid overload, watch closely for these signs of fluid imbalance when the infant you're caring for is vomiting or has diarrhea.

Fluid overload
- Rapid pulse rate
- Hypertension
- Increased urinary output
- Decreased urine specific gravity
- Edema
- Fine rales

Dehydration
- Rapid pulse rate
- Hypotension
- Decreased urinary output
- Increased urine specific gravity
- Dry mucous membranes
- Depressed fontanelles
- Poor skin turgor
- Lethargy
- Refusal to eat
- Distended abdomen
- Weakness
- Absence of tearing and salivation

Remember, each patient's therapy must be adjusted to his individual needs and tolerance levels. When replacing fluids and electrolytes, the type and amounts you'll use may vary from one age-group to another. Nutritional requirements also change with changing growth patterns.

The tables at right contain some guidelines you can follow.

FLUID RECOMMENDATIONS

In Newborn Infants

1st day . . . . 60 to 80 ml/kg	4th day . . . . 100 to 120 ml/kg
2nd day . . . . 70 to 90 ml/kg	5th day
3rd day . . . . 80 to 100 ml/kg	and thereafter . . . . . . 120 to 140 ml/kg

Note: Patent ductus arteriosus or other congenital cardiac conditions may require that fluids be given with greater caution. Also, increased losses may raise fluid requirements.

In Infants and Children

1 to 10 kg . . . . 100 ml/kg/day	20 to 30 kg . . . . .1,500 ml plus 20 ml/each kg over 20
10 to 20 kg . . . . .1,000 ml plus 50 ml/each kg over 10	

Note: Increased losses raise fluid requirements. Also, fluid restriction or concurrent disease may limit fluid intake.

NUTRITIONAL REQUIREMENTS

Protein
1 to 3 g/kg/day

Carbohydrates
Enough to supply necessary calories and, in combination with fat, to supply 20 to 50 nonprotein calories for every gram of protein.

Fats
1 to 4 g/kg/day to provide necessary calories in combination with carbohydrates. If patient's fat intake is restricted, supply 2% to 4% of the calories as linoleic acid to prevent essential fatty acid deficiency.

Electrolytes
Sodium . . . . . . .3 to 4 mEq/kg/day
Potassium . . . . .2 to 3 mEq/kg/day
Chloride . . . . . . .2 to 4 mEq/kg/day
Acetate . . . . .1 to 1.5 mEq/kg/day

Vitamins
Folic acid . . . . . .50 to 75 mcg/kg/day
Vitamin B_{12} . . . .5 to 10 mcg/kg/day
Vitamin K . . . . . .50 to 200 mcg/kg/day
MVI . . . . .0.5 ml/kg/day

Minerals
Phosphate . . . . 1 to 3 millimoles/kg/day
Calcium . . . . . . .300 to 800 mg/kg/day as the gluconate salt
Magnesium . . . .0.25 to 0.5 mEq/kg/day

Trace elements
Zinc . . . . .300 mcg/kg/day in infants less than 3 kg; 100 mcg/day over 3 kg
Chromium . . . . .0.14 mcg/kg/day
Manganese . . . 2 mcg/kg/day
Copper . . . . . . .20 mcg/kg/day

DAILY CALORIC REQUIREMENTS

0 to 1 year . . . . 90 to 120 kcal/kg	7 to 12 years . . . . .60 to 75 kcal/kg
1 to 7 years . . . . 70 to 100 kcal/kg	12 to 18 years . . . . . . .30 to 60 kcal/kg

Caloric requirements may increase:
- 12% for each degree of fever over 37° C. (98.6° F.).
- 20% to 30% with major surgery.
- 40% to 50% with severe sepsis.
- 50% to 100% with long-term failure to thrive.

COMMON DRUG DOSAGES FOR PEDIATRIC EMERGENCIES

This summary is intended only as a guide.
Each emergency requires medical staff discretion.

DRUG OR MIXTURE	HOW SUPPLIED	DOSE BY WEIGHT	DOSE BY VOLUME
albumin, salt poor	25%, 12.5 g/50 ml, 50-ml vial Route: I.V.	0.5 to 1 g/kg	2 to 4 ml/kg
aminophylline	250 mg/10 ml, 10-ml ampul Route: I.V.	2 to 4 mg/kg over 15 to 20 min, then 0.9 mg/kg/hr up to 1.25 mg/kg/hr continuous I.V. infusion	0.08 to 0.16 ml/kg over 15 to 20 min
atropine	1 mg/ml, 1-ml ampul Route: I.V., S.C.	0.01 mg/kg Maximum single dose = 0.4 mg; may be repeated twice in 1 hr	0.01 ml/kg Maximum single dose = 0.4 ml; may be repeated twice in 1 hr
calcium gluconate	10%, 100 mg/ml, 10-ml ampul (4.6 mEq/10 ml) Route: I.V.	60 mg/kg up to 1 g/dose; may be repeated until a maximum of 200 mg/kg has been given *Caution: Do not administer if patient has received digoxin.*	0.6 ml/kg up to 10 ml/dose; may be repeated until a maximum of 2 ml/kg has been given
dexamethasone	10 mg/1 ml, 10-ml vial Route: I.V.	0.6 mg/kg I.V. initially, then 0.3 mg/kg/day given in divided doses (every 6 hr)	0.06 ml/kg I.V. initially, then 0.03 ml/kg/day given in divided doses (every 6 hr)
dextrose	50%, 500 mg/ml, 50-ml vial Route: I.V.	500 mg/kg up to 25 g/dose	1 ml/kg up to 50 ml/dose
dextrose/insulin	dextrose 50%, 500 mg/ml, 50-ml vial Route: I.V. insulin, regular 100 units/ml, 10-ml vial Route: I.V.	Add 8 units of insulin, regular to 50-ml vial of 50% dextrose; 0.5 to 1 ml/kg/dose of the dextrose/insulin mixture	
diazepam	5 mg/ml, 2-ml ampul Route: I.V.	*Acute anticonvulsant dose:* Slow I.V. 0.25 mg/kg at rate not to exceed 2 mg/min; may repeat every 15 min for 2 doses. Maximum dose for infants = 5 mg; maximum dose for older children = 15 mg	0.05 ml/kg slow I.V. Maximum dose for infants = 1 ml; maximum dose for older children = 3 ml
diazoxide	300 mg/20 ml, 20-ml ampul Route: I.V.	3 to 5 mg/kg/dose rapid I.V. push; dose may be repeated in 1 hr; usually recommended not to repeat in less than 1 hr; repeat doses every 4 to 24 hr	0.2 to 0.3 ml/kg/dose rapid I.V. push; dose may be repeated in 1 hr; usually recommended not to repeat in less than 1 hr; repeat doses every 4 to 24 hr

Common Drug Dosages for Pediatric Emergencies (continued)

DRUG OR MIXTURE	HOW SUPPLIED	DOSE BY WEIGHT	DOSE BY VOLUME
digoxin	Pediatric injection: 0.1 mg/ 1 ml, 1-ml ampul (100 mcg/ ml) Route: I.V. *Caution: Never use adult-strength digoxin.*	*Total digitalizing dose (TDD):* **Premature infants** = 25 to 40 mcg/kg	*TDD* 0.25 to 0.4 ml/kg	*Initial dose (0.3 TDD)* 0.08 to 0.13 ml/kg
		Infants 0 to 2 weeks = 35 to 50 mcg/kg	0.35 to 0.5 ml/kg	0.11 to 0.17 ml/kg
		Infants 2 weeks to 2 years = 40 to 65 mcg/kg	0.4 to 0.65 ml/kg	0.13 to 0.22 ml/kg
		Children 2 to 10 years = 35 to 50 mcg/kg	0.35 to 0.5 ml/kg	0.12 to 0.17 ml/kg
		TDD may be divided equally in thirds and given at 8-hr intervals or less; total daily maintenance P.O. = 8 TDD based on original I.V. dosage.	
diphen-hydramine	50 mg/ml, 1-ml syringe Route: I.V.	2 mg/kg slow I.V.	0.04 ml/kg slow I.V.
dopamine	200 mg/5 ml, 5-ml ampul Route: I.V.	*Dilution:* add one ampul to 500 ml dextrose 5% in water (D_5W) to give final concentration of 400 mcg/ml *Dose:* start at 2 to 5 mcg/kg/min and increase by 5 to 10 mcg/kg/min increments after 15-min trial on each dose	*Microdrops/min (200 mg/500 ml D_5W)*

Dopamine dosage table — Microdrops/min (200 mg/500 ml D_5W):

mcg/kg/min	10	20	30	40
20	30	60	90	120
15	23	45	68	90
10	15	30	45	60
5	8	15	23	30
2	3	6	9	12

Patient wt (kg)

Dopamine dosage in microdrops/min (60 drops/ ml minidripper); standard = 200 mg/500 ml D_5W (400 mcg/ml)

DRUG OR MIXTURE	HOW SUPPLIED	DOSE BY WEIGHT	DOSE BY VOLUME
epinephrine 1:1,000 *(anaphylaxis)*	1:1,000, 1-ml ampul (1,000 mcg/ml) Route: S.C.	**Newborns** = 10 mcg/ kg every 15 to 20 min × 3 to 4 (500 mcg/ dose, maximum) **Older children** = 100 to 500 mcg every 15 to 20 min × 3 to 4	0.01 ml/kg (of 1:1,000 epinephrine) 0.1 to 0.5 ml (of 1:1,000 epinephrine)
epinephrine 1:10,000 syringe *(cardiac)*	1:10,000, 10-ml syringe (100 mcg/ml) Route: I.V. or intra-cardiac	**Newborns** = 10 mcg/ kg every 3 to 5 min **Older children** = 100 to 500 mcg every 3 to 5 min	0.1 ml/kg (of 1:10,000 epinephrine) 1 to 5 ml (of 1:10,000)

Common Drug Dosages for Pediatric Emergencies (continued)

DRUG OR MIXTURE	HOW SUPPLIED	DOSE BY WEIGHT	DOSE BY VOLUME
epinephrine 1:1,000 *(infusion)*	1:1,000, 1-ml ampul (1,000 mcg/ml) Route: I.V.	*Dilution:* 3 ml epinephrine in 250 ml D_5W *Final concentration:* 12 mcg/ml *Dose:* 0.25 to 1 mcg/kg/min	*Microdrops/min* (3 mg/250 ml D_5W) (see dose table below)
furosemide	10 mg/ml, 2-ml ampul Route: I.V.	0.5 to 1 mg/kg/dose	0.05 to 0.1 ml/kg/dose
insulin, regular	100 units/ml, 10-ml vial	1 unit for each 3 g (6 ml 50% dextrose) given	0.01 ml for each 3 g (6 ml 50% dextrose) given
isoproterenol	1:5,000, 0.2 mg/ml, 5-ml ampul (200 mcg/ml) Route: I.V.	*Dilution:* 10 ml isoproterenol in 250 ml D_5W *Final concentration:* 8 mcg/ml *Dose:* 0.25 to 1 mcg/kg/min	*Microdrops/min* (2 mg/250 ml D_5W) (see dose table below)
isoproterenol/ levarterenol (norepinephrine) *(alternative mixture)*	Route: I.V.	*Dilution:* 1.25 ml/isoproterenol and 1 ml levarterenol to 250 ml D_5W *Final concentration:* isoproterenol = 1 mcg/ml levarterenol = 4 mcg/ml *Dose:* titrate by blood pressure and heart rate (0.025 ml/kg/min; not to exceed 0.25 ml/kg/min)	
levarterenol (norepinephrine)	1 mg base/ml, 4-ml ampul Route: I.V.	*Dilution:* 1 ml (1 mg) in 250 ml D_5W *Final concentration:* 4 mcg/ml *Initial dose:* 0.1 mcg/kg/min; not to exceed 1 mcg/kg/min	0.025 ml/kg/min; not to exceed 0.25 ml/kg/min; with 60 drops/ml minidripper, instill 2 to 15 drops/kg/min (not to exceed 15 drops/kg/min)
lidocaine	1 g/25 ml, 25-ml vial Route: I.V.	0.5 to 1 mg/kg slow I.V. push; may be repeated every 5 to 10 min as needed; maximum total dose = 5 mg/kg	0.0125 to 0.025 ml/kg slow I.V. push; may be repeated every 5 to 10 min as needed

Epinephrine dose table — Microdrops/min (3 mg/250 ml D_5W)

mcg/kg/min	10	20	30	40
1	50	100	150	200
0.75	38	75	113	150
0.5	25	50	75	100
0.25	13	25	38	50

Patient wt (kg)

Epinephrine dosage in microdrops/min (60 drops/ml minidripper); standard = 3 mg/250 ml D_5W (12 mcg/ml)

Isoproterenol dose table — Microdrops/min (2 mg/250 ml D_5W)

mcg/kg/min	10	20	30	40
1	75	150	225	300
0.75	56	112	169	225
0.5	38	76	113	150
0.25	19	38	56	75

Patient wt (kg)

Isoproterenol dosage in microdrops/min (60 drops/ml minidripper); standard = 2 mg/250 ml D_5W (8 mcg/ml)

Common Drug Dosages for Pediatric Emergencies (continued)

DRUG OR MIXTURE	HOW SUPPLIED	DOSE BY WEIGHT	DOSE BY VOLUME
lidocaine *(continued)*		*Infusion:* 20 to 50 mcg/kg/min; maximum total dose = 5 mg/kg *Dilution:* 1 g in 500 ml D_5W *Final concentration:* 2,000 mcg/ml	*Microdrops/min* (1 g/500 ml D_5W) *mcg/kg/min* 50 : 15 30 45 60 40 : 12 24 36 48 30 : 9 18 27 36 20 : 6 12 18 24 *Patient wt (kg)* 10 20 30 40 Lidocaine dosage in microdrops/min (60 drops/ml minidripper); standard = 1 g/500 ml D_5W (2,000 mcg/ml)
mannitol	25%, 250 mg/ml, 50-ml vial Route: I.V.	*Test dose:* 200 mg/kg I.V. single dose over 3 to 5 min *Edema:* (15% to 20% solution) 1 to 2 g/kg I.V. as slow I.V. infusion over 2 to 6 hr *Cerebral edema:* 1 to 2 g/kg I.V. over 30 to 60 min	*Test dose:* 0.8 ml/kg I.V. single dose over 3 to 5 min *Edema:* 15% solution—6.7 to 13.3 ml/kg I.V. as slow I.V. infusion over 2 to 6 hr; 20% solution—5 to 10 ml/kg I.V. as slow I.V. infusion over 2 to 6 hr *Cerebral edema:* 20% solution—5 to 10 ml/kg I.V. over 30 to 60 min
naloxone *(neonatal strength)*	0.02 mg/ml, 2-ml ampul (20 mcg/ml) Route: I.M. or I.V.	5 to 10 mcg/kg/dose; repeat every 2 to 3 min as needed × three doses	0.25 to 0.5 ml/kg/dose; repeat every 2 to 3 min as needed × three doses
naloxone *(adult strength)*	0.4 mg/ml, 1-ml ampul (400 mcg/ml) Route: I.M. or I.V.	5 to 10 mcg/kg/dose; repeat every 2 to 3 min as needed × three doses; maximum dose = 400 mcg	0.01 to 0.03 ml/kg/dose; repeat every 2 to 3 min as needed × three doses; maximum dose = 1 ml
nitroprusside *(for severe arterial hypertension only)*	50 mg/5 ml vial Route: I.V. *Caution: Solution container should be protected from light with aluminum foil; solution should be discarded after 4 hr*	*Dilution:* 50 mg nitroprusside to 500 ml D_5W *Final concentration:* 100 mcg/ml *Dose:* 0.5 to 2 mcg/kg/min	*Microdrops/min* (50 mg/500 ml D_5W) *mcg/kg/min* 2 : 12 24 36 48 1.5 : 9 18 27 36 1 : 6 12 18 24 0.5 : 3 6 9 12 *Patient wt (kg)* 10 20 30 40 Nitroprusside dosage in microdrops/min (60 drops/ml minidripper); standard = 50 mg/500 ml D_5W
phenytoin *(anticonvulsant);* *therapeutic level = 10 to 20 mcg/ml*	100 mg/2 ml, 2-ml ampul Route: I.V. 100 mg/capsule 50 mg/tablet	*Loading dose:* 8 mg/kg slow IV push at a rate not to exceed 25 mg/min. If seizures persist, another dose of 6 to 8 mg/kg may be administered; total loading dose not to exceed 16 mg/kg	*Loading dose:* 0.16 ml/kg at a rate not to exceed 0.5 ml/min. If seizures persist, another dose of 0.12 to 0.16 ml/kg may be administered; total loading dose not to exceed 0.32 ml/kg

Common Drug Dosages for Pediatric Emergencies (continued)

DRUG OR MIXTURE	HOW SUPPLIED	DOSE BY WEIGHT	DOSE BY VOLUME
phenytoin (continued)	125 mg/5 ml suspension	*Maintenance dose:* 5 to 8 mg/kg P.O. or I.V. given once daily or divided into two equal doses	
phenytoin (antiarrhythmic); therapeutic level = 5 to 18 mcg/ml	100 mg/2 ml, 2-ml ampul Route: I.V.	1 to 5 mg/kg slow I.V. push; rate not to exceed 25 mg/min; repeat as needed; maximum total dose = 500 mg in 4 hr	0.02 to 0.1 ml/kg slow I.V. push; rate not to exceed 0.5 ml/min; repeat as needed; maximum total dose = 10 ml in 4 hr
propranolol (use with extreme caution in congestive heart failure)	1 mg/ml, 1-ml ampul Route: I.V.	0.025 to 0.1 mg/kg slow I.V. push over 10 min every 6 to 8 hr as needed; not to exceed 10 mg/dose (4 mg/dose if patient is anesthetized)	0.025 to 0.1 ml/kg slow I.V. push over 10 min, given every 6 to 8 hr as needed; not to exceed 10 ml/dose (4 ml/dose if patient is anesthetized)
sodium bicarbonate	44.6 mEq/ 50 ml, 50-ml syringe Route: I.V.	1 to 3 mEq/kg I.V. push every 10 min (dosage is empirical only if arterial blood gas data are not available) *Caution: Dilute solution to half strength for use in infants.*	1.1 to 3.4 ml/kg I.V. push every 10 min (dosage is empirical only if arterial blood gas data are not available)

COMMON PROCEDURES FOR PEDIATRIC EMERGENCIES

PROCEDURE	DOSE BY WEIGHT
Defibrillation	1 watt-second/lb (2.2 watt-second/kg)
Cardioversion	2 to 1 watt-second/lb (0.55-2.2 watt-second/kg)

Courtesy of Thomas Jefferson University Hospital, Philadelphia, Pa. Compiled by Harris Koffer, BSc, Department of Pharmacy; Edmond J. Sacks, MD, Department of Pediatrics, and Director, Pediatric Cardiology and Pediatric ICU; Bruce M. Frey, PharmD, Department of Pharmacy.

RECOGNIZING TPN COMPLICATIONS

COMPLICATIONS	SYMPTOMS	TREATMENT
Catheter-related		
Pneumothorax and hydrothorax	Dyspnea, cyanosis, decreased breath sounds, chest pain	Suction; insert chest tube.
Brachial plexus injury	Tingling and numbness along arm in peripheral TPN catheters	Remove catheter.
Air embolism	Dyspnea, chest pain, tachycardia, "mill wheel churning," murmur over precordium	Clamp catheter. Place patient in Trendelenburg's position on left side.
Sepsis	Fever, chills, leukocytosis, erythema or pus at insertion site	Remove catheter and culture tip. Start appropriate antibiotics.
Metabolic		
Hyperglycemia	Polyuria, dehydration, elevated blood and urine glucose levels	Start insulin therapy or adjust flow rate.
Hyperosmolar, hyperglycemic nonketotic coma	Confusion, lethargy, seizures, coma, hyperglycemia, dehydration, glucosuria	Stop dextrose. Give insulin and 0.45% NaCl to rehydrate.
Hypokalemia	Muscle weakness, paralysis, paresthesias, arrhythmias	Increase potassium supplementation.
Hypomagnesemia	Tingling around mouth, paresthesias in fingers, mental changes, hyperreflexia	Increase magnesium supplementation.
Hypophosphatemia	Irritability, weakness, paresthesias, coma, respiratory arrest	Increase phosphate supplementation.
Hypocalcemia	Paresthesias, twitching, positive Chvostek's sign	Increase calcium supplementation.
Metabolic acidosis	Increased serum chloride level, decreased serum bicarbonate level	Use acetate or lactate salts of Na^+ or H^+.
Hepatic dysfunction	Increased serum transaminases, LDH, and bilirubin levels	Change to cyclical schedule. Decrease carbohydrate, add I.V. fats.
Hypoglycemia	Sweating, shaking, irritability when infusion is stopped	Infuse with 5% dextrose.
Mechanical		
Obliteration of catheter lumen	Interrupted flow rate	Reposition catheter. Attempt to aspirate clot.
Air embolism	Apprehension, chest pain, tachycardia, hypotension, cyanosis, seizure, loss of consciousness, possible cardiopulmonary arrest	Place patient in supine or Trendelenburg's position on left side. Have patient perform the Valsalva maneuver. Tape tubing junctions securely.
Thrombosis	Erythema and edema at puncture site; ipsilateral swelling of arm, neck, or face; pain along vein; malaise; fever; tachycardia	Remove catheter promptly. Administer anticoagulant doses of heparin.
Fluid extravasation	Swelling of neck and shoulder area on affected side; pain	Observe patient for cardiopulmonary abnormalities by assessment and chest X-ray.

INDEX

M

P

Page numbers in boldface refer to major entries.

S

Page numbers in boldface refer to major entries.

Page numbers in boldface refer to major entries.

W

NOTES

NOTES

NOTES

NOTES

NOTES